The Practice and Principles of Surgical Assisting

Notice

Medicine is an ever-changing science. As new research and clinical experience broaden our knowledge, changes in treatment and drug therapy are required. The authors and the publisher of this work have checked with sources believed to be reliable in their efforts to provide information that is complete and generally in accord with the standards accepted at the time of publication. However, in view of the possibility of human error or changes in medical sciences, neither the authors nor the publisher nor any other party who has been involved in the preparation or publication of this work warrants that the information contained herein is in every respect accurate or complete, and they disclaim all responsibility for any errors or omissions or for the results obtained from use of the information contained in this work. Readers are encouraged to confirm the information contained herein with other sources. For example and in particular, readers are advised to check the product information sheet included in the package of each drug they plan to administer to be certain that the information contained in this work is accurate and that changes have not been made in the recommended dose or in the contraindications for administration. This recommendation is of particular importance in connection with new or infrequently used drugs.

The Practice and Principles of Surgical Assisting

EDITOR

Rebecca Hall, MS, CRCST, CST, CSA, FAST

The Practice and Principles of Surgical Assisting

1 2 3 4 5 6 7 8 9 DSS 29 28 27 26 25 24

ISBN 978-1-264-26437-7
MHID 1-264-26437-2

This book was set in Minion Pro by MPS Limited.
The editors were Sydney Keen and Peter J. Boyle.
The production supervisor was Richard Ruzycka.
Project management was provided by Karan Rana, MPS Limited.
The interior design was by Mary McKeon.
The cover designer was W2 Design.

Library of Congress Control Number: 2024939783

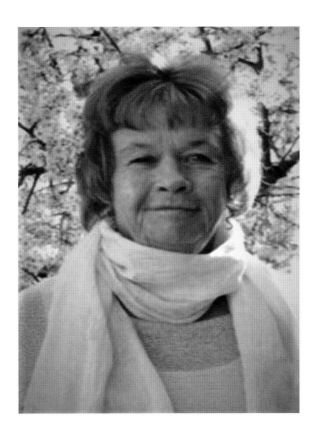

Karen Ludwig
ASA Executive Director
1945–2021

Karen Ludwig became the executive director of the Association of
Surgical Assistants (ASA) upon its creation in 2010. Karen was dedicated to
the promotion of the surgical assisting profession and the development
of an organization that would represent all surgical assistants within the
profession. Her unwavering effort and strategic initiatives provided the
foundation in which the ASA organization quickly became the
premier association for the surgical assisting profession.

It is with great honor and appreciation that we dedicate this textbook,
which would not have been possible without the sincere passion
Karen put forth in its creation and development.

To her husband David and daughter Kristin, thank you for sharing this precious
human being, as she was respected and loved by many.

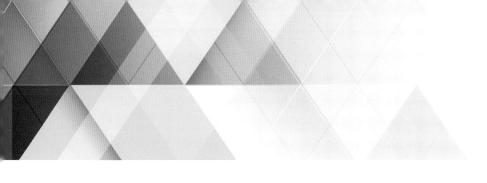

Contents

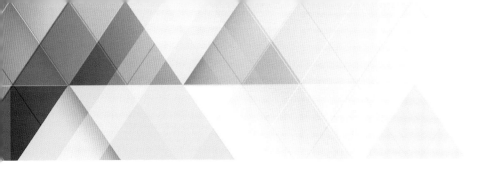

Contributors

Sara Adams, CST, CSFA
Certified Surgical Assistant
American Surgical Professionals, Sunshine Region
Jacksonville, Florida
Chapter 15

David Bartczak, LSA, OPA-C, CSA, OTC
President
Mederi Services, LLC
Sugar Land, Texas
Chapter 3

Jennifer Consorte, BAS, CST, CSFA
Certified First Assistant
Heathtrust Solutions
Miami, Florida
Chapter 18

Kathleen Duffy, CST, CSFA, CSA, FAST
President
KAD Surgical Assisting Inc
Port St. Lucie, Florida
Chapter 15

Brandy Farrington, CST, CSFA
Cardiac Surgical Assistant
Sunrise Hospital
Las Vegas, Nevada
Chapters 5 and 25

Fred Fisher, CSFA, CSA, RSA
President/Owner
Chicagoland Surgical Assisting LLC
Chicago, Illinois
Chapter 3

Sandra Freymuth, CSFA
Certified Surgical Assistant
Fort Lauderdale, Florida
Chapter 16

Rebecca Hall, MS, CRCST, CST, CSA, FAST
Associate Professor
Retired
Chapters 1, 2, 7, 9, 11, 12, and 18

Terry Herring, EdS, CST, CSFA, CSPDT, CSIS, COA, FAST
Division Chair
Surgical Services
Fayetteville Community College
Fayetteville, North Carolina
Chapter 17

Douglas J. Hughes, EdD, CSFA, CST, CRCST
Dean for Health Sciences
Associate Professor for Surgical Technology
Columbia Basin College
Pasco, Washington
Chapters 9, 10, 11, and 12

Jennifer Ickes, CST, CSFA
Certified Surgical Assistant
Wood County Hospital
Bowling Green, Ohio
Chapter 14

Deborah Klaudt
Surgical Assistant
Retired

Dana L. Klope, MD, BSN, RN, CSFA, CST
Certified Surgical Assistant
TRIA Orthopedics
Bloomington, Minnesota
Chapter 23

Cynthia Kreps, BS, CST, CSFA
Program Director
Retired
Chapter 19

David J. Magaster, BS, CST, CSFA
CEO
Surgical Dynamics, LLC
Orthopedic and Trauma Certified
Surgical Assistant
Medical Center of Plano
Parkland Hospital
UTSW Medical Center
Dallas, Texas
Chapter 19

Jeanie Moran, BA, CST, CSFA
Certified Surgical Assistant
Marketing Communications
Port St. Lucie, Florida
Chapter 21

Michael W Morrison, BS, CST, CTP, CSFA, ACLS
CEO, M2 Surgical Concepts, LLC
Cardiac Certified Surgical First Assistant
Transplant Preservationist
University Hospitals—Cleveland Medical Center
Division of Cardiac Surgery, Harrington Heart and Vascular
Institute
Cleveland, Ohio
Chapter 22

**Libby McNaron, MSN, MSHRM, RN, CNOR, CST, CSFA,
FAST**
Panama City, Florida
Chapters 1 and 6

Steven Lee Noyce, CST, CSFA, FAST
Certified Surgical Assistant
Nashville, Tennessee
Chapter 24

Jennifer Paling, TS-C, CSFA
Certified Surgical Assistant
William Beaumont Hospital
Royal Oak, Michigan
Chapter 19

Brenda K. Poynter, MHA, BSW, CST/CSFA, FAST
Associate Professor Educator
Surgical Technology—Program Director
University of Cincinnati—Clermont College
Cincinnati, Ohio
Chapter 13

Margaret H.M. Rodriguez, CST, CSFA, MEd, FAST
Professor
Surgical Technology Program Coordinator
El Paso Community College
El Paso, Texas
Chapters 4 and 8

Jason Ryu, CSFA
Cardiovascular surgery PA
Mayo Clinic School of Health Sciences
Rochester, Minnesota
Chapter 23

Shannon E. Smith, MHSc, CDEI, CST, CSFA, FAST
Surgical Services Program Director
Gulf Coast State College
Panama City, Florida
Chapter 14

**Kerry R. Stanziano-Bradic, MAEd, BSEd, CSFA, CST,
CSPDT**
Associate Professor
Program Coordinator—Surgical Assisting & Medical
Instrument Sterilization Technology
Stark State College
North Canton, Ohio
Chapter 14

Maria Storer Beauchamp, CST, CSFA
Certified Surgical Assistant
University and Hospital Systems
Tampa General Hospital / University of South Florida CVTOR
Team
HCA Healthcare/ West Florida Division Travel First Assist
Team
University of Pittsburgh Medical Center Travel Surgical
Technologist Team
Florida and Pennsylvania
Chapter 26

Jessica Wilhelm, CSA, MSA, LSA, F-PRS
Assistant Professor
Master of Surgical Assisting Program
Eastern Virginia Medical School
Norfolk, Virginia
Chapters 19 and 20

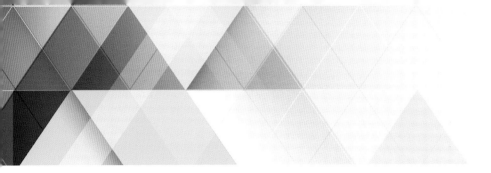

Preface

The inspiration for *The Practice and Principles of Surgical Assisting* is attributable to Karen Ludwig. Her dedication to advancing the profession of surgical assisting led to a discussion about creating a textbook for surgical assisting programs written by surgical assistants. This project would provide a much-needed textbook specific to the role of the surgical assistant. Karen, our biggest cheerleader, was always contemplating ways to promote our profession and build a strong organization well into the future.

This textbook contains the history of surgical assisting, required technical skills, clinical knowledge of surgical specialties, and succinct information for those who wish to embark on the adventure of independent practice.

This is for all future surgical assisting students who have commenced a journey to work alongside surgeons to improve the quality of life for our patients. The authors are a menagerie of assistants with a passion for education and quality patient care. Each of us shared our knowledge and desire to help all surgical assistants have the foundation necessary to be the best of the best in the operating room.

I will be forever grateful to have had the opportunity to work with Karen on this project and so thrilled that we were able to fulfill her dream of a published textbook. I am thankful to all the authors who contributed to making this dream possible.

Introduction to Surgical Assisting

Rebecca Hall and Libby McNaron

DISCUSSED IN THIS CHAPTER

1. The foundation and history of surgery.
2. The history of surgical assisting.
3. The profession of surgical assisting.

HISTORY OF SURGERY

The history of surgery can be traced back to the Stone Age which lasted for roughly 3.4 million years from 8700 BCE to 2000 BCE. Evidence of trephination of the skull, which we can assume was pressure on the brain, has been found from this period.

The Egyptians expanded the knowledge of anatomy when they created mummies. They also treated wounds and broken bones. There is evidence of Egyptians using clamps, sutures, and cauterization. They were the first to realize the benefit of honey to prevent infections.

The ancient Greeks facilitated the advancement of surgery. Herophilus (c. 335-280 BC) has also been called the "Father of Anatomy" as he carried out human dissections in public. The ancient Greeks were known for using wine to prevent infection.

The Roman Empire used the teachings of Galen to advance the techniques of surgery, even though Galen dissected animals to understand human anatomy. For centuries, his writings dominated medicine, even though his writings were inadequate to appropriately describe human anatomy.

The first plastic surgeon recorded in history (600 BC) is Sushruta, who vividly defined the basics of plastic surgery. Sushruta Samhita is one of the oldest treatises dealing with surgery. Although many consider plastic surgery a modern specialty, the origin goes back more than 4000 years to the Indus River Civilization in India (Figure 1-1).

The Sushruta Samhita defines over 120 surgical instruments used at the time. One of the highlights of Sushruta's surgery was "rhinoplasty." The pedicled forehead flap is referred to as the Indian flap even today.

In the 1700s, Dr. Cullen was one of the most respected physicians of his time. He lectured at Edinburgh University where he taught his classes in English. He was also the First Physician to the King of Scotland. John Morgan, one of his students, founded the Medical School at the College of Philadelphia. He treated conditions such as gout, nervousness, fever, and weakness. Some of the medicines Dr. Cullen used included opium and cinnamon.

In 1735, Dr. Claudius Amyand performed the world's first successful appendectomy on an 11-year-old boy. The first successful procedure to treat acute appendicitis was accomplished in 1759 in Bordeaux. Since general anesthesia did not exist until 1846, operations such as appendectomies required many assistants to restrain patients and assist surgeons.

History has taught us much about anatomy and surgery. Although there is no specific documentation, we know that throughout time, every surgeon used a "surgical assistant" to support them during surgery.

HISTORY OF SURGICAL ASSISTANTS

According to the American College of Surgeons, an assistant surgeon should be either a practicing surgeon or a surgical resident if possible. If not available, the role of the surgical assistant may be filled by nonsurgical physicians or allied health professionals.

In 1979, a group of surgical assistants formed the Virginia Association of Surgical Assistants. They established standards of practice and developed a job description. This was the first documented role of the assistant in surgery. In 1983, the

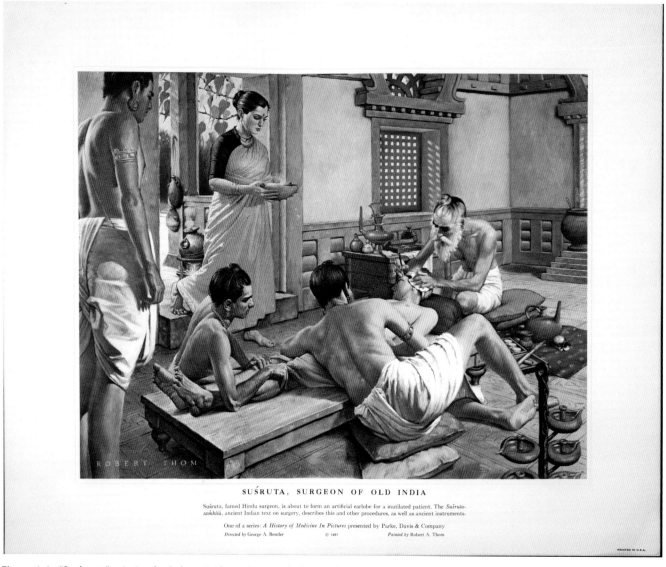

SUŚRUTA, SURGEON OF OLD INDIA

Suśruta, famed Hindu surgeon, is about to form an artificial earlobe for a mutilated patient. The *Suśruta-samhita*, ancient Indian text on surgery, describes this and other procedures, as well as ancient instruments.

One of a series: *A History of Medicine In Pictures* presented by Parke, Davis & Company
Directed by George A. Bender   © 1957   Painted by Robert A. Thom

Figure 1-1 ▪ "Sushruta" painting by Robert A. Thom. (National Library of Medicine. https://collections.nlm.nih.gov/catalog/nlm:nlmuid-101651474-img.) (Used with permission Robert Thom/Alamy Stock Photo.)

Virginia Association of Surgical Assistants became the National Surgical Assistant Association (NSAA), and the first organization in the country to establish standards of professionalism and proficiency for the Non-Physician Surgical Assistant. There are 1400 Certified Surgical Assistants (CSAs) practicing today.

In 1984, the Association of Surgical Technologists (AST) held a meeting to discuss the career ladder for the surgical technologist. In 1986, the First Assistant's Committee was formed to collect information and compose the job description for the first assistant. The AST House of Delegates passed a position statement that included the detailed role of the surgical assistant in 1988. A detailed job description received approval in 1990. Following that, a formal curriculum for the surgical assistant was established along with the first core curriculum that was published in 1993. The fourth edition of the core curriculum was published in 2020 and includes the latest approaches

to surgery. The first Certified Surgical First Assistant (CSFA) exam was administered in 1992. The Commission on Accreditation of Allied Health Education Programs (CAAHEP) accredited the first surgical assisting program in 2003 and today there are 13 accredited programs. The Accreditation Review Council on Education in Surgical Technology and Surgical Assisting (ARC/STSA) works as the liaison between CAAHEP and surgical assisting programs to ensure the program meets the standards set by CAAHEP, and it is the organization that recommends programmatic accreditation to CAAHEP.

FIELD OF SURGICAL ASSISTING

The role of the surgical assistant depends on several facets. One key factor is the training the surgical assistant receives. According to the American College of Surgeons, a surgical assistant should be appropriately trained when it is necessary to have nonphysicians serve as first assistants. "Surgeon assistants (SAs) with additional surgical training should meet national standards and be credentialed by the appropriate local authority." According to Texas law, "'surgical assisting' means providing aid under direct supervision in exposure, hemostasis, and other intraoperative technical functions that assist a physician in performing a safe operation with optimal results for the patient, including the delegated authority to provide local infiltration or the topical application of a local anesthetic at the operation site." The US Bureau of Labor Statistics job classification for surgical assistants, designated the standard occupational classification number of 29-9093, became effective in January 2018. Surgical assistants perform perioperative duties that are outlined in the *Core Curriculum for Surgical Assisting*. Some of the duties include aiding the surgeon with making incisions, manipulating tissues, implanting surgical devices or drains, clamping or cauterizing vessels, closing surgical sites, and applying dressings (Table 1-1). Privileges for the surgical assistant should be clearly delineated as well as the level of surgeon supervision. General supervision means the procedure is furnished under the physician's overall direction and control, but the physician's presence is not required during the performance of the procedure. The training of the nonphysician personnel, under supervision, is the continuing responsibility of the surgeon. For surgical assistants who work in offices, the physician must be present in the office suite and immediately available to provide guidance throughout the

---

TABLE 1-1 • THE SKILLS OF THE SURGICAL ASSISTANT IN THE PERIOPERATIVE ROLE

General Surgical Assistant Skills

1. Demonstrates the ability to communicate the surgeon's preferences and specific patient's needs to surgical team including but not limited to suture needs, specialty supplies and instrumentation, and equipment.
   a. Verifies all implants, supplies, and special procedure equipment are available and functional (ie, microscope, tourniquet, etc.).
   b. Facilitates a cooperative team atmosphere through professional communication.
   c. Listens actively to surgeon, patient, and team to ensure safe patient-centered care.
   d. Maintains awareness of patient monitoring and responds appropriately to potential complications.
2. Demonstrates the ability to apply advanced knowledge of normal and pathological surgical anatomy and physiology.
   a. Describes the assessment and management of acute trauma.
   b. Responds appropriately to emergency conditions.
3. Demonstrates aseptic skills:
   a. Monitors the actions immediately surrounding the sterile field ensuring that the integrity is maintained and/or corrected appropriately.
   b. Evaluates potential causes of surgical site infections, communicating concerns and possible corrective actions to prevent and/or treat potential contamination.
4. Acquires continuing education annually to maintain current competence and credential regarding specific skills and techniques including aseptic technique. Bases decisions on research-based evidence.
5. Participates in the education of allied health personnel including SA and ST students.

Preoperative Role

1. Demonstrates the ability to provide preoperative skills such as assessing patient information, history, preoperative tests (ie, EKG, EEG, EMG, lab values, diagnostic imaging), safety measures, biopsy results, positioning, and draping.
   a. Verifies patient identification, allergies, NPO status, procedure, surgical site, consent, history and physical on chart.
   b. Inspects skin integrity for signs of infection, compromised perfusion, or other signs of potential risk.
   c. Ensures x-rays and applicable diagnostic exams are available for surgeon.
2. Specifics regarding positioning the patient:
   a. Ensures placement of monitoring devices does not interfere with access or prep.
   b. Ensures position of the patient provides the necessary exposure for the procedure, as well as the surgeon preference.
   c. Demonstrates competency in all positioning techniques for the surgeries they are participating in. These competencies include, but are not limited to:
      i. Prevention of nerve damage
      ii. Proper rotation of extremities
      iii. Prevention of circulatory or respiratory compromise
      iv. Prevention of patient sliding on bed due to tilting or Trendelenburg
      v. Proper handling and placement of lines
   d. Demonstrates safe stabilized placement on the appropriate bed/table, with the appropriate operation, set up, safety measures, and utilization of all necessary equipment, stabilizers, padding, wrapping, and/or attachments.
   e. Maintains knowledge of new or upgraded positioning equipment, supplies, and positioning techniques through continuing education.

(Continued)

TABLE 1-1 • (Continued)

3. Specifics regarding surgical skin prep:
   a. Ensures safe placement of tourniquet, extremity padded correctly, safety precautions followed, and the accuracy of the settings for tourniquet inflation.
   b. Ensures skin prep will provide the necessary exposure for the surgical procedure, any possible drain sites and/or possible extension(s) of the operative incision, as well as surgeon preference:
      i. Facilitates clipping or trimming of hair in preop holding and only if necessary
      ii. Demonstrates ability to perform a surgical skin prep selecting the correct prep for the situation (ie, chlorhexidine gluconate/alcohol prep, iodine povacrylex/alcohol prep, chlorhexidine gluconate, povidone-iodine [iodopovidone], etc.) and preparing the appropriate surgical prep site necessary.
      iii. Demonstrates insertion of Foley catheter; prevents potential complications, as indicated.
4. Specifics regarding draping:
   a. Streamlines the establishment of the sterile field.
   b. Coordinates the draping procedure effectively correcting any breaks in aseptic technique.
   c. Supports double gloving/changing outer gloves after establishment of the sterile and periodically (every 90 minutes) during case.
   d. Secures lines and cords in a manner that prevents loss of integrity.
   e. Evaluates and incorporates products to ensure effective barriers are established and maintained that prevent contamination during the entire procedure.

Intraoperative Care

1. Demonstrates the ability to provide intraoperative skills such as visualization, trocar insertion (ie, ASA Trocar Guidelines), injection of local anesthetics (ie, ASA Local Anesthetic Guidelines), hemostasis, tissue handling, placement and securing of wound drains, and closure of body planes.
2. Utilizes the OR equipment pertinent to the surgical procedure. All actions shall facilitate the progress of the surgery, as well as anticipate the preference(s) of the surgeon. This shall include, but not limited to:
   a. Hemostatic equipment and supplies, including monopolar, bipolar, harmonic scalpel, ultrasonic, medications, sponges, etc. Includes appropriate safety precautions such as the placement of grounding pad, assists scrub and circulator with accuracy of counts when necessary, etc.
   b. Knowledge of and use of any and all laparoscopic and robotic equipment necessary for a procedure, such as: Camera, light cord, inserting/removing trocars, graspers, scoops, sprayers, suction/irrigation systems, clamps, tenaculums, etc.
   c. Knowledge of and use of any open procedure equipment necessary for procedures, including, tissue forceps, retractors, clamps, scissors, sponges, suction, irrigation, use of hemostatic agents, etc.
   d. Any further applicable instrumentation or actions deemed necessary by the surgeon.
3. The surgical assistant should be proficient in all pertinent abilities required during a procedure. These shall follow any necessary and appropriate methods applicable to the procedure, as well as surgeon preference. These shall include, but not be limited to:
   a. Clamping, cauterizing, suturing, inserting, injecting, manipulating, retracting, cutting, and ligating tissue as necessary.
   b. Any necessary involvement in hemostasis, including but not limited to the utilization of ties, vessel loops, clip appliers, digital pressure, packing, appropriate manipulation of sutures, etc.
   c. Participation in volume replacement or autotransfusion techniques as necessary and appropriate.
   d. Any further applicable instrumentation or actions deemed necessary by the surgeon.
4. The surgical assistant should be capable of working independently, or codependently with the surgeon, to finalize the surgery, according to the surgeon preference. These actions shall include, but not limited to:
   a. Participates in quality improvement process that includes standardized approaches, checklist interventions such as the Michigan Keystone Surgery Project regarding surgical site infection to improve patient care and Time Out procedures to improve patient safety.
   b. Initiates appropriate actions or instrumentation in collaboration with the surgeon.
   c. Utilizes appropriate suturing techniques, according to surgeon preference, with closure of body planes and utilizing proper manipulation of suture.
      i. Using running, or interrupted suture techniques
      ii. Including absorbable and nonabsorbable sutures, staples, adhesives, strips, etc.
   d. Demonstrates ability to administer a local anesthetic, according to surgeon's preference.
   e. Demonstrates ability to secure drainage systems.
   f. Demonstrates ability to apply dressings, splints, casts, and immobilizers/stabilizers, according to surgeon preference.
   g. Evaluates the patient for any possible damage from positioning. This shall include a skin assessment. Any abnormal condition should be reported to the surgeon, and appropriate treatment be carried out according to the surgeon's instruction.

Postoperative Care

1. Demonstrates the ability to provide postoperative skills in patient care such as dressing application, patient transfer and transport, transfer of care, and monitoring for immediate complications.
2. Collaborates with others to provide continuity of care.

Source: Reproduced with permission from the Association of Surgical Assistants (www.asa.org).

performance of any task or procedure. Personal supervision indicates a physician must be present in the room when the surgical assistant performs any tasks. With the broad scope of practice, the role requires specialized education and training; therefore, on-the-job training is no longer appropriate for the surgical assistant.

EDUCATION

Colleges and technical schools have enrollment requirements that often include specific education outcomes prior to applying for enrollment into a surgical assisting program. Students also must be able to show proof of successful completion of basic science (college level) instruction, including:

- Microbiology
- Pathophysiology
- Pharmacology
- Anatomy and physiology
- Medical terminology

College curriculum for surgical assisting program should include:

- Advanced surgical anatomy
- Surgical microbiology
- Surgical pharmacology
- Anesthesia methods and agents
- Bioscience
- Ethical and legal considerations
- Fundamental technical skills
- Complications during surgery
- Interpersonal skills
- Clinical application of computers

Students entering a surgical assisting program should have prior knowledge of the operating room (OR) and aseptic principles and techniques. Surgical assisting programs have established criteria for those applying to programs. Suggested eligibility criteria must be published on a school's website. All surgical assisting programs require students to "log" cases that include completing the duties of the surgical assisting in order to sit for the national certification exam, whether for the CSFA examination through the National Board of Surgical Technology and Surgical Assisting (NBSTSA) or the CSA examination administered by the National Commission for the Certification of the Surgical Assistants (NCCSA). Continuing education (CE) is required to stay current in the field and for certification renewal.

CAREER DEVELOPMENT

Career development can be broken into two paradigms or viewpoints, one being the perspective of the employer and the other the perspective of the employee. As an employee, career development is very important. This involves managing your career to meet your personal objectives, whether that means higher pay, receiving incentives, or job flexibility and satisfaction. Career development is often a lifelong process and may fluctuate throughout time. All that being said, career development can be described as the ongoing or continuous progression of managing one's life, learning, and work in order to advance forward, toward a desired future. Career development can be broken down into several categories that include experience in a specific profession, education to coincide with the profession, as well as communication of one's skillset as it relates to the job one seeks.

Established career development programs promote equity, allowing employees equal opportunities to improve themselves and advance their careers. This leads to job satisfaction and improved work performance.

Several factors influence career development. These include personality characteristics. Outgoing and assertive people are more likely to advance in their career faster than shy, quiet people. Knowing your personality can make you more successful in achieving career goals. There are self-assessment tests to help recognize personality traits and aid with career planning. Skills and knowledge are important aspects of career planning, especially when specializing in a surgical specialty. Finally, social and economic factors have an impact on whether one is able to pursue their ultimate career choice.

Successful career development involves commitment and a plan. Write down your goals. Studies show that if something is written down, it is more apt to happen. Re-evaluate your goals and objectives regularly. Things can happen and your goals may change with time. Keep your career goals relevant to where you are in your career. It is suggested to pursue career development coaching if you are struggling with your career plan. Choose someone in the same field so that this person understands what you do. Accept your weaknesses. This will give insight into what you need to work on. Develop a timeline for your career goals. This will give you motivation to complete it. Look for skill development opportunities in all places. By stepping outside your comfort zone, the learning process is unforgettable and more apt to be effective.

PROFESSIONALISM

According to the Merriam-Webster dictionary, the word *professionalism* has several meanings: Conduct or qualities that characterize a profession itself, or the following of a profession for gain or livelihood. Either way, every professional has an obligation to demonstrate the following characteristics:

- A professional should be an expert in their field. This includes maintaining certification through CEs, attending educational seminars, and exhibiting a broad set of skills.

- A professional should follow their code of ethics as it relates to their practice and treat all patients and colleagues with the proper decorum.

- A professional exhibits confidence and poise. They remain calm during difficult situations.

- A professional has excellent communication skills and phone etiquette. Listening and relaying information is paramount to good professional behavior.
- A professional promotes patient safety through honesty, respect, and integrity.

Professionalism within the medical community relies on self-regulation, as well as oversight of the medical education discipline. The medical professional places the needs of the patient above all else. Selflessness, competence, and accountability to the patient generate patient trust, which is the foundation of medical professionalism.

Why is professionalism so important to the medical community? A crucial rationale for professionalism is that it promotes patient safety. Healthcare is a team effort that requires excellent communication skills, along with ethical principles of veracity, justice, respect, and confidentiality. Adhering to these principles protects the patient from physical harm. A reference to professionalism should reside within a profession's Code of Ethics, oaths, charters, curriculum, and core competencies.

PROFESSIONAL MANAGEMENT

As a professional facilitator for the case, you are expected to manage your own continuous education regarding anything that could affect the outcome for the patient. This includes any equipment, instrumentation, institution policies, or room turnover. In a leadership role, you set the example for the surgeon's expectations ensuring that everything goes smoothly. Education of others and effective communication techniques are essential for creating a winning team. Take classes, read books to learn how to manage conflict and change, and ensure communication is effective for all types of learners. You cannot communicate the same way with everyone. You must adjust according to the situation, so being flexible with a problem-solving mindset will ensure you are facilitating effectively. The only thing that is constant in our world is "change." Therefore, learning to anticipate, adapt, and manage change is also an essential skill.

- Leadership—what do others expect from you?
  - Teach, coach, and/or mentor others.
  - Take risks or face challenges.
  - Able to negotiate.
  - Able to motivate others.
  - Able to direct others to meet common goals.
  - Demonstrate efficacy—not only efficient but can find ways to improve the system.
  - Look for ways to simplify the process, organize for faster turnover, and check case carts prior to beginning the day.
  - Save time or money.
  - Able to build alliances and partnerships, and work in teams with any coworker.

COMMUNICATION

Effective communication skills can increase the opportunities available to you. Employers appreciate effective communication skills that concisely present information and ideas in a clear and positive manner. Good communication connects people so each person feels understood. A culture of safety environment encourages people to speak up when they identify issues, and it creates a "safe" place where individuals can express their solutions and ideas.

- Active listening skills must be used to truly understand what is being communicated. Each person must look directly at the other, listening carefully and completely, allowing each person to finish talking before responding. It is always good to summarize what was said to verify understanding. For example, "What I heard was …." Then, the other person can verify or clarify what was not clearly understood. In addition, it is okay to jot a note of some point you want clarification about, but refrain from focusing on one issue and formulating a reply until the person is completely finished. You must hear it all to truly understand the who, what, when, where, how, and why about the situation. Once verified, then you can formulate a reply or discuss points of concern.
- Nonverbal communication tips:
  - Learn how to read nonverbal cues (tells). Lack of eye contact can indicate avoidance and too much eye contact aggressiveness. Others include gestures, body movements, posture, and tone of voice.
  - Pay attention to your own tone of voice. Watch others to see how they react. Adjust immediately to ensure your feedback indicates acceptance and/or understanding.
  - Look for incongruence between words and nonverbal actions.
- React promptly: Able to follow directions, verbal and written, correctly.
- Ensure understanding. Restate/Summarize instructions to verify understanding; ask questions to clarify instructions; take notes to ensure accuracy.
- Express ideas and instructions clearly. Ensure to follow directions or understand and respond appropriately.

Teamwork

Teamwork is defined as the collaborative effort of a group with a common goal. In the OR, our common goal is a safe optimal outcome for our patient while completing the schedule in an effective and efficient manner. There are several types of teams but what we need are performing teams. Functional teams utilize synergistic energy and creativity to accomplish more in less time. "Many hands make light work." Dysfunctional teams are those who do not achieve the best outcome in the most efficient and timely manner due to personal conflicts, lack of support for decisions made by the group, and failure to conform to the decisions and processes determined as best practice by the team.

If there are any delays or suboptimal outcomes, then our process and/or our team needs some work to improve.

Key principles for becoming a successful team player:

- Successful teams have a clear goal and all members are willing to identify key requirements that are essential but are willing to compromise on other segments to achieve a win-win solution. All parties must discard personal preferences and focus on achieving the goal. Know the goal and focus on that goal.

- Other teams are formed to achieve specific tasks or goals, such as the turnover team. This team focuses on the processes that will facilitate a fast and safe room turnover to maximize OR productivity. In this case, there may be several objectives that must be met. Safe is one, fast is the second. So, decisions are based on more than one criterion to ensure the final goal is achieved. Safe ensures that we are still able to produce the optimal patient outcome possible. Fast refers to the time frame being measured. We cannot ever lose sight of our first directive in the healthcare field, "To do no harm." Know your strengths and align your role expectations within those strengths.

Some key principles of team development:

- A team is a group of individuals assigned to a common goal.

- A team undergoes stages of development including Forming (initial grouping, and people are getting to know each other), Storming (rules of behavior are being set; differences become apparent, and if not resolved, the team stays in this stage), Norming (rules of behavior have been established, roles have been taken on, and acceptable communication patterns established), and Performing (group is functioning at the highest level with good outcomes and goals are met). There is a final Adjourning stage that occurs when a group has disbanded or achieved the goal. This stage is not applicable to ongoing teams and departments. The length of time for each stage varies with the knowledge, skills, and experience of the team members along with the challenges and management support available.

- Anytime someone is added to or leaves the group, the group will reform through these stages again as roles are shifted and/or the new person is integrated into the team.

- Knowing these principles allows you to merge into a fixed team understanding that you must learn the accepted behaviors of the team, get to know each team member and their role, and understand their expectations from you.

Becoming a productive and respected team member is hard work. It means that you focus on the goal(s) and you work within the team for the good of the institution or goal. When team conflict occurs, it must be addressed. Bad behavior and violated expectations must be handled by the leader. Failure to address those issues in a timely fashion can damage team morale, leading to toxic or dysfunctional teams. If you have any hidden agendas, fail to institute and support the decisions of the team, talk negatively about the decisions, or cannot support the goals of the team, then the team will not be successful because you have become a toxic member. Do the right thing, do what you say you will do, and if you can't support the team then leave the team to find a team you can support. As a team member, you should cultivate a willingness to change, a dedication to evidence-based knowledge, and a commitment to compromise with others in a respectful manner to become a true team player.

ASSOCIATION OF SURGICAL ASSISTANTS

The Association of Surgical Assistants (ASA) represents the interests of more than 5000 surgical assistants throughout the country. The primary purpose is to ensure surgical assistants have the knowledge and skill set to provide quality patient care. ASA works in partnership with the ARC/STSA and the NBSTSA to set standards for education and certification.

"The Association of Surgical Assistants represents a broad coalition of surgical assistant practitioners, who share several common goals, including optimizing surgical patient care, promoting the recognition of all surgical assistants, advancing legislative strategies, and providing relevant continuing education experiences." ASA offers live educational events, malpractice insurance, and insurance discounts through its website.

One of the core responsibilities of the ASA is legislative advocacy. There is legislative recognition in 10 states and ASA is continually working on new state initiatives. Current legislation is as follows:

Licensing:
    Nebraska
    Kentucky
    Virginia
Optional licensing:
    District of Columbia
    Texas
Required registration:
    Colorado
Optional registration/title protection:
    Illinois
    Tennessee
Note: Indiana Surgical Assistants must hold the designation of Certified Surgical First Assistant (CSFA) to perform certain tasks and functions.

The ASA has published a comprehensive guideline as to the role of the surgical assistant (see Table 1-1) and the expectations of the skill set during perioperative care of the patient.

These expectations should be included in a comprehensive job description. When writing a job description, include the following:

- An Introduction: Details about the company and facts about the organization and its mission. The value system of the organization is important to prospective employees.

- Job title and summary of duties: Who will the surgical assistant report to, whether it is a person or department? Is the position full- or part-time? Ten- or 12-hour shifts available? What is the call schedule?

- List key responsibilities: What job responsibilities are expected, especially outside of assisting during operative procedures? What are the hours one can expect to work per pay period?

- Describe core skills: Use bullet points to prioritize the skill set the assistant is expected to master and perform independently.

- Additional skills preferred but not necessary: There may be additional skills that are advantageous to the organization.

- Required qualification and education: List if there is a required certification and/or education level for the position.

- Salary expectations: This will limit applications to those who are truly interested in the position posted, if the salary and benefits are acceptable. It is important to include a contact person or email address where to submit the application/portfolio to.

- Career path: Is there a clinical ladder or any leadership avenues available to the surgical assistant? Is there professional development to maintain certification?

CREDENTIALING

A credential is an attestation of qualification, competence, or authority issued to an individual by a third party with a relevant or de facto authority or assumed competence to do so. The rationale for maintaining a credential is to validate your continued proficiency through CEs.

There are currently two credentials primarily accepted nationwide which include the CSFA sponsored by NBSTSA and CSA sponsored by NCCSA.

Upon graduation from an accredited school of surgical assisting, the individual is eligible to sit for the examination conducted by the credentialing organization. Currently, CAAHEP accredits surgical assisting education programs. The CSFA credential is accepted nationwide and is supported by the ASA which provides CE on an ongoing basis.

CONTINUING EDUCATION

Professional CE is a specific learning activity generally characterized by the issuance of a certificate or CE credits. CE requirements are needed by the certification organizations to renew your certification and continue practicing as a surgical assistant. These requirements are intended to encourage professionals to expand their foundations of knowledge and stay up-to-date on new developments. CE credits are recorded by your professional organization as recognized by the NBSTSA (National Board of Surgical Technology and Surgical Assistants or the National Surgical Assistant Association). CE credits are submitted to the organization which records and reports the number and type of CE credits earned during the renewal period.

As of January 1, 2020, all certification renewal periods are for 2 years. Renewal requires 38 CE credits of which eight credits are identified as advanced level/live CE credits. An alternative is to retest by taking the national certification exam currently in use. The application is submitted to the certification organization along with the fee for renewal prior to the expiration date.

Bibliography

American Board of Medical Specialties. ABMS definition of medical professionalism. www.abm.org. Accessed February 27, 2023.

American College of Surgeons. ACS Releases Seventh Report on Physicians as Assistants at Surgery. https://www.facs.org/media/press-releases/2013/pas1113. Accessed February 27, 2023.

American College of Surgeons. ACS statement on principles. https://www.facs.org/about-acs/statements/stonprin. Accessed February 27, 2023.

Association of Surgical Assistants. Job description. https://www.surgicalassistant.org/about/JobDescription/. Accessed February 27, 2023.

Anatasia. What is career development? https://www.cleverism.com/what-is-career-development/. Accessed February 27, 2023.

National Commission for the Certification of Surgical Assistants. https://www.csaexam.com/. Accessed February 27, 2023.

Bleier J, Kann B. Academic goals in surgery. *Clin Colon Rectal Surg.* 2014;26:212-217.

Ein SH, Amurawaiye E, Ein A. *Recycling the retired surgeon: Surgical assisting—A Canadian's perspective.* https://www.printfriendly.com/p/g/H3TxES. Accessed February 27, 2023.

Medicine in the 1700s: Dr. William Cullen's letters Now Online. https://www.healio.com/hematology-oncology/physicians-life. Accessed February 27, 2023.

National Board of Surgical Technologists and Surgical Assistants. Renewals and Recertification. https://www.nbstsa.org/csfa-certification; https://www.nbstsa.org/renewals-recertification. Accessed February 27, 2023.

Wachter RM. *The Evolution of Patient Safety in Surgery.* https://psnet.ahrq.gov/perspectives/perspective/239/the-evolution-of-patient-safety-in-surgery. Accessed February 27, 2023.

Whitlock J. The evolution of surgery: A historical timeline. https://www.verywellhealth.com/the-hsitory-of-surgery-timeline. Accessed February 27, 2023.

What are key elements for a good job description. https://jobdescriptionimc.wordpress.com/2012/11/01/what-are-the-key-elements-for-a-good-job-description/; and https://www.caahep.org/Students/Program-Info/Surgical-Assisting.aspx. Accessed February 27, 2023.

Burton N. Emotional Intelligence. *Psychology Today.* New York, NY: Sussex Publishers, LLC. https://www.psychologytoday.com/us/basics/emotional-intelligence; and https://www.psychologytoday.com/us/blog/the-brain-and-emotional-intelligence/201310/how-focus-changed-my-thinking-about-emotional. Accessed February 27, 2023.

Minnesota State Colleges and Universities Career and Education Resource. Employability skills. https://careerwise.minnstate.edu/careers/employability-skills.html. Accessed February 27, 2023.

Mastering Soft Skills for Workplace success. Problem solving and critical thinking. https://www.dol.gov/odep/topics/youth/softskills/Problem.pdf. Accessed February 27, 2023.

Key to Lean—Plan, Do, Check, Act!. All about Lean.com. https://www.allaboutlean.com/pdca/. Accessed February 27, 2023.

What is SixSigma.Net. Plan Do Study Act (PDSA). https://www.whatissixsigma.net/plan-do-study-act/. Accessed March 8, 2019.

Planview Leankit. 6 continuous improvement tools and techniques. https://leankit.com/learn/kanban/what-is-value-stream-mapping/. Accessed April 8, 2019.

MindTools.com. Conflict resolution: Using the "interest-based relational" approach. https://www.mindtools.com/pages/article/newLDR_81.htm. Accessed April 8, 2019.

The Balance Careers. Human Resources. (2019) 5 Stages of Team Development. Dotdash Publishing. liveabout.com. Accessed May 8, 2019.

MindTools.com. How to be a great team player: Maximizing your contribution. https://www.mindtools.com/pages/article/newTMM_53.htm. Accessed May 8, 2019.

Riodan C. Forbes Leadership Forum. Why teams turn toxic, and how to heal them. https://www.forbes.com/sites/forbesleadershipforum/2011/09/20/why-teams-turn-toxic-and-how-to-heal-them/#1c7bd0165988. Accessed May 8, 2010.

Legal, Moral, and Ethical Considerations

Rebecca Hall

DISCUSSED IN THIS CHAPTER

1. The surgical assistant scope of practice.
2. Liability as a medical professional.
3. Legal doctrines.
4. Safety organizations.

PATIENT SAFETY

Under the job description of the surgical assistant, you will find "helping the surgeon carry out a safe operation" clearly stated. According to the World Health Organization (WHO), one out of every 10 patients is harmed while receiving hospital care. Iatrogenic events that are the result of unsafe care are associated with one of the 10 leading causes of death. Studies show that improving patient safety leads to better patient outcomes. The Joint Commission has gathered data since 1995 and wrong-site surgery is consistently ranked as the leading cause of surgical errors. Wrong-site surgery can be defined as any procedure completed on the wrong patient, wrong body part, wrong side of the body, or at the wrong level of the correct anatomic site. The importance of communication to prevent wrong-site surgery cannot be understated. Any approach to establishing an algorithm to prevent wrong-site surgery and increase patient safety begins with communication. Hospitals are under increased pressure to reduce sentinel or "never" events and develop a systematic approach to create a safe environment in the operating room for staff and patients. In 2003, the Joint Commission published "Universal Protocol for Preventing Wrong Site, Wrong Procedure, and Wrong Person Surgery." It establishes three components that should be completed prior to the start of any surgical procedure: (1) Pre-procedure verification process, (2) Marking the operative site, and (3) Performing a "time out" before incision. WHO published a Surgical Safety Checklist (Figure 2-1). This checklist is based on the international program "Safe Surgery Saves Lives." This publication contains checklists to be reviewed by the surgical team before induction of anesthesia, before skin incision, and before the patient leaves the operating room. The surgical team should not rely strictly on the surgeon for verification. It is everyone's responsibility to ensure a safe operation for the patient. The risk of any mistake is greatly reduced when the entire surgical team is involved in the verification process prior to incision.

The Safety Checklist can also be described as the OR Briefing and Debriefing. These discussions should be initiated and led by the surgeon. They are designed to mitigate adverse events by improving communication with the surgical team. Team members are encouraged to speak up if they feel there is an issue that may affect patient outcomes. The briefing consists of introductions by first names and the role of each OR team member, a time out that includes the surgical plan, and a conversation of expectations with needed equipment and supplies. The debriefing at the end of the case is intended to discuss any issues that need attention to confirm they will be corrected for future procedures. Studies show that preoperative OR briefings are linked to improved patient safety, as well as a reduction in wrong-site/wrong-procedure surgeries, patient misidentification as well as incorrect positioning of the patient.

Improving patient safety should also be emphasized when privileges are granted for new technology or procedures. In addition to the surgeon being supervised as they master a new procedure, the OR team should be properly trained and well-versed in safety features, including cleaning and sterilizing any required equipment.

Surgical Safety Checklist

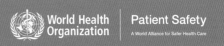

World Health Organization | Patient Safety
A World Alliance for Safer Health Care

Before induction of anesthesia	Before skin incision	Before patient leaves operating room
(with at least nurse and anesthetist)	(with nurse, anesthetist, and surgeon)	(with nurse, anesthetist, and surgeon)

Before induction of anesthesia
(with at least nurse and anesthetist)

Has the patient confirmed his/her identity, site, procedure, and consent?
☐ Yes

Is the site marked?
☐ Yes
☐ Not applicable

Is the anesthesia machine and medication check complete?
☐ Yes

Is the pulse oximeter on the patient and functioning?
☐ Yes

Does the patient have a:

Known allergy?
☐ No
☐ Yes

Difficult airway or aspiration risk?
☐ No
☐ Yes, and equipment/assistance available

Risk of >500 mL blood loss (7 mL/kg in children)?
☐ No
☐ Yes, and two IVs/central access and fluids planned

Before skin incision
(with nurse, anesthetist, and surgeon)

☐ **Confirm all team members have introduced themselves by name and role.**

☐ **Confirm the patient's name, procedure, and where the incision will be made.**

Has antibiotic prophylaxis been given within the last 60 minutes?
☐ Yes
☐ Not applicable

Anticipated Critical Events

To Surgeon:
☐ What are the critical or non-routine steps?
☐ How long will the case take?
☐ What is the anticipated blood loss?

To Anesthetist:
☐ Are there any patient-specific concerns?

To Nursing Team:
☐ Has sterility (including indicator results) been confirmed?
☐ Are there equipment issues or any concerns?

Is essential imaging displayed?
☐ Yes
☐ Not applicable

Before patient leaves operating room
(with nurse, anesthetist, and surgeon)

Nurse Verbally Confirms:
☐ The name of the procedure
☐ Completion of instrument, sponge and needle counts
☐ Specimen labeling (read specimen labels aloud, including patient name)
☐ Whether there are any equipment problems to be addressed

To Surgeon, Anesthetist and Nurse:
☐ What are the key concerns for recovery and management of this patient?

This checklist is not intended to be comprehensive. Additions and modifications to fit local practice are encouraged.   Revised 1 / 2009   © WHO, 2009

Figure 2-1 · WHO surgical safety checklist. (Reproduced with permission from WHO Surgical Safety Checklist, 2009. Geneva: World Health Organization; 2009.)

Medication errors should also be addressed with any safety protocol a hospital incorporates. Staff education is imperative to reduce medication errors and eliminate any confusion in prescribing, administering, or monitoring medication during regular procedures and trauma situations. A sentinel event is considered a patient safety event when it affects a patient and results in any of the following:

- Death
- Permanent harm
- Severe temporary harm and intervention required to sustain life

An event may also be considered a sentinel event even if the outcome was not death, permanent harm, severe temporary harm, or intervention required to sustain life. Such actions include:

- Burns
- Nerve damage
- Muscle strain
- Abandonment

- Improper handling of surgical specimen
- Improper drug administration
- Defective equipment and supplies
- Major breaks in sterile technique
- Documentation errors
- Exceeding authority

Reducing sentinel events such as retained foreign objects can be accomplished by adhering to the accepted standards of practice for counting during surgical procedures. According to the American College of Surgeons, intrinsic distractions such as alarms, noise from surgical devices, communication during shift change as well as extrinsic distractions such as beepers, radios, personal electronic devices, and telephone calls should be minimized in order to eliminate the negative effect on patient safety for the perioperative patient.

SCOPE OF PRACTICE

Advances in healthcare education and healthcare practice have caused a shift in the scope of practice for many professions. It is no longer reasonable to expect each profession to work isolated with a single scope of practice, exclusive of all others. Scope of practice should be reflective of the abilities of each healthcare discipline. The surgical assistant must ask themselves whether they can provide a specified service in a safe and effective manner. This can only be accomplished if they have been properly trained for the task they perform.

A 2005 Federation of State Medical Boards report defined scope of practice as the "Definition of the rules, the regulations, and the boundaries within which a fully qualified practitioner with substantial and appropriate training, knowledge, and experience may practice in a field of medicine or surgery, or other specifically defined field. Such practice is also governed by requirements for continuing education and professional accountability." This mindsight evolves from the trust the public has in healthcare professionals to provide services safely and competently. Healthcare is constantly evolving and changing. These changes can be related to demographic changes, advances in technology, increases between regulation and scope of practice. Regulation within a profession is intended to safeguard the public from incompetent or unethical practitioners. This is accomplished through gatekeeping practices that assure the public any healthcare practitioner is competent to provide services within their scope of practice. Failure to do so could result in fines against a practitioner as well as the revocation of their license to practice. Changes within a healthcare practitioner's scope of practice are intrinsic as our healthcare system continually evolves. No single profession has exclusive rights over a skill or task, nor does one skill or task define a profession. An accumulation of an entire scope of tasks within the practice makes each profession unique. Certification and licensing are essential to demonstrate a practitioner has the vital training and competence to provide a service. Within any profession, there are entry-level skills as well as advanced skills. An entry-level education does not provide a healthcare provider with the skill and knowledge to perform every aspect within their scope of practice. It is the practitioner's responsibility to perform within their scope of practice as well as within their education level. Administration is responsible for ensuring and validating the competence of all individuals performing a task. Individuals have an obligation to limit their scope of practice based on personal knowledge, education, and comfort level performing the task. All three items should be assessed before performing any direct patient care. Scope of practice for surgical assistants varies from state to state and is impacted by employers within that state. It is everyone's responsibility to know and understand their scope of practice and stay within the boundaries of that established scope.

RISK MANAGEMENT

The role of risk management is to initiate action and give advice to avoid or minimize financial loss and legal ramifications for the healthcare provider. It is guided by two standards. First, legal standards are the required standards of action recognized for people in a society. The Constitution of the United States provides the highest judicial authority and provides our operational framework. Second, medical ethics are considered above a legal standard because individuals make a choice grounded on what is the right thing to do, not necessarily what our law dictates. Medical ethics and risk management decisions should be implemented within proper norms and our current moral compass to guide the mission of risk management.

TYPES OF LIABILITY

There are two basic types of law: common law and statutory law. The roots of common law can be traced to judges in England and France over many centuries. Common law was brought to the United States with early settlers. Common law is conclusions made by judges and based on judicial decisions that apply general principles to clearly defined circumstances otherwise known as a precedent. A legal precedent is often the foundation for which future judicial decisions are made. Statutory law is known as legislative rules that congressional and state bodies enact. Statutory laws make up the majority of laws that exist today. Statutory laws may not contradict federal law.

To protect themselves from legal action, healthcare professionals should carry personal liability insurance. Even if you are covered by an employer, it may not fully protect you as an individual healthcare provider if you are accused of negligence. Negligence is the area of tort law that involves harm caused by failing to act in a manner that is expected of a healthcare provider. The core concept of negligence is that people should exercise reasonable care in their actions, by taking into account the potential harm that they might foreseeably cause to other people or property. One doesn't even have to be the primary defendant in a lawsuit for it to be financially devastating. A professional liability insurance policy in your name is important to protect your personal interests.

When a patient enters the healthcare system, they must sign a general consent for treatment. Consent is a voluntary confirmation by a patient to allow touching, examination, or treatment by medically authorized professionals. Without the general consent, any touching, even taking blood pressure readings could be perceived as battery. Consent can be given orally, written, or implied. For any invasive procedure, an informed consent must also be obtained. It is the physician who has the sole responsibility to obtain the informed consent, but it is up to the entire team to ensure the consent is on the patient chart prior to any procedure. An informed consent is intended to ensure the patient understands all the risks and any alternative treatments available that are associated with any procedure. A detailed summary of the procedure and how it will be performed as well as possible results if no treatment is performed should also be part of the informed consent. Uninformed consent occurs when the patient gives authorization but does not understand or comprehend what they are agreeing to.

HIPAA

Along with the general or informed consent for treatment, there is a correlation obligation from healthcare workers to respect a patient's right to privacy and that privacy must be protected.

All healthcare employees sign a memorandum of understanding in regard to their responsibility under the Health Insurance Portability and Accountability Act (HIPAA) guidelines. A major penalty for breach of confidentiality is termination of employment. The breach of patient confidentiality consequences could include a civil lawsuit for medical malpractice. HIPAA was passed by Congress in 1996 to improve the efficiency and effectiveness of the healthcare system. HIPAA requires the following:

- Standardization of electronic patient health data, administrative data, and financial data
- Unique health identifiers for individuals, employees, health plans, and healthcare providers
- Security standards to protect the confidentiality and integrity of the individually identifiable health information, past, present, or future

Physicians are obligated to give patients a notice of their privacy practices that must consist of the following rights:

- Restricts the use of (Protected health information) PHI
- Patients can request confidential communication
- Inspect and obtain a copy of the PHI
- Request any amendment to the PHI
- Receive an accounting of PHI disclosures

LEGAL DOCTRINES

Legal doctrines are most commonly applied in tort law where judicial opinions create the rules or standards that comprise the accepted legal doctrines. Numerous principles and practices today use Latin terms that are very important to those who study law. Legal doctrines have evolved from ancient Roman law, and the Latin form of these legal doctrines is still used in medicine today. The following are the most common Latin doctrines we see in the medical setting.

Respondeat superior: "Let the master respond." This doctrine is associated with malpractice and places ultimate liability with a superior or employer.

Res ipsa loquitor: "The thing speaks for itself." This doctrine allows an inference or presumption that a healthcare provider was negligent based on circumstantial evidence and can be proved without expert testimony.

Primum non nocere: "First do no harm." This Latin term refers to physicians treating their patients. Treatment should always improve the patient to an acceptable baseline or acceptable quality of life. This term is found in the Hippocrates work entitled Epidemics, "either help or do not harm the patient."

In medicine today, there is **the reasonable man doctrine** that refers to a concept where the behavior of an accused individual is equated to how a "reasonable man," would react to the same set of circumstances. This doctrine is used in tort cases, such as personal injury, medical malpractice, or nursing home abuse cases, to show negligence on behalf of the defendant.

The following are legal concepts that relate to the reasonable man doctrine:

- **Negligence**: careless or reckless behavior. The failure to provide the standard of care expected in the situation.
- **Standard of care**: care provided by a reasonable person in the similar set of circumstances.
- **General duty of reasonable care**: the duty that is obligatory for all persons to not place others into foreseeable harm due to their behavior. This duty differs depending on age, experience, and ability.
- **Breach of duty**: when one has failed to provide the standard of care that is expected of a person in his or her position.
- **Statutory standard of care**: where a statute exists in order to govern behavior in order to shield a class of persons from being harmed.
- **Medical malpractice**: negligence by a medical professional.
- **Informed consent**: a patient is fully advised of the risks of medical treatment, alternative treatment and consented to that treatment.
- **Foresight test**: intended to limit recovery in negligence cases to only those harms that were foreseeable and preventable and are the effect of the defendant's negligence.

CIVIL LIABILITY

Caring for patients bears the responsibility of protecting their privacy, but also highlights the fear of litigation for the healthcare provider. Once a professional becomes licensed, they inherit the legal liability for their actions. Civil liability is often associated with healthcare providers. Civil liability recognizes conflicts between individuals, corporations, government bodies, and other organizations. Civil liability addresses breach of contract and torts. Under civil liability, tort law is the largest category. However, under tort law, all personal injury cases fit into one of three primary categories: intentional torts, unintentional torts, and strict liability. Strict liability applies without the need for direct fault. The most common illustration of strict liability is product defect lawsuits. In such cases, the injured patient only has to demonstrate that their injuries were a direct result of the defectiveness of a product. An **intentional tort** is the result of deliberate actions by the healthcare provider.

Examples of Intentional torts:

- Assault and/or battery: assault is placing a person in trepidation of harm and battery is the actual physical contact that harms
- False imprisonment: when someone's freedom is restricted
- Libel or slander: libel is an untrue offensive statement that is made in writing. Slander is an untrue defamatory statement that is spoken orally.
- Defamation: a false statement presented as a fact that causes injury or damage to the character of the person it is about
- Invasion of privacy tort: unjustifiable intrusion into the personal life of another without consent

TABLE 2-1 • EXAMPLES OF MEDICAL NEGLIGENCE
• Failure to diagnose or misdiagnosis
• Misreading or disregarding lab results
• Unnecessary surgery
• Surgical errors or wrong-site surgery
• Improper medication or dosage
• Premature discharge
• Improper patient history
• Failure to order proper diagnostics
• Failure to diagnose symptoms

When a healthcare provider or hospital unintentionally causes a person harm, it is categorized as an **unintentional tort.** Unintentional torts are typically considered negligence, which even though may be accidental, the healthcare provider is held liable. Medical malpractice occurs when a hospital, physician, or other healthcare provider, through negligence, causes injury to a patient. The negligence might be the result of errors in diagnosis, treatment, aftercare, or health management.

Medical negligence is failure to do what a reasonable healthcare provider would do or failing to not do what a reasonable healthcare provider would do (Table 2-1). There are four elements that a plaintiff must prove to win a negligence lawsuit: **duty** (failure to use reasonable care which results in damage or injury), **breach** (a violation of a law or duty), **cause** (breach of duty must have caused harm to the patient), and **harm** (the patient must have suffered harm in order to sue for negligence). In the medical field, negligence is often established

when an iatrogenic injury occurs, meaning damage occurred due to deviation from established standards of care.

SAFETY ORGANIZATIONS

The healthcare industry has the responsibility of improving the quality and safety of patient care within their communities. Healthcare systems are continually developing new models of patient care that include offering new technologies, improving communication between patient and healthcare provider, and record-keeping programs that protect patient privacy and improve transfer of patient care within the system. Within this paradigm, a culture of safety is essential to improve patient outcomes, eliminate medical errors, and reduce patient harm. This leads to patient satisfaction and better patient outcomes.

In 1999, **The Institute of Medicine** (IOM) published *To Err is Human,* which reported that up to 98,000 patients had died in US hospitals every year as a result of preventable sentinel events. Although this report has since been challenged and it is estimated that possibly up to 440,000 patients are injured each year by preventable events, the IOM report resulted in the creation of safety organizations to address the safety of patient care (Table 2-2).

PATIENTS' RIGHTS

Patient rights are the basic rules that incorporate legal and ethical issues in the physician-patient relationship. Included in these rights are the right to privacy, the right to quality medical care, as well as the right of autonomy to refuse medical treatment. The American Hospital Association (AHA) replaced the **"Patient Bill of Rights"** with **"The Patient Care Partnership."**

TABLE 2-2 • SAFETY-RELATED ORGANIZATIONS
Agency for Healthcare Research and Quality (AHRQ): The (AHRQ) mission is to improve the quality, safety, efficiency, and effectiveness of healthcare for all Americans.
American Society for Healthcare Risk Management (ASHRM): ASHRM promotes effective and innovative risk management strategies and professional leadership through education, recognition, advocacy, publications, networking, and interactions with leading healthcare organizations and government agencies.
American Hospital Association (AHA): This organization participates in a range of collaborative actions designed to improve the quality and safety of the care they provide.
Anesthesia Patient Safety Foundation (APSF): The APSF's Mission is to improve continually the safety of patients during anesthesia care.
National Center for Patient Safety (NCPS): The NCPS was established in 1999 to develop and nurture a culture of safety throughout the Veterans Health Administration.
National Patient Safety Foundation (NPSF): The National Patient Safety Foundation has been pursuing one mission; to improve the safety of care provided to patients.
National Quality Forum (NQF): An organization formed to develop and implement a national strategy for healthcare quality measurement and reporting.
Surgical Care Improvement Plan (SCIP): A national quality partnership interested in improving surgical care by significantly reducing surgical complications.
World Health Organization (WHO): The program, WHO Patient Safety, aims to coordinate, disseminate, and accelerate improvements in patient safety worldwide.

This document informs patients what they can expect during their hospital visit concerning their rights and responsibilities. Patients have the right to:

High-quality hospital care	A clean and Safe environment
Involvement in your care	Protection of your privacy
Help when leaving the hospital	Help with your billing claims.

CAREGIVER'S RIGHTS

As we age, all of us will require increased medical care. If we are lucky, a family member may become our caregiver. This can place undue emotional stress or hardship on a person. The American Heart Association reminds us that caregivers have rights that include the right to health and happiness, even when caring for a loved one. There are several websites that provide support that can be found on the American Heart Brochure. The National Alliance for Caregiving at caregiving.org is a group devoted to providing support to family caregivers and the professionals who help them and to increasing public awareness of issues facing family caregivers. The National Family Caregivers Association at Thefamilycaregiver.org provides resource recommendations and information for caregivers. A newsletter and caregiving greeting cards are available to members. It provides free membership to caregivers. The Well Spouse Association at wellspouse.org is a nonprofit group designed to provide support and encouragement for the spouses and children of the chronically ill. It is important for the caregiver to take care of themselves so they can provide care and comfort to their loved ones.

Bibliography

Makary MA, Sexton JB, Freischlag JA, et al. Patient safety in surgery. *Annals of surgery.* 2006;243(5),628-635. doi:10.1097/01.sla.0000216410.74062.0f. https://www.ncbi.nlm.nih.gov/pmc/articles/PMC1570547/#!po=6.52174. Accessed March 1, 2023.

Committee opinion no. 464: Patient safety in the surgical environment. *Obstet Gynecol.* 2010; 116:786-790. https://pssjournal.biomedcentral.com/articles. Accessed March 1, 2023.

Haynes AB, Weiser TG, Berry WR, et al. A surgical safety checklist to reduce morbidity and mortality in a global population. *N Engl J Med.* 2009;360:491-499. https://www.nejm.org/doi/full/10.1056/NEJMsa0810119. Accessed March 2, 2023.

Statement on Distractions in the Operating Room. Online October 1, 2016. This statement was developed by the American College of Surgeons (ACS) Committee on Perioperative Care and approved by the ACS Board of Regents at its June 2016 meeting. https://www.facs.org/about-acs/statements/89-distractions. Accessed March 2, 2023.

Changes in Healthcare Professions' Scope of Practice: Legislative Considerations. National Council on State Boards of Nursing. https://www.ncsbn.org/ScopeofPractice_09.pdf. Accessed March 2, 2023.

Kapp MB. Are risk management and health care ethics compatible? Published Winter 1991. https://onlinelibrary.wiley.com/doi/pdf/10.1002/jhrm.5600110103. Accessed March 2, 2023.

What Are Intentional Torts? FindLaw.

https://injury.findlaw.com/torts-and-personal-injuries/what-are-intentional-torts.html. Accessed March 2, 2023.

What Is Invasion of Privacy? FindLaw. 2019. https://injury.findlaw.com/torts-and-personal-injuries/what-is-invasion-of-privacy-.html. Accessed March 2, 2023.

Introduction to Negligence. LawShelf Educational Media. https://lawshelf.com/coursewarecontentview/introduction-to-negligence. Accessed March 2, 2023.

Sentinel Event Policy and Procedures. The Joint Commission. https://www.jointcommission.org/en/resources/patient-safety-topics/sentinel-event/sentinel-event-policy-and-procedures/. Accessed March 2, 2023.

What Is Medical Malpractice? American Board of Professional Liability Attorneys. https://www.abpla.org/what-is-malpractice. Accessed March 2, 2023.

How PSOs Help Health Care Organizations Improve Patient Safety Culture. Agency for Healthcare Research and Quality. https://www.pso.ahrq.gov/sites/default/files/wysiwyg/npsdpatient-safety-culture-brief.pdf. Accessed March 2, 2023.

Institute of Medicine (US) Committee on Quality of Health Care in America; Kohn LT, Corrigan JM, Donaldson MS, eds. *To Err Is Human: Building a Safer Health System.* Washington, DC: National Academies Press; 2000. https://www.ncbi.nlm.nih.gov/books/NBK225181/. Accessed March 2, 2023.

Study: Medical Error Deaths 4.5 Times More Likely than IOM Estimate. Becker's Clinical Leadership and Infection Control. Published September 20, 2013. https://www.beckershospitalreview.com/quality/study-medical-error-deaths-4-5-times-more-likely-than-iom-estimate.html. Accessed March 2, 2023.

American Hospital Association. https://www.aha.org/system/files/2018-01/aha-patient-care-partnership.pdf. Accessed May 22, 2023.

Nursing Home Abuse and Neglect. Fight Nursing Home Abuse. https://www.nursinghomeabusecenter.org/glossary/reasonable-man-doctrine/. Accessed March 2, 2023.

Business Considerations for Surgical Assistants

Fred Fisher and David Bartczak

1. Hospital and medical staff bylaws.
2. Surgical assistant job description.
3. Informed patient consent.
4. Issues related to independent practice.

Surgical assistants (SAs) serve as an extra pair of hands for the surgeon and can work as a hospital employee or perform as an independent contractor.

Both employment options will be discussed in this chapter but there are several areas that are common to either. It is important to be aware of all opportunities since many SAs begin their careers as hospital employees and later choose to work as independent practitioners in a full- or part-time capacity.

Presently, there are a few states where nonphysician SAs are not allowed to practice due to legislative regulations. Research your state's regulations regarding the use of SAs.

HOSPITAL AND MEDICAL STAFF BYLAWS

The Centers for Medicare and Medicaid Services (CMS) is a federal agency within the United States Department of Health and Human Services that administers the Medicare program and works in partnership with state governments to administer Medicaid, the Children's Health Insurance Program, and health insurance portability standards.

CMS Conditions of Participation ("COP") require an organized medical staff with written bylaws. (42 C.F.R. 482.22). Medical staff bylaws be approved by the Hospital Governing Body. Private accrediting agencies, such as The Joint Commission similarly require written Medical staff bylaws.

Every hospital has developed hospital bylaws that govern the facility's policies and personnel. Bylaws define the rights and responsibilities of the care providers; the rights and responsibilities of the hospital relating to the providers; and the hierarchy of medical staff.

Hospital bylaws govern the hospital. Medical staff bylaws specifically govern providers. The governing body confers powers on the medical staff through the medical staff bylaws. The medical staff is subject to the governing body. Hospital bylaws control if there's a conflict.

If a SA's employment is contingent upon being able to admit, treat, or operate on patients within a hospital setting or you are accepting an employed position with a hospital, it is worthwhile to review the hospital's medical staff bylaws and rules and regulations. The bylaws serve as the formal self-governance structure of the physicians and, if applicable, other licensed and credentialed providers, as delegated by the board of trustees. The rules and regulations outline institutional policies and protocols, such as admitting and emergency room processes; records and charting; and laboratory service orders. Sequentially, you should review the bylaws before accepting an employment opportunity, and you need to review the rules and regulations prior to treating a patient within the hospital.

Beyond the governance structure, including officers and committee responsibilities, the bylaws outline the following items that may affect your job satisfaction or, potentially, your employment status:

- Qualifications for membership and privileges
- Decision-making methods and conflict resolution
- Investigations, corrective action plans, and hearing and appeal plans

- Emergency corrective action
- Automatic suspension and termination
- Hearing and appeal processes
- Final decisions by the board of trustees
- Meeting attendance requirements

When reading the medical staff bylaws and rules and regulations, be sure to pay attention to any item that may directly influence or impact you now or in the future. It is important to know if the privileges are provided to the individual or to the employer.

Example of Medical Staff Bylaws (Figure 3-1)

The following example is found in hospital bylaws from around the country: *Affiliate and/or Active Staff shall live and maintain an office in _____ County.*

Or

For the purposes of providing call coverage — the Affiliate and/or Active Staff shall live within 30 minutes of the hospital's Emergency Department as traveled on town-maintained roads.

This covenant underscores the necessity of reviewing the bylaws and conducting an external cultural assessment prior to accepting an employment offer. Essentially, if you want to move to another county, yet continue your employment at your current practice or hospital, you could have your hospital privileges revoked or nonrenewed based on your place of residence. Why? Because you would be unable to admit, operate, or treat your patients within the hospital setting, and this typically will result in a termination or voluntary resignation if the conflict cannot be remedied to the satisfaction of the hospital.

Job Description

All applicants should be knowledgeable regarding a SA job description that includes the role and responsibilities of the position.

The nonphysician SA should be a formally educated individual who has the proper skills to perform the necessary tasks associated with surgery. SAs should meet national standards and be appropriately credentialed.

A more detailed job description is available at www.surgicalassistant.org.

In addition, requirements in some facilities may also include:

- Current license
- BLS
- Satisfactory performance
- Verification of competency (Figure 3-2)
- Curriculum vitae/resume
- Continuing education
- Fingerprint (criminal background check)
- OIG/GSA
- Sex offender check
- Confidentiality agreement (Figure 3-3)
- Contract (Figure 3-4)
- Drug screening
- EPLS-system for award management/register in the government
- Malpractice insurance
- Disability insurance

Most SAs will apply to medical staffing, but there are some facilities that may utilize human resources. In every instance, be sure that the job description is relevant to your role and responsibilities and that your job title reflects your title as SA and your credential.

BUREAU OF LABOR STATISTICS AND SURGICAL ASSISTANTS

The Bureau of Labor Statistics is the principal data-gathering agency of the federal government in the broad field of labor economics. The bureau collects, processes, analyzes, and disseminates data relating to employment, unemployment, and

---

Medical staff is responsible for administering a privileging process that would include:

- Identifying and approving a procedures list
- Processing the privileging application
- Evaluating applicant information
- Providing recommendations for approving or denying application for privileges
- Notifying applicant and all relevant departments of decision to accept or deny applicant's privileges
- Overseeing the applicant's use of privileges and quality of care issues

Approval or denial of applicant's request for privileges should be judged on the following (selected examples):

- Relevant practitioner-specific data vs aggregate data when available
- Verification of applicant's health status
- Consistency of criteria for all practitioner applicants

Figure 3-1 · Medical staff bylaws sample.

SURGICAL ASSISTANT SKILLS ASSESSMENT

SURGICAL ASSISTANT NAME:_____STATE:_____

    Clinically active as a Surgical Assistant: Yes ☐   No ☐

OCCUPATIONAL TRAINING: Medical School Graduate ☐   Physician Assistant ☐ RNFA ☐ Associate Degree ☐

    Military Trained ☐ RN ☐ ANP ☐ CST/CFA (bridge program) ☐ Accredited Surgical Assistant Program ☐

SURGICAL ASSISTANT FORMAL TRAINING: Robotics (DaVinci) ☐

    EVH (Endoscopic Vessel Harvesting) Maquet ☐ EVH Terumo ☐

CREDENTIALS:

LSA ☐	PA-C ☐
RSA ☐	OPA-C ☐
SA-C ☐	CRNFA ☐
CSA ☐	RNFA ☐
CSFA ☐	RN ☐
KCSA ☐	NP ☐
	ANP ☐

KEY: 1 = Never 2 = Rarely 3 = Sometimes 4 = Very Often 5 = Always

		1	2	3	4	5
A.	1. Compassionate towards patients and respects patients' privacy/confidentiality.					
	2. Participates in "time out" (pause for universal identification protocol) with surgical team.					
	3. Continually demonstrates attention to mental discipline, crisis-management, detail thoroughness, and stamina during the surgical procedure in providing surgical assistance to the surgeon.					
B.	1. Interacts with team positively and communicates relevant information to surgical team members.					
	2. Contributes to minimizing operative time by anticipation, economy of movement, efficiency and advance preparation.					
C.	1. Assists surgical team members with: safe patient transfer, positioning the patient, intubation-cricoid pressure, patient-scrub, foley catherization, shaving, tourniquet application, patient-draping, temperature-control, and dressing application. (based on hospital policy)					
	2. Strictly adheres to principles of aseptic technique, consistent with infection control principles and safe operating procedures.					
D.	1. Demonstrates knowledge of specific surgical procedure and willingness to learn new concepts.					
	2. Anticipates steps in surgical procedure and provides appropriate retraction, exposure and visualization of operative site.					
	3. Demonstrates proper respect and handling of tissue, consistently handling tissues appropriately with minimal damage.					
	4. Uses appropriate suctioning techniques to remove smoke, blood, and fluids from the site to improve visualization and decrease biohazard exposure.					
	5. Demonstrates manual dexterity in the use of surgical instruments and demonstrates appropriate use of instruments, including appropriate instrumentation for required surgical action.					
	6. Provides hemostasis using: electrosurgery, bipolar electrocoagulation, clamps, pressure/sponging, hemostatic agents &, bone wax.					
	7. Proficient in ligating vessels, stapling, securing drains and infiltrating local anesthetic.					
	8. Proficient in one-hand & two-hand knot tying, including Surgeon's, Granny and Square knots with consideration of suture material, displaying correct squaring of the throws and avoiding "air knots."					
	9. Executes appropriate suturing techniques for specific wound closures. Selects appropriate suture material based upon surgeon's preference and the type of closure to be performed.					
	10. Participates in required counts with surgical team.					
	Total Score:		**0**			

SURGICAL ASSISTANT EXPERIENCE

Cardiovascular Surgery: Open ☐ Endoscopic Vessel Harvesting ☐ Open Vessel Harvesting ☐ Minimally Invasive ☐ Robotic ☐

Peripheral Vascular Surgery: Open ☐ Endovascular ☐   **Thoracic Surgery:** Open ☐ Laparoscopic ☐

Plastic & Reconstructive Surgery: Open ☐ Microsurgery ☐ Craniofacial ☐ Cosmetic-Aesthetic ☐ Reconstructive ☐

General Surgery: Open ☐ Laparoscopic ☐ Bariatric ☐ Trauma ☐ Transplantation ☐ Robotic ☐

Orthopedic Surgery: Open ☐ Major Joint Replacement ☐ Spine ☐ Trauma ☐ Arthroscopic ☐

Neurosurgery: Open ☐ Spine ☐ Microsurgery ☐ Trauma ☐   **Otolaryngology & Head-Neck Surgery:** Open ☐ Laparoscopic ☐ Robotic ☐

Urologic Surgery: Open ☐ Laparoscopic ☐ Robotic ☐   **Pediatric Surgery:** Open ☐ Laparoscopic ☐ Robotic ☐

Gynecologic Surgery: Open ☐ Laparoscopic ☐ Robotic ☐   **Obstetrical Surgery:** Open ☐

    Vaginal ☐ Uropelvic ☐

EVALUATOR: Self ☐ Observer ☐ Name (print):_____ **Title:**_____

EVALUATOR Signature:_____**Date:** [_____]

Figure 3-2 · Verification of competency.

Confidentiality Agreement

Name: ____
Last **First** **Middle Initial**

SS#: ____

Workforce Member (circle):

Employee physician volunteer contract/agency student vendor other

I understand that I may be exposed to a variety of clinical, financial, and other types of information generated in the course of business. To assure the integrity of the data, and protect it from accidental loss, alteration, destruction, or tampering by unauthorized individuals, ***I agree to the following:***

1. *I understand that* ***I will refrain from releasing information (verbally, copies, faxes, downloads, or the original record) to individuals who are not authorized to receive this information.*** *This includes refraining from reading the record of or discussing a case/details with coworkers, friends, families, or other associates without a legitimate "need to know" and /or proper authorization.*

2. *Any* ***ID number and passwords*** *for information systems which I may be granted access to are strictly confidential, unique to me, and* ***will not be shared*** *with other users. I understand these computer key codes are equal to my handwritten legal signature.*

3. *I understand these codes have been granted to me under a privileged "right to know" and* ***I will limit my access only to the information pertinent to the care of the patient or within the scope of my job responsibilities.***

4. *If I suspect or have knowledge of someone else inappropriately using my password or sign-on I will report this immediately to security.*

5. *I understand this document will be retained on file and that a violation of this policy and/or releasing any confidential information which I am exposed to in the course of my activities, can result in limited or termination of access to these systems, change in ID number or password assignment, possible disciplinary action, according to hospital policy and/or Medical Staff Rules and Regulations, including termination, and potential liability.*

____
Signature ***Date***

Routing: Employee (Personnel File-Human Resources), Physician (Medical Staff Office), Volunteer (Volunteer Office), Student/Contract/Agency/Vendor (Sponsoring Department

Figure 3-3 • Confidentiality agreement.

other characteristics of the labor force. It also analyzes prices and consumer expenditures, economic growth and employment projections, and occupational health and safety. Most of the data are collected by the bureau, the Bureau of the Census, or state agencies. The basic data are issued in monthly, quarterly, and annual news releases, bulletins, reports, and special publications at https://www.bls.gov/ooh/home.htm.

For many years, there was no separate category for SAs. Practitioners were placed within the surgical technologist category. In 2014, efforts were directed to establish a new job description and occupational code for SAs. By 2016, a new code and independent job description for SAs was developed, 29-9093 and initially published in the 2018 Occupational Outlook Handbook at https://www.bls.gov/soc/2018/major_groups.htm#29-0000.

29-9093 Surgical Assistants

Of most relevance to practitioners is the information published under the Occupational Outlook Handbook which is divided by career categories. Within the healthcare category, statistics related to media pay, number of new jobs projected, entry-level education, and growth rate are published annually. This information is collected from all hospitals and surgery centers nationwide. The information provides employment guidelines

MEDICAL CENTER
PROFESSIONAL SERVICES AGREEMENT

This PROFESSIONAL SERVICES AGREEMENT ("Agreement") is made effective as of this day of _____, ("Effective Date") by and between ____Hospital, and _____ Surgical Assisting LLC, a limited liability company ("Group") and, each a "Party" and collectively the "Parties."

BACKGROUND

1. Hospital owns and operates a general, acute care hospital that provides a variety of services including surgical services.

2. Hospital wishes to engage Group to provide licensed allied health professionals who have the training, experience, and knowledge ("Providers") to provide Surgical Assistant Services (the "Services") to Hospital.

3. Hospital and Group desire to enter into this Agreement for Group's provision of the Services at the Hospital, and Group desires to provide such Services on the terms and conditions set forth in this Agreement.

In consideration of the foregoing, and the terms and conditions set forth herein, the Parties hereby agree as follows:

ARTICLE 1
PROVIDER'S PERFORMANCE OF SERVICES

1.1   Professional Services. During the Term of the Agreement, Group will provide the Services as described in Exhibit A. Group shall provide Services as needed between the hours of 7:00 AM and 3:00 PM Monday - Friday. In addition, Group shall ensure there are two surgical assistants available on-call as follows: (i) Monday through Friday from the hours of 3:00 PM to 7:00 AM and (ii) 24-hours on Saturdays, Sundays, and Hospital holidays.

1.2   Professional Qualifications. Group will at all times during the Term of this Agreement ensure compliance with the following requirements:

(a)   Licensure. Each Provider will hold and maintain a current, valid and unrestricted license to practice his or her respective profession in the State of Illinois.

(b)   Screening. Each Provider shall (i) satisfactorily complete training in infection control, safety and bloodborne pathogens; (ii) successfully pass a pre-employment physical issued within the last twelve months indicating the Group is in good health and free from communicable disease, including, but not limited to, PPD, MMR, varicella, influenza, and Hepatitis B, which will remain valid through the term of the assignment; and (iii) successfully pass a criminal background check.

Figure 3-4 · Hospital contract.

and serves to emphasize the different roles that are within the specific scope of practice for SAs.

THE IMPORTANCE OF UNDERSTANDING RISK MANAGEMENT

Often little known, but one of the most influential departments and executives in a healthcare facility is risk management—and the risk manager.

One responsibility of a hospital risk manager is to identify risks to the hospital. He does this by reviewing past incidents and claims, hospital loss and liability reports, and local and national hospital-related incident or risk data and statistics. The risk manager might also monitor the actions of hospital staff or their work environments to check for issues of compliance with existing policies and procedures or ask hospital department managers to provide risk assessments about staff, patient, or visitor safety.

A risk manager reports his findings and solutions to immediate issues, as well as plans for potential future issues or emergencies, to hospital management. He answers questions and helps develop new policies and procedures. Although a risk manager's recommendations depend on his specific findings, he might recommend that the hospital change the patient privacy policy to make it easier to read or add extra patient account security measures. Additionally, he might recommend giving existing staff additional training and responsibilities designed to prevent errors.

Often enough, SAs can encounter questions about their credentials or facilities using individuals who are not formally educated and appropriately credentialed to perform a SA task.

The best solution is to introduce yourself and explain what you do and how you contribute to patient safety. Many risk managers are not familiar with OR practitioners and their responsibilities. Many risk managers have not visited the OR, so take the initiative and schedule an appointment. Discuss your job description, your education, and your credential—all the reasons why you are qualified to serve as the surgeon's right hand.

Risk issues for SAs include the lack of licensure/registration/appropriate certificate. Many states do not require licensure/registration or even certificate of SAs—but obtaining the highest available level of demonstrated professional competency helps protect you and the hospital, avoids competency questions, and supports scope of practice boundaries.

To reinforce competencies, SAs should keep their license/registration and certification current which is often a hospital requirement. If an adverse event occurs, competency questions could be directed to the SA.

Risk Management—Outside the OR

It is essential to know your sponsoring physician whose actions and ethics are irrevocably intertwined with yours.

Be familiar with your hospital's policies/procedures and where you can find them. These policies will include the medical staff bylaws and rules; scope of practice boundaries; ethical/religious directives and organizational principles. As the saying goes—the more you know, the less risk you will incur—and knowledge demonstrates your respect for your employer and colleagues.

Get to know your team members—and who they are—the staff and the vendors. Ask yourself if you consider them competent. If not, you may be the last line of defense for the patient. Go up the line and introduce yourself to the surgical department leadership—and the risk manager, so you have resources if you need them.

Risk Management—Inside the OR

Be familiar with your facility's policies and procedures that govern working inside the operating room, such as needlestick avoidance, personal protective equipment, single dose/multidose vial usage, safe passing zone, device/equipment sequestration, and data monitoring.

In addition, be sure to treat all team members with respect to facilitate communication, ensure clarity of roles, generate a more stable and safer work environment to reduce stress and anxiety, encourage team accountability and consequently, increased patient safety.

Know your risk manager and ask her/him questions. Your risk manager can be an important ally for you to rely on. Remember—more knowledge is less risk.

ACS		
Never	1802	32%
Sometimes	1689	30%
Always	2101	38%
	5592	
CMS		
	Excluded	
	2089	37%

Figure 3-5 • Physicians as assistants at surgery.

WHICH SURGICAL PROCEDURES UTILIZE SAs

The American College of Surgeons and 15 other surgically related physician groups have identified a list of procedures that will always, sometimes, or never require the use of a SA (Figure 3-5). This list is updated annually and is available at www.facs.org.

Per the CMS list, 63% need an assistant.

Per ACS, considering both the "sometimes" and "always" list, 68% need an assistant. The "sometimes" list most of the time needs medical necessity documentation.

INFORMED PATIENT CONSENT

Under the auspices of CMS, the CMS requires that consent include the name of the hospital where treatment will take place; name of specific procedure to be performed; statement that the procedure/treatment has been explained appropriately as it relates to the risks, benefits, and alternatives; and signature of the patient or his/her representative, along with the date and time.

CMS further indicates that a "well-designed consent form" includes the name of practitioner, date, time, and signatures of the patient and/or representative plus a statement if other practitioners will be performing certain aspects of care.

§482.51(a)(4): Surgical privileges must be delineated for all practitioners performing surgery in accordance with the competencies of each practitioner. The surgical service must maintain a roster of practitioners specifying the surgical privileges of each practitioner.

If the hospital utilizes RN First Assistants, surgical PA, or other non-MD/DO SAs, the hospital must establish criteria, qualifications, and a credentialing process to grant specific privileges to individual practitioners based on each individual practitioner's compliance with the privileging/credentialing criteria and in accordance with Federal and State laws and regulations. This would include surgical services tasks conducted by these practitioners while under the supervision of an MD/DO.

482.51(b)(2): A properly executed informed consent form for the operation must be in the patient's chart before surgery, except in emergencies.

Interpretive Guidelines §482.51(b)(2).

Whether, as permitted by state law, qualified medical practitioners who are not physicians will perform important parts of the surgery or administer the anesthesia, and if so, the types of tasks each type of practitioner will carry out; and that such practitioners will be performing only tasks within their scope of practice for which they have been granted privileges by the hospital. (https://www.cms.gov/media/423601)

The policy of Informed Consent will also play an important role for the SA who is an independent practitioner and will be discussed later in this chapter.

MALPRACTICE INSURANCE

Adverse events during surgery can occur. And the SA, whether hospital employed, working as an independent, or as a student fulfilling clinical requirements, is exposed to possible legal consequences if a patient or patient's family sues.

To protect yourself, it is wise to consider a personal malpractice insurance policy. It can be required by some healthcare employers. These policies are available at different levels of coverage and amounts that are determined by employment status and state.

Compare policies and premiums online. Know what is covered and what is best for your situation.

ISSUES RELATED TO INDEPENDENT PRACTICE

Working in the hospital provides time and invaluable perspectives on surgeons, their working personalities, and case mix. It offers an opportunity to view the business side of surgery. It may be possible at the beginning to clock out of the hospital and work independently and then return to full-time status. (*Verify your state regulations regarding clocking out from a hospital to work independently.*) A word of caution—be sure this does not affect your eligibility for health insurance and other benefits. Another option may be to work independently on weekends and build your relationships with surgeons and meet other surgeons at different healthcare facilities,

Transitioning from working as a hospital-based assistant to an independent practitioner requires time and some detailed planning.

Establishing an Independent Business and Connecting with Surgeons

Starting with a surgeon begins with adding him/her as a sponsoring surgeon through human resources or medical staffing. A sponsoring surgeon assumes responsibility for your performance. This process should be fast if you are currently credentialed at the hospital, but it could require several months if you need to seek credentialing.

When first starting out, finding a surgeon or the right surgeon can be a challenge. Many SAs have previous relationships with surgeons from prior work experience. If that is not the case, then you must find another way. Approaching surgeons cold in the operating room is generally discouraged plus approaching surgeons you do not already know in places like the lounge or parking is not recommended. The best strategy to find a surgeon to help is through networking with surgical technologists, medical sales representatives, SAs, hospital schedulers, or other operating room staff. If a surgeon is looking to find an assistant, the people around them would know first. Alternatively, dropping resumes, brochures, or cards at the surgeons' offices is not usually effective.

If a SA is entering the area as a new independent assistant, it is essential to understand the demographics and the type of surgeries performed. Review information from the Department of Insurance to see which insurances are available in the region. It can also be extremely helpful to look at the city data where the hospital is located. City data details the demographics of potential patients that would be seen in the facility. The better the information about the neighborhood, the more likely you will have patients with better insurance. The types of insurance policies and the volume of cases are key to being successful as an independent SA. Research the surgeons who are credentialed in the facility to see their experience, age, and education. Knowing some of their background will facilitate discussions with them. You can still network through the facility schedulers, the operating room directors, and medical sales representative to see if they know of any surgeons looking for an assistant. Establishing a connection with the hospital or facility OR leadership is recommended when there is a lack of surgeon relationships. They know if there is a need in their operating rooms and they would welcome the extra help if there is staffing shortage. Also, it allows for you to establish contracts with the hospital that will reimburse for those cases that do reimburse for nonphysician SAs.

FACTORS AFFECTING BUSINESS

There are many decisions for SAs to consider when launching an independent practice, including applying for an NPI number, what type of corporate structure is recommended, malpractice insurance, how are you going to bill for your services, accounting guidance, taxes, joining or not joining a network, payor mix, and entering into contracts for nonreimbursable cases.

NATIONAL PROVIDER IDENTIFIER (NPI)

One of the provisions of the Affordable Care Act requires all providers of medical or other items or services & suppliers that qualify for a National Provider Identifier (NPI) to include their NPI number on all applications to enroll in the Medicare and Medicaid programs and on all claims for payment submitted under the Medicare and Medicaid programs.

The **NPI number** is a unique 10-digit number issued by the CMS to healthcare providers in the United States. Since 1996, HIPAA requires the adoption of a standard unique number for healthcare providers (Figure 3-6).

SAs *must* apply for an NPI number to bill insurance companies for patient services. It is important to note that having an NPI number does not mean that you are registered with CMS or Medicare and that you will be eligible for reimbursement or considered an approved provider. Two options for NPI numbers are available and depend on the type of practice established: single or group (Type 1 or Type 2). The application is available online at https://nppes.cms.hhs.gov/#/.

ICD-10

Many countries now use national variations of ICD-10, each modified to align with their unique healthcare infrastructure.

The US version of ICD-10, created by the Centers for Medicare & Medicaid Services (CMS) and the National Center for Health Statistics (NCHS), consists of two medical code sets—ICD-10-CM and ICD-10-PCS.

ICD-10-PCS stands for the International Classification of Diseases, Tenth Revision, Procedure Coding System. As indicated by its name, ICD-10-PCS is a procedural classification system of medical codes. It is used in hospital settings to report inpatient procedures.

ICD-10-CM stands for the International Classification of Diseases, Tenth Revision, Clinical Modification. Used for medical claim reporting in all healthcare settings, ICD-10-CM is a standardized classification system of diagnosis codes that represent conditions and diseases, related health problems, abnormal findings, signs and symptoms, injuries, external causes of injuries and diseases, and social circumstances.

For a medical provider to receive reimbursement for medical services, ICD-10-CM codes are required to be submitted to the payer. While CPT codes depict the services provided to the patient, ICD-10-CM codes depict the patient's diagnoses that justify the services rendered as medically necessary.

MEDICARE AND MEDICAID

Medicare only recognizes four professionals practicing as SAs—surgeons/physicians; physician assistants; advanced nurse practitioners, and nurse midwives. This narrow definition can influence hospital hiring policies, reimbursement for services, and recognition by insurance entities. Independent assistants cannot bill Medicare patients.

Establishing contracts with hospitals for nonbillable cases is one option for the independent assistant which will be discussed in this chapter.

Fees for hospital-employed SAs are included in the diagnosis-related group payment system (DRG) payment to the hospital and reimbursed through the prospective payment system (PPS) with Medicare and contracted rates with commercial insurers.

When a patient is admitted to a hospital and later discharged, a DRG is assigned, based on the care provided. The hospital gets paid a fixed amount for that DRG, regardless of how much money it spends treating the patient. If a hospital can effectively treat a patient for less money than Medicare pays for the DRG, then the hospital makes money on that hospitalization. If the hospital spends more money caring for a patient than Medicare allows for the DRG, then the hospital loses money on that hospitalization.

IN-NETWORK VS OUT-OF-NETWORK

Insurance companies develop a network of contracted providers that include physicians, surgeons, anesthesiologists, SAs, and others who have negotiated a discount on the fees for the services they provide. In return, the insurer provides the SA provider certain guarantees of volume or business to offset the discounted rates. This results in patients paying less; and SA providers must accept the insurer's payment (plus the patient's cost-sharing, such as the deductible, copay, or coinsurance) as payment in full—an in-network provider cannot balance bill a patient. *Note: balance billing occurs when a provider bills you for the difference between the provider's charge and the allowed amount."* https://www.healthcare.gov/glossary/balance-billing.

A SA out-of-network provider can bill a percentage of the surgeon's fee or as Association of Operating Room Nurses (AORN) and American Academy of Physician Assistants (AAPA) recommend to bill at 100% of surgeon's fee with the appropriate modifier indicating that the service was performed by a nonphysician SA and have the payor calculate the discount based on their individual policies. This amount is often higher than the in-network reimbursement, but insurance companies frequently challenge these claims and may issue a denial.

Some health plans only pay for services when the member uses in-network providers, while other health plans will pay at least some of the claim even if the member uses an out-of-network provider.

It is helpful to contact insurance companies and ask if they reimburse independent SAs.

SURPRISE BILLING

Before moving on, another term that is important to the independent SA is surprise billing. **It occurs when out-of-network providers** including anesthesiologists, emergency room physicians, radiologists, pathologists, SAs, and labs may not be contracted with the patient's insurer, even though they provide services at a hospital or facility that is in the patient's health plan's provider network. In this case, the SA may bill at a rate that is higher than what the network allows. The patient's insurance may allow or deny the claim, depending on the type of policy. In the case of denial, the patient may be responsible for the provider's payment. Many states are now supporting legislation to prohibit surprise billing.

Form **SS-4**	**Application for Employer Identification Number**	OMB No. 1545-0003
(Rev. December 2019)	(For use by employers, corporations, partnerships, trusts, estates, churches, government agencies, Indian tribal entities, certain individuals, and others.)	**EIN**
Department of the Treasury Internal Revenue Service	▶ Go to *www.irs.gov/FormSS4* for instructions and the latest information. ▶ See separate instructions for each line. ▶ Keep a copy for your records.	

Type or print clearly.

1 Legal name of entity (or individual) for whom the EIN is being requested

2 Trade name of business (if different from name on line 1)	**3** Executor, administrator, trustee, "care of" name
4a Mailing address (room, apt., suite no. and street, or P.O. box)	**5a** Street address (if different) (Don't enter a P.O. box.)
4b City, state, and ZIP code (if foreign, see instructions)	**5b** City, state, and ZIP code (if foreign, see instructions)

6 County and state where principal business is located

7a Name of responsible party	**7b** SSN, ITIN, or EIN

8a Is this application for a limited liability company (LLC) (or a foreign equivalent)? . . . . ☐ Yes ☐ No	**8b** If 8a is "Yes," enter the number of LLC members . . . . . . ▶

8c If 8a is "Yes," was the LLC organized in the United States? . . . . ☐ Yes ☐ No

9a **Type of entity** (check only one box). **Caution:** If 8a is "Yes," see the instructions for the correct box to check.

☐ Sole proprietor (SSN) _____
☐ Partnership
☐ Corporation (enter form number to be filed) ▶ _____
☐ Personal service corporation
☐ Church or church-controlled organization
☐ Other nonprofit organization (specify) ▶ _____
☐ Other (specify) ▶

☐ Estate (SSN of decedent) _____
☐ Plan administrator (TIN) _____
☐ Trust (TIN of grantor) _____
☐ Military/National Guard   ☐ State/local government
☐ Farmers' cooperative   ☐ Federal government
☐ REMIC   ☐ Indian tribal governments/enterprises
Group Exemption Number (GEN) if any ▶

9b If a corporation, name the state or foreign country (if applicable) where incorporated	State	Foreign country

10 **Reason for applying** (check only one box)

☐ Started new business (specify type) ▶ _____
_____
☐ Hired employees (Check the box and see line 13.)
☐ Compliance with IRS withholding regulations
☐ Other (specify) ▶

☐ Banking purpose (specify purpose) ▶ _____
☐ Changed type of organization (specify new type) ▶ _____
☐ Purchased going business
☐ Created a trust (specify type) ▶ _____
☐ Created a pension plan (specify type) ▶ _____

11 Date business started or acquired (month, day, year). See instructions.	**12** Closing month of accounting year
13 Highest number of employees expected in the next 12 months (enter -0- if none). If no employees expected, skip line 14.	**14** If you expect your employment tax liability to be $1,000 or less in a full calendar year **and** want to file Form 944 annually instead of Forms 941 quarterly, check here. (Your employment tax liability generally will be $1,000 or less if you expect to pay $5,000 or less in total wages.) If you don't check this box, you must file Form 941 for every quarter. ☐

Agricultural	Household	Other

15 First date wages or annuities were paid (month, day, year). **Note:** If applicant is a withholding agent, enter date income will first be paid to nonresident alien (month, day, year) . . . . ▶

16 Check **one** box that best describes the principal activity of your business.

☐ Construction   ☐ Rental & leasing   ☐ Transportation & warehousing
☐ Real estate   ☐ Manufacturing   ☐ Finance & insurance

☐ Health care & social assistance   ☐ Wholesale-agent/broker
☐ Accommodation & food service   ☐ Wholesale-other   ☐ Retail
☐ Other (specify) ▶

17 Indicate principal line of merchandise sold, specific construction work done, products produced, or services provided.

18 Has the applicant entity shown on line 1 ever applied for and received an EIN? ☐ Yes ☐ No
If "Yes," write previous EIN here ▶

Third Party Designee	Complete this section **only** if you want to authorize the named individual to receive the entity's EIN and answer questions about the completion of this form.	
	Designee's name	Designee's telephone number (include area code)
	Address and ZIP code	Designee's fax number (include area code)

Under penalties of perjury, I declare that I have examined this application, and to the best of my knowledge and belief, it is true, correct, and complete.	Applicant's telephone number (include area code)
Name and title (type or print clearly) ▶	
Signature ▶ Date ▶	Applicant's fax number (include area code)

For Privacy Act and Paperwork Reduction Act Notice, see separate instructions.   Cat. No. 16055N   Form **SS-4** (Rev. 12-2019)

Figure 3-6 · Employer identification number.

It is vitally important that SAs who are practicing independently have the patient sign a consent form at least 24 hours prior to the surgery. Many surgeons will include this consent form and provide it to the patient during the preoperative visit.

The consent form should include all the patient's pertinent data, the surgical procedure, the fees that will be billed to the insurance company, and the fee that will be billed to the patient if the claim is denied. The patient will sign the consent form and SAs should keep a record for their own files.

Such a consent form avoids the issue of surprise billing, protects the SA from patients who refuse to pay, and provides valuable documentation if an adverse event occurs.

IMPORTANCE OF CASH FLOW

Not all cases require a SA. It is particularly important for you to know which cases do and which cases do not. Many insurance companies have a list of which cases they will pay an assistant for. These are based on CPT codes (Figure 3-7). These are mostly based on Medicare guidelines. Payment for services varies greatly from state to state. Make sure you check with your state insurance companies. You can download the current CPT code booklet or purchase it. Most insurance companies do not reimburse for the use of a second assistant. Check with insurance company to find out their policy concerning second assisting.

It is important to understand the reality of how long it will take for you to get reimbursement checks and how much money you need to have in reserve. The ballpark figure is around six months of reserves at the minimum. Factors to consider:

- Have you decided to join a network or remain out of network? Typically, in-network payments are received in a timelier fashion than out-of-network payments. Some out-of-network payments go directly to the patients and then you must get the payment from them. Not all insurance networks will offer you an opportunity to be an in-network provider. Many have preset limits and geographic capacity criteria.

- Do not expect to receive the amount that was billed! The amount depends on patient's insurance contract if surgeon was in-network, surgeons negotiated contract with insurance company, and other factors.

- Does the insurance company recognize you as a provider? Do you have state recognition, (registered or licensed)?

- Many surgeons' offices take time to do their billing. Some can take up to three months before you can get codes and charges from their offices. Be prepared for this since it can delay your payment.

- Some insurance companies require timely filing. This means that you have a predetermined time (usually 90 days) to get your claim set in—many of these are health maintenance organizations (HMOs) Again, this goes back to your choice of billing companies and how they handle your claims.

- An initial claim will often be denied, and an appeal will have to be sent to the insurance company. This will delay payment also. This can happen numerous times so just be prepared for this.

CPT Code	Description
59514	Cesarean delivery only
47562	Laparoscopy; surgical; cholecystectomy
27447	Arthroplasty, knee, condyle, and plateau; medial and lateral departments, with or without patella resurfacing
27130	Arthroplasty, acetabular, proximal, and femoral prosthetic replacement (total hip arthroplasty) with or without autograft or allograft
44970	Laparoscopy, surgical, appendectomy
49650	Laparoscopy, surgical, initial inguinal hernia
58571	Laparoscopy, surgical, with total hysterectomy for uterus 250 g or less; with removal of tube(s) and/or ovaries using an endoscope
47563	Laparoscopy; surgical; cholecystectomy with cholangiography
35301	Thromboendarterectomy including patch graft; if performed, carotid, vertebral, subclavian by neck incision
19301	Mastectomy, partial (eg, lumpectomy, tylectomy, quadrantectomy, segmentectomy)
29881	Arthroscopy, knee, surgical; with meniscectomy, (medial or lateral, including any meniscal shaving)
29827	Arthroscopy, shoulder, surgical; with rotator cuff repair
49652	Laparoscopy, surgical, repair, ventral, umbilical, spigelian or epigastric hernia (includes mesh insertion, when performed); reducible
27245	Treatment of intertrochanteric, peritrochanteric, or subtrochanteric femoral fracture; with intramedullary implant, with or without interlocking screws and/or cerclage
43775	Laparoscopy, Surgical, Gastric Restrictive Procedure; Longitudinal Gastrectomy (ie, Sleeve Gastrectomy)
23472	Arthroplasty, glenohumeral joint; total shoulder (glenoid and proximal humeral replacement (eg, total shoulder)
58661	Laparoscopy, surgical; with removal of adnexal structures (partial or total oophorectomy and/or salpingectomy)
22551	Arthrodesis, anterior interbody, including disc space preparation, discectomy, osteophytectomy, and decompression of spinal cord and/or nerve roots; cervical below C2
63030	Laminotomy (hemilaminectomy), with decompression of nerve root(s), including partial facetectomy, foraminotomy and/or excision of herniated intervertebral disc; one interspace, lumbar
33533	Coronary artery bypass, using arterial graft(s); single arterial graft

Figure 3-7 · Most common CPT codes.

- There will be months when the cash flow is good and there will be times when it is limited. Be well equipped for this situation.
- Remember that the money you receive has not been taxed so you are responsible for paying taxes on your reimbursements.
- If you are independent and you are not working—you have no income during that time period.
- What if most of your claims in one month are Medicare? What do you do?

HOSPITAL CONTRACTS

One option to alleviate the burden of nonbillable cases is to establish contracts with hospitals, surgery centers, surgeons, and even insurance companies. One of the first questions to get asked and answered is the hospital payor mix—what percentage of Medicare secondary insurance commercial or self-pay cases can be estimated? Some SAs have a contract with the hospitals that covers Medicare cares and these assistants bill only the hospital. Other SAs or billers who do not have these hospital contracts covering Medicare cases send claims to the secondary insurance. However, you should be careful to file a claim to Medicare for a denial letter as some secondary commercial insurers require as this is prohibited by CMS. ("It is prohibited to file a claim with the sole purpose of obtaining a denial letter.") Assistants cannot bill both.

Find out the hospital payor mix. How much of the payor mix is Medicare, commercial, self-pay, and request a breakdown by surgical specialty. The hospital can provide a spreadsheet that categorizes insurance info on all specialties. General surgery, orthopedic, and any other specialty, % of Medicare, commercial, what cases they used assistants on, etc. This helps to determine if the contract is worth pursuing. They can print it out for you very easily.

Cases will vary if the hospital is a level 1 trauma, level 2 trauma, or community hospital. Are you at a level 1 trauma, level 2 trauma, community hospital? Hospitals are frequently willing to provide a monthly stipend for call, Medicare, self pays, and Medicaid. An annual stipend for coverage has been proven to not be profitable due to the higher percentage of these claims.

Ask how many people the hospital assigns for call duty at one time. Identify what specialties and response time are required. Understand how procedures are scheduled and whether hospital will reimburse if insurance denies claim.

Above all, have a lawyer review any contract before signing.

Surgery Center Contracts

Contracts for SAs working at surgery centers are similar to hospital agreements. Again, the payor mix is an important consideration. Determine the payment for the center's Medicare, self-pay, and Medicaid cases. It is possible there is no reimbursement. Then, ask about options.

SAs may need to explore options for nonbillable cases and whether cases are billed per case or hourly. Be sure that the patient signs a consent form that specifies the use of a SA in the procedure.

For cosmetic cases, tie down how reimbursements are handled—through the surgeon or surgery center.

Above all, have a lawyer review any documents before signing.

CHOOSING A CORPORATE STRUCTURE

A major decision is the type of corporate structure an assistant chooses.

According to the IRS, there are five business structures to choose from:

1. Sole Proprietorship
2. Partnership (general, limited, or limited liability partnerships)
3. Limited Liability Company (single-member or multi-member)
4. Corporation
5. S Corporation

Whichever structure you choose when forming your business, there are some basic questions to consider.

Most nonemployer business structures are sole proprietorships. You can also be in a sole proprietorship with employees.

S corps make up most small employer businesses, usually businesses with less than 500 employees.

Most large businesses are corporations.

Starting a business with someone else?
You can be a partnership, multi-member LLC, or S corporation.

How important is Limited Liability to you?
Are your personal assets at risk?

What kind of tax responsibilities do you want?
What type determines how you are taxed and what tax returns you file.

How do you want to pay yourself?
This depends on what structure you choose

What type of control do you want?
This all depends on the type of corporation you choose.

Do you have the time and money to handle a complex structure?
This is solely depending on you.

What is your business vision and what does it look like?
Look toward the future and where you are heading.
Once you have answered those questions, here are the pros and cons of each type of corporation.

Sole Proprietorship. It is the simplest structure of all to create. It usually involves only one party who owns and operates the business. This is ideal for someone who prefers to work alone. The key advantage of being taxed as a sole proprietorship is that the net income from the business is taxed on personal income tax return of the owner on form 1040. Being at risk for unlimited liability places personal assets at risk.

Partnership. It is a business that is owned and operated by two or more people. It is the least-used structure in the United States. The partners manage the company and are responsible for all debts and obligations. The only advantage is if you need cash to get started.

Corporation. It a separate taxpayer, with income and expenses taxed to the corporation and not to the owners. Profits are distributed to owners as dividends. The owners then must pay personal income tax on these dividends.

Many small businesses do not use this because of the tax feature.

S Corporation. It offers tax benefits, so that profits, losses, and other tax items pass through the corporation to you and are reported on your personal tax return. Major disadvantage is audit from IRS is increased with this type of business

You will have to set it up according to federal and state law.

Limited Liability Company. It is formed under state law and gives you your personal liability protection.

Major disadvantage is you could be paying more tax on your personal income.

Billing: Self-billing vs Third-party. If you decide to perform your own billing, be prepared to devote a great deal of time to paperwork, writing letters, and calling insurance representatives. Billing is a very complex area and not for the faint of heart.

It will be up to you to determine if the time spent understanding the details of insurance regulations is more valuable than hiring a biller.

HOW TO CHOOSE A BILLER

There are numerous billing companies around the country. One of the most important issues is that they know what you do and know how to bill for a SA. Review the contract that they have sent you with an attorney. Discuss any items that you have questions about. Talk to other SAs and see who they recommend. Are they satisfied or have complaints?

Billing companies customarily recommend charging a percentage of the surgeon's fee, such as 20%, 50%, 100%. Confirm how codes and charges are provided to the billing company.

What percentage do they charge? Do you have to get codes and charges and send them to the billing company? What percentage do they bill? Example: 20%, 50%, 100% of surgeon's fee.

Denials of claims are inevitable. Discuss the methods for handling appeals and whether appeals necessitate an additional charge. Updates on the status of claims should be provided regularly: 30 days, 60 days, 90 days.

Complaints from patients and surgeons are part of life too. What is important is how the billing company responds.

Getting paid—what is the procedure? Understand if the billing company deducts their fees and then forwards the payment to you or if a monthly payment to the billing company is preferable.

Deductibles? How is this handled? Do they bill the patient for this?

A length of a contract can vary. Include a reasonable time-frame included in the contract to cancel if the arrangement is not satisfactory.

Make sure that you as a provider have the power to control all your patient's charges, etc.

TAX PREPARATION

As a first step, you will need to apply for an EIN which stands for **employee identification number**. An EIN is also known as a federal tax identification number and is used to identify a business entity. Generally, businesses need an EIN. You may apply for an EIN in various ways, and now you may online at https://www.irs.gov/businesses/small-businesses-self-employed/employer-id-numbers. *This is a free service offered by the Internal Revenue Service and you can get your EIN immediately*. You must check with your state to make sure you need a state number or charter.

One of the most important items for your business. This depends on what type of corporation you have decided that fits your specific needs. Whatever type of corporation you have selected, you need to make sure of the following:

- It should be a reputable CPA or tax firm that has knowledge of surgical assisting.
- They explain to you **exactly** what they need from you in terms of paperwork, receipts, contracts (these may have some language in them that affects taxes), interest on property, rent, etc.
- Listen to them.
- Keep meticulous records and receipts of everything that concerns your business.
- Be prepared to be audited.
- Use a system like QuickBooks to input all your data. Scan all your receipts into categories (mileage, gas, interest, utilities, etc.).
- It is ultimately your responsibility.

BUSINESS ETHICS

Not only are there ethical standards for SAs to follow regarding patient care but there are ethical standards relevant to the business of surgical assisting.

HEALTH INSURANCE PORTABILITY AND ACCOUNTABILITY ACT (HIPAA)

The Privacy Rule standards address the use and disclosure of individuals' health information (known as "protected health information") by entities subject to the Privacy Rule. These individuals and organizations are called "covered entities." The Privacy Rule also contains standards for individuals' rights to understand and control how their health information is used. A major goal of the Privacy Rule is to ensure that individual's health information is properly protected while allowing the flow of health information needed to provide and promote high-quality health care and to protect the public's health and well-being. The Privacy Rule strikes a balance that permits important uses of information while protecting the privacy of people who seek care and healing.

HIPAA is particularly relevant to surgical patient care providers who see patients at their most vulnerable times and have access to their private health information. SAs are obligated to maintain privacy and confidentiality of information except in those circumstances where the patient provides permission, or the law requires disclosure. A word of caution: pay particular attention that all your patient documents (digital and paper) are in a secure location in order to be compliant with HIPAA standards.

Ethical standards also apply to billing practices. SAs should only receive compensation for services rendered ensuring the patient has been properly informed. Surprise billing and balance billing are examples of practices to avoid. SAs should provide accurate, complete, and timely documentation in all financial matters with the patient, insurance, and healthcare financing agencies.

Bibliography

Internal Revenue Service. https://www.irs.gov/. Accessed August 5, 2023.

Executive Medical Board and Governance Advisory Council. Bylaws of the Medical Staff. University of California San Francisco. https://medicalaffairs.ucsf.edu/sites/g/files/tkssra856/f/wysiwyg/UCSF%20Medical%20Staff%20Bylaws.pdf. Accessed August 2, 2023.

US Bureau of Labor Statistics. https://www.bls.gov. Accessed August 5, 2023.

US Department of Labor. Occupational Outlook. https://www.bls.gov/ooh. Accessed May 4, 2023.

American College of Surgeons. https://www.facs.org. Accessed January 25, 2023.

Centers for Medicare and Medicaid Services. https://www.cms.gov. Accessed February 4, 2023.

Forbes Advisor. How to Start a Business in 11 steps (2023 Guide). https://www.forbes.com/advisor/business/how-to-start-a-business/. Accessed March 30, 2023.

NPPES NPI Registry. https://npiregistry.cms.hhs.gov. Accessed February 5, 2023.

National Plan & Provider Enumeration System. https://nppes.cms.hhs.gov. Accessed March 8, 2023.

CMS. Balance Billing: Glossary. HealthCare.gov. Accessed February 5, 2023.

How to Choose an Organizational Structure in Five Steps. https://www.indeed.com/career-advice/career-development/how-to-choose-organization-structure#. Accessed January 25, 2023.

4

Infection Control in the Perioperative Setting

Margaret H.M. Rodriguez

THE INFECTION CONTROL CHALLENGE

The prevention or control of an infection first requires an understanding of it by thoroughly examining its background etiology; characteristics and factors that contribute to its potential for harm; strategies for successful intervention; and ramifications of failure. Throughout history, *Homo sapiens*, better known as humans, have struggled with understanding disease and infection in our species as well as others throughout the natural world. Over the millennia, humans have evolved and developed intricate defenses of innate immune system responses to survive the microbial world's continuous evolution and impact on individual health. Ancient philosophers and curious observers made connections between cause and effect of injury and infection; symptoms and outcomes. World populations grew exponentially and created a need for the scientific professionals to aim their research on community health as well as the impact of disease and the transmissibility of infection among an increasingly urban, interconnected, and global population. Chapter 1 reviewed some of the historical highlights of the practice of surgical intervention, including some of the infection-control strategies used in those historical timelines. This chapter will examine some of the broad impact of disease transmission in the 21st century and, more narrowly, strategies for controlling infection in the perioperative setting.

Surgical assistants and other surgical team members are primarily focused on the prevention of surgical site infection (SSI). Other types of healthcare-associated infections (HAIs) should also be considered for the potentially debilitating or even life-threatening impact that could result from the interactions between patients, the medical professionals, and the surgical environment of care.

MICROBIAL OVERVIEW

Microorganisms or *microbes* are terms used to describe extremely small living beings that are invisible to the naked eye. Microbes may also refer to bits of organic materials such as ribonucleic acid (RNA) or deoxyribonucleic acid (DNA) in the form of viruses that are obligate parasites which do not have the cellular components of living cells and need to invade other cells to make copies of themselves. There are millions of different types of microbes that are ubiquitous—present in every part of the planet. These microbes have lived, reproduced, and evolved over the ages, long before and since the presence of humans and other members of the animal kingdom. There is no way to exclude microbes from our bodies or environment and, luckily for us, most of the microbial populations we encounter are either beneficial to us or coexist with us without causing harm. The endogenous microbes that live in and on us are part of what is termed our normal or resident flora or microbiomes, with which we have a symbiotic relationship that usually benefits us. The human gastrointestinal tract has its own normal microbiome that facilitates the synthesis of nutrients in food that is ingested. Resident microbial populations normally found in human skin layers and mucosal membranes guard against invading transient exogenous microbes that may become pathogenic sources of infection. Even the body's own normal microbes can become opportunistic sources of infection if conditions change or events occur that disrupt the normal human-microbe relationships.

CLASSIFICATIONS OF MICROBES

The Greek philosopher Aristotle was one of the first known historical figures to have developed a classification system of living beings that he based on his observations of the differences and similarities between species of plants (Plantae) or animals (Animalia). Even the Dutch scientist Antonie van Leeuwenhoek, a pioneer of microbiology known for his development of the microscope, referred to the bacterial cells seen under magnification as "animalcules." This two-classification system was used for centuries. Both biologists in the 1800s and more contemporary biophysicists, armed with increasingly complex and sophisticated microscopes and testing methods, added levels of the taxonomic hierarchy, or standardized naming system, to the scientific classification of microorganisms based on their cell structure and genetic sequences. There are separate classification systems and taxonomic hierarchies for eukaryotes, prokaryotes, and viruses.

EUKARYOTES

Eukaryotes are types of living microbes with a cell structure that contains a nucleus. The nucleus is enclosed within a cellular membrane, surrounded by specialized structures called organelles contained in the cellular cytoplasm and within the protective cell wall. Organisms comprised of eukaryotic cells range from single-celled microbes such as protozoa; to multicellular fungi and algae; and even the largest living organisms including plants, animals, and humans. The cellular structure of eukaryotes is more complex than the structure of prokaryotes which include bacteria and archaea.

Eukaryotic organisms including protozoic amoebas and up to 400 species of fungi are capable of causing disease in humans. Various protozoic species, algae (red, green, or brown), and approximately 5000 species of fungi cause disease in plants and animals both on land and in marine environments. *Candida albicans*, a type of yeast, has been documented to be the source of SSIs resulting in osteomyelitis. Root cause tracing for SSIs has identified the source of contamination in some cases as microbial growth under artificial nails worn by surgical staff members.

PROKARYOTES

Prokaryotes are microbes that have a cellular structure which is less complicated than eukaryotes and genetic material contained within the cell without the presence of a cell nucleus. Two forms of prokaryotes, archaea and bacteria, are believed to be the oldest forms of life on the planet. It is estimated that there are millions of species, although only a few thousand have been scientifically identified and classified.

Archaea

Archaea are organisms that are separate from both bacteria and eukaryotes. A new classification system of "archaea" was created in the 1970s to describe prokaryotic microorganisms that had similarities in cell structure and metabolic activity with bacteria; however, the proteins from genetic encoding they produced were more like eukaryotes. Archaea, often termed *extremophiles*, are descendants of anaerobic organisms which emerged approximately 4 billion years ago and thrived in the hot, toxic, oxygen-poor atmosphere. These microbes have been isolated in more modern times in boiling hot springs, volcanic steam vents, salt marshes, and under glacial ice in Antarctica. Archaea have also been isolated in less extreme environments including the ground soil and human intestinal tracts.

Bacteria

A commonly recognized source of infection in the perioperative setting is prokaryotic bacteria, often arising from the patient's own endogenous microbiomes. Bacterial species are categorized by identifying characteristics including:

- Morphology (size, shape, and arrangement)
- Gram-staining studies (determination of cell wall structure)
- Population growth; motility (ability to move)
- Nutritional requirements (oxygen tolerance)
- Pathogenicity (ability to release toxins and cause infection)
- Metabolism (energy and vital processes)
- Proteins (amino acid sequences)
- Genetics (encoding for protein synthesis)

Morphology. Bacterial cultures are examined under the microscope to determine their morphology: size, shape, and arrangement of cells. This basic method of preliminary identification includes the following descriptions:

- Coccus – round-shaped. The plural of coccus is cocci.
- Bacillus – rod-shaped. The plural of bacillus is bacilli.
- Coccobacillus – very short rod which resembles a coccus.
- Spiral or corkscrew – coiled or twisted.
- Pleomorphic or L-form – has the ability to change shape based on adverse conditions.
- Mycoplasma – lobulated "spherules," ring-shaped, or star-shaped.
- Vibrio – comma-shaped.

The arrangement of these shapes is another way that microbiologists identify microbial populations and include the following arrangements of coccus and bacilli bacteria:

- Monococcus (single sphere; also called micrococcus)
- Diplococci (pairs)
- Tetracocci (groups of four)
- Sarcinae (cubic groups of eight)
- Streptococci (chains or filament form)

- Staphylococci (clusters or sheets)
- Monobacillus (single)
- Diplobacillus (paired)
- Streptobacillus (in chains or filament form)
- Palisade (in the shape of a stack of rods)

Gram Staining. Gram staining is a standard method used in the laboratory to provide a preliminary identification of bacterial cultures in order to gauge the potential pathogenicity of the bacteria. Bacterial cell walls that turn purple or dark blue when exposed to the Gram stain are referred to as gram-positive. Those that do not retain the stain and appear red or pink are termed gram-negative. Antibiotics may be prescribed relatively quickly based on the preliminary Gram stain results. Bacterial populations usually demonstrate susceptibility to specific classes of pharmacologic agents. Laboratory examination of cultured bacterial colonies is performed through culture and sensitivity (C&S) techniques that are read in 24- and 48-hour intervals. The antibiotic treatment regimen may be altered based on the completed study and whether those results determine that the bacteria causing the specific infection are or are not sensitive to (killed by) the agent prescribed.

Population Growth and Motility. Bacteria require the presence of specific nutrients and environmental conditions in order to multiply. Bacterial growth refers to the number of cells in a microbial colony not the actual size of the individual cells. A bacterium's ability to move itself is referred to as motility. Cellular movement is seen in bacterial cells which have flagella and axial filaments. Most cocci bacteria are non-motile; only a few species of bacilli are motile; however, most spiral-shaped bacteria are motile.

Nutritional and Oxygen Requirements. Prokaryotes are classified by their nutritional requirements and how they metabolize energy sources. Bacteria, fungi, and algae recycle environmental elements: carbon, oxygen, nitrogen, hydrogen, and sulfur. Bacteria and other prokaryotes are also classified based on their oxygen and carbon dioxide requirements. The three general classes relevant to microbes in the perioperative setting are aerobes (including microaerophiles), anaerobes (including obligate, facultative, and aerotolerant), and capnophiles. Care should be taken to protect the viability of the microbial samples, taken as cultures during surgery, to ensure an accurate identification of the infectious agent sampled.

Obligate aerobic bacteria require approximately 20% oxygen (O_2) in the air in order to thrive and reproduce. *Pseudomonas aeruginosa* and *Mycobacterium tuberculosis* are obligate aerobes. Microaerophile bacteria require low levels of oxygen to reproduce and can tolerate as low as 5% O_2 concentrations with up to 10% carbon dioxide (CO_2). *Helicobacter pylori* which has been identified as a cause of many gastric ulcers is an example of a microaerophile bacterium.

Anaerobic bacteria may be obligate, facultative, or aerotolerant. Anaerobic bacterial colonies are classified as obligate anaerobes if they cannot tolerate even very low concentrations

of oxygen. This type of anaerobe includes *Clostridium perfringens* which causes gas gangrene infections, often requiring a full or partial amputation of an extremity. *Clostridium tetani* (*C. tetani*) causes tetanus infections from traumatic perforation or lacerations with rusty or contaminated objects buried in soil, gaining access into deeper tissues where oxygen is not present. Facultative anaerobes are able to thrive and reproduce in zero-oxygen concentrations or up to the 20% O_2 level found in ambient room air. *Escherichia coli* (*E. coli*) is an example of a facultative anaerobe. Aerotolerant microbes are those that grow well without any oxygen; however, they can thrive in low-oxygen environments with less than 15% O_2 concentration. Some strains of *Clostridium* are aerotolerant bacteria. Capnophile bacteria thrive and reproduce in higher concentrations of carbon dioxide (CO_2), usually in concentrations of 5% to 10%. *Haemophilus infuenzae* and *Neisseria gonorrhoeae* are capnophiles.

Pathogenicity and Spore Formation. Pathogenicity is the ability of a specific type of bacteria to cause infection or disease. Transient microbes or flora and even the resident microbes that normally live in and on us can gain access into body tissues and organs where they are not typically present through various portals of entry. If conditions for their survival and growth are favorable, they may become pathogenic. Exotoxins are a property of pathogenicity secreted by some forms of bacteria that may destroy tissues. The more common factor in pathogenicity is not the presence of microbes, it is the host's compromised immune system that cannot mobilize normal defenses, allowing the infectious agent to proliferate.

Spore or capsule formation may present a special challenge to reducing the potential for infection. Certain types of virulent bacteria possess the ability to utilize a process called sporulation. Bacteria in the genus *Clostridium* and genus *Bacillus* are examples of spore-forming pathogens. When unfavorable environmental conditions are present, the bacteria form an endospore as protection in order to ensure their survival. The bacterium's genetic material is enclosed in a multilayered protein capsule that is highly resistant to heat, desiccation (drying out), and various chemical substances. This dormancy period of spores allows them to survive for extended, even indefinite periods of time until conditions are again favorable for their reproduction.

Bacterial population samples are used as biological indicator (BI) testing of various methods of sterilization. The method of sterilization must be able to kill all of the bacterial spores in order to be an approved, effective method of sterilization. An example of this is *Geobacillus stearothermophilus* used as the BI for steam sterilization. Chemical agents that kill most bacteria but not spores are classified as high-level disinfectants and render items "surgically clean" or disinfected. Based on the Spaulding Classification of Patient Care Items, this method of disinfection may be used for semi-critical patient care items used in natural body orifices such as the nose, mouth, vagina, or anus. All instruments and invasive devices classified as critical patient care items used in surgical procedures or any devices that penetrate the skin, mucosal membranes, or enter blood vessels must be sterile, meaning free from all microbes (pathogenic or nonpathogenic), including spores. Noncritical items include stethoscopes, pulse oximeters, and other noninvasive items that do not come into contact with nonintact skin or mucous membranes and present minimal risk of disease transmission.

Metabolism. The final step in a living organism's metabolic processes, after intake of nutritional and oxygen requirements are met, is that of elimination of waste products. Bacteria secrete waste products and other substances as they grow, including enzymes. Bacterial enzymes invade host tissues, breaking them down, and causing disease. Staphylococcal and Streptococcal bacteria are identified in the laboratory by the enzymes they secrete. These otherwise not harmful bacteria that are part of the body's resident microbiome, may become opportunistic pathogens capable of using their enzyme secretions to break down deeper tissues. The enzymes catalase and coagulase are produced by some species of *Staphylococcus* and contribute to their pathogenicity potential.

The enzyme catalase breaks down hydrogen peroxide (H_2O_2) which is toxic to cells into the separate molecules of water (H_2O) and oxygen (O_2). In a laboratory study for catalase, hydrogen peroxide is placed on a slide or Petri culture dish and observed for a bubbling or effervescing reaction. This indicates the presence of catalase and identifies the bacteria as catalase positive. Typically, staphylococci are catalase positive, although *S. aureus* produces a catalase-negative reaction. Most streptococci are catalase negative.

Coagulase is an enzyme produced by some bacteria that coagulates blood plasma and increases its virulence factor by acting as a protective barrier against the normal inflammatory response of phagocytosis. *Staphylococcus* identified as catalase positive is then further tested to determine whether it is *S. aureus* by demonstrating the presence of coagulase which causes a reaction of clumping together of the bacteria in response to the blood plasma. Bacteria that do not produce the reaction are identified as coagulase-negative staphylococci (CoNS) and include *S. epidermidis*.

Proteins and Genetics. Amino acids linked into single or multiple chains form large organic protein molecules. Certain proteins are specific to microbial species and used as an identifier when the sequencing is then compared to other forms. The synthesis of proteins is determined by the unique instructions encoded in the genes of prokaryotic and eukaryotic cells. The individual cell's structure and physical characteristics are determined by the chemical reactions programmed by those genes and used, along with the other identifiers, to isolate specific microbial populations.

VIRUSES

Viruses are the cause of many diseases in eukaryotes. Viral diseases in humans include the common cold, influenza (flu), acquired immunodeficiency syndrome (AIDS), rotavirus, rabies, herpes, polio, and the novel coronavirus which caused the pandemic outbreak of COVID-19 in late 2019 and continued through 2022, eventually reducing its numbers but remaining present in the population on an ongoing basis. Other frightening viral diseases such as Ebola and Marburg viral hemorrhagic fevers have been covered widely in the media over the past decade.

Viruses defy standard definitions used to describe microbial characteristics and life functions. Each individual virus comprises a genetic component which may be either RNA or DNA that is surrounded by a type of protein coating referred to as a capsid. The capsid is composed of many individual protein molecules called capsomeres that protect the viral genes from protective cellular enzymes. The capsid also has components necessary for attachment to a host cell. Viruses contain the genetic codes required to copy themselves; however, they do not share any of the cellular components present in eukaryotes or prokaryotes that allow for cell division to reproduce. The inability to reproduce on their own forces viruses to be obligate parasites that must invade other eukaryotic or prokaryotic cells to deposit their DNA or RNA into the new host cells. The viral genes are then copied as part of the invaded cells when they reproduce.

Viruses find mechanisms of entry into cells of the body in four basic ways: (1) inhalation of respiratory droplets or aerosolized particles; (2) exchange of body fluids such as blood (eg, sexual contact, sharps injury, open sores, fluid splash into eyes, umbilical cord); (3) ingestion of contaminated food or water; (4) stings or bites by arthropod vectors (eg, mosquitos, biting flies, ticks, fleas). Viruses first attach themselves to the host cell with the aid of receptors on the capsomere. The receptors on the capsomere of corona virus give the now widely recognized spiky or crown-like appearance depicted in images of the novel corona virus responsible for the COVID-19 pandemic.

Acute Viral Infections and Latent Diseases

Viral infections can manifest as acute infections with a quick onset of signs and symptoms or may remain inactive or latent within the body for prolonged periods, reactivating only when conditions are favorable for their replication. Acute viral infections include:

- Gastrointestinal viruses such as rotavirus and norovirus
- Enteroviruses including rhinovirus (the common cold virus) and poliovirus
- Respiratory viruses including paramyxoviruses that cause measles, mumps, and rubella, and the respiratory syncytial virus (RSV) in infants and older adults
- Adenoviruses (influenza A and coronaviruses such as SARS, MERS, and COVID-19)

Herpes Viruses

Virus infections are extremely common in animal populations. The family of viruses called *Herpesviridae*, commonly referred to as the herpes viruses, has over 100 identified strains, eight of which are responsible for disease in humans.

The herpes viral pathogens may remain dormant and emerge, even many years later as latent infections. Examples of common herpes viruses include varicella-zoster virus (VZV) which causes chickenpox and manifests in some individuals as painful shingles infections, usually later in life. Herpes simplex virus 1 and 2 (HSV-1, HSV-2) cause painful open sores known as cold sores in the oral or ocular areas (HSV-1) and genital or anal areas (HSV-2).

Internal activation triggers for HSV include systemic immunocompromise from comorbid conditions treated with chemotherapy or radiation and excessive stress. External triggers may include overexposure to radiation from natural sunlight or other sources. Topical antiviral acyclovir creams may reduce the duration of painful lesions.

Epstein-Barr virus (EBV), another member of the *Herpesviridae* family is the cause of infectious mononucleosis (IM), known as "the kissing disease" or glandular fever, commonly seen in adolescents. The acute infection passed through the exchange of saliva may cause fever, lymphadenopathy (enlarged lymph nodes), and hepatosplenomegaly (enlargement of the liver and spleen). Clinical testing using the Paul-Bunnell (monospot) test confirms the diagnosis of infectious mononucleosis and is based on the detected presence of antibodies. Steroid therapy may be prescribed for localized pharyngeal inflammation. Close monitoring is required in more severe cases involving hepatosplenomegaly. EBV may possibly be linked to chronic fatigue syndrome later in life; although a direct link has not been established. EBV has been identified as a factor in certain nasopharyngeal carcinomas and lymphomas seen mostly in Africa and New Guinea called Burkitt's lymphoma.

The herpes virus Cytomegalovirus (CMV) is an extremely common virus present in 60% to 70% of humans with the ability to invade the majority of human tissue cells. Initial infections most commonly occur in early childhood. Acute CMV infections have been identified as the cause of liver failure, colitis, and retinal inflammation. Passed from mother to fetus through the placenta, the CMV is responsible for birth defects including blindness, deafness, seizures, and cerebral palsy in approximately 1 out of 150 live births in the United States. CMV typically remains dormant until the immune system of the human host becomes compromised. Researchers in recent years identified a specific molecular switch that, under certain environmental conditions or biological cues, sends the signal to the virus to reactivate.

Hepatitis Viruses

Many perioperative infections are caused by viruses commonly known as bloodborne pathogens due to their transmissibility through blood-to-blood contact. Hepatitis B virus (HBV) and Hepatitis C virus (HCV) are transmitted by the parenteral route of blood transfusion, sharing of contaminated needles, or unprotected sexual intercourse. HBV is responsible for acute inflammation of the liver, jaundice, fever, weakness, and nausea. Chronic HBV infection that persists 6 months after acute infection can result in cirrhosis (hardening of the liver) and

hepatic cancer. A vaccine for HBV is available and strongly recommended for all healthcare providers.

HCV infections are often mistaken for influenza infections and become chronic 6 to 10 weeks after exposure. Despite the lack of a vaccine for HCV, newer drug treatments are showing good results in achieving a cure for the disease and preventing cirrhosis or hepatic cancer.

Hepatitis A virus (HAV), unlike the others in this category, is typically transmitted by the fecal-oral route from the ingestion of contaminated food or due to poor hygiene habits.

HIV and AIDS

Another well-known blood-borne viral infection is human immunodeficiency virus (HIV) which is the cause of subsequent acquired immunodeficiency syndrome (AIDS), first definitively identified and named in the early 1980s. The researchers identified significant and decimating reductions in CD4 T-cell (lymphocyte) counts in those infected, leading to opportunistic infections. These infections were most notably diagnosed in homosexual males and intravenous (IV) drug users who developed Kaposi's sarcoma, a rare form of skin cancer that caused large dark lesions.

HIV had become a pandemic by 2000, infecting an estimated 36 million individuals. The Centers for Disease Control and Prevention (CDC) reports that in 2018 there were approximately 1.2 million people in the United States infected with HIV. Approximately 14% or 1 in 7 people were unaware they were infected. Statistically, male-to-male contact was responsible for approximately 68% of infections while 24% were heterosexual individuals and the remainder were from injection drug use. The global impact in 2018 demonstrated nearly 38 million people living with HIV and a rate of nearly 1.7 million new cases.

HIV in the United States has become a manageable long-term, chronic infection for many people. Retroviral pharmaceutical combinations have been developed that help those infected maintain their CD4 T-lymphocyte counts and enjoy relatively good health despite the lack of a definitive cure for the disease.

Prion Diseases

Prions are nonliving proteinaceous agents that are originally normal central nervous system proteins called PrP^c which develop abnormal folds, creating pathogenic prions or PrP^{sc}. The general class of disease caused by prion derangement is called transmissible spongiform encephalopathy (TSE) found in cattle, sheep, and hooved animals like elk, deer, and moose. In humans, TSEs include Creutzfeldt-Jakob disease (CJD), variant CJD (vCJD), Gerstmann-Sträussler-Scheinker syndrome, Fatal Familial Insomnia, and Kuru; all relatively rare, progressive, neurodegenerative prion diseases which are always fatal, with no known cure or treatment. The PrP^c glycoproteins present on the surface of neural tissues such as the brain and spinal cord have no DNA or RNA; however, these are able to replicate themselves without any recognized or understood method used by other living microbes. These deformed protein

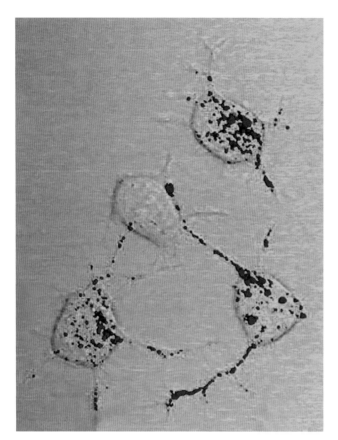

Figure 4-1 · Prion diseases. (US Centers for Disease Control and Prevention, Washington, DC; National Institute of Allergy and Infectious Diseases (NIAID) CDC PHIL #18131, 2011.)

segments create holes in the tissues, destroying them, and resulting in a spongiform (sponge-like) appearance. Researchers have yet to pinpoint the purpose or physiologic functions of the proteins which can become prions (see Figure 4-1).

Creutzfeldt-Jakob Disease. Classic Creutzfeldt-Jakob disease (CJD) is not related to bovine spongiform encephalopathy (BSE), commonly known as "mad cow" disease, according to the CDC. The more recently discovered variant CJD (vCJD), however, does share the same infectious agent responsible for BSE. The age range for the onset of symptoms in classic CJD is between 50 and 75 years of age. A much younger age range of 18 to 41 years of age is seen in vCJD and any cases of onset in an under-50-year-old individual would more likely be confirmed to be vCJD.

The incubation period for CJD and vCJD can be years to decades in length before the initial onset of symptoms of dementia combined with neurologic signs including poor coordination, myoclonus (involuntary muscle jerking), chorea (specific involuntary jerky movements of the face, hips, and shoulders), hyperreflexia (overactivity or exaggerated response to deep tendon physiological reflexes), or signs of visual impairment present. Progression of the various signs and symptoms of CJD and vCJD is relatively rapid once they begin. The destruction of brain and spinal tissue leads to certain death in 12 to 14 months.

Definitive diagnosis of CJD or vCJD is only possible through direct examination of brain tissue through surgical biopsy or during tissue examination at autopsy. Evidence for potential CJD or vCJD infection is obtained through:

* Imaging studies such as MRI
* Electroencephalogram (EEG)
* Tissue biopsy and histology
* Extensive patient history of possible exposure to BSE in the United Kingdom or other geographic areas with known disease
* Family history of CJD
* History of prior surgery with implanted cadaver dura or corneal tissue
* Injection of human pituitary hormone extract

The statistics for transmission of CJD show that less than 10% of cases are familial or inherited. Approximately 90% of infections are acquired or sporadic and only about 1% have been demonstrated to be through person-to-person transmission.

Other TSEs in Humans. Gerstmann-Sträussler-Scheinker syndrome is an inherited prion disease and manifests symptoms typically between 35 and 55 years of age and progresses slowly over 2 to 10 years. Fatal Familial Insomnia is another inherited prion disease likely caused by a mutation of the prion protein gene and once signs and symptoms of untreatable insomnia begin, it is an average 9-month progression to death. Kuru is an acquired TSE seen in the 1950s in the New Guinea Fore tribe who practiced cannibalism of deceased relatives as a sign of respect. The incubation period could be years to decades long; however, it was only 6 to 12 months before death once neurological signs presented.

Prevention of Prion Transmission. The reproductive methods and transmission mechanisms for bacteria and viruses are well-understood by researchers; however, the lethal, nonliving prions present a challenge for infection control, perioperative, and sterile processing professionals. The need for a tissue diagnosis for verification of suspected prion disease requires preplanning for use and subsequent reprocessing of surgical instrumentation as well as containment of contaminated waste in clearly labeled biohazardous materials bags or containers. Special prion disease exposure protocols must be followed for decontamination and sterilization of costly surgical instrumentation. If possible, the better option is to use disposable instruments and discard any items used in verified or suspected cases of CJD or vCJD. When disposal is not possible, current protocols outlined by the Association for the Advancement of Medical Instrumentation (AAMI) for extensive soaking of instrumentation in alkaline cleaning solutions such as sodium hydroxide (NaOH) or lye; sodium hypochlorite (NaOCl) or household bleach; or exposure to vaporized hydrogen peroxide (VHP) should be utilized in conjunction with traditional sterilization methods. Formaldehyde and glutaraldehyde should be avoided as they have been shown to make the prions more resistant to disinfection and sterilization methods by acting as a fixative to inanimate surfaces. Researchers are continuously updating best practices in dealing with the lethal prion proteins; however, no treatment or cure has been developed. Ultimately, thoroughly researched and carefully developed processes to prevent transmission are the best control measures for the prion enigma.

SURGICAL SITE INFECTIONS

According to the CDC National Healthcare Safety Network (NHSN), there were 14.2 million surgical procedures performed in inpatient facilities in 2014. The HAI prevalence survey showed that in 2015 there were an estimated 110,800 SSIs that occurred involving procedures performed in inpatient settings. The "CDC Procedure-Associated Module: Surgical Site Infection (SSI) Event" published in January 2020 reported that from 2015 to 2018 there was a 7% decrease in the standardized infection ratio (SIR) related to the NHSN operative procedures categories as a result of the implementation of the Surgical Care Improvement Project (SCIP). While the report showed that the SCIP measures had produced some benefit, SSIs continue to represent the costliest form of HAIs in terms of monetary loss ($3.3 billion); additional hospital inpatient days (nearly 1 million); and loss of life (3% mortality rate). The Centers for Medicare and Medicaid Services (CMS) consider the majority of SSIs to be preventable events and have implemented policies that deny government-backed insurance reimbursement to facilities in the event of SSI following specific surgical procedures including coronary artery bypass; bariatric procedures; and orthopedic surgeries involving the spine, neck, elbow, or shoulder.

Types of Surgical Site Infections

The CDC's NHSN defines SSIs as superficial, deep, and organ/space infections. Superficial SSIs involve the skin and subcutaneous tissue only and occur within 30 days of the surgical procedure. Purulent drainage is visible, or a culture analysis verifies an infection. The patient must also have signs and/or symptoms indicating acute inflammation: localized pain, erythema or redness, heat, or localized swelling. Superficial SSIs may further be designated as superficial incisional primary (SIP) or superficial incisional secondary (SIS) when there were two incisions made in the same procedural setting. Small areas of swelling or cellulitis related to a localized stitch/suture abscess do not meet the qualifying criteria for the NHSN definition of superficial incisional SSI.

Deep SSIs are those that involve the deeper soft tissues below the level of the subcutaneous layer, including the fascia or muscle layers, and occur from 30 to 90 days following the surgical procedure. There is (1) evidence of purulent drainage from the deep tissues; (2) the wound spontaneously dehisces (separates) or is opened surgically; (3) a culture study is found to be positive for infection; (4) the patient has signs or symptoms of fever or pain/tenderness; and (5) there is evidence of deep tissue infection by gross anatomical, histopathological, or diagnostic imaging studies.

Deep SSIs are also further classified as deep incisional primary (DIP) or deep incisional secondary (DIS) in cases where more than one incision was made in the same surgical setting.

Organ/Space SSI is defined as occurring from 30 to 90 days following the surgical procedure and involves any part of the surgical site deeper than the fascial/muscle layer. Evidence of infection is established by drainage of purulent discharge through wound drains placed at the time of surgery; culture results positive for infection from drainage fluid; or histopathologic or imaging study evidence of organ/space SSI.

SSIs can become superinfections when antibiotic therapy prescribed for the initial SSI is continued for an excessive period, resulting in potential colonization by multidrug-resistant microorganisms, exacerbating the extent of the infection. A 20-month study performed at a teaching hospital from 2014 to 2016 was performed to gather data from 85 patients treated for early SSIs following spinal surgery. The standard 12-week course of antibiotic therapy was shortened to 6 weeks to attempt to demonstrate that reduction of treatment was effective in preventing superinfection of the surgical wound by colonization of drug-resistant bacterial strains. The bacterial populations cultured from the infected surgical sites were split almost equally between facultative anaerobic, gram-positive *Staphylococcus aureus,* and various anaerobic bacteria. The results showed, after a year following the shortened course of antibiotic therapy, only 8% of the SSI infections had failed to be resolved adequately with the 6-week course of antibiotics.

RISK FACTORS FOR SURGICAL SITE INFECTION

The potential risk for SSI is influenced by a number of factors including those involving the patient's own body and health status as well as sources external to the patient but within the perioperative environment of care. Planned elective surgical intervention may allow the surgeon to address patient-specific factors that could reduce risk of SSI; however, certain patient risk factors cannot be effectively mitigated. Examples of patient risk factors include:

- Age – primarily elderly and neonatal patients whose immune systems may be compromised or not fully developed and capable of fending off opportunistic microbial pathogens.

- Body weight – obese and morbidly obese patients have increased risk due to the poor vascularity of excessive adipose fat; potentially larger surgical incisions; and possible comorbidities associated with obesity.

- Nutrition – wound healing requires adequate nutritional intake of protein for the formation of collagen to recreate tissues. Poor hydration, high carbohydrate intake, and inadequate vitamin absorption also inhibit wound healing and increase SSI potential.

- Ambulatory status – early ambulation by the patient has a positive effect for patients to prevent the potential for pneumonia caused by decreased lung function in bed-bound or non-ambulatory patients. Urinary tract infections (UTIs) from indwelling Foley catheters are common in patients unable to void and perform normal hygiene measures. Long-term use of urinary catheters also presents a potential for chronic UTI due to antibiotic-resistant biofilm formation on catheter surfaces.

- Alcohol and illicit drug misuse – although researchers differ in opinion of the influence alcohol intake has as an independent factor for SSI risk, the overuse of alcohol and illicit drugs may reduce an individual's adherence to prescribed postoperative care routines and drug interaction with postoperative pain medications. Use of injection drugs presents an inherent risk of blood-borne pathogen transmission.

- Smoking – nicotine and carbon monoxide present in inhaled tobacco products reduce blood oxygen levels and increase strain on the heart and lungs. Patients should be counseled to discontinue smoking for at least 4 weeks prior to planned surgery to optimize wound healing and reduce risk of SSI.

- Preexisting infection – patients with infections of other parts of the body at the time of surgery are predisposed to SSI of the current area due to circulating bacterial or viral pathogens in the blood. Carriers of drug-resistant pathogens such as methicillin-resistant *Staphylococcus aureus* (MRSA) in the nasal passages are at increased risk of SSI as well as other drug-resistant bacteria discussed in later sections.

- Preexisting disease – patients with preexisting chronic illness on steroid therapy; malignancy requiring chemotherapy or radiation; or organ transplantation requiring immunosuppressive therapy for prevention of rejection present particular challenges to prevent postoperative infection. Normal immune responses to fight opportunistic pathogens are diminished through the use of steroids and other immunosuppressants and tissue and wound healing is delayed in irradiated tissues.

- Duration of hospital stay – the longer patients are required to remain hospitalized, the higher the risk for other HAIs from exposure to other patients, hospital staff, and environmental sources.

Endogenous Sources of SSI

SSIs can be traced to a number of different bacterial strains. These bacteria fall into two broad classifications: endogenous and exogenous. Endogenous bacteria are those found in the skin and mucosal layers and internal tissue layers, spaces, organs, and tracts. Despite aseptic techniques of skin antisepsis, approximately 20% of normal resident skin microflora are found in the sebaceous glands and hair follicles below the superficial epidermis where the antiseptic solutions are unable to reach. The mechanical action of incising the skin or mucous membranes, even with a sterile scalpel blade, hypodermic needle, or other critical patient care device, creates a direct access point for microbial transmission into deeper tissues where

resident skin microbes, commonly known as normal flora, can become opportunistic pathogens when the patient's immune system is compromised. Other transient microbes, including viruses, and resident bacteria present in natural body orifices, as well as those found in the gastrointestinal, biliary, or upper respiratory tracts, may contribute to SSI when opportunity arises to penetrate protective barriers of the intact skin or mucosal membranes.

Exogenous Sources of SSI

Exogenous bacterial contamination causing SSI can come from a variety of sources outside of the patient's own body tissues. These may be microbes circulating in the individual operating room or procedure room as a result of inadequate controls including:

- Lack of recommended 20 to 25 air exchanges per hour

- Lack of positive air pressure through unidirectional flow from ceiling to floor level

- Increased turbulence created by repeated opening of swinging doors and traffic in and out of rooms

- Excessive numbers of individuals present within rooms

- Deviance from recommended temperature and humidity settings

- Lack of proper use of personal protective equipment (PPE) in restricted zones/areas

- Improper disinfection protocols for preoperative, case turnover, or end-of-day cleaning

- Unsterile or contaminated surgical instrumentation or invasive devices

- Breaks in sterile technique by surgical team members

- Failure to confine and contain grossly contaminated instruments, supplies, or waste

Risk Classification for SSI

The CDC created a method of predicting postsurgical outcomes based on important SSI-risk factors including the four-part surgical wound classification, the American Society of Anesthesiology (ASA) Score, and the actual duration of the surgical procedure.

Surgical Wound Classification. The National Academy of Sciences and the National Research Council Cooperative Research study created the original classification system in 1964, with subsequent modifications made by the CDC in 1982. Factors in assignment of surgical wound classification include:

I. Clean: wound is closed with primary suture line under ideal, sterile conditions, with no breaks in sterile technique. Closed wound drainage may be used if necessary. Examples include breast biopsy, inguinal hernia repair, and total hip arthroplasty.

II. Clean-contaminated: wound is closed by primary suture line, with possible open or mechanical drainage, and there was controlled entry into the respiratory, gastrointestinal

(GI)/alimentary, or genitourinary tracts. A minor break in sterile technique may have occurred with immediate corrective action taken.

III. Contaminated: includes traumatic wounds of less than 4 hours since occurrence; penetrating injuries such as gunshot or knife wounds with gross spillage and contamination from GI tract contents, open biliary or respiratory tracts; open, penetrating bone fractures; incidents of major breaks in sterile technique such as use of unsterile instruments; or visible signs of acute inflammation.

IV. Dirty or infected: presence of traumatic injuries of more than 4 hours since occurrence; signs of preexisting infection with purulent drainage and inflammation; perforated viscus (internal organ); presence of necrotic tissue, or foreign material imbedded in tissues.

Due to the possibility of an unintended break occurring during the surgical procedure, the final wound classification (other than Class IV) is not assigned until the end of the procedure (see Figure 4-2).

ASA Patient Physical Status Scores. The ASA score is a mechanism for identifying the adult patient's physical status based on comorbid conditions and assessment by the anesthesia provider on the day of the surgical procedure to be performed. This risk status combined with the surgical wound classification are valuable predictive metrics of risk for surgical patients to develop SSI post-operatively. The ASA scores include:

- ASA I   Normal, healthy patient; little to no alcohol use; non-smoker

- ASA II   Patient with mild systemic disease with no substantive functional limitations; current tobacco user, social alcohol intake, well-managed diabetes mellitus or hypertension, mild lung disease, obesity, or pregnancy

- ASA III Patient with moderate-to-severe systemic disease with substantive functional limitations; poorly controlled diabetes or hypertension, chronic obstructive pulmonary disease (COPD), morbid obesity, alcoholism, end-stage renal disease (ESRD) on regular dialysis, or active hepatitis

- ASA IV   Patient with severe systemic disease that poses constant threat of death; recent myocardial infarction (MI), cerebrovascular accident (CVA), transient ischemic attack (TIA), ESRD not on regular dialysis, sepsis, or disseminated intravascular coagulopathy (DIC)

- ASA V   Patient at immediate risk of death without treatment; ruptured abdominal or thoracic aneurysm; massive trauma; ischemic bowel with multiorgan failure; or intracranial bleed with mass effects

- ASA VI   A patient deemed brain-dead whose organs are to be retrieved for donation

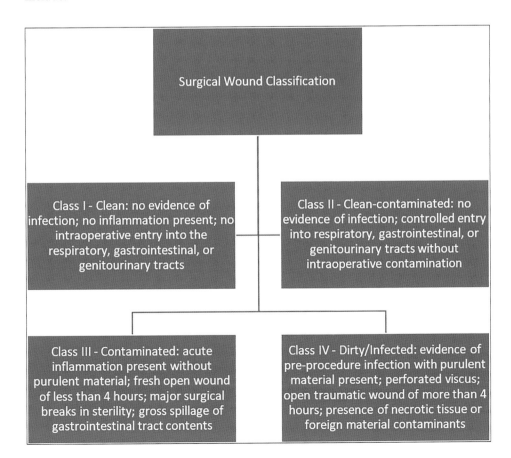

Figure 4-2 · Surgical wound classification.

Prolonged Operative Procedure Time. Research studies of the impact of prolonged surgical procedural times showed a definite increased likelihood of developing SSI in a variety of surgical specialties and types of procedures. The pooled statistical analyses of 81 studies published in a 2017 report published in the journal *Surgical Infections* concluded that patients that underwent longer surgical procedures were twice as likely to develop SSI. The average time between those who suffered SSI and those who did not was approximately 30 minutes longer.

PATHOGENS IN HEALTHCARE-ASSOCIATED INFECTION

Any microbe that is able to gain access into the human body has the potential to create problems if the conditions are optimal. There are certain types of bacteria, fungi, and viruses commonly classified as HAIs and which include SSIs.

Gram-Negative Proteobacteria

Bacteria with the morphological shapes of bacilli (rods) or coccobacilli (short rods that resemble round cocci) that lose the purple crystal violet stain after rinsing with alcohol and take on the red safranin counter-stain in the Gram-staining process are classified as gram-negative and have a pink or red appearance under the microscope.

Bacteria in the phylum Proteobacteria fall into five classes: Alpha (α), Beta (β), Gamma (γ), Delta (δ), Epsilon (ε), and Zeta (ζ). The bacteria in the Delta and Zeta classes are not considered human pathogens. The phylum Proteobacteria includes some of the most pathogenic species of bacteria causing severe infection in humans. The Gamma class contains the bacteria most commonly identified as HAIs and SSIs. All Proteobacteria are gram-negative bacilli or coccobacilli.

Genus Escherichia, Family Enterobacteriaceae. *E. coli*, a part of the resident microbiome of the human gastrointestinal tract is one of the most commonly recognized bacterial species. *E. coli* is included in the class Gamma of the phylum Proteobacteria, family *Enterobacteriaceae*, and genus *Escherichia*. It is a gram-negative rod (GNR), facultative anaerobe that grows as an individual cell which is non–spore-forming and may be motile or non-motile. As a normally harmless commensal microbe residing in the intestines, *E. coli* synthesizes vitamins from ingested food for use in metabolic processes and helps prevent the growth of non-native pathogenic bacteria.

When transmission through the fecal-oral route occurs, for example, *E. coli* is an opportunistic pathogen that can contribute to an endogenous source of SSI as well as UTIs, sepsis, diarrheal disease, and neonatal meningitis. Patients who already have a debilitating condition are at higher risk for infection as compared to healthy persons. The five classes of pathogenic *E. coli* strains are (1) enteropathogenic, (2) enterotoxigenic, (3) enterohemorrhagic, (4) enteroaggregative, and (5) enteroinvasive. The *E. coli* strains responsible for severe diarrheal symptoms are classified according to their specific virulence factors.

Genus Enterobacter, Family Enterobacteriaceae. The genus *Enterobacter* is part of the class Gamma, phylum Proteobacteria, and family *Enterobacteriaceae*. These bacteria are gram-negative, rod-shaped, facultative anaerobes, with motility capability from the presence of peritrichous flagella. *Enterobacter cloacae* and *Enterobacter aerogenes* are the species which are serious human pathogens and major sources of HAI. Bacteria in the family *Enterobacteriaceae* have outer membranes that are endotoxins which stimulate the body's immune system to release cytokines, mediators of systemic inflammation.

Cronobacter sakazakii, formerly called *Enterobacter sakazakii*, in neonates and children under the age of 2 years can be the cause of sepsis and central nervous infections including meningitis, ventriculitis, brain abscess, cerebral infarction, and cyst formation. *C. sakazakii* is characterized by its ability to grow in extremely dry environments. Outbreaks of *C. sakazakii* infections in infants have been associated with contaminated powdered baby formula and other powdered foods.

The spectrum of *Enterobacter* infections, sometimes referred to as "ICU bugs," is responsible for numerous types of HAIs and SSIs including bacteremia, endocarditis, osteomyelitis, peritonitis, and infections involving the lower respiratory tract, central nervous system, urinary tract, eyes, skin, and soft tissues. Specific risk factors in susceptible patients include:

- Intensive care unit (ICU) admission and hospitalization for longer than 2 weeks
- Surgery or other type of invasive procedures in recent days
- The placement and maintenance of a central venous catheter during ICU stay
- Recent broad-spectrum (cephalosporin or aminoglycoside) antibiotic treatment regimen within 30 days
- Older adults and neonates

The primary method of diagnosis for *Enterobacter* infections involves two sets of culture specimens, one aerobic and one anaerobic. These cultures should be obtained from two different sites if possible and spaced 20 to 30 minutes apart. The Gram-staining technique determines the bacterial colony's categorization. Other diagnostic tests to isolate *Enterobacter* include

- Blood sampling
- Urinalysis
- Imaging studies such as x-ray, CT scan, or MRI
- Endoscopic retrograde cholangiopancreatography (ERCP) for possible biliary obstruction
- Soft tissue or bone needle biopsy
- Surgical incision and drainage (I&D) with bacterial cultures
- Lumbar puncture for collection of cerebrospinal fluid samples.

The choice of antibiotic selection and duration of treatment for *Enterobacter* must be carefully considered by healthcare providers due to the bacterial species' ability to quickly develop antibiotic resistance.

Genus Klebsiella, Family Enterobacteriaceae. Klebsiella bacteria is another genus belonging to the family *Enterobacteriaceae*, class Gamma, and phylum Proteobacteria. They are non-motile, gram-negative rod (GNR), facultative anaerobes that have a polysaccharide capsule which gives the bacterium a larger appearance, provides protection against immune system defenses, and enhances antibiotic resistance. Carbapenem-resistant *Enterobacteriaceae* (CRE) has been added to the CDC's list of urgent antibiotic drug-resistant threats.

HAIs from *Klebsiella* involve the biliary, respiratory, and urinary tracts and surgical wounds. The species *K. pneumoniae* is a relatively common cause of bacterial pneumonia. Other species contribute to HAIs involving invasive medical devices, ventilators, indwelling urinary catheters, and prior inappropriate antibiotic treatment. The species *K. oxytoca* has been identified in cases of neonatal septicemia in premature infants in the neonatal intensive care unit (NICU) setting. Other species of *Klebsiella* are responsible for a chronic infection called rhinoscleroma involving the nasopharynx and an ulcerative genital disease called donovanosis or granuloma inguinale seen in developing countries and rarely in the United States.

Genus Proteus, Family Enterobacteriaceae. Another normal member of the class Gamma, phylum Proteobacteria, family *Enterobacteriaceae* is also commonly found in the human intestinal tract is the genus *Proteus*. Community-acquired infections from the species *Proteus mirabilis* account for 90% of Proteus infections. Although less common, two other species, *P. vulgaris* and *P. penneri,* produce the enzyme urease which induces epithelial cell desquamation of urinary tract tissues. The urease hydrolyzes ammonia and creates struvite stones which contribute to urinary tract obstruction. Long-term use of indwelling urinary catheters increases risk of UTI. Soft tissue abscesses unrelated to the urinary tract may require debridement of infected tissues or even amputation of affected extremities. Extensive *Proteus* infections of soft tissues may be fatal, with or without medical or surgical treatment.

Genus Serratia, Family Enterobacteriaceae. The genus *Serratia* also belongs to the large *Enterobacteriaceae* family, class Gamma, phylum Proteobacteria. These bacterial cells are small, motile, gram-negative, and rod-shaped that become opportunistic pathogens. *Serratia* is a common environmental bacterial genus, rarely found in the human intestinal tract; however, identified in a variety of HAIs including:

- Bacteremia or blood sepsis from insertion of venous access lines
- Infective arthritis secondary to intra-articular steroid or local anesthetic injections
- Endocarditis or osteomyelitis in IV drug misuse
- Eye or other soft tissue infections
- Meningitis after epidural anesthesia in C-sections or for chronic pain therapy
- Respiratory infections after intubation or bronchoscopy procedures

- Urinary tract infection from catheter placement or cystoscopy procedures

Serratia marcescens, the most common species in the genus, produces prodigiosin, a pigment that appears deep red to pale pink. Women with postpartum mastitis from *S. marcescens* observe a pink tinge in their breasts due to the prodigiosin pigment. *Serratia* infections are considered HAIs.

Genus Acinetobacter, Family Moraxellaceae. Bacteria in the genus *Acinetobacter* are members of the family *Moraxellaceae*, class Gamma, and phylum Proteobacteria. They have a morphology of bacilli to coccobacilli. These gram-negative, non-motile, aerobic microbes live in soil and water. They do not typically affect healthy humans; however, they may become dangerous opportunistic pathogens in diabetic or immunocompromised individuals and patients with chronic lung disease. It is estimated that *Acinetobacter baumannii* is responsible for 80% of HAIs caused by the genus *Acinetobacter*. The bacterial cells grow well in fluid environments; however, they are able to survive for moderate time periods on dry inanimate surfaces or human skin. Infections in humans are extremely uncommon outside of healthcare environments such as intensive care units (ICUs) or other critical care areas. *A. baumannii* infections affect several body systems and have been cultured from invasive devices such as central venous catheters leading to vascular sepsis or central nervous system infection; tracheostomy tubes causing lung infection; and indwelling urinary catheters resulting in UTIs.

Acinetobacter baumannii has been shown to have the potential for strong antibiotic resistance. Careful consideration must be given to antibiotic therapy for infections involving this type of bacteria. Strict adherence to proper hand hygiene and antiseptic skin preparation prior to invasive procedures must be given to minimize the serious threat of cross-contamination of critically ill patients from healthcare providers or the physical environment.

Genus Pseudomonas, Family Pseudomonadaceae. The family *Pseudomonadaceae* is a member of the class Gamma, phylum Proteobacteria and includes the genus *Pseudomonas,* which is comprised of gram-negative bacterial cells that are short, straight, or slightly curved rods. They are non–spore-forming and motile with some species having flagella at the ends and pili that aid in attachment to tissues of an infected host. Some strains are surrounded by an outer slime layer that may surround individual cells or several cells forming a microcolony. These morphological features add to the virulence of the strains. *Pseudomonas* is found in most areas of the planet and can withstand harsh environmental conditions due to its highly impermeable cell wall and the production of enzymes that destroy toxic substances, even without spore formation capability.

The species *Pseudomonas aeruginosa* is easily identified in the laboratory studies. Colonies produce an extracellular pigment and emit a fruity odor. Bacterial cells are motile and oxidase positive. Strains of non-pigmented motile bacteria require additional laboratory testing due to the difficulty in definitive identification. The *P. aeruginosa* bacteria can live on many hospital surfaces, such as sinks, drinking fountains, cleansing soaps used by the hospital staff, and patient humidifiers. Concerning factors include the bacteria's ability to withstand harsh environments and that the opportunistic pathogen has become highly antibiotic resistant.

Patients with weakened immune systems from conditions such as cystic fibrosis, burns, and leukemia are at high risk for developing *P. aeruginosa* infections as are patients on ventilator assistance or who have a tracheostomy. Primary pneumonia caused by *P. aeruginosa* is more commonly identified in debilitated patients with comorbidities of pulmonary disease or congestive heart failure. The genetic disorder cystic fibrosis causes an accumulation of thick and tenacious mucus in the respiratory tract. These individuals are more prone to pneumonia or tracheobronchitis infections with *P. aeruginosa* as the bacteria colonize the respiratory tract, complicating the underlying disease process, and contributing to the high mortality rate.

Gram-Negative *Bacteroidaceae* Bacteria

Another important gram-negative bacterial family is *Bacteroidaceae* in the phylum Bacteroidetes. The opportunistic microorganism in this group that is normal resident microbe in the human digestive tract is the species *Bacteroides fragilis,* an obligate anaerobe found mainly in the terminal ilium and the large intestine. The bacterial family is important commensals that have beneficial actions of aiding in the biotransformation of bile acids and breaking down carbohydrates for use by the body.

Bacteroides Fragilis. *Bacteroides fragilis* is a small, pleomorphic, bacillus that is non-motile and non-toxin-producing. It is non–spore-forming, although it does have a large polysaccharide capsule that gives the appearance of a spore coating. The capsule resists phagocytosis when it becomes an opportunistic source of abscess formation in the peritoneal cavity. Routes of transmission are through perforated appendix or intestinal ulcer; diverticulitis or inflammatory bowel disease; and through sharp or blunt trauma to the intestinal tract. Following the spillage of intestinal bacteria into the peritoneal cavity, the facultative anaerobic bacteria such as *E. coli* damage internal tissues and consume any oxygen present, allowing the proliferation of the obligate anaerobic *B. fragilis* colonies. This second stage of infection includes abscess formation and resistance to the immune system's mobilization of phagocytes because of the protective capsules around the *B. fragilis* bacteria. The body's attempt to wall off the developing abscess actually shields the bacteria from antibiotic treatment, allowing the abscess to grow and eventually rupture, causing peritonitis which can result in bacteremia, septic shock, and death if not treated aggressively with surgical incision and drainage (I&D) of the peritoneal abscess. Extensive intestinal tissue damage may require bowel resection to remove necrotic areas.

Extraperitoneal abscess formation may be much less apparent and diagnosis can be delayed due to the lack of abdominal symptoms seen in abscesses within the peritoneal space. The retroperitoneum is a space bordered by the peritoneum and the transversalis fascia. The organs located in this space include the kidneys and ureters, pancreas, duodenum, and portions of the ascending and descending large intestine. The source of retroperitoneal abscesses typically involves the kidneys or other renal structures; however, it may be due to ruptured diverticula, gastric ulcer, or retrocecal appendicitis; pancreatitis; inflammatory bowel disease; or osteomyelitis of thoracic or lumbar vertebral bodies. Patients may experience signs and symptoms of pain and swelling involving the groin and in some cases into the hip and upper thigh. Radiologic studies are critical to making definitive diagnosis of retroperitoneal abscess.

Gram-Positive Firmicute Bacteria

Bacteria with the morphological shapes of cocci (round) and bacilli (rods) that retain the purple crystal violet stain after rinsing with alcohol in the Gram-staining process are classified as gram-positive and have a purple or dark blue appearance under the microscope. As with the enteric bacteria in the phylum Proteobacteria, gram-positive bacteria in the phylum Firmicutes are frequently part of the normal intestinal and skin microbiomes of animals and humans as well as in soil around the world. Fortunately, only a few species of staphylococcal and streptococcal bacteria are of significance for surgical site and other HAIs.

Staphylococcal Bacteria. The bacterial genus *Staphylococcus*, a member of the phylum Firmicutes and family *Staphylococcaceae* is an extremely common facultative anaerobe. The two species, *S. aureus* and *S. epidermidis*, found in the deeper layers of human skin, are frequently responsible for SSIs and other HAIs. The bacterial morphology described by the Greek word staphylo is that of a "cluster of grapes" and coccus means "round berries." Colonies of bacteria grown on blood agar culture plates demonstrate a color difference between *S. aureus* which has a yellow coloration and *S. epidermidis* which is whiter in appearance. As discussed in previous sections, catalase and coagulase enzyme tests are also used to distinguish bacterial species from one another. The coagulase-positive bacterial species (CoPS) *S. aureus* has an enhanced virulence factor due to the ability of the bacteria to form a clot (thrombus) around the growing infective microcolony which shields it from destruction from the body's natural inflammatory response of phagocytosis by white blood cells.

S. aureus is considered part of the normal resident microflora of human skin; however, when given access to deeper, subdermal tissues by traumatic injury or surgical incision, it can become an opportunistic pathogen that may cause SSI. *S. aureus* is also responsible for colonizing bacterial biofilms that adhere to surfaces of implantable items and are highly resistant to destruction by antibiotic therapy. Patients on ventilator support are also at increased risk of staphylococcal pneumonia. Methicillin-resistant *S. aureus* or MRSA is widely recognized as an antibiotic-resistant strain of the bacteria that was formerly categorized as a HAI; however, it has become much more common and frequently community-acquired. Signs of infection commonly appear as non-healing skin lesions (see Figures 4-3 and 4-4).

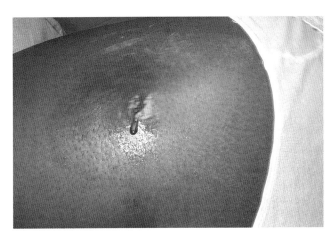

Figure 4-3 · This 2005 photograph depicted a cutaneous abscess located on the hip of a prison inmate, which had begun to spontaneously drain, releasing its purulent contents. The abscess was caused by methicillin-resistant Staphylococcus aureus (MRSA) bacteria. (CDC/ Bruno Coignard, M.D.; Jeff Hageman, M.H.S.)

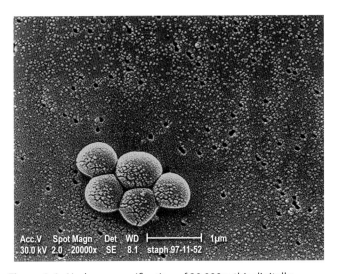

Figure 4-4 · Under a magnification of 20,000×, this digitally-colorized, scanning electron microscopic (SEM) image depicts a grouping of methicillin-resistant Staphylococcus aureus (MRSA) bacteria. See PHIL 617 for a black and white view of this image. These MRSA bacteria are from one of the first isolates in the United States that showed increased resistance to vancomycin as well. (CDC/Jim Biddle/Janice Haney Carr.)

Staphylococcus epidermidis is another species responsible for SSI and creation of biofilms of invasive catheters and implantable devices or prostheses. Unlike coagulase-positive *S. aureus*, *S. epidermidis* is coagulase-negative (CoNS) and produces an extracellular polymeric substance that forms biofilm formation of bacterial colonies contributing to its virulence. The biofilms that coat the surfaces of implanted items such as joint prostheses or heart valves and indwelling long-term catheters are highly resistant to antibiotic therapy and the natural body inflammatory defenses. *S. epidermidis* infection has been documented in cases of subacute bacterial endocarditis infection showing signs up to a year after implantation of artificial heart

valves. Prostheses implanted during total joint arthroplasty present a similar challenge in preventing SSI with *S. epidermidis* or other CoNS species. Prolonged antibiotic therapy and surgical removal of the infected valve or total joint prosthesis may be required to treat the infection. Reimplantation of joint prostheses carries high potential for additional SSI potentially resulting in eventual permanent removal and joint fusion.

Staphylococcus lugdunensis is a less-commonly isolated, virulent CoNS species. Laboratory methods used for identification may mistakenly identify *S. lugdunensis* as *S. aureus*, reducing the accuracy of infection rate reporting. First identified in 1988, researchers and epidemiologists have included *S. lugdunensis* as part of the normal resident human skin flora of the perineal region. Potentially fatal cases of endocarditis complicated by heart failure have been attributed to the lesser-known *S. lugdunensis* and some studies show that the mortality rates for endocarditis from *S. lugdunensis* may be higher when compared with other CoNS infections.

Staphylococcal Disease

Chronic disease processes and acute infections from staphylococcal bacteria are common in humans. The normal resident bacterial populations within the skin layers and mucosal membranes become opportunistic pathogens when conditions are favorable. Concerns are heightened in the healthcare setting when the bacteria that are normally well understood and relatively easily treated evolve to develop resistance to standard antibiotic therapy. Nonsurgical diseases caused by *Staphylococcus* include toxic shock syndrome, impetigo, folliculitis, scalded skin syndrome, osteomyelitis, and food poisoning from poor hand hygiene of food preparers.

Cellulitis. Cellulitis is an infection of the soft tissues and may occur following surgical procedures as superficial SSI. The signs of cellulitis are typically unilateral and may be proximal to the surgical site and with significant warmth, erythema, fever, and inflammation. Other nonsurgical causes of inflammation may be mistaken for cellulitis and should be considered and ruled out prior to initiation of antibiotic treatment.

Venous stasis dermatitis is a chronic condition that is often bilateral and may cause darkening of the skin and pitting edema. There is no evidence of fever or purulent drainage and can be managed with elevation, compression, and topical steroid preparations. Lymphedema is a disruption of the normal lymphatic drainage mechanism and is usually a result of obesity or following lymph node dissection. The signs are typically unilateral and there is little change in skin temperature and no fever. Other causes of swelling not related to an infectious process are gout, peripheral artery disease (PAD), and contact dermatitis.

If signs and symptoms of inflammation appear suddenly, are unrelieved by elevation, and the skin has a shiny, smooth appearance, then cellulitis should be considered, and appropriate diagnostic studies performed to isolate the pathogenic source prior to starting antibiotic therapy.

Nonpurulent cellulitis is most commonly caused by group A streptococcal bacterial. Cellulitis infections with frank pus formation are typically caused by *S. aureus* and may be colonized with MRSA. Surgical debridement of necrotic tissue should be performed to reduce the microbial load. Oral antibiotics may be prescribed in milder cellulitis cases; however, intravenous administration may be necessary in severe cases or when drug-resistant strains are identified.

Skin and subcutaneous abscesses can form following any type of break in the skin, whether surgical or nonsurgical. Localized areas of pus accumulation called furuncles can combine to create larger, painful, edematous lesions called carbuncles. These infections are most commonly a result of opportunistic *S. aureus* or other staphylococcal or streptococcal bacteria gaining access beneath the skin layers where they are resident microflora. Areas of superficial abscess formation in the subcutaneous fat layer following a surgical procedure may be treated with incision and drainage (I&D), with or without placement of plain or iodoform packing materials, oral antibiotics, or topical antibacterial creams.

Toxic Shock Syndrome. Certain strains of *S. aureus* produce toxic shock syndrome–associated toxin (TSST). The exotoxin is a type of super-antigen that causes the disease known as toxic shock syndrome (TSS). Streptococcal bacteria cause a similar infection called toxic shock-like syndrome (TSLS). Risk factors include individuals with history of recent staphylococcal infection such as streptococcal pneumonia, traumatic or surgical wound infection or abscess, and extensive burns. Use of any packing materials (including vaginal or nasal tampons) predisposes patients to potential toxic shock syndrome. Although considered statistically rare, research results vary from 5% to 15% mortality rate with as high as a 50% mortality rate in cases of severe toxic shock, resulting in multiorgan failure.

Osteomyelitis. Osteomyelitis is a bone infection that may originate indirectly at a remote site in the body such as a surgical site or following dental, respiratory, or bladder infection, and travels via the bloodstream to skeletal bones. Direct causes of infection include trauma involving penetrating injury, open fractures, and orthopedic surgical procedures including total joint replacement also known as arthroplasty. *S. aureus* invasion may result in chronic bone marrow and bone infection. Pediatric osteomyelitis is usually an acute infection that involves long bones such as the femur. In adults, the spinal vertebrae and pelvis are most commonly affected and are chronic infections.

Generally, patient risk factors for osteomyelitis include diabetes with or without hemodialysis, peripheral vascular disease, rheumatoid arthritis, alcohol misuse, and immunocompromised status due to prolonged antiviral or steroid use for HIV/AIDS, sickle-cell disease, organ transplantation, or other autoimmune disorders. Procedures used to diagnose osteomyelitis include radiographic tomography and radionuclide bone scanning. Cultures may be obtained through bone biopsy to determine which bacteria are present.

Aggressive high-dose intravenous antibiotics and strict bed rest are ordered for acute infections. Persistent or chronic infection may require surgical debridement of necrotic bone. Even with antibiotic treatment, chronic osteomyelitis can persist for years.

Infective Endocarditis. Infective endocarditis is an infection of the lining of the heart, its valves, or a septal defect. *Staphylococcus* is commonly the infective agent involved; however, fungal infection may also be responsible in less-common cases. The infected heart valves may be native valves or prosthetic implants. The primary effect of infective endocarditis is valvular insufficiency which leads to secondary effects of congestive heart failure and myocardial abscesses. Fatality results if infective endocarditis is not treated.

There are three broad types of infective endocarditis: (1) native valve endocarditis or NVE (acute or subacute); (2) prosthetic valve endocarditis or PVE (early or late); and (3) intravenous drug abuse endocarditis or IVDA. Another cause of infective endocarditis is from implanted cardiac pacemakers. The site of infection may involve the area of the generator or may be at the site of the leads implanted in the heart. Infection may go undiagnosed for a year or more as symptoms may be vague and attributed to other sources. Removal of the infected pacemaker device and leads is usually required in order to clear the microbial colonies that may have developed into biofilms on the implant surfaces.

Acute NVE cases are identified in healthy individuals without a history of valvular disease. *Staphylococcus aureus* or Group B species of *Streptococcus* are the cause of the aggressive, rapidly progressive, acute infection. Remote sites of infection spread bacteria through the vascular system to the heart valves where they quickly infect and destroy heart valve tissue. Death results in a few days to a few weeks if not aggressively treated.

Endocarditis infections that occur within 60 days of implantation called early PVE cases are caused by coagulase-negative staphylococci (CoNS), gram-negative bacilli, or fungal species of *Candida*. The late PVE infections occur more than 60 days after surgical implantation and are most commonly caused by staphylococci, alpha-hemolytic streptococci, or enterococci. Infections from *S. aureus* are the most common cause of early and late PVE and IVDA and which have a 30% to 40% mortality rate.

Healthy heart valve tissue has a light red smooth surface. Following bacterial infection, valvular tissue has a rough, reddened, and inflamed surface that causes the valve opening to narrow and malfunction. The endocardial and pericardial tissues may also be affected by the bacterial infection. Patients may experience chronic fever, heart murmur, splenomegaly, or embolism. Immediate appropriate, bacteria-specific, intravenous antibiotic therapy is critical. Patients with severe heart valve damage from IE may require valve replacement with additional antibiotic infusion treatment.

Streptococcal Bacteria. The sphere-shaped bacterial genus *Streptococcus* belongs to the phylum Firmicutes and family *Streptococcaceae*. The gram-positive, facultative anaerobes are found in many tissues of the human body. They are non-motile, non–spore-forming, and catalase-negative; and they occur in pairs or chains. *Streptococcus* species are divided into broad classes based on their ability to destroy red blood cells, called hemolysis. The use of blood agar in Petri dishes in the laboratory to observe the type or extent of hemolytic has long been used for classification of streptococci as alpha, beta, or gamma.

Streptococci in the alpha (α) class demonstrate minor destruction of red blood cells (erythrocytes) and include the viridans group (VSG) and *Streptococcus pneumoniae.* The beta (β) streptococci bacteria cause complete hemolysis of the erythrocytes in the agar around the colony of bacteria on the culture plate. The beta (β) streptococci also produce toxins that affect blood clotting factors and white blood cells, enhancing the virulence factor of these bacteria. Gamma (γ) hemolytic streptococci do not affect erythrocytes and are classified as non-hemolytic.

A classification system developed in the 1930s, called the Lancefield groups, separates the Beta hemolytic streptococci into lettered groups (A, B, C, D, F, and G) based on specific antigens. Since that time, several streptococci have been found to have several group antigens. Group A streptococci are beta (β) hemolytic while Group B streptococci may be alpha (α), beta (β), or gamma (γ) hemolytic. Most *S. pneumoniae* are α hemolytic but can cause β hemolysis in anaerobic conditions. The A and D groups can be transmitted through contaminated food.

Large colonies of streptococcal bacteria are known as "pyogenic" (pus-forming) groups and have multiple virulence factors.

Cell wall structure and serologic reactions to their antigens provide the definitive laboratory identification of streptococci. All species of streptococci lack the enzyme catalase. Streptococci outside of Group A do not have definite virulence factors. Group A streptococci has been extensively researched due to its multiple virulence factors which include:

- Acids and proteins in the cell wall that aid in bacterial attachment to host cells
- Toxin production including pyrogenic (fever-producing) toxin
- Streptokinase – enzyme that dissolves blood clots
- Streptolysins – toxins that destroy phagocytes
- Protective hyaluronic acid capsule that increases virulence in skin and soft tissues

Streptococcal Disease. Streptococcus is the cause of a wide range of disease in humans from mild to severe and chronic. Group A streptococcal diseases include community-acquired impetigo, strep throat, and scarlet fever. Severe acute diseases include Group A *S. pneumoniae* and *S. pyogenes* infections responsible for life-threatening necrotizing fasciitis, streptococcal meningitis, bacteremia, cellulitis, pneumococcal pneumonia, streptococcal toxic shock syndrome (STSS), and puerperal sepsis.

Necrotizing fasciitis, otherwise known as the "flesh-eating" disease is caused by streptococcal bacteria that produce the enzyme protease which destroys tissue proteins and assists in bacterial invasion of epithelial cells. The portal of entry for the opportunistic pathogen may be an otherwise insignificant break in the skin. Within hours, the individual may experience symptoms of pain similar to muscle strains. Pain progresses in intensity as visible signs of inflammation including redness, heat, and swelling may be observed. The external appearance may not seem to correlate with the extreme pain caused by the progressive destruction of the fascia, leading healthcare providers to miss the underlying infection. The subsequent delay in diagnosis and initiation of aggressive antibiotic therapy may result in the need for surgical removal of infected fascia and adjacent soft tissues (debridement). Extensive tissue destruction may require amputation of an extremity. Hyperbaric oxygen as adjunct therapy may provide some aid in tissue preservation once debridement has been performed to remove necrotic areas. Group A streptococcal strains are the most common cause of necrotizing fasciitis; however, other opportunistic pathogens can also cause severe infection including *E. coli, S. aureus, Klebsiella, Clostridium,* and *Aeromonas hydrophila.* One in three individuals with necrotizing fasciitis infection will die. Patient risk factors include those with diabetes, kidney disease, cirrhosis of the liver, and cancer.

Long-term, chronic diseases referred to as nonsuppurative (non–pus-forming) include rheumatic fever and glomerulonephritis following previous strep throat infection. These chronic sequelae diseases manifest weeks to months after untreated streptococcal infection of other parts of the body. Recurring middle ear infections (otitis media) from *S. pneumoniae* in children often require surgical placement of tiny, pressure-equalizing (PE) drainage tubes called myringotomy tubes to relieve painful pressure by draining the pus.

Gram-Positive Clostridia Bacilli. The genus *Clostridium* is a member of the phylum Firmicutes, family *Clostridiaceae,* and class Clostridia and comprised of over 100 known species of anaerobic, spore-forming, gram-positive bacilli of which the majority are strictly anaerobic; however, some species are aerotolerant. *Clostridium* is found in water, soil, sewage, and often isolated as part of the indigenous normal bacterial flora in gastrointestinal tracts of animals and humans. The majority of species do not cause disease; however, there are a few recognized opportunistic pathogens that cause serious, often fatal disease in humans and the most commonly recognized to be discussed here include:

- Botulism: *Clostridium botulinum*
- Colitis: *Clostridium* (now *Clostridioides*) *difficile*
- Gas gangrene: *Clostridium perfringens*
- Tetanus: *Clostridium tetani*

Virulence factors of *Clostridium* make them powerful pathogens and include spore formation which provides protection from harsh environmental conditions; production of toxins, including enterotoxins and neurotoxins; and rapid growth periods in no or low-oxygen areas.

Clostridium Perfringens. Clostridium perfringens is one of the few nonmotile gram-positive bacilli, although colonies grow rapidly in laboratory cultures. *Clostridium* produces four lethal toxins that are used to subdivide it into five types

(A, B, C, D, and E). Most infections in humans are caused by *C. perfringens* type A, a common member of the normal microbiome of the GI tracts of humans and animals. It is also isolated in water and soil contaminated with feces but gains access to human tissue through traumatic injuries, resulting in gas gangrene or soft tissue infections. Types B, C, D, and E do not survive in the soil and primarily colonize the GI tract of animals and, in rare cases, humans. Type C causes necrotizing enteritis if it gains access to the GI tract.

Toxins.   One of the most serious infections in humans by *Clostridium perfringens* is myonecrosis or muscle tissue death and destruction. Even with rapid medical attention, myonecrosis has a high mortality rate due to the potentially lethal toxins and enzymes the bacteria produce. The alpha toxin produced by *C. perfringens* type A is responsible for increased vascular permeability, massive hemolysis, bleeding, and myonecrosis leading to life-threatening bradycardia (slow heart rate), hypotension, and hepatic toxicity. Other toxins may cause serious GI infections when large quantities are ingested. Necrotizing enteritis is a less common infection that occurs in the jejunum, with a high mortality rate of 50% from the C type of *C. perfringens.*

The prognosis is extremely poor in myonecrosis (gas gangrene) infections, with a reported mortality rate of 40% to 100%. The toxin-releasing microorganism is introduced into the tissue by traumatic injury or surgery. The patient experiences fever; pain and inflammation of tissues; vomiting and jaundice; tachycardia; anxiety; paleness of skin turning grey, brown, or black; air under the skin with a characteristic crackling noise when compressed; and blistering with foul-smelling discharge. Surgical debridement of necrotic tissue is necessary to slow the progression of the infection and tissue loss.

Clostridium perfringens and *C. septicum* also cause cellulitis, a less serious infection, and debilitating fasciitis. As with the gas gangrene of myonecrosis, fasciitis progresses quickly; however, the tissue infected is the fascial layer over skeletal muscle that produces the characteristic gas as tissue is destroyed.

C. perfringens is the third highest cause of food-borne disease, responsible for nearly a million cases per year. Severe infections may produce severe abdominal pain, bloody diarrhea, systemic shock, and peritonitis as the pathogenic bacterial cells create intestinal tissue necrosis and enter the peritoneal cavity.

Clostridium Botulinum Disease.   *Clostridium botulinum* is a gram-positive, rod-shaped, spore-forming, mainly anaerobic bacterial species subdivided into four groups based on toxins produced. The strains of types I and II are the cause of most human diseases. Botulinum toxin is similar to the tetanus toxin that blocks the release of the neurotransmitter acetylcholine at synaptic junctions. Patients recover when nerve endings regenerate.

Botulism is a muscle-paralyzing disease caused by the toxic effects of *C. botulinum*. There are five types of botulism: (1) food-borne, (2) wound, (3) infant, (4) adult intestinal toxemia, and (5) iatrogenic. Food-borne botulism (15% of reported cases) is caused by the ingestion of toxin-contaminated canned foods. Wound botulism (20% of reported cases) is considered relatively rare. Infant botulism (65% of reported cases) is the most common form of the infection and associated with the consumption of contaminated foods, commonly honey. Adult intestinal toxemia botulism and iatrogenic botulism are considered very rare.

In food-borne botulism infection, bilateral flaccid muscle weakness progresses from shoulder level down toward the torso and lower extremities. Diaphragmatic and respiratory paralysis stops breathing as the *C. botulinum* neurotoxin irreversibly blocks neurotransmitters and requires mechanical ventilator assistance until function returns, which may take weeks or up to a year before diaphragmatic function is restored. Food-borne botulism is not transmitted from person to person.

C. botulinum introduced into a traumatic wound either by contaminants in soil through a break in the skin or in the perioperative period is the cause of the relatively uncommon wound botulism infection. The clinical signs and symptoms are similar to food-borne botulism, except the incubation period is longer and there may be no abdominal symptoms.

Infants between the age of one month to six months lack many indigenous intestinal or "gut" microflora, causing infection because *C. botulinum* microbes take over the immature GI tract. Infant botulism signs and symptoms include droopy eyes, weak cry, poor sucking reflex, constipation, lethargy, flaccid paralysis, also called "floppy baby syndrome," and ultimately, respiratory failure. If the cascade of signs is observed in an infant, parents should seek immediate medical attention. Honey, corn syrup, and peanut butter have been identified as potential sources of infant botulism infection and should not be given to children under one year of age.

Clostridium Tetani.   *C. tetani* bacterial spores are easily identified under the microscope. One end is rounded, and a rod extends from the spore, giving a turkey drumstick appearance. Despite the easy identification based on the characteristic appearance, *C. tetani* is difficult to grow due to the anaerobe's extreme sensitivity to any level of oxygen and a low level of metabolic activity.

C. tetani is common in soil and colonizes the GI tracts of humans and animals. *C. tetani* rapidly sporulates (forms a spore coating or capsule) to survive in oxygenated areas of nature. Tetanus is rarely seen in the United States since the development of the tetanus vaccine which may prompt a "booster" dose to be given if an individual suffers some type of penetrating injury with a dirty or rusty item in contaminated soil where *C. tetani* thrives.

Diseases of C. Tetani.   The incubation period for infections from tetanus range between 3 and 21 days, or at an average of 10 days. The closer the site of the infection is to the central nervous system, the quicker the incubation period and appearance of signs. The short time and proximity correlate with increased severity of the infection, higher complication rates, and potential fatality.

Eighty percent of *C. tetani* infections result in generalized tetanus. Trismus, commonly called lockjaw, is a widely recognized sign of tetanus and involves the constant contraction of the masseter muscles of the face resulting in the characteristic "smile" called risus sardonicus. Another sign of tetanus is chronic back spasms referred to as opisthotonos. Autonomic nervous system involvement results in profound sweating that can lead to dehydration, alternating hypertension and hypotension, and cardiac arrhythmias. The rate of fatality for generalized tetanus infections is 10% to 20%. Localized infections involving the muscles at the site of entry are typically mild; however, there is potential for conversion to systemic generalized tetanus in some cases.

Life-threatening cephalic tetanus is relatively rare with the primary site of infection in the head or face, including an association with otitis media infections. Cephalic tetanus causes flaccid cranial nerves (palsies) rather than spasm. The incubation period is very short (1-2 days). Cephalic tetanus can spread to become generalized tetanus.

Neonatal tetanus, also known as tetanus neonatorum, is a deadly infection of a neonate's umbilical stump. After the umbilicus falls off, the umbilical area may become infected and the disease then spreads to become generalized. Incubation is typically between 4 and 14 days (7 days being average) and the mortality rate is close to 100%. The few infants that do survive neonatal tetanus infection often have developmental complications.

Tetanus Treatment and Prevention. Treatments for tetanus infections must be provided as soon as possible and include hospitalization for aggressive surgical wound care if indicated. Generalized tetanus infections may require endotracheal airway, nasotracheal intubation, or tracheostomy with mechanical ventilation and medications to manage autonomic nervous system instability. Severe muscle spasms may be controlled with sedatives and muscle relaxants. Medical treatment includes administration of human tetanus immunoglobulin and antispasm medications. If immunoglobulin is unavailable, a large, single dose of an equine-origin tetanus antitoxin is administered. A tetanus toxoid booster and antibiotics may be sufficient in less severe cases.

The routine prophylactic tetanus vaccine has been available for many years and given in three doses, within the same schedule as the diphtheria and pertussis protection as what is known as the Tdap (tetanus, diphtheria, and pertussis) vaccine. Tdap boosters are recommended every 10 years to maintain immunity status. Individuals with active tetanus infections will be given the tetanus vaccination concurrently with appropriate supportive treatment.

HAI—Clostridium Difficile. Clostridium difficile was reclassified in 2016 to *Clostridioides difficile* and is commonly referred to as "C. diff." As with the other Clostridia bacterial species, it is a gram-positive, rod-shaped, anaerobic, spore-forming bacillus. *C. difficile* has been studied since 1930 when research microbiologists first tried to isolate the bacteria in culture. Due to the difficulty in classifying the bacterial colonies, it was assigned the name *C. difficile*. The Joint Commission, CDC, and state health departments have placed *C. difficile* on their watch lists as an extremely concerning HAI.

Another commensal of the human gastrointestinal tract, *C. difficile* is an opportunistic pathogen with virulence factors that make treatment a challenge for healthcare providers. It is resistant to natural gastric acids and heat. It secretes toxins that cause severe, long-lasting diarrheal disease that damages the colon.

C. difficile colitis has been listed as a HAI due to the predisposing etiology factors of frequent and long-term antibiotic therapy for other comorbid conditions. The antibiotics given to chronically at-risk patients kill off resident gastrointestinal microbial colonies, allowing the virulent opportunistic *C. difficile* to proliferate easily and secrete their toxins in large amounts. *C. difficile* is shed in feces and, in its protective spore state, is able to survive for long periods on inanimate environmental surfaces (fomites) which serve as temporary reservoirs of transmission. Patients acquire the bacteria through direct contact with contaminated surfaces or indirectly as the hands of others who have touched contaminated surfaces and then touch the patient. Indirect transmission of the pathogen from infected to uninfected patients has been linked to poor hand hygiene of healthcare workers (HCWs). The fecal-oral route of transmission is also a common method of infection in patients to themselves or from caregivers and others who do not wash hands after using the restroom then come into contact with the patient.

Patients infected with *C. difficile* experience abdominal pain and tenderness, possible fever, nausea, loss of appetite, and three or more watery diarrheal stools daily leaving them susceptible to dehydration and electrolyte imbalance. Those at highest risk are older adults, infants, and immunocompromised patients. Severe cases of damage to the colon may require colon resection of infected and necrotic bowel.

Treatment and Prevention of C. difficile. Despite the fact that previous inappropriate antibiotic therapy is often the predisposing factor in *C. difficile* infection, treatment with appropriate antibiotics effective in killing *C. difficile* bacteria is recommended. Even with treatment, approximately 20% of infections will recur and may become chronically recurring illness as each new treatment regimen allows the microbes to mutate and develop additional resistance capabilities. Antibiotics for any other conditions are discontinued if possible.

Therapeutic treatments of transplantation of fecal material from healthy donors to severely debilitated patients have proven effective in some cases. The normal commensal bacterial species from the healthy donor repopulate the patient's colon, eliminating the overgrowth of *C. difficile* colonies.

Prevention of *C. difficile* infection is of critical importance. Education for patients, families, and healthcare workers is key to breaking the chain of transmission. There must be strict adherence to proper hand hygiene with routine hand washing or use of antimicrobial skin foams or gels prior to and between each interaction with patients.

Additionally, appropriate use of antibiotic treatment must be evaluated by physicians or other healthcare providers and used only when absolutely necessary. They must also assure that the antibiotic prescribed is tailored to and effective against the patient's specific infection following definitive culture and sensitivity (C&S) studies to reduce risk of creating antibiotic resistance. Patients must also be educated in proper use of prescribed medication as to completion of treatment rather than saving extra for later once symptoms resolve, and to not request antibiotics from multiple healthcare providers for viral or other illness for which they are not effective.

Phylum Actinobacteria

The phylum and class *Actinobacteria* are a group of gram-positive bacteria with various shapes, sizes, and characteristics. The different species may be either aerobes or facultative anaerobes and many have filamentous hyphae that resemble fungal organisms. This mistaken early classification is the reason for the designation of one of the group's most important species, *Mycobacterium tuberculosis*, being given a name that would indicate it is a fungus (myco = fungus) rather than a bacterial species. Actinobacteria make up a sizeable portion of common microbes found in the soil and facilitate the decomposition of organic materials which replenishes the organic nutrients in soil critical to plant life and the carbon cycle. Some species are also relatively insignificant commensals in the human aerodigestive tract; however, some may become significant pathogens.

The genus *Actinomyces* is responsible for dental abscesses that can subsequently invade tissues of the respiratory tract, thoracic cavity, peritoneal cavity, or the brain, most commonly occurring in immunocompromised individuals. Another member of Actinobacteria is *Corynebacterium*. *Corynebacterium diphtheriae* is an important species that causes the respiratory disease diphtheria. All other non-diphtherial species of *Corynebacterium* are referred to collectively as the diphtheroids. The bacteria are normal residents of human skin, GI and GU tracts, and upper respiratory tract; however, as with many resident microbes, they are capable of becoming opportunistic pathogens. Diphtheria has been relatively well controlled in the United States for many years with the successful Tdap trivalent vaccination series administered to infants. Resurgence of the disease has been seen in other areas of the world and incidents may increase in the United States due to the "anti-vaxxer" movement of parents who refuse to vaccinate their children.

Genus Mycobacterium. The family *Mycobacteriaceae*, a member of the phylum and class *Actinobacteria*, has a unique cell wall structure that distinguishes it from other types of bacteria on microscopic examination. The cell wall is composed of waxy mycolic fatty acids that result in the colonies being classified as Gram-variable because the staining results are inconsistent. An additional laboratory analysis using an acid-fast stain to verify the bacterial species. *Mycobacteriaceae* bacteria may have a straight or slightly curved morphology with filaments or branches that grow outward. They are non–spore-forming and nonmotile.

The genus *Mycobacterium* is an important opportunistic human pathogen, especially in immunosuppressed patients. Although not indicated in SSIs or HAIs, surgical personnel are typically required to have annual TB screening to eliminate the possibility of transmission to others. Other species of *Mycobacterium* cause diseases such as leprosy and non-TB respiratory infection. Specimens for study in suspected cases are typically taken from skin lesions, lungs, lymph nodes, or eyes.

Tuberculosis Disease. The bacterial species that causes tuberculosis (TB) is *Mycobacterium tuberculosis*, a very slow-growing, obligate aerobic bacteria with a protective waxy cell wall. The bacteria thrive where the oxygen levels are highest and tend to infect the upper lobes of the lungs. In 2018, nearly one in four (23%) or 1.7 billion individuals in the world were infected with TB with 1.5 million annual deaths according to the CDC's Global Health section. TB is highly contagious, spread by aerosolized particles containing the bacteria through coughing, speaking, or sneezing. Hospitalized patients with active TB disease are isolated in negative-pressure, air-filtered rooms to prevent dissemination of the bacteria.

Exposure to TB does not always result in active disease and not all infected individuals display symptoms, making recognition of latent and active TB challenging. Exposure to and inhalation of *M. tuberculosis* may result in latent TB. These individuals show no signs or symptoms of active TB and are not contagious. Transition to active TB disease occurs when the body's immune system is compromised, and the dormant TB activates and proliferates, creating symptoms including fever, chills, and night sweats; weight loss; weakness or fatigue; severe cough lasting more than 3 weeks, and blood in the sputum.

The initial, primary stage of TB spreads bacteria through the lymphatic system with some lesions creating scar tissues in the lower lobes of the lungs. Bacteria that remain secrete exudate that causes a status of chronic reinfection, causing necrosis of lung tissue that subsequently heals or develops into a small rounded nodule called a tubercle that eventually calcifies. The fibrous capsule around the tubercle is called a Ghon complex and can survive in tissue for many years. Lesions consisting of cells around the bacilli that do not produce exudate are considered productive and called granulomas.

TB Skin Testing. The Mantoux TB skin test utilizes protein antigens to detect *Mycobacterium tuberculosis* by inducing a hypersensitivity reaction. A positive reaction fully develops in 48 to 72 hours after intradermal injection of purified protein derivative (PPD) and must be examined during this time frame for accurate interpretation. A positive TB test reaction indicates (1) latent TB infection (2) active TB disease or (3) the individual has been vaccinated in the past with the Bacille Calmette-Guerin (BCG) vaccine, not commonly administered in the United States. Positive results require chest x-ray, clinical examination, and collection of a sputum or tissue specimen. A negative TB test result indicates no infection; however, it could mean the individual is in the very early stages of infection when the skin test would not yet register the presence of infection.

Drug-Resistant TB. The drugs that are most effective against TB are rifampin, ethambutol, isoniazid, and pyrazinamide. *M. tuberculosis* bacteria can become resistant to these drugs. The strains of TB bacteria that have developed drug resistance then transfer the genes for drug resistance to new bacterial colonies, making TB outbreaks difficult to manage. This tendency toward drug resistance has prompted the CDC to place *M. tuberculosis* in the serious threat level of its "2019 Top Drug-Resistant Threats in the United States." The causes of drug resistance commonly include misuse or mismanagement of prescribed treatment regimens.

Multidrug-resistant TB (MDR TB) is caused by mutated strains that have become resistant to isoniazid and rifampin, the standard treatment drugs for all TB infections. Extensively drug-resistant TB (XDR TB) is a rare type of tuberculosis bacteria that is resistant to isoniazid and rifampin as well as fluoroquinolone and at least one of three second-line drugs, leaving few treatment options. Those with HIV/AIDS or other conditions of severe immunocompromise are much more likely to develop TB disease if exposed and a have higher risk of death from drug-resistant TB.

Side effects of the powerful and extremely expensive drug regimens for treatment of MDR-TB and XDR-TB may be life-threatening and include hepatitis, kidney failure, hearing loss, depression, and psychosis. Duration of drug treatments may be years.

Bacteria-Derived Antibiotics. The species *Streptomyces*, part of the phylum and class Actinobacteria has proven to be of great value in synthesizing over 50 antibiotics, antifungals, and antiparasitics used to treat serious infections from other pathogens and include streptomycin, neomycin, chloramphenicol, tetracyclines, and ivermectin. Isolates from *Streptomyces* have also been used to develop anticancer agents.

Fungal Sources of SSI

Fungi are multicellular eukaryotic heterotrophic organisms that release enzymes to break down organic matter and include yeasts, molds, and mushrooms. Scientists believe there may be more than a million species of which only a few are known to be human pathogens. Fungi do not require sunlight, and most are aerobic; however, some species of yeasts perform the anaerobic function of fermentation used to make bread, beer, and wine. A type of mold, *Penicillium notatum*, was the source of the first antibiotic produced, penicillin.

Candida Yeasts. All species of unicellular yeast microbes are considered opportunistic human pathogens in immunocompromised individuals. Cases of osteomyelitis and diskitis have been linked to transmission of *C. albicans* from surgical team members wearing artificial nails. The species most identified to cause infection are *Candida* species with *C. albicans*, *C. glabrata*, *C. parapsilosis*, *C. tropicalis*, and *C. krusei* being the most common.

Fungal Disease. Fungal disease in humans is termed mycosis and classified for the tissues involved in the infection process. Superficial fungal infections are extremely common and include the cuticle nail beds of hands and feet, soles of the feet in "athlete's foot" infections, and vaginal yeast infections. Systemic fungal infections are more difficult to treat as there are a limited number of effective antifungal medications that can cause toxic effects in humans. Most fungal infections are not life-threatening; however, certain individuals with comorbidities are most at-risk for serious complications. Individuals with HIV/AIDS, those under treatment with corticosteroids for autoimmune disease or organ transplantation, and patients undergoing chemotherapy or extended antibiotic regimens are susceptible to opportunistic fungal infection.

Candidiasis is an infection caused by *C. albicans* and can be localized in the mouth or vagina or travel through the bloodstream resulting in invasive systemic candidemia. The oral form of candidiasis is better known as thrush, an uncommon infection in healthy adults; however, it is more commonly seen in infants younger than one month of age; older adults; and chronically immunocompromised patients. The infection presents as white or yellow patches or plaques on the structures of the mouth and oropharynx which can cause pain, difficulty swallowing, or cracking around the lips. Treatment is available in topical or oral antifungals.

Vulvovaginal candidiasis, better known as a yeast infection, occurs when an overgrowth of *C. albicans* yeast proliferates due to a change in the normal acidity of the vagina, typically following antibiotic treatment for unrelated infection, during pregnancy, or in diabetic individuals. Antifungal vaginal creams or suppositories are usually prescribed for the itching, burning, and discharge produced by the infection.

Invasive systemic candidemia can be caused by several species of *Candida*. Specific at-risk groups include post-operative patients; patients in ICU or other critical care units; premature infants weighing less than 1000 g (2.2 lb); patients with indwelling venous access lines; and HIV or AIDS patients. Treatment with intravenous antifungal medications may take several weeks. Researchers have found a concerning increase of antibiotic resistance and incidence in invasive systemic candidemia from the non–*C. albicans* species including *C. glabrata*, *C. parapsilosis*, *C. tropicalis*, and *C. krusei*. Resistance to the standard treatment with the first-line fluconazole and second-line echinocandin antiviral drugs has prompted the CDC to place *Candida* species in the serious threat level category of its "2019 Top Drug-Resistant Treats in the United States."

MICROBIAL DRUG RESISTANCE

The last decade has seen an increase in the number of multidrug-resistant organisms (MDROs), according to the CDC. The threat levels of urgent, serious, and concerning are assigned to microorganisms, excluding viruses or parasites, identified as clinical causes of HAIs. In its *Antibiotic Resistance Threats in the United States, 2019* (2019 AR Threats Report), the CDC reports, "… more than 2.8 million antibiotic-resistant infections occur in the U.S. each year, and more than 35,000 people die as a result. In addition, 223,900 cases of *C. difficile* occurred in 2017 and at least 12,800 people died."

Antibiotic Resistance

Antibiotics are one of the largest classes of prescribed medications. Due to this frequency of use both in and out of the healthcare setting, pathogenic bacterial species, normally well controlled by administration of antibiotic therapy, have developed mechanisms for acquiring resistance to the drugs, resulting in greater difficulty in effective treatment of infections. Microbial resistance develops when pathogenic microorganisms such as bacteria, fungi, viruses, and parasites are altered by exposure to the broad range of antimicrobial drugs including antibiotics, antifungals, antivirals, antimalarials, and anti-helminths. These resistant pathogens are commonly referred to as "superbugs." Drug resistance can be acquired or intrinsic in the morphology of the bacterial species (see Table 4-1).

Acquired Antibiotic Resistance. New, altered, or mutated strains of multidrug or extensively drug-resistant bacteria have created worrisome trends of serious or life-threatening infections and disease states for which traditional antibiotics or other anti-infectives are ineffective. Genetic changes in bacteria occur naturally; however, these changes can be magnified by frequent exposure to drugs that are inappropriately prescribed for the type of infectious agent responsible for the illness or disease.

One of the chief ways for transmission of genetic encoding for resistance in bacteria is through invasion of bacteria by viral bacteriophages, also known as phages. As the viral phages released from resistant bacterial cells bind to receptors on the new bacterial host cells, they invade the host cell and transfer the genetic coding sequence for the new properties of drug resistance. Bacteriophages make many copies of themselves in the newly infected cell by either the lytic or lysogenic cycles of viral replication. This replication process is called genetic transduction, which is divided into generalized and specialized transduction mechanisms. In 2018, researchers discovered a third method of bacteriophage transfer termed lateral transduction. Their findings described an extremely efficient method of genetic transfer in large quantities between infected and non-infected bacteria which they propose explains the rapid evolution in development of multidrug-resistant bacterial strains (see Figure 4-5).

Intrinsic Antibiotic Resistance. Bacteria and other pathogenic microbes may be intrinsically (naturally) resistant to certain types of antibiotics or other anti-infectives based on their cell wall structure or other physical characteristics. The chemical compounds with larger molecular structure of many anti-infective agents are unable to penetrate the tightly packed fatty acid chains that make up the outer membrane of gram-negative bacterial species. Gram-positive bacterial species are more susceptible than the gram-negative strains to the penicillins and cephalosporins that target the larger mesh structure of the peptidoglycan cell wall. Other intrinsic characteristics for bacterial resistance include the waxy coat produced by *Mycobacterium tuberculosis* as well as glycocalyx capsules or slime layers produced by *Streptococcus pneumoniae*, *Haemophilus influenzae* type b, *Klebsiella pneumoniae*, and *Neisseria meningitidis*.

TABLE 4-1 • 2019 CDC TOP DRUG-RESISTANT THREATS IN THE UNITED STATES				
Microorganism	Type of Organism	Threat Level	Annual Infections	Annual Deaths
Carbapenem-resistant *Acinetobacter*	Bacteria	Urgent	8500 (hospitalized in 2017)	700 (2017)
Drug-resistant *Candida auris*	Fungus	Urgent	373 (2018)	
Clostridioides difficile	Bacteria	Urgent	223,900 annually	12,800 annually
Carbapenem-resistant *Enterobacteriaceae* (CRE)	Bacteria	Urgent	13,100 (2017)	1100 (20170)
Drug-resistant *Neisseria gonorrhoeae*	Bacteria	Urgent	550,000 (annually)	
Drug-resistant *Campylobacter*	Bacteria	Serious	448,400 (annually)	70 (annually)
Drug-resistant *Candida* Species	Fungus	Serious	34,800 (2017)	1700 (2017)
Extended-spectrum β-lactamase (EBSL)–producing Enterobacteriaceae	Bacteria	Serious	197,400 (2017)	9,100 (2017)
Vancomycin-resistant *Enterococcus* (VRE)	Bacteria	Serious	54,500 (2017)	5400 (2017)
Multidrug-resistant *Pseudomonas aeruginosa*	Bacteria	Serious	32,600 (2017)	2700 (2017)
Drug-resistant nontyphoidal *Salmonella*	Bacteria	Serious	212,500 (annually)	70 (annually)
Drug-resistant *Salmonella* serotype Typhi	Bacteria	Serious	4100 (annually)	Less than 5 (annually)
Drug-resistant *Shigella*	Bacteria	Serious	7700 (annually)	Less than 5 (annually)
Methicillin-resistant *Staphylococcus aureus* (MRSA)	Bacteria	Serious	323,700 (2017)	10,600 (2017)
Drug-resistant *Streptococcus pneumonia*	Bacteria	Serious	900,000 (2014)	3600 (20140
Drug-resistant Tuberculosis (*Mycobacterium tuberculosis*)	Bacteria	Serious	847 (2017)	62 (2017)
Erythromycin-resistant Group A *Streptococcus*	Bacteria	Concerning	5400 (2017)	450 (2017)
Clindamycin-resistant Group B *Streptococcus*	Bacteria	Concerning	1300 (2016)	700 (2016)

Source: US Centers for Disease Control and Prevention, Washington, DC. https://www.cdc.gov/drugresistance/biggest-threats.html

How Antibiotic Resistance Spreads

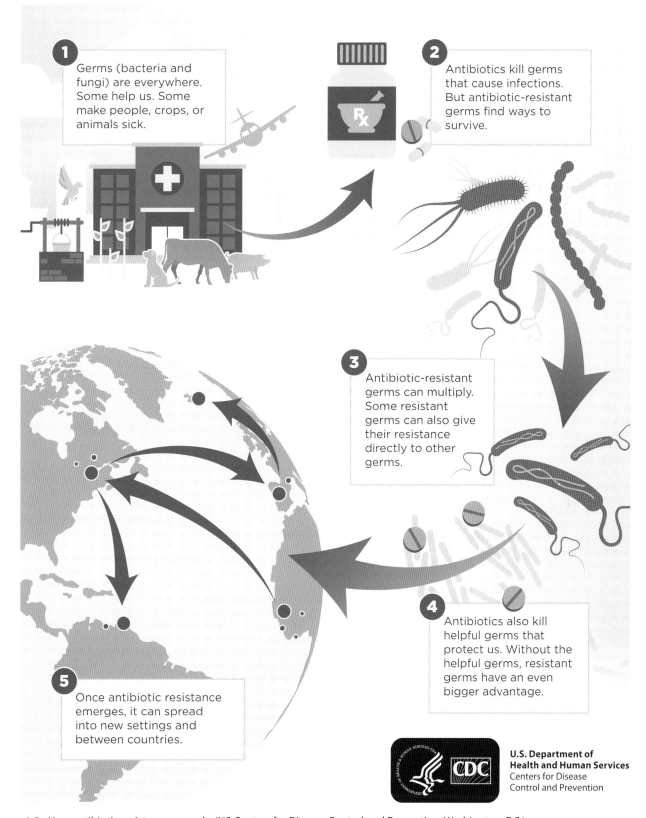

1 Germs (bacteria and fungi) are everywhere. Some help us. Some make people, crops, or animals sick.

2 Antibiotics kill germs that cause infections. But antibiotic-resistant germs find ways to survive.

3 Antibiotic-resistant germs can multiply. Some resistant germs can also give their resistance directly to other germs.

4 Antibiotics also kill helpful germs that protect us. Without the helpful germs, resistant germs have an even bigger advantage.

5 Once antibiotic resistance emerges, it can spread into new settings and between countries.

U.S. Department of Health and Human Services
Centers for Disease Control and Prevention

Figure 4-5 · How antibiotic resistance spreads. (US Centers for Disease Control and Prevention, Washington, DC.)

Patient-Specific Antibiotic Resistance. As previously discussed, misuse and overuse of antimicrobials has been accelerating the progression of antibiotic resistance for many years. Individual patients may gain access to prescription antibiotics or other anti-infectives and inappropriately self-medicate without professional advice or oversight to treat conditions such as viral infections for which antibiotics are not indicated. Community spread of drug-resistant microbes from undertreated infected individual carriers may transmit the new resistance factors to uninfected individuals.

Healthcare providers may contribute to the problem by prescribing antibiotics without waiting for laboratory culture verification of the type of infection present. Re-dosing with additional courses of drug therapy contributes to the development of resistance in the pathogens that may remain dormant or chronically present in the patient's body tissues.

Another factor in patient-specific antibiotic resistance is from ingestion of animal products. Commercial beef, pork, poultry, and dairy producers often administer low-dose antibiotic therapy to animals to enhance their growth and development to maximize production as well as to try to prevent disease outbreaks in overcrowded pens. This dosing given, not for treatment of current infection, contributes to genetic mutations of existing microbes within the animals' tissues. The mutated strains of resistant bacteria may not be killed when undercooked meat is eaten and given entry into the human gastrointestinal tract. Additionally, fertilizer or water supplies contaminated with animal feces seep into the soil and are taken up in crops grown and used for cooked or uncooked food preparation and consumption.

ANTIMICROBIAL AGENTS FOR SURGICAL PROPHYLAXIS

Antimicrobial agents used for prevention of SSI may be topically or parenterally (intravenous, intramuscular injection) administered. Administration of preoperative and intraoperative antibiotics is described as prophylactic use and postoperative antibiotics are for therapeutic use. Initial administration of intravenous preoperative prophylactic antibiotics should occur between 30 and 60 minutes prior to skin incision. Any subsequent doses should be discontinued within 24 hours following surgery. Common antibiotics used for weight-based calculation of prophylactic dose in adult patients include cefazolin, vancomycin, and gentamycin.

Due to increases in antibiotic resistance, the CDC has recommended that acute healthcare facilities create multidisciplinary antibiotic stewardship programs to assess prescribing and administration practices to consider where changes could be made to decrease usage. An area of concern involved use of intraoperative antibiotic wound irrigation. A recommendation was made that intraoperative mixing and preparing of antibiotic irrigation increases the potential for contamination and should be performed in the pharmacy department under strict conditions with a compounding hood. The addition of antibiotics to bone cements for joint prosthesis implantation

was another concern about the possibility for leaching out of antibiotics into tissues or the vascular system over a prolonged period, potentially contributing to microbial resistance (see Figure 4-6).

As described in earlier sections, SSI is an infection that occurs within 30 days after operation or within one year after implantation of a foreign body, graft, or prosthesis. In the United States, the incidence rate of pathogens that cause SSI is 48% gram-negative, 40.8% gram-positive, and 11.2% are fungi-related. Since 2004, antimicrobial drugs have been classified by their biological activity in addition to the previous classifications based on chemical structure, action mode, and antimicrobial spectrum. Based on biological activity, anti-infective drugs are as follows:

- Anti-gram-positive bacteria
- Anti-gram-negative bacteria
- Broad-spectrum antibiotics
- Anti-anaerobic drugs
- Anti-*Mycobacterium tuberculosis*
- Beta-lactamase inhibitors

Mechanical action is another basis for classification of anti-infectives and includes:

- Interference with cell wall synthesis
- Inhibition of protein and nucleic acid synthesis
- Inhibition of metabolic pathways
- Disruption of bacterial membrane structures

Based on their chemical structure, anti-infective drugs are classified and include:

- Aminoglycosides (amikacin, gentamycin, paromomycin, streptomycin, tobramycin): treat gram-negative rods (bacilli), streptococci, and *M. tuberculosis*. Side effects include impaired kidney function and hearing loss due to drug toxicity in higher doses.

- Anti–*M. tuberculosis* (isoniazid, rifampin, ethambutol, pyrazinamide): one or two in combination used for latent TB infection; active TB requires a combination; and MDR-TB requires fluoroquinolone combined with injectable medications (amikacin or capreomycin); side effects of liver toxicity can occur.

- Beta-lactams (penicillins, carbapenems, cephalosporins): inhibit peptidoglycan synthesis for bacterial cell membrane stability; increasing bacterial resistance has caused concern.

- Clindamycin (Cleocin HCl): not for use as a bolus dose, should be infused over 10 to 60 minutes; use caution in patients with history of colitis.

- Macrolides (erythromycin, azithromycin, clarithromycin): inhibit bacterial protein synthesis of aerobic and anaerobic gram-positive bacteria except enterococci.

- Metronidazole and Tinidazole: both inhibit DNA synthesis; oral administration in most cases, effective against obligate anaerobic bacteria (metronidazole), drug of

Antibiotic-Resistant Infections Threaten Modern Medicine

Millions of people in the United States receive care that can be complicated by bacterial and fungal infections. Without antibiotics, we are not able to safely offer some life-saving medical advances.

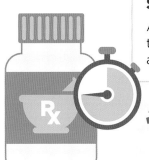

Sepsis Treatment

Anyone can get an infection and almost any infection can lead to sepsis — the body's extreme response to an infection. Without timely treatment with antibiotics, sepsis can rapidly lead to tissue damage, organ failure, and death.

AT LEAST
1.7M adults develop sepsis each year.

Surgery

Patients who have surgery are at risk for surgical site infections. Without effective antibiotics to prevent and treat surgical infections, many surgeries would not be possible today.

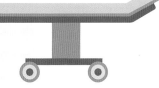

1.2M women had a cesarean section (C-section) in 2017. Antibiotics are recommended to help prevent infection.

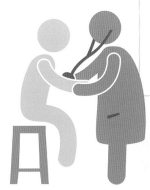

Chronic Conditions

Chronic conditions (e.g., diabetes) put people at higher risk for infection. These conditions and some medicines used to treat them can weaken the immune system (how the body fights infection).

MORE THAN
30M people have diabetes. Antibiotics are used to treat common infections in these patients.

Figure 4-6 · Antibiotic-resistant infections. (US Centers for Disease Control and Prevention, Washington, DC. https://www.cdc.gov/drugresistance/pdf/threats-report/Threat-Modern-Medicine-508.pdf)

Antibiotic-Resistant Infections Threaten Modern Medicine

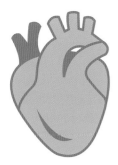

Organ Transplants

Organ transplant recipients are more vulnerable to infections because they undergo complex surgery. Recipients also receive medicine to suppress (weaken) the immune system, increasing risk of infection.

MORE THAN
33,000 organ transplants were performed in 2016. Antibiotics help organ transplants remain possible.

Dialysis for Advanced Kidney Disease

Patients who receive dialysis treatment have a higher risk of infection, the second leading cause of death in dialysis patients.

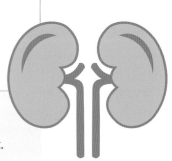

MORE THAN
500,000 patients received dialysis treatment in 2016. Antibiotics are critical to treat infections in patients receiving life-saving dialysis treatment.

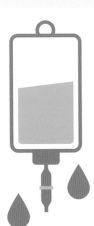

Cancer Care

People receiving chemotherapy for cancer are often at risk for developing an infection during treatment. Infection can quickly become serious for these patients.

AROUND
650,000 people receive outpatient chemotherapy each year. Antibiotics are necessary to protect these patients.

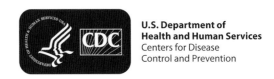

U.S. Department of Health and Human Services
Centers for Disease Control and Prevention

Figure 4-6 • *(Continued)*

choice for bacterial vaginosis; and some protozoan parasites (tinidazole).

- Polypeptides—Polymyxin and Bacitracin (polymyxin B, Neomycin, Neosporin GU irrigant, Colistin, Coly-Mycin® S Otic, Cortisporin ophthalmic suspension): antibiotics mixed with saline for topical wound or bladder irrigation, although some studies demonstrate questionable antimicrobial efficacy and possible cytotoxicity; ointment form for topical skin application; and combined with steroids (hydrocortisone) for otic or ophthalmic drops.

- Quinolones and Fluoroquinolones (ciprofloxacin/Cipro, levofloxacin, norfloxacin): broad spectrum, used only if less toxic antibiotics have failed, may be used for anthrax and plague infections.

- Sulfonamides (sulfadiazine, sulfacetamide, sulfasalazine, mafenide): broad spectrum for gram-positive and many gram-negative bacteria; used topically for burns, vaginosis, or superficial ocular infections, or orally commonly combined with other drugs. Not effective against group A streptococcal infections; antimicrobial resistance is increasing and resistance to one type indicates likely resistance to most all types.

- Tetracyclines (doxycycline, tetracycline, minocycline): inhibits bacterial protein synthesis; effective against many gram-negative rods (GNRs) and a few gram-positive group A streptococcal bacteria.

- Vancomycin: inhibits cell wall synthesis; not well absorbed by the GI tract in oral administration route; however, it is preferred in some cases of *C. difficile* colitis; effective against most gram-positive cocci and bacilli, some enterococci, and some antibiotic-resistant strains including MRSA; resistance to vancomycin by some strains of enterococci has been increasing.

SSI PREVENTION STRATEGIES

Infection control in the perioperative setting is a balance of risk recognition, prevention measures and techniques, and effective response protocols when prevention fails. Previous sections have explored the various aspects of infection risks including a review of common microbes; their potential to become pathogenic and the types of disease or infection they cause; and the mechanisms of bacterial proliferation. Descriptions of patient risk factors; types and descriptions of SSIs; indications for and types of antibiotic or anti-infective medications; and the concerning increases in antibiotic drug resistance have also been discussed (see Figure 4-7).

In 1736, Benjamin Franklin stated, "An ounce of prevention is worth a pound of cure." He was referring to the need for firefighting and prevention strategies in the city of Philadelphia. His wise cautionary comment can be applied to any number of areas in life where disaster preparedness is a critical concept and standard of professional care. Involving all members of the surgical team in effective infection control and empowering the patient and family or other caregivers to take an active role may reduce the risks for surgical site or other HAIs.

Patient Education

Patients and their family members or other caregivers should be given clear instructions for perioperative measures that they can perform to minimize the potential for SSI or HAI.

Patients should be asked to do the following unless directed otherwise by the physician:

- Quit smoking at least two weeks prior to surgery to optimize wound healing.

- Include healthy food choices including adequate protein and water intake.

- Shower or bathe with a surgical soap such as chlorhexidine gluconate the night before and morning of surgery to create a cumulative antimicrobial effect.

- Do not shave the surgical area on the day of surgery because microabrasions can increase the microbial count in the skin layers.

- Practice strict handwashing and require the same from anyone who comes in contact with the patient in or out of the healthcare facility.

- Do not remove surgical dressings unless directed by the physician and do not touch the incisional site or care for a drain without washing hands beforehand.

- Take only prescribed antibiotics and for the period of time and complete course prescribed by the surgeon or treating physician.

- Maintain good glycemic blood levels if diabetic.

- Ambulate if able and use inspirometer-type device to prevent postoperative pneumonia in asthmatic patients or others with diminished lung capacity.

Departmental Environmental Controls

The special environment of the perioperative department or surgical suite is developed by a multidisciplinary group of architects, interior designers, engineers, medical and nursing staff, and hospital administrators. The goals of efficient flow of personnel traffic and zoning measures to prevent the potential for cross-contamination between clean or sterile items with contaminated items or areas must be met for safety of everyone entering the department.

Operating Room Zoning. Specific areas within the surgical suite or operating room department are designated as either unrestricted, semi-restricted, or restricted. In the unrestricted areas, street clothes may be worn and there is no requirement for scrub attire or PPE to be worn. Waiting rooms, administrative offices, staff or physician lounges, locker rooms, outside corridors, and the front desk area are examples of typically unrestricted zones. The preoperative care unit (PCU) and post-anesthesia care unit (PACU) may be considered as part of the surgical department and may also be unrestricted zones.

Surgical Antibiotic Prophylaxis - Adult

Disclaimer: This algorithm has been developed for MD Anderson using a multidisciplinary approach considering circumstances particular to MD Anderson's specific patient population, services and structure, and clinical information. This is not intended to replace the independent medical or professional judgment of physicians or other health care providers in the context of individual clinical circumstances to determine a patient's care. This algorithm should not be used to treat pregnant women. Local microbiology and susceptibility/resistance patterns should be taken into consideration when selecting antibiotics.

Patients scheduled for surgery should have the following antibiotics administered prior to their procedure:

- Vancomycin, ciprofloxacin/levofloxacin, and gentamicin are to be initiated 60-120 minutes prior to incision, and all other antibiotics are to be initiated within 60 minutes of incision
- Carefully evaluate allergy histories before using alternative agents - the majority of patients with listed penicillin allergies can safely be given cephalosporins or carbapenems
- If the patient has multiple known antibiotic drug allergies, is colonized with or has a history of a recent multi-drug infection, administer antibiotics as indicated or consider an outpatient Infectious Diseases referral
- Discontinue all antibiotics within 24 hours of first dose except for: 1) Treatment of established infection, 2) Prophylaxis of prosthesis in the setting of postoperative co-located percutaneous drains, 3) Intraoperative findings that raise the wound classification above 2 (*e.g.*, spillage of enteric contents, purulent fluid, etc.). All of these require appropriate documentation.
- See Appendix A for intraoperative re-dosing recommendations

MRSA screening should be performed on patients hospitalized within 30 days of procedure, transferred from skilled nursing facilities, with percutaneous lines/catheters, or with HIV. Any surgical patient with a history of MRSA infection or positive MRSA screening should receive vancomycin 1 gram IV as part of surgical prophylaxis. If vancomycin is being ordered based on standard disease site recommendations, a second dose is not necessary. Vancomycin prophylaxis should be considered for patients with known MRSA colonization or at high risk for MRSA colonization in the absence of surveillance data (*e.g.*, patients with recent hospitalization, nursing-home residents, hemodialysis patients). *American Society of Health-System Pharmacists (ASHP) guidelines.*

Disease Site	No Penicillin Allergy	Patients with Penicillin Allergy
Breast / Melanoma / Plastics	• Less than 120 kg: cefazolin 2 grams IV • Greater than or equal to 120 kg: cefazolin 3 grams IV	• Less than or equal to 70 kg: vancomycin 1 gram IV • Between 70 kg and 100 kg: vancomycin 1.5 grams IV • Greater than or equal to 100 kg: vancomycin 2 grams IV
Head / Neck (ENT - Clean)	• Less than 120 kg: cefazolin 2 grams IV • Greater than or equal to 120 kg: cefazolin 3 grams IV	• Less than or equal to 70 kg: vancomycin 1 gram IV • Between 70 kg and 100 kg: vancomycin 1.5 grams IV • Greater than or equal to 100 kg: vancomycin 2 grams IV
Head / Neck (ENT - Clean Contaminated)	Ampicillin and sulbactam 3 grams IV	• Levofloxacin 500 mg IV **and** • Less than 70 kg: clindamycin 600 mg IV • Greater than or equal to 70 kg: clindamycin 900 mg IV
Neurosurgery	Skull base ONLY: • Ampicillin and sulbactam 3 grams IV	• Levofloxacin 500 mg IV **and** • Less than 70 kg: clindamycin 600 mg IV • Greater than or equal to 70 kg: clindamycin 900 mg IV
	All other types: • Less than 120 kg: cefazolin 2 grams IV • Greater than or equal to 120 kg: cefazolin 3 grams IV	• Less than or equal to 70 kg: vancomycin 1 gram IV • Between 70 kg and 100 kg: vancomycin 1.5 grams IV • Greater than or equal to 100 kg: vancomycin 2 grams IV **or** • Levofloxacin 500 mg IV **and** • Less than 70 kg: clindamycin 600 mg IV • Greater than or equal to 70 kg: clindamycin 900 mg IV

Department of Clinical Effectiveness V10
Approved by The Executive Committee of the Medical Staff 09/20/2022

Surgical Antibiotic Prophylaxis - Adult

Disclaimer: This algorithm has been developed for MD Anderson using a multidisciplinary approach considering circumstances particular to MD Anderson's specific patient population, services and structure, and clinical information. This is not intended to replace the independent medical or professional judgment of physicians or other health care providers in the context of individual clinical circumstances to determine a patient's care. This algorithm should not be used to treat pregnant women. Local microbiology and susceptibility/resistance patterns should be taken into consideration when selecting antibiotics.

Disease Site	No Penicillin Allergy	Patients with Penicillin Allergy
Vascular	• Less than 120 kg: cefazolin 2 grams IV • Greater than or equal to 120 kg: cefazolin 3 grams IV	• Less than or equal to 70 kg: vancomycin 1 gram IV • Between 70 kg and 100 kg: vancomycin 1.5 grams IV • Greater than or equal to 100 kg: vancomycin 2 grams IV
GI (Clean)	• Less than 120 kg: cefazolin 2 grams IV • Greater than or equal to 120 kg: cefazolin 3 grams IV	• Less than or equal to 70 kg: vancomycin 1 gram IV • Between 70 kg and 100 kg: vancomycin 1.5 grams IV • Greater than or equal to 100 kg: vancomycin 2 grams IV
GI	Gastric, Pancreas, Liver or Colorectal[1]: • Ertapenem 1 gram IV	Gastric, Pancreas, Liver, or Colorectal[1]: • Ciprofloxacin 400 mg IV **and** metronidazole 500 mg IV
Gynecologic	GI procedures unlikely[2]: • Less than 120 kg: cefazolin 2 grams IV • Greater than or equal to 120 kg: cefazolin 3 grams IV GI procedures likely: • Ertapenem 1 gram IV **and** preoperative bowel preparation[1]	GI procedure unlikely: • Ciprofloxacin 400 mg IV **and** metronidazole 500 mg IV GI procedure likely: • Ciprofloxacin 400 mg IV **and** metronidazole 500 mg IV **and** pre-operative bowel preparation[1]
Thoracic / Pulmonary / Esophageal	Ampicillin and sulbactam 3 grams IV	• Less than or equal to 70 kg: vancomycin 1 gram IV • Between 70 kg and 100 kg: vancomycin 1.5 grams IV • Greater than or equal to 100 kg: vancomycin 2 grams IV **and** • Ciprofloxacin 400 mg IV
Orthopedics	Pelvic surgery ONLY: • Ceftriaxone 2 grams IV	• Less than or equal to 70 kg: vancomycin 1 gram IV • Between 70 kg and 100 kg: vancomycin 1.5 grams IV • Greater than or equal to 100 kg: vancomycin 2 grams IV **or** • Less than 70 kg: clindamycin 600 mg IV • Greater than or equal to 70 kg: clindamycin 900 mg IV
	All other types: • Less than 120 kg: cefazolin 2 grams IV • Greater than or equal to 120 kg: cefazolin 3 grams IV	
Endocrine Surgery	• Less than 120 kg: cefazolin 2 grams IV • Greater than or equal to 120 kg: cefazolin 3 grams IV	• Less than or equal to 70 kg: vancomycin 1 gram IV • Between 70 kg and 100 kg: vancomycin 1.5 grams IV • Greater than or equal to 100 kg: vancomycin 2 grams IV

[1] Patients undergoing colorectal resection should be considered for preoperative mechanical and oral antibiotic bowel preparation
[2] Patients with unanticipated GI procedures should receive ertapenem 1 gram IV intraoperatively as soon as need is identified

Continued on next page

Department of Clinical Effectiveness V10
Approved by The Executive Committee of the Medical Staff 09/20/2022

Figure 4-7 • Surgical antibiotic prophylaxis—adult. (Reproduced with permission from the University of Texas MD Anderson Cancer Center. https://www.mdanderson.org/content/dam/mdanderson/documents/for-physicians/algorithms/clinical-management/clin-management-surgical-antibiotic-prophylaxis-adult-web-algorithm.pdf)

Surgical Antibiotic Prophylaxis - Adult

THE UNIVERSITY OF TEXAS
MD Anderson
~~Cancer~~ Center
Making Cancer History®

Disclaimer: *This algorithm has been developed for MD Anderson using a multidisciplinary approach considering circumstances particular to MD Anderson's specific patient population, services and structure, and clinical information. This is not intended to replace the independent medical or professional judgment of physicians or other health care providers in the context of individual clinical circumstances to determine a patient's care. This algorithm should not be used to treat pregnant women. Local microbiology and susceptibility/resistance patterns should be taken into consideration when selecting antibiotics.*

Disease Site	No Penicillin Allergy	Patients with Penicillin Allergy
Pain Surgery	• <u>Less than 120 kg</u>: cefazolin 2 grams IV • <u>Greater than or equal to 120 kg</u>: cefazolin 3 grams IV	• <u>Less than or equal to 70 kg</u>: vancomycin 1 gram IV • <u>Between 70 kg and 100 kg</u>: vancomycin 1.5 grams IV • <u>Greater than or equal to 100 kg</u>: vancomycin 2 grams IV
Genitourinary[1] (Lower Urinary Tract)	Cystourethroscopy with minor manipulation (high risk patients[2]): • Ciprofloxacin 500 mg PO **or** sulfamethoxazole and trimethoprim 800 mg/160 mg PO	Cystourethroscopy with minor manipulation (high risk patients[2]): • Ciprofloxacin 500 mg PO **or** sulfamethoxazole and trimethoprim 800 mg/160 mg PO
	Cystourethroscopy with mucosal break (*i.e.,* TURP, TURBT, laser enucleation/ablation): • Ciprofloxacin 500 mg PO **or** sulfamethoxazole and trimethoprim 800 mg/160 mg PO	Cystourethroscopy with mucosal break (*i.e.,* TURP, TURBT, laser enucleation/ablation): • Ciprofloxacin 500 mg PO **or** sulfamethoxazole and trimethoprim 800 mg/160 mg PO
	Prostate brachytherapy/cryotherapy: • <u>Less than 120 kg</u>: cefazolin 2 grams IV • <u>Greater than or equal to 120 kg</u>: cefazolin 3 grams IV	Prostate brachytherapy/cryotherapy: • <u>Less than or equal to 70 kg</u>: vancomycin 1 gram IV • <u>Between 70 kg and 100 kg</u>: vancomycin 1.5 grams IV • <u>Greater than or equal to 100 kg</u>: vancomycin 2 grams IV
	Transrectal/Transperineal prostate biopsy: • Levofloxacin 500 mg IV or PO **or** gentamicin 1.5 mg/kg IM or IV **or** meropenem 1 gram IV[3]	Transrectal/Transperineal prostate biopsy: • Levofloxacin 500 mg IV or PO **or** gentamicin 1.5 mg/kg IM or IV **or** meropenem 1 gram IV[3]
Genitourinary[1] (Upper Urinary Tract)	Percutaneous Renal Surgery (PCNL): • <u>Less than 120 kg</u>: cefazolin 2 grams IV • <u>Greater than or equal to 120 kg</u>: cefazolin 3 grams IV	Percutaneous Renal Surgery (PCNL): • <u>Less than or equal to 70 kg</u>: vancomycin 1 gram IV • <u>Between 70 kg and 100 kg</u>: vancomycin 1.5 grams IV • <u>Greater than or equal to 100 kg</u>: vancomycin 2 grams IV
	Ureteroscopy (with and without biopsy, laser lithotripsy, etc.): • Ciprofloxacin 500 mg PO **or** sulfamethoxazole and trimethoprim 800 mg/160 mg PO	Ureteroscopy (with and without biopsy, laser lithotripsy, etc.): • Ciprofloxacin 500 mg PO **or** sulfamethoxazole and trimethoprim 800 mg/160 mg PO

TURP = transurethral resection of the prostate   TURBT = transurethral resection of a bladder tumor   PCNL = percutaneous nephrolithonomy

[1] Urology antibiotic prophylaxis recommendations are based on a negative pre-procedure urine culture; prophylaxis should be modified to account for organisms identified from the urine culture
[2] Risk factors to consider are history of recurrent or recent urinary tract infection, immunosuppression, uncontrolled diabetes
[3] Applicable only for cases performed in the outpatient operating room (ACB)

Continued on next page

Department of Clinical Effectiveness V10
Approved by The Executive Committee of the Medical Staff 09/20/2022

Figure 4-7 ▪ (*Continued*)

Semi-restricted zones or areas are those designated by visual markings of red lines on the floor, signs stating restricted access on doors or at entry points. In the semi-restricted zones, proper surgical attire including head covers or hats and clean scrubs must be worn. Shoe covers are not mandated but recommended especially for those scrubbing in and up at the operative field. Masks are not required in the semi-restricted areas unless it is the policy of the individual facility. Internal corridors, sterile supply and equipment rooms, and internal holding areas or medication rooms are examples of semi-restricted areas.

Restricted zones are those areas where there are sterile supplies open, a surgical or other invasive procedure is in progress, or the scrub sink area or substerile room. Masks are required in addition to other proper OR attire in these areas.

Environmental Controls. The ventilation system in each individual operating room must be controlled to create a positive pressure in relation to the peripheral corridors so that when doors are opened, cleaner air under pressure flows out into the adjacent corridors. The filtered air enters the operating room from the ceiling in a unidirectional flow and is vented out near the floor. This top to bottom airflow reduces the potential for turbulence picking up dust or other inanimate carriers of microbes called fomites from becoming airborne and settling onto open, exposed sterile items. The rate of air exchanges in each room should be a minimum of 15 per hour (most will be set at 15-25) with a recommended 3 being with outside air. Room temperature should range between 68°F and 73°F and

the humidity should be between 30% and 60% to reduce microbial growth and contribute to static electricity buildup.

Walls, floors, doors, and ceilings must be nonporous and able to withstand constant cleaning with disinfectant agents. Tile floors or walls are not recommended because porous grout lines can harbor microbes. Sliding doors create less turbulence when opened; however, this requires adequate wall space allocations to allow for thorough cleaning of both sides. Pocket doors cannot be adequately cleaned and are not recommended. Track lighting systems are also not recommended due to the difficulty in adequate cleaning of the tracks and potential dissemination of dust over the surgical field. Storage cabinets should have doors to prevent potential splash contamination of items from the operative field or cleaning measures.

Standard and Transmission-Based Precautions

Standard precautions were created by the CDC and combined the former "body substance isolation" (BSI) measures with "universal precautions" used in non-medical settings to create a clear plan for prevention of disease transmission in healthcare settings. The categories of potentially infectious materials in standard precautions include:

- Blood
- All body fluids, secretions, and excretions (except sweat) regardless of whether or not there is visible blood present
- Mucous membranes
- Nonintact skin

Proper personal protective equipment (PPE) must be used by surgical personnel. The Occupational Safety and Health Administration (OSHA) mandates that healthcare facilities provide personnel with adequate PPE appropriate to the potential for exposure to possible infection during performance of their professional duties.

Transmission-based precautions are an additional measure of precaution measures taken when there is a known patient diagnosis of an infection that can be transmitted by contact, direct or indirect (eg, MRSA, VRE, and *C. difficile*); droplet propulsion (eg, influenza, diphtheria, and the mumps); or airborne dissemination (eg, tuberculosis, measles, and chicken pox).

Surgical Team Measures

The most critical and easiest way to prevent infection by breaking the chain of transmission in the perioperative environment of care is through proper hand hygiene in the form of handwashing with soap and water or use of surgical alcohol-based skin preparations. Surgical personnel should be required to don (put on) clean, facility-laundered scrub attire when entering the semi-restricted and restricted areas of the department.

In addition to the surgical scrubs, surgical personnel must use PPE as dual barriers that protect the patient from exposure to staff and to protect team members from exposure to the patient's blood, body fluids, or other potentially infectious materials (OPIMs). Components of PPE include disposable bouffant-style caps or wrap-around hoods that must cover and contain all head and sideburn hair to prevent shedding. Skull-cap-type hats may be worn if hair is short and does not extend beyond the borders of the hat. Disposable surgical masks must fit snugly and not gap at the sides of the face and fully cover the nose and mouth of the wearer. Special N-95 respirator masks must be fit-tested for the individual prior to use and should be worn when airborne precautions are required.

Prior to entering the sterile field, surgical team members must perform surgical skin antisepsis by either the traditional scrub brush and water technique or the brushless, waterless hand rub procedure to achieve surgical cleanliness of their hands and arms. Living skin cannot be sterilized as there are always resident microbes in the deeper skin layers that can be reduced in numbers, but not entirely eliminated. Sterile gowns and gloves are donned by team members allowing them to enter the sterile field and work within it. Once scrubbed, it becomes the responsibility of all sterilely attired team members to protect and maintain the integrity of the sterile field and take corrective action should contamination occur (see Table 4-2).

Surgical team members must utilize proper and careful tissue handling techniques to prevent tissue damage that might delay wound healing and contribute to potential SSI. Placement of retractors without excessive force prevents ischemia of wound edges. Properly functioning surgical instruments prevent shredding or tearing of tissues from dull edges. Careful suturing technique approximates wound layers and edges, eliminates dead space where microbial growth can proliferate, and keeps from strangulation of incised tissues resulting in ischemia and necrosis.

Instrument Sterilization Methods

The highest level of assurance against disease transmission is sterility. All surgical instrumentation and other supplies that enter into the bloodstream such as hypodermic needles and vascular access catheters must be sterilized in order to prevent transmission of pathogenic microbes directly into the body bypassing its innate protection of intact protective skin and the normal inflammatory response. Surgical instruments and devices can be classified as heat-stable or heat-sensitive and moisture-stable or moisture-sensitive. High-grade stainless-steel surgical instruments are both heat and moisture stable and are sterilized by the most commonly used method of sterilization: steam under pressure. Steam sterilization is inexpensive, reliable, quick, and leaves no toxic residues and has been the method of choice for many years. Not all items, however, can be steam sterilized. Delicate rigid laparoscopes may be damaged by the high heat of 250°F to 270°F for most steam sterilization cycles.

Heat-sensitive and moisture-sensitive items were formerly routinely sterilized by ethylene oxide (EO) gas; however, ethylene oxide is an explosive, flammable, carcinogenic, and toxic chemical agent that presents a real threat to sterile processing

TABLE 4-2 • WHO TECHNIQUE FOR APPLICATION OF ALCOHOL-BASED HAND RUB PRIOR TO SURGERY
• Surgical hand antisepsis should be performed using either a suitable antimicrobial soap or suitable ABHR, preferably with a product ensuring sustained activity, before donning sterile gloves.
• If the quality of water is not assured in the OR, surgical hand antisepsis using an ABHR is recommended before donning sterile gloves when performing surgical procedures.
• When performing surgical hand antisepsis using an antimicrobial soap, scrub hands and forearms for the length of time recommended by the manufacturer, typically 2-5 minutes. Long scrub times (eg, 10 minutes) are not necessary.
• When using an alcohol-based surgical handrub product with sustained activity, follow the manufacturer's instructions for application times. Apply the product to dry hands only. Do not combine surgical handscrub and surgical handrub with alcohol-based products sequentially.
• When using an ABHR, use a sufficient amount of the product to keep hands and forearms wet with the handrub throughout the surgical hand preparation procedure.
• After application of the ABHR as recommended, allow hands and forearms to dry thoroughly before donning sterile gloves.

personnel exposed to the fumes. Manufacturers of medical goods use EO for sterilization; however, very few hospital sterile processing departments have EO sterilizers any longer due to the hazards they pose.

A widely used alternative to EO is the hydrogen peroxide gas plasma(eg, Sterrad) method of sterilization which uses the fourth state of matter (plasma) combined with radiofrequency energy at low-temperature settings to sterilize items which cannot withstand the heat of steam.

Liquid chemical sterilant solutions can be used for heat-sensitive, moisture-stable items that can withstand immersion. The peracetic acid (eg, Steris) method of sterilization may be used for some endoscopic instruments with narrow channels and lumens. Complex-powered instrument motors should never be immersed in liquid and are incompatible with liquid chemical sterilization methods.

Monitoring of the different sterilization methods is a critical step in infection prevention and includes the use of chemical indicators/integrators that change color when exposed to the sterilizing agent; mechanical printouts from the sterilizers that verify process parameters were met; and biological test doses of bacterial spores that are highly resistant to the type of sterilizer being used. Assurance that the instruments are actually sterile is achieved only after adequate exposure to the sterilization process and proper incubation of the test dose to verify no evidence of bacterial colony growth. The last of the process monitoring methods is the administrative record-keeping of all pertinent activities and test results that demonstrate proper sterilizer functioning, maintenance logs, and departmental personnel performance.

SUMMARY

Despite planning and protocols, SSIs remain a reality and must be continuously analyzed for the root causes and lessons to be gained for prevention in the future. Surgical assistants play an important role in the fight against infection through a comprehensive knowledge of the mechanisms of transmission; the various characteristics of pathogens associated with SSI; the scope of preventative measures available, and the potential impact of HAIs and SSIs on the patients under our care.

Bibliography

AHRQ Safety Program for Improving Antibiotic Use, Best Practices in the Diagnosis and Treatment of Cellulitis and Skin and Soft Tissue Infections—Acute Care. https://www.ahrq.gov/sites/default/files/wysiwyg/antibiotic-use/best-practices/cellulitis-facilitator-guide.pdf. Accessed August 30, 2020.

American Society of Anesthesiologists Guidelines, Statements, Clinical Resources ASA Physical Status Classification System. https://www.asahq.org/standards-and-guidelines/asa-physical-status-classification-system. Updated October 23, 2019. Accessed August 29, 2020.

Berríos-Torres SI, Umscheid CA, Bratzler DW, et al. Centers for Disease Control and Prevention guideline for the prevention of surgical site infection, 2017. *JAMA Surg.* 2017;152(8):784-791. doi:10.1001/jamasurg.2017.0904. https://jamanetwork.com/journals/jamasurgery/fullarticle/2623725 Accessed 7-26-2020.

Centers for Disease Control and Prevention. Antibiotic-Resistant Infections Threaten Modern Medicine. https://www.cdc.gov/drugresistance/pdf/threats-report/Threat-Modern-Medicine-508.pdf. Accessed August 2, 2020.

Centers for Disease Control and Prevention. Biggest Threats and Data 2019 AR Threats Report. https://www.cdc.gov/drugresistance/biggest-threats.html. Accessed August 2, 2020.

Centers for Disease Control and Prevention. HIV Basic Statistics. https://www.cdc.gov/hiv/basics/statistics.html. Accessed July 26, 2020.

Centers for Disease Control and Prevention. Global Health, Tuberculosis. https://www.cdc.gov/globalhealth/newsroom/topics/tb/index.html#:~:text=In%202018%2C%201.7%20billion%20people,1.5%20million%20lives%20each%20year. Accessed August 23, 2020.

Centers for Disease Control and Prevention. MRSA Fact Sheet. https://www.cdc.gov/mrsa/community/posters/index.html. Accessed August 14, 2020.

Centers for Disease Control and Prevention. Prion Diseases. https://www.cdc.gov/prions/index.html. Accessed August 2, 2020.

Cheng H, Chen BP, Soleas IM, Ferko NC, Cameron CG, Hinoul, P. Prolonged operative duration increases risk of surgical site infections: A systematic review. *Surgical infect.* 2017;18(6):722-735. https://doi.org/10.1089/sur.2017.089. Accessed August 29, 2020.

Cleveland Clinic Health Essentials. Is a Hidden Pacemaker Infection Making You Sick? Complications Related to Device Leads May Go Unnoticed. May 4, 2017, https://health.clevelandclinic.org/hidden-pacemaker-infection-making-sick/. Accessed August 30, 2020.

Crader MF, Varacallo M. *Preoperative Antibiotic Prophylaxis.* [Updated 2020 March 30]. In: StatPearls [Internet]. Treasure Island, FL: StatPearls Publishing; 2020. https://www.ncbi.nlm.nih.gov/books/NBK442032/. Accessed August 30, 2020.

Fookes C. Quinolones. Drugs.com. https://www.drugs.com/drug-class/quinolones.html. Accessed August 23, 2020.

Fernandez-Gerlinger M-P, Arvieu R, Lebeaux D, et al. Successful 6-week antibiotic treatment for early surgical-site infections in spinal surgery. *Clin Infect Dis.* 2019;68(11):1856-1861. https://doi.org/10.1093/cid/ciy805. Accessed August 22, 2020.

Forastiero A, Garcia-Gil V, Rivero-Menendez O, et al. Rapid Development of *Candida krusei* Echinocandin Resistance during Caspofungin Therapy. *Antimicrob Agents Chemothera.* 2015;59(11):6975-6982. doi: 10.1128/AAC.01005-15. Accessed August 22, 2020.

Goswami K, Cho J, Foltz C, et al. Polymyxin and bacitracin in the irrigation solution provide no benefit for bacterial killing in vitro. *J Bone Joint Surg Am.* 2019;101(18): 1689-1697. doi: 10.2106/JBJS.18.01362. Accessed August 23, 2020.

The Lancet Infectious Diseases. *C. difficile*—a rose by any other name…. *Lancet Infect Dis.* 2019;19(5):449-558, e148-e186. doi: https://doi.org/10.1016/S1473-3099(19)30177-X. Accessed August 29, 2020.

Mallia AJ, Ashwood N, Arealis G, Galanopoulos I. Retroperitoneal abscess: An extra-abdominal manifestation. *BMJ case reports, 2015.* https://doi.org/10.1136/bcr-2014-207437. Accessed August 30, 2020.

Mayo Clinic. Patient Care and Health Information, Tuberculosis. https://www.mayoclinic.org/diseases-conditions/tuberculosis/diagnosis-treatment/drc-20351256. Accessed August 23, 2020.

MD Anderson Surgical Antibiotic Prophylaxis—Adult. https://www.mdanderson.org/content/dam/mdanderson/documents/for-physicians/algorithms/clinical-management/clin-management-surgical-antibiotic-prophylaxis-adult-web-algorithm.pdf. Accessed August 23, 2020.

Medscape. Drugs and Diseases—clindamycin. https://reference.medscape.com/drug/cleocin-clindesse-clindamycin-342558#5. Accessed August 23, 2020.

Merck Manual Professional. Bacteria and Antibacterial Drugs, Macrolides. https://www.merckmanuals.com/professional/infectious-diseases/bacteria-and-antibacterialdrugs/macrolides?network=g&matchtype=b&keyword=&creative=436945397179&device=c&devicemodel=&placement=&position=&campaignid=10050999304&adgroupid=100873967413&loc_physical_ms=9028693&loc_interest_ms=&gclid=EAIaIQobChMIn7f-w18Sy6wIVlxatBh2xRwbbEAMYASAAEgKP4_D_BwE. Accessed August 23, 2020.

Merck Manual Professional. Bacteria and Antibacterial Drugs, Metronidazole and Tinidazole. https://www.merckmanuals.com/professional/infectious-diseases/bacteria-and-antibacterial-drugs/metronidazole-and-tinidazole. Accessed August 29, 2020.

Merck Manual Professional, Bacteria and Antibacterial Drugs, Sulfonamides. https://www.merckmanuals.com/professional/infectious-diseases/bacteria-and-antibacterial-drugs/sulfonamides. Accessed August 23, 2020.

Merck Manual Professional, Bacteria and Antibacterial Drugs, Tetracyclines. https://www.merckmanuals.com/professional/infectious-diseases/bacteria-and-antibacterial-drugs/tetracyclines. Accessed August 23, 2020.

Merck Manual Professional, Bacteria and Antibacterial Drugs, Vancomycin. https://www.merckmanuals.com/professional/infectious-diseases/bacteria-and-antibacterial-drugs/vancomycin. Accessed August 23, 2020.

Mu Y, Edwards JR, Horan TC, Berríos-Torres SI, Fridkin SK. Improving risk-adjusted measures of surgical site infection for the National Healthcare Safety Network. *Infect Control Hosp Epidemiol.* 2011;32(10):970-986. https://www.jstor.org/stable/pdf/10.1086/662016.pdf. Accessed July 26, 2020.

National Healthcare Safety Network, Centers for Disease Control and Prevention. Surgical site infection (SSI) event. http://www.cdc.gov/nhsn/pdfs/pscmanual/9pscssicurrent.pdf. Published January 2017. Accessed July 26, 2020.

National University of Singapore, Yong Loo Lin School of Medicine. New route of acquiring antibiotic resistance in bacteria is the most potent one to date. *ScienceDaily.* 2018. www.sciencedaily.com/releases/2018/10/181011143101.htm. Accessed August 23, 2020.

Onyekwelu I, Yakkanti R, Protzer L, Pinkston CM, Tucker C, Seligson D. Surgical wound classification and surgical site infections in the orthopaedic patient. *J Am Acad Orthop Surg Glob Res Rev.* 2017;1(3):e022. https://doi.org/10.5435/JAAOSGlobal-D-17-00022. Accessed August 29, 2020.

Pandey N, Cascella M. *Beta Lactam Antibiotics.* [Updated 2020 July 4]. In: StatPearls [Internet]. Treasure Island (FL): StatPearls Publishing; 2020. https://www.ncbi.nlm.nih.gov/books/NBK545311/. Accessed August 23, 2020.

Rodriguez MR. *Microbiology for Surgical Technologists.* 2nd ed. Boston, MA: Cengage Learning; 2017.

Rothrock JC. *Alexander's Care of the Patient in Surgery.* 16th ed. St. Louis, MO: Elsevier; 2016.

Shabanzadeh DM, Sorensen LT. Alcohol drinking does not affect postoperative surgical site infection or anastomotic leakage: A systematic review and meta-analysis. *J Gastrointest Surg.* 2014;18:414-425. doi: 10.1007/s11605-013-2275-5. Accessed August 9, 2020.

Sizar O, Unakal CG. *Gram Positive Bacteria.* [Updated 2020 Jun 27]. In: StatPearls [Internet]. Treasure Island (FL): StatPearls Publishing; 2020 January. https://www.ncbi.nlm.nih.gov/books/NBK470553/. Accessed August 1, 2020.

Umscheid CA, Mitchell MD, Doshi JA, Agarwal R, Williams K, Brennan PJ. Estimating the proportion of healthcare-associated infections that are reasonably preventable and the related mortality and costs. *Infect Control Hosp Epidemiol.* 2011;32(2):101-114. https://scholar.google.com/scholar_lookup?title=Estimating%20the%20proportion%20of%20healthcare-associated%20infections%20that%20are%20reasonably%20preventable%20and%20the%20related%20mortality%20and%20costs.&author=CA%20Umscheid&author=MD%20Mitchell&author=JA%20Doshi&author=R%20Agarwal&author=K%20Williams&author=PJ%20Brennan&publication_year=2011&journal=Infect%20Control%20Hosp%20Epidemiol&volume=32&pages=101-114. Accessed July 26, 2020.

World Health Organization Newsroom. Antibiotic Resistance. https://www.who.int/news-room/fact-sheets/detail/antimicrobial-resistance. Accessed August 23, 2020.

World Health Organization Newsroom. Smoking Greatly Increases Risk of Complications After Surgery, January 20, 2020; https://www.who.int/news-room/detail/20-01-2020-smoking-greatly-increases-risk-of-complications-after-surgery. Accessed August 9, 2020.

Yang X, Xiao X, Wang L, et al. (2018). Application of antimicrobial drugs in perioperative surgical incision. *Ann Clin Microbiol Antimicrob.* 17(1):2. https://doi.org/10.1186/s12941-018-0254-0. Accessed August 23, 2020.

Perioperative Patient Management

Brandy Farrington

DISCUSSED IN THIS CHAPTER

1. Preoperative patient education.
2. Perioperative patient assessment.
3. History and physical.
4. Preoperative checklists.
5. Laboratory values.
6. Diagnostic images.
7. Fluid and electrolyte balance.
8. Patient monitoring.
9. Handling specimens.
10. Postoperative patient care, pain management, and alternative therapies.

Perioperative care takes place in hospitals, surgery centers, endoscopy suites, interventional radiology departments, healthcare providers' offices, and other patient care facilities. Perioperative care involves surgeons, anesthesiologists, nurse anesthetists, perioperative nurses, nurse practitioners, surgical assistants, surgical technologists, radiology technicians, and others working together to achieve scientific, evidence-based, professional care. The primary objective in perioperative care is to provide the best conditions for the patient before, during, and after surgery. Perioperative patient management includes preoperative patient education, perioperative assessment of patient history, labs, imaging, fluid and electrolyte balance, patient monitoring, patient positioning, tissue and specimen handling, and postoperative patient care.

PREOPERATIVE PATIENT EDUCATION

The goals of preoperative patient education and discharge planning are to increase patient safety, decrease fear and anxiety, decrease length of stay, decrease postoperative complications, decrease hospital costs, decrease the amount of perceived pain, increase self-esteem by increasing self-efficacy, and prepare the patient for what to expect before, during, and after surgery, allowing the patient to take an active role in their recovery and feel more in control. Education for the patient's family and support members alleviates fear and anxiety, reduces costs, reduces complaints about care, speeds the return to normal functioning, and develops support for the caregivers' efforts. Patient and family education helps increase nursing job satisfaction, increases self-esteem, and reduces the nurse's stress level. Institutionally, benefits include increased patient and family satisfaction, decreased length of stay, fewer re-hospitalizations, and compliance with Joint Commission requirements.

One of the most important education provided to the patients, families, and relatives is preoperative education. Ideally, this education should be an ongoing process that begins with the pre-admission visit. Adequate time should be allowed for the patients to ask questions and ensure the information is understood. Information may need to be repeated several times due to the patient's anxiety, which can make information retention difficult. The patient's age and mental status should also be considered when teaching. Information should be presented in a way that is age appropriate and easy to understand.

Printed information should be provided to the patient whenever it is available. Selected information should be written at a sixth- to eighth-grade reading level.

Surgical team members' roles should be explained to the patient. The surgeon is responsible for explaining the procedure and risks and benefits to the patient as well as obtaining surgical consent. The anesthesia provider should explain their role and what to expect from the type of anesthesia administered. The nurse should explain preprocedural preparations, what to expect in the operating room, and what to expect postoperatively. Such things include, but are not limited to, fasting, medication usage, insertion of intravenous catheters, application of monitors, sensations, drains, urinary catheters, deep breathing, pain control, bowel movements, and wound care.

All patients have the right to accurate, easily understood information that allows them to participate and make decisions regarding treatments and procedures. Most patients need to know enough to obtain informed consent. Informed consent is defined as permission granted in the knowledge of the possible consequences. Most patients need to know enough to cooperate intraoperatively, provide self-care at home, and to survive until more teaching can be provided.

Several factors influence a patient's ability to learn. The first of these factors is physical (pain, nausea, itching, fatigue, hunger, or a need to urinate or defecate) and psychological (fear, anxiety, worry, grief, anger, guilt) comfort. The appropriate intervention is to attempt to relieve the discomfort in order to provide a better learning environment. The second factor is the amount of energy currently available to the patient. A patient fighting for their life will have a difficult time focusing on learning. The third factor is motivation. Leaning forward, asking for more complete explanations, taking notes, and requesting additional written information are indications that the patient is motivated to learn. The fourth factor is the patient's capability to learn. Learning can be inhibited by vision and hearing deficits, limited manual dexterity, language limitations, and neurological deficits.

Discharge planning is about not only discharging the patient but preparing the patient for movement from one level of care to another within or outside the current care facility. It should include helping the family create a supportive environment at home, arranging referrals for financial and social services and home health care, as well as evaluating the need for caregiver support. The patient and family should be ready to assume care of the patient on discharge. They should know how to take a temperature, look for signs of infection, and when to contact the physician. They should understand home medications and medical devices needed. An appointment for a return visit and the importance of that appointment should be conveyed to the patient. Preoperative education and discharge planning will help eliminate the patient's stress and anxiety by alleviating the fear of the unknown.

PERIOPERATIVE PATIENT ASSESSMENT

Perioperative patient assessment consists of preoperative, intraoperative, and postoperative assessment. It is a collection of relevant health information about the patient to help determine if the patient is at risk for adverse effects. Preoperative assessment may include information from the preoperative interview, the medical record, vital signs including height and weight, results of diagnostic studies, and physician consultations. Assessment should focus on the patient's current diagnosis, physical and psychosocial status, previous hospitalizations, and surgical interventions. The patient and family's understanding of the procedure and the ability to participate in correct site/side marking is of utmost importance in the concept of patient-centered care. Deviations in diagnostic studies should be reported to the surgeon and anesthesiologist. The Surgical Care Improvement Project (SCIP) protocol as well as Enhanced Surgical Recovery (ESR) protocol should be followed throughout the preoperative, intraoperative, and postoperative periods. Adjustments should be made based on the assessment findings to reduce risks of anesthetic, surgical, and postoperative complications.

The goals of intraoperative patient assessment are to keep the patient safe and prevent injury due to surgical errors, positioning, and temperature. Surgical errors are preventable but occur for reasons such as incompetence, insufficient preoperative planning, improper work processes, poor communication, fatigue, drug/alcohol use, and neglect. Examples of errors include but are not limited to nerve injury, medication mistakes, wrong site/side surgery, retained foreign objects, and wrong patient surgery. Patient positioning should provide optimal surgical site exposure and anesthesia access while maintaining circulatory, respiratory, and neurologic function. According to the Guideline Statement for the Maintenance of Normothermia in the Perioperative Patient from the Association of Surgical Technologists (AST), "Measures to monitor and maintain body temperature should begin in the pre-operative phase and continue into the postoperative phase of the surgical procedure. The monitoring of patient temperature is the responsibility of all surgical team members and not just the anesthesia provider." Maintenance of normothermia (36°C–38°C) decreases morbidity, mortality, and risks for surgical site infections.

Postoperative patient assessment occurs when the patient arrives in the post-anesthesia care unit (PACU) or intensive care unit (ICU). Immediate assessment begins with the adequacy of the airway, breathing, and circulation (ABCs). Once the ABCs are accessed, a handoff report between the anesthesia provider, PACU nurse, and operating room nurse should commence. Information should include vital signs, temperature, labs, oxygen saturation, allergies, medications, disabilities, substance abuse, prosthetics, catheters and drains, relevant pediatric birth and developmental history, length and type of anesthesia, operative procedures, fluid and blood loss/replacement, and complications. Once the PACU nurse accepts the patient a more thorough assessment can be performed. This assessment includes the integration of data received at the transfer of care, vital signs, temperature, pain control assessment, level of consciousness, pressure readings, position of the patient, condition and color of the skin, patient safety needs, neurovascular exam, condition of dressings, condition of suture line, drains and catheters, amount and type of drainage, muscle strength and response, pupillary response, intravenous fluid therapy, level of physical and emotional comfort, and procedure-specific assessment. The PACU nurse also completes an assessment before discharge or transfer to a surgical unit.

HISTORY AND PHYSICAL

The preoperative history and physical contains the same components as a standard history and physical with the addition of anesthesia- and surgery-specific topics. The Joint Commission (TJC): PC 01.02.03 states, "A history and physical exam must be performed on the patient and completed within a 30 day window of any surgical procedure that requires anesthesia." In an emergency, when there is no time to complete a history and physical exam, a progress or admission note describing a brief history and appropriate physical findings and the preoperative diagnosis should be recorded in the medical record before surgery. The history and physical should be completed by a licensed physician, physician assistant, or nurse practitioner. The following outlines the structure of the history and physical as described by Louisiana State University Medical School.

1. The Chief Complaint: Should tell why the patient came to the hospital in the patient's own words.

2. History of Present Illness: A chronologic account of the problems that the patient is seeking care for. Symptoms should be described by location, quality, severity, timing, setting in which they occurred, what aggravates or relieves symptoms, and associated symptoms. Also, a review of the organ system involved in the complaint should be included.

3. Past Medical History: Should include medical conditions and comorbidities, congenital conditions, physical disabilities, cognitive ability, and anything that limits the activities of daily living.

    A. Childhood illness: Ask about measles, mumps, rubella, polio, chicken pox, whooping cough, rheumatic fever, and scarlet fever.

    B. Immunizations: Ask about diphtheria, pertussis, tetanus; were they completed during childhood and when was the last booster? Ask if polio, measles, mumps, and rubella vaccinations are up to date. Ask if the patient has received any other vaccinations such as pneumococcal, hepatitis B, and influenza.

    C. Adult illness: Include the type of illness, the date it occurred, whether hospitalization was required (where?), and give a brief summary of the illness.

    D. Operations: Include what procedures were done, why was it done, if they have implants, when and where it was done, and whether there were complications with surgery or anesthesia.

    E. Allergies: What medications are they allergic to? What was the reaction and how soon did it occur after the medication was given? What foods are they allergic to and what type of reaction did they have? Are they allergic to latex? What was the reaction and when did the sensitivity begin?

    F. Medications: List the names and dosages of current medications. How long and with what frequency have they taken the medications? What conditions were the medications prescribed for?

    G. Complimentary treatments: Ask about massage therapy and acupuncture. Do they take herbals and vitamins? What kind do they take and how often?

4. Family History: Include information about parents, siblings, grandparents, aunts, and uncles. Major diseases of interest are diabetes, hypertension, heart disease, cancer, stroke, kidney disease, tuberculosis, blood disorders, arthritis, and mental disease.

5. Social History: Include education, occupation, travel, financial and living situation, smoking (how many, how long), alcohol use (what, how much, how long), illicit drug use (what, how often, how long), sexual history. If they quit smoking, drinking, and drug use, how long ago did they quit?

6. Review of Systems:

    A. General: Include usual weight, weight change, weakness, fatigue, fever, night sweats, eating disorders, and malaise.

    B. Skin: Include color changes, pruritis, bruising, petechiae, infection, rash, sores, changes in moles, and changes in hair and nails.

    C. Head: Include headaches and head injuries

    D. Eyes: Include vision changes, pain, redness, excessive tearing, diplopia, floaters, and loss of vision fields. Ask for date of last eye exam and if there is history of cataracts or glaucoma.

    E. Ears: Include hearing loss, change in hearing, tinnitus, and ear infections.

    F. Nose and sinuses: Include frequent colds, nasal stuffiness, hay fever, epistaxis, sinus trouble, obstruction, discharge, pain, change in ability to smell, sneezing, post-nasal drip, and history of polyps.

    G. Mouth and throat: Include soreness, dryness, pain, ulcers, sore tongue, bleeding gums, pyorrhea, caries, abscesses, extractions, dentures, sore throat, hoarseness, and history of recurrent strep throat or rheumatic fever.

    H. Neck: Include lumps, swollen lymph nodes or glands, pain, and goiter.

    I. Lymphatics: Include swollen lymph nodes in neck, axillae, epitrochlear areas, and inguinal area.

    J. Breasts: Include lumps, pain, nipple discharge, self-examination, and gynecomastia.

    K. Pulmonary: Include change in chronic cough, dyspnea, wheezing, hemoptysis, pleuritic chest pain, cyanosis, recurrent pneumonia, and environmental exposure to irritants. Ask for duration and sputum production associated with cough. Ask about exposure and history of tuberculosis. Ask about TB skin test and results.

L. Cardiovascular: Include dyspnea, paroxysmal nocturnal dyspnea, chest pain described in detail, orthopnea, edema, palpitations, hypertension, known heart disease, history of murmur and rheumatic fever, syncope and near syncope events, claudication, varicosities, thrombophlebitis, and history of abnormal electrocardiogram.

M. Gastrointestinal: Include dysphagia, odynophagia, nausea, vomiting, hematemesis, food intolerance, indigestion, heartburn, changes in appetite, early satiety, frequency and consistency of bowel movements, change in bowel pattern, rectal bleeding, melena, constipation, diarrhea, jaundice, liver or gallbladder problems, and history of hepatitis.

N. Urinary: Include hematuria, dysuria, frequency, suprapubic pain, costovertebral angle tenderness, nocturia, polyuria, stones, inguinal pain, incontinence, history of urinary tract infections, and trouble initiating urinary stream.

O. Genitals: (Males) Include penile discharge, lesions, history of sexually transmitted disease (STD), testicular pain or swelling, scrotal mass, infertility, impotence, change in libido, sexual difficulties, and hernias. (Females) Include age of menarche, last menstrual period, length of cycle and amount of bleeding, intermenstrual bleeding, postcoital bleeding, dyspareunia, vaginal discharge, pruritis, contraceptive use, history of STD, last PAP smear and results, age at menopause, postmenopausal bleeding, infertility, change in libido, and sexual difficulties. Ask about pregnancies, including live births and abortions, both spontaneous and induced. Ask if complications from pregnancies are due to diabetes or hypertension.

P. Musculoskeletal: Include joint pain, stiffness, arthritis, gout, back pain, joint swelling, tenderness, or effusion, limitation of motion, and history of fractures.

Q. Neurologic: Include fainting, blackouts, seizures, paralysis, local weakness, numbness, tingling, tremors, memory changes, headaches, vertigo, and muscle atrophy.

R. Psychiatric: Include anxiety, nightmares, nervousness, irritability, depression, insomnia, hypersomnia, phobias, and tension. If there are any clues that the patient may be suicidal, or have criminal or other sociopathic behavior, this should be pursued.

S. Endocrine: Include thyroid trouble, heat or cold intolerance, excessive sweating or flushing, diabetes, and excessive thirst, hunger, or urination.

T. Hematologic: Include anemia, easy bruising or bleeding, past transfusions and reactions, and history of bleeding disorders.

7. Physical Examination:

A. Vital signs: Compare blood pressure on right and left arm. Measure on one arm while standing and sitting. Check pulses. Are respirations regular or irregular? Document temperature and if taken orally or by another route.

B. General appearance: Does the patient appear acutely ill and is the patient oriented to time, place, and person?

C. Skin: Describe texture, turgor, skin lesions, icterus, pallor edema, and cyanosis if present.

D. HEENT (Head, Eyes, Ears, Nose, Throat): Skull (normocephalic, atraumatic, deformities?), scalp, hair, and distribution. Eyelids (ptosis?), sclera (icterus, muddy appearance?), conjunctivae (pale, injected, red?), cornea (opacified?), pupils (pupils equal, round, react to light and accommodation), light reflexes (direct and consensual), visual acuity, fundoscopic exam (describe optic disc, retinal vessels, and lesions). External auditory canal and tympanic membrane. Nasal septum and whether turbinates are enlarged or reddened, sinus tender to palpitation and percussion. Lips, tongue, teeth, gums, oral mucosa, and breath odor. Tonsils, posterior pharyngeal injection or exudates, uvula (midline, moves?).

E. Neck: Supple (mobile?). Thyroid (palpable, nodules, masses, tender?). Trachea (midline, stridor?). Carotids (volume, upstroke, bruits?). Jugular venous distention.

F. Nodes: Submandibular, submental, pre- and post-auricular, occipital, anterior and posterior cervical triangle, and supraclavicular nodes should be checked during the HEENT and neck exams. The following node groups should be checked during the remainder of the physical: axillary, epitrochlear, and inguinal. You can also examine these while examining that region of the body.

G. Breasts: Inspect and palpate for masses, discharge, and tenderness.

H. Chest: Inspect for symmetry of respiratory excursions and deformities. Palpate for fremitus. Check percussion for resonance, hyper resonance, or dullness. Check auscultation for normal breath sounds, crackles, wheezes, rhonchi, and rubs.

I. Heart: Inspect for normal outward pulsations and visible point of maximal impulse (PMI). Palpate for lifts, heaves, palpable heart sounds, and murmurs. PMI should be described in reference to the location on the chest, whether it is discreet or generalized, and if it is abnormally sustained. Check auscultation for rate, rhythm, heart sounds, murmurs, gallops, rubs, and clicks.

J. Abdomen: Inspect size, contour, scars, and abnormal venous patterns. Check auscultation of bowel sounds and bruits before palpitation. Check percussion for

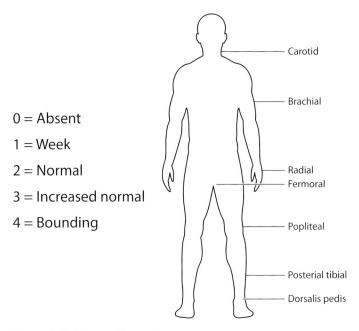

0 = Absent

1 = Week

2 = Normal

3 = Increased normal

4 = Bounding

Carotid

Brachial

Radial
Fermoral

Popliteal

Posterial tibial

Dorsalis pedis

Figure 5-1 · Pulse grading scale.

tympany, shifting dullness, fluid wave, and liver size. Palpate for tenderness (rebound, guarding?), liver, spleen, masses, aortic pulsations, and hernias.

K. Back and spine: Check mobility, curvature, posture, and tenderness.

L. Extremities: Examine upper and lower extremities for symmetry, moisture, nails, cyanosis, clubbing, edema, and tremor. Examine joints for tenderness, warmth, erythema, effusions, and range of motion. Check the following pulses and grade using Peripheral Pulse Grading Scale (see Figure 5-1): carotids, brachial, radial, femoral, popliteal, dorsalis pedis, and posterior tibial.

M. Genitalia: In males, check distribution and amount of pubic hair, penile lesions or discharge, circumcision, scrotum, and testes for masses and tenderness, epididymis, and inguinal canal. In females, check the distribution and amount of pubic hair, external genitalia for lesions, discharge, or evidence of inflammation, vagina, cervix, uterus and adnexa for masses and tenderness, and rectovaginal.

N. Rectal: Check for external lesions, hemorrhoids, fissures, fistulae, sphincter tone, prostate for size, masses, and tenderness, and stool for color, consistency, and occult blood.

O. Neurologic: Mental status: check the level of consciousness, behavior, attention and concentration, language, memory, drawings, and abstract reasoning (proverb interpretation, similarities, calculations). Cranial nerves: check nerves II-XII and list the manner in which they were checked. Motor: check gait, balance, involuntary movements, limb tone, contracture, strength graded using Muscle Strength Grading Scale (Table 5-1), and muscle bulk and tenderness. Sensory: check pinprick, light touch, graphesthesia, stereognosis, and double stimulus touch. Cerebellar: check gait for ataxia, finger to nose, heel to shin, rapid alternating movements, and standing with feet together and eyes open. Posterior column: check vibratory sensation, position sense, and Romberg sign. Reflexes: check deep tendon, biceps, triceps, brachioradialis, knee jerk and ankle jerk using Reflex Grading Scale (Table 5-2). Pathologic reflexes: check Babinski, digital reflexes, grasp reflexes, and snout reflexes.

8. Problem List: This is a list of all abnormal findings from the history and physical exam, organized so the most serious problems are listed first.

9. Differential Diagnosis: A list of diseases that can explain the major problems on the problem list, organized so the most likely diagnoses are listed first.

In addition to the history and physical, special attention should be placed on the physical analysis of the preoperative patient. This includes vital statistics such as blood pressure,

TABLE 5-2 • DEEP TENDON REFLEXES: GRADING	
Grade	DTR Response
4+	Very brisk, hyperactive, with clonus
3+	Brisker than average, slightly hyperreflexic
2+	Average, expected response; normal
1+	Somewhat diminished, low normal
0	No response, absent

TABLE 5-1 • MANUAL MUSCLE STRENGTH GRADING			
Grade	Percentage (%)	Qualitative Value	Muscle Strength
5	100	Normal	Complete range of motion (ROM) against gravity with full resistance
4	75	Good	Complete ROM against gravity with some resistance
3	50	Fair	Complete ROM against gravity with no resistance
2	25	Poor	Complete ROM with gravity omitted
1	10	Trace	Evidence of slight contractility with no joint motion
0	0	Zero	No evidence of muscle contractility

Source: Reproduced, with permission, from Prentice WE. *Principles of Athletic Training: A Guide to Evidence-Based Clinical Practice.* 17th ed. New York, NY: McGraw Hill; 2021.

heart rate, pulses, respiratory rate, and pulse oximetry. Also, attention should be given to central venous pressures, arterial pressures, and any other pressures being monitored. Laboratory tests such as CBC (complete blood count), chemistry, PT/PTT (prothrombin/partial thromboplastin time), urinalysis, toxicology, serology, and other pertinent tests should be reviewed before surgery. Ensure all relevant imaging films are available and have been reviewed before surgery begins. Examples are x-rays, computed axial tomography (CT/CAT) scans, magnetic resonance imaging (MRI), ultrasound, and positron emission tomography (PET) scans. Other diagnostic tests pertaining to patient's procedure should also be reviewed before surgery. These include, but are not limited to, pulmonary function tests, electrocardiogram, and stress tests.

Preoperative Checklist

Preoperative preparation of patients undergoing surgical procedures is an important part of perioperative care. A preoperative checklist is a list of important patient care measures that is carried out preoperatively. The checklist is usually completed in the patient care unit, preoperative holding area, or in the pre-admission area for ambulatory surgery patients. Preoperative checklists help promote patient safety and enhance effective communication and teamwork. Checklists also help to reduce decision fatigue by not forcing you to remember every single detail. Checklists reduce the potential for oversights, omissions, and sentinel events, and drive consistency. They also ensure that everything that needs to be completed gets done. The preoperative checklist can be broken down into three main categories: patient and procedure verification, patient assessment, and patient preparation.

Patient and procedure verification should be conducted following the national patient safety goals set forth by the Joint Commission on Accreditation of Healthcare Organizations (JCAHO). Patient and procedure verification should be conducted with the patient and/or caregiver whenever possible. Ensure that the patient's armband is on the patient and contains the correct patient name, date of birth, and any other pertinent information. Two of these identifiers should be checked before any test or treatments are administered. Acceptable patient identifiers may be the individual's name, an assigned identification number, telephone number, birth date, or other person-specific identifier. The patient's room number or physical location is not used as an identifier. Ensure that the patient's allergy band is on the patient and contains the correct allergy information. This information should be verified by the patient and/or caregiver as well. Blood bands should be secured and verified as well. Make sure that the correct surgery is done on the correct patient and at the correct place on the patient's body. The surgeon, along with the patient, should mark the correct place on the patient's body where the surgery is to be done. The procedure to be performed, including the operative site, side, and surgical approach should be verified with the patient and correspond to the surgical consent and the surgical schedule. Anesthesia consent forms and blood product consent/refusal forms should be signed, witnessed, and verified by the patient as well.

Patient assessments on the preoperative checklist include verification of an updated history and physical exam, vital signs, relevant laboratory results, and other relevant examinations or diagnostic results such as blood and urine testing, chest x-ray, and ECG. Preoperative patient teaching, physical and mental challenges, mobility needs, and healthcare directives should be addressed and documented. Religious, cultural, spiritual, or ethnic preferences must be carefully noted. All preoperative orders concerning skin preparation, medication administration, and elimination should be reviewed. SCIP protocol requires prophylactic antibiotics be received within 1 hour prior to surgical incision, correct prophylactic antibiotic be selected for surgical patients, and prophylactic antibiotics be discontinued within 24 hours after surgery end time. Preoperative dietary and fluid restrictions should be maintained to prevent aspiration of gastric content during anesthesia induction. Patient medical/surgical implants and allergies should be documented. A current list of all patient medications and supplements should be included and verified. Supplements are often overlooked but can affect bleeding and anesthesia. The *Journal of the American Medical Association* (*JAMA*) and the American Society of Anesthesiologists list kava root, St. John's wort, and valerian as herbs that might interfere. Kava and valerian were said to possibly increase the effects of anesthesia, while St. John's wort might increase the metabolism of drugs used before and after the operation. Ephedra, ginseng, garlic, and vitamin E are also on the list. Allergies should include previous unfavorable reactions to anesthesia (ie, anaphylaxis, malignant hyperthermia), blood product transfusions, medications, IV contrast media, food, and latex.

IV contrast media is used widely in the United States for a variety of radiological studies, such as angiograms, x-rays, magnetic resonance imaging (MRI), and computed tomography (CT) scans. Adverse reactions to contrast media are common, though allergies are much rarer. The two major types of contrast used are iodinated contrast (used in most CT scans) and gadolinium-based contrast (used in most MRI scans that use contrast media). The two types are quite different and are not thought to cross-react. Symptoms range from nausea and vomiting to anaphylaxis. Treatment of an acute reaction may include injectable epinephrine and antihistamines, as well as the use of intravenous fluids for hypotension and shock. Patients with a history of non-severe reactions should be treated with a combination of oral corticosteroids, such as prednisone, and antihistamines, such as diphenhydramine, before any future contrast administrations.

Latex allergy is the immunoglobulin E (IgE)–mediated reaction to certain proteins in latex rubber. Latex has been the material of choice for surgical gloves and thousands of other medical and consumer products. Increasing exposure to latex proteins increases the risk of developing allergic symptoms. Symptoms range from contact dermatitis, respiratory symptoms, such as rhinitis, itchy eyes, scratchy throat, or asthma, to more severe manifestations such as anaphylaxis, shock, respiratory, and cardiac arrest. Therapeutic management of latex allergies includes epinephrine, beta-agonist inhalers, prednisone, and other anaphylactic life-supporting medications. Latex-sensitive individuals should avoid exposure to latex products.

In preparing the preoperative patient for surgery, multiple tasks need to be accomplished and documented. Patients should shower or receive a bath the night before surgery. Bowel preps, if indicated, should also be accomplished the night before surgery. Patient's personal clothing should be removed as well as any personal belongings. Prosthesis, eyeglasses, contacts, dentures, partials, retainers, hearing aids, makeup, nail polish, and hair clips should be removed to reduce risks of damage or injury. All SCIP and ESR protocols should be carried out. Blood products should be arranged to be picked up. IV catheters of appropriate size should be placed, and functionality verified. Preoperative medications should be given. Anti-embolic stockings and sequential compression devices should also be applied if indicated. The preoperative nurse is responsible for the safe handling and proper disposition of the patient's property and valuables. Patients should be encouraged to leave property and valuables with the accompanying caregiver if present. Some facilities offer security services to secure inpatient belongings or temporary lockers for outpatient surgery.

Any discrepancies or omissions noted on the preoperative checklist should be corrected and communicated with the entire surgical team as soon as possible to help prevent surgical and medication errors and provide a safe environment for the patient. Upon completion, the preoperative checklist is signed by the preoperative nurse and becomes part of the patient's medical record.

Laboratory Values

Preoperative lab tests are often performed before surgical procedures. The results of these tests can be helpful to stratify risk, direct anesthetic choices, and guide postoperative management. Risk stratification is defined as an estimate of the probability of a person succumbing to a disease or benefiting from a treatment for that disease. It is measured by a variety of scoring systems depending on the diagnosis. The decision to perform preoperative testing should be based on the history and physical examination findings, perioperative-risk assessment, and clinical judgment. Most preoperative lab test results should be recent, within 30 days; however, each patient and their condition are unique. Some lab tests may need to be more recent based on overall patient health and procedure being performed. The following recommendations were formulated by the American Society of Anesthesia (ASA) and the American College of Cardiology/American Hospital Association (ACC/AHA). The recommendations are based on the ASA Physical Status classification system (Table 5-3) and the ACC/AHA risk stratification score (Table 5-4). The following is a description of the most commonly ordered laboratory tests.

Preoperative urinalysis is indicated for patients undergoing urologic procedures or implantation of foreign material. Preoperative urine pregnancy testing is automatically ordered on female patients of potential child-bearing age that have not undergone hysterectomy or tubal ligation. Urinalysis examines urine for certain physical properties, solutes, cells, casts,

crystals, organisms, or particulate matter. Urine culture and urine electrolyte levels are part of urinalysis. There are three basic components to urinalysis include gross examination, chemical evaluation, and microscopic examination. Gross examination uses criteria that can be quantified with the naked eye (or other senses), including volume, color, transparency, odor, and specific gravity. Chemical evaluation uses urine test strips to quantify leukocytes, nitrite, protein, erythrocytes, specific gravity, glucose, bilirubin, and ketones. Microscopic examination measures the numbers and types of cells and/or material, such as urinary casts (indicative of kidney disease), in the urine. It offers a great deal of information and may suggest a specific diagnosis. Hematuria is associated with kidney stones, infections, tumors, and other conditions. Pyuria is associated with urinary infections. Eosinophiluria is associated with allergic interstitial nephritis and atheroembolic disease. Red blood cell casts are associated with glomerulonephritis, vasculitis, and malignant hypertension. White blood cell casts are associated with acute interstitial nephritis, exudative glomerulonephritis, and severe pyelonephritis. Granular casts are associated with acute tubular necrosis. Crystalluria is associated with acute urate nephropathy. Calcium oxalatin is associated with ethylene glycol and kidney stone disease.

Preoperative electrolyte, blood urea nitrogen (BUN), and creatinine testing should be reserved for patients at risk of electrolyte abnormalities or renal impairment, diabetics, patients using diuretics, digoxin, or steroids, and patients with pacemakers, implantable cardioverter defibrillator (ICD), or cardiac resynchronization therapy (CRT) devices. These tests are usually consolidated, along with glucose, into a basic metabolic panel (BMP). It consists of a set of seven or eight biochemical tests and is one of the most common lab tests ordered by healthcare providers in the United States. The BMP includes electrolyte levels for calcium (Ca^{2+}), sodium (Na^+), potassium (K^+), chloride (Cl^-), and bicarbonate (HCO_3^-) or CO_2. Abnormal calcium levels are associated with malnutrition, osteoporosis, and malignancy, especially of the thyroid. BUN, creatinine, and glucose, along with the other four electrolytes, are indicative of dehydration/hypovolemia, water intoxication, diabetic shock (either ketoacidosis, hyperglycemia, or hypoglycemia), congestive heart failure, kidney failure or liver failure, and various substance overdoses and adverse reactions. The basic metabolic panel is a simpler version of the comprehensive metabolic panel, which includes tests for kidney function, liver function, diabetic and parathyroid status in addition to the values included in the BMP. Preoperative glucose and A1C testing should be considered on patients with endocrine, renal, and hepatic disorders and patients on whom an abnormal result would change the perioperative management. Preoperative liver function testing should be done in patients with liver disease or a history of alcohol abuse. Preoperative thyroid testing should be done in patients with active thyroid disease or in those exhibiting signs of hyper- or hypothyroidism.

A preoperative complete blood count (CBC) is indicated for patients with a history of anemia, chemotherapy, renal failure, bleeding disorders, and in those patients of advanced age and

TABLE 5-3 • ASA PS CLASSIFICATION

ASA PS Classification[†]	Definition	Adult Examples, Including, But Not Limited to:	Pediatric Examples, Including But Not Limited to:	Obstetric Examples, Including But Not Limited to:
ASA I	A normal healthy patient	Healthy, non-smoking, no or minimal alcohol use	Healthy (no acute or chronic disease), normal BMI percentile for age	
ASA II	A patient with mild systemic disease	Mild diseases only without substantive functional limitations. Current smoker, social alcohol drinker, pregnancy, obesity (30<BMI<40), well-controlled DM/HTN, mild lung disease	Asymptomatic congenital cardiac disease, well controlled dysrhythmias, asthma without exacerbation, well controlled epilepsy, non-insulin dependent diabetes mellitus, abnormal BMI percentile for age, mild/moderate OSA, oncologic state in remission, autism with mild limitations	Normal pregnancy,* well controlled gestational HTN, controlled pre-eclampsia without severe features, diet-controlled gestational DM
ASA III	A patient with severe systemic disease	Substantive functional limitations; One or more moderate to severe diseases. Poorly controlled DM or HTN, COPD, morbid obesity (BMI ≥40), active hepatitis, alcohol dependence or abuse, implanted pacemaker, moderate reduction of ejection fraction, ESRD undergoing regularly scheduled dialysis, history (>3 months) of MI, CVA, TIA, or CAD/stents	Uncorrected stable congenital cardiac abnormality, asthma with exacerbation, poorly controlled epilepsy, insulin dependent diabetes mellitus, morbid obesity, malnutrition, severe OSA, oncologic state, renal failure, muscular dystrophy, cystic fibrosis, history of organ transplantation, brain/spinal cord malformation, symptomatic hydrocephalus, premature infant PCA <60 weeks, autism with severe limitations, metabolic disease, difficult airway, long term parenteral nutrition. Full term infants <6 weeks of age	Preeclampsia with severe features, gestational DM with complications or high insulin requirements, a thrombophilic disease requiring anticoagulation
ASA IV	A patient with severe systemic disease that is a constant threat to life	Recent (<3 months) MI, CVA, TIA or CAD/stents, ongoing cardiac ischemia or severe valve dysfunction, severe reduction of ejection fraction, shock, sepsis, DIC, ARD or ESRD not undergoing regularly scheduled dialysis	Symptomatic congenital cardiac abnormality, congestive heart failure, active sequelae of prematurity, acute hypoxic-ischemic encephalopathy, shock, sepsis, disseminated intravascular coagulation, automatic implantable cardioverter-defibrillator, ventilator dependence, endocrinopathy, severe trauma, severe respiratory distress, advanced oncologic state	Preeclampsia with severe features complicated by HELLP or other adverse event, peripartum cardiomyopathy with EF <40, uncorrected/decompensated heart disease, acquired or congenital
ASA V	A moribund patient who is not expected to survive without the operation	Ruptured abdominal/thoracic aneurysm, massive trauma, intracranial bleed with mass effect, ischemic bowel in the face of significant cardiac pathology or multiple organ/system dysfunction	Massive trauma, intracranial hemorrhage with mass effect, patient requiring ECMO, respiratory failure or arrest, malignant hypertension, decompensated congestive heart failure, hepatic encephalopathy, ischemic bowel or multiple organ/system dysfunction	Uterine rupture
ASA VI	A declared brain-dead patient whose organs are being removed for donor purposes			

Source: ASA Physical Status Classification System, American Society of Anesthesiologists 2020, is reprinted with permission of the American Society of Anesthesiologists, 1061 American Lane, Schaumburg, Illinois 60173-4973.

*Although pregnancy is not a disease, the parturient's physiologic state is significantly altered from when the woman is not pregnant, hence the assignment of ASA 2 for a woman with uncomplicated pregnancy.

[†]The addition of "E" denotes Emergency surgery: (An emergency is defined as existing when delay in treatment of the patient would lead to a significant increase in the threat to life or body part.)

TABLE 5-4 • CARDIAC RISK STRATIFICATION FOR NONCARDIAC SURGICAL PROCEDURES

High (reported cardiac risk often >5%)
Emergent major operations, particularly in the elderly
Aortic and other major vascular surgery
Anticipated prolonged surgical procedures associated with large fluid shifts and/or blood loss (eg, liver transplantation)
Intermediate (reported cardiac risk generally 1–5%)
Carotid endarterectomy surgery
Head and neck surgery
Intraperitoneal and intrathoracic surgery
Orthopedic surgery
Peripheral vascular surgery
Prostate surgery
Low (reported cardiac risk generally <1%)
Endoscopic procedures
Superficial procedure
Cataract or other eye surgery
Breast surgery

Source: Reproduced, with permission, from Crawford MH, ed. *Current Diagnosis & Treatment: Cardiology*. 5th ed. New York, NY: McGraw Hill; 2017.

TABLE 5-5 • NORMAL COAGULATION LABORATORY VALUES

Laboratory findings

Test	Value	Reference Range	Units
PT	12.5	10-13	seconds
aPTT	70	25-36	seconds
Fibrinogen	145	130-330	mg/dL
Hemoglobin	11	12-15	g/dL
Hematocrit	34	36-44	percent
WBC	9,000	4,000-10,000	per L
Platelet count	145,000	150,000-450,000	per L

Source: Olson JD, Addressing clinical etiologies of a prolonged aPTT. *CAP today*, 1999;13(9). Copyright, College of American Pathologists, Used with permission.

where significant blood loss is anticipated. The CBC indicates the amounts of white blood cells, red blood cells and platelets, the concentration of hemoglobin, and the hematocrit percentage. Also included are the red blood cell indices, which indicate the average size and hemoglobin content of red blood cells, and a white blood cell differential, which counts the different types of white blood cells. Abnormal complete blood counts are indicative of anemia and thrombocytopenia. The red blood cell indices provide information about the cause of a person's anemia such as iron deficiency and vitamin B12 deficiency. The white blood cell differential can help to diagnose viral, bacterial, and parasitic infections and blood disorders such as leukemia. The CBC aids in diagnosis when there is suspicion of an infection, a bleeding disorder, or some cancers.

Preoperative coagulation testing (Table 5-5) should be reserved for patients who are taking anticoagulants, who have a history of bleeding, or who have medical conditions, such as liver and renal disease, that predispose them to coagulopathy. Coagulation panels usually include international normalized ratio (INR), prothrombin time (PT), partial thromboplastin time (PTT), platelets, and fibrinogen. INR is calculated based on PT test result and is used to monitor how well the anticoagulant warfarin is working to prevent blood clotting. The PT and INR are used to determine the clotting tendency of blood, in the measure of warfarin dosage, liver damage, and vitamin K status. The PT measures the coagulation factors I (fibrinogen), II (prothrombin), V (proaccelerin), VII (proconvertin), and X (Stuart–Prower factor). The PT is the time it takes plasma to clot after addition of tissue factors by means of the extrinsic

pathway. The PT can be prolonged as a result of deficiencies in vitamin K, warfarin therapy, malabsorption, lack of intestinal colonization by bacteria (such as in newborns), poor factor VII synthesis (due to liver disease), or increased consumption (in disseminated intravascular coagulation). The PTT is used to detect blood clotting times by means of the intrinsic pathway and to monitor the treatment effect of heparin. The PTT measures the coagulation factors I (fibrinogen), II (prothrombin), V (proaccelerin), VIII (anti-hemophilic factor), X (Stuart–Prower factor), XI (plasma thromboplastin antecedent), and XII (Hageman factor). Prolonged PTT may indicate the use of heparin, antiphospholipid antibodies, coagulation factor deficiencies and consumption (sepsis), and the presence of antibodies against coagulation factors. Platelets (thrombocytes) are a component of blood that reacts to bleeding from blood vessel injury by clumping and initiating a blood clot. Along with von Willebrand factor and fibrin, platelets interact with thrombin, factors X, V, VII, XI, IX, and prothrombin to complete clot formation via the coagulation cascade. A low platelet count (thrombocytopenia) is due to either decreased production or increased destruction of platelets. An elevated platelet count (thrombocytosis) is either congenital, reactive (to cytokines), or due to unregulated production of myeloid neoplasms. Fibrinogen (factor I) is made in the liver. During vessel injury, fibrinogen is enzymatically converted by thrombin to fibrin to help produce blood clots. Fibrinogen disorders, such as congenital afibrinogenemia, congenital hypofibrinogenemia, fibrinogen storage disease, congenital dysfibrinogenemia, acquired dysfibrinogenemia, congenital hypodysfibrinogenemia, and cryofibrinogenemia, may lead to pathological bleeding and/or blood clotting or the deposition of fibrinogen in the liver, kidneys, or other organs and tissues.

Diagnostic Imaging

Diagnostic imaging is non-invasive and does everything from confirming the presence of disease and determining the severity of an injury to providing a strategy for surgical procedures. The five most common modalities for imaging tests are x-rays, computed axial tomography (CT/CAT) scans, magnetic resonance imaging (MRI), ultrasound, and positron emission tomography (PET) scans. The American College of Radiology (ACR) Appropriateness Criteria (AC) are the largest body of evidence-based guidelines in medical imaging. The AC have aided physicians and other providers with resources for appropriate utilization of medical imaging. The Radiological Society of North America (RSNA) and the American College of Radiology (ACR), as well as multiple government agencies, indicate safety standards to ensure that radiation dosage is as low as possible. Lead is the most common shield against x-rays because of its high density, stopping power, ease of installation, and low cost. Lead gowns and shields should be used to protect medical staff, as well as areas of the patient that do not need exposure. A radiation dosimeter should be worn by all medical staff who are exposed to radiation. The dosimeter badge does not provide protection from radiation but detects and measures exposure.

X-rays (see Figure 5-2) are the most common diagnostic imaging tests performed in medical facilities. They are quick painless tests that produce images of the structures in the body, especially bones. X-rays are performed to diagnose the cause of pain, determine the extent of injuries, check the progression of diseases, and the effectiveness of treatment. Examples include bone fractures, arthritis, osteoporosis, infections, breast cancer, retained items, and digestive tract problems. An x-ray is a penetrating form of high-energy electromagnetic radiation that has an extremely short wavelength of less than 100 Å and has the properties of penetrating various thicknesses of all solids, of producing secondary radiations by impinging on material bodies, and of acting on photographic films and plates. X-ray photons carry enough energy to ionize atoms and disrupt molecular bonds making a type of ionizing radiation that is harmful to living tissue. An extremely high radiation dose over a short period of time can cause radiation sickness, while lower doses can give an increased risk of radiation-induced cancer. In medical imaging, this increased cancer risk is greatly outweighed by the benefits of the examination.

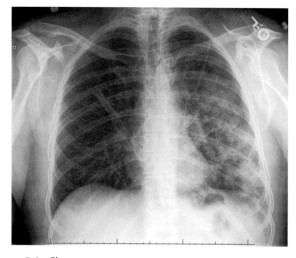

Figure 5-2 · Chest x-ray.

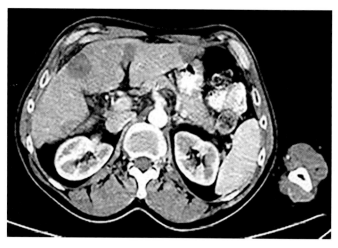

Figure 5-3 · Axial CT image of the abdomen.

The CT scan (see Figure 5-3) is a medical imaging procedure that uses computer-processed combinations of many x-ray measurements taken from different angles to produce cross-sectional images of specific areas, including soft tissue, blood vessels, and bones. CT scans can be used to guide biopsies and diagnose injuries from trauma, fractures, tumors, cancers, vascular and heart disease, and infections. CT scanning of the head is typically used to detect infarction, tumors, calcifications, hemorrhage, and bone trauma. Contrast CT is the study of choice for neck masses in adults and plays an important role in the evaluation of thyroid abnormalities and cancer. CT scan of the thorax can be used for detecting both acute and chronic changes in the lung parenchyma, nodules, and visualization of the arteries and veins using contrast media. CT is the preferred modality for diagnosis of abdominal diseases. This includes diagnosis and staging of cancer, as well as follow-up after cancer treatment to assess response. It is also used to investigate acute abdominal pain. CT is also used to image complex fractures around joints. The major advantages of CT scans are that it eliminates the superimposition of images of structures outside the area of interest, the high-contrast resolution shows differences between tissues that differ in physical density by less than 1%, and data from a single CT imaging procedure consisting of either multiple contiguous or one helical scan can be viewed as images in the axial, coronal, or sagittal planes. The ionizing radiation used in CT scans can damage DNA molecules which can lead to radiation-induced cancer. Compared to the lowest dose x-ray techniques, CT scans can have 100 to 1000 times higher dose than conventional x-rays. In the United States, half of CT scans require the use of contrast media. Common reactions to contrast media range from nausea and vomiting to kidney damage and anaphylaxis.

MRI (see Figure 5-4) is a medical imaging technique used to form pictures of the anatomy and the physiological processes of the body. They are used to diagnose aneurysms, multiple sclerosis, stroke, spinal cord disorders, tumors, blood vessel issues, and joint and tendon injuries. MRI scanners use strong magnetic fields, magnetic field gradients, and radio waves to

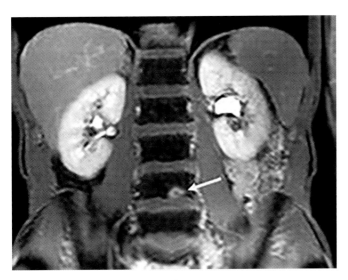

Figure 5-4 · MRI image of the lumbar spine.

generate images of the organs in the body. The magnetic field temporarily realigns water molecules in your body. Radio waves cause these aligned atoms to produce faint signals, which are used to create cross-sectional MRI images. MRI is the examination of choice for neurological cancers and is used in guided stereotactic surgery and radiosurgery for treatment of intracranial tumors, arteriovenous malformations, and other surgically treatable conditions. In the musculoskeletal system, applications include spinal imaging, assessment of joint disease, and soft tissue injuries and tumors. Other specialized configurations include magnetic resonance spectroscopy (MRS) which is used to measure the levels of different metabolites in body tissues, real-time MRI which refers to the continuous imaging of moving objects (such as the heart) in real-time, and magnetic-resonance-guided-focused ultrasound in which high frequency focused ultrasound is used for tissue ablation using MR thermal imaging. MRI requires an extraordinary strong magnetic field which causes magnetic material to move at great speeds posing a projectile risk. Contraindications to MRI include cochlear implants, cardiac pacemakers, metallic artificial joints and heart valves, intrauterine devices, bone plates, pins, and screws, shrapnel, and metallic foreign bodies in the eyes unless they have been certified as MRI safe.

Medical ultrasound (sonography) uses sound waves to develop ultrasound images of what is going on inside the body. A transducer emits high-frequency sound, inaudible to human ears, and then records the echoes as the sound waves bounce back to determine the size, shape, and consistency of soft tissues and organs. This information is relayed in real-time to produce images on a computer screen. Ultrasound can be used to diagnose gallbladder disease, breast lumps, genital/prostate issues, joint inflammation, and blood flow problems. It is also used in monitoring pregnancy and guiding biopsies. Anesthesiologists use ultrasound to guide the placement of needles when placing nerve blocks, arterial lines, and central venous lines. Vascular medicine uses duplex ultrasound to diagnose arterial and venous disease. Echocardiography is an essential tool in

cardiology, assisting in evaluation of heart valve function, and the strength of cardiac muscle contractions. Abdominal and endoanal ultrasounds are frequently used in gastroenterology and colorectal surgery. Ultrasound is the preferred imaging modality for thyroid tumors and lesions and is critical in the evaluation, preoperative planning, and postoperative surveillance of patients with thyroid cancer. Expansions in ultrasonography include Doppler, contrast, molecular, interventional, compression, and panoramic ultrasound, as well as elastography. Ultrasound has several advantages. It provides images in real-time, it is portable and can be brought to the bedside, it is lower in cost than other imaging modalities, and it does not use harmful ionizing radiation. Disadvantages include limits on its field of view, need for patient cooperation, dependence on physique, difficulty imaging structures behind bone and air or gases, and the necessity of a skilled sonographer.

PET (see Figure 5-5) is an imaging modality that uses radioactive substances to visualize and measure metabolic processes in the body. PET is mainly used in detecting or measuring changes in physiological activities like metabolism, blood flow, regional chemical composition, and absorption. PET scans use radioactive materials (tracers) which are injected into the body and get trapped within the tissues of interest. The unstable nucleus emits positrons, which combine with electrons to produce gamma rays in the opposite direction at 180° to each other. These gamma rays are detected by the detector placed within the scanner. The energy and location of these gamma rays are recorded and used to reconstruct three-dimensional (3D) images of tracer concentrations within the body. PET is especially useful in the imaging of tumors and the search for metastases within the field of clinical oncology, and for the diagnosis of certain diffuse brain diseases such as dementia and Alzheimer. PET scans are also useful in the diagnosis of heart disease, coronary artery disease, seizures, epilepsy, and Parkinson disease.

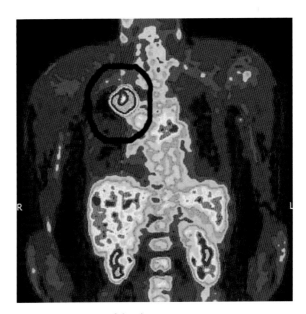

Figure 5-5 · PET image of the thorax.

Fluid and Electrolyte Balance

Homeostasis is the state of steady internal conditions needed to maintain proper body functioning. Body fluids and electrolyte balances play a key role in maintaining homeostasis, transporting oxygen and nutrients to the cells, removing waste products from the cells, and maintaining normothermia. Electrolytes help transmit nerve impulses, regulate water distribution, contract muscles, generate adenosine triphosphate (ATP), regulate pH, and help with blood clotting. The gastrointestinal (GI) tract, the kidneys, and the endocrine system (pituitary-thyroid-adrenals) maintain fluid and electrolyte balance and the respiratory system helps to maintain pH balance. Electrolyte imbalance leads to a fluid imbalance that in turn, leads to a pH imbalance. Fluid and electrolyte imbalances in the surgical patient may occur due to preoperative dietary restrictions, intraoperative fluid/blood loss, or the stress of surgery.

The human body is approximately 60% water but varies with age, gender, and body mass. The elderly adult averages 45% to 55% water, whereas infants average 70% to 80% water. Both age groups have a decreased ability to compensate for fluid shifts. The core principle of fluid balance is that the amount of water lost from the body must equal the amount of water taken in. Body fluids are distributed between intracellular fluid (ICF) and extracellular fluid (ECF). Approximately 70% of the body's fluid is contained in the ICF along with dissolved substances essential to fluid and electrolyte balance and metabolism. ICF functions as a stabilizing agent for parts of the cell, helps maintain cell shape, and assists with nutrient transport across the cell membrane. Approximately 30% of the body's fluid is in the ECF, including plasma, intravascular fluid, cerebrospinal fluid (CSF), and fluid in the gastrointestinal (GI)tract. Fluid spacing is used to classify water distribution in the body. First spacing is the normal distribution of fluid. Second spacing is an excess accumulation of edema. Third spacing occurs when fluid accumulates in areas that generally have little to no fluid. This occurs with burns, ascites, peritonitis, and small bowel obstruction. Third spacing results in a deficit of extracellular fluid.

Electrolyte levels in both intracellular and extracellular fluids are a determinant of fluid balance. Electrolytes are substances that when dissolved in water dissociate into ions and carry a positive (cation) and negative (anion) charges. Electrolytes found in the ICF and ECF are the same, but the concentrations are different. In the ICF, the primary cation is potassium and the primary anion is phosphate. In the ECF, the primary cation is sodium and the primary anion is chloride. Fluids and electrolytes shift across the cell membrane to facilitate pH balance, oxygenation, and responses to drug therapies and illnesses. Movement across the cell membrane is accomplished through diffusion, active transport, and osmosis.

Diffusion is the movement of molecules from an area of higher concentration to an area of lower concentration across a permeable membrane until equilibrium is achieved. In active transport, the molecules are moved across the cell membrane, against a gradient by use of pumps to maintain equilibrium. The sodium-potassium pump moves three sodium ions out for every two potassium ions moved into the cell. ATP is the energy source for the sodium-potassium pump. Osmosis is the movement of fluid across a semipermeable membrane from an area that has a lower concentration of solute to an area of higher concentration. The membrane prevents the movement of the solute. Osmolality expresses the concentration of a solution in milliosmoles per kilogram (mOsm/kg) of water. Isotonic solutions, those having the same osmolality as plasma, prevent fluid and electrolyte shifts from intracellular compartments. Examples include 0.9% sodium chloride and lactated Ringer's solution. A hypotonic solution has a lower concentration of solutes than plasma and moves water into the cells. Examples include 0.45% saline and 2.5% dextrose. A hypertonic solution has a greater concentration of solutes than plasma and moves water out of the cells. Examples include 5% dextrose in saline or in lactated Ringer's solution.

During surgical procedures, fluid requirement increases by increased evaporation, fluid shifts, or excessive urine production. Minor surgical procedures may cause a fluid loss of approximately 4 mL/kg/h, and larger surgical procedures of approximately 8 mL/kg/h. The most common problems associated with fluid and electrolyte shift during surgery include fluid volume deficit (hypovolemia) and potassium imbalances. Hypovolemia occurs when the loss of ECF exceeds fluid intake. The effect of fluid loss during surgery depends on the rate at which it is lost. Patients experiencing rapid fluid loss can exhibit signs of shock and require immediate fluid replacement. Slow fluid loss can be treated with IV fluids, albumin, and erythropoiesis. Blood products such as packed red blood cells, fresh frozen plasma, platelets, and cryoprecipitate can be used to treat hypovolemia. Plasma expanders may also be used. Plasma expanders increase the oncotic pressure in the intravascular space. Water moves from the interstitial spaces into the intravascular space, increasing the circulating blood volume. This increase in volume leads to an increase in central venous pressure, cardiac output, stroke volume, blood pressure, urinary output, and capillary perfusion. It also causes a decrease in heart rate, peripheral resistance, and blood viscosity. Fluid volume excess (hypervolemia) refers to an isotonic expansion of the ECF caused by water and sodium retention. Signs of hypervolemia include edema, distended jugular veins, and lung crackles.

Sodium helps maintain the pH balance in the body. The sodium-potassium pump plays a vital role in neuromuscular activity. Patients undergoing certain gynecologic and urologic procedures are at risk of dilutional hyponatremia and fluid overload due to the absorption of non-electrolytic irrigation fluids used during those procedures. Potassium is necessary for contraction of smooth, skeletal, and cardiac muscle, as well as peristalsis. It helps transmit nerve impulses by regulating neuromuscular excitability and in the formation of muscle proteins by transporting glucose into the cells along with insulin. It also aids in maintaining pH balance and intracellular osmotic pressure. Hypokalemia can occur during surgery due to diuretics and fluid loss. Symptoms include ectopy, dysrhythmias, muscle weakness, gastric distention, paralytic ileus, and urinary retention. Treatment includes IV replacement therapy of potassium when the deficit is severe. Hyperkalemia can be caused during surgery due to massive transfusion of stored blood, decreased excretion of potassium caused by hypovolemia or renal failure, and potassium shifts caused by acidosis. Drugs such as anti-inflammatory agents, beta-blockers, succinylcholine, heparin, and the penicillins can cause hyperkalemia. Symptoms include muscular weakness and paresthesia, diarrhea, abdominal distention, ventricular dysrhythmias, heart block, and asystole. Cardiac effects are treated with calcium gluconate, sodium bicarbonate, and insulin-glucose.

Perioperative fluid balance has been highlighted as a major contributing factor in postoperative morbidity and mortality. Preoperative laboratory analysis of electrolyte levels (Table 5-6) should be reviewed with discrepancies corrected prior to surgery unless the patient's condition is a threat to life or limbs. Pre-existing conditions such as diabetes and liver or renal disease may be exacerbated by the stress of surgery,

increasing the risks of fluid and electrolyte imbalance. Diagnostic tests requiring the administration of contrast media can cause osmotic diuresis. Preoperative steroids, diuretics, enemas, laxatives, and dietary restrictions also cause shifts in fluids and electrolytes.

Patient Monitoring

Vital signs are a group of four main measurements of the body's life-sustaining functions. These measurements give information of the individual's overall health, give clues to possible diseases, and show progress and decline in recovery. The normal ranges of the vital signs vary with age, weight, gender, exercise capacity, and overall health of the individual. There are four primary vital signs. They are heart rate (pulse), blood pressure, respiratory rate, and body temperature. Surgery also requires monitoring of pulse oximetry. Multimodal monitors

TABLE 5-6 • ELECTROLYTES	
Electrolyte	**Information Regarding Supplements**
Sodium (NA^+) • Major electrolyte in extracellular fluid • Normal range 135-145 mEq/L	• Administer Isotonic IV therapy of 0.9% normal saline or ringer's lactate
Potassium (K^+) • Essential for maintaining electrical excitability of muscle, conduction of nerve impulses, and regulation of acid/base balance • Normal range 3-5 – 5.0 MEg/L	Potassium chloride (K-Dur) • Oral or IV administration • NEVER give IV push to avoid fatal hyperkalemia • Dilute potassium and give no more than 40 mEq/L per IV to prevent irritation of vein • Administer no faster than 10 mEq/L per IV • Concurrent use with potassium-sparing diuretics or ACE inhibitors can cause hyperkalemia • Administer Kayexalate for hyperkalemia with serum potassium • > 5.0 mEq/L
Calcium (Ca^{2+}) • Essential for normal musculoskeletal, neurological, and cardiovascular function • Normal range: 9.0-10.5 mEq/L	Calcium citrate (Citrical) • Calcium carbonate or calcium acetate • Oral or IV administration • Implement seizure precautions during administration and have emergency equipment on hand
Magnesium (Mg^{2+}) • Regulates skeletal muscle contraction and blood coagulation • Normal range: 1.3-2.1 mEq/L	Magnesium sulfate • Magnesium gluconate or magnesium hydroxide • Monitor BP, pulse and respirations with IV administration • Decreased/absent deep tendon reflexes indicates toxicity • Have injectable calcium gluconate on hand to counteract toxicity when giving magnesium sulfate via IV
Bicarbonate (HCO_3^-) • Maintains blood pH to prevent metabolic acidosis • Normal pH range: 7.35-7.45	Sodium bicarbonate • Given orally as an antacid or via IV • Numerous incompatibilities with IV form

Sources: What happens when your body is low on electrolytes? - Kokoro Nutrition (mykokoronutrition.com). https://mykokoronutrition.com/electrolytes-needed-for-runners/; A Clinician's Guide to Inpatient Electrolyte Replacement—tl;dr pharmacy (tldrpharmacy.com). https://www.tldrpharmacy.com/content/a-clinicians-guide-to-inpatient-electrolyte-replacement; Electrolytes—Enteral-and-Intravenous—Adult—Inpatient-171222.pdf (uwhealth.org). https://www.uwhealth.org/cckm/cpg/medications/Electrolytes—Enteral-and-Intravenous—Adult—Inpatient-171222.pdf; Adult Electrolyte Replacement Protocols. https://surgicalcriticalcare.net/Guidelines/Electrolyte%20replacement%20 2018.pdf; https://www.ausmed.com/learn/articles/normal-electrolyte-levels.

that measure and display the relevant vital signs are commonly integrated into the bedside monitors in ICUs and the anesthetic machines in operating rooms. These allow for continuous monitoring of a patient.

Heart rate or pulse is a measurement, recorded in beats per minute, of the rate in which the heart pumps blood through the arteries. On a monitor, heart rate will be displayed in conjunction with an electrocardiogram, which can alert healthcare providers to arrhythmias. The pulse should be evaluated for strength and arrhythmias as well as rate. The pulse rate may vary due to age, exercise, fitness level, disease, emotions, and medications. Radial, brachial, carotid, femoral, popliteal, dorsalis pedis, and posterior tibial pulses are among the most common areas measured and can be accomplished by applying slight pressure with the index and middle finger and counting for 60 seconds. Normal pulse ranges for children and adults are displayed in Tables 5-7 and 5-8.

Blood pressure is the pressure of blood pushing against the arterial walls. Blood pressure varies throughout the day, depending on body position, breathing rhythm, stress level, physical condition, medications you take, what you eat and drink, and the time of day. It is measured as systolic pressure over diastolic pressure (ventricular contraction/relaxation) and is measured in millimeters of mercury (mm Hg). The difference between the systolic and diastolic pressure is known as the pulse pressure which measures the force generated by the heart with each contraction. A blood pressure of less than 120/80 mm Hg is considered within normal range. High blood pressure, hypertension, puts patients at risk for heart attack, stroke, and chronic kidney disease. Some contributing risk factors for hypertension are high salt intake or salt sensitivity, smoking, being overweight or obesity, lack of physical activity, too much of alcohol consumption, stress, being above age 40, and genetics. Blood pressure greater than 140/90 mm Hg on average (measured several times over several days) is defined as hypertension. Low blood pressure, hypotension, is a blood pressure measurement of 90/60 mm Hg or less. Hypotension can be caused by medications, pregnancy, heart problems, endocrine problems, dehydration, blood loss, septicemia, anaphylaxis, and a lack of nutrients in your diet. Even moderate forms of low blood pressure can cause dizziness, weakness, fainting, and a risk of injury from falls. Severely low blood pressure can deprive your body of enough oxygen to carry out its functions, leading to damage to your heart and brain.

TABLE 5-7 • NORMAL VITAL SIGNS BY AGE

Age	Heart Rate/Min	Respirations/Min	Systolic Blood Pressure	Weight in Kilos	Weight in Pounds
Newborn	120-160	30-50	50-70	2-3	4.5-7
Infant (1-12 months)	80-140	20-30	70-100	4-10	9-22
Toddler (1-3 years)	80-130	20-30	80-110	10-14	22-31
Pre-schooler (3-5 years)	80-120	20-30	80-110	14-18	31-40
School-age (6-12 years)	70-110	20-30	80-120	20-42	41-92
Adolescent (13+ years)	55-105	12-20	110-120	>50	>110

TABLE 5-8 • RESTING HEART RATE CHARTS FOR MEN AND WOMEN

Resting Heart Rate Chart for Men							
Age	Athlete	Excellent	Good	Above Average	Average	Below Average	Poor
18-25	45-55	56-61	62-65	66-69	70-73	74-81	82+
26-35	49-54	55-61	62-65	66-70	71-74	75-81	82+
36-45	50-56	57-62	63-66	67-70	71-75	76-82	83+
46-55	50-57	58-63	64-67	68-71	72-76	77-83	84+
56-65	51-56	57-61	62-67	68-71	72-75	76-81	82+
65+	50-55	56-61	62-65	66-69	70-73	74-79	80+
Resting Heart Rate Chart for Women							
18-25	54-60	61-65	66-69	70-73	74-78	79-84	85+
26-35	54-59	60-64	65-68	69-72	73-76	77-82	83+
36-45	54-59	60-64	65-68	70-73	74-78	79-84	85+
46-55	54-60	61-65	66-69	70-73	74-77	78-83	84+
56-65	54-59	60-64	65-68	69-73	74-77	78-83	84+
65+	54-59	60-64	65-68	69-72	73-76	77-84	84+

Respiratory rate is defined as the number of breaths taken per minute. A normal respiratory rate for adults is 12 to 20 breaths per minute. The normal respiratory rate for children varies by age (see Table 5-7). Respiration is the metabolic process of taking in oxygen and releasing carbon dioxide. Oxygen is critical for cellular metabolism and carbon dioxide is crucial for maintaining adequate pH levels. In response to blood gas changes, the pulmonary system adapts by adjusting breathing patterns to meet the body's metabolic demand. The respiratory control system drives respiratory cycles which consist of three components: the neural central control, sensory input, and muscular effect. The rate and strength in which the diaphragm contracts depend heavily on the pacemaker cells in the brainstem. The sensory input sends signals to the brain to adjust respiratory patterns to meet metabolic demands. The muscular system moves the lungs in accordance with signal inputs. Factors affecting respiratory rate include stroke, narcotics, alcohol, hypothyroidism, sleep apnea, COPD, heart conditions, drug overdose, infections, anxiety and panic attacks, and transient tachypnea. Low respiratory rate can cause low blood oxygen, acidosis, and respiratory failure. Tachypnea may occur with dyspnea, cyanosis, and sucking in of the chest muscles with breathing (retracting). Treatment of respiratory problems depends primarily on determining the underlying cause.

Maintaining patient normothermia is a critical element in preventing surgical site infections and other complications such as metabolic acidosis, cardiovascular effects, increased respiratory distress, and surgical bleeding. Normal core body temperature, normothermia, in a typical adult, ranges from 97.7°F to 99.5°F (36.5°C–37.5°C). Babies and children range from 95.9°F to 99.8°F (35.5°C–37.7°C). Hypothermia in surgery can be intentional or unintentional. Hypothermia is a core body temperature below 35°C (95°F). Unintentional hypothermia can cause discomfort, cardiac events, adrenergic stimulation, impaired platelet function, altered drug metabolism, and impaired wound healing. Children under 2 years of age, the elderly, and burn patients tend to be the most vulnerable. Other contributing risk factors include co-morbidities, length of surgery, cachexia, fluid shifts, cold irrigating and intravenous solutions, and general and regional anesthesia. Anesthetic agents interfere with shivering mechanisms and autonomic reflexes that would ordinarily autoregulate body temperature. Vasodilation from anesthetic agents enhances heat transfer from the core to the periphery where heat is easily lost to the environment. The use of cold, unhumidified inhalation gases also promotes hypothermia. Many things can be done to help prevent hypothermia in the perioperative patient. Such things include warming the room, using forced air blankets, using warming lights, lowering fresh-gas flow rates, using a heat/moisture exchanger, and using blood, intravenous, and irrigation fluid warmers.

Hyperthermia, a body temperature greater than 37.5°C to 38.3°C (99.5°F–100.9°F), occurs when the body's heat-regulating mechanisms do not work effectively, mainly due to environmental conditions. Hyperthermia occurs when the body temperature rises without a change in the heat control centers.

Body temperatures above 40°C (104°F) can be life-threatening. This is mainly due to heat stroke or adverse drug reactions. Malignant hyperthermia is a rare complication of some types of general anesthesia using inhalation agents and succinylcholine. It begins with a hypermetabolic condition in the skeletal muscle cells that involve altered mechanisms of calcium function in the cells. Symptoms include muscle rigidity, hypercarbia, tachypnea, tachycardia, hypoxia, metabolic and respiratory acidosis, cardiac dysrhythmias, and body temperature elevation occurring at a rate of 1°C to 2°C every 5 minutes. Complications can include rhabdomyolysis, hyperkalemia, and organ failure. Treatment of malignant hyperthermia includes administration of dantrolene, diuretics, and medication to correct acidosis, electrolyte imbalance, and cardiac dysrhythmias, cooling the patient, monitoring fluid intake and output (I&O), and hyperventilating the patient. Patients known or suspected to have malignant hyperthermia can be anesthetized safely if appropriate precautions are taken. Patients suspected of having malignant hyperthermia should be sent for muscle biopsy prior to receiving anesthesia.

Oximetry is a procedure for measuring the concentration of oxygen in the blood using a probe attached to the fingers, toes, or earlobes. Oximeters are commonly called pulse oximeters because they respond only to pulsations, such as those in pulsating capillaries. Pulse oximetry is an undisputable standard of care in clinical monitoring. It combines a spectrometer to detect hypoxemia with a plethysmograph for the diagnosis, monitoring, and follow-up of cardiovascular diseases. A pulse oximeter works by passing a beam of red and infrared light through a pulsating capillary bed. The ratio of red to infrared blood light transmitted gives a measure of the oxygen saturation of the blood.

The oximeter works on the principle that the oxygenated blood is a brighter color of red than the deoxygenated blood, which is darker. First, the oximeter measures the sum of the intensity of both shades of red, representing the fractions of the blood with and without oxygen. The oximeter detects the pulse, and then subtracts the intensity of color detected when the pulse is absent. The remaining intensity of color represents only the oxygenated red blood. This is displayed on the patient monitor as a percentage of oxygen saturation in the blood. The pulse oximeter is extremely useful for assessing respiratory and circulatory status and for monitoring the ventilated patients. On the one hand, the key spectrography-derived function of pulse oximetry is to evaluate a patient's gas exchange by continuously and noninvasively measuring arterial hemoglobin saturation (SpO_2). This information helps to maintain patients above the hypoxemic levels, leading to appropriate ventilator settings and inspired oxygen fractions. On the other hand, the photoplethysmography-derived oximeter function has barely been used in monitoring hemodynamics in mechanically-ventilated patients. Analysis of the photoplethysmography curve provides useful real-time and noninvasive information about the interaction of heart and lungs during positive pressure ventilation. Normal pulse oximeter readings usually range from 95% to 100%. Values under 90% are considered low and require supplemental oxygen. Exceptions include babies and children with certain congenital heart defects.

It may be necessary to monitor other pressures and saturations depending on the patient's medical condition or type of surgery being performed. These include peripheral arterial pressure, pulmonary artery pressure, central venous pressure, and cerebral oximetry. All critically ill patients need monitoring of intravascular volume status. I&O, to include drain output, must regularly be observed and recorded. Invasive peripheral arterial pressure monitoring is done by inserting a cannula most commonly into the radial or femoral artery to directly measure blood pressure. The cannula is connected to an electronic transducer which can record beat-to-beat pressure changes. Blood pressure monitoring can be done accurately and continuously over long periods. Blood samples can also be obtained directly from the arterial line. Pulmonary artery (PA) pressure monitoring is measuring the pressure in the pulmonary artery leading to the lungs. It allows for indirect measurement of left heart pressures and collects the information needed to calculate cardiac output and resistance. The PA catheter assesses all three components of stroke volume: preload, afterload, and contractility. It is used to guide the management of the patient with heart and lung disease and shock of all types, and to monitor hemodynamic pressures during fluid resuscitation and inotropic, vasoconstrictor, and vasodilator drug infusion therapy. Normal pulmonary artery pressure is 8 to 20 mm Hg at rest. Central venous pressure (CVP) is a measure of the blood pressure in the vena cava, near the right atrium of the heart. CVP is often a good approximation of right atrial pressure. CVP monitoring helps to assess cardiac function, evaluate venous return to the heart, and indirectly gauge how well the heart is pumping. The central venous (CV) catheter also provides access to a large vessel for rapid, high-volume fluid administration and allows frequent blood withdrawal for laboratory samples. Normal CVP ranges from 5 to 10 cmH$_2$O or 2 to 6 mm Hg. Cerebral oximeters consist of a monitor that is connected to oximeter probes which are attached to the patient's forehead. Cerebral oximeters enable continuous non-invasive monitoring of cerebral oxygenation. Cerebral oximeters utilize similar physical principles to pulse oximeters. Cerebral oximetry differs from pulse oximetry in that tissue sampling represents primarily (70%-75%) venous, and less (20%-25%) arterial blood. Cerebral oximetry monitoring is also not dependent upon pulsatile flow. Baseline cerebral oximetry values should be obtained before induction of anesthesia. Normal values range from 60% to 80%. Lower values of 55% to 60% are not considered abnormal in some cardiac patients. Cerebral oxygenation is dependent upon adequate cerebral blood flow and oxygen content. Factors affecting either of these will result in a reduction in cerebral oxygenation. Patients undergoing carotid artery and/or cardiac surgery are at risk of adverse perioperative neurological events. Cerebral oximetry monitoring can be used to help reduce the incidence of these devastating events.

Accurate assessment of intravascular volume remains one of the most challenging and important tasks for clinicians. Intravascular volume status refers to the volume of blood in a patient's circulatory system and is essentially the blood plasma component of the overall volume status of the body, which otherwise includes both intracellular fluid and extracellular fluid. Signs of intravascular volume depletion, hypovolemia, include a fast pulse, infrequent and low-volume urination, dry mucous membranes, poor capillary refill, decreased skin turgor, a weak pulse, orthostatic hypotension, and cool extremities. The most common causes of hypovolemia are diarrhea, vomiting, overuse of diuretics, trauma or disease of the kidney, bleeding, burns, and any causes of edema such as congestive heart failure and liver failure. The most indicative sign of intravascular volume overload is increased venous pressure. Intravascular volume overload can occur during surgery if water rather than isotonic saline is used to wash the incision. It can also occur if there is inadequate urination associated with certain kidney diseases. Monitoring of central pressures and cardiac output are combined to assess the patient's intravascular volume and determine clinical interventions such as fluid or diuretic administration.

It is important to measure the patient's I&O to determine fluid and electrolyte (sodium) gains and losses, and loss of plasma proteins. Excess fluid volume increases isotonic fluid retention. Isotonic overhydration causes circulatory overload and interstitial edema in patients with poor cardiac function, congestive heart failure (CHF), and pulmonary edema. Hypertonic overhydration, though rare, occurs with too much ingestion of sodium, rapid infusion of hypertonic saline, and unmonitored sodium bicarbonate therapy. Hypotonic overhydration (water intoxication) and electrolyte imbalances occur with early renal failure, CHF, syndrome of inadequate antidiuretic hormone secretion (SIADH), unmonitored IV fluid therapy, using hypotonic IV fluids to replace isotonic fluid loss, and irrigating wounds and body cavities with hypotonic fluids.

Deficient fluid volume decreases intravascular, interstitial, and/or intracellular fluid. This refers to dehydration, water loss alone without change in sodium. Isotonic dehydration, hypovolemia, is the most common type of dehydration with water loss that causes a decrease in circulating blood volume and inadequate tissue perfusion. It occurs with vomiting, diarrhea, GI suctioning, and actively draining GI drainage tubes. Conditions that produce polyuria such as hyperglycemia and patients getting hyperosmolar tube feeding are also at risk for hypovolemia. Fever increases urine output as well as insensible fluid loss through the lungs due to hyperpnea. Other conditions that produce insensible fluid losses include sweating, and third spacing. Third spacing is the sequestration and trapping of fluid from the vascular space to another portion of the body such as the pleura, peritoneum, pericardium, joints, bowels, and interstitial spaces after burns or trauma. This fluid for all intents and purposes is considered lost and cannot be directly measured. Third spacing can cause an increase in body weight, intestinal obstruction, ascites, peritonitis, pancreatitis, pericarditis, and hemothorax.

In hypertonic dehydration, more water than electrolytes is lost. This occurs with excessive sweating, hyperventilation, ketoacidosis, prolonged fevers, uncontrolled diarrhea, early stage of renal failure, and diabetes insipidus. In hypotonic dehydration, more electrolytes than water are lost. This occurs with chronic illness, over-infusing too much hypotonic IV fluid, renal failure, and chronic malnutrition. Accurate measurement and documentation of I&Os are important because medications, intravenous and fluid administration, dietary decisions, and tube feeding physician orders are based on I&O 24-hour totals. The numbers provide real-time data that guides daily care of the patient.

Bispectral index (BIS) monitoring monitors the depth of anesthesia. Titrating anesthetic agents to a specific bispectral index during general anesthesia allows the anesthetist to adjust the amount of anesthetic agent to the needs of the patient, resulting in a faster emergence from anesthesia. It is a measure of the level of consciousness by algorithmic analysis of a patient's electroencephalogram during general anesthesia. The BIS monitor provides a number, which ranges from 0 (equivalent to EEG silence) to 100 (equivalent to fully awake and alert). A BIS value between 40 and 60 indicates an appropriate level for general anesthesia. The bispectral index is prone to artifacts. Its numbers cannot be relied upon in all situations, including brain death, circulatory arrest, or hypothermia.

Electrophysiologic monitoring, or neuromonitoring, can be used during surgery to assess the functional integrity of the brain, brainstem, spinal cord, or peripheral and cranial nerves. The goal of monitoring is to alert the surgeon and anesthesiologist to impending injury in order to prevent permanent damage. Neuromonitoring can include the recording of spontaneous activity (electroencephalogram and spontaneous electromyogram) or evoked response to stimulus (somatosensory evoked potentials, motor evoked potentials, triggered electromyography, and brainstem auditory evoked potentials). Multiple techniques are used together in order to increase the utility of monitoring and to overcome the limitations of individual techniques. Electroencephalography (EEG), electrocorticography (ECoG), electromyography (EMG), somatosensory evoked potentials (SSEPs), brainstem auditory evoked potentials (BAEPs), and motor evoked potentials (MEPs) are electrophysiologic monitoring techniques that are commonly used in the operating room to improve surgical decision-making and possibly reduce neurologic complications.

Specimen Handling

Accurate specimen handling requires effective communication, minimized distractions, and awareness of the potential for errors. Errors in specimen handling can lead to inaccurate or incomplete diagnosis and the need for additional procedures or unnecessary surgery. In a survey commissioned by the Association of Directors of Anatomic and Surgical pathology, 53% of respondents indicated that errors in surgical pathology occur before the specimen reaches the laboratory for examination. Examples of these errors include pathology requests/orders, patient identification, specimen identification, no specimen in the container, collection and handling methods, wrong preservatives, and transport methods. Errors in specimen management may be classified as a near miss, adverse event, or sentinel event. Specimen errors may be attributed to poor communication, fatigue, inadequate education/competency, the environment, equipment failure, and inadequate policies and procedures. However, most errors are a result of human errors. Double checking the steps in specimen management has the potential to significantly reduce errors.

Specimen collection refers to the act of obtaining a biopsy or specimen, whereas specimen handling involves holding, securing, moving, and manipulating the specimen. Proper specimen handling is crucial to the safe outcome of the patient's surgical experience. Blood, body fluids, soft tissue to include lymph nodes, organs, bone, and foreign bodies are among the most common handled specimens. Specimens should be handled in a manner that preserves and protects the integrity of the specimen. Facility policies and procedures should be followed when handling radioactive specimens and specimens collected for forensic analysis.

Collected specimens should be passed off the sterile field as soon as possible to reduce the potential for the integrity of the specimen to be compromised or the specimen to be lost. Specimens should be kept moist until they are transferred from the sterile field, as air exposure can lead to tissue desiccation. Specimens should never be crushed, twisted, or otherwise damaged. Maintaining the cellular and molecular structure of specimen important for complete and accurate diagnosis. If preservatives cannot be added in a timely manner, the specimen should be placed in a sterile basin and kept moist with sterile saline or wrapped in saline-dampened sponges until the specimen can be properly placed in preservatives. Certain biopsies may need special handling and should be confirmed with the surgeon and pathology. All unpreserved specimens should be transported to the pathology laboratory as soon as possible and refrigerated until placed into appropriate preservative. Some specimens may be "tagged" or marked with sutures or markers in order to orient the specimen. Specimens transferred between surgical team members should be verbally identified and verified using the "write down, read back" method. Sterile technique and standard precautions should always be used when transferring specimens.

Containing specimens in a manner that prevents exposure of personnel to blood, body fluids, and other infectious materials is a regulatory requirement. Regulations also require containers to be labeled to communicate chemical preservatives and biohazard information. Containers must be leakproof, puncture-resistant, and of the correct size and type to fully secure the specimen and preservative fluids. Specimen containers may be sterile or clean, depending on the specimen type and collection requirements. Specimens should be labeled with a facility sticker containing unique patient identifiers, the source of the specimen including laterality, type of tissue, clinical diagnosis, and additional pertinent information such as location of suture tags. Labels should be placed on the container, not the lid.

Confirmation and identification of the surgical specimens should take place during the debriefing. This should include visual confirmation that specimens are in the containers, verification of correct patient information and specimen labeling, and confirmation of the use of preservatives or chemical additives for tissue preservation. Formalin is a commonly used combustible liquid containing formaldehyde, a hazardous substance. Formaldehyde should be stored in a well-ventilated location with posted signs warning of use, and eyewash stations available in the immediate area. Care must be taken to avoid exposure to skin and the respiratory tract. Gloves, eye shields, and masks should be worn when handling formaldehyde.

A frozen section is used when immediate tissue or malignancy identification is needed. A frozen section consists of specimens being quickly frozen, sliced, stained, and examined under a microscope. A specimen sent for frozen section is never placed in saline or formalin, but should be placed in a sterile, dry specimen container. The results of the examination are communicated to the surgeon intraoperatively. Often the pathologist will communicate with the surgeon directly; however, the circulating nurse may need to communicate findings to the surgeon. In this instance, it is considered a critical test result and the nurse should "read back" the results to the pathologist to verify correct communication of the results.

Postoperative Patient Care

As discussed previously, postoperative patient care begins when the patient arrives in the PACU or ICU. Immediate assessment begins with the adequacy of the ABCs. Once the ABCs are accessed, a hand-off report is given. Once the PACU nurse accepts the patient a more thorough assessment can be performed. Respiratory assessment includes rate, rhythm, auscultation of breath sounds, and oxygen saturation. Cardiovascular assessment includes monitoring heart rate and rhythm, monitoring body temperature, and checking peripheral pulses. Neurologic function is assessed by observation and patient participation. Is the patient conscious and oriented? Do they follow commands? Can they move all extremities and lift the head? Are there deviations from the preoperative status? Is the patient unconscious or exhibiting and altered levels of consciousness? These include confusion, delirium, lethargy, obtundation, stupor and coma. Renal function is assessed by the measurement of I&Os. The surgical site is assessed for drainage and bleeding. The patient is also assessed for signs and symptoms of pain.

Life-threatening changes can occur rapidly in the immediate postoperative period. Patients are vulnerable to several post-anesthetic complications. Preservation of the patient requires prompt recognition and treatment of the complications. Respiratory complications include airway obstruction, laryngospasm, and bronchospasm. Treatment of respiratory complications includes encouraging deep breathing, using supplemental oxygen, using a chin lift or jaw thrust, using the recovery position, positive pressure ventilation, medication therapy, and inserting an artificial airway. Cardiovascular complications include hypo/hypertension, hypovolemia, and dysrhythmias. Postoperative hypotension is usually the result of hypovolemia and can be treated with fluid and/or blood replacement. Hypertension should be treated with antihypertensive drugs. Most postoperative cardiac dysrhythmias have causes unrelated to myocardial infarction such as hypovolemia, hypoxemia, and pain. Common dysrhythmias include sinus tachycardia, sinus bradycardia, and pre-ventricular contractions (PVCs). Treatment includes identifying and resolving the underlying cause and administering anti-dysrhythmia drugs. Other postoperative complications include hypo/hyperthermia, disturbed thought processes, nausea and vomiting, aspiration, and acute pain.

Pain control is of utmost importance in the postoperative patient and should be assessed on admission to the PACU or ICU and reassessed at frequent intervals. Pain should be assessed every 2 hours during the first postoperative day. If pain is poorly controlled, the frequency of assessments should increase. It is important to remember that not all patients respond to pain in the same manner. Patients of different cultures respond to and express pain in different ways. The most reliable indicator of the existence and intensity of pain is the patient's self-report. Clinicians should never allow their opinions to drive practice. Even with severe pain, physiologic and behavioral adaptations can lead to periods of minimal to no pain. There is no predetermined opioid dose that is effective for all patients. Pain is a complication or risk of surgery, not a consequence. Untreated or delayed pain control can delay healing and contribute to life-threatening complications.

Opioids (narcotics) are a class of drugs that include the illegal drug heroin, synthetic opioids such as fentanyl, and pain relievers available legally by prescription, such as oxycodone, hydrocodone, codeine, morphine, and many others. Opioids are effective for the treatment of acute pain following surgery. Opioids are frequently the treatment of choice for immediate relief of moderate-to-severe acute pain. A clear risk of prolonged opioid use exists when opioid analgesics are initiated for an acute pain management following surgery or trauma. Multimodal pain control helps reduce this risk.

Multimodal pain control employs multiple classes of pain medications or therapies, working with different mechanisms of action, to treat acute pain instead of relying on opioids alone. Opioids continue to be important in pain management, but they should be combined with other classes of medications to help relieve postoperative pain. These include:

1. Non-steroidal anti-inflammatory drugs (NSAIDs): Examples include ibuprofen, diclofenac, ketorolac, celecoxib, nabumetone. NSAIDs act on the prostaglandin system peripherally and work to decrease inflammation. Using NSAIDs in combination with opiates can reduce opioid requirements by 20% to 40%.

2. Ketamine: When administered in low dose, ketamine acts on the N-methyl-D-aspartate receptors in the central nerve system to decrease acute pain and hyperalgesia.

3. Acetaminophen: Acetaminophen acts on central prostaglandin synthesis and provides pain relief through multiple mechanisms.

4. Gabapentinoids: Examples include gabapentin and pregabalin. These medications are membrane stabilizers that essentially decrease nerve firing.

5. Regional block: The ASA strongly recommends the use of target-specific local anesthetic applications in the form of regional analgesic techniques as part of the multimodal analgesic protocol whenever possible.

6. Local anesthetics: Injection of local anesthetic in or around the surgical site by the surgeon is one example. Examples include lidocaine, bupivacaine, ropivacaine, polocaine, and many others. The use of bupivacaine liposome injectable suspensions and BKK (bupivacaine, ketorolac, and ketamine) allows for long-acting analgesia.

Types of regional blocks include spinal anesthesia, epidural anesthesia, and peripheral nerve blocks. Local anesthetic solution is given as close to the nerve as possible without entering the nerve itself. The procedure blocks the nerves, ensuring pain control during and immediately after surgery. Depending on the local anesthetic used, the effects of the block can last even longer, ranging from hours to days. This can provide pain relief as well as blocking motor function. Locating nerves is made easier by using a nerve stimulator or a portable ultrasound device. Single injections or catheters may be used, depending on the purpose of the nerve block.

Spinal anesthesia is a form of neuraxial regional anesthesia involving the injection of a local anesthetic or opioid into the subarachnoid space, generally through a fine needle. It is a safe and effective form of anesthesia commonly used in surgeries involving the lower extremities and surgeries below the umbilicus. The local anesthetic or opioid injected into the cerebrospinal fluid provides anesthesia, analgesia, and motor and sensory blockade. Contraindications to spinal anesthesia are rare, but include infection at the injection site, bleeding disorders, severe aortic stenosis, increased intracranial pressure, space-occupying lesions of the brain, anatomic disorders of the spine, hypovolemia, Ehlers-Danlos Syndrome, and other disorders causing resistance to local anesthesia. Complications from spinal anesthesia range from mild to severe and include mild hypotension, bradycardia, nausea and vomiting, transient neurological symptoms, urinary retention, post-spinal headache, nerve injuries, cardiac arrest, severe hypotension, spinal epidural hematoma, epidural abscess, and infection.

Epidural anesthesia is a form of neuraxial regional anesthesia involving the injection of a local anesthetic through a catheter placed into the epidural space. Differences between spinal and epidural anesthesia are as follows:

1. A spinal delivers drug to the subarachnoid space and into the cerebrospinal fluid, allowing it to act on the spinal cord directly. An epidural delivers drugs outside the dura and has its main effect on nerve roots leaving the dura at the level of the epidural.

2. A spinal gives a profound block of all motor and sensory functions below the level of injection, whereas an epidural blocks a band of nerve roots around the site of injection, with normal function above, and close-to-normal function below the levels blocked.

3. The injected dose for an epidural is larger, being about 10 to 20 mL compared to 1.5 to 3.5 mL in a spinal.

4. In an epidural, an indwelling catheter is placed that allows for redosing injections, while a spinal is almost always a one-shot only. Therefore, spinal anesthesia is more often used for shorter procedures relative to procedures which require epidural anesthesia.

5. The onset of analgesia is approximately 25 to 30 minutes in an epidural, while it is approximately 5 minutes in a spinal.

6. An epidural may be given at a cervical, thoracic, or lumbar site, while a spinal must be injected below L2 to avoid piercing the spinal cord.

Peripheral nerve blocks are injections of local anesthesia that interrupt the signals traveling along a nerve for the purpose of pain relief. Peripheral nerve blocks can be performed in several locations on the body and can provide analgesia lasting hours to days depending on the medications injected.

The National Center for Complementary and Alternative Medicine (NCCAM) categorized complementary and alternative medicine (CAM) into five categories. Alternative medical systems are based on alternative tradition and may aid in decreasing anxiety and the perception of pain. Many of these therapies are based on cultural, spiritual, and religious beliefs. Examples include homeopathic medicine (based on the principle that like cures like) and naturopathic medicine (based on the belief that disease is a manifestation of alterations to the body's natural healing process). Mind and body interventions include cognitive behavioral approaches, meditation, hypnosis, prayer, mental healing, and art therapy. Biologically based therapies include biologically and naturally based practices and products. Examples are herbal, orthomolecular, and dietary-based treatments. Manipulative and body-based methods are based on the movement and manipulation of the body. Examples include chiropractic, osteopathic, and massage therapies. Energy therapies are categorized into biofield therapies (focuses on fields believed to originate within the body) and electromagnetic fields (those that originate from other sources).

CAM is finding its place in surgery as many progressive medical centers embrace a holistic patient focus. Therapeutic touch (TT) is the interpretation of several ancient healing modalities. It consists of learned skills in the manipulation of energies. Medical hypnotherapy allows a patient to explore emotions without judgment of those feelings. Imagery is used by the autonomic nervous system (controls unconscious body functions) as a primary mode of communication. Guided imagery in the form of tapes and/or monotone speech can help decrease anxiety and pain perception, increase sense of control, and allow for faster recovery. Music is used in surgery to decrease anxiety and discomfort. Psychoneuroimmunology seeks to analyze the relationship between the brain and the immune system. An example is a reduction in perioperative stress improving the immune system functions. Herbal and botanical products are commonly used in today's society. Unfortunately, use of these products is not always conveyed to the healthcare providers. Use of herbal supplements can produce coagulation interactions, sedative interactions, and cardiovascular interactions. Healthcare providers can use a blend of traditional and nontraditional therapies to enhance the overall patient experience.

Bibliography

AORN. *2020 Guidelines for Perioperative Practice*. Denver, CO: AORN, Inc; 2020.

BELLEZA M. Fluid and Electrolytes, Acid-Base Balance. *Nurseslabs*. https://nurseslabs.com/fluid-and-electrolytes/. Accessed May 16, 2023.

CT Scan. Wikipedia. https://en.wikipedia.org/wiki/CT_scan. Accessed May 16, 2023.

History and Physical—Update Requirements. 2020. The Joint Commission. http://www.jointcommission.org/standards/standard-faqs/critical-access-hospital/provision-of-care-treatment-and-services-pc/000002112/.

Magnetic Resonance Imaging. Wikipedia. https://en.wikipedia.org/wiki/Magnetic_resonance_imaging. Accessed May 16, 2023.

Makary MA, Epstein J, Pronovost PJ, Millman EA, Hartmann EC, Freischlag JA. (2007). Surgical specimen identification errors: A new measure of quality in surgical care. *Surgery*. 2007;141(4):450-455.

Medical Dictionary. 2009. https://medical-dictionary.thefreedictionary.com/risk+stratification. Accessed May 16, 2023.

Neuromonitoring in Surgery and Anesthesia. UpToDate. 2020. https://www.uptodate/contents/neuromonitoring-in-surgery-and-anesthesia#!

Perioperative. (n.d.) Farlex Partner Medical Dictionary. 2012. https://medical-dictionary.thefreedictionary.com/perioperative. Accessed May 16, 2023.

Rothrock JC. *Alexander's Care of the Patient in Surgery*, 13th ed. St Louis, MO: Mosby/Elsevier; 2007.

Spinal Anaesthesia. Wikipedia. https://en.wikipedia.org/wiki/Spinal_anaesthesia. Accessed May 16, 2023.

Standard of Practice for Handling and Care of Surgical Specimens. AST. http://www.ast.org/uploadedFiles/Main_Site/Content/About_Us/Standard_Handling_Care_Surgical_Specimens.pdf#:~:text=AST%20developed%20the%20Standards%20of%20Practice%20to%20support,the%20perioperative%20setting%20can%20use%20to%20develop%20and. Accessed May 16, 2023.

The History and Physical. 2020. https://www.medschool.lsuhsc.edu/medical_education/undergraduate/spm/SPM_100/documents/HistoryandPhysical_000.pdf. Accessed May 16, 2023.

The Right Plasma Volume Expander. *Nursing Times*. 2001. https://www.nursingtimes.net/clinical-archive/tissue-viability/the-right-plasma-volume-expander-05-07-2001/. Accessed May 16, 2023.

6

Pharmacology and Anesthesia Principles

Libby McNaron

DISCUSSED IN THIS CHAPTER

1. Basic pharmacology concepts.
2. Perioperative principles of patient assessment.
3. Goals, risks and adverse effects of anesthesia.
4. Principles of local anesthetic agents.

INTRODUCTION TO PHARMACOLOGY

History of Pharmacology

Pharmacology originated in the 19th century, and is the study of the origin, history, uses, and properties of drugs. A drug is a substance that is used to treat, cure, or prevent a disease. It is also used to enhance a component of physical or mental health.

The medicinal chemist creates the compound. Pharmacologists are scientists who develop, test, and evaluate new drugs regarding the physiological activity. However, a pharmacist who is a medical professional dispenses drugs. The Father of Modern Pharmacology is Oswald Schmiedeberg who was a Baltic German Pharmacologist that studied the measurement of chloroform, later publishing a classic pharmacology textbook and training most of the men who became professors. Once a promising drug compound's therapeutic effect is identified, then toxicologists, microbiologists, or clinicians will further investigate for safe usage and administration.

The role of the Food and Drug Administration (FDA) in drug development as a consumer watchdog is primarily filled by the Center for Drug Evaluation and Research. They employ their own team of physicians, statisticians, chemists, and pharmacologists among other scientists to evaluate the efficacy and safety of the drug by reviewing the drug's benefits versus known risks and conducting some limited research regarding quality, safety, and effectiveness. Human Research is of special interest and requires strict adherence to human subject protection (HSP) through the agency's bioresearch monitoring program (BIMO). This process could be quite lengthy, and the United States lagged in the approval process.

The process of drug discovery and development begins with the drug discovery and preclinical trials (3-6 years), followed by clinical trials which can take another 6 to 7 years in phase 1 (20-100 volunteers), phase 2 (100-500 volunteers), and finally phase 3 (1000-5000 volunteers) are using a process known as double-blind studies. This process randomizes the trials so that neither the patient nor the physician knows who is receiving a control placebo (non-treatment) or the actual drug to prevent any possibility of bias regarding the results reported. Then, it is sent to the FDA which could take from 6 months to 2 years. Finally, approval leads to large-scale manufacturing and the final phase 4 postmarketing surveillance. In 1992, the Prescription Drug User Fee Act (PDUFA) authorized the collection of fees from the pharmaceutical industry to facilitate this process so that performance benchmarks were met thereby speeding up the process. It continues today along with other acts to facilitate faster development and response times such as the 2020 COVID-19 pandemic response. The FDA provides a Health

Professional Section that provides information on product safety, product recalls, adverse event/problem reporting, and other resources. The FDA-approved *Drug Products with Therapeutic Equivalence Evaluations* book commonly known as THE ORANGE BOOK identifies products approved on an annual basis.

Pharmacology has two major branches known as pharmacokinetics and pharmacodynamics. Pharmacokinetics is concerned with the absorption of drugs via capillary action or directly intravenous, distribution by the circulatory system, metabolism by the liver, and excretion by the kidneys—basically, what the body does to a drug after it is administered. While pharmacodynamics is concerned with the drug's mechanism of action—what are the molecular, biochemical, and physiological effects on the target tissue. The mechanisms of action (MOA) refer to the specific biochemical interaction through which the drug produces the pharmacological effect. Currently, developing research and knowledge of cell receptors is leading to new drugs that inhibit, treat, or cure.

Finally, to understand your patient, you need to understand that patients can develop allergies to drugs at any time even though they may have taken them before or over a long period of time. One of two reactions can lead to an immediate (anaphylactic) reaction causing respiratory or cardiovascular distress or a delayed reaction. In addition, tachyphylaxis is an acute drug tolerance to a medication or similar medication (cross-tolerance) and over time may require a higher dose to achieve the same response.

Medications taken should be reviewed for potential interactions. Medications such as those prescribed by the surgeon, certain foods ingested, or alternative remedies such as herbal medications, home remedies, or other over-the-counter (OTC) medications may produce any one or a combination of the following events: (1) therapeutic effect which produces a desired improvement in the condition or prevents a poor outcome; (2) side effect which is mildly harmful such as nausea or vomiting but does not hinder the intended therapeutic effect; (3) adverse effect which can hinder treatment and lead to complications; (4) additive effects which usually allows the two similar drugs given to produce an overall improvement (1 + 1 = 2 times as good); and (5) potentiation when a second drug is given that enhances the action of the therapeutic drug but no additional action (1 + 0= 3), or synergistic effects when an additional drug is added that results in a much better effect of both drugs (1 +1= 3). Careful attention should be given to analyze all the medications or routine supplements for potential drug and food interactions which can affect the outcome. For example, certain herbal drugs can affect the patient's ability to clot such as St. John's Wort, Garlic, Ginger, Ginkgo Biloba, Ginseng, Omega-3-fatty acid (high dose), and Vitamin E (high dose). Some can work against the medications prescribed such as CoQ10 which interferes with warfarin (Coumadin) leading to blood clots. Others are very

dangerous for the liver since it is responsible such as acetaminophen (Tylenol), other nonsteroidal anti-inflammatory drugs (NSAIDs), amoxicillin/clavulante, Dilantin (phenytoin), and amiodarone, among others.

PHARMACOLOGY BASICS

Review of Basic Pharmacology Concepts

Drug Sources. The major drug sources include natural (pharmacognosy), synthetic (man-made/altered), or biotechnology engineered. Researchers are ready to investigate local or home remedies for new medications that can be explored. Knowledge over the last few centuries that has been lost or not recognized for its importance can lead to the next breakthrough treatment.

Natural sources include plants, animals, and minerals. Laboratory chemical synthesis includes synthetics which are chemically created in the lab and semi-synthetics which are designed from altered natural resources. The last major source relies on DNA biotechnology and recombinant DNA technology.

Plant-sourced medications include atropine sulfate from belladonna which dilates eyes, increases heart rate, and is a treatment for toxic nerve gases; morphine sulfate from opium seeds that is used as an analgesic; digitalis from purple foxglove which is used for the treatment of congestive heart failure as a cardiotonic; and Taxol (paclitaxel) from Taxus baccata which is used to treat breast cancer.

Animal drug sources include bovine (cattle), porcine (hogs), and equine (horses) sources. These can include such medications as thrombin (thrombogen) as a bovine topical hemostatic, proloid (thyroglobulin) as a porcine thyroid hormone replacement, and Premarin (conjugated estrogen) which is an equine replacement (urine of pregnant horses).

Mineral drug sources include antacids made from calcium (tums) or magnesium (Mylanta) and silver found in silver sulfadiazine (Silvadene) used in the treatment of burns.

Laboratory chemical synthesis includes both synthetic Demerol (meperidine) and semi-synthetics such as an altered natural penicillin called amoxicillin.

Biotechnology recombinant DNA technology can include genetically altered bacteria such as *E. coli* to produce insulin, nutropin, activase, and thyrogen. Genetically altered mammalian cells such as Chinese hamster ovary (CHO) can produce hormones at a higher volume.

Drug Forms. The form of the drug is chosen to meet the needs of the patient at that time and the preferred method of administration. They are formulated for the most effective dosage and administered via the drug form as determined safe and effective. Solid, liquid, semi-solid, and gases. Solids can include pills, tablets, capsules, powders, and formulated sheets or granules. Liquids can include solutions, emulsions, suspensions, elixirs, and syrups. Semi-solids can include ointments, creams, and suppositories (see Table 6-1).

TABLE 6-1 • DRUG FORMS

Form	Example 1	Example 2	Example 3
Pills are given sublingual, buccal, po, crushed, and mixed in solution for administration via NGT or tube feeding.	Tablets are compressed powder(s) which may be scored for easy breaking. Chewable tablets and medications or supplements that are gummy based.	Capsules containing the medication in liquid or powder form.	Time-released granules in a capsule; never removed from capsule and administered.
Solutions: Injection, infusion, irrigation, flushing or pulsed irrigation	IV Fluids Irrigations solutions Vials	Elixir – sweet alcohol and water solution that contains the medication. An emulsion is a mixture of two liquids that do not fully combine. An emulsion may look like a single liquid, but it is made of particles of one liquid distributed throughout another liquid which may or may not contain an emulsifying agent. An emulsifying agent keeps the oily (lipid) solution mixed with an aqueous solution.	Suspension has fine solid particles in an aqueous liquid. Effervescent granules dissolve in liquid, which makes the medication easier to absorb, gentler for the patient's stomach and it markets well. Due to limited stability in liquid form, the effervescent method was developed.
Powders are applied topically, mixed as a paste, and applied topically, mixed in solution and injected, infused or used for irrigation.	To be applied dry or mixed in solution. That is, collagen powder/Avitene is placed in a dry asepto syringe and blown into the wound.	Vials of powders to be mixed with injectable 0.9% saline or sterile water. That is, dantrium (Dantrolene) mixed with sterile water to treat malignant hyperthermia	Combination vials: powder on bottom, stopper, solution on top. Pressed upper plunger to push separating stopper inward allowing you to mix solution
Topical applications	Lotions	Ointment medication mixed with oil. Crème medications are water-based and applied topically to mucous membranes or skin.	K-Y Jelly as a lubricant
Respiratory inhalation forms	Anesthetic gases absorbed via respiratory tract	Emergency medication via endotracheal tube (ETT) when IV or IO cannot be accessed. That is, (NAVEL) Narcan, Atropine, Vasopressin, Epinephrine, Lidocaine	Aerosolized nebulizer delivery such as normal saline to liquefy secretions, aminophylline, or other bronchodilators. Inhaler delivery of medications for asthma such as a bronchodilator or cortisone treatment.

Routes of Administration. The route of administration and form of drug administered affects the onset of the medication (time that a medication initiates the desired effect). Enteral routes (Gastrointestinal tract) of administration include (1) by mouth (PO), (2) sublingual (under the tongue), (3) buccal (in the pocket between the cheek and gum), (4) topical sprays (back of throat, organ, etc.), and (5) rectal (suppository or enema). Sublingual absorption via the mucous membranes includes nitroglycerin to treat angina. Medications swallowed must be dissolved in the stomach making it the slowest route of absorption. Time-released granule coatings are designed to dissolve at different rates to provide longer therapeutic times.

Parenteral routes of administration include injections into various tissues including (1) subcutaneous (SC), (2) intramuscular (IM), (3) intrathecal (spinal), (4) injections such as a local or epidural, (5) intradermal (allergy test/tuberculin skin test), (6) interosseous (IO), or (7) intravenous (IV). Intravenous is systemically circulated the fastest and is, therefore, the most common route of administration in surgery. Intraosseous can be used for pediatrics or when intravenous access cannot be obtained in emergencies. Intramuscular injections are usually absorbed faster than subcutaneous because of the vascular supply. For emergencies, it is common to administer a large dose (bolus) which may or may not be followed by an intravenous drip (IV) of the medication. For example, a xylocaine

(Lidocaine) bolus is given to treat the ventricular tachycardia, followed by a lidocaine intravenous drip calculated to maintain a therapeutic blood level. Last but not least is the instillation of ophthalmic eye drops or ointments and otic ear drops to the external ear canal. Medications must be labeled for "Ophthalmic Use" which means they are preservative-free and are safe for application. This means great care must be taken to prevent contamination of the dropper or tip of bottle.

Drug Classifications. There are many ways to classify drugs and a single drug may be classified in several ways. Since there may be multiple drug classifications for one drug, it is helpful to identify the most common reason(s) for administration. Specifically, medications are classified as therapeutic (what do they do), the physiological mechanism (how do they do it), the chemical type (what are they made of), how they are dispensed (controlled drugs, prescription, over-the-counter, FDA controlled (dispensed by a pharmacy), and those not approved by the FDA as an alternative medication distribution (herbal or nutritional supplements).

The World Health Organization Anatomical Therapeutic Chemical Classification System is widely used. There are five levels within the first level (parent level) which relate primarily to anatomical usage (Table 6-2). For examples of therapeutic action classification by purpose or expected used in surgery (Table 6-3). For examples of physiologic action which are classified by what they do in the body (Table 6-4). For examples of chemical classification which are classified according to composition (Table 6-5). Medications can also be classified by how they are administered such as inhalation agents: (1) nasal sprays, (2) anesthesia gases, and (3) respiratory inhalers or nebulizer aerosolization. Controlled substances include those that have the potential for abuse or addiction either physical or mental (for safety or overdose prevention). There are five classes of controlled substances that include stimulants, depressants, narcotics (opium-related analgesics), hallucinogens, and anabolic steroid. See further discussion under section "Medication Distribution."

TABLE 6-2 • ANATOMICAL SYSTEM CLASSIFICATION BY THE BODY SYSTEM TARGETED OR AFFECTED

Anatomical System— Level 1 of the World Health Organization's ATC System	Action	Common Medications	Key Considerations

Alimentary Tract and Metabolism
 	
Gastric medications
1. Antacids
2. Antisecretory drugs
 	
Metabolism
1. Insulin
2. Glucagon
	Gastric
	1. Neutralizes HCL (pH 1-3)
	2. Prevents secretion of HCL.
	  A. H2 Receptor Blockers
	  B. Proton pump blockers (H+)
	
	Metabolism
	1. Insulin replacement to ensure glucose entry into the cell for ATP production. It is also used for emergency protocols.
	Diabetes treatment
	  A. Type 1: Insulin-dependent
	  B. Type 2: Adult onset, Noninsulin drugs
	2. Glucagon treatment for hypoglycemia. Causes liver and muscles to release stored glycogen as glucose.
		Gastric
		1. Citric acid/bicitra, (sodium citrate)
		2. A. Ranitidine/zantac, famotidine/pepcid, cimetidine/tagamet
		2. B. Omeprazole: prevacid, protonix, nexium
		
		Metabolism
		1. A. Insulin types: rapid-acting humalog; short-acting/regular insulin humulin R; intermediate-acting NPH humulin N; long-acting Lantas; combination doses of NPH and rapid or short-acting.
		1. B. Noninsulin Type 2 Tx: 6 types including sulfonylureas, ie, glucotrol/glipizide, acts by increasing insulin production. Others have a variety of actions, ie, increase glucagon production, decrease glucagon secretion; increase secretion of glucose in urine; decrease glucose release from liver, increase storage in liver, muscles & fat.
		2. Glucagon used in Tx of severe hypoglycemia (diabetic coma—took insulin, unable to eat or digest food, coma, seizures)
			1. Bicitra used prn when NPO status is questionable.
			2. Patients with GERD may need their medications to reduce HCL production.
			3. Common to use Cricoid pressure (Sellick maneuver) to prevent regurgitation and aspiration.
			
			Metabolism
			1. Monitor glucose levels.
			2. Ensure balance for healing and infection prevention.
			3. Insulin has other uses including organ preservation, wound healing, management of septic shock, etc.

TABLE 6-2 • *(Continued)*			

Blood and Blood-forming Organs
1. Volume expanders (IV)
2. Blood substitutes
3. Blood products
	1. Volume expanders draw fluid into the circulatory system to increase circulating volume for treatment of hypotension.
	2. Provides oxygen transportation for Tx of hypoxia.
	3. Autotransfusion: cell saver recovery of blood.
	4. Blood bank products, autologous donation prior to surgery; or homologous match using Type & crossmatch.
		1. Can include dextran or He span solutions, crystalloids (RL, NS, or Hypertonic saline), albumin.
		2. Blood substitute products in research. Hematopoietic stem cells (autologous or allogenic) to restore immune function.
		3. Cell recovery via cell saver (CS): autologous blood salvage during surgery or orthopedic or chest tube recovery postop via smaller units to drains. Two methods to recover: (1) RBC recovery washes/removes all other components. (2) Hemofiltration returns all components. Note: contraindicated with liposuction (too much fat for filtration device. Since effects unknown, for titanium alloy prothesis that causes blue/green/black discolored tissue or clots around the prosthesis, resume CS recovery after removal and irrigation with NS.
		4. Blood products: whole blood, packed RBC, fresh frozen plasma (ffp), platelets, and cryoprecipitate
			1. Can increase blood pressure, treatment of hemorrhagic shock.
			2. Potential stem cell-generated blood products from Umbilical cord in development.
			3. Washed with NS 0.9, Concentrated, can be used up to 6 h at room temp or 24 h chilled. Not used with malignancy, infection, or contaminated with urine, feces, bone fragments, or amniotic fluid.
			    Hemostat agents should not be aspirated; cell saving resumed after copious NS irrigation. If fat present, use a lipofilter for transfusion.
			4. Transfusion reactions include Agglutination, Hemolysis or Febrile reactions. Other complications include circulatory overload and transfusion-related acute lung injury (TRALI
			   • Transfusions or cell saver recommended anytime 20% blood loss anticipated or Hgb 8 or less.

Cardiovascular System
Cardiac Agents
1. Antiarrhythmics (5 classes below)
2. Sodium channel blockers (Class 1)
3. Beta blockers (Class II)
4. Potassium channel blockers (Class III)
5. Calcium channel blocker (Class IV)
6. Inotropic agents and vasodilators (Class V – Other)
7. Antispasmodics
8. Coronary dilators
9. Statins
10. Other medications used:
   A. Anticoagulants
   B. Fibrinolytics
	1. Controls dysrhythmias; Classes 1-5.
	2. Class I: Na. channel blockers slow HR.
	3. Class II: beta blocker: decrease heart rate (HR) and cardiac output (lowering blood pressure) by blocking adrenalin and vagus nerve stimulation.
	4. Class III: K+ channel blocker: prolongs QT interval; refractory period (repolarization of cell) to slow HR; Tx SV and ventricular arrhythmias
	5. Class IV: Ca+ channel blocker: relaxes muscle and relieves angina, treat irregular heartbeats, high blood pressure.
	6. Inotropic: improves cardiac contraction strength and blood flow to the kidney. Vasodilator used for stress test.
	7. Used during CABG arterial grafts for anastomosis.
	8. Improves coronary blood flow to relieve hypoxia and resultant angina.
		1. Examples: Sotolol /betapace (AFIB/AF, V-tach), procainamide (Ventricular, supraventricular Tachycardias), Xylocaine/lidocaine/IV only then last resort amiodarone (V-tach), atropine (symptomatic bradycardia), etc.
		2. Na+: Xylocaine/lidocaine, pronestyl/procainamide quinidine
		3. Beta: propranolol/inderal, metoprolol/lopressor, atenolol/tenormin, etc.
		4. K+: Amiodarone/cordarone, sotalol/betapace, etc.
		5. Ca+: Verapamil/callan or diltiazem /cardizem.
		6. Other: digitalis Tx CHF and AF, dopamine (in low doses).
		    Adenosine for heart stress test only or to restore heart rhythm.
		7. Papaverine (pavatine), 30-60 mg Tx: instilled into internal thoracic artery (CABG) prior to beginning anastomosis.
		8. Nitroglycerin (NTG) to treat angina/AMI, sublingual or IV; nitroprusside Na (Nipride), vasodilator, antihypertensive.
		9. Pravastatin (Pravachol, simvastatin (Zocor), atorvastin (lipitor), etc.
			Congestive heart failure (CHF) is characterized by shortness of breath upon exertion, water retention which can lead to pitting edema in lower extremities and eventually pulmonary edema (PE). Diuretics such as furosemide (Lasix), anticoagulants (AFIB or AFL) and KCL potassium replacement are common. Acute Myocardial Infarction (AMI) or heart attack presents differently for males and females. Typical signs/symptoms include angina (chest pain), lasting more than a few minutes (chest, arm, back or jaw, may radiate), shortness of breath, dizziness, N &/or V, diaphoresis (cold sweats), cough, anxiety, tachycardia, etc. 45% of individuals have atypical signs "like the flu." With feelings of pressure, fullness or discomfort in the chest and "heartburn like symptoms. Silent heart attacks also cause fatigue, lightheadedness, and shortness of breath.

(Continued)

TABLE 6-2 • ANATOMICAL SYSTEM CLASSIFICATION BY THE BODY SYSTEM TARGETED OR AFFECTED *(Continued)*

	9. Lower cholesterol levels to prevent atherosclerosis and resultant obstruction (atherosclerosis) or embolus formation (CVA, pulmonary embolus, AMI, etc.) 10. A. Prevent blood clots with atrial fibrillation (AF) and artificial heart valves given to prevent thrombus or embolism, angina, or acute myocardial infarction (AMI/heart attack). 10. B. Dissolves blood clots (treatment of DVT, PE, PAO, AMI, and thrombolytic CVA (stroke). Contraindicated: Hx of surgery, GI tract or GU bleeding in past 10 days or increased risk of bleeding due to clotting disorders, thrombocytopenia, etc.	10. A. Coumadin (warfarin) as a vitamin K antagonist given oral (severe mitral valve stenosis or artificial heart valve) and Heparin given subcutaneous injection. Also used aspirin (ASA) or clopidogrel/plavix as antiplatelet drugs. NOACs (novel oral anti-coagulants) recommended for routine use include rivaroxaban/Xarelto or apixaban/Eliquis. 10. B. Streptokinase (SK), tissue plasminogen activator/Activase (tPA), and Urokinase (UK). Administered within 3 h of event streptokinase (steptase) Tx: AMI, pulmonary embolism, and acute arterial embolism. urikinase (Abbokinase) Tx: pulmonary embolism, deep vein thrombosis (DVT), clearing IV catheters, acute arterial embolism. Alteplase (activase). Tx: AMI coronary thrombolysis, extensive pulmonary embolism.	An AMI can occur anytime during any surgery. Being alert to changes in patient condition is essential since the patient is not alert to report pain. The younger a person is, the higher risk for a major arterial obstruction. Older patients who have had chest pain can develop collateral circulation due to the episodes of hypoxia that can stimulate angiogenesis. This provides alternate blood flow and increases survival rates. Thrombus prevention is monitored closely to prevent overdose (heparin PTT and coumadin PT). Clue to remember which each makes 10 letters.
Dermatological Agents 1. Antihistamines 2. Anti-inflammatory agents 3. Anti-infectives include: antifungal, antibiotic	1. Reduce allergic reactions including rash and itching. 2. Steroid agents used to reduce the symptoms of inflammation—pain, redness and swelling. 3. Used to treat common skin infections.	1. Minor reactions: benadryl; severe reactions: adrenaline 2. Steroids: celestone, corticosporin, hydrocortisone, solumedrol 3. Silvadene, penicillin, tetracycline, erythromycin or cephalosporins.	1. Benadryl may be given as a prophylactic to prevent minor allergy symptoms. 2. Steroids reduce the body's naturally protective defense mechanism (inflammation) and can lead to infection. 3. Anti-infectives to prevent or treat infections.
Genito-urinary System and Sex Hormones Obstetrical agents 1. Oxytocic 2. Nonconductive irrigation solutions Urinary system 1. Diuretics 2. Sulfonamides 3. Irrigation solutions—water 4. Irrigation solutions—normal saline 5. Nonconductive irrigation solutions 6. Transplant preservative solutions Sex hormones	GYN/Obstetrical Agents 1. Pitocin or Oxytocin; 10 U/mL IM postdelivery; hormone naturally produced by the posterior pituitary gland (neurotransmitter) that is known as the LOVE hormone. It is released during the first stages of romantic attachment, sexual activity, let down of milk, contraction of uterus, and movement of sperm. Used to induce labor or control hemorrhage. Uterine stimulant, vasopressive, and antidiuretic 2. RH: mother prevents RH immunization. RH antibodies from human plasma to prevent the patient development of circulating B memory lymphocyte cells which could prevent future pregnancies.	GYN/obstetrical agents 1. For induction, requires fetal heart monitor and intrauterine pressure due to potential adverse effects including hypotension, bradycardia, tachycardia, permanent CNS damage, death due to asphyxia, fluid overload/water intoxication, uterine rupture; neonatal seizure, fetal death, low Apgar score at 5 min; fetal hypoxia. Fundal massage may be performed to stimulate contractions also. 2. RHOGAM administered postdelivery IM. Urinary agents 1. Lasix (furosemide, loop of Henle action), Diamox (diuril) 2. Bactrim, Septra, sulfadiazine 3. Hypotonic Irrigation solution for Cystoscopy Tx TURBT; causes any residual tumor cells to swell and burst due to osmosis.	GYN/OB 1. Monitor contractions/dose to prevent uterine rupture; fetal heart tones to prevent fetal distress/demise. 2. RhoGAM given after birth of baby. UA 1. Monitor K+ levels KCL replacement prn. 2. C&S provides best coverage. 3. For fluids numbered 3-5 from column one, Genito-urinary System and Sex Hormones: use fluid warmers to prevent hypothermia prn for large volumes. 4. Contains electrolytes and therefore conduct electricity used for thermal hemostasis.

TABLE 6-2 • (Continued)

	Urinary Agents 1. Diuretics increase fluid excretion to prevent or treat fluid overload (CHF, pulmonary edema, pitting edema, etc.) 2. Common antibiotic for UTI. 3. Water for bladder tumors. 4. Conductive fluids used for routine cystoscopy. 5. Nonconductive solutions used to maintain a full bladder and for irrigation when electrocautery is used to prevent electrical shock. 6. Electrolyte and pH balanced to preserve tissue. Sex Hormones 1. Estrogen used for HRT, Gender reassignment, alleviate menopause symptoms, etc. 2. Progesterone for ovulation and menstruation regulation. Prevents overgrowth of endometrium when paired with estrogen for HRT. 3. Used for Hormone-replacement therapy (HRT); gender reassignment; hypogonadism, gender dysphoria and certain types of breast cancer. • Unethical use of testosterone: to increase athletic ability.	4. Isotonic conductive solutions: Normal Saline (0.9%), Ringers lactate. No change to cells due to similarity to plasma/body fluids. Not used with electrocautery Cystoscopy cases. 5. Slightly hypotonic, nonconductive solutions: Glycine 1.5% (amino acid solution) is an inhibitory neurotransmitter used for TURP Tx of BPH/inhibits muscle tone) or Sorbitol 2.7% (glucitol—fruit/plant sugar alcohol) used as an artificial sweetener or laxative, or Mannitol 0.54% are commonly used as an osmotic diuretic to treat elevated ICP or IOP. 6. University of Wisconsin Solution (UW) primarily; Euro-Collins or Collins Solution was used prior to development of UW Solution. Sex Hormones 1. Estrogen: systemic pill, skin patch, ring, gel, cream, or spray. Low-dose vaginal products. 2. Progesterone: some forms contain peanut oil (allergy alert). 3. Testosterone: injections or buccal/nasal patches or skin gels.	5. Safe for use with electrocautery. With large amounts of Glycine absorbed by the large venous process of prostate, CNS toxicity can develop (transient blindness and/or encephalopathy). Sorbitol and Mannitol are more costly and can lead to fluid overload. NOTE: Height of bag (hydrostatic pressure) and length of procedure determines absorption rate (Average varies from 10-30 mL/min). Adverse effect: TURP syndrome due to hypervolemic hyponatremia (<120 mEq/L). 6. UW solution can be used to limit cold storage damage up to 2 days. Hormones: 1. Estrogen or progesterone therapy may increase risk of blood clots, breast cancer, stroke, or heart disease. 2. Testosterone contraindicated for males with cancer of prostate, male breast cancer, serious heart condition, severe liver, or kidney disease. Injection can cause POME (Pulmonary oil micro embolism; fatal)

Systemic Hormones (does not include sex hormones or insulin)
1. Adrenal cortical steroids
  A. Corticosteroids
  B. Glucocorticoids
  C. Mineralocorticoids
2. Antidiuretic hormones
3. Calcitonin
4. Parathyroid hormone
5. Thyroid
6. Other(s) include: adrenal corticosteroid inhibitors, calcimimetics, growth hormone, somatostatin, etc.
	Hormone replacement therapy postsurgical removal or disease
	1. Corticosteroids include:
	  A. Corticotropin (ACTH) produced by anterior pituitary gland—Stress response. Stimulates adrenal gland to release glucocorticoids.
	  B. Glucocorticoids: Reduces inflammation. Used to prevent postop swelling and resultant pain or disturbance of implants. Treatment of Addison's disease.
	  C. Mineral corticosteroids: aldosterone which regulates salt absorption and water thereby affecting blood pressure. Tx: Addison's disease.
		1. Corticosteroids
		  A. ACTH (corticotropin): used to test adrenal gland function.
		  B. Glucocorticosteroids: anti-inflammatory action. Includes hydrocortisone, dexamethas-one, prednisolone, prednisone, methyl-prednisolone (Solu-Medrol or Depo-Medrol); betamethasone (Celestone).
		  C. Mineral corticosteroids: Fludrocortisone (Florinef).
		2. Antidiuretic hormone: Vasopressin (pitressin and desmopressin).
		3. Calcitonin level can be elevated with medullary thyroid cancer or other thyroid diseases. Replacement therapy or given to women (5 y postmenopause) to increase bone density (Tx Osteoporosis).
			All require monitoring.
			1. Steroid anti-inflammatory drugs also increase chances of surgical site infections or postop wound infections.
			2. ADH hormones: Take care with sound-alike drugs: Pitressin (vasopressin—vasoconstriction) and pitocin (uterine contractions)
			3. Taken with vitamin D and calcium. Monitor calcium levels. Care is taken to find and ensure safe placement of the parathyroid gland(s) during total thyroidectomy.
			4. Parathyroid hormone (PTH) increases the blood level of calcium via osteoclast activity.
			5. Thyroxine levels are monitored to ensure a therapeutic level is maintained. Hyperthyroidism may require surgery to remove the goiter or carcinoma.

(Continued)

TABLE 6-2 • ANATOMICAL SYSTEM CLASSIFICATION BY THE BODY SYSTEM TARGETED OR AFFECTED (*Continued*)

	2. Antidiuretic hormone: vasopressin (produced by the posterior pituitary gland) increases reabsorption of water in kidney (vasoconstrictor). Tx: diabetes insipidus 3. Calcitonin secreted by C cells of thyroid lowers blood calcium levels; used to treat hypercalcemia and Paget's disease of the bone. 4. PTH—Parathyroid hormone—Controls calcium blood levels 5. Thyroid: T4/thyroxine and T3/triiodothyronine. T4 converts to T3 in bloodstream. Controls cellular metabolism.	4. Parathyroid hormone (PTH): (natpara), Tx: hypoparathyroidism S&S include paresthesia (tingling numbness), tetany, muscle aches/cramps, muscle spasms, fatigue, etc.) 5. Thyroxine: levothyroxine sodium (Synthroid)Tx: Hypothyroidism/myxedema	
Anti-infectives: anything that can prevent the spread of an infectious organism by killing the organism.	Antibiotic Antifungal Antituberculosis Antivirals	1. Amebicides (pyrantel) (Flagyl/metronidazole) 2. Antibiotics: 　A. Aminoglycosides: "mycin" tobramycin, kanamycin, neomycin, amikacin, gentamycin, 　B. Carbapenems include thienamycin, doripenem (doribax), silastin (imipenem) (primaxin) IM. 　C. Cephalosporins (cephalexin cefazolin (ancef or kefzol), cefadroxil/ duracef, rocephin/ceftriaxone, etc.) 　D. Fluoroquinolone Tx of plague/anthrax, iprofloxacin (Cipro), levofloxacin (Levaquin), etc. 　E. Penicillin (amoxicillin), 　F. Strepto sulfonamides 　G. Tetracyclines (doxycycline) 3. UTI anti-infectives 4. Antifungals or antimycotics (nystatin, amphotericin b, (Flagyl) 5. Antituberculosis (isoniazid, rifampin, capreomycin, etc.) 6. Antivirals (interferons, tenofovir, acyclovir, ribavirin, etc.)	1. Worm infestations can lead to bowel obstruction. 2. A. Toxic: Monitor kidney function & hearing loss 　B. Carbapenems – considered a last line defense and used for high-risk known or suspected multidrug-resistant (MDR) bacteria. Potential carbapenem-resistant organisms (CRO) include carbapenem-resistant Enterobacteriaceae (CRE) such as *Klebsiella* species (K. pneumoniae). *E. coli,* and others such as *Pseudomonas* species. 　C. Cephalosporins are a broad-spectrum fungal derivative from cephalosporin acremonium. Developed five (5) generations of structural changes to increase effectiveness. Contraindicated in those with penicillin Type 1 anaphylaxis reactions. 　D. Fluoroquinolones can cause severe peripheral neuropathy leading to disability, can also cause tendon damage/rupture. Not used with patients on benzodiazepines, can lead to acute withdrawal symptoms.

TABLE 6-2 • (*Continued*)

Antineoplastic and Immunomodulating Agents 1. Antineoplastic agents can be used in conjunction with surgery and/or radiation therapy. 2. Immunomodulating agent affect specific parts of the immune system.	1. Antineoplastic or anticancer drugs can be used prior to surgery to shrink tumor or after surgery to ensure eradication. Dosage is calculated based on body surface area (BSA) to reduce the toxicity and resultant side-effects. 2. Immunomodulators (IMiDS) improve patient outcomes and can slow disease progression. Used to treat sarcoidosis, myeloma,	1. Includes alkylating agents, anthracyclines taxanes, vinca alkaloids, and anti-metabolites. Examples: breast cance— methotrexate & 5-fluorouracil; bladder cancer—methotrexate & doxorubicin; colorectal cancer 5 fluorouracil, & folinic acid; lung cancer doxorubicin & cyclophosphamide; etc. 2. Includes thalidomide 1st-generation, lenalidomide 2nd-generation, and apremilast 3rd-generation treatment for cancer and inflammatory diseases. With each generation the drugs were better tolerated and provided more active effects. Examples include Crohn's disease Azathioprine/Imuran; multiple sclerosis with glatiramer that prevents the body from damaging nerve cells; osteosarcoma with mifamurtide; and lenalidomide for multiple myeloma to kill abnormal bone marrow cells and produce normal blood cells, etc.	1. Side effects include damage to rapidly growing cells (epidermal and bone marrow) causing hair loss (alopecia). 2. Side effects of IMiDS include teratogenic side effects and other adverse side effects. Care is taken with any history of kidney disease. There is a risk of secondary malignancy.
Musculo-skeletal System 1. Muscle relaxants 2. Benzodiazepines 3. SNRIs: serotonin and norepinephrine reuptake inhibitors 4. Gene therapy drugs 5. Antisense therapeutics	1. Relaxes muscles relieving spasms, pain, and stiffness due to strains, sprains, and injury. Action CNS level. Used Tx of multiple sclerosis and cerebral palsy. 2. Anti-anxiety, relax muscles, treat seizures. 3. SNRIs are used to elevate mood to treat depression, anxiety, diabetic neuropathy, fibromyalgia, ADHD, OCD, musculoskeletal conditions, and panic disorder. They work by increasing levels of serotonin and norepinephrine in the brain. 4. Tx of Spinal muscular atrophy (SMA, not a cure) 5. Used to treat genetic disorders or infections by turning off a particular gene to treat muscular dystrophy and musculoskeletal conditions.	1. Robaxin (methocarbamol), cyclobenzaprine, metaxalone, dantrium (dantrolene) 2. Valium/diazepam 3. Cymbalta. Duloxetine. 4. Zolgensma 5. Tegsedi/Inotersen or 6. Used to treat duchenne muscular dystrophy	1. Cyclobenzaprine can cause serotonin syndrome which includes hallucinations. Metaxalone is not used with liver/kidney disease 2. Addiction, overdose, and death can occur.

(*Continued*)

TABLE 6-2 • ANATOMICAL SYSTEM CLASSIFICATION BY THE BODY SYSTEM TARGETED OR AFFECTED (*Continued*)

Nervous System
1. Stimulants
  A. Analeptics
  B. Neuroleptics
    i. Cortical
    ii. Medullary
    iii. Spinal
  C. Emetics
2. Hallucinogens
3. Depressants
  A. Sedatives
    i. Induce calm/sleep/tranquilize
    ii. Hypnotics produce sleep.
  B. Narcotics
  C. General anesthesia
	1. Stimulants
	  A. Analeptics: CNS stimulant, used for anesthesia recovery and to treat respiratory distress/apnea, especially in infants.
	  B. Neuroleptics: antipsychotics treatment of schizophrenia, bipolar, delusions, etc.
	2. Hallucinogens: used for anesthesia.
	3. Depressants are commonly used for anxiety, pain control, conscious sedation induction agents, and maintaining general anesthesia for surgery (Sedative/Hypnotics usually grouped together; not used for pain).
	4. Narcotics relieve pain (analgesic) and produce narcosis (state of stupor or sleep). Can be used medically or classified as an illegal recreational drug. Can be called opiates or opioid analgesics; binds to opioid receptors in brain to control pain, pleasure, and addictive behaviors.
		1. A. Analeptics: Doxapram, caffeine, and theophylline
		1. B. Neuroleptics
		  i. cortical: amphetamine, ephedrine, aminophylline, caffeine.
		  ii. medullary: adrenalin, picrotoxin, nikethamide
		  iii. Spinal- strychnine, brucine
		2. Hallucinogens: ketamine
		3. A. sedatives such as benzodiazepine include diazepam (valium), midazolam (versed). Other sedative-hypnotics include propofol (diprivan), etomidate (amidate). barbiturates such as sodium thiopental, secobarbital and phenobarbital are used in surgery, assisted suicide, and epilepsy. Nonaddictive include ambien (zolipidem), etc. Melatonin (hormone produced pineal gland) promotes sleep.
		3. B. Narcotic used for postop pain control, end-of-life care or palliative care for cancer. Include three classes: Class 1. phenanthrenes such as naturally produced morphine (duramorph) semisynthetic dilaudid (hydromorphine), heroin, hydrocodone, oxycodone; Class 2. Phenylpiperidines such as the synthetic opioids meperidine, sufentanil, alfentanil or fentanyl which is 80-100 times stronger than morphine; and Class 3. Phenylheptylamines such as methadone does not produce a 'drug' high.
			1. A. Can be used to increase the speed of recovery from propofol, remifentanil, sevoflurane.
			1. B. Caution: Neuroleptic malignant syndrome causing hyperpyrexia (high fever)
			2. Ketamine: used for pediatrics as an IM or IV anesthetic can stimulate hallucinations (over 15). Care with conversation. Does not affect laryngeal or pharyngeal reflexes.
			3. A. Valium and Versed also provide amnesia and can be used for seizure activity. Can cause hypotension and Respiratory depression. Can be habit-forming. Benzodiazepine overdose reversal agent is flumazenil (Mazicon, Romazicon) which can put patient into withdrawal symptoms/cause seizures. Propofol also has anticonvulsive effects, stings on injection. Etomidate useful in hypotensive patient/trauma; Risk is N&V.
			3. B. Danger of respiratory depression; opioid-use disorder and potentially fatal overdose. Controlled substance. Addictive. Side effects include itchiness, miosis (constrict pupil), N & V, drowsiness/ dizziness and/or constipation. Reversal agent is Narcan (naloxone).

Antiparasitic, Insecticides, and Repellants	Antiparasitic 1. Anthelmintic or Anthelmintic 2. Antimalarial 3. Antiprotozoals	1. Antimalarial (quinine, chloroquine, hydroxychloroquine, etc.). 2. Anthelmintics (worm treatment) mebendazole for worm infestations 3. Rx malathion or ivermectin for lice/mite infestations.	Parasitic infections can be significant for travelers and immigrants and can require surgical removal. Examples include biliary liver fluke from eating raw fresh-water fish, brain tapeworm infections from undercooked pork and intestinal worms causing intestinal obstruction.
Respiratory System	1. Nasal preparations 2. Throat drugs 3. Drugs for obstructive airway diseases 4. Cough and cold drugs 5. Antihistamines systemic use 6. Other respiratory system	1. Nasal decongestants and antihistamines, corticosteroids, antiallergic, etc. Example: Oxymetazoline/Afrin, ephedrine, etc. 2. Throat preparations include antiseptics, antibiotics, local anesthetics, and other preparations.	1. Neosynephrine (Afrin) commonly used as a vasoconstrictor for nasal surgery, replaces cocaine previously used for septorhinoplasty. Mupirocin is helpful for eliminating nasal colonization of strep, staph, or MRSA.

TABLE 6-2 • (*Continued*)

		3. Obstructive airway disease includes adrenergic inhalants, glucocorticoids, anticholinergics such as atropine to dry secretions, bronchodilators such as albuterol, aminophylline, and theophylline, mucolytics. Note: Bronchospasm is a reversible spasm of the smooth muscles located within the bronchioles. Symptoms include wheezing, decreased breath sounds, dropping oxygen saturation (desaturation), and increased difficulty ventilating patient. Causes can include asthma, emphysema, exercise, foreign body, allergies, irritants, upper respiratory infections, and bronchitis. Medications include bronchodilators, inhaled steroids, and anticholinergics to relieve the spasm. 4. Cough and cold preparations include combination medications with analgesics, anti-inflammatory, anti-infectives, expectorants, mucolytics, antihistamines, adrenergics, bronchodilators, cough suppressants, and antipyretics.	2. Surgical throat applications may involve local anesthetics with vasoconstrictors or astringents such as sodium bismuth to control the gag reflex and control bleeding. 3. Surgical considerations for respiratory obstructive airway diseases include positioning to prevent orthopnea, shortness of breath, chest constriction, and hypoventilation. Prevention of postop pneumonia includes alternate methods of anesthesia (no general anesthesia), use of spirometry postop, and early ambulation. 4. Patients with respiratory infections/colds should delay elective surgery until well.
Sensory Organs Ophthalmic agent 1. Enzymes 2. Miotic 3. Mydriatics 4. Viscoelastics 5. Others	1. Enzymes used include Zolyse used to dissolve the ciliary body ligaments called zonules. Hyaluronidase additive used to spread local anesthetic evenly through tissue. 2. Miotics stimulate the iris to constrict reducing the size of the pupil. This can also increase flow of aqueous humor to the trabecular meshwork/Canal of Schlemm decreasing IOP (intraocular pressure) as seen with Glaucoma. 3. Mydriatics paralyze the iris to dilate causing enlarged pupils. Most mydriatics are also cycloplegics which paralyze the intrinsic muscles (ciliary body and iris).	1. Alphachymotrypsin (Zolyse) in cataract surgery. Hyaluronidase additive for retrobulbar or peribulbar anesthesia to disperse evenly. 2. Carbacol (Miostat), or pilocarpine hydrochloride (pilocar, isopto carpine), solution is absorbed by hazel/brown eye pigment and may require more solution. acetylcholine chloride in mannitol (Miochol-E), used for laser iridectomy. 3. Atropine, phenylephrine (neosynephrine), tropicamide (Mydriacyl), and cyclopentolate (Cyclogyl) dilate and paralyze. 4. Sodium hyaluronate (provisc, amvisc, healon), sodium chondroitin/sodium hyaluronate combination (Viscoat, DisCoVisc).	1. Must be labeled for Ophthalmic Use/no preservatives. Medications soaked pledgets may be used after eye is anesthetized in the cul de sac. 2. Instillation of eye drops should begin with a wipe (cotton ball with normal saline) once from inner to outer canthus to cleanse the eyelid/lashes. Tilt head back slightly; pulldown lower lid with finger gently, instruct patient to look upward; DO NOT touch any surface, squeeze gently to instill the appropriate number of drops into conjunctival sac (NOT ON Cornea). Wipe off any excess. The blood-eye barrier prevents systemic absorption, inner canthus obstruction can be used to prevent systemic medications such as cycloplegics/ atropine from entering the nasolacrimal duct.

(*Continued*)

TABLE 6-2 • ANATOMICAL SYSTEM CLASSIFICATION BY THE BODY SYSTEM TARGETED OR AFFECTED (*Continued*)

	4. Viscoelastic: instilled to maintain the shape of the eye, protect the cornea endothelium, stabilize the vitreous, and maintain the chamber depth. It can also fill the anterior chamber to make a bed for the corneal transplanted tissue. Can be used with detached retina in the vitreous chamber.
	5. Others: anesthetics, irrigation
		5. Anesthetic: tetracaine (Pontocaine), proparacaine (Alcaine, Ophthaine).
		    Irrigation: Balanced salt solution (BSS).
		    Dye for corneal abrasions or foreign body: Fluorescein sodium with a Wood's lamp (ultraviolet light); abrasions appear a bright green.
		    Dye for Conjunctival stains: Rose Bengal or lissamine green is used primarily for identification of devitalized cells due to Keratoconjunctivitis sicca (KCS).
		    Dye for Ophthalmic angiography: Indocyanine green (IC-Green given IV after reconstitution with sterile water. Contains sodium iodide, Care is taken with iodine allergies. Use within 10 h)
		    Anti-inflammatory agents: Steroids: betamethasone (Celestone), dexamethasone (Maxidex), Prednisolone (Pred Forte), or antibiotic combination drugs such as PRED-G or TobrDex.
		    NSAIDS (non-steroid): ketorolac (Acular), Bromfenac (Bromday). Others that also prevent miosis intraop include flurbiprofen (Ocufen)
			3. Eye precautions: prevent loud noises that may startle physician or team, strict aseptic technique to prevent infections or toxemia, ointments should have the first ¼ inch discarded prior to instillation.

Various	1. Antidotes 2. Iron chelating agents 3. Drugs tx of hyperkalemia & hyperphosphatemia 4. Detoxifying agent for antineoplastic treatment 5. Drugs tx hypercalcemia 6. Tx of hypoglycemia 7. Tissue adhesives 8. Embolization drugs 9. Medical Gases 10. Other therapeutic nerve depressants	1. Examples: naloxone, flumazenil, Sugammadex (reverses rocuronium/vecuronium Nondepolarizing muscle blockers), etc. 2. Chelating agent (Metal-binding medication): iron, copper, aluminum, and zinc. Used to treat iron overload due to blood transfusions. 3. Used to bind to K+: Sodium zirconium cyclosilicate (Lokelma) oral suspension (Kayexalate discontinued in the US) 4. Detoxifying Antineoplastic: Example Dexrazoxane is used to treat severe side effects from chemotherapy. 5. Tx Hypercalcemia and secondary hyperparathyroidism: Sodium cellulose Phosphate (Cinacalcet 6. Tx Hyperinsulinism/hypoglycemia: Dizoxide (proglycem, Hyperstat)	Evaluation of all medications, over-the-counter medications, herbal remedies, and supplements including possible interactions, side effects, or potential adverse effects should be considered during the preop assessment.

TABLE 6-2 • (*Continued*)			
		7. Tissue adhesives: Example: Cyanoacrylate (Dermabond) 8. Chemoembolization with drug-eluting loaded: doxorubicin (DEBDOX) is used for treatment of hepatocellular carcinoma, **irinotecan** beads (DEBIRI) are used for metastatic colon cancer. 9. Medical Gases: Oxygen (green tank), carbon dioxide (grey tank), helium (brown tank). Nitrogen tank (black tank), Medical Air (yellow tank) 10. Nerve depressants: Dehydrated Alcohol injection 98% (Ethanol) used for nerve ablations such as celiac plexus neurolysis, trigeminal neuralgia (tic douloureux), peripheral nerve sheath tumor, etc.	

TABLE 6-3 • EXAMPLES OF THERAPEUTIC ACTION CLASSIFICATION BY PURPOSE OR EXPECTED USE IN SURGERY			
Classification	**Definition**	**Common Medications**	**Key Considerations**

Analgesic	Relieves pain.
	
	Used as an induction agent or to maintain general anesthesia providing pain management during surgical procedure.
	
	Types:
	1. Narcotic Analgesics
	  A. Natural opioid agonist
	  B. Synthetic opioid agonists
	2. NSAIDS (nonsteroidal anti-inflammatory drugs) effects include:
	  A. Analgesic
	  B. Anti-inflammatory
	  C. Antipyretic
	  D. Reversible inhibition of platelet aggregation
		1. Opioids
		  A. Natural: Morphine Tx: Premedication and postop pain.
		  B. Synthetic Opioid Agonist
		    i. Fentanyl (Sublimaze) High doses: primary anesthetic agent.
		    ii. Fentanyl and droperidol (Innovar). Tx: Long lasting Has antiemetic properties. No liver or kidney toxicity. Long lasting.
		    iii. Remifentanil (Ultiva)- Tx: induction agent, maintain general anesthesia, MAC analgesia and postop analgesic; synergistic with sedative/hypnotics and gas inhalation agents.
		    iv. Alfentanil (Alfenta): induction agent/ maintain anesthesia.
		    v. Sufentanil (Sufenta): High doses—primary anesthetic agent. Adjunct to general anesthesia.
		    vi. Hydromorphone (Dilaudid) Tx: Postop pain
		    vii. Meperidine (Demerol) Tx: Premedication and postop pain, not used with convulsive disorders or undiagnosed abdominal pain.
			1. Opioid Reversal Agent, Opioid Antagonists: Narcan (Naloxane) reversal of opioid-induced respiratory depression and sedation. Note the action of morphine will outlast the action of Narcan (relapse of respiratory depression). Naltrexone (Trexon) used for Tx of detoxified formerly opioid-dependent individuals. Nalmefene (Reve) used for complete or partial opioid "overdose" and Tx of side effects caused by epidural opioids postop.
			2. Opioid agonists can cause nausea and vomiting, decreased peristalsis, gastric emptying, and dizziness. When combined with N2O can cause CV depression. Combined with Benzodiazepine can increase risk of CV and Respiratory depression.
			3. NSAIDS: Postop regime Acetaminophen and Ibuprofen for pain control every 2 h. Concurrent use of other NSAIDS increases risks of nephropathy (Kidney damage) or GI side effects. Acetaminophen overdose or taken with alcohol can increase risk of acetaminophen hepatotoxicity. When taken with methotrexate, lithium or digoxin can cause toxicity as NSAIDs reduces excretion of those medications.

(Continued)

TABLE 6-3 • EXAMPLES OF THERAPEUTIC ACTION CLASSIFICATION BY PURPOSE OR EXPECTED USE IN SURGERY *(Continued)*			
		viii. Methadone (Dolphine) Tx: Used for narcotic abstinence syndrome suppressant and antitussive. C. Opioid Agonist-Antagonist i. Butorphanol (Stadol) used as analgesia during L&D; Can reverse respiratory depression of pure opioid agonist. ii. Nalbuphine (Nubain) Used for patients with heart disease or Obstetric analgesia during L& D. 2. NSAIDS A. Toradal (Ketorolac Tromethamine) Injection IM/IV 20-60 mg, then 15-30 mg q6 h. Max dose 150 mg daily. Limit 5 days. PO dose pediatrics. B. ASA—Aspirin C. Acetaminophen D. Ibuprofen (Motrin, Advil, Nuprin) E. Naproxen (Naprosyn)	
Anesthetic Inhalation	Inhaled agents that eliminate sensation	1. Nitrous Oxide N2O Adjunct to IV anesthesia, has analgesic properties. Safe for MH protocols. 2. Halothane Inexpensive, Good cerebral flow and bronchodilator. Use with caution possible Liver Hypoxia. Possible rare postop autoimmune hepatitis. 3. Isoflurane inexpensive. 4. Desflurane Strong pungent odor; Possible bronchiole irritant. Most rapid onset. Requires heated vaporizer. 5. Sevoflurane Best choice for inhalational anesthesia (MAC); least pungent; fast onset and offset. Questionable nephrotoxicity (+ for animals).	1. N2O rapidly diffuses into and expands into air spaces. Shut off prior to insertion of tubes; avoid with middle ear and retinal procedures. Monitor ETT cuff/PAC Balloon for expansion. 2. All "ane" inhalation anesthetics have the potential to trigger MH.
Anesthetic Intravenous	Eliminates sensation by producing rapid induction of general anesthesia.	1. Propofol (Diprivan): Induction agent; CV depression. Reduce dose for elderly or those unstable 2. Amidate-etomidate induction agent: unconscious in less than 1 min, no analgesia Favored for unstable (B/P, CV) 3. Methohexital sodium: Brevital— barbiturate—Unique: used for identification of seizure foci during ablative surgery. 4. Ketamine (Ketalar) Dissociative agent 5. Dexmedetomidine (Precedex) Good for procedure sedation, minimal respiratory depression.	1. Diprivan is a lipid solution supporting bacterial technique (Sepsis). Prolonged use linked to lethal syndrome of arrhythmia, lipemia, metabolic acidosis and rhabdomyolysis. 2. *Thiopental sodium – Pentothal – barbiturate Favored for Neuro protection during decreased cerebral perfusion.*

TABLE 6-3 • (Continued)

Anticoagulant	Prevention of clots Used for patient in atrial fibrillation, prevention of DVT, or treatment of thrombophlebitis and pulmonary embolism.	1. Heparin sodium or heparin calcium which activates antithrombin III which inhibits thrombin and factor Xa preventing the final stages of a blood clot. 2. Coumadin—Warfarin: Inhibits the enzyme that recycles oxidized vitamin K, thereby preventing the activation of coagulating factors. 3. Apixaban, edoxaban, fondaparinux, and rivaroxaban are all Factor Xa inhibitors which prevent clot formation. 4. Direct Thrombin inhibitors (DTI) inactivate free thrombin and thrombin that is bound to fibrin. Includes IV bivalirudin (Angiomax) and oral dabigatran (Pradaxa) among others. Used when heparin-induced thrombocytopenia with thrombosis (HIT) is suspected.	1. Heparin lab tests include the aPTT (activated partial thromboplastin time) and INR. Note: LMWH (low molecular weight heparin) Fragmin **(dalteparin)** and Lovenox (enoxaparin) do not require monitoring and are given SC. 2. Coumadin lab test is the PT/INR. Requires dietary restrictions. 3. Factor Xa inhibitors do not require routine coagulation monitoring. If needed, plasma levels can be measured. 4. DTI prolongs PT, PTT, TCT (Thrombin clotting time), and ACT, (activated clotting time) monitored usually with the PTT or for surgery the ACT. Antidote 1. Protamine Sulfate; Heparin antagonist. 2. Vitamin K
Anti-arrhythmic	Used in emergency treatment dysrhythmia	1. Amiodarone (Cordarone) Ventricular tachycardia and SVT 2. Digoxin (Lanoxin) Tx: CHF, AFib, or AFlutter with slow ventricular rate. 3. Lidocaine (Xylocaine) Tx: VTach, VFib, PVC > 6/min Amino Amide potential for toxicity. 4. Verapamil (Calan, Isoptin)	
Anti-inflammatory, steroid	Hormone that reduces inflammatory response.	Dexamethasone acetate (Decadron); used intra-articular (joint) to reduce postop swelling.	Can increase glucose levels. Monitor glucose levels for Diabetics.
Antiemetic	Given to prevent vomiting.	1. Transdermal Scopolamine (Anticholinergic) Tx: Presurgical prevention NV, motion sickness, vertigo, parkinsonism. Sedative, amnesic, 2. Droperidol (Inapsine), Tranquilizer, antianxiety, N&V prevention, and sedative 3. Metoclopramide HCL (Reglan) Tx: GERD, N & V, Preop med to prevent aspiration. 4. Ondansetron HCL (Zofran) 5. Prochlorperazine (Compazine), sedative too 6. Promethazine (Phenergan) Potentiates effects of Demerol when mixed. 7. Hydroxyzine (Vistaril) Tx: anxiety, N & V, sedative, vertigo. Can cause dizziness, hypotension.	Contraindicated with narrow-angle glaucoma.
Antipyretic			
Blood replacement • Autologous blood • Donated blood • Whole blood Plasma expanders			

TABLE 6-3 • EXAMPLES OF THERAPEUTIC ACTION CLASSIFICATION BY PURPOSE OR EXPECTED USE IN SURGERY *(Continued)*

Coagulant	Tx of heparin overdose or reverse heparinization after extracorporeal circulation.	Protamine sulfate (fish roe derivative).	Can cause hypotension, pulmonary edema, and anaphylaxis.
Diuretics	Increase urine	1. Furosemide (Lasix) Tx: edema, pulmonary edema, CHF, hypertension. 2. Mannitol (Osmitrol) Tx: elevated ICP or IOP, treatment of oliguria, prevent oliguria and renal failure. Can be used during TURP for irrigation to prevent abnormal fluid retention. For ocular surgery, administered 60-90 min prior.	Insert Foley catheter to aid in measurement of output.
Hemostatic	Used to control capillary bleeding and/or cancellous bone oozing.	1. Cellulose – oxidized (Oxycel, Surgicel) 2. Collagen – microfibrillar (Avitene), compressed pad or powder. Powder can be placed inside dry asepto and blown into crevices. 3. Gelatin-absorbable (Gelfoam), Sponge/powder swells. Mechanical obstruction. 4. Thrombin (bovine origin) used for capillary/venule bleeding; never injected IV. 5. Fibrin glue (Floseal Matri) gelatin matrix includes thrombin to facilitate clotting.	1. Collagen: must be handled dry; not used with cell saver. 2. Gelfoam can be cut, pressed and applied either dry or saturated with thrombin or a sodium chloride solution.
Fluids for irrigation, intravenous, instillation, and organ preservation	Classified according to their osmolality, their electrolyte content, and their viscosity: Isotonic (same concentrations as the body), hypotonic (lower concentrations than the body), or hypertonic (higher concentrations than the body). Fluids and those with minerals or other medications given for therapeutic treatment, ie, hydration replacement fluids, treatment of shock (low blood pressure), fluids as carriers for drug administration, etc.	1. Sodium chloride 0.9% (Normal Saline) Isotonic Fluid with electrolytes sodium (Na+) and chloride (Cl−) replacement or for medication 1.5. 2. Lactated Ringer's: isotonic solution for fluid and electrolyte replacement. Can be used for renal failure patient. 3. Plasmalyte A: balanced isotonic electrolyte solution used primarily for pediatrics and infants. Studies indicate useful for adults also. Contains sodium chloride sodium gluconate, sodium acetate trihydrate, potassium chloride, and magnesium chloride. 4. Normosol R: replacement of acute extracellular fluid volume losses in surgery, trauma, burns, or shock. 5. 3% Sorbitol: nonelectrolyte hypotonic solution used when cautery is used for cystoscopy or hysteroscopy. 6. 5% Mannitol: nonelectrolyte solution used when cautery is used for cystoscopy or hysteroscopy. Used IV Mannitol as an osmotic diuretic Tx for increased cerebral pressure (ICP). 7. 32% Dextran 70 (Hyskon): hypertonic nonelectrolyte with high viscosity used for tubal reanastomosis to prevent strictures or for hysteroscopy.	1. IV solutions are used with care in patients with renal failure. 2. Potential for fluid overload when too much is administered, fluid administered too fast, fluid absorbed due to vascularity of uterus or prostate, or can cause fluid and/or solute overloading resulting in dilution of serum electrolyte concentrations, overhydration, congested states, or pulmonary edema. 3. Potential for precipitate formation (crystals, haziness, or turbidity) in the IV fluid from (precipitated medications injected or medication interactions due to compounding or flushing errors in which the wrong diluent, flush or base solution, or concentration/dose was used. If precipitate formation is observed, the injection should be stopped immediately to prevent precipitate pulmonary embolization. 4. Other complications can include infiltration, extravasation (medication into the tissue causes tissue damage, necrosis, even amputation), phlebitis, infection, and hypersensitivity.

TABLE 6-3 • *(Continued)*			
		8. Dextrose 5% (D5W): isotonic for hysteroscopy; for IV use until dextrose is utilized, becomes hypotonic at that time. 9. Other hypertonic solutions include: D5NS (dextrose 5% in 0.9% saline), D5 ½ NS (dextrose 5% in 0.45% saline), D5LR. 10. Dextran: high-molecular weight (Dextran 75). Used for Plasma expander. 11. Hetastarch (Hespan): plasma expander which can be used in combination with blood products. 12. Sodium bicarbonate: given IV during hypoxic emergencies to treat acidosis based on ABG results. 13. Organ preservation fluids used with hypothermia include: EuroCollins Solution (Heart, liver, and lung), University of Wisconsin Solution (lung, heart, and all abdominal organs, ie, kidney, pancreas, liver, small bowel; Trade names: Belzer & Viaspan), Celsior (heart).	5. Note: UW solution has adenosine and allopurinol added just prior to use to improve oxygen scavenging and improve function after transplantation.

Neuromuscular blocking agents (potent muscle relaxers)	Used for endotracheal intubations and skeletal muscle relaxation during surgery or mechanical ventilation.
	
	Blocks neuromuscular transmission causing paralysis of muscles. Used only as an adjunct to anesthesia when artificial ventilation is available.
	
	Types:
	1. Depolarizing agents
	2. Non-depolarizing agents
	3. Non-depolarizing Neuromuscular blockade (antagonists) reversal agents
		Types:
		1. Depolarizing agents.
		  A. Succinylcholine (Anectine, Quelicin): also used rapid sequence inductions. No prolonged duration with Liver or Renal disease.
		2. Nondepolarizing agents
		  A. Pancuronium bromide (Pavulon)
		  B. Rocuronium bromide (Zermuron) *Does not cause histamine release.*
		  C. Vecuronium bromide (Norcuron) *Does not cause histamine release. Avoid long-term use due to residual muscle weakness.*
		  D. Atracurium besylate (Tracrium) *Not prolonged with renal or hepatic failure.*
		  E. Cisatracurium (Nibex) *Not prolonged with renal or hepatic failure.*
		3. Nondepolarizing Reversal agents
		  A. Cholinesterase inhibitors
		    i. Edrophonium chloride (Tensilon, Enlon)
		    ii. Neostigmine (Prostigmine)
		    iii. Pyridostigmine bromide (Regonol, Mestinon)
		    iv. Glycopyrrolate (Robinul). Used with Neostigmine and/or Pyridostigmine.
		    v. Atropine sulfate. Used with edrophonium or neostigmine.
		  B. Used for reversal of rocuronium and vecuronium (encapsulates molecule/Binds it).
		    1. Suggammadex (Bridion)
			1. Depolarizing agent: Monitor for MH symptoms. Monitor extremities during induction to ensure no injury occurs. Use with digitalis may cause arrhythmia. Not used for patients with Hx of MH or genetic disorders of plasma cholinesterase. Increases ICP and IOP. Can increase K+ levels. Possible vagal stimulation causing bradycardia or asystole, possible cardiac arrest with denervation patients (disease, injury, or intentional interruption of nerves results in muscle atrophy).
			2. Nondepolarizing agent: prolonged action with inhalation agents. Probable prolonged effects with some antibiotic and anticonvulsant medications. Histamine release causes tachycardia and hypotension.

(Continued)

TABLE 6-3 • EXAMPLES OF THERAPEUTIC ACTION CLASSIFICATION BY PURPOSE OR EXPECTED USE IN SURGERY *(Continued)*

Distention Media	Used to establish pneumoperitoneum for laparoscopic surgery and hysteroscopy to distend uterus.	Carbon Dioxide: CO_2, grey gas tank, ensure sufficient tank pressure to prevent interruption during procedure. Should be warmed to prevent hypothermia and filtered to prevent contamination from any tank "trash" such as rust or debris.	Danger of CO_2 embolus. Establishment of the abdominal pneumoperitoneum can cause pressure on diaphragm with resultant referred shoulder pain and dysrhythmia. Abdominal pneumoperitoneum is released at end of procedure to reduce pressure and postop pain/complications.
Vasopressors	Vasopressor and Adrenergic Agonist. *(Also increases cardiac contractility; bronchiole relaxation and increased renal, mesentery, and coronary blood flow.)*	Vasopressor and Adrenergic Agonist 1. Metaraminol (Aramine) Tx: *Hypotension during anesthesia.* 2. Norepinephrine (Levophed, Levarterenol) *Tx: Hypotension with anesthesia and septic shock* 3. Epinephrine (Adrenaline) *Tx: Cardiac arrest, Bronchospasm/ Anaphylaxis, heart failure, hypotension, severe bradycardia* 4. Dopamine (Intropin)*Tx: Hypotension, Acute CHF, used with renal failure.* 5. Dobutamine (Dobutrex) *Tx: Heart Failure, cardiac decompensation after cardiac surgery;* Short-term Tx: hypotension. 6. Isoproterenol (Isuprel) *Tx: Heart Block, Bronchospasm/ Anaphylaxis, Heart Failure, Hypotension, Severe Bradycardia.* 7. Vasopressin (ADH, Pitressin) *Tx: Diabetes insipidus, abdominal distention, Pulseless V-tach of V-fib* 8. Phenylephrine *(Neosynephrine) Tx: Hypotension, shock, SVT, Tetralogy of Fallot,* prolonged duration of local anesthesia.	Emergency medications utilized for patients in shock. Extravasation (IV out of vein) with dopamine and norepinephrine can lead to tissue sloughing. Tx: Phentolamine (Regiline). Premature labor after 20 weeks: Tx: Ritodrine (Yutapor) inhibits uterine contraction.

TABLE 6-4 • EXAMPLES OF PHYSIOLOGIC ACTION: CLASSIFIED BY WHAT THEY DO IN THE BODY

Physiological Classification	Action	Common Medications	Key Considerations
Antihistamine (histamine receptor antagonist)	Blocks histamine release.	Benadryl (used for local reactions with urticaria/hives and itching) Epinephrine (used for Anaphylaxis allergic reactions including bronchodilation	Monitor symptoms. Allergic reactions can occur when taking a medication for the first time or any subsequent dosage. When patient states allergic, it is good to identify what type of reaction including the signs and symptoms. If an anaphylactic reaction, you should identify any similar medications that may stimulate this same reaction.

TABLE 6-4 • (*Continued*)

Autonomic agents
1. Adrenergic agents sympat-homimetics
   A. Alpha-adrenergic blocker
   B. Beta-adrenergic blockers
   C. Both alpha- and beta-ad-renergic blockers.
2. Cholinergic agents mimic the action of acetylcholine and affect smooth muscle, digestion, and heart function.
3. Anticholinergic (cholinergic blockers) includes some antidepressants, antihistamines, antipsychotics, etc.
	Drugs that mimic the actions of autonomic nervous system.	Examples:
		1. A. Tx: BPH and Hypertension. ie, Terazosin
		1. B. Tx: heart failure, bronchial dilator: ie, metoprolol (Lopressor)
		   2. Tx: shock. epinephrine, Norepinephrine, Dobutamine
		   3. Tx: pilocarpine Tx glaucoma; miotic. Tx: Myasthenia gravis, ie, neostigmine (prostigmine)
		   4. Tx: Parkinson's, mydriatic, ie, atropine
			Drugs used for the autonomic system have either an agonist (stimulate) or antagonist (prevent) effect.

Contrast Media
 	
Note: Iodine is not an allergen. The risk of reaction to contrast administration is low, even in patients with a history of "iodine allergy," seafood allergy, or prior contrast reaction. Allergies to shellfish do not increase the risk of reaction to intravenous contrast any more that of other allergies.
	Used to see structural anatomical details, locate stones or blockages, etc.	1. Hypaque 50 lowest iodine content; highest osmolarity.
		2. Lower Osmolarity:
		   A. Isovue 370
		   B. Omnipaque 350 (iohexol)
		   C. Visipaque 320
			Used diluted or full strength.
			
			Lower osmolarity contrast media has fewer toxic effects.
			
			Due to increased use of CT scans, possible side effects include contrast-induced hyperthyroidism, iodine-induced hypothyroidism, which is usually transient.

Dye or stains	Used to mark skin, locate orifices (ureteral openings when cut), and check for tubal patency.
	
	Ophthalmic dyes are used to detect damage, perforating injury (Seidel's test), nasolacrimal duct patency, fundus angiography (retina vasculature), etc.
		1. Gentian violet topical
		2. Indigo carmine (ampule)
		3. Methylene blue (ampule)
		4. Ophthalmic use:
		   A. Fluorescein with wood's lamp (UV)
		   B. Lissamine green
		   C. Rose Bengal
			When preop skin marking is completed, care is taken not to remove during skin prep.
			
			IV use for Ophthalmic dyes requires that a crash cart be available due to potential allergic reactions.

Diuretic	Used for treatment of high blood pressure, fluid retention, Congestive heart failure, and pulmonary edema.	Lasix (furosemide) works on the Loop of Henle to prevent reabsorption of salt-causing diuresis. Hydrochlorothiazide (Hydrodiuril) Mannitol is an osmotic diuretic preventing reabsorption of water in the kidney. Diamox is used to treat acute glaucoma. Potassium-sparing diuretics: Amiloride Triamterene, Spironolactone (Aldactone) Eplerenone (Inspra)	Lasix can cause potassium depletion and may require replacement. Osmotic diuretic used for acute sudden renal failure, increased cerebral pressure/cerebral edema (ICP), Increased ocular pressure (IOP). Not used when kidneys have already shut down with no urination.

(*Continued*)

TABLE 6-4 • EXAMPLES OF PHYSIOLOGIC ACTION: CLASSIFIED BY WHAT THEY DO IN THE BODY *(Continued)*			
Thrombolytics	Dissolve clots. Used in treatment of Pulmonary embolism, thrombosis occurring in cerebrovascular accident (CVA), or acute myocardial infarction (AMI).	Alteplase (Activase), Reteplase (Retavase), Streptokinase (Streptase), Urokinase (Kinlytic), Tenecteplase.	Reversal agent for thrombolytics is Amicar (Aminocaproic acid); also used for treatment of DIC (disseminated intravascular coagulation or intravascular clotting. Contraindications: any prior intracranial hemorrhage, suspected aortic dissection, <3 weeks major surgery, peptic ulcer, current use of anticoagulants.
Vasoconstrictor	Epinephrine Others include: Norepinephrine (Levophed), vasopressin, phenylephrine, pseudoephedrine	Additive to local anesthetic to prolong retention, Emergency treatment of anaphylactic shock.	Dosage is dependent on the strength of the solution. 1:100,000 or 1:200,000 is utilized for local anesthesia. Treatment of asystole is 1:10,000. Solutions available to treat shock via IV drip use a mixture of 1:1000 in IV fluids titrated to elevate the blood pressure.

TABLE 6-5 • EXAMPLES OF CHEMICAL CLASSIFICATION: CLASSIFIED ACCORDING TO COMPOSITION			
Classification	**Actions**	**Common Medications**	**Key Considerations**
Barbiturate	Sedative hypnotic anesthetic adjunct (induction agent)	Phenobarbital (Luminal) Pentobarbital (Nembutal) Brevital Thiopental Secobarbital sodium (Seconal) sedative	CNS depressant; no antidote; used for capital punishment and assisted suicide.
Benzodiazepine	Anti-anxiety, amnesia, sedation, tranquilizer, anticonvulsant, Skeletal muscle relaxant	1. Diazepam (Valium) Tx: Status epilepticus, reduce anxiety, sedation. 2. Midazolam (Versed) 3. Lorazepam (Ativan)	Used for conscious sedation, preop sedation, cardioversion and to reduce anxiety. Hypotension
Hormones 1. Oxytocin 2. Corticosteroids 3. Insulin/glucagon 4. Prostaglandins 5. Sex hormones	Hormone replacement	Oxytocin: uterine contractions Cortisone Insulin Synthyroid Testosterone Estrogen	When used for replacement therapy, blood levels used to titrate for effectiveness

Medication Orders

Medication orders can be written by medical doctors (surgeons), physician assistants as defined by state and hospital policy, and advanced registered nurse practitioners. As identified by state law, a pharmacist can also prescribe medications, adapt prescriptions or vaccines, and make recommendations for over-the-counter medications for common ailments.

• A prescription order can be a written order or prescription, a standing order to be enacted for certain situations, a verbal order, a stat order (usually given during an emergency or in response to a complication), or a written pro re nata (PRN) order usually found on preop and postop orders. Written prescriptions must include the drug enforcement agency (DEA) number of the person writing the prescription. Medication orders in surgery can be received via standing orders such as those found on the preference cards in the operating room, verbal orders given during surgery, stat orders such as those during an emergency, PRN orders which are using written in the postoperative orders or given as prescriptions for the patient to self-administer. The prescription includes the drug, dose, form, route, and time (dosing schedule) for administration.

When a verbal order is given, it is always confirmed by repeating the order back to the surgeon or medical doctor. When passing medications, the medication is confirmed when the scrub surgical technologist passes the medication, syringe, or solution. It is your responsibility to listen and mentally confirm that the appropriate medication is being given to either you or the physician. Knowledge of allergies reviewed during the time out is essential to prevent anaphylactic life-threatening reactions.

Important points of prescriptions include the following key points:

- Medication – drug must be identified; form may also be needed depending on the route of administration and forms available.
- Dosage must be clear, if it is a tenth or hundredth dosage, a leading zero must be utilized to clearly locate the decimal point.

Important points of medication administration core knowledge:

- Patient Allergies
- Maximum or usual dosage (usually identified on the label or is a known amount per kilogram of patient weight)
- Expiration date – medications can deteriorate or lose potency over time
- Potential hazards or precautions for administration
- Medication abbreviations and the ability to read and interpret the standing orders, physician orders, or prescription given to the patient is an essential skill

Medication Distribution. Drug distribution is controlled by institution policy and state pharmacy distribution requirements. Typically, a pharmacist must dispense medications for administration so that an audit trail can be established. Systems used include centralized unit-dose drug distribution systems, satellite pharmacies, and automated dispensing cabinets (pyxis). There are mixing solutions for medications that may be dispensed as floor stock such as irrigation or IV solutions. Medications may also require refrigeration or protection from light to prevent loss of potency.

Controlled substances may require additional handling measures to prevent abuse or theft of the medication due to their potential for physical and/or mental dependency. Controlled substances are categorized into Schedules from I to V as follows: Schedule I Controlled substance with no accepted use, ie, heroin, bath salts, etc.; II Controlled substance that is highly addictive, ie, demerol/meperidine, sublimaze/fentanyl, etc.; III Controlled substance with moderate or low dependency, ie, ketamine, steroids, codeine, Vicodin, etc.; IV Controlled substance with lower dependency possibility, ie, Valium/diazepam, Versed/midazolam; or V Controlled substance with the lowest potential for abuse, ie, low-dose codeine with Phenergan or Robitussin. Controlled substances that are wasted must meet local or state requirements such as two licensed witnesses or return to the pharmacy. The DEA requires that they be disposed of so that they are rendered "non-retrievable." In addition, local or state laws may prohibit medication disposal into sewers (down the drain). The preferred methods for wastage include either a neutralizing media such as a solidifier for liquids or a neutralizing media such as Cactus Smart Sink/Rx Destroyer, containment in a nonhazardous pharmaceutical waste container which is sent out for incineration. Finally, it is recommended that there be two witnesses to any wastage, signatures for wastage should include the licensed circulator as per institution policy.

Medication Administration Supplies. Medications come in a variety of delivery systems including vials, ampules, intravenous piggyback pouches, intravenous bags of solution (250, 500, 1000, 3000, and 5000 mL bags), pour bottles of solutions (100, 250, 500, and 1000 mL), and a variety of dispensers such as ophthalmic drops, otic drops, nasal sprays, inhalers, aerosols, etc. (Table 6-6).

TABLE 6-6 • SUPPLIES		
Supply	**Types/Uses**	**Tip for practice**
Syringe tips	Used for specific functions. 1. Luer lock 2. Slip tip (plain) 3. Catheter tip 4. Toomey tip	1. Luer lock – for locking the needle tip in place. 2. Slip tip for easy attachment and removal for use with catheters or Seldinger technique. 3. To irrigate catheters and drains. 4. For use in cystoscopy to attach to equipment
Syringe sizes Parts include tip, calibrated barrel, flange (finger control), rubber stopper, and plunger.	Used for medications, diagnostic agents, and saline drips. 1. Insulin syringe 2. Tuberculin or 1 cc syringe 3. 3 cc syringe 4. 5 or 6 cc syringe 5. 10- or 12-mL syringe 6. 20 mL syringe 7. 30 mL syringe 8. 60 mL syringe 9. Asepto syringe (catheter tip)	1. Calibrated in units. 2. Calibrated in tenths 0.1 mL/cc with each hashmark worth 0.01 mL 3–5. Calibrated in ½ cc with each hashmark work 0.1 cc/mL or 1 cc/mL with each hashmark worth 0.2 cc/mL. 6–7. Calibrated in 5 cc/mL increments with each hashmark worth 1 cc/mL (Note: 30 mL may also be calibrated for an ounce.) 8–9. Calibrated in 10 mL with each hashmark worth 1 cc/mL

(Continued)

TABLE 6-6 • SUPPLIES (Continued)		
Emesis basin	Used for medications, passing sharps, specimens, or cottonoids.	Can vary in size from 12 oz to 20 oz. Calibrated on inside edge.
Bowls	Used for irrigation fluids, rinse basins, and to moisten lap sponges.	Typically, 2 bowls on set, 1 for irrigation solution and 1 to moisten lap sponges. (Do not want cloth fibers in your irrigation fluid as it can cause adhesions.)
Specimen cups	Calibrated according to size. May be sterile (used on sterile field) or unsterile (used only for specimens).	Size may vary. Typically, 2 on a setup to utilize for medications and smaller specimens.
Needles Parts include tip, lumen, shaft, hilt, and hub.	Types of tips: 1. Bevel tip 2. Blunt tip 3. Huber non-coring needle (slit) (straight or 90-degree angle) 4. Tonsil needle (angled) 5. Spinal needle 3.5-8 in (Quickne or pencil tip) 6. Intravenous needle (catheter over a needle) 7. Peel-away catheter dilator sheath	1. Standard injection needle 2. Used to attach to catheters for irrigation. 3. Used to access ports (silicone) for medication administration (self-seals). 4. Tonsil needle used for medication administration during T & A. 5. Spinal needles may be utilized for various markers or securing tissue. 6. Catheter is left when the needle is removed for IV access. 7. During Seldinger vessel access, needle is inserted into vessel, guide wire inserted, needle removed, and catheter sheath inserted over guidewire; vessel access enlarged enough for a catheter or pacemaker to be inserted within the sheath. Usually confirmed access via fluoroscopy.
Needle sizes Measured "Gauge"	1. 14-16 g 2. 18 g 3. 16-24 g 4. 22-25 g 5. 27-30 g	1. Largest size typically used for IV or injections. Preferred for Trauma IV access; used for administering large amounts of fluids. 2. 18 g used for drawing up medications- faster to draw up with. 3. Safe for blood administration (smaller the gauge the slower the blood administration). 4. 22-25 g used typically for local infiltration or IM injections. 5. 27-30 g used for plastic surgery facial local administration. Careful, easily broken.
Needle lengths	1. ½ in 2. 1 in 3. 1½ in 4. 3½-8 in (average 5 in)	1. Utilized for subcutaneous and intradermal injections. 2. Utilized for 27-30 g needles due to fragility of longer lengths. 3. Utilized for IM and infiltration injections. 4. Used for spinal needles. (needle with stainless steel obturator to stiffen needle for insertion)

Medication Administration. When administering the drug, the six rights of drug administration must be adhered to. They include right drug, right dose, right time, right patient, right route, and right documentation. The confirmation process for a medication order begins with transcription of the order for the patient. A medication error can occur at any point in the medication administration process from the time that the physician provides the order, unit transcription, pharmacy preparation, and then the actual patient administration process. Proper identification of the patient, their allergies, and any medications or herbal/nutritional supplements they utilize cannot be overemphasized. Overdosage of medications can lead to toxic reactions including seizures, coma, cardiac

or respiratory arrest, and shock. All of which can result in death ultimately.

Drug interactions, contraindications, and dosage limits are evaluated by both the pharmacist and the nurse during a routine assessment. If you are part of taking a history and physical, resources such as the drug insert, medication handbooks, the physician desk reference, and other medication references can provide up-to-date information regarding the medication ordered. Knowing your medications, reason for administration, usual dosage, and route is essential to ensure medication errors do not occur. Medication administration errors continue to occur despite the many safety precautions taken. These are usually a result of the work environment issues such as persistent staff shortages or turnover, too many distractions and interruptions, poorly designed medication safety protocols, and failure to adhere to policies and guidelines. Other issues include *look-alike and/or sound-alike* (LASA) and High alert medications including insulin, opiates and narcotics, injectable potassium chloride (or phosphate) concentrate, intravenous anticoagulants (heparin), and sodium chloride solutions above 0.9%, according to the Institute for Safe Medication Practices (ISMP). When names, packaging, various strengths/types, or administration device design are similar, these medications can be mistaken for each other. Being aware of this allows you to take extra care when these issues are occurring to prevent said medication errors.

During surgery, medications are ordered via the preference card and verbal orders from the physician. Common back table medications include diagnostic aids, antibiotics, irrigation fluids, hemostatics, anticoagulants, anti-inflammatories, analgesics, and local anesthesia. Verification of the medication includes not only the correct patient but correct physician and procedure when selecting the correct preference cards. Maintaining an up-to-date preference card is an essential element of the process. The administration of local anesthetics is a skill permitted by most institutions for the surgical assistant. Part of that process includes the preparation and planning including local anesthesia dosage calculations per kilogram to prevent local anesthesia systemic toxicity (formerly called lidocaine toxicity).

Ophthalmic Administration: When instilling eye drops, the medication must be labeled for "Ophthalmic" use. Because it does not contain preservatives, if contaminated, there is nothing to restrict microbial growth. Make sure the tip of the dropper does not inadvertently touch the eyelashes or conjunctiva. Instruct the patient to look up and pull down on the lower eyelid and instill the drops into the lower conjunctival pouch created. To prevent systemic absorption, compress the inner canthus with gauze to prevent the medication from entering the nasolacrimal duct system. ie, atropine sulfate (used for mydriatic and cycloplegic effects) which can affect the heart rate. Have the patient close the eyelids and blink to distribute the solution. For ophthalmic ointment, squeeze a thin strip of ointment from the inner canthus to the outer canthus, then have the patient roll his eye behind closed eyelids to distribute the ointment.

Otic Administration: Ensure ear medication is at room temperature not cold (can cause pain and vertigo). Warm prn by rolling between hands. For children less than 3 years and infants, pull on the earlobe down and back to straighten the ear canal and then instill the into the open canal. For adults and older children, pull auricle back and up, to straighten correct number of ear drops of the external ear canal and instill the ear drops. Tragus can be manipulated to ensure solution flows toward the middle ear.

Medication Conversions. Essential conversions include knowledge of the apothecary and metric systems, temperature conversions from Fahrenheit to Celsius or vice versa, and conversion of body weight from pounds to kilograms to calculate drug dosages (Tables 6-7 and 6-8).

TABLE 6-7 • ESSENTIAL CONVERSIONS

Fluid Unit	Conversion	Additional Conversion
1 milliliter (mL)	12 gtt old apothecary medical dropper. 20 gtt new pharmacy metric gtt—0.05 mL. Varies according to size and shape of a dropper. IV Macrodrip 10-20 gtt/mL—see box for specific calculations. IV Microdrip 60 gtt/mL	16 minims (m)
1 milliliter (mL)	1 cubic centimeter (cc)	1 gram (g)
1 Ounce (oz)	30 milliliters (mL)	30 cubic centimeters (cc)
1 Liter (L)	1000 milliliters (mL)	1000 cubic centimeter (cc)
Weight Unit	**Conversion**	**Additional Conversion**
1 milligram (mg)	1000 micrograms (mcg)	
1 gram (g)	1000 milligrams (mg)	
1 kilogram (kg)	1000 grams (g)	2.2 pounds (lbs.)
Length	**Conversion**	**Additional Conversions**
1 inch (in)	2.54 centimeter (cm)	
Solutions (Local Anesthetics)	**Dosage Equivalence**	**Solution**
0.25%	2.5 mg/mL	1000 mg / 100 mL

(Continued)

TABLE 6-7 • ESSENTIAL CONVERSIONS (*Continued*)

0.5%	5 mg/mL	1000 mg / 100 mL
0.75%	7.5 mg/mL	1000 mg / 100 mL
1%	10 mg/mL	1000 mg / 100 mL
2%	20 mg/mL	1000 mg / 100 mL
Concentration (Epinephrine)	**Dosage Equivalence**	**Solution**
1:1000	1 mg/mL	1000 mg / 1000 mL
1:50,000	0.02 mg/mL or 20 mcg/mL	1000 mg / 50,000 mL
1:100,000	0.01 mg/mL or 10 mcg/mL	1000 mg / 100,000 mL
1:200,000	0.005 mg/mL or 5 mcg/mL	1000 mg / 200,000 mL
Temperature	**Fahrenheit to Celsius F° to C°**	**Celsius to Fahrenheit C° to F°**
Using Decimals	$C° = (F° - 32) \div 1.8$	$F° = (C° \times 1.8)$ plus 32
Using Fraction	$(F° - 32) \times 5 \div 9 = C°$	$F° = (C° \div 5) \times 9$ plus 32

TABLE 6-8 • TYPICAL TEMPERATURES

°C	°F	Description
100	**212**	Water boils
40	**104**	Hot bath or fever
37	**98.6**	Body temperature
35	**95**	Hypothermia
25	77	Room temperature
21	70	Room temperature
0	**32**	Freezing point of water
−17.77778	**0**	Values

Note: **Bold temperatures** are exact.

Facility policy may require the use of a 24-hour military clock with midnight recorded as 2400 or 0000 as per institutional policy. This prevents errors in time stamps that are missing AM or PM (Table 6-9).

TABLE 6-9 • MILITARY 24-HOUR TIME VERSUS 12-HOUR STANDARD TIME

Time (12 h)	Military Time (24 h)	Time (12 h)	Military Time (24 h)
Midnight	0000 or 2400 h	Noon	1200 h
1:00 am	0100 h	1:00 pm	1300 h
2:00 am	0200 h	2:00 pm	1400 h
3:00 am	0300 h	3:00 pm	1500 h
4:00 am	0400 h	4:00 pm	1600 h
5:00 am	0500 h	5:00 pm	1700 h
6:00 am	0600 h	6:00 pm	1800 h
7:00 am	0700 h	7:00 pm	1900 h
8:00 am	0800 h	8:00 pm	2000 h
9:00 am	0900 h	9:00 pm	2100 h
10:00 am	1000 h	10:00 pm	2200 h
11:00 am	1100 h	11:00 pm	2300 h

Emergency Medications. Crash carts are typically stocked with all the emergency drugs commonly used for a medical emergency (Table 6-10). The only exception is dantrolene used for malignant hyperthermia which requires a recovery room or operating room malignant hyperthermia cart.

TABLE 6-10 • COMMON COMPLICATIONS AND EMERGENCY MEDICATIONS

Complication	Cause	Symptoms	Treatment
1. Allergic reaction simple versus anaphylactic shock	Causes: neuromuscular blocking agents, latex, antibiotics, bone cement, chlorhexidine, and vascular grafts. Contrast media, codeine, morphine sulfate (MS), demerol, and thiopental. Most common drugs include penicillin, codeine, contrast media, morphine, meperidine, atracurium, and thiopental.	1. Rash: simple, may itch; urticaria (wheals) petechiae. 2. Sudden or progressive changes in level of consciousness (LOC) (anxiety, restlessness, confusion, disorientation, sleepiness, unconscious, coma, death) 3. Bronchospasm, dyspnea, labored breathing, tachypnea, respiratory obstruction laryngeal edema, cardiac or resp arrest. 4. (B/P ↓) 1st sign with general anesthesia	1. IV fluids, medications to raise B/P such as dopamine or dobutrex. 2. Benadryl for minor reactions or early stages (25-50 IV) 3. Epinephrine for anaphylactic shock 4. Transfusion reaction (febrile nonhemolytic, allergic or hemolytic); stop blood —control hypotension, diuretics
2. Atelectasis: A. Pneumothorax, B. Hemothorax C. Empyema, D. Pleural effusion	Collapsed lung: potential causes A. Air either from perforated lung or perforated chest wall. B. Blood fills cavity. C. Pus fills cavity. D. Painful area of plural space leads to inflammation with fluid accumulation.	1. Surgical cause, perforation of the pleura during insertion of IV subclavian, life port, or vascular access catheter 2. Shortness of breath, dyspnea, labored breathing, tracheal deviation as lung collapses and another lung begins to collapse. 3. Crepitus of skin (air crackles) around site	1. Thoracostomy: insertion of chest tube until it heals to allow expansion of lung. 2. Pleural effusion may require thoracentesis.
3. Cardiac dysrhythmias	Heart block Frequent PVC (premature ventricular contraction) Ventricular tachycardia Ventricular fibrillation Asystole	1. No relationship between atrial and ventricular contraction. 2. PVC occurring greater than 6/min or multifocal. 3. V-tach: irritable focus in ventricle 4. V-fib: chaotic muscle contraction with no pulse or mechanical action 5. Asystole: no pulse, no rhythm on EKG	1. Heart block: pacemaker 2. PVC: lidocaine or po medication 3. V-Tach: lidocaine if pulse; if no pulse CPR and lidocaine. 4. V-fib: Defibrillate 5. Asystole: CPR—Epinephrine CPR steps - Airway - Breathing - Circulation

(Continued)

TABLE 6-10 • COMMON COMPLICATIONS AND EMERGENCY MEDICATIONS (*Continued*)

4. Cardiac arrest	LOC, No resp or cardiac function	1. Causes include arrhythmias from medications, AMI, CHF, Anaphylaxis; etc. 2. Symptoms include pale, cold, clammy with resp distress, hypotension, or no vital signs 3. Treatment with medications to stimulate heart rate, treat dysrhythmias, improve force of muscle contraction—inotropics	1. Code Blue or Code 99 2. ABCD 3. Duties vary with role: Scrub usually stays sterile to provide any sterile assistance. 4. Drugs include adrenaline, 1 mg bolus q 3-5 min; ADH vasopressin (Pitressin 40 units can be given to adults); amiodarone (Cordarone) or xylocaine (lidocaine), atropine, Mag Sulfact if hypomagnesia; sodium bicarbonate to treat acidosis from buildup of CO_2; calcium for hypocalcemia. 5. Tx: cause: hypotension and low cardiac output especially due to bradycardia includes dopamine (Intropin); dobutrex or dobutamine to treat CHF and shock along with Lasix; Isuprel (isoproterenol can be used for bradyarrhythmia's and bronchodilator, increases HR and contractility; neosynephrine and vsoxyl to treat vasoconstriction and hypotension. If respiratory emergency use albuterol and brethine; inotropic to improve cardiac muscle contraction such as digoxin, dopamine, dobutamine, epinephrine, or norepinephrine. Also, pronesterol; vasodilators such as nitroglycerine and nipride to treat hypertension, angina, or cardiogenic shock.
5. DIC – disseminated intravascular collapse	Processes of coagulation and fibrinolysis lose control, and the result is widespread clotting with resultant bleeding.	1. Multiple traumas with massive blood transfusion. 2. Pregnancy: amniotic fluid embolus or fetal demise 3. Gram-negative sepsis: release of enzyme	1. Usually not successful: may use FFP and platelets. 2. Infusion with antithrombin (AT) synthesized in the liver and is the major inhibitor of blood coagulation. 3. A reversal agent for thrombolytics is anti-fibrinolytic - Amicar (Aminocaproic acid) Tx: Bleeding due to systemic hyperfibrinolysis.
6. Drug interactions	Overdose Patient Sensitivity Size of patient Failure of drugs to be broken down (liver) and excreted (kidneys	1. Drop in blood pressure. 2. Respiratory arrest 3. Cardiac arrest 4. Prolonged anesthesia	1. Stop the drug; give antidote if possible. 2. For narcotic OD, give Narcan. 3. For valium or versed give Mazicon or Romazicon 4. Support ventilation and circulation (CPR)

TABLE 6-10 • (Continued)			
7. Laryngospasm (potential complication of laryngospasm treatment can include pulmonary edema.)	Involuntary constriction of vocal cords/larynx	1. High-pitched crowing or stridor 2. No air exchanges. 3. Oxygen Desaturation ↓oxygen level pulse oximetry, bradycardia	1. Forced continuous positive airway pressure (CPAP) utilizing ambu bag with mask/100% Oxygen. 2. Anectine/ succinylcholine to allow re-intubation. 3. Cricothyroidotomy (Emergency Trach prn)
8. Local anesthetic systemic toxicity (LAST) originally known as lidocaine toxicity.	Overdose of Amino Amide local anesthetic such as xylocaine (lidocaine), bupivacaine (Marcaine), or ropivacaine	1. CNS symptoms: drowsy, excitement, or agitation. Tinnitus, tremors, blurred vision, seizures. 2. N&V 3. CV symptoms: Hypotension, bradycardia, arrhythmias. Cardiac arrest	1. Stop drug; give IV fluids, maintain airway, Oxygen, Valium to treat seizures, drugs to raise B/P prn. 2. 20% Lipid emulsion Infusion: fat cells absorb the medication. 3. Lidocaine 5 mg/kg, max. 350 mg; with epinephrine up to 7 mg/kg, max 500 mg. 4. Bupivacaine 2 mg/kg, max 175 mg; with epinephrine 3 mg/kg, max 225 mg. 5. Ropivacaine 3 mg/kg, max 300 mg; with epinephrine 3 mg/kg; max 500 mg.
9. Malignant hyperthermia Definitive dx: Muscle biopsy reaction to halothane Genetic family history; pediatric with history of rheumatoid arthritis; musculoskeletal diseases	An anesthesia triggers a response: calcium causes muscle contraction thereby raising patient's temperature as heat is generated. Due to genetic predisposition. Trigger: Anesthesia drug: Gas inhalation agents (ending -ane) halothane, forane, enflurane, suprane and 1 depolarizing muscle relaxer—Anectine (Succinylcholine)	1. Tachycardia, tachypnea 2. Rise in end-tidal CO_2 monitoring Capnography. 3. Masseter jaw rigidity (Trismus); skeletal muscle rigidity 4. Metabolic and respiratory acidosis 5. Cardiac arrhythmias 6. Signs of shock 7. Pyrexia: increase as much as 1-2°C q 5 min. Can get as high as 108°F.	1. Stop the anesthesia trigger. 2. Change out the breathing circuit hyperventilate 100% O_2. 3. Give dantrolene (skeletal muscle relaxant) mixed in H_2O via large bore IV or central line if possible (36 vials on hand); sodium bicarbonate IV. 4. Iced lavage, everywhere including an open abdomen. 5. Diuretics to keep kidney working; insulin for ↓ K. 6. Best method – screening and prevention by muscle biopsy: (in vitro contraction test, IVCT or caffeine-halothane contracture test [CHCT]), then use thiopental sodium and pancuronium prn. droperidol or benzodiazepine and type local anesthetic
10. Paralytic ileus	Absence of peristalsis of the bowel leading to obstruction; may be a side effect of the anesthesia (when all other muscles relaxed these do too)	1. Absent bowel sounds 2. Retention of air, feces, etc.	1. NPO, provide stimulants 2. Salem Sump NGT to suction to prevent N&V 3. Ambulation to stimulate peristalsis
11. Pulmonary edema	Fluid overload, circulatory overload, or congestive heart failure (CHF) causing a buildup of fluid in the lungs	1. Frothy sputum 2. Visible on chest x-ray 3. Shortness of breath, tachycardia	1. Lasix to remove fluid. 2. Oxygen; HOB elevated. 3. Insert Foley; measure I & O along with weight. 4. Cardiac drugs such as digoxin or verapamil to treat CHF.

(Continued)

TABLE 6-10 • COMMON COMPLICATIONS AND EMERGENCY MEDICATIONS (*Continued*)			
12. Pulmonary embolism	Clot breaks off and travels to lungs where it obstructs blood flow. If large enough will cause death due to obstruction of a major vessel and sudden hypoxia.	1. Chest pain 2. Shortness of breath 3. Visible on arteriogram	1. Treatment is prevention of venous stasis of lower limbs using TED hose and SCD stockings. 2. Heparin IV or SC to thin blood and prevent clots. 3. Streptokinase can be given if no recent surgery to dissolve clots.
13. Respiratory arrest	Obstruction: tongue, teeth Medulla oblongata compression due to increased cranial pressure (ICP) greater than 20). Diaphragm paralysis (spinal too high)	1. Progressive peripheral cyanosis (nail beds) progressing to central cyanosis (circumoral) 2. Hypoxia or hypercapnia (breathing too shallow and fast) 3. Change in LOC, restlessness, anxiety, etc. 4. Rapid shallow breathing, dyspnea, or Cheyne Stokes respirations (episodes of tachypnea with apnea) 5. Physical signs or complaints of shortness of breath	1. Open airway 2. ABG's to determine pH status of blood. Normal pH 7.35-7.45. CO_2 35-45 %. 3. Respiratory Acidosis Tx. Oxygen, Sodium bicarbonate IV, intubate, ventilator prn. 4. Treat cause

14. Shock	Drop in blood pressure with resultant changes in level of consciousness, if not reversed leads to death.
	
	Caused by a variety of causes including:
	1. Hypovolemic shock from hemorrhage or dehydration
	2. Cardiogenic when heart unable to circulate the blood.
	3. Neurogenic when nerves fail and there is pooling of blood and fluids in the extremities.
	4. Fluid leaving circulatory system into the body such as with extensive burns.
		1. Drop in B/P of 20 or more points.
		2. Pale cold, clammy skin (Diaphoresis)
		3. Oliguria
		4. Progressive changes in level of consciousness (LOC) (dizziness, fainting, weakness, disorientation, confusion, unconsciousness, coma)
		5. Initial Tachycardia (rapid weak pulse) with slowing to Bradycardia and cardiac arrest as it progresses.
			1. Trendelenburg position: modified Trendelenburg may be used whereby feet and lower legs are level with head down to prevent cardiac and/or respiratory stress.
			2. Variations according to cause include:
			  A. IV fluids may include dextran (plasma expander to increase circulating volume) or blood and normal saline.
			  B. Medications to increase blood pressure such as dopamine, dobutamine, epinephrine (adrenaline)m norepinephrine (Levophed), milrinone, phenylephrine,
			3. Treat underlying cause of the shock.

15. Transfusion reaction (hemolytic)	1. Types: febrile nonhemolytic, allergic, or hemolytic	1. Febrile causes by antibodies binding to WBC or platelets, rarely seen. 2. Allergic: usually mild, caused by meds taken by donor or additives used to prepare the blood product. 3. Hemolytic: hypotension, hemoglobinuria, anuria or oliguria, fever, and DIC.	1. Febrile treated with acetaminophen 2. Allergic treated same as above. 3. Hemolytic: incompatible blood. Stop blood, treat hypotension, and give mannitol diuretic

Routes of Administration. There are four major routes of administration including topical, inhalation, enteral (GI tract), and parenteral. The route of administration is selected for effectiveness, the form of the drug available, and how soon the drug onset/peak action is needed. The forms include solids (powdered drugs to be reconstituted, tablets, and capsules), semisolids (creams, foams, gels, ointments, and suppositories), liquids (solutions, nasal sprays, suspensions, emulsions, elixirs syrups, and lozenges), and gas (oxygen, anesthesia gases, etc.).

Topical applications work locally at the site of application. Topicals placed on intact skin have little to no penetration of the skin. Topicals can include semisolids, liquids, and reconstituted powders. In surgery, topical examples include those drugs applied to wounds or imbedded in dressings (xeroform), hemostatic agents such as collagen (Avitene, Thrombin, etc.), and local anesthetic sprays such as those to eliminate the gag reflex during bronchoscopy.

Inhalation drugs are administered via the lungs which are absorbed immediately into the bloodstream and can be an effective substitution for emergency drugs when an intravenous line has not been established yet. Drugs administered via inhalation include gases of which oxygen is the most common first-line drug treatment and liquids and anesthetic agents. Emergency drugs that can be administered via endotracheal tube include Narcan (naloxone, an opioid reversal agent), atropine sulfate (symptomatic bradycardia, nerve gas), lidocaine (ventricular tachycardia), epinephrine (vasoconstrictor, treatment of shock), and midazolam (versed for sedation or seizures). Vasopressin can also be given via ETT. The dose is usually 2 to 2½ times the IV route and is diluted with 10 mL of saline.

Enteral drugs are those that are absorbed by the GI tract. Onset varies by route and form. For example, sublingual, buccal, or rectal are absorbed by the mucous membrane directly into the bloodstream and include such drugs as nitroglycerin (treatment of angina/chest pain to increase blood flow to area of hypoxia). Other oral drugs can be coated with agents for time-released capsules to spread absorption over an expected length of time and eliminate multi doses.

Parenteral drug routes include transdermal, intravenous, intramuscular, and subcutaneous. Transdermal discs or patches contain compounds that increase medication penetration through the stratum corneum for systemic or deeper tissue effects. Typical time for onset of an oral drug that is not coated is approximately 1 hour.

Role of the Surgical Team. The surgical team has a unique role in the administration of medications for the patient. The anesthesia provider is responsible for maintaining surgical anesthesia, analgesia, and homeostasis for the patient as appropriate to the surgical procedure and condition of the patient. Vital signs are monitored routinely including blood pressure, temperature, respiratory rate, pulse oximetry for oxygen saturation, end-tidal carbon dioxide measurements via capnography, and EKG heart monitoring for arrhythmias and rate. Anesthesia administers medications to maintain the patient safe, stable, and free from psychological or physical trauma. BiSpectral Index Monitoring

(BIS) is aimed at the prevention of anesthesia awareness during general anesthesia. A goal of 40 to 60 ensures that the patient is under hypnosis and is not aware of sensations including pain and hearing.

The circulator as the unsterile member of the team provides the team with assistance as needed during the surgical procedure. Coordination of the team with the control desk and other departments is essential to ensure resources are available to the team as needed. This includes the medications used intraoperatively during the surgical procedure. The circulator selects the appropriate medications and solutions providing them to the sterile team member.

The sterile team member receives the medication. Both team members are responsible for identifying the correct medication, strength, any additives, and expiration date. The medication is inspected for any problems such as precipitates, glass particles, etc., and transferred in a manner that sterility is maintained. Transfer devices, syringes, and pouring of solutions can be utilized.

When receiving the medication, the circulator reads the information, and the sterile team member repeats/confirms the medication as they read it too. The label is made and applied to the receiving container and the medication received.

Receiving a medication via syringe: The labeled syringe is fitted with an 18-gauge needle and the circulator cleans the medication vial/ampule with alcohol, then holds the vial (air is drawn into the syringe in the amount to be received and injected into the sealed vial) or broken ampule steady with two hands to allow the sterile team member to enter the opening. Once entered, the needle tip is turned so the bevel is down and in the neck of the container. Solution is withdrawn. 18-gauge needle (may be filtered) is removed from the syringe and placed in the sharps container as per hospital policy. If to be injected the appropriate size needle 22 to 25 gauge (1½ in needle usually or 27 to 30 gauge (1/2-in needle usually to limit breakage within the skin) is applied and syringe is stored until needed.

Receiving a medication or solution poured or transferred via transfer device: The labeled container is placed at edge of table to prevent an unsterile hand from passing over the table. The circulator pours the solution or medication into the container ensuring that all is poured at once and the lip of the container does not cross the vertical plane of the table edge.

Some medications are packaged in a manner for the circulator to flip or present the item to the sterile team member. Transfer of the item should always be completed in a manner that prevents an unsterile hand from passing over the sterile field.

Receiving a medication such as K-Y Jelly. According to hospital policy, a multi-use container may have a small amount discarded to ensure no contamination. Single-dose medications such as ointments and cremes are utilized by dispersing an amount at the end of the procedure just prior to dressing application once the skin is closed.

Receiving medications such as ointment-impregnated dressings, Vaseline gauze, the sterile team member utilizes a pair of rat tooth or smooth dressing forceps to pick up the item from the opened package held firmly by the circulator.

Sterile Team Member Medication Administration

- Demonstrates the ability to prepare and safely administer medications intraoperatively.
  - Demonstrates ability to identify the medication(s) to be used intraoperatively or in an emergency including the classification, usage, precautions, and potential hazards of the medication.
  - Verifies patient identification, allergies, NPO status, procedure, surgical site, consent, history and physical on chart.
  - Ensures ordered medication(s) are available for surgeon.
  - As appropriate to procedure/surgeon, designates the neutral zone according to hospital policy. Typically, even if the surgeon may need the sharp item placed in the surgeon's hand, it is returned to the neutral zone for the sterile team member to retrieve and secure safely.
  - Local anesthesia administration
    - Identifies types of local anesthesia, dosage per kilogram, and safety precautions.
    - Maintains knowledge of signs and symptoms of local anesthesia systemic toxicity (LAST, formerly known as lidocaine toxicity).
    - Confirms total amount safe for administration to the patient either by consulting anesthesia or calculating dosage according to the patient's weight in kilograms just prior to start of surgical procedure.
- Specifics regarding preparation of the medication:
  - Ensures medication is identified correctly and safely. Reads and confirms medication with the circulator including expiration date. Ensures label is correctly prepared and placed so calibrations are not covered.
  - Ensures medication is correct for the patient including considerations for age, weight, type of anesthesia, site of procedure, and allergies as well as the surgeon preference.
  - Demonstrates competency in passing medications to the surgeon or surgical assistant:
    - Labeled correctly.
    - Passes safely as per hospital policy. (Needle tip protected, no recapping of needles, double-gloving, the neutral (safe) passing zone also known as hands-free-technique (HFT), and appropriate use of blunt-tip suture needle technology.)
    - Confirms medication while passing to surgeon by stating out loud the medication, strength or dose, and any additives.
    - Identifies syringe calibrations correctly. Tracks and reports amount utilized correctly. Notifies circulator for documentation at end of procedure.
    - Recaps as necessary using scoop and pop technique.

ASA GUIDELINES FOR INJECTION OF LOCAL ANESTHETICS

Guideline I

Injection of local anesthetics should only be performed by surgical assistants with documented training in sterile technique, administration of local anesthetics, and monitoring techniques that will allow the surgical assistant to identify signs and symptoms of adverse reactions to the medication(s).

1. Surgical assistants should possess a thorough knowledge of surgical anatomy to prevent errors and patient injury.

2. Surgical assistants should know, and practice sterile technique related to the injection of local anesthetics.

3. Surgical assistants should perform local anesthetic injection techniques under the supervision of the surgeon.

   A. Injection techniques to be performed under the surgeon's supervision include intradermal, subcutaneous, deep tissue, and intra-articular.

      i. The surgical assistant should be able to demonstrate the ability to select the correct size of hypodermic needle for intradermal, subcutaneous, deep tissue and intra-articular injections.

4. Surgical assistants should know and practice knowledge of the maximum doses with and without epinephrine of all local anesthetic drugs.

5. Surgical assistants should be knowledgeable of the surgical pharmacological.

   A. Surgical assistants should know and practice knowledge of the pharmacodynamics of all local anesthetic drugs.

   B. Surgical assistants should know and practice knowledge of the pharmacokinetics of all local anesthetic drugs.

   C. Surgical assistants should know and practice knowledge of the indications and contraindications of all local anesthetic drugs.

6. Surgical assistants should be knowledgeable of patient monitoring techniques to identify signs and symptoms of adverse local anesthetic reactions.

   A. Surgical assistants should know the cardiovascular and neurologic signs and symptoms of adverse local anesthetic reactions, to assist the surgical team in treating the patient.

      i. Surgical assistants should know the patient treatment principles of recognition, immediate management, treatment, and follow-up.

      ii. The surgical assistant should have the necessary skills to perform specific duties including CPR; assist with airway maintenance and oxygen administration; establishing additional vascular access, ie, assist with swan ganz or intravenous insertion.

      iii. The surgical assistant should know treatment protocols regarding the administration of drugs used to treat local anesthetic reactions including types, concentrations, and dosage of drugs, ie, benzodiazepines and IV lipids.

Guideline II

The surgical assistant should be knowledgeable and have the training to determine the timing of the local anesthetics effects and identify when the localized area is numb.

1. The surgical assistant should take the appropriate measures to determine when the localized area is numb.

Guideline III

The surgical assistant should practice the principles of sharps safety when handling hypodermic needles.

1. The surgical assistant should be familiar with policies regarding establishment and use of the neutral zone; recapping of hypodermic needles; use of various types of sharps containers within the sterile field and off the field; use of mechanical devices to remove needles from syringes; and double gloving.

   A. It is recommended the surgical assistant become familiar with the AST Guidelines of Practice for Sharps Safety and Use of the Neutral Zone (2006).

Guideline IV

The surgical assistant should practice positive communication skills when coordinating the care of the local anesthetic patient with the surgical team.

1. Miscommunication between physicians, pharmacists, and other healthcare providers including surgical technologists, surgical assistants, and nurses is one of the most common causes of medication errors. It is essential the surgical team practices the principles of verifying drug information as well as positive communication skills that eliminate communication barriers (Institute for Safe Medication Practices, 2013).

2. Coordinating care of the local anesthetic patient begins during the preoperative phase; the surgical assistant should confirm the following with the surgical team:

   A. Six rights of safe medication handling practices

      i. Right patient

      ii. Right drug, including name, concentration, with or without epinephrine

      iii. Right dose

      iv. Right route of administration

      v. Right time and frequency

      vi. Right labeling

   B. Patient allergies if present

3. Coordinating care of the local anesthetic patient continues during the intraoperative phase.

   A. The surgical assistant should coordinate verification of the name of the drug, concentration, and with or without epinephrine, each time the local anesthetic is used intraoperatively.

4. Coordinating care of the local anesthetic patient continues during the postoperative phase.

   A. The surgical assistant should communicate the name of the drug, whether it contains epinephrine, concentration of the drug, and the amount of the drug administered to other healthcare providers who will be providing postoperative patient care.

Guideline V

Documentation of the competency of the surgical assistant regarding injection of local anesthetics should be kept current.

1. The surgical assistant should have completed training in the injection of localized anesthetics in a simulated environment under the instruction of a surgeon.

2. The surgical assistant should complete an annual competency assessment that is confirmed by the surgeon for the injection of local anesthetics.

   A. The competency assessment should be conducted by a surgeon.

3. The surgical assistant should complete continuing education to remain current in his/her knowledge of the techniques for the injection of local anesthetics.

4. The surgical assistant should complete continuing education to remain current in his/her knowledge of new local anesthetic drugs. Please note, surgical assisting is prohibited in a few states. Given the variation between surgical assistants' related state statutes, rules, and regulations, it is essential that surgical assistants have a clear understanding of how their scope of practice is defined by their state's laws and regulations, as well as any opinions promulgated by the state regulatory agency. Local surgical assistant scope of practice is usually defined by the supervising surgeon, the hospital credentialing body, the state's board of medicine, and applicable state statute and regulation.

LOCAL ANESTHESIA COMPETENCY STATEMENT

Criteria 1. The surgical assistant possesses the knowledge and skills to inject local anesthetics to include application of sterile technique and patient monitoring.

Measurable Criteria:

1. Educational Guidelines as established in the current edition of the Core Curriculum for Surgical Assisting.

2. The subject of local anesthetics to include types, indications, contraindications, patient reactions, and treatment protocols of adverse reactions is included in the didactic studies of the surgical assistant student.

3. The subject of sterile technique regarding injecting local anesthetics is included in the didactic studies of the surgical assistant student.

   A. Surgical assistant students demonstrate their knowledge of the use of sterile technique and injection of local anesthetics during simulated operating room practice and clinical rotation.

   B. Surgical assistant practitioners implement proper sterile and injection techniques when injecting local anesthetics in the perioperative setting.

   C. Surgical assistants complete continuing education to remain current in their anesthetics, including annual review of the healthcare facility's policies and procedures.

Local Anesthetics

Due to the potential for complications, the surgical assistant must have a good working knowledge of the medication to be administered via infiltration (Table 6-11). The mechanism of action for local anesthetics is the blocking of nerve conduction near the site of administration, thereby producing temporary loss of sharp pain sensation in a limited area. Nerve impulse conduction is blocked by inhibition of sodium channels at the nerve endings and along the axon. This causes a decrease in nerve cell membrane permeability to sodium ions, possibly by competing with calcium-binding sites that control sodium permeability. This change in permeability results in decreased depolarization and an increased excitability threshold that ultimately prevents the nerve action potential from forming. Local anesthesia does not eliminate pressure sensation. The two types include the amino amides which are metabolized by liver and the amino esters which are metabolized by plasma.

Adverse events include symptoms of central nervous system (CNS) and cardiovascular (CV) collapse. Adverse CNS effects include circumoral numbness, facial tingling, vertigo, tinnitus, restlessness, anxiety, dizziness, seizure, and coma. CV effects include hypotension, arrhythmia, bradycardia, heart block, cardiac arrest. Bupivacaine is not injected intra-articular (into a joint space) since it can cause chondrolysis.

LAST is treated with an 20% intralipid infusion (Intralipid, Liposyn, Medialipid). When symptoms begin, no further local is injected, oxygen is administered (if not already in place), and the symptoms treated such as IV fluids may be increased to dilute and treat hypotension, head of bed lowered to increase blood pressure, etc.

As you can see calculating the maximum dosage is essential to preventing LAST. To calculate drug dosage using concentration, remember that Percentage is measured in grams per 100 mL (ie, 1% is 1 g/100 mL [1000 mg/100 mL], or 10 mg/mL). Calculate the mg/mL concentration quickly from the percentage by moving the decimal point 1 place to the right. (ie, bupivacaine 0.25% translates to 2.5 mg/mL, lidocaine 2% translates to 20 mg/mL, and ropivacaine 0.5% translates to 5 mg/mL).

Consequently, when 8 mL of 0.25% bupivacaine is administered, the total dose would be calculated as 2.5 mg × 8 mL which equals 20 mg.

Epinephrine overdose can result in cardiac arrhythmia, cardiac arrest, and death. Epinephrine as an additive can also be calculated when necessary. When epinephrine is combined in an anesthetic solution, the result is expressed as a dilution (ie, 1:100,000). Calculations:

1. 1:1000 means there is 1 mg or 1000 mcg/mL (ie, 0.1%)
2. 1:50,000 epinephrine concentration means that the solution contains 0.02 mg/mL or 20 mcg/mL.
3. 1:100,000 epinephrine concentration means that the solution contains 0.01 mg/mL or 10 mcg/mL.
4. 1: 200,000 epinephrine concentration means that the solution contains 5 mcg/mL.

Calculation Example:

1. 50 mL of 1% lidocaine with epinephrine 1:200,000 contains 500 mg of lidocaine and 250 mcg or 0.25 mg of epinephrine.

For the awake or monitored anesthesia care/IV sedation patient, another additive to local anesthesia can include sodium bicarbonate to change the pH to a more neutral solution reducing the painful "sting" as the medication is injected. Typically, the ratio for lidocaine is 9:1 mL of injectable sodium bicarbonate and for bupivacaine 19:1 mL of injectable sodium bicarbonate. A useful modification is to give the first prick intradermally, at right angles to the surface and a small quantity infiltrated to raise a wheal. After waiting for 2 minutes, a subsequent prick is given through the anesthetized area. Repetitive rapid rubbing and shaking of the skin proximal to the site of injection during infiltration also reduced the level of pain and discomfort. This is an application of the gate control theory of pain which states that nonpainful sensations can override and reduce painful sensations from being transmitted. The gate has been "closed" by the non-painful sensation transmission. A final method of preventing pain is to warm the local anesthetic solution prior to administration to 25°C to 40°C prior to infiltration.

TABLE 6-11 • LOCAL ANESTHETICS					
Local Anesthetic	**Strengths**	**Dosage**	**Classified as**	**Onset**	**Duration**
Lidocaine (least expensive) (Xylocaine) Kerns Law-	0.5%, 1%, 2%, and 4% gel	3-5 mg/kg not to exceed 300 mg	Amino amide / intermediate acting	1-2 min Rapid onset	30 min to 1 h
Lidocaine with epinephrine (Xylocaine with Epi)	0.5%, 1%, 1.5%, 2%, and 4% gel Epinephrine strengths: 1:100,000 (1% or 2%) 1:200,000 (0.5%, 1%, 1.5%, 2%)	7 mg/kg not to exceed 500 mg	Amino Amide / intermediate acting Epinephrine vasoconstriction decreases the risk of toxicity; slows absorption increasing duration of action.	1-5 min rapid onset	1½-2 h

TABLE 6-11 • *(Continued)*

Bupivacaine (Marcaine) Note: Implantable version of collagen & bupivacaine approved 2020: Xaracoll. Postop Pain management liposomal formulation: Exparel. Subacromial Space injection Posimir.	0.125% 0.25% 0.5% 0.75%	2-3 mg/kg maximum dose: 175 mg Not recommended for children under 12 y	Amino amide / long acting Analgesia without motor blockade (popular for labor)	4-8 min Slow onset	2-4 h
Bupivacaine with epinephrine (Marcaine)	0.25% 0.5% 0.75% Epinephrine strengths: 1:200,000	2-3 mg/kg Maximum dose: 225 mg	Amino amide / long acting Epinephrine vasoconstriction decreases the risk of toxicity; slows absorption increasing duration of action.	4-8 min Slow onset	3-8 h
Ropivacaine (Naropin)	0.2%, 0.5%, 0.75%	4 mg/kg 5-200 mg	Amino amide / long acting	Slow onset 1-15 min	4-9 h (2-6 h)
Cocaine Hydrochloride (Goprelto, Numbrino) Not used for Local infiltration, may be used for nasal topical packing or pledgets ½ in × 3 in 1-2 per nasal passage up to 20 mins.	4% (40 mg/mL)	40-160 mg Maximum dosage is 3 mg/kg	Amino ester / intermediate acting	Seconds to minutes	45 min to 1.5 h
Procaine (Novocaine)			Amino ester		
Tetracaine (Pontocaine HCL, Niphanoid, Ophthaine) Regional, topical, or ophthalmic usually	1%	1.5 mg/kg	Amino ester	Slow onset 10 min	3-8 h

Infiltration of Local Anesthetics. The field block technique includes infiltration along the wound edges of an open laceration or traumatic wound, encircling technique, and fan-shaped technique. Typically, a 22- to 25-g 1½ in needle with a 10-cc syringe is utilized for routine infiltration. Anything smaller can break easily within the skin and become a retained surgical item (RSI) that must be retrieved. If a 27- to 30-g needle is utilized for facial injections/plastic surgery, 1 in to ½ in needle should be utilized with a 3-cc syringe for control. A nerve block injection is injected around a sensory nerve that supplies the area. For the awake patient, insert the needle and inject a small amount intradermal. Then, continue to insert the needle up to the hub or depth of anticipated dissection parallel to intended incision line, aspirate prior to injection to avoid inadvertent intravenous administration. Then, inject as you slowly withdraw the needle. Inject until you see skin begin to swell. Stop withdrawal just prior to dermis exit, adjust angle, and infiltrate in a circular pattern around the wound (encircling technique) or fan-shaped technique.

Bibliography

American Heart Association. Cardiac Medications. 2020. https://www.heart.org/en/health-topics/heart-attack/treatment-of-a-heart-attack/cardiac-medications. Accessed April 3, 2023.

Association of Surgical Assistants. Job Description. Guidelines for Injection of Local Anesthetics. https://www.surgicalassistant.org/about/JobDescription/ and ASA_Guideline_Injection of Local Anesthetics_4.2.18 (surgicalassistant.org). Accessed April 3, 2023.

Association of Surgical Technologists. Guidelines for Best Practices for Treatment of Surgical Patients Experiencing Malignant Hyperthermia in the Operating Room. Approved October 2005. Revised April 9, 2018

AST Guidelines of Practice for Sharps www.ast.org. Safety and Use of the Neutral Zone (2006). Accessed January 2022.

Cave G, Harrop-Griffiths W, Harvey M, et al. AAGBI Safety guideline management of severe local anaesthetic toxicity. 2010. http://www.aagbi.org/sites/default/files/la_toxicity_2010_0.pdf. Accessed April 14, 2014.

Core Curriculum for Surgical Assisting. 3rd ed. Littleton: CO Association of Surgical Assistants; 2014.

Cox B, Durieux ME, Marcus MAE. Toxicity of local anaesthetics. *Best Pract Res Clin Anaesthesiol.* 2003;17(1):111-136.

Drug Specifics for Each Table (2019-2021). Drugs.com. https://www.drugs.com/professionals.html and https://www.drugs.com/pro/. Accessed April 3, 2023.

Eggleston ST, Lush LW. Understanding allergic reactions to local anesthetics. *Ann Pharmacother.* 1996;30(7-8):851-857.

El-Boghdadly K, Pawa A, Chin KJ. Local anesthetic systemic toxicity: Current perspectives. *Local Reg Anesth.* 2018;11:35-44. https://doi.org/10.2147/LRA.S154512. Accessed April 3, 2023.

Food and Drug Administration. Clinical Trials and Human Subject Protection. 2020. https://www.fda.gov/science-research/science-and-research-special-topics/clinical-trials-and-human-subject-protection. Accessed November 11, 2020.

Food and Drug Administration. Development and Approval Process. 2020. https://www.fda.gov/drugs/development-approval-process-drugs. Accessed November 11, 2020.

Food and Drug Administration. FDA for Health Professionals. 2020. https://www.fda.gov/health-professionals. Accessed November 11, 2020.

Food and Drug Administration. How Drugs Are Developed and Approved. 2020. https://www.fda.gov/drugs/development-approval-process-drugs/how-drugs-are-developed-and-approved. Accessed November 11, 2020.

Galen N. How to Select the Correct Needle Size for an Injection. 2009. http://pcos.about.com/od/medication1/qt/needlesize.htm. Accessed April 14, 2014.

Ghofaily LA, Simmons C, Chen L, Liu R. Negative pressure pulmonary edema after laryngospasm: A revisit with a case report. *J Anesth Clin Res.* 2013;3(10):252. https://doi.org/10.4172/2155 6148.1000252. Accessed April 3, 2023.

Institute for Safe Medication Practices. Frequently asked questions (FAQ). 2013. http://www.ismp.org/faq.asp. Accessed April 14, 2014.

Medicine Net.Com. What Drugs Are Used for Conscious Sedation? (medicinenet.com). 2021.

Medscape. Organ Preservation. Organ Preservation: Practice Essentials, Pathophysiology of Organ Preservation, Preservation Solutions and Their Pharmacology (medscape.com). Updated November 7, 2020. Accessed March 3, 2021.

Nagelhout J. Basic Principles of Pharmacology. 2015. https://clinicalgate.com/basic-principles-of-pharmacology/. Accessed November 11, 2020.

National Skin Centre. Dermatological Drugs. https://www.nsc.com.sg/Patient-Guide/Health-Library/List-of-Dermatological-Drugs/Pages/List-of-Dermatological-Drugs.aspx. Accessed May 26, 2020.

North Carolina General Assembly Report: The Role of the FDA and PDFA in Drug Development. https://www.ncleg.gov/documentsites/committees/senatejudiciaryi2011/Subcommittee%20on%20Pharmaceutical%20Liability/April%2025,%202012%20Meeting/Documents%20Submitted%20by%20Speakers%20and%20Interested%20Parties/PhRMA%20Publication%20-%20Role%20of%20FDA%20and%20PDUFA%20in%20Drug%20Development.pdf. Accessed November 11, 2020.

Open Anesthesia Organization. Bronchospasm: acute treatment (openanesthesia.org) Bronchospasm: acute treatment (openanesthesia.org). 2021.

Pharmacology Education Project. https://pharmacologyeducation.org/drugs/gastrointestinal-system. Accessed May 26, 2020.

Samama MM, Amiral J, Guinet C, Le Flem L, Seghatchian J. Monitoring plasma levels of factor Xa inhibitors: How, why, and when? *Expert Rev Hematol.* 2013;6(2):155-164.

University of Denver, School of Medicine, Department of Pharmacology. A brief History of Pharmacology. www.ucdenver.edu/. Accessed April 3, 2023.

7

Technical Sciences

Rebecca Hall

DISCUSSED IN THIS CHAPTER

1. Principles of electricity and electrosurgery.
2. Minimally invasive surgical concepts and equipment.
3. Robotic surgery principles.

PRINCIPLES OF ELECTRICITY

Benjamin Franklin did not invent electricity. He did, however, conduct experiments on electricity to prove that electricity consisted of a common element which became the basis for his work titled "single fluid theory." Franklin believed electricity flows from a positive body, that with an excess charge, to a negative body, that with a negative charge. Electricity is the movement of electrical energy and one of our most widely used forms of energy.

All matter is formed of atoms, including the human body. Atoms are made up of protons, neutrons, and electrons. The center of the atom contains the nucleus and where the protons and neutrons reside. Protons are positively charged; neutrons are void of any electrical charge; electrons maintain a negative charge as they revolve around the nucleus. Each chemical element has a set number of protons and electrons. Electrons occupy valence shells around the nucleus. The electrons in the shells closest to the nucleus have a strong force of attraction to the protons. The electrons in the outermost shells can be pushed out of their orbit and the application of any force will cause them to move from one atom to another. The moving electrons are electricity. Electrical current is the movement of electrons due to a force which is driven by a change in voltage. Electrical current is directly proportionate to the voltage relative to the electrical resistance in a circuit.

Background of Electrosurgery

Electrosurgery and electrocautery are terms often used interchangeably; however, these different modalities have different applications. Electrocautery uses a direct electrical current to heat a metal wire that is used as an electrode. It is the electrode that will burn or coagulate tissue. In surgery, we use low-temperature and high-temperature cautery on tissue. The direct electrical current for electrocautery is produced by a battery. Electrocautery is often used in dermatologist offices, plastic surgery offices, and pediatric cases.

During electrosurgery, the electrical current passes through biological tissue utilizing a high-frequency alternating current that allows for cutting or coagulating tissue, reducing blood loss, and decreasing procedure times. Surgical diathermy was developed by electrophysicist William Bovie in 1926. The electrosurgical generator is the source of the electron flow and voltage. Temperatures over 45°C disrupt normal cell function and between 45°C and 60°C coagulation takes place, and the cell protein begins to solidify. Temperatures of 100°C will cause desiccation of the cell and beyond 100°C cells are reduced to carbon. The normal frequency of electrosurgery is as high as 500,000 cycles per second.

The power setting has a direct correlation on tissue effect. The higher the setting on the generator, the more extensive effect on the tissue. Extensive activation of electrical current increases the thermal effect on tissue and may have a larger thermal spread causing damage to unintended tissue.

Types of Electrosurgery

Monopolar electrosurgery devises use blades, round balls, needle tip, and loop configurations to initiate an effect on tissue. A complete circuit will allow for the flow of electrons and consists of the generator, active electrode, patient, and patient return electrode. The alternating current passes through tissue creating heat by the

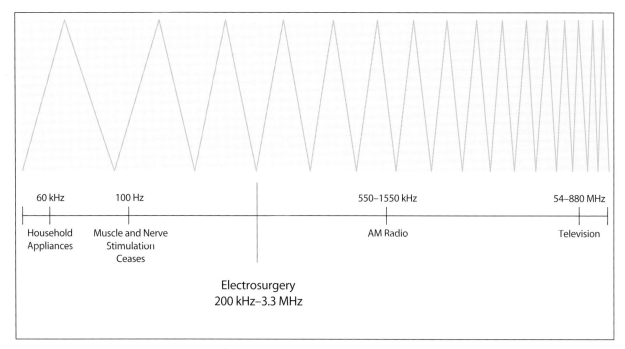

Figure 7-1 · Radiofrequency spectrum.

resistance of the tissue to the electrical current (Figure 7-1). The return electrode is positioned on the patient away from the surgical site, covering a large surface area. Low impedance is used to disperse the electrical current back to the generator, which completes the circuit and will prevent alternate burn sites as the high-frequency AC current leaves the patient's body.

With bipolar electrosurgery, the active and return electrodes are within the instrument tips, usually in the form of bayonet forceps. The current pathway is confined to the tissue grasped between the forcep tines with one tip being the active electrode and the other being the return electrode resulting in no need for a patient return electrode, or grounding pad to complete the circuit. During bipolar diathermy, the movement of electricity will stop if a specific impedance level is reached, most commonly 100 ohms. Bipolar electrosurgery is used for coagulating delicate tissue and does not damage adjacent tissue due to the lack of any electrical arc or spread of high-frequency current.

Electrical Terminology

Term	Definition
Current	The flow of electrons measured in amperes or amps
Voltage	The force or push that moves the electrons
Impedance	Obstacle to the flow of current
Resistance	Measured in ohms
Circuit	Pathway for the uninterrupted flow of electrons
Ohm	The SI unit of electrical resistance
Coulomb	Unit of electrical charge
Ampere	Unit of electric current

Surgical diathermy reacts differently on the different tissue types. Adipose tissue is not well vascularized, thereby presents more impedance requiring a higher power setting to produce an effect. Muscle tissue, however, is highly vascularized and does not require as much power to attain tissue effect.

Electrosurgical Waveforms

Electrosurgical units (ESUs) produce a variety of electrical waveforms which will produce a range of tissue effects.

- The pure cut mode means the electrical flow is continually applied to the tissue. The constant waveform produces heat very quickly cutting or vaporizing the selected tissue. The heat generated will dissipate as steam when the cell is vaporized. The current is high, but the voltage is low. The cut mode is a continuous barrage of electrons on the tissue, heat is produced, cells rupture, and the tissue is cut. To utilize the cutting mode in a monopolar bovie, the electrode should be held slightly away from the tissue to produce a spark gap and discharge arc.

- An intermittent waveform will generate a coagulation effect on tissue. The interrupted waveform is modified and delivers less heat to the target area. During the coagulation mode only 6% of the time electrons are flowing and 94% of the time there is no flow to the targeted tissue. With the absence of electrons flowing, the voltage is increased to produce the required wattage. The higher voltage allows for a spraying effect that will coagulate a large tissue area, collapse the cells, and produce a clot.

- A blended waveform will alternate from blend 1 to blend 3 waveform. Blend 1 will vaporize tissue with little hemostasis and blend 3 allows for maximum hemostasis without vaporizing tissue.

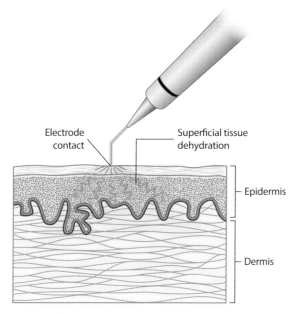

Electrode contact   Superficial tissue dehydration

Epidermis

Dermis

Figure 7-2 · Fulguration.

- Fulguration will coagulate and char tissue over a large area. The coagulation waveform has a higher voltage than the cutting current (Figure 7-2).
- Electrical desiccation occurs when the needle is in direct contact with tissue using the cutting current. Less heat is produced and there is no cutting action. The cell basically dries out and forms a clot.

Electrosurgical Units

Electrosurgical units (ESUs) have changed since their introduction to surgery in the 1920s. The first ESUs were grounded units. The grounded ESU provides electrical energy from the generator to the patient, and sends energy to the ground, which is intended to be the generator. Patients experienced burns from electricity seeking the path of least resistance, which may include alternative path sites as it seeks to return to ground.

In 1968, the isolated ESU transformed surgery. The integrated transformer only allows the current to return to the generator as the ground and not any alternative pathway that might be in the operating room. The current flowing through the patient must return to the ground (the generator) to complete the circuit. This safety feature works well to prevent alternative site burns to the patient.

Dispersive electrode monitoring was launched in the 1980s. Dispersive monitoring protects the patient from dispersive electrode site burns caused by inadequate contact with the dispersive electrode pad. Correct placement of a dispersive electrode pad is essential to avoid patient injuries. The pad should be placed over an area that is well vascularized, such as a muscle mass.

Advanced technology uses **capacitance** that works on the principle of bulk resistivity. A capacitor is described as two conductors split by an insulator. A large capacitive pad consists

of a flexible conductive fabric bordered by a non-latex urethane insulating material. The layer of insulation prevents the direct flow of electricity between the two plates. Current from the active electrode produces a charge that accumulates on the first conductive plate. This causes an equal but opposite charge to develop on the second conductive plate. The charge on the second plate produces current that returns to the generator which completes the circuit. The interaction between the two plates happens through an electromagnetic field. The capacitive pad removes the need for an individual adhesive dispersive electrode pad, which is problematic if an ESU is used without dispersive electrode monitoring capabilities and the pad tents during a procedure.

Tissue response monitoring uses a computer-controlled tissue feedback system that detects resistance of the tissue and instinctively adjusts current and voltage output to provide a constant surgical effect. Tissue Response monitoring allows usage at a lower power setting thereby reducing the risk of patient injury.

ESU Complications during Endoscopic Surgery

Stray currents can cause injury to vessels or viscera by way of defective insulation on laparoscopic instrumentation. The two general causes of insulation failure are the use of high-voltage currents and the repeated re-sterilization of instruments, which will weaken and break the insulation. It is very important that insulated instrumentation is checked prior to sterilization. The coagulation waveform utilizes high-voltage currents to achieve its effect. However, using the cutting mode while holding the tip directly on the tissue will also coagulate at a lower voltage, thereby reducing the chances of insulation failure.

Direct coupling occurs when the active electrode is accidentally activated when it is near another metal instrument allowing electrical energy to flow and cause sparking as the energy seeks an alternative pathway to complete the circuit.

Capacitive coupling occurs when a nonconductive material such as insulation on a laparoscopic instrument separates two metal conductors. A capacitor creates an electrostatic field between the two conductors. The electrostatic field allows the current in the one conductor to jump to the second conductor. This is observed when monopolar ESUs are used with metal suction irrigators or even the laparoscope itself, leading to alternate site burns. These burns are not immediately detected but later when the patient presents with postoperative complications. The risk of capacitive coupling and insulation failure can be reduced or eliminated by using **active electrode monitoring** (AEM) instrumentation with shielding and the ability to monitor RF current to prevent ESU burns (Figure 7-3). The protective shield of the AEM instrument offers a neutral path for capacitive coupled energy and sends it to the ESU. AEM is the only technology available designed to address insulation failure and capacitive coupling and guarantees that 100% of electrosurgical energy is distributed at the intended location. The use of AEM technology on a patient must be documented in the patient chart for liability and risk management.

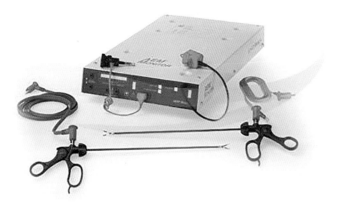

Figure 7-3 · AEM instrumentation.

Surgical assistants should be familiar with the various types of electrosurgery utilized in the surgical setting to assist the surgeon. The assistant will be across the surgeon when the initial incision is made, the first layer visible is the subcutaneous level containing adipose tissue, blood vessels, nerves, and lymphatics located in the tissue layer. As the surgeon applies electrocautery dissecting through the subcutaneous fat layer, the assistant must be ready to offer equal and opposite countertraction as the surgeon reaches deeper into the wound. Working across the surgeon mirroring his actions during the dissection is called "walking down the wound." As the surgeon adjusts his hand, he is applying traction to the area of tissue he plans to dissect next. The assistant should be ready to imitate the surgeon's new actions. While the surgeon continues the dissection into deep tissue, the assistant should continue the application of countertraction to aid the surgeon to stay on midline by visualizing the wound and identifying vessels that may need ligation. The assistant may be in the situation to coagulate bleeding vessels with the ESU. The assistant should place the end of the tip against the point in the tissue where the blood is deriving from, depress the coagulation switch or cutting mode, and stop the bleeding.

MINIMALLY INVASIVE SURGERY

History

Minimally invasive surgery is one of the most widely used modalities in surgery today. In 1805 the Italian-German Physician, Philip Bozzini took concepts of optical technology and expanded them to generate a light transmitting apparatus called "the lichtleiter" (Figure 7-4) and hence "modern endoscopy" was established. His attempt to visualize the interior body granted him the title, "the father of endoscopy." Laparoscopic surgery started at the beginning of the 20th century when Von Ott examined the abdominal cavity of a pregnant woman in 1901 and Georg Kelling achieved a "koelioscopie" procedure. Jacobeus published an article on "Laparothorakoskopie" that same year. Kurt Semm from the University of Kiel used a laparoscopic approach to treat gynecological disorders in the 1970s. He created instruments and explained techniques for ovariectomy, adenectomy, and myomectomy. Semm is thought to be the father of "modern Laparoscopy." It was not until 1982 when Semm

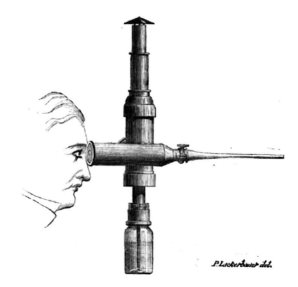

Figure 7-4 · The lichtleiter.

completed a laparoscopic appendectomy that general surgeons started to take notice. In 1985 Eric Muhe of Germany performed a laparoscopic cholecystectomy using what he called a "galloscope." When French gynecologist Phillip Mouret performed a laparoscopic cholecystectomy using four trocars in 1987, laparoscopic surgeries became the preferred method of surgery among general surgeons. Performing minimally invasive surgery has improved patient outcomes through shorter hospital stays and improved cosmetic outcomes leading to higher patient satisfaction. See Table 7-1.

Overview

Laparoscopic surgery begins with the insertion of gas in the peritoneal cavity (**pneumoperitoneum**). An open or closed technique can be used to create pneumoperitoneum using carbon dioxide. A spring-loaded Verres needle is used along with a trocar in a closed method.

Steps in a closed method:

1. The abdominal fascia is elevated with two towel clips or hands to protect the intra-abdominal organs.

2. A small incision is made in the umbilicus and the Veress needle is passed through abdominal wall fascia and the peritoneum.

3. The abdomen is inflated with an insufflator and CO_2 to a pressure of around 14 to 15 mm Hg.

4. The Verres needle is removed and a 5- or 10-mm bladed trocar is inserted to provide direct access to the abdomen. The trocar must be pointed away from the **sacral promontory** and the great vessels. Once through the peritoneum, the trocar is removed, forming the first port.

Steps in an open method:

1. In an open technique, the first port is introduced into the peritoneal cavity under direct vision reducing possible injury to blood vessels, bowel, or bladder.

TABLE 7-1 • MINIMALLY INVASIVE SURGERY WITH ADVANCED TECHNOLOGY HAS IMPROVED PATIENT OUTCOMES	
Shorter hospital stay	Reduced postoperative pain
Lower infection rates	Decreased blood loss
Faster recovery	Decreased need for postoperative medication

TABLE 7-2 • LAPAROSCOPIC EQUIPMENT	
Camera box	Camera
Insufflator	Light cord
Light box	Insufflation tubing
Printer	Scope
Video screen	

2. A small incision is made just below the umbilicus. The surgeon uses blunt dissection of the subcutaneous tissue to locate the abdominal fascia and clamps the linea alba with two Kocher clamps.

3. The Kocher clamps elevate the tissue, and a 1-cm vertical incision is made into the linea alba.

4. Blunt dissection is used to enlarge the opening and a finger is inserted to confirm the intraperitoneal space and to clear away any adhesions.

5. Stay sutures are inserted into the superior and inferior aspects of the fascial incision. A blunt-tipped Hasson trocar is inserted under direct vision into the peritoneum. The stay sutures are attached around the suture wings of the cannula to make certain an airtight seal. Insufflation tubing is attached to introduce 14 to 15 mm Hg of CO_2 into the abdomen. The stay sutures are used to help close the incision at the end of the procedure.

Once pneumoperitoneum is achieved, the surgeon will insert the camera into the first port and scan the peritoneal cavity. The surgical assistant will aid the surgeon in placing subsequent ports. The camera is aimed toward where the next port will be placed. If requested, the surgical assistant will inject local anesthetic at the incision site. Incisions for port sites are made away from the procedure site to facilitate control of instruments and provide traction as needed, commonly at a 30° to 60° angle creating a symmetrical triangle or a diamond. Skin incisions are made in Langer's line and just large enough for the cannula diameter. The trocar is inserted under direct vision with the camera, with slow, steady pressure while being mindful of the viscera in the peritoneal cavity. Once the blade of the trocar is visible, the surgical assistant should tilt the trocar at an angle to protect any viscera or large vessels that may be in the space. This step is repeated for all remaining port sites dependent on the surgical procedure. The consequence of improper trocar placement includes major vascular injury, intestinal injury, or possible air embolism.

Ergonomic Challenges of Laparoscopic Surgery

There are some limitations to minimally invasive surgery. Laparascopic surgery requires additional equipment, and it should be checked before the patient is brought into the room. See Table 7-2. Laparoscopic surgery only offers two-dimensional vision and there is a loss of depth perception to some degree. Laparoscopic instruments offer only four degrees of freedom. Additional limitation is loss of peripheral vision caused by the limited view and loss of tactile feedback achieved during open procedures. Tactile feedback presents a level of dexterity often associated with competence in surgery. In laparoscopic surgery, coordination of hand movements is difficult with a limited range of motion to the target, making it more difficult to achieve the efficiency often seen in open cases.

The Role of the Assistant in Laparoscopic Surgery. The role of the surgical assistant in laparoscopic surgery varies demographically as well as procedurally. However, surgical assistants will often control the camera. A surgical assistant may also help retract critical structures out of the way by introducing instruments into the ports, passing sutures, and suctioning/removing specimens, with the assistance of the endoscopic camera that displays the view onto the monitor. Blunt dissection can be achieved by the surgical assistant using retractors to stabilize tissues and establish mild tension. They may also be required to apply monopolar diathermy to seal or disrupt tissues or vessels. When the procedure is completed, it is typically the surgical assistant's task to remove the ports and suture the incisions.

ROBOTIC SURGERY

History

Minimally invasive techniques have transformed operative surgery. Computer-aided surgery and robotic surgical systems attempt to advance minimally invasive surgery and open new horizons. A robot is a sophisticated machine developed to perform specific tasks. The term "**robot**" can be traced back to a play written in 1923 by Czech playwright Karel Capek. The play was entitled *Rossum's Universal Robots* (the Czech word "robota" means heavy labor) and the name became commonplace for describing complex machines. The first industrial robot was developed in the United States in 1961.

A machine is defined as a robot if it features some degree of mobility, and once programmed, operates automatically and performs a large variety of tasks. Most robots are used in factories, but with advances in technology, robots are functioning in agriculture, construction, retailing, and other services.

The use of robots in surgery has only been in existence for the past 30 years. The concept of robotic telepresence was created through the mutual efforts of the Stanford Research Institute, the Department of Defense, and the National Aeronautics and Space Administration. This movement was prompted by the need to provide immediate operative care to wounded soldiers on the battlefield. Initial prototypes involved robotic arms that could be mounted on armored vehicles to facilitate surgery via remote access. Almost immediately, the technology was commercialized and robots became devices that are actively controlled in operating rooms today. Performing a surgical procedure in real-time at a distance is termed **telesurgery.** One major problem in telesurgery has been the time delay between the surgeon's hand movements and the robotic arms response.

Geometry

Manipulators (robotic arms) are categorized by geometrical design. If the arm resembles a human arm, then the joints may be referred to as shoulders, elbow, and wrist. Cartesian coordinate geometry, or rectangular coordinate geometry, is a manipulator design derived from the Cartesian system for graphing mathematical functions. An arm with Cartesian geometry moves along x, y, and z axes (up-down, right-left, and front-back). The manipulator has a definite number of degrees of freedom and rotation. Spatial positioning involves three degrees of freedom (DOF): first, z-axis or up-down movement, and the second and third are x-axis and y-axis movements that allow for motion in the horizontal plane. An up and down movement of the jaw(s) is known as "pitch" while the right and left movement of the jaw(s) is called "yaw." A rotating movement of the instrument shaft is the "roll."

Other manipulator geometry designs include cylindrical coordinate geometry, a manipulator design that incorporates a plane polar coordinate system with an elevation dimension added; and revolute geometry, or design that allows an arm to move in three dimensions with 360° rotation and 90° elevation from the shoulder. An elbow joint moves through 180° (from a straight position to double back on itself), and a wrist joint revolves and flexes like the elbow.

Hearing and Vision

Sound arrives at each ear at a different level of intensity. Because of binaural hearing, the brain processes sound waves to enable an individual to locate the source of the sound and interpret it. Machine hearing is analogous to human hearing. A robot can distinguish from which direction sound originates and the actual type of sound, such as a human voice. To accomplish these functions, robots are built with binaural hearing, the same type of hearing humans possess.

Robots, particularly voice-controlled units employed in surgery, are equipped with two sound transducers to provide the robot with binaural hearing. Utilizing microprocessors installed in the computer connected to the manipulator, the robot can differentiate various voice patterns and waveforms. This makes it possible for the robot to determine the source of the sound and its origin. Each human voice produces a unique waveform. The robot will be able to analyze the waveform and interpret commonly spoken commands issued by specific individuals.

Two important concepts must be understood when discussing robotic vision: sensitivity and resolution. Sensitivity is the ability of the robot to see in dim light. In some instances, a high level of sensitivity is necessary. For example, during endoscopic procedures, the lights in the operating room, including the surgical overhead lights, are either dimmed or turned off. A robot would require a level of sensitivity to see in such dim light.

The term resolution may be familiar since its application with the microscope is the same as robotics. Resolution is the ability to differentiate between two objects, and the level of resolution can vary. A higher resolution indicates better vision. However, sensitivity and resolution exert a negative effect on each other. If the resolution is improved, the vision function of the robot will decrease in dim light; and vice-versa, improved sensitivity causes a decrease in resolution.

Like binaural hearing, binocular machine vision is similar to binocular human vision, also referred to as stereovision. Binocular vision allows for depth perception. A distinct advantage of current robotic systems is the existence of stereoscopic vision. With the incorporation of three-dimensional robotic vision, the number of errors in robotic surgery versus laparoscopic surgery in two dimensions is significantly lower. The word "stereo" comes from the Greek word "stereos" which means firm or solid. With stereo vision, you see an object as solid in three spatial dimensions—width, height, and depth or x, y, and z. It is the added perception of the depth dimension that makes stereo vision so rich and special.

Robotic Design

Robots are classified by generations. **First-generation robots** are simple mechanical arms without artificial intelligence (AI). They perform precise repetitive motions at high speeds for industrial applications and require consistent oversight. **Second-generation robots** incorporate a level of artificial intelligence. Characteristically, these machines may include pressure or tactile sensors and some type of vision and hearing. While not requiring constant supervision, occasional monitoring is necessary. **Third-generation robots** include autonomous and insect robots. An autonomous robot works independently, without human supervision or an overseeing computer. The insect robots are controlled by a larger central AI computer, much like bees in a hive and a queen bee. Their collective intelligence is greater than their individual intelligence. The original surgical robot consisted of three arms: one to hold the camera and two for working instruments. The newest technology consists of a fourth arm version to allow for additional retraction as well as an enhanced system that incorporates a motorized cart, increased arm rate of motion, and high-definition vision.

Automated Endoscopic System for Optimal Positioning-HERMES Ready (AESOP-HR®) originally manufactured by Computer Motion was the first widely used robotic arm. AESOP-HR guides the lens of a surgical camera via an endoscope. Voice-activated software permits the physician to position the camera with his/her hands free to continue operating on the patient. Automated endoscopic system operative positioning (AESOP) is a voice-activated robotic arm. It took over the task of endoscope positioning and provided the surgeon with direct control and a stable view of the internal surgical field. AESOP was acquired by Intuitive in 2003 and is no longer being produced.

The Zeus Surgical Robot originally designed by Computer Motion uses three robotic arms that manipulate instruments and the endoscope. Zeus was designed to perform minimally invasive surgery (MIS). Robotic instruments were created to aid in MIS. In 2001, surgeons in New York, Dr. Jacques Marceau and Dr. Michel Ganer, used a satellite link to operate Zeus by remote control, successfully removing the gallbladder of a patient in Strasbourg, France. The Zeus system has now been phased out as a result of the merger of Computer Motion with Intuitive Surgical in 2003.

The *da Vinci* Surgical System uses 3D visualization along with enhanced dexterity, precision, and control. With *robotic surgery,* as with traditional methods, the patient is under the care of at least two medical professionals: The surgeon at the console and an assistant at the sterile field. The assistant is responsible for tasks such as switching between instruments, placing mesh through the cannula, and retracting tissue. As the surgeon maneuvers the controls, *da Vinci* scales, filters, and translates his or her wrist and finger movements into precise movements of the instruments in real time. Any hand tremor the surgeon may have is removed from the instrumentation. Some of the technical features of the *da Vinci* Robot include endoscopic instrumentation with seven DOF which allows for optimal results in any anastomosis of tissue.

Endowrist instruments are available in 5-mm and 8-mm shafts and are specifically designed for the *da Vinci* systems and are not interchangeable between the various da Vinci systems. These instruments are designated by their housing color, length, and graphics. The use of 5-mm articulating wrist instruments mimics open surgery movements in endoscopic procedures.

The advantage of the *da Vinci* robot offers improved patient outcomes. There is reduced trauma to the body, reduced blood loss with less need for transfusions, decreased postoperative pain and discomfort, less risk of infection, shorter hospital stays, faster recovery and return to normal activities, less scarring, and improved cosmesis.

Mako robotic-arm assisted total joint arthroplasty has surpassed the typical knee and hip replacement surgery. The robot is designed with haptic feedback to prevent soft tissue trauma. Surgeries performed with the Mako have produced a reduction in postoperative pain, increased patient satisfaction, improved flexion, less opioid drug use, and a decrease in complications and hospital readmissions. With a CT scan of the patient's joint, the system converts it into a three-dimensional model including damaged surfaces due to arthritis. The surgeon finalizes his plans pre-operatively and they are uploaded onto the robot. The surgeon can compare the plan to the individual patient's motion, such as bending the knee, flexion, and extension while it is replicated on the robot's screen. Positioning of the robot can be adjusted to millimeters to ensure correct cutting of any bone. The surgeon still performs the surgery; however, with the Mako System, there is an increased accuracy and precision to the repair of the hip or knee joint.

Viking 3D Vision System (Viking Systems, Inc. San Diego, CA) has a 10-mm camera that transmits the image to a processor. The processor translates the image to a stereotactic view made available to the surgeon from displays mounted on a headrest.

Cambridge-Endo handheld articulating instruments (Cambridge Endoscopic Devices, Inc. Framingham, Maryland) include needle holders, bipolar scissors, and Maryland dissectors with seven degrees of freedom. Their design facilitates difficult cases, such as prostates or tight spaces, with the advantage of maintaining tactile perception.

Radius Surgical System (Tuegingen Scientific, Tuebingen, Germany) consists of two mechanical manipulators providing rotating and deflectable tips that permit six degrees of freedom.

Erbe Hydro Dissector System (ERBE-USA, Inc. Marrieta, GA) consists of a pressure source and a laparoscopic tip that delivers a high-pressure helical water jet. The device aids in cautery-free mobilization of the neurovascular bundles.

PAKY-RCM is the percutaneous access to the kidney remote center of motion developed by John Hopkins Hospital in Baltimore, Maryland. It allows remote operation of a robotic arm which is designed to percutaneously puncture a kidney.

Mazor X Stealth Edition Robot is a robotic guidance system that permits pre-operative or intra-operative planning and robotic and image-guided trajectories for spine surgery. Using an innovative imaging cross-modality registration process, each vertebral body registers independently, and the robotic system analyzes and pairs images from different modalities, such as matching a preoperative CT with intraoperative fluoroscopy or 3D surgical imaging.

Hansen's Senser X2 robotic catheter system utilizes robotically steerable catheters for electrophysiological (EP) and peripheral vascular procedures. Robotic catheterization facilitates and improves the performance of minimally invasive procedures (endovascular procedures using catheters). Hansen's systems are intuitive, have six degrees of freedom of movement, and offer 3D live views of the internal vasculature during catheter navigation. Robot-steered catheters shorten procedure times, reduce exertion by the catheter tip on vessels, and augment accuracy in positioning of the catheter and remote operation that eliminates the operator from radiation exposure. The robotic arm is attached to the patient's bed and works with Ensite NaVx, CARTO, as well as standard mapping and ablation catheters. The Sensei system includes the Sensei X and Sensei X2 generations of systems and is comprised of three components: the physician control console, robotic catheter manipulator (RCM), and the electronics frame. The control console has three imaging monitors that integrate data from the EKG, image source, and catheter navigation. The RCM is attached to the operating table and electromechanically controls the Artisan Extend catheter in response to the physician's hand movement.

Corindus Vascular Robotics – Corpath®200 enables the placement of coronary guidewires and balloon/stent devices through a radiation-protected, interventional control center. The articulating arm interprets physician directions into precise movements and manipulations of guidewires and balloon/stent catheters. The Arm extends the physician's dexterity with 1-mm distinct movements with sub-millimeter measurement capabilities.

Stereotaxis' Niobe Epoch Robotic Surgery System provides remote catheter navigation with a magnetically-guided catheter and offers a clear benefit over traditional pull-wire catheters. The catheter is guided by magnets, is soft and flexible, and eliminates the possibility of injuries caused by rigid pull-wire-based catheters. It is nearly impossible to injure an organ or damage blood vessels with the magnetically-guided catheter. The goal of remote magnetic navigation is to treat ventricular arrhythmias, and potentially to treat atrial fibrillation.

Rosa® Brain/Rosa® Spine Robot by Zimmer Biomet is a "GPS" for the skull, and may be used for several kinds of cranial procedures necessitating surgical planning based on preoperative data, precise location of the patient's anatomy, and accurate positioning and handling of instruments. The robot assists the surgeon with numerous surgical interventions such as biopsies, electrode implantation for functional procedures (stimulation of the cerebral cortex, deep brain stimulation), open skull surgical procedures requiring a navigation device, endoscopic interventions, and various other "key-hole" surgeries. Some of the diagnosis treatable with ROSA include: **Hydrocephalus**, Generalized **Dystonia,** Parkinson disease, and **Cavernoma**.

Transenterix Senhance robot-assisted surgery is a robot used in minimally invasive laparoscopic surgery. The company, Transenterix also created the SPIDER device and the SurgiBot system, a single port, robotically enhanced laparoscopic surgical platform. It utilizes haptic feedback and eye-sensing camera control as well as 3-mm instruments for performing a microlaparoscopy. The Senhance Ultrasonic System is an energy device that pairs with the Senhance robotic surgery platform. The use of ultrasonic energy assists in the flexibility of the system for numerous procedures. The Senhance Ultrasonic System functions similarly to other ultrasonic devices by creating high-frequency vibration that denatures proteins, causing hemostasis. Ultrasonic energy has the advantage of minimizing thermal spread during dissection. The Senhance Ultrasonic System is comparable to the Harmonic Scalpel. The Senhance Surgical System is approved for use in minimally invasive gynecological surgery, colorectal surgery, cholecystectomy, and inguinal hernia repair.

Medtronics Hugo RAS Minimally Invasive Robotic System is developed to compete with Intuitive's da Vinci robot and based on a modular and upgradeable design. The Hugo system includes an operating console, central tower, and multiple, cart-based robotic arms. Surgical specialties that the robot is designed for include general, gynecology, urology, bariatric, thoracic, and colorectal.

Robotic Surgery Terminology

Term	Definition
Articulated	Broken into sections by joint. Many robot arms have articulated geometry and the versatility is measured in degrees of freedom.
Binaural hearing	The ability of humans and robots to determine the direction from which sound is coming. Humans have two ears that provide this ability; robots are given two sound transducers that provide a similar ability.
Cartesian coordinate geometry	Refers to the 16th century philosopher Renes Descartes who invented coordinate geometry. Principles of his Cartesian system are used for graphing mathematical functions. Axes are always perpendicular to each other, also called rectangular coordinate geometry.
Cylindrical-coordinate geometry	A robot arm in which a reference plane is used in combination with a plane coordinate system and elevation.
Degrees of freedom	The number of ways that a robot manipulator can move. The majority of manipulators move in three dimensions but have six or seven degrees of freedom.
Degrees of rotation	The extent that a robot joint or a set of joints moves clockwise or counterclockwise about an axis. A reference point is established and the angles of the joint are stated in degrees.
Endowrist instruments	Multiple use endoscopic instruments are used in conjunction with the da Vinci Surgical System. These include scissors, scalpels, forceps, needle drivers, and electrocautery.
Expert systems	A method of reasoning in artificial intelligence used to control smart robots. The expert system consists of facts or data supplied to the robot about the robot's environment; also called a rule-based system.

Term	Definition
Machine hearing	Advanced "hearing" by a robot that picks up and amplifies the sound, and determines the direction where the sound originates.
Manipulators	Technical term for robot arms.
Resolution	The extent to which a machine, microscope, human, or robot visually differentiates between two objects. A higher resolution indicates sharper image.
Revolute geometry	A robot arm that moves in three dimensions resembling the movements of a human arm, such as rotating in a full circle (360°).
Sensitivity	Ability of a machine or robot to see in dim light or detect weak impulses at invisible wavelengths.
Telechir	The name given to remotely controlled robots.
Telepresence	Refers to the operation of a robot at a distance, meaning the operator is situated in one location, and the robot is performing at a distant site.

Bibliography

What Are the Basic Principles of Electricity? https://electricalapprentice.co.uk/what-are-the-basic-principles-of-electricity/. Accessed May 16, 2023.

History of Electricity. Institute for Energy Research. https://www.instituteforenergyresearch.org/history-electricity/. Accessed May 16, 2023.

The Electric Ben Franklin. https://www.ushistory.org/franklin/science/electricity.htm. Accessed May 16, 2023.

Bovie. http://www.boviemedical.com/2016/09/05/3-key-differences-between-electrosurgery-electrocautery/; Prinicpals_in_electrosurgery.pdf. Covidien; Rigel_Electrosurgical-Guidance-Booklet_WEB.pdf. Accessed May 16, 2023.

Megasoft Return Electrode – Johnson & Johnson. https://www.jnj-medicaldevices.com/sites/default/files/user_uploaded_assets/pdf_assets/2019-10/MEGA-SOFT-Technology-White-Paper-090233-180417.pdf. Accessed May 16, 2023.

Huang H-Y, Yen C-F, Wu M-P. Complications of electrosurgery in laparoscopy. ScienceDirect. https://www.sciencedirect.com/science/article/pii/S221330701400029X. Accessed May 16, 2023.

Blum CA, Adams DB. Who did the first Laparoscopic Cholecystectomy?. *J Minim Access Surg.* 2011;7(3):165-168. doi:10.4103/0972-9941.83506. https://www.ncbi.nlm.nih.gov/pmc/articles/PMC3193755/. Accessed May 16, 2023.

Society of Laparoscopic and Robotic Surgery. Chapter 23. http://sls.org/nezhats-history-of-endoscopy-chapter-23/. Accessed May 16, 2023.

The Historical Evolution of Endoscopy. Sarah Ellison Western Michigan University, https://scholarworks.wmich.edu/cgi/viewcontent.cgi?article=3580&context=honors_theses. Accessed May 16, 2023.

R Vecchio R, MacFayden BV, Palazzo F. History of Laparoscopic Surgery. *Panminerva Med.* 2000;42(1):87-90. https://pubmed.ncbi.nlm.nih.gov/11019611/. Accessed May 16, 2023.

Supe AN, Kulkarni GV, Supe PA. Ergonomics in laparoscopic surgery. *J Minim Access Surg.* 2010; 6(2): 31-36. doi:10.4103/0972-9941.65161.

Metronic Mazor X Stealth Edition Spine Robots. https://www.medtronic.com/us-en/healthcare-professionals/therapies-procedures/spinal-orthopaedic/spine-robotics.html. Accessed May 16, 2023.

Dushyanth A. HNSN: Revolutionizing Physicians' Capabilities with Robotics! January 28, 2016. https://www.yahoo.com/entertainment/news/hnsn-revoutionizing-physcians-capabilities-robotics-220000034.html. Accessed May 16, 2023.

Corindus Corpath®200; robot assisted PCI system. https://www.usa.philips.com/healthcare/product/HC722362/corinduscorpath-200roboticassistedpci. Accessed May 16, 2023.

Weiss P. Time to Take Another Look at Robotics in Electrophysiology. Diagnostic and Interventional Cardiology. December 23, 2019. https://www.dicardiology.com/article/time-take-another-look-robotics-electrophysiology. Accessed May 16, 2023.

Costa AD, Guichard JB, Roméyer-Bouchard C, Gerbay A, Isaaz K. Robotic Magnetic Navigation for ablation of human arrhythmias. Published online September 19, 2016. NCBI. https://www.ncbi.nlm.nih.gov/pmc/articles/PMC5034914/. Accessed May 16, 2023.

Zimmer Biomet. ROSA ®Brain. https://www.medtech.fr/en/rosa-brain. Accessed May 16, 2023.

Transenterix Senhance Robot. https://transenterix.com/about/our-history. Accessed May 16, 2023.

Miller R. Medtronics Launches Hugo to Rival Intuitive's Robotic Surgery System. Informa Pharma Intelligence. Issue 164. October 7, 2019. https://medtech.pharmaintelligence.informa.com/-/media/supporting-documents/mti-issue-pdfs/mt191007.pdf. Accessed May 16, 2023.

https://www.eia.gov/energyexplained/electricity/how-electricity-is-generated.php

https://www.medtronic.com/us-en/healthcare-professionals/products/neurological/surgical-navigation-systems/stealthstation.html

8

Preoperative Patient Preparation

Margaret H.M. Rodriguez

DISCUSSED IN THIS CHAPTER

1. **Preparing the patient for surgery.**
2. **Patient positioning.**
3. **Patient draping.**

INTRODUCTION

Once the patient has been transported to the operating room, there are a number of tasks that must be performed before the actual surgical procedure can commence. In most situations, the patient is transferred to the operating table, also referred to as the OR bed, prior to administration of anesthesia. If the procedure requires prone positioning, the patient must be anesthetized and intubated on the transfer stretcher or gurney prior to being placed face-down in the prone position on the OR table. Following proper positioning and prior to application of the sterile draping components, the patient's skin around the planned incisional area must be prepped with antiseptic agents to reduce the potential for surgical site infection (SSI). The circulating nurse or surgical assistant may also place a urinary drainage catheter if ordered by the surgeon as part of the prep and before draping. Procedures on the extremities may require placement of a pneumatic tourniquet around the arm or leg prior to the skin prep and draping procedure. The final preoperative step is the application of sterile surgical draping materials that delineate the areas included in the sterile field of which the patient is the center, and in which the scrubbed members of the surgical team function.

TRANSFER TO THE OPERATING ROOM TABLE

The process of moving the patient from the transport stretcher or bed requires a coordinated effort by several surgical team members to assure that the patient is protected from injury from unintended falls, skin abrasions, dislodgement of indwelling devices, or muscle strain in those with limited range of motion (ROM). The stretcher should be positioned adjacent to the OR table and both must be locked to prevent movement during transfer which may allow the patient to fall between them. Any positioning devices attached to the OR table such as arm boards or stirrup holders on the side where the stretcher is positioned must be removed to allow for close approximation of the table and transport stretcher. Both OR table and stretcher should be positioned at the same height prior to the patient moving over.

Before transfer, any indwelling devices in the patient must be positioned to move easily with the patient. Examples of these include the patient's intravenous (IV) or other vascular access tubing, urinary catheter and collection bag, chest tubes attached to pleural drainage systems, wound drains and collection devices, or preoperative needle localization (PNL) needles. Other possible items attached to the patient rather than indwelling devices may include electrocardiographic (ECG) leads, anti-DVT devices such as plexi-pulses or sequential compression devices (SCDs), neuromonitoring wires, or traction cables. Ties of patient gowns should also be loosened or untied before transfer to prevent binding up and facilitate removal prior to prepping.

Conscious, mobile patients should be empowered to move themselves over from stretcher to OR table; however, a team member must be present on the contralateral side of the OR table to ensure the patient does not go over the edge. Obese or very large patients may cause the stretcher to tip as they move over; therefore, a team member should exert force against the stretcher to help stabilize it. The anesthesia provider at the head of the bed should guide the patient to place their head on the pillow or foam cushion on the OR table and move any IV bags to an adjacent IV pole.

Once transferred to the OR table, patients should be asked to feel the sides of the table and center themselves. Application of the safety strap should be done after advising the patient that it is a reminder of how narrow the bed is. It is better to create a positive therapeutic mindset for the patient by allowing them to do as much as they are able to do, with guidance and protection of their dignity and privacy during the transfer. Any mention of the safety strap as a restraint may leave a negative connotation in the patient's mind and should not be done even in a facetious manner. Referring to the safety strap as a necessity to prevent their legs from falling off the bed, while a true statement, may cause apprehension in the already frightened and nervous patient who will focus on the danger of injury from their legs falling off the bed. Using the positive phrasing of being just a reminder for them that the bed is narrow is less threatening and concerning in their vulnerable state. Advising the conscious patient about other measures being taken beforehand also provides a sense of comfort and care. Patients should be kept warm with blankets if possible until anesthetized to maintain normothermia.

Conscious, immobile, or unconscious patients will require additional team members to transfer them from stretcher to OR table safely. A minimum of four team members with addition of transfer devices such as patient rollers, slide boards, air-filled hover mats, or lift hoists may be required to move immobile, frail, or morbidly obese patients. The patient's spine, head, and legs must be kept in a neutral alignment to prevent potential spinal nerve injury during transfer. The anesthesia provider should direct the transfer process and give the okay for transfer to commence. The conscious, immobile patients should also be advised of steps taken on their behalf to protect them during transfer and positioning on the OR table. The dignity and privacy of all patients, whether conscious or unconscious, must be protected by all members of the surgical team.

Patients who will be placed in the prone position for the surgical procedure will undergo anesthesia induction and intubation on the transport stretcher prior to transfer and positioning on the OR table. Positioning devices such as laminectomy frames, chest rolls, or specialized spinal procedure tables may be used. A minimum of four team members is required to safely move the anesthetized patient into the prone position and onto these devices or tables. More team members may be required if the patient is obese. Additional positioning devices such as pillows, foam pads, axillary rolls, gel pads, straps, arm boards, or other items may be necessary to complete the process upon transfer into prone position (Table 8-1).

CONSIDERATIONS FOR SURGICAL PATIENT POSITIONING

The need for surgical access to virtually every part of the human body requires specific positioning maneuvers to reach the areas in need of intervention. As important as access is, safely achieving that access without causing harm to the surgical patient is paramount because a surgical procedure may otherwise go well, however, if the patient suffers lasting damage due to inadequate precautions to prevent improper positioning, it cannot be considered a successful outcome. The broad goals of proper surgical patient positioning include:

- Adequate access to the specific anatomical areas, organs, or structures in need of surgical treatment.

- Maintenance of correct alignment and ROM of the patient's body in all phases of surgical care including when patients are anesthetized and cannot complain of discomfort or distress from positioning.

- Prevention of dislodgement of IV access lines, indwelling catheters, or monitoring equipment during transfer to the OR table or when the table is manipulated, and various positioning devices are attached to the table.

- Appropriate padding of all bony prominences or other body parts to prevent skin breakdown or pressure necrosis.

- Protection from skin touching the metal rails of the OR table or other conductive metal surfaces or equipment, to prevent potential alternate exit pathway burns with use of the electrosurgical unit (ESU).

- Careful consideration of the choice of surgical patient position taken and the impact on all body systems.

Impact on Body Systems

The five general anatomical and physiological body systems impacted by choice of surgical position are circulatory, respiratory, integumentary (soft tissue and skin), musculoskeletal, and peripheral nervous systems. The acronym CRIMP may be helpful in remembering to protect and monitor the crucial body systems and not crimp them and cause injury.

Circulatory System. The circulatory system must be protected to ensure that arterial and venous return blood flow is adequate for normal blood pressure regulation and oxygen perfusion of tissue. Elderly patients and those with compromised cardiac status or inadequate vascularity are at particular risk of injury from positioning. Positions that keep the extremities elevated such as lithotomy alter the hemodynamic status of the patient. Postoperative return to supine position from lithotomy may have an adverse impact on blood pressure as blood readily flows back into the legs as they are lowered and level with the torso. Legs should be lowered slowly from lithotomy back to supine.

Hyper-rotation of the neck may cause diminished blood perfusion to the brain with compression of the carotid artery on one side. Patients with carotid stenosis have preexisting vascular insufficiency and excessive rotation or compression exacerbates the risk of dangerous blockage. Prolonged periods of compression of soft tissues may contribute to loss of blood supply to the skin and subcutaneous tissue layers, depriving areas of oxygen resulting in ischemia and formation of decubitus (pressure) ulcers.

TABLE 8-1 • SURGICAL POSITIONING ACCESSORIES AND EQUIPMENT

Accessory	Description and Use
Arm board	Attachment to OR table side rail for positioning arms laterally to the patient; adjustable angles used range from 0° (parallel to bed) to 90°
Arm board (double)	Two-tiered attachment used in lateral position to support and separate both arms on one side of OR table
Arm brace (sled, toboggan)	Curved panel of clear plastic; one long end inserted under mattress used to keep a tucked-in arm secured against patient's side without arm board
Arm cradles	Long curved foam or gel pads used on arm boards to stabilize arms
Arm table	Attachment to OR table side rails or rolling, padded table placed perpendicular to OR table for use in hand and upper extremity cases
Arthroscopy leg holder/brace	Rounded foam or gel padded, circular-shaped brace attached to OR table side rail on operative side to support leg when foot section is lowered; facilitates manipulation of leg and knee in arthroscopy
Axillary roll	Small pad or roll made of sheets or gel used to elevate dependent chest off OR table to facilitate respiration and prevent compression of axillary artery and brachial plexus when placed in lateral position
Beach chair device	Large OR table attachment used to support back and head with operative side at table edge to facilitate arm and shoulder manipulation during shoulder arthroscopy or other procedures
Bean bag	Device filled with small beads used to conform to patient contours when air suctioned from device to prevent rolling or movement
Bracing system	Padded devices attached to OR table side rails with special holders to support various anatomical areas rigidly in lateral position
Chest rolls	Tubular-shaped rolled sheets, gel pads, or foam rolls used to elevate chest and abdomen to prevent compression of aorta and vena cava and facilitate chest expansion; should extend from shoulders to hips
Footboard/brace	Flat, padded device attached to OR table side rails with special holders; used in reverse Trendelenburg or Fowler to keep feet perpendicular
Headrests	Foam squares or gel donuts for stabilization of the head with minimal pressure
Heel pads	Foam or gel wrap pads or stabilizers to prevent pressure on heels of feet
Laminectomy frames	Wilson (double-curved) or Relton Hall type (4 posts) frames placed on OR table top used to support patient in prone position to facilitate respiration and reduce pressure on ventral surfaces and major vessels; flattens lower back; may be radiolucent for lateral fluoroscopic imaging
Mayfield skull fixation clamp	Sterilized device with adjustable torque handle for insertion into outer skull bone layer for rigid head positioning when OR table head removed
Pegboard system	Rigid flat board with multiple holes for insertion of padded pegs or posts; used to maintain lateral or semi-lateral position without rolling
Shoulder braces	Small, padded, C-shaped devices attached to OR table side rails bilaterally to prevent patient sliding in Trendelenburg position
Shoulder roll/thyroid pillow	Small towel roll, gel device, or inflatable pillow used under scapula area or lower cervical spine in supine to increase neck extension
Stirrups – candy cane type	Hooked devices attached to OR table side rails with stirrup holders to elevate and abduct legs for access to vaginal, perineal, anal areas
Stirrups – half boot calf support type	Allen or Yellowfin type of half boot devices attached to OR table with special stirrup holders; elevates and abducts legs with adjustable height ability from low-lithotomy to high-lithotomy in combined access procedures such as low-anterior colon resection, laparoscopic or robotic-assisted vaginal or perineal procedures
Stirrups – knee crutch/support type	Padded devices attached to OR table side rails placed under knees in some gynecological or urological procedures
Wedges	Foam or gel square, curved, or triangular-shaped blocks used to maintain elevation of various anatomical areas in multiple positions

Respiratory System. The airway must be patent and accessible regardless of the patient's position. There must be adequate movement and function of the diaphragm to prevent hypoxia or compromise the reoxygenation of venous blood passing through the pulmonary system before being returned to the body's arterial system. Prone and lateral positions present increased risk for compromise of adequate chest expansion or mechanical excursion, especially in the anesthetized patient. Even in simple supine position, there is a normal decrease in respiratory tidal volume, a measurement of the functional movement of air with each single breath. Arms should not be crossed over the patient's chest and positioned out to the sides on arm boards or safely tucked in at the patient's side. If arms must be placed across the chest, care must be taken to ensure adequate chest expansion.

The lateral position places excess stress on the dependent or lower, non-operative side lung due to the pressure of the body from the contralateral side. A small axillary roll is routinely placed transversely under the dependent chest wall, caudal to the axilla to slightly elevate the dependent side and facilitate chest expansion on that side while not compressing the brachial plexus. The prone position also requires placement of chest rolls or positioning frames to allow full forward chest expansion. The chest rolls should span the distance from the acromioclavicular joint to the iliac crest bilaterally in order to lift the patient's torso off the OR table surface slightly and enhance bilateral lung function.

Patients with pre-existing conditions such as pulmonary disease, history of smoking, or morbid obesity may have increased respiratory compromise. The elevation of the patient's head and torso facilitates respiration and is often done after extubation when the patient is transferred back onto the transport stretcher on the way to the post-anesthesia care unit (PACU).

Integumentary System. The integumentary system is comprised of the skin, the largest organ of the human body, and the underlying soft tissues of the subcutaneous fat layer that overlies the muscles and fascial coverings. Skin is normally a thick and tough tissue layer; however, in the elderly, underweight, undernourished, obese, diabetic, or immunocompromised, skin is at greater risk for injury from mechanical compressive forces if not adequately padded and protected. Elderly patients may have very thin, fragile, loosely adhered skin that is susceptible to tearing from shearing forces of being pulled across surfaces, including bed linens. These patients must be carefully lifted rather than pulled during transfer or positioning to prevent skin injury.

Prolonged periods of pressure on bony prominences such as the occiput of the skull, shoulders, scapulae, elbows, hips, knees, and heels can cause initial ischemic changes that continue and progress to formation of decubitus ulcer or pressure sore, even postoperatively. The subcutaneous fat layer is friable, poorly vascularized, and easily damaged in obese or morbidly obese patients whose own anatomical structures may produce compressive forces against other tissue areas when the patient is paralyzed under general anesthesia or immobilized and unable to shift positions. Two hours is the approximate recognized time frame beyond which even healthy individuals may begin to suffer skin breakdown if padding is inadequate or not provided.

Care must be taken to provide padding to all anatomical areas at risk of excessive pressure during surgery. The head is frequently positioned on a foam headrest or gel donut in the supine position to pad the occipital area of the scalp. The facial areas and the endotracheal tube may be protected by use of a foam headrest or gel horseshoe-type frame in the prone position. Pressure on the heels of the feet may be reduced by use of a small pillow, roll, or gel donut under the ankles in the supine position. Pillows or foam padding should be placed between the legs of patients placed in the lateral position to prevent pressure of the weight of the operative side leg on the dependent side. The ears must also be adequately padded to prevent breakdown of the external ear. The breasts of female patients and the male genitalia must be protected from compression for extended periods of time in the prone position. The perineal post, used to prevent a patient from sliding off the fracture table when lower extremity traction is applied, must be adequately padded to prevent compression of male and female external genital structures and perineal tissues.

Musculoskeletal System. The musculoskeletal system is comprised of the bony skeletal framework of the body and its accompanying muscles, articulation joints, and attachments of ligaments and tendons. Patients under general anesthesia cannot express discomfort; therefore, it may be helpful to ask the patient about limitation of movement prior to induction. The patient's spinal column must be maintained in a neutral or straight alignment during transfer or positioning to prevent excessive stress on spinal nerves which could cause pain, numbness, or other nerve disruption postoperatively (Figure 8-1). Elderly, osteoporotic, malnourished, or paralyzed patients have higher risk of bone fracture from even moderate pressure or manipulation beyond their individual normal ROM. A pillow may be placed

A

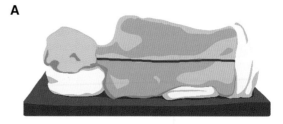

B

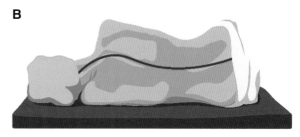

Figure 8-1 · **(A)** Proper neutral or straight spinal alignment to prevent excessive stress on spinal nerves. **(B)** Improper spinal alignment.

under the knees for slight flexion or under the concave lumbar curvature in the supine position to reduce lower back strain.

The safety strap is placed across the patient's legs about 2 in above the knees in the supine position. The placement of the safety strap prevents possible disarticulation of a hip if one leg falls off the bed during the excitement phase of general anesthesia. The strap should not be overly tight and can be checked by flatly placing a hand between the strap and the patient to ensure proper application and to prevent a tourniquet-type effect.

Peripheral Nervous System. Limited ROM is due not only to the amount of muscle mass, but to peripheral motor and sensory nerve functions. Excessive stretching or compression of peripheral nerves can contribute to loss of function or sensation postoperatively which may be transient or permanent. Areas of nerve bundles called plexuses are at particular risk for injury from surgical positioning and include the cervical, brachial, lumber, and sacral plexuses. Other frequently injured peripheral nerves include the facial, peroneal (leg), ulnar (elbow), and radial (wrist).

The cervical plexus is injured by excessive rotation of the head and neck. The brachial plexus located in the axillary area is most commonly injured by hyperextension of the arms when positioned laterally on arm boards beyond a 90° configuration in the supine position. The patient may suffer loss of sensation or strength in the arm or hand due to intraoperative brachial plexus injury related to improper positioning.

The lumbar plexus in the lower back and hip area may be injured when the patient is positioned in lithotomy with legs in stirrups. The buttocks must not be positioned beyond the border of the table break edge. The lack of support and hanging of the lower buttocks off the edge of the table break causes an undue lordotic curvature of the lumbar spine and stretching of the sciatic or other spinal nerves during surgery. A padded footboard placed against the soles of the feet should be used for procedures performed in the reverse Trendelenburg position to prevent sliding. Lengthy procedures performed in the supine or sitting position may utilize a padded footboard to reduce risk of postoperative foot drop, or loss of the ability to dorsiflex the foot, caused by prolonged plantar flexion (pointing of toes) of the feet and stretching or compression of the peroneal nerves which are branches of the sciatic nerves bilaterally.

Positioning Supplies

Prior to the patient entering the operating room, the surgical team members should have all necessary positioning supplies available in the room. The supplies and equipment should have been checked for proper working order; cleanliness; completeness of all parts and attachments; and instructions for use. A wide array of positioning devices are available for use in the operating room to safely position patients preoperatively and are discussed within the following sections.

Surgical Positions

Surgical intervention may be required anywhere on the human body and requires positioning that facilitates the required access to the operative area utilizing all possible safety considerations to mitigate the potential for injury to the patient. The three general positions are supine (facing up/forward), lateral (facing to the side), and prone (facing downward). Numerous variations to those basic positions provide a more targeted approach to the relevant anatomical structures.

Supine Position. The supine position, also referred to as dorsal recumbent, is that of the patient's anterior or ventral surface on top and the posterior or dorsal surface beneath resting on the OR table. The supine position is the most commonly used position, providing access to the head, face, anterior neck and chest, the abdominal and pelvic cavities, and the upper and lower extremities. Supine is required for induction and intubation in general anesthesia prior to placement into other positions. The bony prominences at risk for pressure sore formation include the occiput of the posterior skull, both scapulae, olecranon and thoracic spinal processes, sacrum, and calcaneus bones of the feet. Very thin or elderly patients with little subcutaneous fat and fragile skin are at particular risk for injury to these areas. The arms are routinely positioned outstretched laterally on arm boards at less than a 90° angle to the OR table to prevent excessive stretching and tension on the nerves of the brachial plexuses. There are three main peripheral nerves of the arm that descend from the brachial plexus: the median, radial, and ulnar nerves. Foam arm cradles or gel pads may be used to reduce pressure and maintain arms in position. Palms are usually supinated (facing up) unless the IV site is located on the dorsum of the hand and access to it is required (Figure 8-2).

The surgeon may request that the arms are tucked in at the sides using a draw sheet wrapped around the arms on both sides and then tucked in under the patient's back. The tucked-in arms should have the palms resting flatly against the patient's sides. The draw sheet should not be tucked in between the mattress pad and the tabletop, as this may allow the sheet to slide

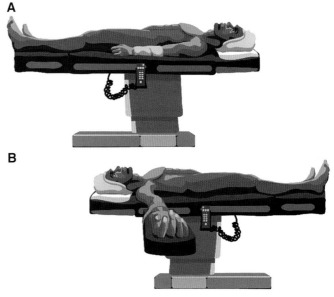

Figure 8-2 · **(A)** Supine position with arms secured at patient's sides. **(B)** Supine position with arms on arm boards at less than 90° angle.

out; causing the draw sheet and arms to sag and possibly fall or rest against the metal side rails of the OR table. The draw sheet secured under the weight of the patient's torso, secured in a manner without slippery surfaces, keeps the arms securely fastened at the sides. Compression and postoperative neuropathy of the ulnar nerve that runs behind the elbow may occur if the arm is not properly padded and protected. Arms may be tucked in at the sides when the surgical team members will need to stand adjacent to the sides of the OR table at or near the level of the shoulders, where the presence of one or both arm boards would obstruct access. Caution must be used to prevent undue pressure being exerted on the arms by team members leaning against the table edge and arms. Tucking the arms should be done only if necessary.

Blood volume in the heart is increased in the supine position as compared to the upright or standing position. Cardiac output is also increased, requiring more work for the heart muscle. A slight compromise to respiratory function in the supine position is due to lessened tidal volume as compared to the Fowler (sitting) position or standing. Obese and pregnant patients or those with large intra-abdominal masses may have decreased venous return to the heart due to compression of the vena cava, which leads to decreased blood pressure.

Trendelenburg Position. The Trendelenburg position, also referred to as the shock position, is a modification of supine in which the head is lowered, and legs are elevated. The gravitational forces of dropping the head lower than the level of the heart improves blood flow to the brain when there is a critical drop in blood pressure or massive blood loss creating hypovolemia and systemic shock.

The patient's knees should be positioned over the table break between the back and foot sections to allow for articulation at the knee joints to provide a counterbalance of the lower legs and the torso, reducing sliding of the body toward the head (Figure 8-3). Alternately, the patient's legs may be placed in half-boot type stirrups that bend the knees and abduct the legs for access to the perineal area. Steep Trendelenburg in excess of 15° may require use of a vacuum pressure bean bag device under the patient's torso to prevent sliding of the head and

torso toward the head of the bed and potentially causing shearing of the integumentary tissues against the sheets of the OR table. Shoulder brace attachments are sometimes used in positioning for specific procedures performed laparoscopically or with robotic assistance involving the pelvis or lower abdominal cavity; however, may contribute to brachial plexus stretching and injury in steep Trendelenburg.

Respiration and chest expansion may be reduced due to the shift of the abdominal viscera against the diaphragm. Although Trendelenburg is beneficial in cases of systemic shock, prolonged Trendelenburg may contribute to dangerous increase in intraocular and intracranial pressure and decreased respiratory tidal volume and should be used for as short a time as possible to mitigate risk of potential injury.

Reverse Trendelenburg Position. Reverse Trendelenburg is another modification of supine in which the head of the OR table and patient's head and upper body are elevated while the foot section of the bed and lower extremities are lowered. Attachment of a padded footboard is critically important to support the patient's body weight and prevent shearing forces of the integumentary system structures from the patient sliding down toward the foot of the bed (Figure 8-4).

Elevation of the head and upper torso facilitates respiration and chest expansion as abdominal viscera shift downward toward the pelvic cavity and is the most similar to the respiratory dynamic of standing upright. Venous return from the lower extremities may be reduced in prolonged procedures and consideration should be given to preoperative placement of anti-DVT stockings or sequential compression devices to facilitate vascular return.

Positioning devices such as a shoulder roll or thyroid pillow may be used to extend the anterior neck for enhanced exposure in procedures involving the neck and upper shoulders. Reverse Trendelenburg is often used in laparoscopic cholecystectomy with a slight lateral tilt to the patient's left in order to allow gravity to separate the abdominal viscera away from the right upper quadrant.

Lithotomy Position. Lithotomy position is another variation of supine in which the dorsal torso is lying on the OR table with

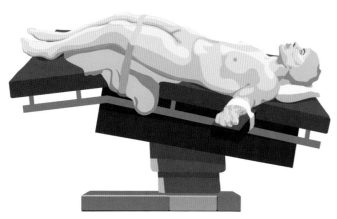

Figure 8-3 · Trendelenburg position with arms extended laterally on arm boards and knees positioned over table break.

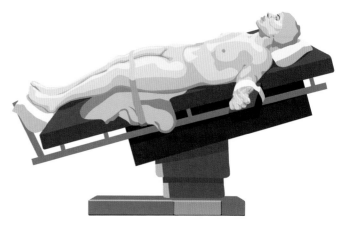

Figure 8-4 · Reverse Trendelenburg position with attached footboard and arms extended laterally on arm boards.

lower extremities elevated and abducted to provide exposure to the genitourinary structures, perineum, and anal area. Various types of positioning stirrups may be used including candy-cane type, knee brace, and half-boot calf supports. Each device requires special attachments to the OR table side rails. All stirrup devices are adjustable to modify the degree of leg elevation ranging from low, standard, high, to exaggerated, depending on the approach to the anatomical area to be operated, the surgical method used (endoscopic, robotic-assisted, or combination open and minimally invasive), procedure scheduled, and patient-specific considerations.

The head of the OR table may be removed prior to patient transfer and added to the foot section. This allows the patient to be placed on the OR table with buttocks oriented at the edge of the cut-out buttocks notch/break and keeps the feet and ankles supported until the legs are positioned in the stirrups. Preplanning reduces the need for additional team members to assist in moving the anesthetized patient down toward the break, potentially causing shearing of the skin. The buttocks must not extend beyond or hang over the table edge, as this would cause lumbosacral strain of the lumbar plexus and potential postoperative neuropathy.

Stirrup holders must be checked to ensure secure attachment of stirrups to prevent legs from falling and resulting in potential musculoskeletal injury, fracture, or even hip dislocation. Once the legs are secured in the stirrups, the head section piece previously added to the foot is removed first, then the foot section of the OR table is lowered to at least 90° toward the floor or removed if that is a feature of the OR table. Care should be used when dropping the foot section to prevent OR table platform and mattress pad from falling off once perpendicular to the tabletop. Arm boards should be used if possible (Figure 8-5). The fingers may be crushed if they extend over the lower edge of the back section, adjacent to the buttocks break, when the patient is positioned farther toward the end

of the OR table and the foot section is returned to a horizontal position or reattached following completion of the procedure. Arms may alternately be crossed loosely over the upper abdomen and secured with sheets or tape if the procedure does not require abdominal cavity access and respiration is not restricted.

The degree of flexion of the hips increases from approximately 30° in low-lithotomy, 90° in standard lithotomy, and well in excess of 90° in high and exaggerated lithotomy. The knees should not be flexed beyond 90° due to a potential risk of compartment syndrome from restricted venous return from the lower legs. Anti-DVT devices should be used in procedures lasting more than 2 hours. Two team members must slowly and simultaneously elevate the patient's legs, flexing the hips, and positioning them in stirrups in a coordinated fashion to prevent undue stretching of the obturator nerve or lumbosacral strain. Patients with pre-existing spinal pathology such as herniated disc or sciatic nerve impingement are at particular risk of injury from muscle strain or exacerbation of nerve irritation. Patients with limited ROM or hip replacement prostheses may require a lesser degree of flexion to prevent possible disarticulation of the femoral head from the acetabulum.

The lateral aspects of the knees and calves must not lean against candy-cane type stirrups as foot drop or other neuropathy may result from compression of the common peroneal or the saphenous branch of the femoral nerve, even if stirrups are covered with foam or gel padding. Use of wide straps, foam or gel wraps, or pads over the foot and ankle may prevent injury to the plantar and sural nerves. Knee brace type stirrups may compress the common peroneal and posterior tibial nerves and the popliteal artery due to the weight of the entire extremity being supported by the posterior aspect of the knee. The padded half-boot type stirrups including Allen and Yellowfin devices may be preferred over either candy cane or knee brace stirrups due to the even pressure distribution to the entire surface of the lower legs. The additional advantage of these types of stirrups is the ease of modification of height and degree of leg abduction by handles which can be operated even with sterile legging drapes in place.

Elevation of the lower extremities increases blood flow to and potential pooling in the trunk of the body. Exaggerated or high lithotomy positions with extreme flexion of the hips may compromise respiration by pushing abdominal viscera against the diaphragm and reducing tidal volume. At completion of the procedure, the foot section of the OR table must be elevated back to horizontal or, if removed, reapplied. The platform and mattress pad must be replaced as well if previously removed. The head section should also be reattached to support the ankles and feet. Removal of the legs from lithotomy and return to supine position must be performed slowly with both legs lowered simultaneously, at equal levels. Leveling of the body results in the pooled volume of blood from the trunk returning back into the legs and may cause significant decrease in blood pressure until hemodynamic equilibrium can be reestablished.

Fowler's Position. The modification of supine position in which the patient is in a modified or semi-sitting to full sitting

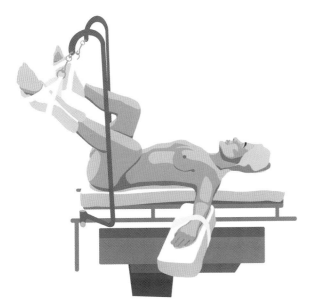

Figure 8-5 · Lithotomy position using candy-cane type stirrups and arms positioned laterally on arm boards.

position is also known as modified or semi-Fowler's and Fowler's position. Procedures in the semi-Fowler's position include procedures of the face such as rhytidectomy, anterior neck such as thyroidectomy, or neck reconstruction as well as others based on surgeon's preference. The OR table is articulated to slightly elevate the back section and drop the foot section into a beach or recliner chair configuration. This position is the most normal for respiration, especially for patients with lung disease who may not tolerate the flat supine position. Hamstring tightness can be alleviated by use of pillows under the knees. The arms are usually placed over the lower abdominal area and secured to prevent falling off the sides of the table.

Full sitting or Fowler's position is a complicated procedure to achieve safely. Posterior cranial or upper cervical spine procedures may be performed in Fowler's position but will require use of cranial fixation devices such as a Mayfield skull brace and arch-bar attachment to the side rails. The most dangerous complication of the sitting or Fowler's position is release of an air embolus into the venous system, into the right ventricle of the heart, then into the pulmonary system. The anesthesia provider will place a central venous catheter into the right atrium preoperatively and listen with a Doppler device for any potential air bubbles which could then be aspirated via the catheter, maintaining cardiac and pulmonary function. In cases where a central venous line may not be in place, an emergency procedure to treat an air embolus is known as the Durant maneuver. Upon recognition of an air embolus, the patient is repositioned immediately into left lateral position with steep Trendelenburg, head-down tilt. This causes the air bubble to hopefully stay in the right atrium. If it does get into the lungs, the Trendelenburg should help keep the air embolus from traveling from the lungs to the brain through the arterial system.

Other potential positioning complications include venous stasis of the lower extremities for which anti-embolic stockings or sequential compression devices should be used. A padded footboard may be placed to support the feet and prevent foot-drop. Procedures of long duration increase the risk of pressure sores formation of ischial tuberosities and sciatic nerve compression.

Newer beach chair shoulder positioning attachments are popular for orthopedic procedures including shoulder arthroscopy, rotator cuff repair, and reverse shoulder arthroplasty. These attachments are placed on the OR table to orient the patient's torso and upper extremity to the operative side edge of the table while supporting the head and neck in neutral alignment. The operative arm and shoulder are free for manipulation during the procedure. Other safety precautions described for sitting or semi-sitting procedures may also be used in addition to the beach chair device.

Fracture Table Positioning. The fracture table provides a small surface area for the patient's torso and has adjustable extensions for placement of the lower extremities in traction or abducted away from the midline and supported in a low-lithotomy, half-boot type stirrup. The arms are placed laterally on arm boards if the operative side arm board does not obstruct access to the operative area. In most procedures, the surgical assistant

or circulating nurse is responsible for positioning the patient; however, in patients with un-splinted, unstable hip, or femoral fractures, the surgeon is responsible for the final positioning on the fracture table and determination of appropriate degree of traction of the operative leg, abduction of the non-operative leg, and orientation of the C-arm prior to the skin prep. A perineal post is part of most fracture tables and prevents the patient from being pulled off the back section of the table when traction is applied to the operative leg. The perineal post must be well-padded to ensure the external genitalia and perineal tissues are not overly compressed during the procedure.

Prone Position. The prone position is used for surgical procedures involving the posterior or dorsal areas of the body. The patient is face-down; therefore, anesthesia induction and intubation is performed prior to positioning with the patient in supine position on the stretcher or other transport device. Careful attention to protection of the endotracheal tube and breathing circuit as well as any additional indwelling lines (eg, IVs, urinary catheters, neuromonitoring leads) must be taken during the transfer of the patient into the final prone position. Extra personnel may be required to keep the patient's spine in neutral alignment during the log-roll turning and placement on positioning devices including chest rolls or bolsters, laminectomy frames, pillows or padding, or specialty tables.

The weight of the patient's body resting on the anterior chest compromises anterior chest expansion during inspiration. Cardiac filling and vital capacity may be reduced due to the pressure against the rigid surface of the OR table. Breasts of females and genitals of males may suffer pressure injury after extended periods in the prone position if not padded or elevated. Chest rolls made of gel material, blankets, or encased foam may be used to lift the torso off the table surface to facilitate respiration, reduce hypotension, improve venous return from the femoral veins and inferior vena cava, and reduce pressure on anterior surfaces. The chest rolls should extend bilaterally from the acromioclavicular joint to the iliac crest to adequately elevate the anterior torso. The arms should be placed laterally on arm boards positioned parallel to the OR table sides with arms oriented beside the head and palms down to reduce potential musculoskeletal strain or brachial plexus compromise. Adequate padding must be used to protect the airway and hyper-rotation of the neck avoided to prevent injury to the cervical plexus, lateral face, and ear of the dependent side. Pillows may be placed under the calves to reduce stress on the sciatic or peroneal nerves.

Spinal positioning devices including the Wilson or Hall frames and specialty spine tables may be used for procedures including laminectomy/laminotomy, spinal fusion and instrumentation, vertebroplasty, or other procedures of the spinal column. The frames or tables reduce the amount of lumbar concavity to provide a more flattened lower spine curvature as an adjunct to access and visualization of the surgical area. These devices or tables provide the same or enhanced elements of positioning safety mentioned for use of chest rolls (Figure 8-6).

The jackknife or Kraske position is a variation of the prone position and used most commonly for rectal area procedures

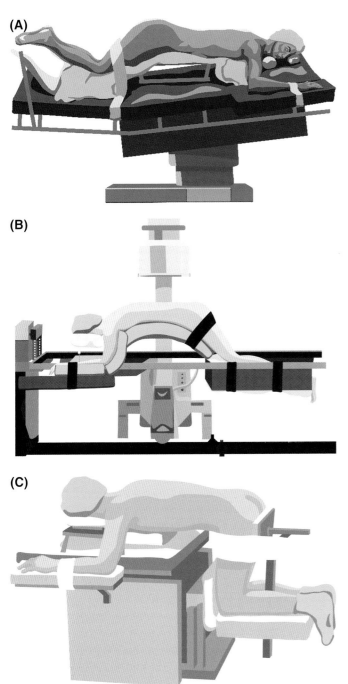

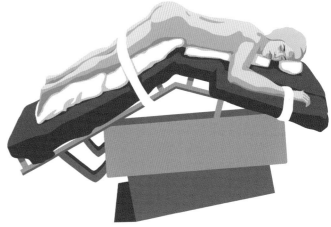

Figure 8-7 · Kraske or jackknife position variation of prone.

(A)

(B)

(C)

Figure 8-6 · **(A)** Prone/Laminectomy position utilizing specialty frame. **(B)** Prone/Spinal position utilizing specialty table with fluoroscopy compatibility. **(C)** Prone/Spinal position utilizing Andrews-type specialty table.

such as excision of pilonidal cyst or hemorrhoidectomy. The patient's hips are positioned over the middle break or flex-point of the table to elevate the area of the superior buttocks for access to the anatomical area to be operated. The other steps for safe positioning described for use of chest rolls in straight prone position are utilized for jackknife/Kraske. Tape may be used to laterally retract the buttocks for exposure of the operative area (Figure 8-7).

Lateral Positions. The lateral position, also referred to as lateral decubitus or lateral recumbent requires additional team members to safely achieve the final position of the patient. Surgical procedures performed in the lateral position include unilateral open or laparoscopic/robotic/MIS kidney procedures, thoracic procedures, total hip arthroplasty, or combined anterior-posterior thoracoabdominal spinal fusion. The positioning process may be complicated due to the challenge of keeping the body in the lateral position as it tends to roll forward or backward if not carefully stabilized. A coordinated effort of at least four team members is needed to prevent injury to the patient. As with all positioning, the anesthesia provider supports the head, protects the airway, and gives permission before any steps are initiated. A draw sheet is extremely useful to move the patient and prevent shearing of the skin. The patient is first moved from supine position onto the appropriate side. This turning places the patient at the very edge of the narrow OR table. Team members then together lift the patient with the draw sheet to the middle of the OR table-top before proceeding with application of other devices. The postoperative return to supine from the lateral position also requires carefully coordinated steps to again bring the patient to the edge of the table before placing back into supine in the center of the table.

As with the prone position, respiration involving the dependent (downward-facing) lung is compromised by the weight of the remaining torso on that side. Use of a gel or fabric roll placed inferior to the axilla reduces compression of the dependent brachial plexus and elevates the dependent chest wall to facilitate chest expansion. Commonly referred to as the axillary roll, care should be taken not to place it directly under the axilla which would exacerbate the pressure against the peripheral nerve structures. The dependent lateral face and ear are also at risk of soft tissue injury from prolonged compression if not adequately padded. The arms should be positioned outstretched and separated by either a padded double-level arm board, stacked pillows between arms, or placed on a padded Mayo stand, taking care that no metal surfaces are touching the patient and the operative side arm is not out of neutral forward position. Pillows or foam padding is used to prevent soft tissue or peripheral nerve compression of the dependent leg by the upper, operative side leg.

Bean bag-type vacuum devices may be used to help keep the patient's torso from shifting to the front or back. The device must be placed on the OR table prior to the patient's transfer onto the table. Once placed in the lateral position, the bean bag is held against the patient to conform to the anatomical areas and suction is applied to the bag which becomes rigid when air is removed. Care should be taken to not open the suction valve, or the bag will lose its rigidity and not maintain the patient in position. Kidney braces are table attachments that connect to the kidney elevator/bridge to prevent the patient from tilting out of position. They may be used in conjunction with the bean bag device. The shorter brace is typically used on the side of the body plane (anterior or posterior) where the incision extends the farthest to prevent obstruction of the operative field.

Peg-board systems are utilized for orthopedic procedures of the hip when a posterolateral approach is used. A gel pad may be placed over the board which is placed on the OR table. After transfer of the patient onto the covered peg board, various pegs are inserted into holes in the board to stabilize the patient in the appropriate position based on surgical access and patient anatomy. Padded stabilizing braces that attach to the side rails of the OR table may also be used to hold the patient in place without shifting or tilting.

The lateral position referred to as lateral kidney position utilizes steps to enhance access to the anterior to posterolateral areas of the operative side retroperitoneal space to reach the kidney, upper ureter, or adrenal glands. After anesthesia administration and placement in the lateral position with the patient's waist area over the middle table break, the dependent (lower) leg is flexed, and the operative (upper) leg is left mostly straight with pillows between them. The flexing of the dependent leg causes the operative leg to hang over it, increasing the stretch of the tissues of the operative anatomical area. The axillary roll is placed inferior to the axillary area to facilitate dependent chest expansion. The arms are separated and placed on double arm boards or pillows and the patient is secured with safety straps or other stabilizing devices. Prior to incision, the OR table is flexed at the mid-point and the kidney elevator bridge is raised to apply pressure against the dependent side and increase the distance between the lower rib on the operative side and the iliac crest, maximizing access to the operative area. The steps must be reversed prior to the start of wound closure so that tissue layers are brought back into normal position for careful suture approximation. The kidney elevator bridge is lowered, and the table is unflexed. A wound, closed prior to return to normal flat lateral, would be closed under excess tension and, then after return to a flat table level, would then gap from release of tension, leaving dead space and failure of adequate tissue approximation (Figure 8-8).

Lateral chest position is used most commonly for posterior or combination thoracotomy or thoracoscopic procedures. The same steps are used as described for lateral kidney with a few exceptions. The operative side arm may be oriented upward toward the head to allow access to the subscapular area. The

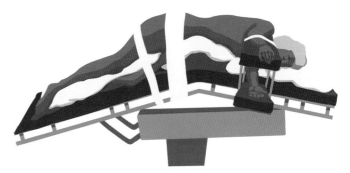

Figure 8-8 · Lateral kidney position utilizing double arm board, kidney elevator/bridge, axillary roll, pillows between legs (lower flexed, upper straight), and safety straps.

OR table is not flexed, and the kidney elevator bridge is not raised. There is no need to increase the distance between lower rib and iliac crest for access to the thoracic cavity. Rib spreaders or other surgical instruments are used rather than gravity and positioning measures. The operative side, upper leg may be flexed with the dependent leg more or less straight to help prevent the patient from tilting forward by using the flexed knee as a stop. All other safety measures for lateral positioning should be followed.

The Sims or lateral recumbent position is a mix of prone and lateral position mainly used for lower GI diagnostic procedures such as colonoscopy under moderate sedation. The patient is placed usually with left side down and the upper leg flexed to provide access to the anal area for insertion of the colonoscope. Additional padding and safety measures taken for lateral or prone positioning for surgical procedures under general anesthesia are not required with the much shorter-duration endoscopic procedures.

INDICATIONS FOR URINARY CATHETERIZATION

Patients scheduled for surgery may be asked to void to empty the urinary bladder as part of their preliminary preparation in the preoperative care unit (PCU), also known as the holding area. Surgical procedures that are expected to last for a prolonged period may require placement of an indwelling urinary drainage catheter to prevent bladder distention as well as to keep an accurate count of the amount of fluid input from IV fluids and output of urine through the urethral catheter, also known as the I&O (input and output) to prevent fluid overloading. Surgical procedures performed in the abdominal or pelvic cavities may require bladder decompression to prevent potential trauma to the bladder during manipulation or dissection of internal organs. This decompression may also be accomplished for shorter-duration procedures by insertion of a sterile, non-retaining urinary drainage catheter such as a Red Robinson, prior to or in conjunction with the skin prep.

Surgical procedures involving genitourinary system structures such as the kidneys, ureters, bladder, prostate, urethra, or vagina may require temporary indwelling catheter placement to facilitate wound healing. These catheters are not typically

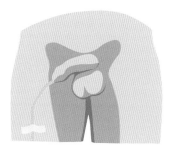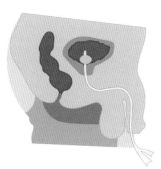

Figure 8-9 · Urethral catherization in a male.

inserted preoperatively, only post-procedurally and may include percutaneous insertion of Malecot, Pezzer, Bonanno, or other suprapubic urinary drainage catheters. Large balloon three-way Foley catheters are inserted for mechanical hemostasis and continuous fluid irrigation to flush the bladder of blood clots following transurethral resection of the prostate (TURP) or transurethral resection of bladder tumor (TURBT) procedures. These catheters should be removed as soon as possible following surgery when postoperative bleeding and clot formation has decreased significantly or ceased.

Preoperative urinary catheterization may be performed prior to or after final positioning for the surgical procedure and may be part of the antiseptic skin preparation. Temporary flexing of the knees, also known as frog-legging, may be necessary for access to the perineal area and placement of the catheter when patient is in supine, also known as dorsal recumbent position. Procedures performed in the lateral or prone position require urinary catheter insertion prior to positioning. For procedures performed in supine or lithotomy, positioning is performed prior to catheterization (Figure 8-9).

The process of inserting a urinary catheter is an invasive procedure, whether indwelling, or for in-and-out bladder drainage, and requires use of a sterile catheter placed by a trained individual wearing sterile gloves, and after cleansing of the perineum and urethral meatus with an antiseptic skin prep agent. A sterile, water-based lubricant gel is used to facilitate easy passage of the catheter into the urethral meatus and along the length of the urethral canal. Many newer catheters are coated with a lubricant to facilitate easy insertion without the need for an added lubricant gel. Preassembled catheters have the drainage bag attached to the Foley and some catheter manufacturers, including Bard, do not recommend pretesting of the inflation balloon as they state it is part of the prepackaging routine.

Characteristics of Urethral Catheters

The diameter of the urethral catheter is measured in French or Fr. units with 1 Fr. = 0.33 mm, rounded up to the nearest tenth. For example, 6 Fr. is 0.33 mm multiplied by 6 = 1.98 mm rounded up to 2.0 mm. The first indwelling, two-way catheters with the inflation balloon were designed by a Boston surgeon named Fredric Foley in the 1930s and developed by C. R. Bard, Inc. A 14 Fr. (4.62/4.7 mm) Red Robinson-type catheter

is typically adequate for straight catheterization and bladder decompression in adults prior to shorter-duration surgical procedures. A 16 Fr. (5.28/5.3 mm) Foley catheter is a standard size for average adults requiring indwelling catheterization intraoperatively or for the immediate postoperative period. Pediatric patients may require 6 Fr. (1.98/2.0 mm) catheters for neonates and infants. Catheter size increases in diameter as patient age and size increases. The smallest possible size that provides adequate drainage is preferred to reduce potential trauma to delicate meatal mucosal tissues by compression which can lead to potential necrosis or stricture of the bladder neck. Leakage of urine around the outside of the catheter may require insertion of a larger diameter replacement.

The materials used for short-term urinary drainage catheters are polyvinylchloride (PVC), a type of plastic, latex with or without antimicrobial or PTFE (Teflon) coating, and 100% silicone with or without antimicrobial coating. PVC catheters contain a plasticizer DEHP or Di(2-ethylhexyl) phthalate used to soften the rigid plastic catheters and make them more flexible. The European Union (EU) banned DEHP in consumer products in 2015. In 2018, the EU expanded its ban to include four classes of phthalates: BBP, DBP, DIBP, and the previously banned DEHP due to research findings indicating a possible damaging effect on reproductive health. In the United States, California now requires warning labels on all PVC catheters.

Latex catheters have long been the routine material of choice for urethral catheters due to their excellent flexibility and low cost when compared to PVC or silicone. The problem with latex has been the increase in patients with latex allergy or sensitivity to the natural rubber product. Long-term use of latex catheters in patients with chronic conditions such as paralysis from spinal injury or deformity predisposes patients to develop an allergy to latex. Healthcare workers have similar risk of latex sensitivity or allergy following years of use of natural latex gloves in the workplace. Some surgical departments and even hospitals have opted to be totally latex-free facilities to prevent potential adverse hypersensitivity reactions in these individuals.

Silicone catheters are gaining in popularity and use due to the issues with PVC and latex. Silicone is totally free of latex and relatively flexible and provides smooth passage through urethral tissue, whether coated or uncoated. Clear catheters also allow for ease of visualization of urine in the catheter and tubing; however, they are comparatively more expensive than the other materials. Manufacturers of silicone catheters do not recommend pretesting silicone balloons due to a risk that the additional inflation test might create a folding of the stiffer material that could potentially form a cuff at the neck of the balloon which might abrade delicate mucosal tissue during insertion or removal of the catheter.

Urethral Catheterization

1. Open sterile Foley catheter kit or other sterile supplies using proper sterile technique.

2. Position the patient for access to the perineal area and urethral meatus.

3. Perform hand hygiene by traditional hand washing or alcohol-based hand rub agent.

4. Don sterile gloves using the open-gloving technique.

5. Organize sterile items for easy access and test the Foley catheter balloon with the pre-filled syringe of sterile water to verify balloon is not ruptured.

6. If catheter is covered with a thin plastic cover, open partially to expose only the catheter tip and leave the remainder of the tube covered.

7. Many catheter kits have urethral catheter already connected to the urine drainage collection device. Do not disconnect unless there is a need to change the catheter out. If disconnected, protect the connection ports of the catheter and tubing from contamination.

8. Open and squeeze out the lubricant into a compartment of the tray unless the catheter is pre-lubricated. Open and pour the antiseptic prep solution into a compartment of the tray.

9. Place sterile towels or paper drapes to isolate the perineal area and urethral meatus.

10. Moisten sterile gauze pads, sponges, or cotton balls with antiseptic solution and cleanse the urethral meatus. In female patients, the labial folds may be retracted with the gloved fingers of the non-dominant hand. In uncircumcised male patients, the penile foreskin may be pulled down with the gloved non-dominant hand to expose the meatus.

11. Obtain catheter with the dominant hand and dip the Foley tip in the sterile lubricant gel.

12. Insert the tip of the catheter into the urethral meatus and advance the catheter through the urethral canal. For adult females the average distance is approximately 2 in or 5 cm; in pediatric females, it would be approximately 1 in or 2.5 cm. For adult males, length would be approximately 7 to 9 in or 17.5 to 22.5 cm. In pediatric males, approximately 2 to 3 in or 5 to 7.5 cm.

13. Watch tubing for evidence of urine flow. In females, lack of flow could indicate misplacement of the catheter tip into the vagina rather than the urethra. A new sterile catheter should be obtained, lubricated if appropriate, and inserted while leaving the misplaced catheter in the vagina until the Foley is in correct position, then removed from the vagina (Figure 8-10).

14. Once flow of urine is observed, retracted tissues (foreskin or labia) are released, and the balloon inflation syringe is attached. The syringe plunger is slowly and gently pushed with the dominant hand, and the balloon is filled with the pre-measured amount of sterile water. If resistance is felt, pull back plunger and readjust the catheter and try again.

15. Pull the catheter gently to verify the balloon is inflated, and maintains its position within the bladder.

16. Remove the syringe from the balloon-inflation collet.

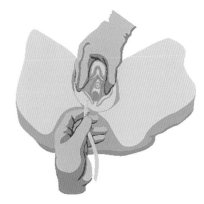

Figure 8-10 · Insertion of a urethral catheter in female.

17. If collection device tubing is not already connected, carefully connect to the funnel end of the Foley catheter without contaminating either opening.

18. Remove draping materials used to isolate the area for insertion.

19. If patient is frog-legged, legs are repositioned on the OR table and safety strap reapplied 2 in above the patient's knees.

20. Catheter-tubing connection should be adjusted depending on patient's position and secured to prevent possible dislodgement. Tubing may be positioned under the patient's leg if in the supine position.

21. The urine collection bag or device should be attached to the OR table and not left sitting on the floor.

Steps for preoperative in-and-out, non-indwelling catheterization are similar to those listed with exclusion of balloon inflation and attachment to tubing of collection device. A sterile basin should be used to collect the urine flow from the Red Robinson–type urinary drainage catheter.

Catheter-Associated Urinary Tract Infections

Despite the value of urinary catheterization, there are recognized risks that must be considered, and the cost-benefit ratio examined before use in surgical patient preparation. Recommendations from the CDC's Healthcare Infection Control Practices Advisory Committee (HICPAC) and the World Health Organization (WHO) were published in their report, *Guideline for Prevention of Urinary Catheter-Associated Urinary Tract Infections 2009*. In the June 2019 update to the 2009 report, the recommendations applicable to surgical patients include:

- The use of urinary catheters and the duration of time left in place should be minimized for all patients in general and in particular for patient populations most at risk for catheter-associated urinary tract infection (CAUTI) including female patients, the elderly, and immunocompromised individuals.

- Use indwelling urinary catheters in surgical patients only when necessary rather than routinely.

- Surgical patients with an indication for use of an indwelling catheter should have it removed as soon as possible postoperatively or within 24 hours unless there are strong indications for continued use.

- Urinary catheters placed due to prolonged duration of surgical procedure or use of large volumes of intraoperative fluids or diuretics should be removed in the PACU.

- Sterile urinary catheters should be inserted using strict aseptic technique by a trained individual following proper hand hygiene, wearing sterile gloves, and using sterile drapes, appropriate antiseptic cleansing solution with sterile sponges or cotton pads, sterile lubricant gel for coating the tip of the catheter, and syringe of sterile water for balloon inflation.

- After aseptic insertion of urethral catheter, a closed drainage system must be maintained.

- Kinks in the catheter or closed drainage bag or urometer tubing should be avoided to prevent backing up of urine.

- Straight in-and-out, non-indwelling, preoperative catheterization for bladder decompression of surgical patients is preferable to indwelling catheters to reduce the potential for CAUTI.

The CDC estimates that between 15% and 25% of hospitalized patients have placement of short-term, indwelling urinary catheters. Nearly all acute care cases of urinary tract infections are catheter-associated, therefore are CAUTIs; constituting the most commonly recognized type of healthcare-associated infections (HAIs) and representing an estimated 30% of all categories of infections in acute care facilities.

There are two recognized sources of microbial contamination leading to CAUTI, endogenous and exogenous. Endogenous contamination involves the patient's own bacteria-colonized tissues including the urethral meatus, anal or rectal area, and vagina. Exogenous contamination results most commonly from contamination of the hands of healthcare personnel or the items used during catheter placement. Opportunistic resident or pathogenic transient bacteria can enter the urinary tract during catheter insertion by way of the inside of the catheter (intraluminal route) or along the outside surface (extraluminal route).

The most common pathogens isolated in CAUTI reported by the CDC were *Escherichia coli*, species of *Candida*, various *Enterococcus* species, *Pseudomonas aeruginosa*, *Klebsiella pneumoniae*, and species of *Enterobacter*. Other Gram-negative bacteria and staphylococcal bacteria were seen in a smaller number of infections. Increasing incidents of antimicrobial resistance seen in CAUTI have raised concern in health agencies as multidrug-resistant bacterial and fungal strains have been detected more frequently. Recommendations for enhanced surveillance and review of antibiotic protocols have led to changes in routine orders for antibiotic prophylaxis in patients with urinary catheters and revising of traditional practice guidelines.

PREOPERATIVE SKIN PREPARATION

The aseptic practice of cleansing the area for insertion of a urethral catheter with an antimicrobial agent is an important measure to reduce the possibility of CAUTI. Similarly, the aseptic technique of performing preoperative skin preparation over and adjacent to the planned incisional site with antimicrobial agents is an important factor in reducing SSI. As discussed in Chapter 4, many bacterial and microbial species are normal residents of the human body and only become pathogenic invaders when the opportunity presents itself to gain entry beyond the strong protective barrier of our intact skin layers and mucosal membranes. Surgical interventions present such an opportunity, disrupting the skin by sharply incising through the superficial and deep layers of tissue where most skin bacteria cannot otherwise access.

Skin Preparation Goals

The three major goals of an effective preoperative surgical skin prep are: (1) to remove all transient surface microbes, oils, and secretions on the surface of the skin as well as dirt or other inorganic environmental contaminants by use of mechanical friction with antiseptic solutions and prep sponges, (2) to reduce the resident skin microbial count to the smallest possible, irreducible number, and (3) to delay rebound microbial colony growth through chemical suppression. The National Institutes of Health (NIH) Human Genome Project found that there are trillions of bacterial cells within us, outnumbering human cells 10:1. Therefore, these measures represent aseptic (without infection) principles because living human skin cannot be sterilized, meaning free of all living microorganisms, pathogenic or non-pathogenic, including spores.

Preoperative Hair Removal

The presence of hair growth in or around the incisional site was long believed to be a potential source of SSI; however, newer research has determined that infection rates are not increased by leaving hair in place. Methods of hair removal such as shaving actually contribute to SSI risk by causing microabrasions of the skin that increase the microbial count in the area and produce greater inflammation. Patients are instructed not to shave at home the night before or day of a scheduled surgery.

Depilatory creams have been recommended in the literature; however, due to the requirement of a patch test for allergy assessment needed at least 24 hours prior to surgery and the inconsistent results and prolonged time required for depilatory creams to work, they are not generally considered practical for routine hair removal in the perioperative setting. Patients should be instructed not to use a depilatory cream the night before or day of surgery due to similar potential for increased microbial growth seen in shaving.

If hair must be removed, it should be clipped using single-use sterile clipper heads or trimmed with scissors. The ideal place to perform hair removal is in the preoperative care unit (PCU) or holding area when standard or routine physician orders are on file for the procedure. Hair that interferes with adhesion of electrocardiographic (ECG) leads or the electrosurgical patient return electrode may need to be removed to ensure proper electrical conduction and prevent burns. This may not be practical in the PCU and may be performed in the operating room by the circulating RN after anesthetic induction, final positioning, and prior to the skin prep procedure. Stray hairs should be removed from the area using adhesive tape to pick up the clipped hairs and prevent risk of migration onto the surgical site or sterile drapes. Patients with excessively oily skin may additionally require preparation of areas with degreasing sheets to ensure proper adherence to ECG leads and ESU ground pads.

Pubic hair may be clipped if ordered and likely to get caught in the incision during skin closure. Patients should be advised not to wax, shave, or use depilatory creams the night before or day of surgery to reduce inflammation and increased microbial rebound growth.

Long eyelashes may require trimming by small, delicate scissors dipped in lubricant gel to catch cut lashes and prevent falling onto the surface of the eye. Eyebrows are rarely trimmed unless under surgeon's orders. Scalp hair clipped in preparation for cranial surgery should be collected, bagged, labeled with patient sticker, and kept as patient property. If the surgeon prefers to leave the scalp hair in place, it may be cleansed, combed, and secured with ties and coated with water-based sterile lubricant gel to create parted areas for incision. Mustaches are normally left in place for procedures involving the nose or mouth unless otherwise ordered by the surgeon.

Antiseptic Skin Prep Solutions

The antiseptic or antimicrobial agents used for preoperative skin antisepsis should be broad-spectrum and safe for use. Patients can still have a sensitivity or allergy to certain prep solutions.

Alcohol. Isopropyl alcohol is most commonly added to other prep agents such as chlorhexidine gluconate and iodophors to enhance their antimicrobial effectiveness, cumulative action, and facilitate evaporation. Alcohol denatures microbial cell proteins to neutralize them. It is effective against both gram-positive and gram-negative bacteria including antibiotic-resistant pathogens such as MRSA and VRE, as well as *Mycobacterium tuberculosis* and fungal pathogens. As a prep agent, it is effective in degreasing oily areas; however, it is very drying to mucosal tissues and not recommended in those areas. The advantage of the clear, uncolored agent is that it does not leave any residue or coloration on areas such as the face; however, it does not have a cumulative effect as a stand-alone agent and should be used following skin cleansing with a plain soap solution then dried prior to the alcohol wipe. Isopropyl and ethyl alcohol are extremely flammable and volatile and must be allowed to completely evaporate and fumes dissipate prior to application of sterile drapes.

Iodine and Iodophors. Iodine and iodophor solutions have been used for wound care since the 1830s. Iodophors are broad-spectrum prep agents considered generally non-toxic and non-irritating. Surgical skin prep agents are supplied in 1% and 2% concentrations combined with water (aqueous) or 70% isopropyl or ethyl alcohol (alcoholic). These prepping agents are commonly used in a two-step process. Iodine used for preoperative antiseptic skin cleansing is frequently combined with povidone, a detergent surfactant (wetting and dispersive agent) in an aqueous solution scrub which produces a foaming action. The 10% solution is a common strength; however, diluted concentrations as low as 0.3% are available for use in the eyes and vagina. Many who work in the operating room are familiar with the brand Betadine® which has long been almost synonymous with iodine/iodophor skin preps.

The first step of the two-step prep involves the povidone-iodine agent applied topically to the patient's skin with soft foam sponges supplied in disposable prep kits. Following blotting of the soap lather with sterile absorbent towels, the aqueous, non-foaming, brown paint solution is applied to the anticipated incisional site and in an expanding circumference around the incisional site in the same manner as the prep agent. This colored paint solution provides a helpful visible demarcation of prepped areas in case of need to expand the surgical field to accommodate extension of the original incision, additional incisions for access trocars, or postoperative drain placement. Some surgeons will use isopropyl alcohol over the paint to facilitate evaporation for application of an adhesive incise drape directly to the patient's skin.

Duraprep™ from 3M™ is a commonly used, one-step prep solution in a tubular, sponge-tip applicator of a combination of 0.7% iodine povacrylex and 74% isopropyl alcohol with water. The solution creates a film on the skin following drying that is visible and resistant to removal from exposure to blood, body fluids, and irrigation solutions. Care should be used to lightly paint clean, dry skin surfaces and not exert pressure in a scrubbing motion during application. Adhesive incise drapes can be applied directly over prepped areas given time to dry and alcohol evaporate. Removal of the incise drape commonly removes the Duraprep™ film as well.

Another iodophor in a one-step applicator is Prevail® from CareFusion 2200 Inc. The concentration of the skin prep agent is 5.0% combined with 62% ethanol in a viscous gel. The application, precautions, and risks are similar to those of Duraprep™.

Iodine and iodophors have been used less frequently for surgical skin preps due to fears of possible iodine allergy or sensitivity. Patients are preoperatively screened for history of known allergies to prep solutions, latex, and medications. If no allergies are known, further screening questions about food allergies such as shellfish are asked to assess the possibility of a correlation between a sensitivity and actual allergy to shellfish which usually contain iodine. Researchers differ in opinion as to the actual relevance of shellfish allergy to topical use of iodine or iodophor prep solutions; however, most clinicians will err on the side of caution and opt for other types of prep agents.

Caution should be taken when iodine-containing prep agents are used in the highly vascular mucosal tissues of the vaginal vault due to potential for absorption of excess iodine into the bloodstream from pooled solution. Neonatal patients also have a higher risk of excessive skin irritation and transient hypothyroidism due to absorption of the iodine through the highly permeable skin. Iodine and iodophors combined with alcohol are highly flammable and must be allowed to completely dry before activation of energy sources such as the electrosurgical unit or lasers. Wet hair can take up to 1 hour to dry and presents a fire hazard if drapes are applied over hair wet with alcohol-containing prep solutions.

Chlorhexidine Gluconate. First developed in England in the 1950s, chlorhexidine gluconate (CHG) is a broad-spectrum, fast-acting, and generally nontoxic surgical antiseptic used for preoperative skin preps available in concentrations of 0.5% to 2.0% chlorhexidine combined with 70% isopropyl alcohol or as a 4% chlorhexidine gluconate solution. CHG is available in lightly tinted and non-tinted solutions.

CHG is also used by surgical personnel as a preoperative surgical scrub agent to cleanse hands and forearms prior to donning sterile gown and gloves. The activity of CHG is diminished by the presence of organic matter, detergents, and shampoos. Patients directed to use CHG preoperatively the night before and morning of surgery should be advised to use their normal soaps and shampoos first, rinse thoroughly, then wash with the CHG and rinse. This initiates the cumulative effect that enhances the antiseptic action of the skin preparation.

Brands familiar to surgical personnel include Bactoshield, Betasept, Dyna-Hex 4, Hibiclens®, Scrub Care Exidine-4 CHG, as well as numerous generic liquid solutions, all 4% CHG solutions used for preoperative patient skin antisepsis. Several of these agents are available in 2% concentrations as well as the 4%.

A single-use foam-tipped device containing the skin antiseptic combination of 2% CHG and 70% alcohol is available as Chloraprep® applicators of various sizes and amounts. The Chloraprep® solution is applied as a light painting motion over all appropriate incisional site areas and allowed to air dry fully prior to application of sterile drapes or activation of ignition sources such as monopolar electrosurgical instruments or laser devices. Hairy areas should not be prepped with the alcohol-containing agent due to the excessive (1-hour minimum) time to allow for full dissipation of fumes and drying of solution.

Although not a two-step prep utilizing detergent and paint agents as in iodophors, manufacturer recommendations for use state that the CHG skin antiseptic solution should be swabbed on the patient's skin for at least two minutes, blotted off with a sterile towel, then swabbed again for another two minutes and dried with another sterile towel prior to application of sterile draping materials. CHG is also used as a mouth rinse in oral surgical procedures and impregnated in foam sponges for surgical personnel use for traditional surgical skin scrub processes.

Chlorhexidine is contraindicated for use on the head or face due to serious risk potential for corneal abrasions or chemical burns and possible ototoxicity resulting in sensory deafness if allowed to pool in the ear canal if there is a non-intact tympanic membrane. Additionally, CHG should not come in contact with meninges or the genital area. Caution should be taken if used on infants under the age of 2 months due to potential for chemical burns. Application of CHG on open wounds should be minimal and rinsed thoroughly if used for wound care.

As with other CHG preparations in solution, Chloraprep® should not be used around the head or face, perineal region, on meningeal tissues, or on neonates.

General Considerations for Surgical Skin Preparation

The benefit and effectiveness of the preoperative skin prep is determined by the level of skill and techniques used by the surgical team members responsible for performance of the procedure. Several factors must be considered by the circulating RN, surgical assistant, or other team members for patient safety and include:

- Appropriate selection of prep solution to prevent allergic or sensitivity reactions.
- Surgical skin preps are performed after final positioning has been achieved.
- Hospital-prepared prep trays may include plain gauze sponges, cotton balls, cotton-tipped applicators, towels, small metal bowls, and non-disposable sponge forceps for application of the skin prep scrub and paint agents.
- Prep solutions must be prevented from pooling under the patient, under the ESU patient return pad, or pneumatic tourniquets to prevent chemical or thermal burns.
- Prep solutions containing alcohol should be allowed time to evaporate prior to application of sterile draping materials to prevent potential ignition of trapped fumes during use of electrosurgical or laser energy.
- Preoperative skin markings should not be removed during the mechanical action of cleansing the skin.
- Excessive pressure should be avoided during prepping over areas of malignancy, abdominal aneurysms, carotid artery narrowing or obstruction from arterial plaque formation, or traumatic wounds with foreign body contamination.
- Assistance may be required from support devices or additional team members to elevate and perform circumferential (360°) preps of extremities.
- Draping materials such as under-buttocks drapes in lithotomy positioning; U-drapes placed prior to the skin prep to prevent soaking of the OR table beneath the patient, isolate non-operative extremities, or other contaminated anatomical areas such as the perineum; or to prevent pooling of prep solutions under pneumatic tourniquet placed on an extremity.
- Separate skin preps may be required for multiple anatomical areas such as planned donor and recipient sites.

Skin Prepping Involving Contaminated Areas. The general rule of preoperative prepping that includes clean and contaminated areas is that the contaminated areas are prepped either separately or last. The following includes various examples of contaminated areas within the surgical field and how they should be handled in general.

Umbilicus: The umbilicus is typically a depressed area in the center of the abdomen that may contain an accumulation of organic debris and lint and has a higher microbial count than the surrounding abdominal skin surfaces. It is at the anatomical midpoint of the abdomen so cannot be excluded or fully isolated during most laparotomy or laparoscopy procedures. Many surgeons will instead incise above (supraumbilically), below (infraumbically), or laterally around the umbilicus rather than through the center of it. Preoperative skin antisepsis for abdominal procedures begins with dripping the prep agent from the one-step applicator device into the umbilicus or dipping cotton-tipped applicators supplied with a traditional skin prep kit into the solution, then cleansing the umbilicus thoroughly to remove any detritus from its folds and depressions. Following that, the remainder of the abdominal prep is performed in the usual manner, starting at the incision site and working out in a circular motion toward the periphery, using a new sponge each time in the same sequence.

Stomas: Non-native openings, referred to in general as stomas, are contaminated areas and include colostomy, ileostomy, gastrostomy, or tracheostomy. Stomas located within the planned surgical area are either isolated from the remainder of the surgical area or prepped if included as part of the planned surgical procedure. Isolation can be achieved with placement of a sterile adhesive impervious drape adjacent to the stoma prior to the start of the skin prep. A stoma, included as part of the procedure, as in colostomy "take down" reanastomosis surgery, is prepped last as the final step in the skin prep process. A stoma incorporated into the operative area may have a prep sponge soaked with antiseptic agent initially placed over the stoma. A surgeon may choose to pack a stoma with a counted radiopaque povidone-iodine–soaked sponge. Following completion of the prep of the clean incisional area, the previously placed sponge is discarded into the kick bucket as a countable item, and the contaminated stomal opening is gently prepped last without returning to any previously prepped clean areas.

Natural Body Orifices: The mucosal membranes of natural body orifices include nasal, oral, vaginal, and anal mucosa. Surgeons will direct whether and with what agent body orifices will be prepped. Some may routinely leave orders to not prep the mouth or anus and only prep the adjacent areas. Many will request a vaginal prep; however, the vagina is considered contaminated in relation to the external genitalia and prepped after the suprapubic area, vulva, labia, and inner thighs. If sponges are used to swipe prep solution over the anus after use in the vagina, they must be discarded as the anus is more contaminated than the vagina.

Surgeons may inject epinephrine into the nasal mucosa or soak compressed cotton patties (cottonoids) soaked in liquid cocaine or other vasoconstrictive agents and insert into the nares before they scrub, gown, glove, and drape the patient. A small separate table should be used for that setup. A facial prep may or may not be performed prior to nasal procedures and is based on the surgeon's preferences. Extensive maxillofacial procedures may require use of an antiseptic periodontal agent swabbed over oral structures in addition to an outer facial prep, depending on where incisions will be located.

Procedures involving structures around the ear, as in mastoidectomy or cochlear implant surgery, may require the skin and scalp around the ear to be prepped routinely; however, a sterile cotton ball should be placed in the external ear canal to prevent pooling of prep solutions in the ear canal. Chlorhexidine is contraindicated for ear preps due to the potential for ototoxicity.

Combination Preps: Procedures requiring both abdominal and vaginal or perineal preps require two separate prep kits or sets of sponges and prep agents. If only one individual is available to perform both the abdominal and vaginal preps, the vaginal or perineal prep is typically performed first, despite it being more contaminated than the abdomen. The reason for this is that if the cleaner abdominal area was prepped first and then the vaginal or perineal prep done to follow, there is a high likelihood of contamination of the prepped abdomen by disseminated aerosolized particles of prep solution used in the less clean vaginal vault or perineal/perianal area settling onto the abdomen. The vagina or perineal area may be covered with a sterile towel prior to starting the abdominal prep. When two individuals are available to perform simultaneous abdominal and vaginal or perineal preps, the potential for contamination of the cleaner abdominal prep is lessened; however, care must be taken to not prep the vagina or perineal area vigorously enough to spray droplets onto the clean abdominal prep areas.

Tissue Graft Sites: The guidelines governing combination preps involving clean and contaminated areas can be similarly applied to procedures requiring tissue grafting from one anatomical site to another area. Tissue grafts taken from one area of the patient's body and transferred to another are called autografts. Homografts are tissues taken from another human and xenografts are tissues taken from another non-human species such as heart valves or skin from pigs. Use of these types of grafts would not require additional prepped areas. Autografting of split-thickness or full-thickness skin, muscle, tendon, vessel, or bone from an intact, non-injured area to a non-intact, burned, or denuded area requires two separate skin preps. The donor (non-injured) area is cleaner than the less clean traumatized site; therefore, the donor site is prepped first, and the recipient site is prepped last. Non-tinted prep agents are preferred to allow for assessment of vascular flow of pedicle flaps following tissue grafting and repositioning.

Grossly Contaminated and Traumatic Wounds: Draining infected sinus tracts or skin ulcers are grossly contaminated areas and must be prepped last, gently, and with separate sponges that do not touch clean areas adjacent to the contaminated areas.

Traumatic wounds may be gently irrigated with saline and a bulb syringe to try to remove embedded foreign debris. Care must be taken to not drive foreign materials or macerated tissues deeper into wounds by use of forceful irrigation or mechanical pressure exerted with prep sponges. Copious amounts of irrigation of a traumatic wound require placement of a basin under or adjacent to the wound to prevent soaking the OR table linens under the patient. An impervious-backed absorbent pad or drape may be used to isolate non-involved areas and contain irrigation fluids. The surgeon may request scissors and tissue forceps from the sterile setup to excise devitalized and nonviable tissue that would become necrotic postoperatively if left in place. Alcohol, CHG, and iodine prep agents can cause tissue irritation and should not be used in open traumatic, denuded (stripped of covering), or burn wounds unless directed by the surgeon.

Skin Preparation for Specific Anatomical Areas

The previous sections have discussed general preoperative routines of and steps for urethral catheterization; indications for and methods of hair removal; characteristics of various skin prep agents, including uses and contraindications; and special considerations for contaminated areas within the planned surgical area. In this section, steps for performing preoperative surgical skin preparation of specific anatomical areas will be discussed.

Torso: Abdomen, Chest, and Breasts. The anterior or ventral surface of the patient's torso is preoperatively prepped for surgical procedures involving anatomical sites from the face and anterior neck down to the chest or breasts, abdomen, and pelvis. The supine position is also used for procedures performed on the anterior surface of the lower extremities. The areas of the chest, breasts, abdomen, and pelvis are relatively flat when the patient is positioned in the supine position, although the lateral aspects of the patient down toward table level may be included as part of the prepped area. A typical preoperative abdominal skin prep with a two-step prep agent such as Betadine follows the following general steps:

1. Expose the areas to be prepped, to include a broad perimeter area, based on the scheduled surgical procedural approach.

2. Open the disposable sterile skin prep kit or sterile nondisposable prep tray on a small prep table.

3. Plastic forceps may be included in commercially prepared prep kits that allow for organization of the kit components (sterile gloves, paper towels, compartmentalized trays, cotton-tipped applicators, foam sponge pads and sponge sticks, and prep agent bottles). The wrapped kits prepared in the hospital sterile processing departments will typically have plain gauze sponges, cotton-tipped applicators, woven cloth towels, non-disposable basins, ring forceps, and dressing forceps.

4. Dispense the prep agents (iodophor scrub and iodine paint or chlorhexidine solution) into the appropriate basins or trays.

5. Don sterile gloves using the open-gloving technique.

6. With a protective cuff over sterile gloves, place and gently tuck in paper or cloth towels alongside the patient's lateral sides to catch runoff and prevent pooling of prep solutions under the patient.

7. Prior to starting the prep, dip cotton-tipped applicators into the scrub agent and clean the umbilicus to remove and dirt, lint, or other detritus and set aside on prep table.

8. Wet the foam sponges in the scrub solution which may have been mixed with warm sterile water and squeeze to produce a lather. Many sponges have slits to provide "handles" to prevent touching the patient's skin during application. Plain gauze sponges wet with scrub solution are used with one gloved hand to scrub the skin.

9. Start at the center of the prep area (umbilicus for most laparotomy procedures) using mechanical friction to scrub the skin in a circular configuration and widen the circle out toward the peripheral areas, laterally to table level where the towels were placed; superiorly to nipple level; and inferiorly to upper thighs. Each sponge is discarded if it touches the patient's gown, blankets, or towels placed to define the prep borders, and not brought back toward the center.

10. Continue in the same manner, starting every time at the center and working outward for 2 to 5 minutes or until all plain foam or gauze sponges have been used and discarded.

11. Absorbent paper or cloth towels are used to blot the scrub soap from the patient's skin then carefully removed by lifting up without dragging edges across prepped areas and discarded.

12. Foam sponges on sticks or plain gauze sponges mounted on ring forceps are wet with the iodine paint solution and applied to the skin, starting at the center, and working outward in the same manner as the scrub solution (Figure 8-11). Mechanical friction is not necessary as the paint provides the chemical film for prevention of microbial rebound growth during the procedure. Iodine paint and tinted chlorhexidine create the visible demarcation of the expanded prepped areas.

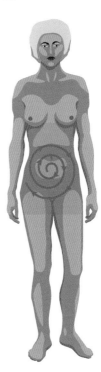

Figure 8-11 · Abdominal skin prep starting at incisional site and extending toward periphery.

13. Following the application of the paint solution, the towels placed at the beginning to catch prep solution runoff at the lateral sides, as well as those placed at the superior and inferior borders if used, are carefully removed without touching and contaminating the prepped areas.

14. All prep supplies are discarded or removed from the area, soiled gloves are removed, and hand hygiene is performed prior to proceeding with subsequent tasks.

15. Importantly, prep solutions containing alcohol must be given time to evaporate and dissipate prior to placement of sterile drapes, to prevent possibility of ignition of pooled agents or fumes trapped under drapes when electrosurgery or laser energies are used.

Procedures involving the chest or breasts require the prep borders to shift upward on the patient's anterior surface and may be modified to include the axillary area and upper extremity of one or both sides of a bilateral procedure. The superior border is typically the mandible, includes the shoulders, and the inferior border is the level of the iliac crest or suprapubic area. Unilateral procedures that include the axillary area on the operative side extend medially and to the anterior axillary line on the contralateral side, however, do not include the contralateral axilla or arm. Breast or chest procedures that involve the axillary area require elevation of the operative side arm by an assistant for access during the prep procedure and until sterile drapes are applied (Figure 8-12).

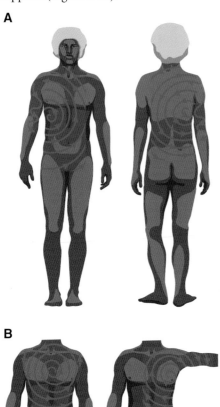

Figure 8-12 ▪ **(A)** Upper anterior or combined lateral position chest prep. **(B)** anterior chest or bilateral breast or unilateral breast and axillary preoperative skin prep.

Chest procedures with midline incisions may not include the axillary areas. The routine preoperative skin prep for open heart procedures such as coronary artery bypass with grafting (CABG) spans from the mandible superiorly, laterally bilaterally as far as possible to table level and inferiorly downward to the toes of both lower extremities which are prepped circumferentially. The genital area and the feet may be isolated with towel drapes prior to the prep. An assistant wearing sterile gloves or table attachment for temporary leg elevation is required to lift and abduct the lower extremities for the circumferential application of the prep agent to all surfaces.

Posterior Torso Prep. Similar to the steps for an abdominal prep, procedures performed on the dorsal or posterior surface of the torso require preoperative skin preparation that liberally extends beyond the planned surgical incision site. Antiseptic skin preps for midline procedures such as spinal procedures extend superiorly to the neck and shoulders, inferiorly to the upper buttocks, and laterally to the sides of the patient with care being taken to prevent runoff solutions pooling under the patient or onto the OR table beneath the spinal positioning frame or device on which the patient might be placed.

Rectal procedures performed in the Kraske or jackknife position may require measures to separate the buttocks prior to initiation of the prep. This may include application of adhesive tape to the medial buttocks bilaterally and pulling the tape laterally and attaching to the side of the OR table. This keeps the perianal area open and visible for the prep as well as for the surgical procedure to be performed. A towel may be placed between the legs under the perineum to catch any runoff solutions from pooling in the genital areas. The adjacent buttocks and perineum inferiorly are prepped first and as the sponge is crossed over the anus, it is discarded, and a new sponge is used to prep the surrounding areas first and anus last.

Head, Neck, and Face Prep. Surgical skin preps for head procedures may require special handling of the hair as discussed previously. The scalp prep is performed using the surgeon's choice of prep agent; however, hair saturated with alcohol prep solutions may require up to an hour for fumes to dissipate. Aqueous solutions may be preferred, and hair blotted dry with sterile towels prior to draping. Long hair may be braided or combed with a water-based lubricant to contain it out of the way of the planned incisional line.

Care must be taken to prevent pooling of any prep solutions in the ear canals or in the eyes. Chlorhexidine is contraindicated for use in the eyes due to the potential for chemical corneal damage or in ears due to the potential for sensory deafness if the tympanic membrane is not intact and solutions reach the middle or inner ear. A dry cotton ball may be placed in the ear to catch any potential prep solution and adhesive eye shields, or impervious towel drapes may be used to isolate the eyes during a scalp or upper face prep.

Hair removal for eye procedures, as previously discussed, is performed only if deemed essential by the surgeon. Antiseptic cleansing of the eyelids, eyelashes, and periorbital areas must be done with a non-irritating cleanser such as 10%

povidone-iodine. The eye may be cleansed with povidone-iodine diluted with balanced salt solution (BSS) to a 5% concentration. Baby shampoo or body wash may be mixed with BSS as a facial prep around the eye for patients allergic to iodine. Soft gauze sponges are used with the prepping agent and applied starting at the inner canthus of the eye and swabbed across the upper and lower lids in a crescent-shaped arc. Extend the prep outward to include the forehead, cheek, and side of the nose of the operative side. The conjunctiva of the eye should be flushed gently with sterile water in a small bulb syringe and runoff contained by sterile gauze sponges or towels.

The nares may not be prepped at all or may have a small amount of prep solution on a cotton-tipped applicator gently swabbed over the nasal mucosa. Alcohol is contraindicated for use on mucosal tissues. Mustache or other facial hair is removed by electric clippers only if ordered by the surgeon. Used clipper heads are disposed of in the sharps container.

Skin preps of the anterior neck include the area from mandible superiorly, laterally to table level or where towels are placed to catch runoff, and over the shoulders, and inferiorly to clavicles or mid-sternum. Care is taken to not exert excessive mechanical pressure over the carotid arteries of the neck in elderly patients undergoing carotid endarterectomy. Unilateral neck procedures may require neck rotation; however, care must be taken to not hyper-rotate the head and neck which could diminish cerebral blood flow on that side or cause nerve impingement (Figure 8-13).

Shoulder Prep. Patients undergoing shoulder surgery may be placed in a sitting or semi-sitting position often called beach chair position with the operative side of the patient at the edge of the OR table and the arm left loose in order to manipulate it during the procedure. No tourniquet is placed, and the prepped areas include the operative side shoulder and axilla, laterally to mid-chest, superiorly to the mandible, posteriorly to the scapula, and inferiorly to the elbow or fingers, depending on surgeon's preference. An assistant may or may not be used to elevate the arm during the prep and until placement of sterile drapes (Figure 8-14).

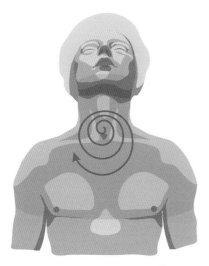

Figure 8-13 · Preoperative skin preparation of anterior neck or upper chest.

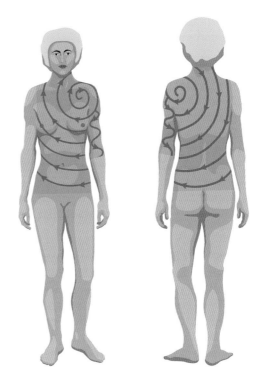

Figure 8-14 · Unilateral shoulder preoperative skin prep extending anteriorly and posteriorly as far as possible.

Extremity Preps. The operative side upper extremity is frequently positioned out to the side on an operative hand table or double arm boards. If the procedure is performed with use of a pneumatic tourniquet, the tourniquet is placed prior to the prep and an absorbent towel or impervious U-drape may be placed around the arm just below the tourniquet before the prep to prevent pooling of solutions under the tourniquet which could cause chemical burns. An absorbent drape or towels may be placed on the hand table or arm boards to catch the dripping solutions during the prep. A sterile, soap-impregnated, soft-bristled scrub brush and water may be used to clean the subungual (under the nails) space if gross soil is present. The prep may begin at the fingers and hand, even when not the planned incision site, in order for the arm to be elevated by the individual performing the prep or by an assistant with sterile gloves and grasping the hands and fingers to keep the arm elevated off the table so that the prep can be applied circumferentially around the entire arm up to the level of the tourniquet. Once the hand is elevated, the prep sponges are applied at the planned incision site and around up toward the tourniquet and down to the fingers.

Lower extremities also may or may not have a tourniquet placed prior to the skin prep. An impervious U-drape may be used to isolate the non-operative leg and prevent pooling of prep solutions under it or the pneumatic tourniquet. For foot procedures, this may be placed at mid-calf, and for knee or ankle procedures, the tourniquet is placed on the upper thigh. The leg must be elevated off the OR table in order for the prep to be applied to all surfaces in a circumferential manner (Figure 8-15). Unless a small child, it is advisable to have an assistant elevate the patient's leg. As with the fingernails, if

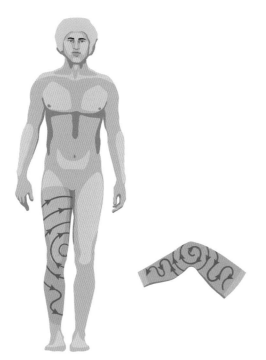

Figure 8-15 · Preoperative circumferential skin prep for knee or mid-leg procedure.

the procedure involves the toes, a soft bristle scrub brush may be used to clean under the toenails to remove any gross dirt or debris. Prep solution may be first placed over the toes so the positioning assistant can lift the foot, then the heel, sole, and ankle are prepped so the assistant can grasp the back of the foot to keep elevated during the remainder of the prep. The prep then begins at the planned incision site and extends in one direction, completely covering every surface around the leg to the toes. Starting again at the incision site with a new sponge, it proceeds upward to the level of the tourniquet covering all surfaces. This process is followed until the sponges are used up. The lower extremity is kept elevated by the prepping assistant until the surgical team members apply a sterile stockinette over the foot to begin the sterile draping process.

If a one-step paint applicator is used, initially paint the area to be grasped then start at the incision site and outward and around to cover the entire extremity. Keep the extremity elevated until sterile surgical drapes are applied by the scrubbed team members. If no tourniquet is used, the prep may include the axillary or groin area on that side. Minimally, extremities should be prepped to one joint above the planned surgical site and one joint below; however, more commonly for ease of draping, the entire extremity is prepped.

Lateral Position Preps. Procedures such as lateral thoracotomy, nephrectomy, or anterior spinal fusion require access to the dorsal (posterior) and ventral (anterior) surfaces of one side of the body in the same procedure. The preoperative skin prep must cover an area adequate for surgical access and any additional placement of drains or trocar port sites. Care must be taken to prevent pooling of prep solutions under stabilization devices such as bean bags, axillary rolls, peg boards, or various

other table attachments or protective patient padding placed during positioning. Paint applicators with antiseptic gels may be preferred for safety in these circumstances.

Total hip arthroplasty procedures performed in the posterolateral position also require prepping of the hip area, anteriorly to the mid-abdomen, posteriorly as far as possible, and inferiorly to the foot, covering the entire lower extremity circumferentially to allow for manipulation during disarticulation of the femoral head. Placement of an impervious U-drape under the operative leg to isolate the perineal region and to prevent soaking of the non-operative leg is commonly done after positioning and before the commencement of the skin prep (Figure 8-16).

Vaginal and Perineal Preps. Procedures performed in the lithotomy position may involve the vagina, urethral meatus, perineum, or anus. An impervious drape laminated with an absorbent layer is commonly placed under the patient's hips prior to the preoperative prep to catch runoff solutions and prevent soaking of the OR table linens and pooling under the patient. This drape is removed at the end of the prep and a separate sterile under-buttocks drape placed as part of the draping process.

The prep for vaginal procedures begins with the surrounding areas of the cleaner pubis, inner thighs, vulva, labia, and perineum then over the contaminated anus. The pubis is scrubbed first, transversely to the iliac crests bilaterally. The vulva and labia are prepped next then downward over the perineum. As each sponge is used from cleaner areas and finishing with the anus, it is discarded. A new sponge is used starting at the labia and vulva, moving laterally outward over the inner thigh on one side then discarded. The same is done for

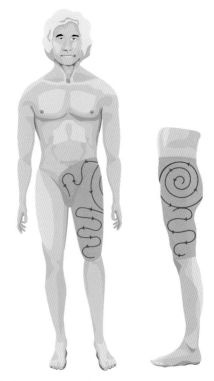

Figure 8-16 · Preoperative skin prep for posterior hip procedure in the lateral position.

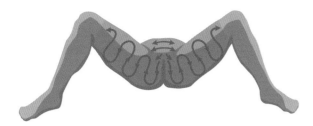

Figure 8-17 · Vaginal/perineal area skin prep.

the contralateral labia, vulva, and thigh. The vagina, considered a contaminated area, is prepped last. Foam sponges on sticks or plain gauze sponges mounted on ring forceps are dipped in the prep agent and used to cleanse the cervix and vaginal vault liberally due to the many folds of the mucosal tissues. This should be done several times and a dry sponge used as the final step to absorb excess prep solution to prevent mucosal irritation or vascular absorption of the prep agent (Figure 8-17).

Policies for vaginal preps differ by facility. In some cases, a sponge stick with antiseptic agent is inserted into the vagina initially before the cleaner outer anatomical areas are prepped. The vaginal sponge stick is removed following prep of the outer structures and additional sponges used to complete the vaginal prep. Steps for placement of the Foley catheter also vary. In some cases, a vaginal sponge stick is inserted first, to assist in preventing inadvertent insertion of the catheter into the vagina. The Foley may be placed prior to or following the vaginal prep, depending on the potential for contamination of the catheter during the vaginal prep process.

Perianal preps cleanse the tissues surrounding the anus first, and as each sponge passes over the anus, it is discarded, and a new sponge used on surrounding areas before the anus. The anus is not penetrated with prep sponges or sticks.

Preps of the penis, scrotal area, and perineum follow similar steps to a vaginal prep and may require the legs to be flexed in the frog-legged position. The pubis is scrubbed first, extending outward to the inguinal creases bilaterally then downward over one inner thigh. A new sponge is used to repeat the steps and downward over the contralateral inner thigh area. The penis is prepped next, retracting the foreskin if present and repositioned over the glans following the prep to prevent vascular constriction. The scrotum is prepped with a new sponge and downward over the perineum and the anus is last. The sponge is discarded.

Documentation. The circulating nurse documents the details pertaining to the preoperative antiseptic skin preparation including:

- Any patient allergies to prep agents
- Method of hair removal if performed
- Condition of the skin before and after the prep procedure
- The antiseptic prep agents, solvents, irrigants, or degreasers used
- Anatomical areas prepped
- Postoperative condition of the areas prepped
- Name of the individual or individuals who performed the prep

SURGICAL DRAPING

Surgical draping is the final step in the preoperative preparation of the patient. The placement of sterile draping materials is a way to create a barrier between unsterile items and surfaces and establish a sterile field in which the sterilely attired team members function during the surgical procedure. These drapes should have characteristics that establish their use as effective barriers.

- Sterile with no toxic dyes or laundry residues
- Lint-free to reduce potential transfer into the wound resulting in potential granuloma formation
- Porous and breathable to vent heat buildup and maintain normothermia of the patient
- Fluid and puncture resistant unless used as an impervious plastic cover over inanimate furniture or equipment or absorbable layers around wound edges
- Fire retardant and antistatic, meeting National Fire Protection Agency standards
- Drapable around patient, furniture, or equipment within the sterile field
- Packaged and folded to maintain sterility and barrier effectiveness when applied

Types of Surgical Drapes

Draping materials are comprised of the following general types:

- Woven, also referred to as cloth, linen, non-disposable, reusable, or muslin
- Non-woven, as referred to as compressed fiber, cellulose, paper, or disposable
- Synthetic materials including:
  - Plastic impervious furniture covers
  - Adhesive incise drapes applied directly to prepped incisional sites
  - Specialized equipment drapes for robots, microscopes, drills, endoscopes, and imaging transducers
  - Polypropylene laser–resistant drapes
  - Plastic fluid collection or instrument pouches
  - Thermal, aluminum-coated rolls or covers

There are advantages and disadvantages of both woven and non-woven draping materials. Surgical facilities must weigh the cost–benefit ratio when deciding which types of materials to use in the surgical department. Woven reusable drapes may be less expensive than non-woven disposable drapes; however, costs associated with the commercial laundering, monitoring for barrier integrity, proper folding, sterile packaging materials, and sterilization processes, plus eventual repair or replacement costs may make their use less cost-effective.

Non-woven disposable drapes are supplied in a wide variety of styles and are reliably prepared and sterilely packaged in sealed impervious plastic packages. They do create a substantial amount of material medical waste that contributes to landfill volume or air pollution from incineration processes.

Both types of drapes are frequently used in combination to provide the best qualities of both types within the same procedure's sterile field. An important point to remember is that all drapes are flammable and even flame-retardant drapes and synthetic plastic drapes may melt when exposed to high heat sources such as laser beams, fiberoptic light cables, electrosurgical energy, or open flames. All draping materials are at risk of puncture from sharp objects such as scalpel blades, suture and hypodermic needles, K-wires or Steinman pins, and perforating surgical instruments. They may be impervious to fluid penetration, referred to as strike-through, but not impenetrable to mechanical penetration.

Drape Configurations. Draping materials are available in a variety of styles and configurations. The two major categories of sterile drapes are non-fenestrated and fenestrated. Fenestrated drapes have a specific opening area in the drape which is placed over and exposes only the surgical or incisional area and covers the remainder of the patient to allow for placement of sterilely draped Mayo stands over the patient and creates the center of the sterile field. The opening (fenestration) in a fenestrated drape is bordered on all sides by draping material. Aperture drapes are a type of fenestrated drape used over smaller, specific anatomical areas, typically the eyes and ears.

Most fenestrated drapes are named for the anatomical area they cover or the surgical procedure to be performed. Some drapes may be used for other procedures than what the name indicates if the size and shape of the fenestration match the planned incisional size and location. An example is using a laparotomy drape which has a midline, vertical fenestration for a midline abdominal procedure or for a lumbar laminectomy in which the patient is in the prone position. The areas of exposure on the dorsal and ventral surfaces of the body are similar enough to make the drape useful for both.

Other fenestrated drapes have a unique-shaped fenestration and location within the drape, making use in other anatomical locations inappropriate. Fenestrated drapes may also have special features incorporated into the design including arm board extensions, additional absorptive layers bordering the fenestration edges, adhesive incise sheets matching the fenestration size, anti-skid mats, fluid collection or instrument pouches, and straps or tabs for securing tubing or cords on the field without use of instruments. Fenestrated drapes used on upper or lower extremities may have a stretchy impervious material that conforms around the limb to isolate non-operative, unsterile areas and prevent seepage of fluids under the fenestration edges.

Drape manufacturers may vary in the names used for their fenestrated drapes; however, the names are usually self-explanatory. In addition to the name, most will include an image of the drape on the content sheet, including the special features of the drape and specific dimensions for size of the fenestrated opening as well as the overall measurements of the drape. Most drapes have application directions, arrows, or prompts to assist in proper orientation and unfolding to maintain sterility. Examples of fenestrated drape sheet names include, but are not limited to:

- Laparotomy drape/sheet
- Adolescent laparotomy drape/sheet
- Pediatric laparotomy drape/sheet
- Transverse laparotomy drape/sheet
- Pfannensteil drape/sheet
- Laparoscopy drape/sheet
- Laparoscopic Cholecystectomy drape/sheet
- Kidney drape/sheet
- C-section drape/sheet
- Breast/Chest drape/sheet
- Thyroid drape/sheet
- Craniotomy drape/sheet
- Peri/GYN drape/sheet (with or without attached leggings)
- Cystoscopy drape/sheet
- Upper Extremity drape/sheet
- Hip drape/sheet
- Lower extremity drape/sheet
- Bilateral limb drape/sheet
- Knee arthroscopy drape/sheet

Non-fenestrated drapes do not have a specific-size or -shaped opening in the drape sheet and include:

- Flat sheets and table covers are fan-folded drapes without any openings in the drape used to cover large flat furniture or as additional coverage in combination with other specialty drapes.

- Towel drapes of either woven materials for absorbable purposes or non-woven materials for creating the definition of borders or isolation of contaminated areas. Plastic isolation drapes may have an adhesive edge to maintain placement on the patient's skin or on other draping materials.

- Plastic adhesive incise drapes are used to seal the resident microbial population present in the skin layers in place and prevent them from being transferred into the open wound from adjacent areas. As the name indicates, the skin incision is made through both the adhesive drape and the patient's skin simultaneously. The incise drapes are commonly impregnated with iodine as a barrier to microbial rebound growth during the duration of the procedure. Large, flat incise drapes commonly referred to as "shower curtain" drapes are suspended from a transverse rod attached to two rolling stands. The clear drape has an adhesive area that is applied to the area of the hip or upper portion of the lower extremity for hip or femoral fracture fixation procedures when the patient is positioned on a fracture table. The large vertical drape provides a barrier mechanism in which the C-arm can be rotated for imaging during fracture reduction and placement of hardware without contaminating the operative field.

- Split sheets are large drapes with an adhesive-edged split end that allows placement around anatomical structures such as the face or upper extremity while still covering the remainder of the body.

- Impervious plastic U-drapes have adhesive strips along the edges of the U-shaped split and are used to wrap around operative extremities to isolate non-operative areas or surfaces to prevent strike-through fluid penetration. U-drapes are also commonly used to isolate pneumatic tourniquets placed on upper or lower extremities and prevent prep solutions from seeping under the tourniquet, causing chemical irritation of the skin beneath.

- Stockinettes are tubular drapes of woven material or a combination of woven laminated with plastic impervious outer layer to cover upper and lower extremities.

- Leggings are split tubular drapes used to cover lower extremities placed in stirrups for lithotomy positioning.

- Mayo stand covers are tubular drapes similar to large pillowcases that create sterile coverage of the stand placed over the sterilely draped patient even on the underside of the drape, creating circumferential sterile barrier protection.

- Under-buttocks drapes are cuffed flat sheets which are often impervious and may have a soft, absorptive layer laminated over the plastic. These drapes are placed under the hips and buttocks of patients in lithotomy position to prevent fluid accumulation under the patient and cuffed at one end to protect the sterile gloves of the team member placing it.

- Plastic impervious drapes used to line powered irrigation fluid warmer units are usually large and flat to accommodate various sizes and shapes of warming devices. Care must be taken with sharp instruments to guard against mechanical perforation of the drape which is only impervious to fluid penetration, not punctures.

- Cassette covers are clear bags large enough to accommodate placement of a large x-ray film cassette to be used within the sterile field.

- C-arm covers are available in single or double arms to cover one or both sides of the fluoroscopic imaging machine brought into or adjacent to the sterile field. The attached straps provided are used to prevent sagging of the excess drape material.

- Plastic impervious fluid collection pouches may be built into fenestrated drape sheets or as separate pouches with adhesive edges to allow placement on the patient's skin or onto other draping materials. Fluid pouches may have a suction port for attachment of suction tubing to remove accumulated fluid and prevent excessive weight of the pooled fluid from pulling the drape down or the supplemental pouch falling off the drape and spilling contents.

- Microscope drapes are large, complicated drapes that are specific to certain microscopes and not interchangeable due to the importance of the objective lens cover fitting correctly. Drapes are typically configured to include three sets of ocular lens eyepieces with removable tabs to expose the ocular lenses without contamination of the gloves. As with C-arm covers, attached straps and adhesive tabs provide a way to keep excess drape material or unused ocular lens openings from sagging or obscuring the operative field.

Draping Techniques

After final positioning and prior to draping, the circulating nurse must apply the patient return electrode (grounding pad) of the electrosurgical unit (ESU) or Bovie. Placement prior to positioning may cause derangement or shifting of the pad and potential for patient burns. Lack of placement prior to draping may require maneuvering underneath drapes and potential for contamination of prepped and draped areas of the sterile field. In addition, a final check by the surgical assistant or circulating nurse should be made to ensure all lines, catheters, and positioning devices and equipment are secure before being covered with sterile drapes.

There are general common principles and techniques for draping that can be applied to various anatomical areas.

- Draping materials should be kept at or above table level when manipulating or applying over the patient, furniture, or equipment.

- Keep distance between the front of sterile gowns and unsterile areas such as the patient's blankets, OR table, or other surfaces.

- Do not unfold fan-folded or fenestrated drapes until ready for application.

- Most large fenestrated drape sheets should be applied by two persons in unison to maintain sterility and not drop edges of the drape below table level until fully applied. Edges of drapes that fall below table level cannot be subsequently elevated without contamination of the surface of the drape and the gloves of the person applying it.

- Cuff ends of drapes over sterile gloves for protection when extending drape ends or handing to other unsterile team members such as the anesthesia provider for securing the upper end to IV poles or anesthesia screen; covering the C-arm or microscope with sterile drapes; raising up the vertical "shower curtain" drape for securing to the curtain rod. Unsterile team members may assist sterile team members by reaching inside or under sterile drapes to help support or cover hard-to-reach areas.

- Drapes must not be repositioned once placed on the patient.

- Mechanical perforation of sterile drapes violates the integrity of the barrier and must be covered with a sterile drape.

- Any exposed areas within the sterile field should be covered by additional drapes to maintain the integrity of the sterile field.

- Fluid penetration of non-impervious drapes placed on furniture or equipment results in strike-through contamination by transferring microbes from the surface area below the drape through the non-impervious material by wicking action.

- Unsterile team members should maintain a minimum of 12 in from sterilely draped areas or equipment when passing.

- Accessory equipment such as C-arms and microscopes should be kept within the sterile field and not left unattended and unobserved at the periphery without risk of contamination.

- Many surgeons require removal and replacement of outer gloves following the draping process and prior to initial incision.

- Use of lasers may present additional risk of potential ignition of drapes. Woven towels may be soaked in water or saline, any excess squeezed out, and the wet towels placed over the fenestrated drape around the edges of the incisional area as a precaution if any sparks or embers land around the incisional area.

As previously discussed, disposable fenestrated drape sheets provide directional markings to facilitate proper placement. Due to the large variety of draping materials available and the broad range of possible individual surgeon preferences, the following section outlines general steps for application of sterile drapes over specific anatomical areas.

Squaring Off the Incisional Site. The first step of draping for many procedures involves placement of towels around the incisional area after the skin prep which narrow and define more specifically the operative site. These towels referred to as wound towels, usually made of absorbent woven materials, square off the area and may be held in place with perforating or non-perforating (preferred) towel clips at the corner junctions. If no clips are used, a plastic adhesive incise drape may be applied over the wound towels and skin to hold the towels securely in place. The towels are often turned under at the edge closest to the incision site to add a double layer.

Laparotomy Draping. The process of draping for a laparotomy also applies to draping for procedures of the back or spine as the surface areas and incisional locations are very similar only on opposite sides of the body. Following the skin preparation and appropriate drying or evaporation of any alcohol used, the surgeon or surgical assistant will often square off the incisional area. Some prefer to use a plain sheet below the incisional area and covering the lower part of the body and another plain sheet starting at the superior border of the incisional area, covering the upper part of the body. This may be preferred when woven drape sheets are used to provide an additional layer. The fenestrated drape is placed directly over the planned incisional area in the proper orientation indicated on the drape. One sterile team member on each side of the patient unfolds the drape laterally keeping it at or above table level and without contaminating their gowns on the unsterile blankets or arm boards. With gloved hands cuffed under the inferior edge of the drape, they simultaneously unfold the drape to cover the lower part of the patient and let it fall over the feet. Switching hands, they unfold the drape upward and cover the upper half, taking care to not release the drape until the anesthesia provider attaches the superior edge to both IV poles, or covers the anesthesia screen if used instead. Grasping the edge of the lateral side of the drape folded inward, they orient the arm board cover flap to ensure it covers the arms completely before finally releasing the drape. Any paper covering the fenestration is removed and handed off the field.

Draping for a spinal procedure may include placement of an impervious adhesive incise drape as the first step or applied over wound towels to hold them in place after squaring off. Alternately, a plastic towel drape may be placed at the level of the gluteal cleft to isolate the area prior to application of the fenestrated drape sheet. Instrument pouches may be applied to the fenestrated drape sheet to hold suction, bipolar forceps, and ESU pencils. These should not be placed in areas that might interfere with intraoperative fluoroscopic imaging of the spine.

Lithotomy Draping. Draping for the lithotomy position often requires the use of an under-buttocks drape to provide an impervious barrier between the patient's buttocks and perineal area and the sheets covering the OR table under the patient. The under-buttocks drape may have an absorptive layer laminated onto the outer impervious plastic layer to prevent sticking to or heating of the patient's skin and allow for easier sliding under the patient during placement. The drape is cuffed to protect the sterile gloves of the team member applying the drape sheet. The end of the drape is unfolded down toward the floor and may be placed into a kick bucket to collect any fluid dripping from the surgical area during the procedure. If the procedure does not involve the anal area, an adhesive towel drape, woven wound towel, or plastic fluid pouch may be placed to isolate the more contaminated anal area during the vaginal or perineal surgery. Leggings are applied over the extremities whether in low, moderate, or high lithotomy position in half-boot, knee brace, or candy-cane type stirrups. Some Peri/GYN drapes consist of a one-piece fenestrated drape sheet with attached leggings. Directions and prompts are included to facilitate placement of the complicated drape and maintain sterility during the process. It is often more efficient for two persons to apply the drape. This is frequently the surgical assistant and surgical technologist and working together but may be the surgical assistant and surgeon.

Extremity Draping. Surgery on extremities often includes use of a pneumatic tourniquet to achieve a bloodless field during the procedure. An impervious table cover may be placed under the operative extremity and over the non-operative leg or over the hand table to prevent dripping and pooling on the table, bed, or other extremity. A U-drape may be placed around the extremity just distal to the tourniquet to isolate unsterile, non-operative areas and to prevent prep solutions from seeping under the tourniquet. A sterile woven or impervious stockinette is usually placed over the extremity and then the foot or hand is inserted into and through the fenestrated portion of the drape which is unfolded to cover the entire patient.

Gravity helps drain blood from the extremity, so arms or legs are typically kept elevated during the preoperative skin prep and sterile draping process. Additional removal of blood from the extremity is achieved by tightly wrapping an elastic Esmarch bandage around the extremity from fingers or toes up to the level of the tourniquet in a process called exsanguination. This squeezes and compresses the elevated extremity from the most distal point down to the tourniquet, which is then inflated to prevent backflow of blood into the extremity (Figure 8-18). The Esmarch bandage is removed, and the extremity is placed on the sterilely draped arm board or OR table.

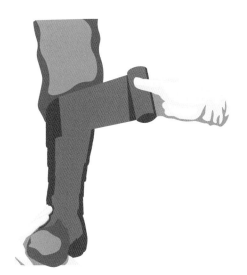

Figure 8-18 · Wrapping of an extremity with Esmarch bandage for exsanguination.

The surgeon and surgical assistant are responsible for this procedure. Exsanguination is not necessary in a procedure in which a pneumatic tourniquet is not used and not in all cases when it is used. The surgeon must determine the best course based on the patient's health status and the condition of the extremity on which surgery is to be performed.

Once exsanguinated, the stockinette may be cut with bandage or straight Mayo scissors to expose the incisional area of the extremity. Impervious stockinettes may be placed and the edge sealed in place with sterile roller tape such as Coban to isolate non-operative areas such as the hand or foot. Alternately, many orthopedic surgeons performing total joint replacement procedures prefer to use extra-large plastic adhesive incise drapes wrapped circumferentially around the extremity. These processes are typically performed by the surgical assistant with or without the surgeon.

Cranial Procedure Draping. In some cases, overhead instrument tables or Mayo stands may be placed over the patient prior to the skin prep and drapes applied over the patient and tables together. The OR table may be turned 180°, with the patient's feet toward anesthesia or 90° with one side toward anesthesia, depending on surgeon's preference, number of assistants, and types of equipment used within the sterile field including the microscope or C-arm. The surgeon may square off the incisional area using clips or skin staples to prevent shifting of the wound towels. Separate plain sheets may be applied laterally, covering any instrument tables or stands. A fenestrated cranial drape may have an adhesive incise area as the drape opening. The incise cover is removed prior to placement directly on the patient's head. Following the drape's arrows or directions, the drape is unfolded to cover the lower body first, then the flap is unfolded downward toward the floor. A fluid collection pouch may be attached to that portion of the drape to collect any fluid runoff from the wound. A final plain cloth drape may be placed over the instrument table per surgeon's preference if using spring-loaded scalp or dural hooks which might otherwise tear paper drapes. Instrument pouches may be applied to the

fenestrated drape on one or both sides of the head to hold suctions and bipolar forceps or ESU pencils. Some surgeons may choose to place an additional set of wound towels following use of the craniotome and before opening the dura to isolate any bone dust that might be pulled into the exposed brain.

Facial Draping. The surgeon may choose to wrap the patient's head and hair with sterile towels and plain sheets that also cover the head section of the OR table. Following the skin prep and allowing adequate time for evaporation of any alcohol in the prep solutions, the circulator or anesthesia provider may elevate the patient's head so the drapes can be placed over the table and under the head. The towel may be wrapped around the head first, and then the small plain drape sheet in similar fashion and secured with a clip. Alternately, only a towel is used to wrap the head and the other sheet remains under the head, covering the OR table (Figure 8-19). A large split sheet is applied with the inferior edge of the split at the patient's jawline and the drape unfolded by two team members, one on each side, down toward the feet, covering the entire body. The strips over the adhesive edges of the tails are removed and each side is placed around the face, leaving the appropriate areas of the face exposed. Alternately, instead of a split sheet, a large plain drape sheet may be used to cover the patient's body with the upper border of the drape covering the patient's shoulders.

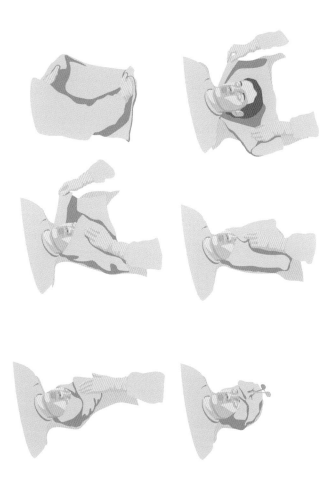

Figure 8-19 · Wrapping the head with a sterile towel or plain sheet to expose the operative area and isolate the OR table under the head.

SUMMARY

The preoperative patient care routines of positioning, skin preparation, and draping are critical steps to ensuring positive patient outcomes. The surgical assistant has a responsibility to understand and coordinate the performance of these procedures with the appropriate surgical team members to prevent SSIs or other injury to the patient. Any breaks in sterile techniques must be identified and corrective actions be taken to protect the patient.

Terminology Used in Surgical Positioning

Term	Definition
Abduct/abduction	To move away from the midline
Adduct/adduction	To move toward the midline
Anterior	Frontal surface of the body or anatomical area.
Beach chair position	Sitting with operative arm at edge of OR table, semi-Fowler
Caudal	Tail or lower part of the body
Cephalad	Head or upper part of the body
Cervical	Neck (spine or uterus)
Contralateral	Opposite side
Corpus, corpor/o	Body
Cubital	Elbow or forearm
Dorsal, dorsum	Back or posterior surface or anatomical area
Epi-	On, above, superficial layer
Extend/extension	Straighten at a joint, increase an angle to decrease a bend
Fascia, fasci/o	Tough membrane attached to and support for muscle tissue
Flex/flexion	Bend at a joint, reduce an angle to make less straight
Fowler position	Sitting position, semi-Fowler–reclined sitting position
Fracture table position	Modification of supine on orthopedic table for hip or femoral access
Hemi, semi, demi	Half
Hyper-	Above, excessive
Infra-	Below, beneath, lesser
Inter-	Between
Intra-	Within
Lateral/later/o	On the side, adjacent to, lateral recumbent (right or left), Sims
Lateral chest position	Lateral recumbent for access to thoracic cavity (right or left)
Lateral kidney position	Lateral recumbent for access to kidney or retroperitoneal space
Lithotomy	Legs raised and abducted, modification of supine
Medial/medi/o	Middle, toward the center
Posterior	Back surface of the body or anatomical area, dorsal
Pronate/pronation	Rotate the wrist so palm of hand faces backward
Prone	Position of lying face down
Recumbent	Resting on, lying down
Retro-	Behind, back, before
Reverse Trendelenburg	Head elevated, modification of supine
Rotation	To turn, medial rotation (turn inward), lateral rotation (turn outward)
Sims recumbent	Modified left lateral recumbent for lower GI endoscopy
Sub-	Under, below
Supinate/supination	Rotation of the wrist so palm of hand faces forward
Supine	Position of lying face up, also called dorsal recumbent
Trendelenburg position	Head down, modification of supine, shock position
Ventral/ventr/o	Front side, belly, abdominal

Bibliography

AST Guidelines for Best Practices for Patient Transportation, revised April 14, 2017; Guideline III. https://www.ast.org/webdocuments/ASTGuidelinesforPatientTransportation/#4. Accessed September 13, 2020.

Association of Surgical Technologists Standards of Practice for Skin Prep of the Surgical Patient. https://www.ast.org/uploadedFiles/Main_Site/Content/About_Us/Standard_Skin_Prep.pdf. Accessed September 27, 2020.

Bard Medical. A Guide for Nurses—Bard Comprehensive Care Management of Catheters and Collection Systems. http://media.bardmedical.com/media/1679/a-guide-for-nurses.pdf. Accessed September 26, 2020.

Centers for Disease Control and Prevention, Infection Control, Catheter-Associated Urinary. Tract Infection, Background, page reviewed May 11, 2015. https://www.cdc.gov/infectioncontrol/guidelines/cauti/background.html. Accessed September 26, 2020.

Charles D, Heal CF, Delpachitra M, et al. (2017). Alcoholic versus aqueous chlorhexidine for skin antisepsis: the AVALANCHE trial. *CMAJ*. 2017;189(31):E1008-E1016. https://doi.org/10.1503/cmaj.161460. Accessed October 3, 2020.

FDA, 3M Duraprep Surgical Solution. https://dailymed.nlm.nih.gov/dailymed/fda/fdaDrugXsl.cfm?setid=c951336f-9cb2-40cc-98f3-b5c4d9f5e27d&type=display. Accessed October 3, 2020.

Fortunato N. *Berry & Kohn's Operating Room Technique*. 9th ed. St. Louis, MO: Mosby, Inc.; 2000.

Gould CV, Umscheid CA, Agarwal RK, Kuntz G, Pegues DA; the Healthcare Infection Control Practices Advisory Committee (HICPAC). Guideline for Prevention of Catheter-Associated Urinary Tract Infections, 2009. https://www.cdc.gov/infectioncontrol/pdf/guidelines/cauti-guidelines-H.pdf. Accessed September 26, 2020.

Healio. *Durant's maneuver*. Cardiology Topic Reviews. https://www.healio.com/cardiology/learn-the-heart/cardiology-review/topic-reviews/durants-maneuver. Accessed December 8, 2021.

Healthgrades, Inc. Betasept Antiseptic Surgical Scrub. https://www.healthgrades.com/drugs/betasept. Accessed October 3, 2020.

Ideal Medical Solutions, What Are Urinary Catheters Make of? Blog, August 14, 2019. https://www.ideal-uroshield.com/blogs/what-are-urinary-catheters-made-of/. Accessed September 26, 2020.

Kaoutzanis C, Kavanagh CM, Leichtle SW, et al. Chlorhexidine with isopropyl alcohol versus iodine povacrylex with isopropyl alcohol and alcohol- versus nonalcohol-based skin preparations: the incidence of and readmissions for surgical site infections after colorectal operations. *Dis Colon Rectum*. 2015;58(6):588-596. https://doi.org/10.1097/DCR.0000000000000379. Accessed October 3, 2020.

Maki DG, Tambyah PA. Engineering out the risk for infection with urinary catheters. *Emerg Infect Dis*. 2001;7(2): 342-347.

National Institutes of Health (NIH). News Release, NIH Human Microbiome Project defines normal bacterial makeup of the body, 2012. https://www.nih.gov/news-events/news-releases/nih-human-microbiome-project-defines-normal-bacterial-makeup-body#:~:text=Methods%20and%20Results,vital%20role%20in%20human%20health. Accessed September 26, 2020.

Newman DK. Indwelling Catheter Types. *UroToday*, 2013. https://www.urotoday.com/urinary-catheters-home/indwelling-catheters/description/types.html. Accessed September 26, 2020.

Pei Diana M, Poison Control—National Capital Poison Center. Povidone-iodine Safe Use of a Common Antiseptic. https://www.poison.org/articles/povidone-iodine-safe-use-of-a-common-antiseptic-193. Accessed October 3, 2020.

Rank DS. Patient Positioning an OR Team Effort, *OR Nurse*. 2008;2(1)21-23. https://www.nursingcenter.com/journalarticle?Article_ID=762266&Journal_ID=682710&Issue_ID=762253. Accessed October 31, 2020.

Swenson BR, Hedrick TL, Metzger R, Bonatti H, Pruett TL, Sawyer RG. Effects of preoperative skin preparation on postoperative wound infection rates: A prospective study of 3 skin preparation protocols. *Infect Control Hosp Epidemiol*. 2009;30(10):964-971. https://doi.org/10.1086/605926. Accessed October 3, 2020.

Winnipeg Regional Health Authority. Surgical Skin Preparation. 2018. https://professionals.wrha.mb.ca/old/extranet/eipt/files/EIPT-005-001.pdf. Accessed October 4, 2020.

World Health Organization. Prevention of catheter-associated urinary tract infection (CAUTI): Student Handbook. May 2018 version, *Advanced Infection Prevention and Control Training* Handout 5. Supplementary information related to quiz 1, page 15. https://www.who.int/infection-prevention/tools/core-components/CAUTI_student-handbook.pdf. Accessed September 20, 2020.

9

Intraoperative Tissue Care and Handling

Douglas J. Hughes and Rebecca Hall

DISCUSSED IN THIS CHAPTER

1. Surgical incisions.
2. Halsted's principles of tissue handling.
3. Handling connective tissue.
4. Instrument handling.

Successful postoperative healing of the surgical wound hinges largely on how the wound and body tissues are handled by sterile team members during the operation. The type and location of incision utilized, methods of tissue dissection employed, achievement of adequate hemostasis, and proper closure of the surgical wound are each a key element that must be addressed.

SURGICAL INCISIONS

Described as the intentional cutting of intact body tissue, the incision is an integral part of any operative intervention and is often the first step in the exposure, repair, or removal of anatomic structures. A well-planned and expertly-executed incision allows for the best possible access to the operative field, the ability to extend the incision in the event of an unforeseen complication, and the most effective closure of the wound. Therefore, the surgeon will choose the most appropriate approach based on several considerations. Niederhuber states that "An incision becomes a balance between a wound that will heal rapidly with minimal scarring and disfigurement and a wound that offers ample access to the task at hand." For the surgeon and surgical assistant, access in the form of exposure and visualization are critical to carrying out a safe and successful operation and is directly impacted by the location, size, length, and direction of the incision. Incisions should be long enough to provide effective access to operative field, but small enough to allow for the rapid and complication-free recovery of the patient postoperatively.

Consideration should be given to the quality and consistency of the patient's tissues and their anticipated healing with regard to wound tensile strength, breaking strength (load required before a wound breaks regardless of its geometry), and burst strength (measurement of the pressure needed to rupture an internal organ). Each of these values differs from tissue to tissue and from structure to structure. Incisions should be planned so that primary wound closure adequately approximates tissue while wound strength is regained.

The use of well-planned surgical incisions made in a conscientious and conservative manner will greatly enhance the likelihood of proper, complication-free wound healing in the surgical patient. It is important to remember that the patient must live with the scar of the incision and see it each day. It should therefore stand as a mark of quality and provide the patient with a sense of confidence that the work performed internally was carried out in just as precise a manner.

The direction of the incision should be made in the direction of the tissue fibers to ensure the best cosmetic result after the wound has healed. Many surgeons prefer to make such incisions along the natural skin tension lines of the body, or Langer lines (Figure 9-1). Incisions should also be made in areas that are easily concealable, such as along normal skin wrinkle lines, whenever possible. While making the incision, the surgeon should be mindful of the fact that the wound will heal from side-to-side, rather than from end to end.

Generally speaking, the location and length of the surgical incision are most often dictated by the type of anticipated

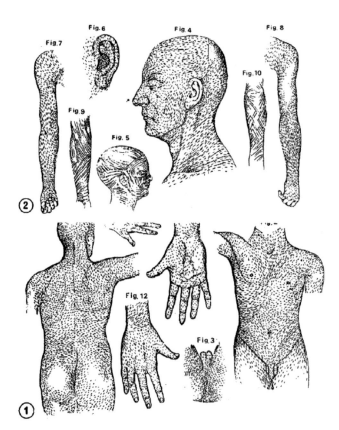

Figure 9-1 · Langer lines. (Reproduced, with permission, from Brunicardi FC, Andersen DK, Billiar TR, et al, eds. *Schwartz's Principles of Surgery*. 11th ed. New York, NY: McGraw Hill; 2019.)

surgical intervention. Therefore, various, different incision options are available depending on the area of the body and anatomic structures involved (Figure 9-1). Langer lines of the skin represent normal skin tension. Incising along Langer's lines decreases tension upon wound closure and results in minimal scarring.

Abdominal Incisions

Incision of the abdominal wall, or laparotomy, may be performed via a variety of techniques. Collectively, laparotomy incisions are the most commonly utilized surgical wounds. Such wounds are created to access intra-abdominal and abdominopelvic structures including the small and large intestines, stomach, pancreas, spleen, liver, gall bladder and biliary tract, urinary bladder, female reproductive anatomy, and appendix. The retroperitoneal space may also be reached through laparotomy.

In order to enter the abdominal cavity, dissection must be carried through each layer of the abdominal wall (Figure 9-2) located under the selected incision site. Careful consideration must be given to choosing the best incision through which to carry out a specific operative intervention, ensuring that the nerves, blood vessels, and muscles suffer the least amount of tissue trauma possible.

Regardless of incision chosen, the general structures involved in laparotomy of the anterior abdominal wall include the layers of the skin, subcutaneous fat and superficial fascia,

abdominal musculature, transversalis fascia, preperitoneal fat (extraperitoneal fascia), and the parietal peritoneum which lines the entire abdominopelvic cavity. Blood supply to the abdominal wall is provided by the superior and inferior epigastric arteries, deep and superficial circumflex iliac arteries, and the superficial epigastric arteries. Innervation is provided by branches of the T7-L1 spinal nerves, specifically the thoracoabdominal, subcostal, iliohypogastric, and ilioinguinal nerves. When choosing the appropriate site and approach for laparotomy, the following considerations must be made: the certainty of the diagnosis with regard to the planned surgical intervention; the speed with which the operation must be completed (affected by trauma or the presence of another emergent condition such as hemorrhage); the physical characteristics (habitus) of the patient (such as size and obesity) that may affect exposure, visualization, postoperative healing, and cosmesis; the patient's medical history and previous surgeries; the necessity for abdominal stoma creation (incision placed as far from the stoma site as possible); and the surgeon's preference.

Each of the various approaches to laparotomy is classified into one of three primary abdominal incision categories: vertical, transverse and oblique, and abdominothoracic.

Vertical Incisions.   Vertical abdominal incisions offer excellent exposure and visualization of the operative site and are widely utilized for a variety of procedures including exploratory laparotomy, surgical management of cancer, and procedures of the digestive tract.

Midline Incision: The most commonly performed of all surgical incisions is the midline vertical incision. This approach allows for quick entry into the abdominopelvic cavity and retroperitoneum and access to each anatomic structure located therein.

Virtually all abdominopelvic procedures can be performed via this incision. It is particularly useful when emergent conditions such as hemorrhage, traumatic injury, and sepsis are present. With this approach, achievement of hemostasis is less complicated and dissection is much faster than with alternative incisions because fewer layers of the abdominal wall are divided. Dissection of the abdominal musculature is avoided and damage to the nerves is greatly minimized as the incision is carried directly through the abdominal aponeurosis at the linea alba. Adding to its usefulness, the vertical midline incision can be carried from the xiphoid process to the pubis by incising around the umbilicus.

The incision may also be readily extended into the thoracic cavity and mediastinum. This allows for easy extension of the surgical wound and excellent exposure of the abdominal and abdominothoracic contents. The location and healing of the incision also facilitate reentry into the abdominal cavity if repeat surgery is anticipated, making it an ideal approach for the management of cancer and other recurring pathologies.

Although commonly chosen for its simplicity and ease, use of the midline vertical incision carries with it an increased risk of postoperative complications such as burst abdomen and incisional hernia (particularly epigastric) when compared to alternative approaches. Therefore, if the patient's condition

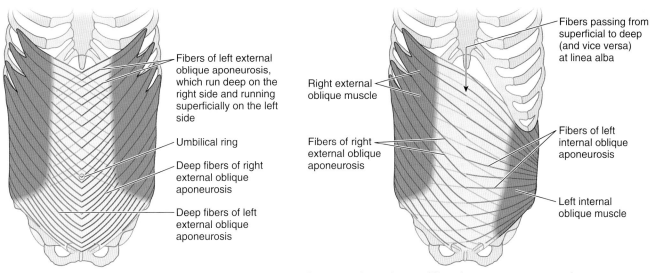

A Anterior views

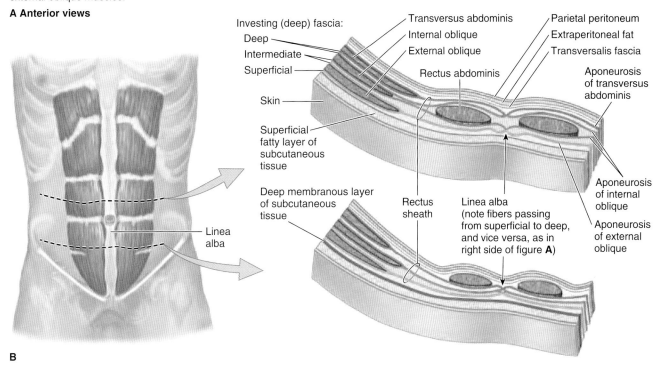

B

Figure 9-2 · Abdominal wall layers. Fiber direction and cross-sectional anatomy of the abdominal wall. **A.** Muscular and aponeurosis fiber direction of external and internal obliques. **B.** Crosssectional anatomy of the anterior abdominal wall above and below the arcuate line. The posterior leaf of the rectus sheath exists above the arcuate line. Below this line, all aponeurotic sheaths converge and travel anterior to the rectus muscles, leaving the posterior rectus uncovered by a fascial layer. (**A-B (left):** Reproduced with permission from Brunicardi FC et al, eds. *Schwartz's Principles of Surgery*. 11th ed. New York, NY: McGraw Hill; 2019. **B (Right):** Reproduced with permission from Moore KL, Agur AM. *Essential Clinical Anatomy*. 5th ed. Philadelphia, PA: Lippincott Williams & Wilkins; 2014.)

allows for slower and more careful dissection, use of a more specialized incision is typically preferred for specific surgical interventions. Operative steps common to the performance of the midline vertical incision are found in Table 9-1. It is important to remember that these steps are provided as a reference and that individual techniques may vary based on the surgeon's preference.

Paramedian Incision: The paramedian, or rectus incision is created approximately 1 to 2 in (2.5-5 cm) lateral to the midline of the abdomen (upper or lower) over the bulge of the rectus muscle. The incision can be extended superiorly and curved medially toward the xiphoid process in order to gain additional access, a procedure known as the Mayo-Robson modification. As the dissection is carried through the

TABLE 9-1 • COMMON INTRAOPERATIVE STEPS IN THE PERFORMANCE OF MIDLINE VERTICAL LAPAROTOMY
Incision and Exposure
1. The surgical wound is planned to accommodate exposure of the anticipated operative site and may be marked prior to the incision.
2. The skin incision is made at the desired level of the midline anterior abdomen and carried to the fascia with a #10 blade on a #3 knife handle. The lower midline incision extends from the umbilicus to the pubic symphysis inferiorly. The upper midline incision extends from the xyphoid process to the umbilicus inferiorly. Full midline exposure is possible by extending the incision from xyphoid to pubis, skirting around the umbilicus.
3. Hemostasis may be achieved by clamping and ligating bleeding vessels (using curved hemostats and fine nonabsorbable ties) or via the application of electrosurgery.
4. Superficial retractors appropriate to the size and depth of the wound may be placed to retract the skin and subcutaneous tissues, exposing the linea alba of the abdominal aponeurosis.
5. The incision is carried through the fascia to the preperitoneal fat with the deep scalpel or electrosurgical hand piece. Decussation of the right and left medial aspects of the rectus muscle indicates dissection through the midline.
6. Preperitoneal fat is divided to the level of the peritoneum at the lower extremity of the wound.
7. A clear fold of peritoneum is tented with curved hemostats, palpated to rule out the presence of bowel or other viscera, and nicked with the scalpel.
8. Two fingers are placed under the peritoneum to add traction and protect underlying structures as the abdominal cavity is opened.
9. The peritoneal incision is extended in time with the patient's expirations to decrease the likelihood of visceral perforation. Care must be taken to avoid the falciform ligament. Division of the ligament may be necessary and should be completed via clamping and ligation. Special attention should also be paid to loops of bowel and tissue adhesions that may interfere with dissection (Ellis, et al., 1985; Patnaik, et al., 2001; Wind & Rich, 1987).
10. Once the peritoneum is entered, the bowel is protected using moist laparotomy sponges and a self-retaining retractor may be placed to maintain exposure.

abdominal wall, the rectus muscle is typically dissected free from the anterior sheath and retracted laterally. A muscle-splitting technique may be employed in the presence of scar tissue from a previous paramedian incision. However, muscle splitting is generally avoided during these incisions as it may result in damage to the muscular blood and nervous supply leading to atrophy of the rectus abdominis medial to the incision site. Extension of the muscle-splitting approach superiorly is limited by the costal margin. This limits its usefulness in accessing the cephalad-most recesses of the abdominal cavity. In theory, paramedian incisions are beneficial because they provide access to lateral anatomic structures (such as the kidney and spleen) and can be closed more securely with a decreased risk of ventral hernia formation because the wound can be buttressed with the rectus abdominis muscle. However, the risk of postoperative herniation is increased the farther lateral the incision is made. Paramedian incisions are less commonly employed than vertical midline incisions as much more painstaking dissection is required to achieve visualization and exposure of the operative site.

Transverse and Oblique Incisions. Transverse and oblique abdominal incisions are generally performed for access to specific intra-abdominal structures and provide the benefit of localized exposure and visualization.

McBurney Incision: First described by Charles McBurney in 1894, the gridiron muscle-splitting (McBurney) incision is

often the incision of choice for the performance of open appendectomy. It is also commonly employed to facilitate Meckel's diverticulectomy. The incision is typically made obliquely over the appendix at McBurney's point, which can be located one-third the distance along a line drawn between the right anterior superior iliac spine and the umbilicus (Figure 9-3). Although this is the normal anatomic position of the appendix,

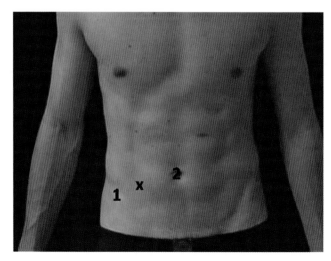

Figure 9-3 · McBurney's point. (Reproduced, with permission, from Brunicardi FC, Andersen DK, Billiar TR, et al, eds. *Schwartz's Principles of Surgery.* 11th ed. New York, NY: McGraw Hill; 2019.)

the location of the incision may be modified as warranted by patient-specific conditions or the presence of a palpable abdominal mass upon physical examination under anesthesia. If a mass is present, the incision should be placed directly over its location.

The McBurney incision offers the benefits of excellent access to the appendix and ileocecal anatomy with quick uncomplicated closure and little to no risk of postoperative herniation or wound disruption.

However, exposure to other structures may be limited and medial extension of the incision requires ligation of the inferior epigastric vessels and transverse incision of the rectus sheath. Because the incision is small (averaging only 8 cm) and typically placed in the natural skin crease, a good cosmetic result is expected once wound healing is completed.

To perform the incision, the placement of the wound is carefully planned and may be outlined with a skin marker. The skin is incised and dissection is carried through the subcutaneous tissues. Blunt dissection of the external oblique muscle and fascia is performed in the direction of the fibers and the muscle is retracted. Splitting and retraction of the internal oblique, transverse muscle, and fascia are then completed. This method of splitting the muscles along their fibers allows for secure wound closure and reduces the risk of postoperative herniation. A transverse incision is then made through the peritoneum, and the abdominal cavity is entered.

When performed on the left side, an extended version of this muscle-splitting incision can provide adequate access for surgery of the sigmoid colon. A horizontal variant of the McBurney approach, known as the Lanz incision, has increased in popularity due to its desirable cosmetic result.

The Rutherford-Morrison incision is an oblique muscle-cutting approach that is an extension of the McBurney incision. During dissection, the oblique fossa is divided and the resulting exposure can be used to access the colon for right or left colectomy, cecostomy, or sigmoid resection.

Rockey-Davis Incision: The Rockey-Davis incision is an alternative to the McBurney incision for the performance of open appendectomy and is characterized by a straight, transverse, muscle-splitting wound located in the right lower quadrant. Although used with less frequency, the incision can be hidden in a normal skin wrinkle for a better cosmetic result.

Subcostal Incision: Introduced by Nobel Prize-winning surgeon Theodor Kocher (1841-1917), the right Kocher subcostal incision is widely utilized to gain access to the gall bladder and biliary system during open cholecystectomy and related procedures. When performed on the left side of the abdomen, exposure of the spleen is facilitated.

The right subcostal approach begins with the incision placed in the right upper quadrant, approximately 2.5 to 5 cm below the xiphoid process, beginning at the midline and extending laterally and caudally to 2.5 cm below the costal margin. Branches of the superior epigastric blood vessels are coagulated. The rectus sheath is incised in the direction of the skin and the muscle is divided to the length of the incision. The oblique abdominal

muscles are divided outwardly. The large ninth thoracic nerve is identified and preserved to prevent postoperative abdominal muscle weakness; however, the smaller eighth thoracic nerve is typically sacrificed. The incision is carried deeper and the peritoneal cavity is entered.

Chevron Incision: If extensive exposure of the upper abdomen is indicated (as in the case of liver transplantation, total abdominal gastrectomy, total esophagectomy, and other procedures of the upper abdomen), the subcostal approach can be carried bilaterally across the patient's abdomen in an inverted "V" fashion, connecting both right and left Kocher incisions. This modification is known as a chevron or roof-top incision (Figure 9-4). It is

important to note that there is an increased risk of abdominal musculature weakness associated with this approach as both left and right eighth thoracic nerves are lost and potential injury to the ninth thoracic nerve is increased during dissection.

Mercedes-Benz Incision: The Mercedes-Benz modification adds the benefit of further exposure to the chevron incision by adding a superior midline limb toward the xiphoid process. The resulting wound resembles a Mercedes-Benz automobile logo. This approach is particularly useful during procedures requiring open access to the diaphragmatic anatomy and esophageal hiatus.

Transverse Muscle-Dividing Incision: The approach used in the creation of the transverse muscle-dividing incision resembles that of the Kocher subcostal incision. This technique is utilized when abdominal access is needed in infants and short, obese adults. Better exposure is offered in these patients when compared to midline laparotomy because their abdomens do not provide adequate length to accommodate vertical access to the operative site.

Pfannenstiel Incision: The Pfannenstiel incision is a low transverse laparotomy developed by German gynecologist, Hermann Johannes Pfannenstiel (1862-1909). Originally, it was

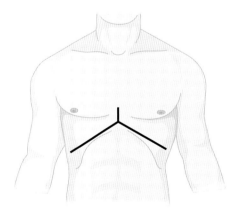

Figure 9-4 · Chevron incision. (Reproduced, with permission, from Singh D, Holton L, Antognoli L, Choudhry S. Strategies for operative management of abdominal wall hernia after solid organ transplant. *Plastic and Aesthetic Research*. 2020;7:39.)

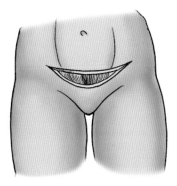

Figure 9-5 · Pfannesteil incision. (Reproduced, with permission, from Zinner MJ, Ashley SW, Hines OJ, eds. *Maingot's Abdominal Operations.* 13th ed. New York, NY: McGraw Hill; 2019.)

intended to decrease the risk of postoperative herniation associated with the surgical management of female pelvic disorders. Since that time, the approach has become popular among both gynecologists and urologists alike and is commonly used for procedures such as cesarean section total abdominal hysterectomy, open retropubic (see Figure 9-5) prostatectomy, and open surgery of the urinary bladder. The approach begins with a 12-cm-long transverse skin incision placed approximately 5 cm above the pubic symphysis in the natural folds of the skin. Dissection is carried to the fascia with the scalpel or electrosurgery. Once exposed, the anterior fascia is incised at the midline and the incision is carried bilaterally with curved Mayo scissors. Blunt dissection of the rectus muscle from the posterior fascia is followed by separation of the aponeurosis. Separation begins at the midline and is carried upward toward the umbilicus and downward toward the pubis. Lateral retraction of the abdominal musculature reveals the peritoneum, which is incised and stretched longitudinally. Once the abdominal cavity is exposed, care must be taken to protect the urinary bladder. In females, it is dissected free from the uterus and retracted caudally. In addition to excellent exposure of the pelvic organs, the abdominal vasculature is unaffected when the deep inferior epigastric artery is preserved. Postoperative healing often results in a strong, cosmetically acceptable scar that is hidden in the pubic hair.

Transverse Muscle-Cutting Incision: The transverse muscle-cutting, or Maylard, incision is an alternative approach to surgery of the pelvic organs and is placed more superior than the Pfannenstiel incision. The Maylard incision is particularly useful when extensive exposure of the pelvis is needed.

The skin incision begins at the anterior superior iliac spine, slopes downward over the mons pubis, and curves back upward toward the contralateral anterior superior iliac spine. Rather than lateral retraction of the rectus muscles, the rectus abdominis fascia and muscles are exposed and transversely cut. The transection is continued laterally and the internal and external oblique muscles are divided. The transverse abdominis and transversalis fascia are then divided along their fibers and the peritoneum is opened.

The lower oblique inguinal incision is the typical incision used to facilitate inguinal herniorrhaphy. Oblique inguinal incisions are also utilized by endovascular and urologic surgery specialists. The skin is incised obliquely, superior, and parallel to the inguinal crease extending from the pubic tubercle to the anterior iliac crest. The external oblique muscle is incised, allowing exposure of the cremaster muscle, inguinal canal, and spermatic cord.

Gibson Incision: The Gibson incision is commonly used by urologic surgeons for procedures of the distal ureter or for donor kidney implantation. Although the incision is made in the abdominal wall (, the approach is retroperitoneal and the abdominal cavity is not entered. The incision can be made on the right or left and begins 2 cm medial to the anterior-superior iliac spine 3 cm above and parallel to the inguinal ligament, continues to the lateral border of the rectus abdominis muscle. The incision is continued obliquely along the lateral margin of the rectus sheath toward the symphysis pubis.

After dissection through the subcutaneous tissues, the external oblique fascia is incised and the muscle is split along its fibers. The internal oblique and transverse abdominis muscles are cut in the direction of their fibers. The lateral margin of the rectus sheath is exposed.

The peritoneum is elevated using blunt dissection and retracted superior and medially to gain access to the iliac vessels and ureter. The rectus muscle can be transected following ligation and division of the inferior epigastric vein and artery if additional exposure is needed.

Flank Incision: Like the Gibson incision, the flank incision is widely used by urologists for exposure during procedures of the retroperitoneum. This approach offers the benefit of direct access to the proximal ureter, kidney, and adrenal gland. Depending on the anticipated operative site or location of the kidney, three modifications are available: subcostal, transcostal, or intercostal.

Thoracoabdominal Incisions. When simultaneous access to both the abdominal and pleural cavities is indicated, exposure can be gained via the use of a thoracoabdominal approach. Such exposure is often necessary to carry out surgical interventions of the distal esophagus, proximal stomach, and anterior spinal column.[1] When performed on the right, hepatic resection is facilitated. With the patient in lateral corkscrew position, the incision is made midline over the middle superior abdomen between the umbilicus and xiphoid process. After careful examination of the abdomen to assess the need for further exposure, it is continued posteriorly along the edge of the eighth costal interspace just distal to the inferior scapular pole. The latissimus dorsi, serratus anterior, and external oblique muscles are incised. Electrosurgical dissection of the intercostal muscles is followed by entry into the pleural cavity. The lung is collapsed to protect it from damage during the procedure. The costal cartilage is divided in a "V" shape, which facilitates secure closure as the two ends interdigitate upon re-approximation. A chest retractor is placed, the phrenic vessels are ligated, and the diaphragm is divided in radial fashion. Because wound healing can become rather complicated due to prolonged pain and the risk of infection within two body cavities, elective use of the thoracoabdominal incision has fallen out of favor except in incidences of retroperitoneal pathology or hepatic and thoracic trauma.

Thoracic Incisions

Incisions into the thoracic cavity are most often performed for procedures of the heart, great vessels, and lungs. Mediastinal anatomy such as the esophagus, trachea, thymus, and regional lymph nodes can also be reached. The two primary incisions associated with thoracic surgery are the median sternotomy and posterolateral thoracotomy. The layers of the thoracic wall and anterior thoracic anatomy are illustrated in Figure 9-6.

Median Sternotomy. Access to the thoracic cavity via median sternotomy provides excellent exposure of the mediastinum, thymus, pericardial tissues, heart, aorta, and venae cavae. The left and right pleural cavities are also accessible. The incision begins by incising the skin directly over the midline of the sternum from the sternal notch to just above the xiphoid process inferiorly. Hemostasis is achieved by electrosurgery. Dissection is carried to the sternal bone. The sternum is opened using a sternal saw (or Lebsche knife and mallet if power is not available) and a self-retaining retractor is placed to maintain exposure of the chest cavity. Retraction must not damage the sternal halves and care must be taken to avoid overspreading of the retractor blades and subsequent injury to the C_8-T_1 brachial plexus components. The pericardial sac may be incised and retracted with sutures for access to the heart.

Posterolateral Thoracotomy. With the exception of lung biopsy, posterolateral thoracotomy is the preferred incision for most pulmonary resections. It is also useful as an approach to the esophagus, posterior mediastinum, and thoracic vertebrae. The skin is incised at the line of the anterior axilla inferior to the areolar level. The incision continues posteriorly around the inferior scapular tip (following the rib) and curves cephalad to the midpoint between the scapula and vertebrae. The latissimus dorsi muscle is divided and the serratus anterior, trapezius, and rhomboid major muscles are retracted. The intercostal muscles of the selected interspace are divided in order to gain access to the pleura. Posterior rib division facilitates retractor and rib spreader placement with minimal risk of fracture or costochondral separation. Because of the risk of brachial plexus injury and damage to axillary neurovasculature associated with this approach, excess displacement of the shoulder during positioning must be avoided.

Head and Neck Incisions

When planning incisions of the head and neck, it is important to remember that a cosmetically acceptable scar is a major concern for the surgical patient. While adequate operative exposure is the concern of the surgeon and surgical assistant, Deitch (1997) states that when operating on the head and neck "a slightly different balance may need to be struck between optimal exposure and an optimal cosmetic result" (p. 45).[2] Placing incisions along normal skin creases and wrinkles provides a good cosmetic result as scars are usually well hidden. These natural wrinkles are the result of the skin's intimate connection to the underlying muscles that animate the face. As these muscles move, the skin contracts and gathers perpendicular to the pull of the underlying musculature. Therefore, postoperative scarring is reasonably concealed. Additionally, incisions can be made in areas such as the hairline, behind the ear, in the folds of the nose and eyelids, or under the mandible. Once planned, the intended wound should be drawn with a skin marker. To ensure that the facial incision is clean, consistent, and produces minimal decrease in vascular supply, Kruger in 1989 suggested that the skin be stretched and positioned so that it rests over a solid bone.[3] The incision should be made with a sharp blade through all of the layers of the skin in one complete motion and avoid jagged wound edges that complicate healing and scar formation. Further dissection should be performed carefully to avoid disruption of complex facial nervous and vascular structures.

Extremity Incisions

Incisions of the upper and lower extremities are typically made directly over the area of surgical interest. When operating on a long bone, nerve, artery, or vein, it is often best to utilize longitudinal incisions because they are easily extendable and offer superb exposure. These incisions must be carefully planned due to the presence of peripheral motor and sensory nerves that can be easily damaged. When incising over a joint, it is important to remember that adhesions may cause deep structures to adhere to the scar, forming restricting bands of tissue that impede movement and function. Therefore, incisions should not be made across joints or in the line of long muscles. Incisions over the extensor side of the joint may be paramedian and axial. However, when incising through the flexor side, such as within the antecubital or popliteal fossae, the incision should be made transversely, following the flexor crease in an S-shape fashion. The flexor creases are also followed as closely as possible when incising the palmar surface of the hand. Because of the intricate nature of hand anatomy, some incisions can be rather complex (Figure 9-7).

DISSECTION OF TISSUE

As operative dissection is carried out by the surgeon, the primary role of the surgical assistant is to ensure and facilitate proper exposure and visualization of the wound. It is vital that the assistant use proper techniques for tissue handling to promote the patient's successful recovery. Excessive tissue manipulation, overuse of electrocoagulation, lack of proper asepsis, and improper utilization of surgical instrumentation with regard to actions such as grasping, clamping, and retracting all directly impact the integrity of the wound and affect postoperative healing. In addition to case-specific operative anatomy and physiology, the assistant should study and understand

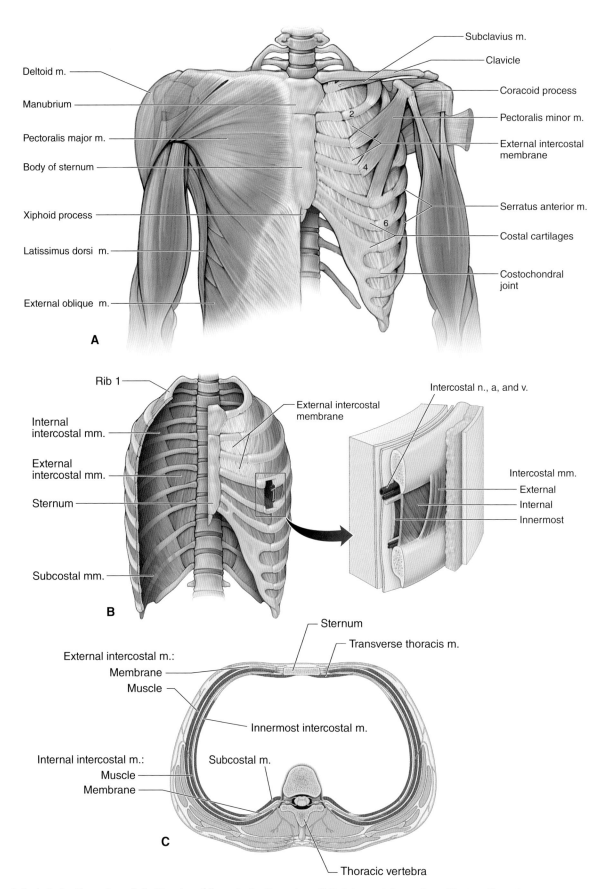

Figure 9-6 · Anterior thoracic wall. **A.** Muscles of the anterior thoracic wall. **B.** Intercostal muscles with step dissection. **C.** Cross-section of intercostal muscles and nerves. (Reproduced, with permission, from Morton DA, Foreman KB, Albertine KH. *The Big Picture: Gross Anatomy.* 2nd ed. New York, NY: McGraw Hill; 2019.)

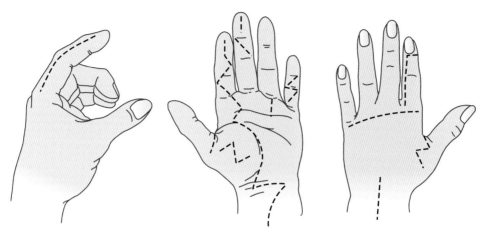

Figure 9-7 · Incisions for hand surgery. (Reproduced, with permission, from Doherty GM, ed. *Current Diagnosis & Treatment: Surgery.* 15th ed. New York, NY: McGraw Hill; 2020.)

appropriate intraoperative tissue handling techniques and implement them accordingly. The incision is one of the most important factors in gaining adequate exposure of the surgical site. Incisions should be made with a clean, sharp blade in one stroke of the hand while applying even pressure on the scalpel. The blade should remain perpendicular to the skin and downward pressure is achieved with the arm's passive weight. The index finger may be placed on the back of the blade for stability. The edges of traumatic wounds or those lined with scar tissue should be trimmed conservatively. As surgical exposure is achieved, the assistant should maintain adequate lighting by adjusting the intensity and direction of overhead operating room lights. Skin traction, sponging or suctioning of superficial bleeding vessels, and assistance with hemostasis may be needed as the wound is extended.

Once the incision is made, further dissection is ideally completed using sharp dissection. This may be accomplished using a deep knife blade, scissors, or other means such as electrosurgery. Sharp dissection is also recommended in the presence of scar tissue. Blunt dissection is best used to separate tissues along natural anatomic planes and may be performed using the fingers, a blunt instrument, or with the aid of a sponge. Care must be taken as improper blunt dissection leads to increased tissue injury when compared to sharp dissection. While dissecting tissue, the identification of tissue planes is facilitated using traction and countertraction. Additional structures may be identified by pressing the tissue between the thumb and index finger.

Grasping forceps are used to facilitate tissue dissection and are available in a wide range of styles and configurations. Tissue forceps are held in the non-dominant hand with a gentle, balanced grip between the thumb and index finger. The middle finger is placed on the shaft of the instrument for stabilization. Movement of the instrument is initiated by the wrist. The surgical assistant must become knowledgeable of the specific tissue indications for each type of forceps available at their facility. For example, Adson tissue forceps are finely-toothed and generally used to manipulate the skin and other

moderately dense tissues. Heavy toothed forceps such as a Ferris-Smith are indicated for use on tough connective tissues. Vessels may be grasped with the fine serrations of the DeBakey vascular forceps.

Various other instruments may also be used to aid in the dissection of tissues and body structures. In loose areolar tissue, blunt dissection may be facilitated in part through the use of hemostatic clamps. The blunt tips of hemostats are useful when dividing tissue perpendicular to vessels. Small spreading movements are used to separate planes and expose structures. Toothed clamps such as the Kocher may be used to grasp and retract fascia. Allis clamps are ideal for use in breast and adipose tissue. The non-crushing Babcock is designed for manipulation of luminated structures such as the appendix and fallopian tubes. Retractors are placed to maintain exposure of the surgical site. The preservation of underlying blood vessels and nerves is a vital component of successful postoperative healing.

Ischemia, blockage of lymphatics, and neurological compromise may result when excessive pressure is placed on the wound edges and internal structures, therefore retraction should be done with great care. The type and direction of retraction used will be determined by the nature of the wound, surgical anatomy, and surgeon's preference. When placed by the surgeon, retractors should not be moved or repositioned, especially during fine dissection and critical procedural steps. The surgical assistant must also ensure that the type of retractor utilized is appropriately sized and that its configuration (ie, toothed, smooth, sharp, or dull) will not cause additional trauma to the wound edges and other body tissues. For this reason, the best retractor may be the assistant's hands. Digital retraction during fine dissection facilitates proper pressure and precise handling of the tissues. The non-dominant hand is typically used to retract the viscera away from the field. Wide retraction can be facilitated by the administration of muscle-paralyzing agents. Moistened laparotomy sponges are often used to pad retractors and protect the wound edges. Desiccation may develop as a result of factors such as over-sponging or suctioning the operative site, inadequate irrigation, or prolonged exposure of the tissues to room air. Cells along the wound edges desiccate and lose blood supply continually. Shortened operative times reduce this and other cellular damage.

Removal of necrotic tissue (including electrosurgical char) and foreign infectious material is also vital, especially in the case of traumatic injury, and serves to greatly reduce the risk of postoperative infection and other wound complications. The assistant can further aid in dissection by providing traction and countertraction to tissues being divided. This technique involves gently pulling or retracting tissues in order to facilitate their division and identify tissue planes between anatomic structures. Additional considerations for the exposure of the surgical site include the removal of blood and body fluids by sponging or suctioning the wound and ensuring that the surgeon's direct line of sight remains clear. The assistant can avoid obstructing the surgeon's view by keeping her arms close to her body, working within a small area, and maintaining her hands and instruments around the perimeter of the surgeon's direct line of sight as much as possible. A good rule of thumb is, *if the assistant can't see, neither can the surgeon.* The assistant should also avoid crossing hands when manipulating tissue or using instrumentation and be prepared to react promptly as needed.

HEMOSTASIS

The achievement and maintenance of thorough intraoperative hemostasis is important for three primary reasons: (1) to minimize blood loss (leading to possible shock) and the need for blood volume replacement, (2) to increase visibility by providing a relatively bloodless field, and (3) to limit the formation of clots, hematomas, and seromas that may increase the risk of infection once the wound is closed. There are several types of bleeding (hemorrhage) that may occur intraoperatively: oozing (typically from capillaries), punctate hemorrhage (spotty bleeding from small vessels), and significant hemorrhage from large vessels. Hemorrhage may also be characterized as deep, superficial, or inaccessible depending on its location within the wound. When bleeding is controlled, the technical accuracy of the surgeon is greatly enhanced as clear visualization of the operative field is facilitated. The surgical assistant should respond promptly to bleeding as long as the associated vessels are located within noncritical tissue and the method of hemostasis utilized is within the assistant's clinical competency level. Achievement of hemostasis may be complicated by patient-related factors such as congenital or preexisting bleeding disorders; hemophilia is most common. Hemostatic disorders may also be acquired as a result of hepatic pathology, heparin or warfarin anticoagulant therapy, aplastic anemia, or liver failure related to alcohol consumption. Drug-induced coagulopathies affecting platelet function are the most common cause of bleeding disorders during surgery. Routine tests are performed preoperatively to rule out such potential complications.

A number of different mechanical, thermal, and chemical means are available to achieve and maintain intraoperative hemostasis. The most appropriate method will be dictated by factors such as the source and location of bleeding, the type of vessels involved, the amount of hemorrhage, the nature of nearby tissues, the need for permanent or temporary hemostasis, and patient-specific physiologic factors. Table 9-2 lists recommended hemostatic interventions according to hemorrhage source and location. Because of the complexity of many of these techniques, the surgical assistant must be properly educated and trained in their correct implementation. Common methods and techniques of intraoperative hemostasis include the following.

Mechanical Hemostasis

The use of instruments, physical devices, or direct pressure on bleeding tissues is referred to as mechanical hemostasis. Once mechanical hemostasis is applied, bleeding will cease as a result of the body's natural clotting mechanisms.

TABLE 9-2 • METHODS OF ACHIEVING HEMOSTASIS BY SOURCE AND LOCATION OF HEMORRHAGE

Hemorrhage Source	Location	Methods of Hemostasis
Capillaries	Any	Direct pressure
Small vessels (1-2 mm)	Any	Electrosurgery/ligate
	Deep/inaccessible	Direct pressure
Medium vessels (2-3 mm)	Any	Clamp and ligate
	Deep	Ligate/hemoclip
Large vessels (>3 mm)	Any	Clamp and ligate
	Deep	Hemoclip as secondary option
Named vessels	Any	Clamp and ligate
		Suture ligate
Raw tissue surfaces	Any	Direct pressure
		Topical hemostatic agent
		Electrosurgery

Source: Reproduced, with permission, from Deitch EA, ed. *Tools of the Trade and Rules of the Road: A Surgical Guide.* Philadelphia, PA: Lippincott-Raven; 1997.

Direct Pressure. The oldest and simplest method of achieving mechanical hemostasis is via the application of direct pressure to a bleeding wound. One type, digital pressure, involves placing a finger over or within the site of hemorrhage. The finger should be left in place until bleeding stops or until another means of hemostasis is ready to be applied. Pressure with the gloved finger is advantageous because it does not disrupt or remove formed clot when the finger is retracted. The palm of the hand may also be used for larger surfaces. Direct pressure can also be facilitated through the use of surgical sponges. For control of diffuse venous oozing from friable tissues or raw organ surfaces, sponges such as laparotomy sponges are moistened with cold saline and packed within the body. The packs may be left in place for 10-20 minutes while a fibrin clot is formed against the interlacing of the sponge's fibrous material matrix. A folded ray-tec may be clamped within the jaws of a Foerster sponge stick to apply direct pressure on deep vessels.

Hemostatic Instrumentation. Various types and sizes of hemostatic instruments are available depending on the characteristics of individual bleeding structures and the surgeon's preference. Examples include general hemostatic clamps, vascular clamps, vascular tourniquets, vascular staples, vessel loops and tapes, and specialty permanent clips such as those used in the operative management of aneurysms. General hemostatic clamps are applied to vessels to temporarily compress vessel walls in anticipation of ligature placement. Intact vessels can be doubly clamped, cut, and ligated for bloodless division. For routine vessels, electrosurgical current may be applied to the shaft of a hemostatic clamp to aid in the achievement of thermal hemostasis. During arteriotomy, vessels may be temporarily cross-clamped with vascular clamps or occluded with vessel loops or tapes using proximal-distal control. Permanent clips are implanted into the patient's tissues for long-term maintenance of hemostasis.

Ligatures (ties)

Ligation refers to the application of a binding or tying material such as a suture and is intended to constrict or fasten a blood vessel. Many different types of suture materials exist for ligation. It is vital that the surgical assistant have a comprehensive knowledge of each. Suture material is foreign matter and its selection is based on its properties, the characteristics of the patient's tissues, the patient's allergy status, availability, and the surgeon or assistant's personal preference.

Once a vessel is clamped, a ligature is placed at the base of the clamp and tied securely to prevent hemorrhage. The clamp is removed and the ligature is left in place with the ends cut as close to the knot as possible depending on the material used. For monofilament suture, tails should be cut to approximately ¼ in. To avoid adverse tissue reactions, the smallest diameter ligature strong enough to maintain hemostasis should be used. Depending on the suture material utilized, the ligature may reside permanently within the tissue or be absorbed by the body once healing is complete. Ligatures are available in several configurations.

Free Ties. Precut, single ligature strands without attached needles are known as free ties. Free ties are used for the ligation of small and medium blood vessels and luminated structures that do not require transfixion. Various lengths are available depending on the location of the vessel to be tied, whether superficial or deep.

Tie on a Pass. A tie on a pass is a free tie with one end loaded into the jaws of a hemostat or other clamp. This technique is utilized to reach vessels that are otherwise inaccessible with free-hand ties. The Schnidt tonsil clamp is most commonly used because its long shaft enables placement of the tie around deep vessels. A right-angle clamp is often used to facilitate ligation within deep cavities such as the abdomen and thorax and is placed under the vessel to receive the tie.

Ligature Reels. Ligature reels are longer ties that are preloaded onto dispensing reels to facilitate easy application without tangling. They are commonly used on superficial bleeding vessels of the subcutaneous tissue. Additionally, ligature reels are ideal for applications requiring placement of multiple ties in sequence, such as during open tubal ligation. The most common suture materials available in the ligature reel are chromic and plain gut, polyglactin 910, and silk. The number of holes on the dispenser indicates the diameter of the suture. Typical diameters are 2-0, 3-0, and 4-0.

Suture Ligatures. A suture ligature, or stick tie, is a ligature preloaded onto a swaged needle for passage (transfixion) through a large vessel. Transfixion of the suture material prevents slippage once the ligature is securely tied in place. Large vessels are clamped proximally and distally with appropriately sized hemostats and sharply divided using fine scissors. The suture ligature needle is passed through the center of the vessel at the base of the clamp. Passage through the vessel prevents dislodging of the ligature due to pulsatile action. The ends of the suture are passed around the vessel to doubly ligate the lumen. A single throw can be placed following transfixion prior to wrapping the suture around the vessel and securing the knot on the contralateral side. Large vessels may be double-ligated by placing a free tie proximal to the suture ligature. Figure-of-eight suture configurations are used for occlusion and to control bleeding. Figure-of-eight configurations are also indicated for occlusion of vessels that lie within friable tissues or planes that are difficult to reach by clamping (Figure 9-8).

Suture ligatures are available in a myriad of different materials and diameters. The most widely used are size 2-0 and 3-0 silk sutures. The smallest diameter suture that can effectively occlude the vessel without breakage should be used. Deitch suggests using a 2-0 diameter suture for large vessels, a 3-0 suture for vessels effectively occluded with a Kelly clamp, and a 4-0 for those vessels that can be occluded using a mosquito. If the appropriate-diameter suture breaks during knot tying, it is likely that too much pressure was applied and the knot was pulled too tightly. Because silk has been associated with the formation of granulomas, many surgeons prefer polyglactic materials, although they do not handle as well within the tissue. For superficial vessels,

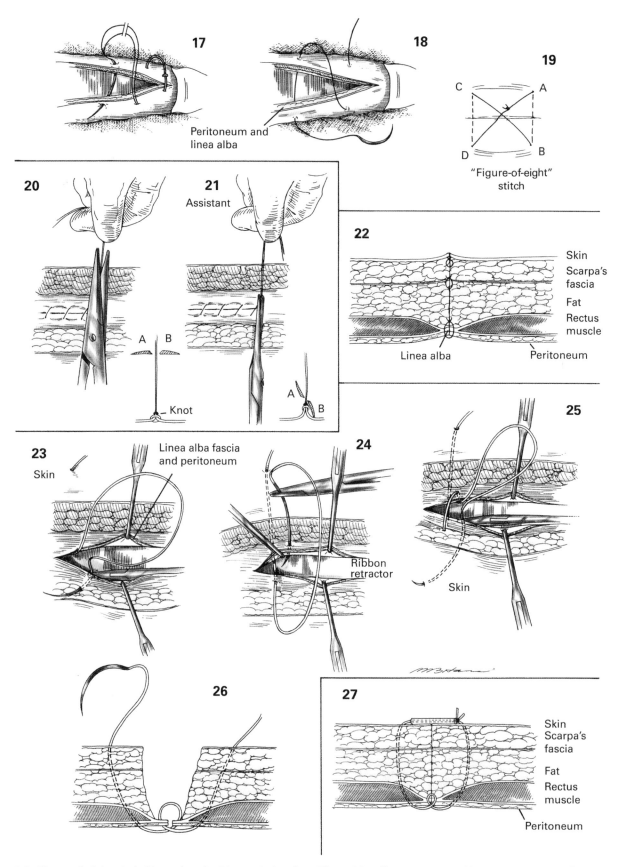

Figure 9-8 · Figure-of-eight stitch. (Reproduced, with permission, from Ellison EC, Zollinger Jr RM, Pawlik TM, Vaccaro PS. *Zollinger's Atlas of Surgical Operations.* 11th ed. New York, NY: McGraw Hill; 2022.)

18-in-long ligatures are sufficient. Deep vessels require the use of 27-in-long ligatures to ensure that enough strand length is available to tie, seat, and secure deep knots.

Pledgets. When vessel anastomosis is performed with suture, swaged needles leave anastomosis is performed with suture; swaged needles leave small puncture holes in the vessel wall that may cause postoperative hemorrhage. To prevent bleeding and promote clotting at these sites, small pieces of Teflon known as pledgets are sewn in place to buttress the suture line. Pledgeted sutures are also used to prevent hemorrhage along suture lines in tissues or organs at risk of suture cut through. Some examples include wounds of the liver, spleen, and heart.

Hemoclips. Hemoclips are small vessel ligating clips that are an alternative to suture ligatures or free ties. Hemoclips are advantageous because they can be applied quickly and easily using a dispensing applicator that provides ready access to areas of the body where suturing and knot tying may be difficult to perform. Hemoclips are available in sizes small (3 mm), medium (4 mm), and large (6 mm) and may be permanent or absorbable. They may be made from such materials as titanium, stainless steel, or plastic. Applicators are available in various configurations such as reusable, manually-loaded, single-fire instruments or preloaded, multi-fire, disposable appliers. Laparoscopic applicators are also available. Use of hemoclips should be carefully considered as they can easily become dislodged during blunt dissection, sponging, or retracting. Dislodged hemoclips may result in postoperative hemorrhage and significant complications. Once applied, the clips should be verified for proper placement.

Bone Wax. Oozing from cut bone edges may be sealed using refined, sterilized beeswax commonly referred to as bone wax. To apply bone wax, a small piece is pinched from the package, rolled into a ball, and placed on the end of a spatulated instrument for application. The Freer elevator is commonly used for this purpose. Using the applicator, the bone wax is gently packed into the bone to wall off the site of bleeding. Because bone wax is a foreign material, its use should be minimal.

Suction. During the course of the operation, blood and body fluids are aspirated from the surgical site by the surgical assistant. Appropriate suctioning allows the surgeon a clear view of the field and is used to facilitate dissection, exposure, and approximation of tissue. Without adequate aspiration of blood, locating bleeding vessels is problematic and achievement of hemostasis is difficult at best.

Thermal hemostasis

Thermal hemostasis involves the application of heat energy to arrest bleeding within the wound. Several devices for thermal hemostasis exist and include the electrosurgical unit, surgical lasers, argon plasma coagulator, and ultrasonic scalpel.

Electrosurgery. Hemostasis may be achieved through the induction of thermal energy using an alternating electrical current, a widely-used technique known as electrosurgery. The electrosurgical handpiece delivers heat to the target tissues and coagulation results as proteins within tissue cells are denatured. Several handpiece options are available and include monopolar pencils for general hemostasis and bipolar forceps for more precise applications.

Monopolar devices offer both coagulation and tissue-cutting functions. Amplitude settings should be set as low as possible to effectively coagulate bleeding vessels while avoiding excess tissue necrosis due to collateral tissue damage and eschar formation. Deitch warns that the presence of electrosurgical eschar within the wound increases the risk of postoperative infection. However, when used carefully electrosurgery decreases total operating time due to its rapid effectiveness and ease of use. Electrosurgery is most effective when used to coagulate vessels of 2 mm in diameter or smaller. Multiple small vessels may be coagulated rapidly by applying electrosurgery to an instrument such as such as hemostatic clamp or tissue forceps.

To utilize this method, the vessel is occluded in the jaws of the instrument and lifted away from the skin and other adjacent tissues. The assistant may gently squeeze the vessel with a sponge to force blood away from the clamp and minimize electrical current transmission. The tip of the electrosurgical handpiece is then touched to the instrument and activated to direct the current toward the vessel within its jaws. The current is removed immediately once coagulation is effective. The surgical assistant should become proficient at removing clamps with both right and left hands. Electrosurgical current may also be applied to Frazier and other small metal suction tips for the simultaneous evacuation of field-obscuring blood and vessel coagulation. This technique is especially useful in the presence of brisk bleeding from a vessel that cannot be visualized without constant suction.

If the handpiece is used frequently, eschar accumulation may need to be scraped or wiped clean from the tip regularly. It is important to note that clots formed by electrocoagulation may be easily disrupted by retraction, so care must be taken. According to Wind and Rich, correct application of electrosurgery results in less tissue trauma than ligature use.

Lasers. Surgical lasers provide precise simultaneous cutting and coagulation of tissue via a highly concentrated light beam. Laser use minimizes collateral damage to tissues adjacent to those targeted for surgical intervention. Several types of lasers are available and each requires adherence to specific safety protocols in order to prevent injury to the patient and members of the surgical team. When laser use is anticipated, the surgical assistant should prepare by donning appropriate personal protective equipment and ensure that additional safety precautions are taken such as the utilization of anti-reflective instrumentation and the availability of sterile water and moist sponges.

Argon Plasma Coagulation. Argon plasma coagulation (APC) is commonly employed to arrest bleeding from superficial tissue erosions of such organs as the liver and spleen. This form of thermal hemostasis combines argon gas with a monopolar electrical current to create a white light beam that emits from a handpiece and coagulates delicate surface tissues without contact. The lack of direct contact minimizes tissue adherence to the handpiece as well as eschar formation within the wound.

Ultrasonic Scalpel. The ultrasonic (harmonic) scalpel is a device that consists of a single-use handpiece connected to a generator that converts electrical energy into mechanical energy. Mechanical action is transferred to the jaws and blade of the instrument resulting in ultrasonic vibrations of 55,000 movements per second. These movements cause localized protein denaturation leading to the precise, simultaneous coagulation and cutting of tissue. Continuous protein denaturation produces heat that is directed toward deeper tissues, thus increasing the depth and penetration of coagulation while minimizing damage to nearby structures. The harmonic scalpel is useful during laparoscopic procedures because it does not char tissues or produce smoke plume that may obscure the endoscope or camera.

Chemical Hemostasis

Chemical hemostatic agents control bleeding by one of three pharmaceutical mechanisms: (1) vessel occlusion via the formation of a bulky plug, (2) induced coagulation, or (3) vasoconstriction. Depending on the nature and location of hemorrhage, the surgeon may choose between a myriad of different agents, each with its own specific indications, advantages, and disadvantages. Table 9-3 outlines the action, usage, and additional characteristics of several commonly used topical absorbable agents.

Other chemical hemostatic agents, including epinephrine and silver nitrate, are routinely utilized.

Epinephrine. Epinephrine (adrenaline) is a natural hormone from the adrenal gland that causes local vasoconstriction when

TABLE 9-3 • ACTION, USAGE, ADVANTAGES, AND DISADVANTAGES OF COMMON TOPICAL ABSORBABLE HEMOSTATIC AGENTS

	Collagen	Gelatin Sponge	Oxidized Cellulose	Thrombin
Proprietary Name	Sponges: Collastat, Superstat, Helistat Microfibrillar: Avitene	Gelfoam	Surgicel, Oxycel	Evithrom, Recothrom, Thrombin-JMI
Origin	Bovine collagen	Purified porcine gelatin	Water insoluble cellulose product	Bovine protein
Action	Reaction with blood causes platelet aggregation and sticky clot formation	Direct contact with bleeding capillaries causes fibrin deposit and clot formation	Direct contact with whole blood causes rapid clotting	Joins with fibrinogen to accelerate coagulation and clotting for control of capillary bleeding
Usage	Apply dry using direct pressure to vascular suture lines or oozing surfaces of the liver or spleen	May be soaked in thrombin or epinephrine, for plain use dip in saline and squeeze to remove air, mix powdered gelatin with saline for cancellous bone or denuded skin	Apply dry to oozing tissue surfaces, may be sutured, wrapped, or firmly held in place to achieve hemostasis	Dry powder applied directly to oozing surfaces, may be used to saturate a gelatin sponge, can be sprayed onto denuded areas, should not be used on large vessels
Onset of Hemostasis	1-5 min	Not specified	2-8 min	>1 min depending on concentration
Absorption Time	8-12 weeks	4-6 weeks	Oxidized regenerated cellulose knit: 1-2 weeks Oxidized gauze: 3- 4 weeks	Immediate
Advantages	Conforms well to tissues, sponges dissolve as hemostasis occurs, ideal for friable tissue	Various pad sizes can be cut easily	Conforms well to tissues, absorbs 10 times its weight with minimal reaction, bactericidal	Rapid coagulation, ideal for denuded areas
Disadvantages	Contraindicated for use in infected tissues and in the presence of pooled blood or fluids, causes scarring and healing complications if placed within the skin incision	Slows wound healing	Slows wound healing, contraindicated for bone unless removed prior to closure	Loses potency after 3 hours
Special Characteristics	Sponges: Good wet integrity	Absorbs 45 times its weight in blood	Inactivated by thrombin	Mix just before time of use

Source: Adapted, with permission, from Schwartz SI, ed. *Principles of Surgery.* 7th ed. New York, NY: McGraw Hill; 1999.

applied topically to bleeding tissues. When added to local anesthetics such as marcaine and lidocaine at concentrations of 1:100,000 or 1:200,000, epinephrine's vasoconstricting properties prolong the effects of these agents and may counteract their cardiovascular depressant actions.

Epinephrine is commonly used to manage oozing from small vessels and vascular tissues such as the oral mucosa during tonsillectomy. For control of bleeding during ear and microsurgical procedures, gelatin sponges may be soaked in a 1:1,000 concentration. Extensive use and application of epinephrine should be avoided as systemic effects such as cardiac dysrhythmia and hypertension may result from excess absorption. It is widely accepted that the injection of epinephrine into end-arterial fields (ie, digits, nose, pinnae, and penis) should be avoided as vasoconstriction within these structures may lead to ischemia.

Silver Nitrate. Silver nitrate is an organic compound with hemostatic, astringent, and antimicrobial properties. As a chemical hemostatic agent, silver nitrate crystals may be mixed into 20% to 50% solution or combined with silver chloride and formed onto the tip of topical applicator sticks. Common indications for the use of silver nitrate include burns, moist wounds, cervical and nasal hemorrhage, and as a sealant for wound healing by second intention. To apply, the applicator is placed in direct contact with the bleeding surfaces. Silver nitrate is contraindicated for wounds of the face because it stains the skin black and may negatively impact cosmesis.

TISSUE APPROXIMATION

Tissue approximation refers to the bringing together (coaption) and alignment of disrupted body tissues and is usually performed via the use of sutures, staples, tapes, or liquid adhesives. Precise tissue approximation, leak-proof anastomosis, and the secure closure of the surgical wound are all vital elements in ensuring proper, disruption-free healing with minimal risk of postoperative complication. When performing tissue approximation within the body (ie, vessel or bowel anastomosis, repair of lacerated viscera, or suturing of graft material), careful consideration should be given to the type of approximation utilized, the material (suture, staples, etc.) used to facilitate approximation, as well as the specific nature of the individual tissues.

Appropriate suture materials, suture gauges, and needles should be chosen carefully to ensure minimal tissue reaction, adequate wound support, and acceptable cosmesis. Remember that suture, although designed for use within body tissues, is a foreign substance, and improper suture choice, handling, and knot tying may cause adverse tissue reactions. The surgical assistant should be cognizant of the number of throws indicated to secure knots of different suture materials in order to limit the amount of foreign body in the wound. Also, over-tightening of suture and knots may lead to strangulation (ischemia) and subsequent necrosis may develop.

For this reason, a common slogan of tissue handling and suturing is *approximation not strangulation*. After tying, suture should be cut so that tails are of the appropriate length.

When closing the wound, tissue approximation techniques should eliminate dead space without causing ischemia to the wound edges. The presence of dead space in the wound often results from inadequate closure and consequent air pocket formation. This causes tissue layers under the skin to separate as air pockets are filled with fluid (blood or serum) during the inflammatory response phase. Fluid accumulation provides an ideal environment for the colonization of microorganisms, leading to infection and wound disruption. For instances in which some bleeding is expected postoperatively, a drain may be inserted or a pressure dressing may be utilized to place direct pressure on the wound and limit the formation of dead space and accumulation of blood or tissue fluids.

HALSTED'S PRINCIPLES

One of the most influential surgeons and healthcare educators in the history of medicine, William S. Halsted (1852-1922), is credited as setting "the tone for modern American surgical training" (Figure 9-9). Several of his innovations, including the Halsted stitch and the wearing of gloves to reduce infection, are still central to operative technique today. Halsted's Principles of Tissue Handling are perhaps his greatest legacy and many of the considerations mentioned in other sections of this manual were heavily influenced by his theories. Some of the key components of his theories with regard to wound management and closure are outlined as follows:

- The use of interrupted sutures leads to greater wound strength during healing and if one knot slips or breaks, the others serve to maintain integrity and prevent dehiscence.

- Interrupted sutures are a barrier to infection as microbial contamination wicks along continuous suture lines.

- The selection of suture material and its diameter should be consistent with wound security and the strength of the closure should match the strength of the tissues.

- Long suture tails left after tying and cutting can cause inflammation and irritation of the adjacent tissues, therefore suture should be cut close to the knot.

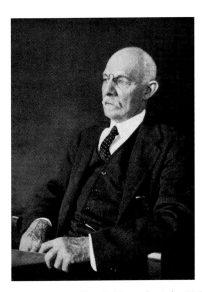

Figure 9-9 · William Stewart Halsted. (Photo by John H. Stocksdale, 1922.)

- A separate needle should be used for each skin stitch to minimize tissue drag and needle penetration trauma.
- Dead space within the wound must be eliminated by thorough approximation of the tissues under the skin.
- Two fine sutures are preferred over one large suture.
- The use of silk suture in the presence of infection must be avoided.

Approximation of the wound edges must be secure without applying undue pressure to the tissues, as doing so leads to ischemic strangulation. Thus, tissue approximation under tension should be avoided whenever possible. Although advancements in suture materials, their properties, and operative wound closure techniques have occurred over the years, these practical considerations are still applicable today. The surgical assistant should be mindful of Halsted's Principles when assisting in tissue approximation and performing closure of the surgical wound.

TISSUE HAN DLING

All soft tissue dissection should be approached with a thorough foundational knowledge of anatomy. The key to successful dissection is the locating the surgical plane and staying within that plane. Any disruption of soft tissue is considered damaged, even with careful dissection. However, harmful effects of tissue adherence can be minimized with attentiveness when using sharp or traumatic instrumentation. It is important for the surgical assistant to acquaint themselves with the anatomical structure of the tissue, distinguishing the texture, strength, and fragility. Also important is the age, nutritional status and health of the patient, and the affect any of these variables may have on the tissue during handling.

Connective Tissue

Connective tissue is found in between other tissues everywhere in the body, including the nervous system. Connective tissues are specialized soft tissues, which provide support to hold the body's other tissues together. Connective tissue surrounds blood vessels and nerves, and offers a scaffold for most organs. The texture and structure of connective tissue varies from flimsy areolar tissue to tough ligaments, tendons, and aponeuroses. Although there is limited vascularity to connective tissue, a surgical assistant should be aware of any blood vessels that cross connective tissues when dissecting it.

Areolar Tissue. In addition to binding structures and holding them in their anatomical spaces, areolar connective tissue stores fat and helps the body conserve heat. Dissecting areolar tissue should be accomplished with a scalpel or scissors sealing any fine vessels with diathermy or a harmonic scalpel. Stripping can also be done through blunt dissection using your finger.

Aponeuroses. An aponeurosis is a sheet of pearly-white tendinous tissue which is the site of attachment of flat muscles or intercepts where there is a separation of flat muscles. The aponeurosis is comprised of dense fibrous connective tissue containing fibroblasts and bundles of collagenous fibers. Dissecting through any aponeuroses should be parallel if possible. This lends itself to

minimal or no repair as the muscle tone pulls the fibers straight closing the gap. If a cut is made across the fibers, it is recommended to close the gap with horizontal stitches to ensure the sutures hold. Healing of the aponeuroses is a slow process.

Tendons. Tendons are composed of dense fibrous connective tissue and attach muscle to other body parts, usually bones. Tendons are responsible for transmitting the mechanical force of muscle contraction to the bones. They are considered to have the highest tensile strengths among soft tissue. If tendons are split into the fiber lines, they will heal without losing their strength. However, if they are divided transverse to the fibers, the ends will retract. Tendon repair should be accomplished with a braided polyester utilizing a mattress stitch. It is important to remember that tendon ends will damage with forceps making the surface rough. Tendons should be manipulated with a straight Keith needle. Tension on the tendon repair can be achieved by immobilizing joints in a position that brings the muscle origin and insertion point as close as possible.

Ligaments. Ligaments are fibrous bands of connective tissue that connects bone to bone and supports our internal organs. There are two major types of ligaments; white ligaments of collagenous fibers that are inelastic and tough yellow ligaments abundant with elastic fibers. Ligaments form a capsular sac at the joint to enclose the articulating bone ends and the lubricating membrane known as synovial membrane. Ligaments like the cruciate ligament are difficult to repair, although some can be repaired by employing the same technique as repairing tendons. Repair of the cruciate ligaments of the knee can be repaired using either tendons of hamstring muscle or the central portion of the patellar tendon with a piece of the tibia and the patella at each end attached through tunnels within the femur and tibia.

Nerves. The nervous system is an intricate group of nerves and specific cells known as neurons that transmit signals between different areas of the body. It is basically the body's electrical wiring. Structurally, the nervous system has two components: the central nervous system and the peripheral nervous system. The central nervous system is made up of the brain, spinal cord, and nerves. The peripheral nervous system consists of sensory neurons, ganglia outside of the brain, spinal cord, and nerves that connect the central nervous system to the limbs and organs.

There are three layers to nerve fibers: the epineurium, the perineurium, and the endoneurium. When repairing a nerve, it is important to align the severed nerve fibers perfectly without tension or rotation. The microvascular repair should begin with a bloodless exposure with the aid of a tourniquet. Nerve ends should be trimmed with a sharp scalpel if necessary, before uniting the ends utilizing an 8-0 to 10-0 nylon suture. If nerve repair involves a limb, immobilization will become necessary to ensure proper fusion of the nerve endings.

Skeletal Muscle. According to Britannica, skeletal muscle is considered voluntary muscle and one of the most common of the three types of muscle in the body. Skeletal muscles are attached to the bone by tendons, and they create movements of all the body parts in their relation to each other. Completely different from smooth or cardiac muscles, skeletal muscles are considered voluntary muscles. However, like cardiac muscle, skeletal muscle is striated; its appearance is long, thin, with multinucleated fibers that are intersected with a pattern of thin red and white lines, giving the muscle a characteristic appearance. Skeletal muscle fibers are bound together by connective tissue and communicate with nerves and blood vessels.

Skeletal muscle is strongly resistant to injury if it is healthy. However, if the motor nerve supply is lost, the muscle will become paralyzed and will atrophy. It is important when carrying out a cutdown, to attempt to bypass the muscle to reach your surgical target. However, extreme displacement of any muscle may result in disruption of the nerve and blood supply. Dissection should keep in mind the external fascia that enables the layered muscle to glide over each other without friction. Repair of skeletal muscle is accomplished by reapposing the parallel muscle fibers and separated muscle fibers with absorbable sutures swaged on round-bodied needles. Kessler stitches, horizontal mattress, and figure-of-eight stitches are some suture techniques utilized for lacerated or transected muscle repair, although horizontal mattress sutures are known to cut out after reapposition (Figure 9-10). Although skeletal muscle is the predominant tissue in our limbs, it is most vulnerable to ischemia. If ischemia is not relieved, the muscle atrophies and will be replaced with fibrous tissue, resulting in shortened muscles and contractures.

Volkmann contracture has been identified by Richard Volkmann in 1872. This occurs when there is a lack of blood flow and swelling of muscle within the inelastic fascia (ischemia) to the limb. Relief to the compromised muscle is achieved through an open fasciotomy to allow the muscle to bulge through. In the lower leg, all four muscle compartments must be released. This is accomplished under general anesthesia through an anterolateral incision.

Cartilage. Cartilage is made up of specialized cells called chondrocytes. It is an avascular, flexible connective tissue that provides support and cushioning for adjacent tissues. Cartilage lacks blood vessels; therefore, nutrients diffuse through the perichondrium surrounding the cartilage and into the central

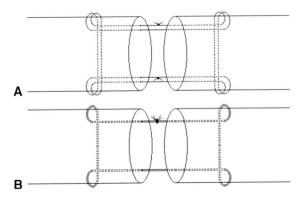

Figure 9-10 · Schematic of 4-stranded modified Kessler core suture configurations, single-stranded (**A**) and looped (**B**). (Reproduced, with permission, from Bernstein DT, Alexander JJ, Petersen NJ, Lambert BS, Noble PC, Netscher DT. The impact of suture caliber and looped configurations on the suture-tendon interface in zone II flexor tendon repair. *J Hand Surg Am.* 2019;44(2):156.e1-156.e8.)

portion. There are three types of cartilage: hyaline, fibrocartilage, and elastic cartilage. It is found in many areas of the body including the ends of ribs, between the vertebra in the spine, ears and noses, bronchial tubes and the joints between bones. With a lack of blood vessels, cartilage grows and repairs at a slower rate than other tissue. Fibrocartilage is found in the pubic symphysis, the annulus fibrosus of intervertebral discs, menisci, and the temporal mandibular joint. Fibrocartilage can be relocated from one position to another as part of a composite graft. It can also withstand being cut, sutured, and drilled. Repairs of fibrocartilage located in areas such as the menisci of the knee joint can be repaired arthroscopically.

Mucoperiosteum. The hard palate forms the roof of the mouth and is covered with keratinized epithelium. Mucoperiosteum is a layer of connective tissue covering the bone and forms the mucosal lining of the maxillary sinuses along with the hard palate. The mucoperiosteum can be elevated from the bone as a flap to repair bony defects such as a congenital cleft palate. Suture material for repairs should consist of 3-0 black silk or black monofilament nylon on a reverse cutting needle. Anatomical repairs that would make suture removal difficult can be performed with a 4-0 synthetic absorbable suture.

Breast. The female breast is mostly made up of different types of fibrous tissue, glandular tissue as well as fatty tissue called adipose. This tissue extends from the collarbone down to the underarm and across to the middle of the ribcage. The glandular tissue includes the breast lobes and breast ducts. The fibrous or connective tissue is the same tissue that comprises ligaments. Adipose tissue fills in the spaces between the glandular and fibrous tissue. It is the adipose tissue that determines your breast size. A healthy female breast is made of 12 to 20 sections called lobes. Each lobe is made up of smaller lobules, the gland that produces milk in nursing women. Both the lobes and lobules are linked by milk ducts, which act as stems or tubes to transport the milk to the nipple.

When operating on the breast, it is important to consider the radial distribution of the lobules, mainly because they drain centrally to reach the nipple. Incisions should be planned to achieve the finest cosmetic effect making incisions parallel to Langer's Lines. Judicious attention to achieving perfect hemostasis will prevent hematomas.

Lymph Nodes. The lymphatic system is an intricate network of thin vessels, valves, ducts, nodes, and organs. There are hundreds of lymph nodes found throughout the body and are part of your immune system. Lymph vessels connect lymph nodes to each other. Clusters of lymph nodes are found in the neck, axilla (underarm), chest, abdomen, and groin and play a significant part in the body's defense against infection. Swollen lymph nodes can appear as a lump beneath your skin. They often become swollen and infected after exposure to bacteria or viruses.

When removing lymph nodes for pathology, ensure you have adequate exposure and a clear view of the anatomy. Incisions to remove lymph nodes should be made in a skin crease if possible, to allow for aesthetic skin closure. Lymph nodes can be very fragile and if crushed will upset the accuracy of any diagnosis.

They should not be grasped with forceps as it could damage the tissue. Leaving connective tissue attached to the lymph node will allow you to grasp the node without damaging it.

Sentinel Node Biopsy. With the diagnosis of breast cancer, a sentinel node biopsy can isolate the first lymph nodes into which a tumor drains (called the "sentinel" node). The sentinel node is typically located in the axillary nodes, under the arm. A positive biopsy result indicates that cancer is present in the sentinel lymph node and that it may have spread to other nearby lymph nodes and, possibly other organs. Intraoperative evaluation of tumor cells within the sentinel node is a routine procedure which uses isosulfan blue/patent blue V combined with radioactive colloid tracer, although Methylene blue (MB) is a less expensive and readily available alternative dye. The surgeon then uses a probe to find the sentinel lymph node(s) containing the radioactive substance or looks for the lymph node(s) stained with dye. The surgeon then removes the sentinel node(s) to check for the presence of cancer cells.

Abdominal Wall Midline Incision. A cutdown utilizing a midline incision will divide the skin, linea alba, and peritoneum. Right-handed people should stand on the right side of the patient to make an incision. The incision should be planned with the patient's needs in mind and should follow Langer's lines when possible for a better cosmetic outcome. The skin is separated by holding the knife in a manner so it cuts vertically. If the midline incision includes the umbilicus, care is taken by creating a semicircle around the umbilicus leaving a 2 to 3 mm margin. Another method for a midline incision that goes around the umbilicus is to grasp the edge of the umbilicus with an Allis tissue forceps holding the forceps with your nondominant hand. The umbilicus should be pulled towards you pulling the umbilicus out of the way of the straight-line incision while making the incision in a straight line down the midline. Hemostasis should be achieved with the initial incision before continuing the cutdown through the vertical fibrous line of the aponeuroses of the rectus abdominus or linea alba and stopping when reaching the layer of fat that superimposes the fused fascia transversalis and peritoneum. Once the initial skin incision is made, a diathermy can be used instead of a scalpel to complete the cutdown. Above the accurate line located at the umbilicus in the abdomen, the rectus sheath contains both an anterior and posterior portion. Below the accurate line, the sheath is only on the anterior side with transversalis fascia only in the posterior portion.

From there, the final layer is grasped with the tips of a hemostat to tent the tissue up, and grasped again next to the first hold. Release the first hemostat only and re-grasp the tissue to allow any viscus that may have been picked up to be released before re-attaching the hemostat. Tension should be placed on the peritoneum as you pull both hemostats up and a small incision is made between the two hemostats. Air will enter the abdomen further pushing viscera clear of the incision. To ensure no viscera is in danger of being injured, place a finger into the peritoneal cavity moving it to verify no viscera is in

the locality of the incision. Once you are assured there is no viscera in the space, mayo scissors are used to complete the peritoneum incision. The peritoneum is a thin membrane made of cells called mesothelium and supported by a thin layer of connective tissue. Many surgeons believe the peritoneum is a layer that can be left to heal without closure. The layers will heal on their own without significance. There does not appear to be any evidence for a short-term or long-term advantage in peritoneal closure in operations not related to childbirth. If the peritoneum is closed, a thin absorbable suture is used for this task. A running closure stitch of the peritoneum requires the assistant to "follow" the suture. If the surgeon decides on interrupted stitches for the closure of the peritoneum, the assistant should be prepared to tie the stitches and cut them as they are placed. Typically, most surgeons will incorporate the anterior and posterior rectus sheath along with the transversalis fascia and close them as one layer. If there is a concern of dehiscence or evisceration, the surgeon may opt to close this layer with interrupted stitches to provide strength to the closure. A figure-of-eight stitch will distribute the pressure to more of the surface area. The linea alba is closed with either a running or an interrupted stitch. When closing the subcutaneous layer, it is important to incorporate Scarpa's fascia to strengthen the closure. The subcutaneous layer is closed to eliminate dead space and relieve tension off the skin edges which will promote healing. Utilizing the over-and-under stitch will take care of the deep and superficial subcutaneous layers while incorporating Scarpa's fascia between the two. The skin can be closed with a variety of suture or methods, including staples, skin tape, or skin glue. The main goal should keep pressure to a minimum and promote wound healing. Surgeons will often employ a subcuticular stitch with an absorbable suture if suturing the epidermis. This will give the wound an aesthetic closure with minimal scarring.

References

1. Smith CE. General surgery. In: Rothrock JC, McEwen DR (eds.), *Alexander's Care of the Patient in Surgery.* 10th ed. St. Louis, MO: Mosby Elsevier; 2007:297-355.

2. Deitch EA, ed. *Tools of the trade and rules of the road: A surgical guide.* Philadelphia, PA: Lippincott-Raven; 1997.

3. Patnaik VVG, Singla RK, Sanjus B. Surgical Incisions—Their Anatomical Basis: Part 1—Head and Neck. *J Anat Soc India.* 2006;49(1). https://vdocument.in/surgical-incision-head-neck.html?page=1. Accessed September 13, 2023.

Bibliography

Price P, Smith C. Chapter 10: Wound healing, sutures, needles, and stapling devices. In K. B. Frey & T. Ross (Eds.), *Surgical Technology for the Surgical Technologist.* Cengage Publishing; 2008.

Caruthers B, May M, Ward-English L. *The Surgical Wound.* Englewood, CO: Association of Surgical Technologists; 1995.

Dunn DL, ed. *Wound Closure Manual.* Somerville, NJ: Ethicon, Inc; 2007.

Niederhuber JE. Incisions, wound closure, & the healing process. In: Niederhuber JE, Dunwoody SL, eds. *Fundamentals of Surgery.* Stamford, CT: Appleton & Lange; 1998:79-92.

Ellis H, Bucknall TE, Cox PJ. Abdominal incisions and their closure. *Curr Probl Surg.* 1985;22(4):4-51.

University of Michigan Medical School. *Dissector Answers: Abdominal Wall*. 2000. http://anatomy.med.umich.edu/gastrointestinal_system/abdo_wall_ans.h tml. Accessed May 24, 2023.

Patnaik VVG, Singla RK, Bansal BK. Surgical incisions their anatomic basis part IV abdomen. J Anat Soc India. 2001;50(2):170-178.

Wind GG, Rich NM. *Principles of Surgical Technique: The Art of Surgery*. 2nd ed. Baltimore, MD: Urban & Schwarzenberg; 1987.

Association of Surgical Technologists. *Surgical Technology for the Surgical Technologist: A positive care approach*. 3rd ed. Clifton Park, NY: Delmar Cengage Learning; 2008:278-303.

Allen G, Caruthers B, Ross T. Obstetric and gynecologic surgery. In: Frey KB, Ross T, eds. *Surgical Technology for the Surgical Technologist: A Positive Care Approach*. 3rd ed. Clifton Park, NY: Delmar Cengage Learning; 2008:496-575.

Junge T, Ross T. Genitourinary surgery. In Frey KB, Ross T, eds. *Surgical Technology for the Surgical Technologist: A Positive Care Approach*. 3rd ed. Clifton Park, NY: Delmar Cengage Learning; 2008:769-827.

Manski D. *Gibson incision*. 2011. Retrieved from http://www.urology-textbook.com/gibson-incision.html. Accessed May 24, 2023.

Rousch VW, Ginsberg RJ (1999). Chest wall, pleura, lung, and mediastinum. In: Schwartz SI, Shires GT, Spencer FC, Daly JM, Fischer JE, Galloway AC, eds. *Principles of surgery*. New York, NY: McGraw Hill; 1999: 667-790.

Price P, Zacharias R. Cardiothoracic surgery. In: Frey KB, Ross T, eds. *Surgical Technology for the Surgical Technologist: A Positive Care Approach*. 3rd ed. Clifton Park, NY: Delmar Cengage Learning; 2008:912-972.

Fischer JE, Fegelman E, Johannigman J. Surgical complications. In: Schwartz SI, Shires GT, Spencer FC, Daly JM, Fischer JE, Galloway AC, eds, *Principles of surgery*. New York, NY: McGraw Hill; 1999:441-483.

Dharmananda S. Abdominal Adhesions: Prevention and Treatment. 2003. Retrieved from http://www.itmonline.org/arts/adhesions.htm. Accessed May 24, 2023.

Solomkin JS, Wittman DW, West MA, Barie PS. (1999). Intraabdominal infections. In: Schwartz SI, Shires GT, Spencer FC, Daly JM, Fischer JE, Galloway AC, eds. *Principles of surgery*. New York, NY: McGraw Hill; 1999: 1515-1550.

Green DP. Exposure and Soft Tissue Dissection. *Oper Tech Sports Med*. 2011;19(4). https://www.sciencedirect.com/science/article/pii/S1060187211000293. Accessed May 24, 2023.

Aponeurosis anatomy. https://www.britannica.com/science/aponeurosis. Accessed May 24, 2023.

Functional Atlas of Human Fascial System, 2015. *Loose connective Tissue*. https://www.sciencedirect.com/topics/medicine-and-dentistry/loose-connective-tissue. Accessed May 24, 2023.

Chhabra T. 7 types of Connective Tissue. Published March 13, 2018. https://sciencing.com/7-types-connective-tissue-8768445.html. Accessed May 24, 2023.

Myint F. *Kirk's Basic Surgical Techniques*. 7th ed. Elsevier Publishing; 2019.

Tendon anatomy. https://www.britannica.com/science/tendon. Accessed May 24, 2023.

Newmarker C. Stryker Strives for Market Share in Orthopedic Surgery Robots. Published May 2019. https://www.therobotreport.com/stryker-leads-orthopedic-surgery-robots/. Accessed May 24, 2023.

Zimmermann KA. Nervous System: Facts, Function & Diseases. Published February 14, 2018. https://www.livescience.com/22665-nervous-system.html. Accessed May 24, 2023.

The Editors of Encyclopedia Britannica. *Skeletal Muscle Anatomy*. https://www.britannica.com/science/skeletal-muscle. Accessed May 24, 2023.

Olivia F, Via OG, Kiristi O, Foti C, Maffulli N. Surgical Repair of Muscle Laceration: Biomechanical Properties at 6 Years Follow-up. Published February 24, 2014. https://www.ncbi.nlm.nih.gov/pmc/articles/PMC3940505/. Accessed May 24, 2023.

Mandal A. What Is Cartilage? https://www.news-medical.net/health/What-is-Cartilage.aspx. Accessed May 24, 2023.

Anatomy of the breast. https://www.mskcc.org/cancer-care/types/breast/anatomy-breast. Accessed May 24, 2023.

Breast Anatomy. https://www.nationalbreastcancer.org/breast-anatomy. Accessed May 24, 2023.

Lymph Nodes. Published through the NIH, U.S. Library of Medicine. https://medlineplus.gov/ency/anatomyvideos/000083.htm. Accessed May 24, 2023.

Lymph Nodes. Published through the NIH, National Cancer Institute. https://www.cancer.gov/publications/dictionaries/cancer-terms/def/lymph-node. Accessed May 24, 2023.

Breast Cancer and the Sentinel Node Biopsy. https://www.webmd.com/breast-cancer/sentinel-node-biopsy. Accessed May 24, 2023.

Sentinel Node Biopsy. National Cancer Institute. https://www.cancer.gov/about-cancer/diagnosis-staging/staging/sentinel-node-biopsy-fact-sheet. Accessed May 24, 2023.

Methylene blue dye—a safe and effective alternative for sentinel lymph node localization. Breast Unit, St Bartholomew's Hospital, Queen Mary University of London, United Kingdom. https://www.ncbi.nlm.nih.gov/pubmed/18186867. Accessed May 24, 2023.

Gursusamy KS, Delia EC, Davidson BR. Peritoneal closure versus no peritoneal closure for patients undergoing non-obstetric abdominal operations. Published July 4, 2013. https://www.cochranelibrary.com/cdsr/doi/10.1002/14651858.CD010424.pub2/full. Accessed May 24, 2023.

Abdominal anatomy photo, accurate line. https://accessmedicine.mhmedical.com/content.aspx?bookid=399&aid=56715037. Accessed May 31, 2023.

Lymph Node photo. https://www.cancer.org/cancer/cancer-basics/lymph-nodes-and-cancer.html. Accessed May 24, 2023.

The Surgical Wound

Douglas J. Hughes

Although access to the operative site is accomplished via a myriad of different methods and approaches, each shares an often overlooked and misunderstood commonality: the surgical wound. According to Taber's Cyclopedic Medical Dictionary (21st ed.),[1] a wound is defined as a "break in the continuity of body structures caused by violence, trauma, or surgery to tissues." While there is certainly a break in body structure continuity associated with surgical wounds, they differ from other wound types in that they are made intentionally and under controlled circumstances for the purpose of operative intervention. Great care must be taken to ensure that an appropriate wound—either incisional or excisional—is created and managed to facilitate a safe and effective operation for the surgical patient and help ensure their successful postoperative recovery. To accomplish this task, the surgical assistant must have an in-depth understanding of the fundamentals of the surgical wound.

THE SURGICAL WOUND

Disruption of normal body tissues by intentional (surgical) or accidental (traumatic) means results in a wound. Surgical wounds involve the intentional incision or excision of tissues and are performed to facilitate the process of surgical diagnostic or therapeutic intervention. Once tissue damage ensues, the body immediately begins to heal itself. Healing takes place in many stages and begins with localized inflammation at the site of injury.

Depending upon the amount of microbial contamination present, surgical wounds may be classified as clean, clean-contaminated, contaminated, or dirty. This classification system plays a major role in postoperative healing, as do many patient and surgical team-related factors.

The Inflammatory Process

Localized activation of the humoral and cellular immune responses by damaged or infected body tissue is known as the inflammatory process. Inflammation functions to neutralize or destroy invading foreign agents, minimize tissue damage, alert the body to threat, and initiate healing. Without inflammation, wound healing would not be possible. This acquired immune response begins with increased blood flow to the target tissues and may be marked by the presence of four clinical signs: pain (dolor), swelling (tumor), redness (rubor), and loss of function (functio laesa). There are two major classifications of inflammation: **acute** and **chronic**.

Acute Inflammation. Acute inflammation is characterized by a rapid onset at the time of injury and may last up to 2 weeks. As the process begins, complement proteins and cytokines cause blood vessels to dilate and white blood cells (leukocytes) are attracted to the target tissues. Devitalized tissue and foreign material within the wound are removed by leukocytes which release additional chemicals and histamines to increase and perpetuate the inflammatory response.

Invading microorganisms are destroyed by the release of leukocytic enzymes and other cellular substances in order to prevent infection.

Phagocytic leukocytes continue to debride the wound during healing (resulting in the formation of pus) and play an active role in the restoration of disrupted tissues. Typically, the inflammatory response is localized but may spread **systemically** as a result of infection or systemic disease processes.

Chronic Inflammation. If the inflammatory response is prolonged it is classified as chronic inflammation. This condition may last from several weeks to many years as a result of persistent stimulus at the target tissues, repeated injury, or complications in the healing process such as the presence of toxic substances, or tubercular, viral, and autoimmune disease. Tissue damage as a result of chronic inflammation occurs in many debilitating diseases, these include **rheumatoid arthritis**, chronic lung diseases, and tuberculosis.

Types of Wound Healing

Under normal circumstances, surgical and traumatic wounds follow a relatively predictable pattern of healing. Based upon the condition of the patient's tissues, the manner in which those tissues were handled intraoperatively, and the presence of contamination, the surgeon will decide which of the three methods is the best approach to wound healing. The three types of wound healing that occur are healing by first intention, second intention, and third intention.

First-Intention Wound Healing. Healing by first intention, also known as primary union, occurs when disrupted tissue is closed using primary wound approximation methods such as sutures, staples, liquid skin adhesive, or specialty dressings. The wound edges must be properly approximated to ensure the removal of dead space (see Figure 10-1), leaving the wound to heal normally from side to side. Over time, the tensile strength of the wound increases and reaches 70% to 80% by the third postoperative month. Wound tensile strength refers to the load applied per unit cross-sectional area at the time of breaking.

The amount a wound will stretch before breaking is known as **extensibility** and is largely dependent on collagen. Collagen is a strong, fibrous protein found in connective tissues and plays a major role in healing. **Primary union** is the most common type of surgical wound healing and is indicated for class I and II wounds. There are three phases of first-intention wound healing (see Figure 10-2).

Phase I, the Inflammatory Response Phase: Immediately following the disruption of normal tissue, the body initiates phase I—the substrate or inflammatory response phase—of the wound-healing process. This phase lasts between 1 and 5 days and is characterized by the achievement of hemostasis through platelet aggregation and the activation of the body's immune response system and inflammatory process. As mentioned previously, immune responses may be marked by the presence of heat, redness, swelling, pain, and loss of function. Localized inflammation leads to increased arterial blood supply to the healing area and results in the accumulation of tissue fluids, cells, and fibroblasts in the wound. Damaged tissue and foreign objects are debrided through the actions of phagocytic leukocytes and proteolytic enzymes. A scab is formed over the wound to seal in tissue fluids and protect it from microbial contamination.

Cumulatively, these processes prepare the damaged tissue for the second phase in first-intention wound healing.

Phase II, the Proliferative Phase: Once the debridement system of phase I is well underway, the tissues can begin the process of repair or proliferation. The proliferative phase is the second phase in normal wound healing. Phase II typically begins around the third day following tissue damage and can take between 5 and 20 days to complete. **Fibroblasts** begin the formation of a network of collagen fibers (granulation) between the edges of the wound. The collagen works to form connective tissue and bridge the wound together. **Epithelialization** of the wound occurs, and the collagen matrix is filled with new blood vessels which supply rich nutrients to the proliferating tissue. As this process continues, the pliability of the wound is increased, and the tensile strength is restored to approximately 25% to 30%. Wound contraction may develop depending on the area of the body affected and is typically found on the buttocks, back, and posterior neck. With the tissues pulled tightly together, the sutures can be removed during this phase of wound healing.

Phase III, the Remodeling or Maturation Phase: The third phase of first-intention wound healing, known as the remodeling or **maturation phase,** typically begins around the 14th to 21st day following tissue disruption and can last as long as 1 year. During this phase, the wound fully regains tensile strength, and wound contraction from **myofibroblasts** is completed.

The maturation of the wound causes a decrease in local vascularity resulting in a paler, more mature scar or cicatrix.

Second-Intention Wound Healing. Secondary wound healing, or spontaneous wound closure, results from self-generated closure of the wound margins through the normal biologic processes of tissue granulation and contraction which take place from the bottom up. In this type of healing, the wound edges are not approximated (as in first intention healing) following a wide **debridement** or due to the presence of infection or tissue necrosis. When infectious or **devitalized** tissues are present, suturing or stapling traps contaminate material within the wound causing further infection and other complications. Also, the inflammation present in the various phases of wound healing through first intention cause sutures placed within the wound to break down as a result of **phagocytic** and **enzymatic** activity. Therefore, the wound is left open during healing.

As the wound heals, it may need to be packed with a moist dressing to minimize **tissue desiccation** and facilitate debridement. As moistened dressing materials dry, they adhere to adjacent infected and necrotic tissue which is then removed during dressing changes. Healing through the second intention typically lasts an extended period while infection subsides and the body fills the wound with granulation tissue. Once healing is complete, the result is weak tissue union with an irregular scar. **Re-epithelialization** may be hindered by excess granulation tissue (proud flesh) that develops and protrudes above the margins of the wound.

Third-Intention Wound Healing. Third-intention wound healing, or delayed-primary wound closure, is a combination of primary and secondary wound closure methods and is utilized when suturing of the wound must be delayed. In this form of wound healing, the wound is left to heal by second intention or **granulation** for 3 to 5 days, after which it is approximated

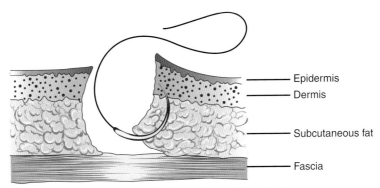

Epidermis
Dermis
Subcutaneous fat
Fascia

A. The strength of the closure lies in the dermis. Occasionally, the subcutaneous fat is incorporated to obliterate dead space.

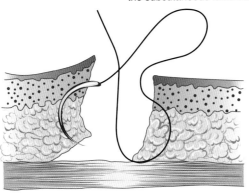

B. The suture is placed so that the knot will lie in the deepest part of the wound. Take care to avoid incorporating the epidermis with this suture, since epithelial cysts will form and result in suture extrusion.

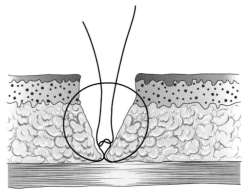

C. The dermal suture is tied just tightly enough to approximate the wound margins. Synthetic absorbable sutures are most commonly used for closure of the dermis.

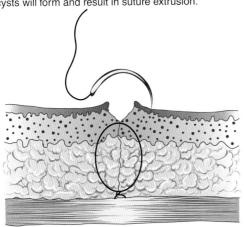

D. After the dermis is approximated, a fine "epidermal" suture is placed to align the wound edges. This suture adds little to the tensile strength of the wound closure.

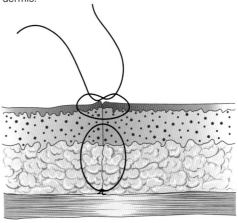

E. The epidermal suture is tied just tightly enough to approximate the epidermal edges of the wound. Since the strength of this closure lies in the dermis, the epidermal suture can be removed after 2-3 days. Skin tapes are often used to support the wound for an additional 7-10 days.

Figure 10-1 · Wound dead space. (Reproduced, with permission, from Saunders CE, Ho MT. Current Emergency Diagnosis & Treatment, 4th ed. New York, NY: McGraw-Hill Education; 1992.)

using sutures as in primary closure. This method is particularly useful in the management of wounds requiring frequent irrigation, those with significant microbial contamination, or in the presence of foreign bodies, extensive tissue damage, or dehisced wound edges. Dehisced wounds typically present with weakened margins that need time to heal before being reapproximated. Other examples of wounds typically managed through third-intention wound healing techniques are those related to motor vehicle trauma and tissue damage from gunshots and penetrating knife wounds.

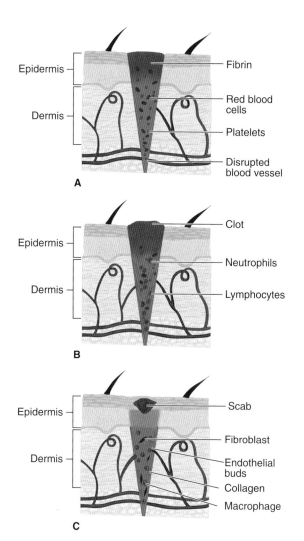

A

B

C

Figure 10-2 · First-intention wound healing. The phases of wound healing viewed histologically. **A.** The hemostatic/inflammatory phase. **B.** Latter inflammatory phases reflecting infiltration by mononuclear cells and lymphocytes. **C.** The proliferative phase, with associated angiogenesis and collagen synthesis. (Reproduced, with permission, from Brunicardi FC, Andersen DK, Billiar TR, et al, eds. *Schwartz's Principles of Surgery*. 11th ed. New York, NY: McGraw Hill; 2019.)

Wound Classifications

Depending upon several factors, such as the area of the body accessed and the care in which that access takes place, the degree of microbial contamination within the wound will vary. Therefore, surgical wounds are classified into four categories or classes to describe the level of contamination present. The following wound classification system was developed by the US Centers for Disease Control and Prevention (CDC) using a schema outlined by the American College of Surgeons (ACS).

Class I Wounds.   Approximately 75% of surgical wounds can be classified as class I or clean wounds. These consist of an incision or excision made under ideal sterile circumstances with no break in aseptic technique during the operation. In addition, entry into the aerodigestive, biliary, or urinary tracts

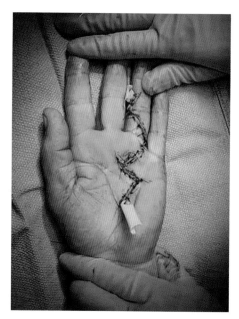

Figure 10-3 · Class II clean-contaminated wound.

is avoided as these areas contain high numbers of microbial contaminants. Class I wounds can be approximated or closed using primary wound closure techniques and carry a low infection rate of approximately 1% to 5%. Therefore, class I surgical wounds offer the lowest risk of infection-related postoperative complications.

Class II Wounds.   Class II wounds (see Figure 10-3), described as clean-contaminated, include surgical wounds in which a minor break-in sterile technique occurs, a wound drain is placed, or controlled access into the aerodigestive, biliary, or genitourinary tract occurs. These wounds carry an inherently higher risk of infection—approximately 10% due to the higher microbial count—yet may be approximated using primary wound closure techniques.

Class III Wounds.   Contaminated wounds are categorized as class III wounds. These are the result of factors such as a major break in sterile or aseptic technique, traumatic injuries or other microbial contamination before the start of the procedure, acute inflammation, or surgical incisions resulting in gross spillage of contents from the aerodigestive, biliary, or genitourinary tract. Contaminated wounds contain high levels of microbial contamination and can become actively infected within 6 hours. The infection rate of a class III wound is approximately 15% to 20%.

Class IV Wounds.   Finally, class IV wounds (see Figure 10-4), also known as dirty or infected wounds, are wounds in which an open traumatic injury older than 4 hours is present, there is gross microbial contamination before the start of the procedure, or in which unintentional visceral perforation has resulted in the presence of infected foreign material in the wound. Class IV wounds are associated with infection rates as high as 40%.

Considerations.   Solid understanding of the wound classification system coupled with proper application of sterile and

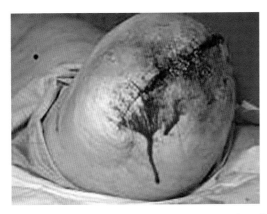

Figure 10-4 · Class IV wound: Necrosis on AKA. (Reproduced from Harker J. Wound healing complications associated with lower limb amputation. World Wide Wounds. September 2006. Copyright Surgical Materials Testing Laboratory (SMTL), Bridgend, South Wales, UK.)

aseptic techniques, minimal and appropriate tissue handling following concepts such as Halsted's Principles, and the use of antibiotic prophylaxis can serve to significantly lower the risk of infection associated with each class of surgical wound. It is important to note that the wound class can change at any moment during the operation depending on a myriad of factors including the actions of surgical team members and the presence of infectious material. Therefore, the final classification of the surgical wound is not established and documented until the end of the operative procedure. The outcome of this final classification in conjunction with several other patient-related and surgical-team-related factors plays a major role in the healing of the surgical wound and directly impacts the patient's postoperative recovery and prognosis.

Factors That Affect Wound Healing

Healing of the surgical wound is a naturally occurring phenomenon that can be described as the return of body tissues to a healthy state. Body tissues are defined as groups of similar cells that work in tandem to carry out a specific function and are classified into four basic categories: epithelial, connective, muscular, and nervous tissue. The restoration of the continuity and function of each of these tissues is dependent upon a myriad of factors, some patient-related, and others under the direct control of the operative team members. Each of these factors can have a direct impact on the rate of wound healing, the tensile tissue strength of the wound, and the risk of associated postoperative infection.

Patient-Related Factors. Important patient-related factors that affect wound healing includes the patient's age, weight, nutritional status, level of dehydration, blood supply to the surgical wound, and general health including the presence of comorbid diseases or conditions. It is also necessary to consider whether the patient is a smoker, undergoing radiation treatment or therapy, or is otherwise in an immunocompromised state.

For the elderly patient, wound healing is slowed due in part to changes that occur in the vascular system. As individuals age, the body's ability to produce new blood vessels (angiogenesis) deteriorates. Emerging evidence has linked this deterioration with a decline in the function of macrophages necessary in the production of vascular endothelial growth factor (VEGF). Additional studies have also linked a decrease in insulin-like growth factor (ILGF) produced by platelets to slowed healing. As levels of these and other related growth factors decrease, so does the production of new vessels within the wound and subsequent blood flow and oxygenation to damaged tissues. Thus, the wound-healing process is complicated when compared to similar wounds in younger patients. Wound healing is also complicated in patients lacking proper nutrition. For example, protein is necessary during the inflammatory and immune responses and throughout the development of granulation tissue. Fats and carbohydrates also play an integral role. To ensure optimal collagen synthesis, nitrogen must be balanced through the intake of sufficient calories and amino acids. Vitamin C is vital to collagen formation and is necessary for vascular ingrowth. Regeneration of epithelial tissue is directly affected by vitamin A, as is the function of B and T lymphocytes. Other nutrients, vitamins, and minerals are also necessary. Examples of these include Zinc, vitamin D, vitamin E, copper, and manganese. Hypovolemia due to dehydration is also a major concern.

Comorbid patient conditions and illnesses that affect wound healing include endocrine and metabolic disorders (ie, diabetes mellitus (see Figure 10-5), adrenal insufficiency, obesity, and uremia), hematologic disorders (anemia, leukocytopenia, arterial disease, and systemic circulatory pathologies), hemorrhagic disorders (coagulopathy, vitamin K deficiency, and thrombocytopenia), immunocompromising conditions, and malignancy. Additionally, healing of the surgical wound can be complicated by the presence of foreign bodies and wound contaminants which may lead to infection.

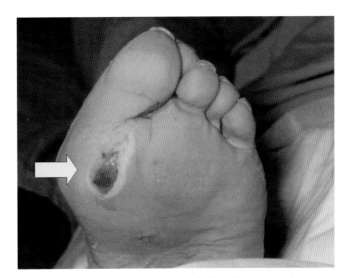

Figure 10-5 · Nonhealing diabetic foot ulcer. (Reproduced, with permission, from Dean SM, Satiani B, Abraham WT, eds. *Color Atlas and Synopsis of Vascular Diseases*. New York, NY: McGraw Hill; 2014. Fig. 5-1.)

Surgical Team–Related Factors. Factors under the control of the surgical team members include the use of strict sterile and aseptic technique, the length of the surgical procedure, and the use of proper intraoperative tissue handling techniques and wound closure methods. These factors are discussed in detail in the following section.

WOUND CLOSURE MODALITIES

Throughout recorded history, techniques and approaches to wound closure and healing have taken many forms. While some approaches may seem bizarre by today's standards, others may seem quite modern and sophisticated. Some of the earliest medical records from ancient Hindu and South African societies document the use of insect mandibles to effect complete tissue approximation. Insects such as large black ants were made to bite wound edges and bridge them together. Once their jaws were tightly clamped, the bodies were removed by twisting them free from the head, leaving the jaws in place to hold the tissues. Early attempts at ligature use can be found in classical Indian and Greek writings. Physicians of this era used sutures made from hair, flax, silk, linen, cotton, hemp, and bark fiber in much the same fashion as modern practitioners. Such sutures were dipped in oil and wine to decrease tissue drag (resistance) and minimize infection; however, knowledge of infectious disease etiology was dreadfully limited and post-surgical mortality rates were high. The suturing of cuts was widely practiced in ancient Greece. The practice involved the use of a curved needle made from bronze with a thread placed through the eye. The sutured wound was covered in a solution of copper oxide and honey followed by wine-soaked padding as an antiseptic, a dry sponge for absorption, and a handful of leaves to create a bulky pressure dressing. The Greek physician Galen (ca.130– ca. 200 ad) first described the use of sheep intestine as a suture material in his ancient texts.

The first use of surgical gut for the closure of abdominal wounds is credited to the Persian Physician and Philosopher Rhazes, who first described its use in 900 AD. While each of these antiquated techniques may have proven successful, modern advances in tissue approximation and wound closure have far exceeded much of their practicality and usefulness. In fact, advances in wound closure over the past two to three decades have far surpassed those of the previous 2000 years. Today, the objective of wound closure is to reapproximate wound edges with sufficient tension to hold them together with minimal tissue compression and reduce the risk of disruption and infection during healing. Meeting this goal is often difficult given the type of tissue, nature of the wound, and other wound healing factors previously mentioned. Therefore, modern research and practice have yielded several useful materials and techniques.

Suture

Generically speaking, suture can be defined as any material that is used in the approximation of severed body tissue to hold that tissue together until adequate healing has occurred. A single strand of suture material used to seal bleeding vessels and achieve hemostasis or localize tissue for excision is known as a ligature. Many different types of suture materials are available for ligation, tissue approximation, and wound closure. Selection of the preferred material is based on the following factors:

- The patient's history and physical with special attention paid to any preexisting conditions that may directly impact the rate and quality of wound healing
- The surgical procedure being performed and the type of tissues involved
- The desired method of tissue re-approximation
- Suture material availability
- Cost of the product
- The surgeon's preference (influenced by the area of specialization, knowledge of suture characteristics, professional experience, and influence during training)

Regarding disease processes, pathologies that directly impact suture choice include diabetes mellitus, dysfunction of the pituitary gland, immunological diseases, and localized and systemic infection. Each of these disorders alters the patient's normal metabolic function and can affect body tissues and retard the natural healing process. Additionally, the patient's age, weight, metabolism, nutritional status, level of hydration, tissue thickness, presence of edema, amount of necrotic tissue or foreign body in the wound, and incision type are considered.

Ideal Suture Characteristics. Due to the many variables that are considered during wound closure and suture selection, sutures are available in a myriad of configurations, materials, sizes, and textures. The search is still underway for the perfect suture type whose characteristics are ideal for all applications. In a perfect world, the ideal suture material would have the following characteristics:

- High tensile strength and a small diameter to minimize the amount of foreign body in the wound yet provide enough strength to adequately hold wound edges together during healing
- Rapid absorption of the suture material once healing has occurred
- A diameter that is uniform and consistent
- Sterile to prevent the introduction of microbial contaminants into the wound
- Pliable and easy to handle to allow for smooth passage through the tissues with minimal cellular damage and secure knot tying
- Inert without risk of inflammatory, allergic, infectious, or other reaction
- Inexpensive

Though this ideal suture material does not exist, combinations of many of these characteristics can be found in available materials. The general properties of suture materials are grouped into three categories that include physical, handling, and tissue reaction characteristics.

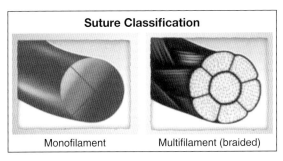

Suture Classification

Monofilament   Multifilament (braided)

Figure 10-6 · Monofilament (**A**) and multifilament (**B**) sutures. (Reproduced with permission from Needles & Sutures in Ophthalmic Plastic. Sheriff Elwan.)

Physical Characteristics. The physical characteristics of suture are those properties that affect its size, strength, and presentation. Such characteristics can be measured or objectively determined and are outlined by the United States Pharmacopeia (USP) as follows:

Configuration: Suture configuration plays an important role in determining such properties as its tensile strength, tissue reactivity, and handling within the wound. Individual sutures are classified by the number of fibers they contain. There are two types of suture configurations: monofilament and multifilament.

Monofilament sutures: Monofilament sutures (see Figure 10-6A) consist of a single filament or strand of fiber along their entire length. When passed through wound layers and body structures, the consistent, uniform nature of the strand elicits minimal resistance and enables these sutures to glide almost effortlessly through the tissues. Because monofilament sutures have a smooth, nonporous surface, bacteria are unable to wick along the suture line. As a result, postoperative wound infection risks are minimized. Wicking is the process by which tissue fluids and microorganisms are absorbed into the suture and carried along the length of the strands in much the same manner as lamp oil is carried along a wick.

Although these sutures are relatively inert and perform well within the body, they are difficult to handle because of increased memory.

Knot security is a concern due to slippage. Handling of monofilament suture materials with instruments such as hemostatic clamps or needle holders should be avoided as the strands are more prone to crushing than multifilament configurations. Crushing of the strand compromises its integrity and tensile strength, leading to breakage and wound disruption. Sutures of this configuration are preferred in vascular surgery.

Multifilament sutures: Sutures comprised of multiple filaments or strands that are braided or twisted together along their length are categorized as multifilament sutures (see Figure 10-6B). Combining several strands together in this manner increases the tensile strength, pliability, and flexibility of the suture material. Multifilament sutures drag when passed through body tissues and may be coated to decrease resistance. The uneven surface of the suture may also cause the strands to saw and cut through tissues if tied under excess pressure. Additionally,

bacteria can easily wick across the braided strands. For this reason, multifilament suture use should be avoided in the skin (due to the presence of resident and transient microbes) or in the presence of infection. Coated multifilament sutures are commonly used during procedures involving the intestines.

Absorption: Sutures are also classified by their ability or inability to absorb within the body. Absorption involves the process by which the suture material is digested by enzymatic activity or broken down by water within the tissue fluids, a chemical reaction known as hydrolyzation.

Absorbable sutures: Absorbable sutures are derived from mammalian collagen, surgical gut, or synthetic polymers such as glycolic acid. The general principle behind absorbable sutures is to provide temporary support for the wound until it is able withstand disruption and dehiscence. Strands may be treated to withstand absorption over an extended period and effectively retain their tensile strength during the critical stages of wound healing. Absorbable sutures may also be colored or dyed for visibility within the tissues. Synthetic absorbable suture materials are absorbed through the process of hydrolyzation. This form of absorption offers reduced tissue reactivity when compared to the enzymatic breakdown of natural absorbable materials. Maintenance of suture strand tensile strength during healing is not necessarily dependent on the rate of absorption. Some materials lose tensile strength rapidly and absorb slowly, while others retain tensile strength until the wound is healed and absorbed quickly thereafter. Regardless of the specific mechanism, complete absorption leaves no visible trace of the suture within the wound. Some limitations of absorbable suture include the following:

- Acceleration of absorption rate is noted in patients with protein deficiency and active infection.
- Premature absorption can ensue if sutures are wet or moistened prior to use.
- Absorption rate is retarded in patients suffering from physiologic conditions that cause delayed healing.

Nonabsorbable sutures: Nonabsorbable sutures resist enzymatic and hydrolytic activity and remain within the body for an indefinite period of time. These nonbiodegradable materials are walled off by fibroblasts and become encapsulated within the tissues. Nonabsorbable materials may be coated to reduce capillarity and resistance when passing through tissue layers. Coating options include Teflon, silicone, and polymers. Like absorbable varieties, they may be dyed to increase strand visibility in the presence of blood and tissue fluids. Nonabsorbable sutures are commonly used for skin closure and the stitches must be removed postoperatively. Additional applications include patients who are sensitive to absorbable materials, those with a history of keloid formation, and the attachment of prosthetics. The various nonabsorbable suture materials are classified into three distinct categories by the USP.

- Class I nonabsorbable sutures consist of silk and synthetic monofilament or multifilament fibers.
- Class II nonabsorbable sutures include cotton, linen fibers, natural coated fibers, and synthetic fibers. Added coating

USP Size	11-0	10-0	9-0	8-0	7-0	6-0	5-0	4-0	3-0	2-0	0	1	2	3	4	5	6
TABLE 10-1 • METRIC MEASURES AND USP SUTURE DIAMETER EQUIVALENTS																	
Natural Collagen	-	0.2	0.3	0.5	0.7	1.0	1.5	2.0	3.0	3.5	4.0	5.0	6.0	7.0	8.0	-	-
Synthetic Absorbables	-	0.2	0.3	0.4	0.5	0.7	1.0	1.5	2.0	3.0	3.5	4.0	5.0	6.0	6.0	7.0	-
Nonabsorbable Materials	0.1	0.2	0.3	0.4	0.5	0.7	1.0	1.5	2.0	3.0	3.5	4.0	5.0	6.0	6.0	7.0	8.0

Note: Metric conversions are provided in millimeters. For example, size 9-0 natural collagen suture has a diameter of 0.3 mm.

may augment the diameter of these sutures but may not contribute significantly to their tensile strength.

- Class III nonabsorbable sutures are monofilament or multi-filament metal wire such as surgical stainless steel.

Capillarity: The ability of fluid to travel along suture strands is known as suture capillarity. The wicking of infectious microorganisms is directly related to capillarity.

Suture Tensile Strength: Suture tensile strength refers to the amount of pressure (breaking load) that can be applied to a strand before it breaks. This measurement differs by suture material and diameter.

Diameter: Commonly referred to as size, diameter is a measurement of the thickness of the suture. As stated by Halsted, the smallest diameter suture capable of providing sufficient tensile strength during wound healing should be used. This logic is based on the idea that minimal foreign suture material left inside the wound will decrease the risk of tissue reactivity. Also, smaller suture diameters cause less cellular trauma when passed through tissues. Suture diameter is expressed numerically in USP sizes 11-0 (smallest diameter) to #7 (largest diameter). Table 10-1 provides a chart of USP numeric diameter values and their relationship to metric measurements by suture type.

Knot Strength: The tensile strength of the knot is a measurement of the force (in pounds) that can be applied to the tied suture before disruption or breakage of the knot occurs.

Elasticity: The ability of suture to regain its original form and length after stretching is referred to as its elasticity.

Memory: Suture memory is the inherent ability of the material to return to its previous shape following manipulation and reformation. Sutures with high memory are difficult to knot securely because the suture tends to unravel back to its original shape following tying.

Handling Characteristics. Properties related to the manner in which the suture bends (pliability) and passes through the tissue (friction coefficient) are referred to as handling characteristics. Handling of the suture is an important factor in reducing the amount of cellular damage within tissues due to resistance or tissue drag and the ability to tie and seat secure knots.

Pliability: The ability of the suture to bend while being manipulated and tied is referred to as its pliability. Pliability is directly related to the nature of the suture material, its diameter, and the type of filament. Pliable sutures offer significant advantages such as ease of handling and the ability to secure and adjust knot tension.

Friction Coefficient: Suture friction coefficient refers to the amount of friction or tissue drag that is experienced as the suture is passed through the wound layers. High friction coefficient sutures have increased drag and require the application of additional force to pull them through the tissue. Such resistance causes friction against tissue cells which can lead to localized damage. Additionally, knot tying is more difficult when the friction coefficient of the suture material is high. To reduce these complications and improve handling, suture strands may be coated. It is important that the correct balance between low and high friction coefficients is met because sutures with too little resistance are prone to unraveling the knot.

Tissue Reaction Characteristics. Once suture material is introduced into the body it is recognized as foreign invading material by the body's natural immunologic defense mechanisms. As such, each one of the various suture materials elicits varying degrees of tissue reactivity as the body attempts to neutralize it. From the moment the suture passes through the tissues, cell destruction occurs, and the inflammatory response system is activated. By the seventh postoperative day, chronic inflammation ensues and lasts until the material is either absorbed or encapsulated. Suture materials with the highest degree of tissue reactivity include nonabsorbable silk and cotton and absorbable gut. Minimal reactivity is noted with polypropylene (nonabsorbable) and poliglecaprone (absorbable) materials.

Suture Material: As noted previously, suture materials are classified by configuration and into two broad categories based on how they react to body tissues: absorbable and nonabsorbable. Suture materials are further divided into synthetic or natural groups depending on the source of the material used to construct them. Natural sutures include those created from raw materials found in nature, for example, natural metals, animal products (cellulose), and natural fibers such as cotton and silk. Man-made materials are classified as synthetic materials. Examples of these include petroleum-based polymers.

Tables 10-2 and 10-3 list additional information related to widely utilized suture materials and their individual properties. A brief description of each is provided here.

TABLE 10-2 • COMPARISON OF ABSORBABLE SUTURE TYPES AND CHARACTERISTICS	
Absorbable Sutures	
Suture Type	**Characteristics**
Plain gut	**Trade name:** None **Configuration:** Monofilament **Raw Material:** Natural – beef and sheep intestinal collagen **Tensile strength:** Complete loss at 7-10 days depending on the presence of tissue fluids and patient- related factors **Absorption:** Proteolytic enzymatic action – complete around 70 days **Level of tissue reactivity:** Moderate **Contraindications:** Patients with known allergy or sensitivity, wounds requiring long-term support, cardiovascular and neurological tissues **Frequent uses:** General ligation and soft tissue approximation, ophthalmic procedures **Handling:** Fair **Knot security:** Poor **Package color:** Yellow
Chromic gut	**Trade name:** None **Configuration:** Monofilament **Raw Material:** Natural – beef and sheep intestinal collagen treated with chromium salt solution **Tensile strength:** Complete loss at 10-14 days depending on the presence of tissue fluids and patient- related factors **Absorption:** Proteolytic enzymatic action – complete around 90 days **Level of tissue reactivity:** Moderate **Contraindications:** Patients with known allergy or sensitivity, wounds requiring long-term support, cardiovascular and neurological tissues **Frequent uses:** General ligation and soft tissue approximation, ophthalmic procedures **Handling:** Fair **Knot security:** Fair **Package color:** Tan

(Continued)

TABLE 10-2 • COMPARISON OF ABSORBABLE SUTURE TYPES AND CHARACTERISTICS (*Continued*)	
Polyglactin 910	**Trade name:** Vicryl (Ethicon) **Configuration:** Coated monofilament and multifilament **Raw Material:** Synthetic – lactide and glycolide copolymer coated with 370 and calcium stearate **Tensile strength:** Approximately 75% remaining at 14 days, 50% at 21 days, 25% at 28 days **Absorption:** Hydrolysis – complete around 56-70 days **Level of tissue reactivity:** Minimal acute inflammation **Contraindications:** Wounds requiring long-term support, cardiovascular and neurological tissues **Frequent uses:** General ligation and soft tissue approximation, ophthalmic procedures **Handling:** Good **Knot security:** Good **Package color:** Violet
Fast-absorbing polyglactin 910	**Trade name:** Vicryl *Rapide* (Ethicon) **Configuration:** Multifilament **Raw Material:** Synthetic – lactide and glycolide copolymer coated with 370 and calcium **Tensile strength:** Approximately 50% remaining at 5 days, 0% at 14 days **Absorption:** Hydrolysis – complete by 42 days **Level of tissue reactivity:** Minimal to moderate acute inflammation **Contraindications:** Patients with known allergy or sensitivity; wounds requiring long-term support beyond 7 days; ophthalmic, cardiovascular, and neurological tissues **Frequent uses:** Approximation of skin and mucosa specifically **Handling:** Excellent **Knot security:** Good **Package color:** Red

TABLE 10-2 • (*Continued*)	
Poliglecaprone 25	**Trade name:** Monocryl (Ethicon) **Configuration:** Monofilament **Raw Material:** Synthetic - glycolide and epsilon-caprolactone copolymer **Tensile strength:** Approximately 50-60% remaining at 7 days, 20-30% at 14 days, 0% at 21 days **Absorption:** Hydrolysis – complete by 91-119 days **Level of tissue reactivity:** Minimal acute inflammation **Contraindications:** Wounds requiring long-term support, undyed contraindicated for fascial closure, ophthalmic and microsurgical applications, cardiovascular and neurological tissues **Frequent uses:** General ligation and soft tissue approximation **Handling:** Excellent **Knot security:** Good **Package color:** Coral
Polydioxanone	**Trade name:** PDS II (Ethicon) **Configuration:** Monofilament **Raw Material:** Synthetic – polymer of polyester **Tensile strength:** Approximately 70% remaining at 14 days, 50% at 28 days, 25% at 42 days **Absorption:** Hydrolysis – significant absorption delayed until day 90, complete by 6 months **Level of tissue reactivity:** Slight **Contraindications:** Wounds requiring long-term support, fixation of prosthetics, adult cardiovascular tissues, neurological tissues, microsurgical applications **Frequent uses:** All soft tissue approximation, pediatric ophthalmic and cardiovascular applications **Handling:** Good **Knot security:** Good **Package color:** Silver

TABLE 10-3 • COMPARISON OF NONABSORBABLE SUTURE TYPES AND CHARACTERISTICS	
Nonabsorbable Sutures	
Suture Type	**Characteristics**
Silk	**Trade name:** Perma-Hand (Ethicon), Sofsilk (Syneture) **Configuration:** Multifilament **Raw Material:** Natural – organic fibrin protein **Tensile strength:** Lost over time due to progressive degradation of fibers **Absorption:** Hydrolysis – gradual encapsulation by fibrous connective tissue **Level of tissue reactivity:** Acute inflammation **Contraindications:** Patients with known allergy or sensitivity **Frequent uses:** General ligation and soft tissue approximation; cardiovascular, neurologic, and ophthalmic procedures **Handling:** Good **Knot security:** Good **Package color:** Light blue
Surgical stainless steel	**Trade name:** None **Configuration:** Monofilament, multifilament **Raw Material:** Natural – 316L stainless steel **Tensile strength:** Indefinite **Absorption:** None **Level of tissue reactivity:** Minimal acute inflammation **Contraindications:** Patients with known allergy or sensitivity to stainless steel, chromium, or nickel **Frequent uses:** Closure of the abdominal wall and sternum, orthopedics including tendon repair and cerclage **Handling:** Poor **Knot security:** Good **Package color:** Yellow-ochre (mustard)

TABLE 10-3 • (Continued)	
Nylon	**Trade name:** Ethilon (Ethicon) **Configuration:** Monofilament **Raw Material:** Synthetic – long-chain aliphatic polymers of Nylon 6 or Nylon 6,6 **Tensile strength:** Lost over time due to progressive degradation of fibers **Absorption:** Gradual encapsulation by fibrous connective tissue **Level of tissue reactivity:** Minimal acute inflammation **Contraindications:** Wounds requiring long-term support **Frequent uses:** General ligation and soft tissue approximation; ophthalmic, cardiovascular, and neurosurgical procedures **Handling:** Poor **Knot security:** Poor **Package color:** Mint green
Braided nylon	**Trade name:** Nurolon (Ethicon); Dermalon, Surgilon, Monosof (Syneture) **Configuration:** Multifilament **Raw Material:** Synthetic – long-chain aliphatic polymers of Nylon 6 or Nylon 6,6 **Tensile strength:** Lost over time due to progressive degradation of fibers **Absorption:** Gradual encapsulation by fibrous connective tissue **Level of tissue reactivity:** Minimal acute inflammation **Contraindications:** Wounds requiring long-term support **Frequent uses:** General ligation and soft tissue approximation; ophthalmic, cardiovascular, and neurosurgical procedures **Handling:** Fair **Knot security:** Fair **Package color:** Mint green

(Continued)

TABLE 10-3 • COMPARISON OF NONABSORBABLE SUTURE TYPES AND CHARACTERISTICS (*Continued*)	
Polyester fiber	**Trade name:** Mersilene (Ethicon), Surgidac (Syneture) **Configuration:** Monofilament, multifilament **Raw Material:** Synthetic – poly (ethylene terephthalate) **Tensile strength:** Significant loss not noted **Absorption:** Gradual encapsulation by fibrous connective tissue **Level of tissue reactivity:** Minimal acute inflammation **Contraindications:** None known **Frequent uses:** General ligation and soft tissue approximation; ophthalmic, cardiovascular, and neurosurgical procedures **Handling:** Good **Knot security:** Good **Package color:** Turquoise
Excel polyester fiber	**Trade name:** Ethibond (Ethicon), Ti-Cron (Syneture) **Configuration:** Multifilament **Raw Material:** Synthetic – polybutilate-coated poly (ethylene terephthalate) **Tensile strength:** Significant loss not noted **Absorption:** Gradual encapsulation by fibrous connective tissue **Level of tissue reactivity:** Minimal acute inflammation **Contraindications:** None known **Frequent uses:** General ligation and soft tissue approximation; ophthalmic, cardiovascular, and neurosurgical procedures **Handling:** Good **Knot security:** Good **Package color:** Orange

TABLE 10-3 • (*Continued*)
Polypropylene	**Trade name:** Prolene, Pronova (Ethicon); Surgipro, Surgipro II (Syneture) **Configuration:** Monofilament **Raw Material:** Synthetic – isotactic crystalline stereoisomer of polypropylene **Tensile strength:** Not affected by enzymatic degradation **Absorption:** None **Level of tissue reactivity:** Minimal acute inflammation **Contraindications:** None known **Frequent uses:** General ligation and soft tissue approximation; ophthalmic, cardiovascular, and neurosurgical procedures **Handling:** Poor **Knot security:** Poor **Package color:** Deep blue

Natural absorbable suture materials: Natural absorbable sutures include monofilament surgical gut and collagen sutures made from highly purified animal collagen.

Surgical gut: During the manufacture of surgical gut sutures (commonly and erroneously referred to as catgut), collagen ribbons from beef intestinal serosa or sheep submucosal intestinal tissue are spun and formed into strands at concentrations of 97% to 98%. Tensile strength is determined by the total amount of collagen contained within each strand. Strands consisting of high levels of purified collagen are more inert than noncollagenous materials and less likely to cause foreign body tissue reactivity within the wound. However, the overall reactivity of surgical gut sutures is moderate to high. Because it is difficult to ensure a smooth, consistent diameter when spinning collagen into suture, uneven areas often appear on the surface of the strand and can fray during knot tying. Careful refinement during processing minimizes fraying and helps to ensure even tensile strength along the entire length of the suture. Plain and chromic varieties are available, each with different absorption rates and operative applications.

Plain gut sutures are made from untreated collagen ribbons that are rapidly absorbed within the body via enzymatic activity. During wound healing, tensile strength is maintained up to 7 to 10 days following implantation depending on the presence of tissue fluids (which speed absorption) and the patient's habitus. The absorption process is fully completed in approximately 70 days. Because of the rate at which plain gut is absorbed, it is ideal for approximation of the rapidly-healing tissues of the subcutaneous fat and for the ligation of superficial blood vessels. During healing, a marked inflammatory response is noted and sinus tract formation may result.

Chromic gut suture: It is treated with chromium salts that slow absorption by making the suture resistant to enzymatic breakdown. Tensile strength is extended to 10 to 14 days with total absorption of the material taking place around 90 days. However, absorption is increased in the presence of infection. Despite this increased timeframe, strands of chromic gut are less reactive than plain strands during early wound healing. Chromic gut is commonly used during approximation of the peritoneum and fascia, superficial vessel ligation, and procedures of the biliary and urinary tracts. Additional indications for chromic gut include vessel suture ligation and closure of the epidermis, oral mucosa, and tongue. Both plain and chromic gut sutures are packaged in alcohol solution to protect the strands from drying and maintain their integrity until the time of use. Surgical gut sutures can be dipped in tepid saline or sterile water just before use to reduce memory and restore pliability.

Collagen sutures: Collagen sutures have superior properties to surgical gut and are manufactured from refined collagen harvested from cattle tendon. They are commonly used during ophthalmic procedures.

Synthetic absorbable suture materials: Because they are specifically engineered to exhibit a wide range of desired characteristics, synthetic absorbable suture materials are utilized across all specialty surgical areas and for several diverse applications.

Polyglactin 910 (Vicryl): It is a coated copolymer of lactide and glycolide that has been routinely used throughout many specialties since its introduction in 1974. Its popularity is based primarily on its ability to retain tensile strength, up to 50% at 21 days postimplantation, for tissues requiring longer healing times. Its good handling characteristics, low friction coefficient, minimal tissue reactivity, ease of tying, and unparalleled knot security are also highly noteworthy. Polyglactin 910 is ideal for use in general soft tissue approximation and vessel ligation. A fast-absorbing variant, known as Vicryl *Rapide*, offers lower tissue reactivity than chromic gut and is best suited for applications in which tissues quickly heal such as episiotomy repair and skin closure. Like surgical silk, polyglactin 910 may cause suture spitting if placed too close to the surface of the skin.

Poliglecaprone 25: Poliglecaprone 25 (Monocryl), a copolymer of glycolide and epsilon-caprolactone, is a popular material that is absorbed predictably and is virtually inert within body tissues, causing minimal tissue reactivity. Its high initial tensile strength makes it an ideal suture for subcutaneous wound closure as well as soft tissue approximation and vessel ligation. It is contraindicated for use in microsurgical applications and procedures of the neural, vascular, and ophthalmic tissues.

Polydioxanone: Polydioxanone (PDS II) is a well-balanced suture for approximation of many types of soft tissue and can retain approximately 50% of its tensile strength by the fourth week following implantation. The slow absorption rate of polydioxanone makes it ideal for the closure of wounds requiring longer healing times. Common indications for its use include procedures of the digestive tract, colon, female pelvic anatomy, orthopedic and ophthalmic applications, plastic surgery, and pediatric cardiovascular intervention.

Polyglytone 6211: Polyglytone 6211 (Caprosyn) is a monofilament polyester material derived from glycolide, caprolactone, trimethylene carbonate, and lactide. This material offers the advantages of low tissue reactivity, 10-day wound support, and total absorption at 56 days. Polyglytone 6211 is commonly used as a subcuticular skin suture and is appropriate for general soft tissue approximation excluding cardiovascular, neurologic, ophthalmic, and microsurgical applications. Its use should be carefully considered in wounds requiring more than the indicated 10 days of tensile support as postoperative wound dehiscence is a concern.

Glycomer 631: Synthesized from glycolide, dioxanone, and trimethylene carbonate, glycomer 631 (Biosyn) is a monofilament polyester fiber that maintains adequate tensile strength and wound support through the 21st postoperative day. Complete absorption of the material is anticipated between 90 and 110 days following implantation once hydrolysis is complete. Glycomer 631 is indicated for general approximation and ligation of soft tissues and for use in ophthalmic tissues. As with any absorbable material, wound dehiscence is possible if tissue healing is delayed.

Polyglyconate: Polyglyconate (Maxon) is a monofilament suture material consisting of glycolic acid and trimethylene carbonate copolymer. It is commonly used to approximate soft tissue, pediatric cardiovascular structures, and tissues of the peripheral vascular system. Its use is contraindicated in adult cardiovascular applications. Polyglyconate provides extended wound support for up to 6 weeks and is completely absorbed in approximately 6 months.

Polyglycolic acid: A similar material to polyglactin 910, polyglycolic acid (Dexon, Dexon II) sutures maintain 50% tensile strength for up to 21 days with minimal tissue reactivity. Absorption is minimal for up to 40 days postoperatively and complete within 60 to 90 days. Because polyglycolic acid retains tensile strength and withstands apportion for an extended time, it is very popular and widely utilized for the approximation of tissues requiring long-term wound support and eventual absorption of the suture material. Introduced in 1970, polyglycolic acid is the oldest of the synthetic absorbable sutures. Common uses are general soft tissue approximation, vessel ligation, skin closure, and approximation of mucosa. Multifilament strands are most commonly used, though monofilament varieties are also available.

Natural nonabsorbable suture materials: Commonly used natural nonabsorbable suture materials include surgical silk, cotton, and surgical stainless steel. Given their nonabsorbable characteristics, these materials provide sustained support and tensile strength during each of the phases of wound healing.

Surgical silk: Surgical silk (Perma-Hand, Sofsilk) is unique to the nonabsorbable category. Rather than becoming indefinitely encapsulated by fibrous connective tissue once wound healing is complete, surgical silk is hydrolyzed and loses most or all of its tensile strength by 1 year following implantation. By the second postoperative year, it is virtually undetectable in the wound. Surgical silk suture is derived and processed from silkworm moth cocoons. Natural waxes and sericin gums are removed and the suture is braided or twisted, scoured, stretched, and colored black with vegetable dye to improve its visibility against the tissues. Strands are coated with waxes or silicone to improve handling. The characteristics of surgical silk make it the gold standard for handling and a formidable suture material by which many others are judged. Despite great handling, however, silk lacks significantly in tensile strength and knot security when compared to newer synthetic materials. Common applications include gastrointestinal serosa, infection-free fascia, and vessel ligation.

Although surgical silk is treated to decrease its capillarity, wicking of infectious microorganisms is a concern. Also, tracts may form within the wound during healing and cause suture migration. This phenomenon is referred to as suture spitting because the material will eventually be expelled from the body as the tracts reach the skin's surface. Suture spitting is not limited to silk; however, its reactive properties increase the likelihood of this occurrence.

Cotton: The use of surgical cotton as a suturing material has fallen out of favor as other newly introduced fibers have rendered it virtually obsolete. Cotton umbilical tapes are still utilized for the retraction and manipulation of anatomic structures and the isolation of vessels or ducts.

Surgical stainless steel: Surgical stainless steel (316L) is a very minimally reactive and flexible suture material that offers the advantages of extremely high tensile strength and secure knotting in the form of a fine wire that is compatible with many surgical implants and prostheses. It is widely used throughout orthopedics and neurosurgery for applications such as cerclage wiring of the femur and fixation of osteotomies. Additional uses include sternal wiring following midline sternotomy and abdominal wound closure. Despite its advantages, surgical stainless steel exhibits poor handling characteristics. The use of specialty instrumentation such as pliers and wire cutters is required to manipulate and place sutures and properly seat knots. Stainless steel wires may barb or break, posing an injury risk to adjacent tissues and surgical team members. Because it does not display elastic properties within the tissues, cutting, tearing, or pulling of the wire through the wound layers is possible. Buckling may result from asymmetrical fracture fixation. Due to the possibility of metallurgic reaction, stainless steel should not be used in the presence of other metals such as titanium.

Synthetic nonabsorbable suture materials: Synthetic nonabsorbable sutures include various options derived from polymers such as nylon, polyester, and polypropylene.

Nylon: Surgical nylon (Ethilon, Nurolon, Dermalon, Surgilon, Monosof) is synthesized from polyamide polymers and offers limited tissue reactivity and superb elasticity. Monofilament varieties are frequently used for skin closure and preserving of suture lines. Multifilament nylon sutures lend intermediate tensile strength to healing tissues and handle in much the same way as surgical silk but with less reactivity. Most configurations display characteristics of poor to fair handling due to high memory and difficult-to-achieve knot security. Some products are coated or pre-moistened to improve handling. Hydrolytic activities at the site of suture implantation cause nylon strands to degrade at a rate of approximately 15% to 20% per year, stabilizing around 2 years. Retained tensile strength at 11 years postimplantation has been estimated at two-thirds in some studies. Nylon is manufactured in sizes as small as 11-0, making it ideal for tissue approximation during ophthalmic procedures.

Polyester fiber: Polyester fiber sutures (Dacron, Ethibond, Mersilene, Polydek, Surgidac, Tevdek, Ti-cron) are the strongest nonabsorbable suture materials next to surgical stainless steel. In addition to their strength, they are minimally reactive, easy to handle (though not as easy as silk), provide excellent knot security, and resist the absorption of tissue fluids. Sutures are available as untreated strands or may be coated with Teflon or impregnated with silicone to decrease tissue drag by lowering the friction coefficient. Knot security is compromised in treated varieties. Common usage includes general soft tissue approximation requiring extended wound support, tendon repair, fascial closure, and cardiovascular, ophthalmic, and neurosurgical procedures.

Polypropylene: Polypropylene (Prolene, Pronova, Surgipro, Surgipro II) is a monofilament polymer of isotactic crystalline stereoisomer of polypropylene. Usage includes approximation of the soft tissues, cardiovascular applications including vessel anastomosis, ophthalmic procedures, and nervous tissues. Polypropylene sutures are monofilament, extremely inert, cause very little tissue reactivity, and are not affected by enzymatic activity. Thus, their use is ideal in the presence of infection.

Polybutester: Polybutester (Novafil, Vascufil) is a monofilament suture material consisting of glycol and butylene copolymers. High tensile strength with low tissue reactivity and the greatest elasticity of any suture are the hallmarks of this material. Polybutester strands are capable of stretching 50% of their length under a mere 25% of their knot-breaking level. This makes them very useful for wound closure in the presence of swelling and edema. Other typical applications include tissue requiring long-term tensile strength, anastomosis of blood vessels, and for subcuticular skin closure.

Barbed suture: The latest barbed, or knotless suture, was originally designed by Dr. John H. Alcamo, who presented his concept to the US Patent office on August 13, 1956, receiving US Patent number 3,123,077 on March 3, 1964, for a suture that would not slip. In 1967, Dr. A.R. McKenzie described its use in vitro in human cadavers and in vivo in dogs for the repair of long flexor tendons. Dr. Harry J. Buncke received US Patent 5,931,855 on August 3, 1999, for "several surgical procedures for binding together living tissue using one-way sutures having barbs on their exterior surfaces and a needle on one or both ends." His patents were obtained by Quill Medical. Quill™ Knotless Tissue-Closure Device (Angiotech Pharmaceuticals), received approval by the US Food and Drug Administration (FDA) in 2004. In 2009, Covidien announced V-Loc™ (Covidien Healthcare, Mansfield, Massachusetts) a unidirectional barbed suture with a fixed loop, and in 2013 both Angiotech Pharmaceuticals and Ethicon Endo-Surgery (Cincinnati, Ohio) introduced unidirectional barbed sutures with a variable loop at the end for facilitated fixation.

Suture Handling. Adherence to certain recommendations will prolong the life of suture materials and help to ensure their proper function within the wound. Recommended guidelines for the handling of sutures are as follows:

- Before opening packages, be sure to read all labels and verify that the correct suture is chosen for the task at hand.
- Make certain that sutures are not expired, and that on-hand stock is rotated regularly.
- Avoid waste by only opening those sutures that will be needed for the procedure.
- Do not rub or crush suture strands as doing so can cause damage to the fibers and may lead to suture breakage and wound disruption.
- Avoid excessive handling and sawing of suture strands against each other.
- Keep surgical gut away from heat during storage.
- Surgical gut may be moistened to restore pliability, but soaking causes suture degradation.
- Keep rapidly absorbing sutures dry to avoid premature breakdown.
- Silk must also remain dry until the time of implantation.
- Wetting sutures and tapes made from linen or cotton augments their strength.

TABLE 10-4 • GENERAL GUIDELINES FOR SUTURE REMOVAL BY ANATOMIC LOCATION	
Anatomic Location	**Removal by Number of Days Post Implantation**
Eyelid	2–3
Face	4–5
Neck	3–5
Scalp	7
Trunk	6–14
Extremities	10–21
Joints	14

- Bending of stainless-steel wire should be avoided.

- Synthetic monofilament sutures such as nylon may be drawn between the thumb and index finger to reduce memory.

- Proper loading of the needle holder is essential to minimizing suture and needle damage that can increase cellular insult and complicate wound healing.

Suture Removal. Once the wound regains sufficient tensile strength and can maintain integrity on its own, nonabsorbable skin sutures and some epidermal absorbables are removed. The timing of suture removal (see Table 10-4) is dependent on several factors that affect the rate of wound healing and include the amount of tension on the wound edges, the patient's nutritional status, prior history of radiation treatment or chemotherapy, and steroid use. Wound edges may need temporary reinforcement with adhesive surgical tapes to reduce tension as healing continues.

To reduce the risk of infection, sutures should be removed under aseptic and sterile conditions. Since many patients have their sutures removed during a postoperative follow-up visit at their doctor's office, suture removal trays are available to facilitate the process. The general procedural steps for the removal of sutures are as follows:

Step 1 – A sterile field is created in anticipation of the procedure and sterile gloves are donned.

Step 2 – The wound is prepped with an antiseptic skin prep solution and dried serum may be removed using hydrogen peroxide.

Step 3 – The suture is grasped with forceps at the end opposite to the knot and elevated away from the skin.

Step 4 – Scissors are used to cut the suture as close to the skin as possible.

Step 5 – Grasping the suture with forceps at the side containing the knot, the suture is gently pulled through the skin. Note: Portions of the suture that have resided outside the skin should not be pulled back through the wound. Doing so causes flora from the skin's surface to be transplanted into the wound.

Step 6 – A sterile dressing is applied according to preference.

Surgical Needles

The general purpose of the surgical needle is to provide a medium for the passage of suture strands through body tissues. The ideal needle facilitates tissue approximation with minimal trauma. Surgical needles are manufactured from high-quality surgical stainless steel to provide rigidity and withstand manipulation by surgical instrumentation. Additionally, needles must be:

- Sharp and able to pass through tissue multiple times with minimal resistance;

- Strong and firm to resist deformation yet pliable enough to bend and resist breakage under excessive force;

- Of the smallest diameter possible to decrease cellular damage when passing through tissue;

- Thick enough in diameter to carry the desired suture and maintain rigidity;

- Appropriate in size, shape, and configuration for the intended tissues;

- Smooth and consistent without surface burrs or pits that can transport bacteria into the wound;

- Stable and firm within the jaws of the needle holder; and

- Corrosion-resistant and able to withstand sterilization processes.

Needle Size. Needles are available in many different sizes and lengths and are measured according to their chord length, needle length, radius, and diameter (see Figure 10-7).

Chord Length: The distance from the point of a curved needle to its eye or swage is referred to as its chord length.

Needle Length: Needle length is the total length of the needle along its body or shank from eye to point.

Radius: The radius of the needle is used to describe its total curvature. It is measured from the theoretical center of the curvature (if the needle were a complete circle) to the body of the needle.

Diameter: Needle diameter is used to describe the thickness or gauge of the needle. A general principle of needle selection is to choose a diameter that matches the size or thickness of the tissues to be sutured. For example, very fine diameters are typically used for microsurgical small vessel and nerve procedures, and very large diameters are used for approximation of heavy tissues such as the abdominal wall and sternum.

Needle Performance. The ability of a needle to exhibit each of the characteristics mentioned above is known as its

Surgical Needle

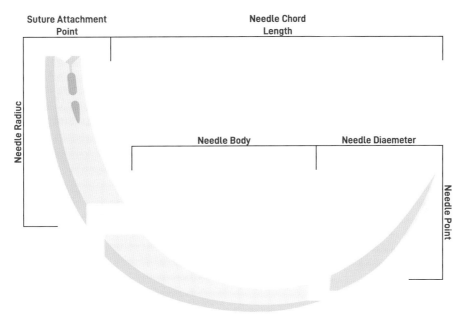

Figure 10-7 · Surgical needle anatomy. (Used with permission from Inspiring.team/Shutterstock)

performance. Needle performance is judged based on strength, ductility, sharpness, and clamping moment.

Strength: The ability of a needle to pass through tissue multiple times while resisting deformation and breakage is known as its strength. Strength is measured by two factors: the needle's ultimate moment and its surgical-yield moment.

Ultimate moment: The ultimate moment is the moment at which sufficient force is applied to the needle to bend it to 90°. The measurement of the amount of force required to reach this point determines the needle's maximum strength. Bending during approximation can lead to compromised wound closure, tissue trauma, and increased risk of needle stick injury.

Surgical-yield moment: The surgical-yield moment is determined by the amount of angular deformation the needle can withstand before being permanently damaged. This is the most important measure of strength to the surgeon and surgical assistant. Typical needles can withstand 10° to 30° of angulation. Reshaping deformed needles is contraindicated as this practice renders them more likely to break. Broken needles may cause excessive tissue trauma. Pieces of the needle may become lodged within tissue or lost within the wound. Although intact needles are detectable with radiography, small portions of needles are less likely to be found.

Ductility: Ductility is the needle's ability to bend (pliability) without breaking. Ductile needles are rigid and resistant to breakage, yet pliable enough to bend in the presence of excessive force. The ductility of a needle can be increased by heat treatment during manufacturing.

Sharpness: The sharpness of the needle is affected by its angle, type of point, and taper ratio. Taper ratio is a comparison of the length of the taper to the diameter of the needle. Sharp needles resist friction and drag when passing through body tissues and are more likely to leave a cosmetically acceptable scar in their wake. Decreased resistance helps minimize tissue damage caused as the needle cuts, dissects, or pushes its way through the wound layers. Some needles are coated with silicone to increase sharpness and maintain the point during repeated use.

Clamping Moment: Needle clamping moment is a measurement of the needle's interaction with the needle holder and stability in its jaws. Needles must be easy to manipulate, grasp, and push to ensure ease of handling, accurate placement, and minimal tissue damage. A poor clamping moment causes the needle to slip, twist, rock, or turn during tissue approximation. Many needles have flattened bodies that facilitate their manipulation with surgical instruments. Heavier needles are also ribbed to allow for cross-locking within the jaws of the needle holder.

Needle Components. No one universal needle exhibits the ideal requirements and characteristics for every tissue within the body. Just as many suture varieties and configurations abound to fulfill a number of specific purposes, surgical needles are equally as varied. Despite their many differences, each surgical needle has the following major components: eye, body, and point (see Figure 10-8).

Eye: The eye of the needle is the point of fixation for the suture strand. Needle eyes are available in three configurations including closed eye, French eye, and swaged or eyeless.

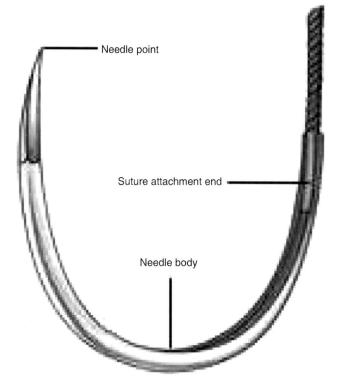

Figure 10-8 · Needle components. (Reproduced with permission from Wu K, Ni J, Wu D, Wang L. Design and Selection of Surgical Suturing Materials. In: Tang P, Wu K, Fu Z, Chen H, Zhang Y, eds. *Tutorials in Suturing Techniques for Orthopedics.* Springer; 2021.)

Closed-eye needle: Closed-eye needle has a round, oblong, or square opening through which the suture is threaded in the same manner as a household sewing needle. Threading is accomplished by pulling one end of the suture strand 5 to 10 cm through the eye until it is approximately one-sixth the length of the opposite end. Threading the needle is a tedious process, especially when using multifilament sutures that can fray. There are several disadvantages to the use of closed-eye needles. The most significant disadvantage is that passing double-stranded suture through the wound increases resistance and leaves a tunnel through the tissues that are wider than the diameter of the suture strand. This may lead to bleeding or leakage of body fluids at the site of needle puncture. Closed-eye needles are not well suited for use with more than one suture strand because they become dull and weakened if used repeatedly. Although utilized to some degree in orthopedics and other specialties, the use of closed-eye needles has fallen out of favor since the advent of swaged needles.

French-eye needle: The French-eye or spring-eye needle improves upon the closed-eye needle design by incorporating a split or slitted eye that is quick and easy to load with suture. However, these needles are still bulky and subject to the same major disadvantages as closed-eye needle.

Swaged needle: Single-use needles that are pre-attached to suture strands by the manufacturer are known as swaged

needles. These needles are joined to the suture strand by one of two methods. For large-diameter needles, a hole is drilled into the needle and the suture is fitted within the needle to create a continuous unit with less bulk and minimal tissue resistance. Smaller diameter needles are attached to the suture via a channel that is crimped around the strand to secure it in place. Some swaged needles incorporate a control release feature that enables them to be quickly removed from the suture with a gentle tug, thus eliminating the need to cut the suture to remove the needle. Advantages of swaged needles include the following:

- Pre-attachment of the suture eliminates the need to choose a separate needle when selecting wound closure materials.
- Swaged sutures may be loaded directly from the package with minimal handling as eyes do not have to be threaded. Tissue trauma is reduced because the needle diameter is equal to or smaller than the diameter of the suture, minimizing bulk.
- A new, sharp, and reliable needle accompanies each strand of suture material.
- Premature unthreading during suturing is eliminated.
- Dropped needles are easily found by identifying the tail of the suture strand.
- Personnel and equipment costs are reduced as swaged needles do not require reprocessing and sharpening.
- Swaged needles allow for rapid wound closure, especially when control-release sutures are used.
- Fraying of suture material is reduced.

Body: Located between the eye and the point, the body or shaft is the part of the needle that is grasped within the jaws of the needle holder. Ideally, the body of the needle should be smaller or of the same diameter as the suture strand to prevent leakage from vessel and bowel anastomoses, suture lines of the urinary and alimentary tracts, and needle puncture sites of other fluid-filled structures. Many different diameters are available to facilitate the placement of each size, type, and configuration of suture. The body may have a round, oval, flat, or triangular configuration that matches the shape of the point. Body characteristics vary depending on their curvature.

Straight needle: Straight needles have the appearance of typical sewing needles and are indicated for the closure of tissues that are easy to access and manipulate manually. Straight needles are designed to be held in the hand and passed through tissue without the aid of a needle holder. Direct finger manipulation gives the user added control and stability. Thus, straight needles are preferred by some microsurgeons for the repair of small nerves and vessels. Examples of this needle body type include the Keith needle, a cutting needle used primarily for abdominal wound skin closure, and the tapered Bunnell needle for gastrointestinal procedure.

Half-curved needle: Half-curved (ski) needles feature a curved point, straight body and eye, and a low profile that enable their easy passage through laparoscopic trocars. They are also used to a limited degree during skin closure; however, they are difficult to handle without bending or causing unnecessary tissue trauma as the straight portion of the body is pushed through the path cut by the curved tip.

Curved needle: The most widely utilized of all body types is the curved needle. The popularity of these needles is due to their versatility, maneuverability, predictable tissue turnout, and even distribution of tension on the tissue edges during wound closure. Curved needles require the use of a needle holder to manipulate and push them through tissue. They are passed through tissues following the curve of the needle body by gently pronating the wrist once the tip pierces the desired tissue. Many of these needles have longitudinal serrations that cross-hatch with the jaws of the needle holder for added security.

Others may be flattened through the body to facilitate proper placement of the needle during reloading of the needle holder. Curved needles are available in 1/4-, 3/8-, 1/2-, and 5/8-inch circle configurations. The skin is most commonly approximated using 3/8-circle needles. These needles are not generally used intra-abdominally because too much space is needed to manipulate the curve of the needle. Approximation within confined areas is best achieved using the 1/2-circle needle, although the tip is easily obscured within deep body cavities and thick tissues. Therefore, the most common application for the 5/8-circle needle is pelvic genitourinary procedures, closure of fascial incisions following laparoscopy, and for use within deep structures such as the anus and oral cavity. Choosing a curvature that is great enough to match the thickness of the tissues and allow for the tip of the needle to be seen when passed through the wound layers is the key principle of curved needle selection.

Compound curve needle: Used in ophthalmic surgery for procedures of the anterior segment of the eye, the compound curve needle ensures even closure of the corneal-scleral junction and decreases postoperative incidence of astigmatism.

Point: The point of the needle is located opposite the eye and is the portion used to pierce or penetrate tissue. Points vary in sharpness and configuration and are designed to match the consistency of the tissues for which they are intended to perforate. Surgical needles are available with either cutting, tapered, or blunt points (see Figure 10-9).

Cutting point: The razor-sharp point of the cutting needle is specifically designed to penetrate tough, thick, irregular, and highly dense connective tissues such as the skin, oral mucosa, tendon sheath, periosteum, perichondrium, and sclera. Care should be taken when approximating tendon and oral mucosa as the highly sharpened edges of the needle can cut through more tissue than desired. Cutting needles are available in several configurations, each having at least two opposing cutting edges.

Conventional cutting needles are triangular. The sharpness of the two cutting edges of the point is augmented by a third

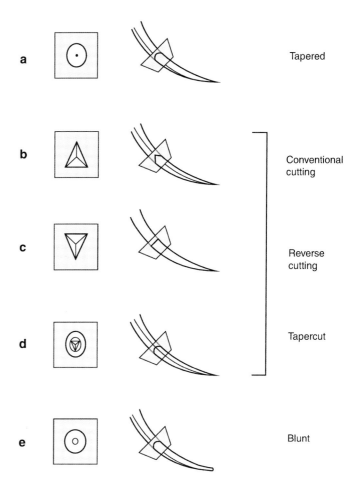

Figure 10-9 · Basic needle point options. (Reproduced with permission from Latona JA, Tannouri S, Palazzo F, Pucci MJ. Fundamentals of Sutures, Needles, Knot Tying, and Suturing Technique. In: Palazzo F, eds. *Fundamentals of General Surgery*. Springer; 2018.)

cutting surface along its inner concave curvature. The body of the needle is flattened to facilitate manipulation within the jaws of the needle holder and reduce bending. The streamlined design allows for the creation of a small, rapidly-healing tunnel through which the suture is pulled. This enhances cosmesis and makes the conventional cutting needle ideal for skin closure. The sternum is commonly closed with a conventional cutting needle with properties that reduce bending and enhance sharpness to ease its passage through bone. A disadvantage of the conventional cutting needle is the possibility of suture pullout. Because the edges of the point cut toward the wound edges, excess tension on the sutures can cause them to pull through the tissues. The risk of suture pullout is significantly reduced when reverse-cutting needles are used.

Reverse-cutting needles are similar in design to conventional cutting needles but with one distinct difference. Rather than on the inside, the third cutting edge follows the outer convex curve of the needle. Since the third edge is away from the wound edges, a wall of tissue is left to protect against pullout.

Additional advantages include increased needle strength and excellent wound cosmesis, making them the needle of choice for many plastic surgeons. Reverse cutting needles are commonly used on the tough tissues of the skin, tendons, oral mucosa, and eye.

Side-cutting needles, also known as spatula needles, are designed for use in ophthalmology. Because they are relatively flat with the opposing cutting edges located on the sides of the needle, they are able to penetrate the tough tunics of the eye and separate the layers into planes without damaging deeper structures. Trocar point needles have three highly sharpened edges located directly at the point. They are designed to provide maximum cutting action with minimal trauma to the tissues.

Tapered point: Rather than cutting, tapered point needles penetrate and spread tissue. The round, tapered tip flattens to a rectangular shape along the body to prevent twisting in the needle holder and provide a firm gripping surface. These needles are ideal for softer tissues with minimal resistance, including abdominal viscera, bowel, dura mater, myocardium, peritoneum, and subcutaneous tissues. A variation of the tapered point needle, known as the taper-cut needle, adds the benefits of a cutting point to the round, tapered body design. Taper-cut needles are used for closure of dense connective tissues such as fascia, periosteum, and tendon.

Blunt point: Blunt point needles are specially designed tapered needles that are rounded at the tip to separate tissue without cutting or damaging cells. Blunt needles are indicated for use on friable tissues that tear or bleed easily such as the liver and kidneys. The atraumatic nature of the tip may also reduce the risk of needle-stick injury and is therefore preferred by some gynecologic and pelvic surgeons when working within deep cavities where space and visibility are limited.

Needle Identification. Surgical needles are classified by their differing characteristics. Needles vary according to size, configuration, point, and eye. For identification purposes, manufacturers assign codes to each needle class. Needle codes may be followed by whole numbers indicating their size. For example, the Ethicon needle code FS (For Skin) represents a class of 3/8-circle curved reverse-cutting needles with swaged eyes commonly used for skin approximation. Needle sizes in the FS series from largest to smallest include FSLX (For Skin Extra Large), FSL (For Skin Large), FS, FS-1, FS-2, and FS-3. Table 10-5 lists each of the Ethicon needle codes and their meanings. A conversion chart comparing common Ethicon and Syneture needle codes is found in Table 10-6.

Skin Staplers

The appeal of surgical skin stapling devices is neat, accurate, and uniform approximation of the skin edges with minimal tissue trauma in much less time than suturing. A variety of different stapler options is available and includes devices that deliver stainless steel epidermal or bioabsorbable subcuticular staples; however, each variation functions in much the same manner.

To close the wound using a standard epidermal skin stapler, the skin edges are grasped with Adson tissue forceps (or other fine forceps) by the assistant, carefully lined up, and slightly everted. The stapler operator then places the centerline indicator of the stapler directly over the midline of the incision at the level of the forceps. Ensuring that the stapler is level and perpendicular to the wound, the operator squeezes the handle and fires the staple across the skin edges. The assistant then advances the forceps and the process continues until the entire length of the wound is closed. Proper staple placement is indicated by a well-centered appearance and precise apposition of the wound edges. To facilitate closure of loose or wrinkly skin, the stapler operator may continue to hold pressure on the handle after the staple is fired and pull gentle axial traction to straighten the skin as the assistant replaces his forceps in anticipation of the next staple.

As the stapler fires, the legs of the staple puncture the skin and form a rectangular shape that maintains the integrity of the wound until sufficient tensile strength has been regained. Once adequate healing is achieved, the staples are removed. Staple removal is typically performed between the fifth and seventh postoperative day (depending on the location of the staples) and is facilitated by a special instrument. When using the staple remover (see Figure 10-10), complete crimping of the staple crossbar (portion bridging the wound edges) is required to reduce patient discomfort or pain. Because surgical skin staples do not stick to the skin as readily as suture, removal is often less painful. Cross-hatching of the skin is expected to be minimal because the staple is designed to float above the wound without placing downward pressure on the skin. Surgical skin staple use is indicated for the closure of uncomplicated scalp lacerations and non-facial linear lacerations caused by sharp objects (ie, surgical incisions).

Adhesive Tapes

Adhesive tapes are sterile strips used to approximate the edges of a minor laceration without the need for local anesthesia and suture placement. They are also commonly utilized in place of an epidermal suture line following subcuticular skin closure or to maintain tensile strength when skin stitches are removed

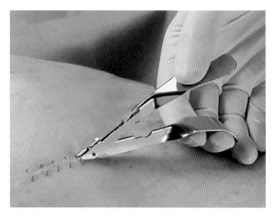

Figure 10-10 · Staple remover.

TABLE 10-5 • ETHICON NEEDLE CODES AND THEIR MEANINGS

Code	Meaning	Code	Meaning	Code	Meaning
BB	Blue Baby	FSLX	For Skin Extra Large	STB	Straight Blunt
BIF	Intraocular Fixation	G	Greishaber	STC	Straight Cutting
BN	Bunnell	GS	Greishaber Spatula	STP	Straight Taper Point
BP	Blunt Point	J	Conjunctive	TE	Three-Eights
BV	Blood Vessel	KS	Keith Straight	TF	Tetralogy of Fallot
BVH	Blood Vessel Half	LH	Large Half	TG	Transverse Ground
C	Cardiovascular	LR	Larger Retention	TGW	Transverse Ground Wide
CC	Calcified Coronary	LS	Large Sternotomy	TN	Trocar Needle
CCS	Conventional Cutting Sternotomy	M	Muscle	TP	Taper Pericostal/Point
CE	Cutting Edge	MF	Modified Furgusan	TPB	Taper Pericostal/Point Blunt
CFS	Conventional for Skin	MH	Medium Half (Circle)	TS	Tendon Straight
CIF	Cutting Intraocular Fixation	MO	Mayo	TQ	Twisty Q
CP	Cutting Point	MOB	Mayo Blunt	UCL	5/8 Circle Collateral Ligament
CPS	Conventional Plastic Surgery	OPS	Ocular Plastic Surgery	UR	Urology
CPX	Cutting Point Extra Large	OS	Orthopaedic Surgery	URB	Urology Blunt
CS	Corneal-Scleral	P	Plastic	V	Tapercut Surgical Needle
CSB	Corneal-Scleral Bi-Curve	PC	Precision Cosmetic	VAS	Vas Deferens
CSC	Corneal-Scleral Compound-Curve	PS	Plastic Surgery	X or P	Exodontal (Dental)
CT	Circle Taper	RB	Renal (Artery) Bypass	XLH	Extra Large Half (Circle)
CTB	Circle Taper Blunt	RD	Retinal Detachment	XXLH	Extra Extra Large Half (Circle)
CTX	Circle Taper Extra Large	RH	Round Half (Circle)		
CTXB	Circle Taper Extra Large Blunt	RV	Retinal-Vitreous		
CV	Cardiovascular	S	Spatula		
DC	Dura Closure	SC	Straight Cutting		
DP	Double Point	SFS	Spatulated for Skin		
EN	Endoscopic Needle	SH	Small Half (Circle)		
EST	Eyed Straight Taper	SIF	Ski Intraocular Fixation		
FN	For Tonsil	SKS	Sternotomy Keith Straight		
FS	For Skin	SM	Spatulated Module		
FSL	For Skin Large	ST	Straight Taper		

early. Because adhesive tapes bridge the wound edges without piercing the skin, they are associated with very low infection rates and tissue reactivity when compared to skin suturing or stapling. Adhesive tapes are contraindicated for wounds closed under tension or as the sole mechanism of wound closure.

Adhesive tapes are placed using sterile technique (see Figure 10-11). Once removed from the packaging, the card containing the tapes is cut if desired and the tab is removed to expose the end of the tapes. The tapes are peeled from the card diagonally using the fingers or a tissue forceps. The skin is dried, and the tapes are placed individually by adhering one end of the strip to the skin on either side of the wound at its midpoint. The opposing side of the wound is then brought into apposition and the remaining end of the tape is adhered to the skin under slight tension. Complete wound approximation is achieved by placing the tapes at 1/8-in intervals along the length of the incision. Additional tapes are applied parallel to the wound to prevent shearing and tape dislodgement. To ensure precise approximation and because the effectiveness of adhesive tapes is determined by the quality of the skin-to-tape

TABLE 10-6 • NEEDLE CONVERSION CART			
Ethicon	**Syneture**	**Ethicon**	**Syneture**
BB	CV-15	OS-4	HOS-10
BV	CV	OS-6	HOS-11
BV-1	CV-1	P-1	P-10
BV-75-4	MV-70-4	P-2	P-21
BV-100-4	MV-100-4	P-3	P-13
BV-130-5	MV-135-5	PC-1	PC-13
BV-175-6	MV-175-8	PC-3	PC-11
C-1	CV-11	PS-1	P-14
CC	KV-1	PS-2	P-12
CC-1	KV-11	PS-4	P-24
CCCS	SCC	PS-5	P-22
CP	GS-12	RB-1	CV-23
CP-1	GS-11	RB-2	CV-22
CS-160-6	SE-160-6	S-2	SS-2
CT	GS-24	S-14	SS-14
CT-1	GS-21, HGS-21	S-29	SS-29
CT-2	GS-22	SH	V-20, GS-22
CTX	GS-25	SH-1	CV-25
FN-2	GS-23	TF	CVF-21
FS	C-15	TG-140-8	SE-140-8
FS-1	C-14	TP-1	GS-26
FS-2	C-13	UR-5	GU-45
FSL	C-16	UR-6	GU-46
G-1	HE-1	V-4	KV-15
G-3	HE-3	V-5	KV-5
G-6	HE-6	V-7	KV-7
KS	CS-2	V-34	KV-34
MH	V-26	V-37	KV-37
MO-4, CT-1	GHS-21	V-40	KV-40
MO-6	HGS-22	X-1	C-23

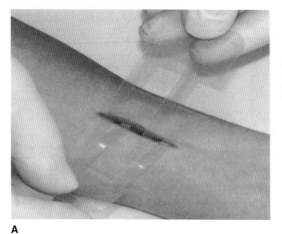
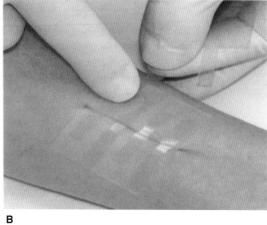

A   B

Figure 10-11 • Adhesive tape application. (Reproduced, with permission, from Tintinalli J, Stapczynski J, Ma O, Cline D, Cydulka R, Meckler G. *Tintinalli's Emergency Medicine: A Comprehensive Study Guide.* 8th ed. New York, NY: McGraw Hill; 2020.)

bond, adhesive adjuncts such as tincture of benzoin or Mastisol are frequently used. Once wound healing is deemed adequate, the tapes can be left to slough off or removed by peeling each end inward toward the incision and gently lifting away from the skin.

Liquid Adhesive

Liquid tissue adhesives (Dermabond, Indermil) are an effective alternative to the closure of uncomplicated lacerations and surgical incisions that are not subject to movement or excess tension (ie, skin over joints or areas subject to repetitive motion). Liquid adhesives are applied topically to glue the edges of intact skin together and seal the wound from microbial contamination. The wound edges must be held in adequate apposition during application to avoid adhesive entering the wound. Liquid adhesive creates a barrier to wound healing when used internally.

References

Venes D. *Tabor's Cyclopedic Medical Dictionary*. 21st ed. Philadelphia, PA: FA Davis Company; 2009.

Bibliography

Caruthers B, May M, Ward-English L. *The Surgical Wound*. Englewood, CO: Association of Surgical Technologists; 1995.

Cohen IK, Diegelmann RF, Yager DR, Wornum IL, Graham MF, Crossland MC. Wound care and wound healing. In: Schwartz SI, Shires GT, Spencer FC, Daly JM, Fischer JE, Galloway AC, eds. *Principles of surgery*. New York, NY: McGraw-Hill; 1999:263-295.

Deitch EA, ed. *Tools of the Trade and Rules of the Road: A Surgical Guide*. Philadelphia, PA: Lippincott-Raven; 1997.

Dunn DL, ed. *Wound Closure Manual*. Somerville, NJ: Ethicon, Inc; 2007.

Ellis H, Bucknall TE, Cox PJ. Abdominal incisions and their closure. *Current Problems in Surgery*. 1985;22(4):4-51.

Frey KB, Ross T, eds. *Surgical Technology for the Surgical Technologist: A Positive Care Approach*. 4th ed. Clifton Park, NY: Delmar Cengage Learning; 2014.

Fuller JK. Sutures and wound healing. In: Fuller JK, Ness E, eds., *Surgical Technology Principles and Practice*. St. Louis, MO: Elsevier Saunders; 2005:321-346.

Greenburg J, Goldman RH. Barbed suture: a review of the technology and clinical uses in obstetrics. *Rev Obstet Gynecol*. 2013;6 (3-4):107-115. https://www.ncbi.nlm.nih.gov/pmc/articles/PMC4002186/. Accessed May 25, 2023.

Junge T, Price B, Ross T. Hemostasis and emergency situations. In: Frey KB, Ross T, eds. *Surgical Technology for the Surgical Technologist: A Positive Care Approach*. 3rd ed. Clifton Park, NY: Delmar Cengage Learning;2008:185-202.

Junge T, Ross T. Genitourinary surgery. In: Frey KB, Ross T, eds. *Surgical Technology for the Surgical Technologist: A Positive Care Approach*. 3rd ed. Clifton Park, NY: Delmar Cengage Learning; 2008:769-827.

Lai SY, Becker DG, Edlich RF. Sutures and Needles. 2010. http://emedicine.medscape.com/article/884838-overview#aw2aab6b3. Accessed May 25, 2023.

Langenburg SE, Hanks JB. Principles of operative surgery. In: Sabiston, Jr DC, Lyerly HK, eds., *Sabiston Essentials of Surgery*. 2nd ed. Philadelphia, PA: Saunders; 1994: 98-103.

Nandi PL, Rajan SS, Mak KC, Chan S, So YP. Surgical wound infection. *Hong Kong M J*. 1999;5(1):82-86.

Niederhuber JE. Incisions, wound closure, & the healing process. In: Niederhuber JE, Dunwoody SL, eds. *Fundamentals of Surgery*. Stamford, CT: Appleton & Lange; 1998: 79-92.

Patnaik VVG, Singla RK, Sanju B. Surgical incisions their anatomic basis part I head and neck. *J Anat Soc India*. 2000;49(1):69-77.

Phillips N. *Berry & Kohn's Operating Room Technique*. 11th ed. St. Louis, MO: Mosby Elsevier; 2007.

Pieknik R. *Suture and Surgical Hemostasis: A Pocket Guide*. St. Louis, MO: Saunders Elsevier; 2006.

Price P, Smith C. Wound healing, sutures, needles, and stapling devices. In: Frey KB, Ross T, eds. *Surgical Technology for the Surgical Technologist: A Positive Care Approach*. 3rd ed. Clifton Park, NY: Delmar Cengage Learning; 2008:278-303.

Shmaefsky BR. *Applied Anatomy & Physiology: A Case Study Approach*. St. Paul, MN: Paradigm Publishing; 2007.

Smith CE. General surgery. In: Rothrock JC, McEwen DR, eds. *Alexander's Care of the Patient in Surgery*. 10th ed. St. Louis, MO: Mosby Elsevier; 2007:297-355.

University of Michigan Medical School. *Dissector answers: Abdominal wall*. 2000. http://anatomy.med.umich.edu/gastrointestinal_system/abdo_wall_ans.html. Accessed May 25, 2023.

Wind GG, Rich NM. *Principles of Surgical Technique: The Art of Surgery*. 2nd ed. Baltimore, MD: Urban & Schwarzenberg; 1987.

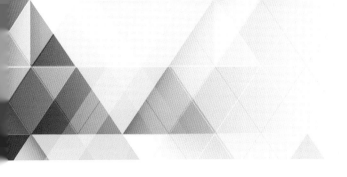

11

Wound Closure Techniques

Douglas J. Hughes and Rebecca Hall

DISCUSSED IN THIS CHAPTER

1. Wound closure considerations.
2. Basic suture techniques.
3. Surgical site infections.
4. Wound healing complications.

Suturing is the most commonly employed method of wound closure. It involves the placement of suture material within the layers of the wound to effectively hold them in approximation until sufficient healing has occurred and the wound is able to maintain its own tensile strength without disruption. There are many techniques for closing the wound with sutures and several considerations that must be understood to use each technique appropriately.

ABDOMINAL WOUND CLOSURE CONSIDERATIONS

Although it is widely accepted that wound strength and **cosmesis** are the two primary concerns regarding the closure and postoperative healing of abdominal laparotomy wounds, the most effective way to achieve these ends is a matter of much debate. A great deal of disagreement surrounds the choice of suture material, the most appropriate method of fascial closure, and the best cosmetic approach to skin approximation. As a result, differences in technique, style, and preference abound. Many surgeons prefer mass closure of the abdominal wall (closure of all internal layers simultaneously), while some still use a layered technique (closure of each layer individually). There are also differing opinions on the use of running versus interrupted primary suture lines. Ultimately, use of a technique that ensures strong fascial closure is of utmost importance. For the most part, many suture types have proven effective in achieving this goal; therefore, their selection is of secondary concern to the overall technique employed. General considerations related to the closure of each layer of the abdominal wall follow.

Peritoneum

The decision whether to close the peritoneum or not is one based on theory and preference. While some surgeons prefer to suture this layer, it is generally agreed that its closure is not necessary. Approximation of the peritoneum does not significantly reduce the incidence of incisional hernia in the presence of a strong closure of the posterior fascia. Studies have indicated that unsutured defects within the peritoneum heal spontaneously by rapid mesothelial differentiation from underlying connective tissues within days after surgery. Additionally, it has been hypothesized that peritoneal suturing may lead to localized **ischemia** and even increase the risk of herniation. If approximated, the peritoneum heals very quickly. Placement of a running suture line using absorbable material is generally preferred. Recommended sutures include the following: 0 polydioxanone (PDS II), 0 or 2-0 polyglactin 910 (Vicryl), or 0 chromic gut.

Fascia

Because fascia is the main supportive structure within the body, its meticulous closure is critical to ensuring secure, disruption-free healing. Following surgery, closure of the fascia must be strong enough to withstand changes in intra-abdominal pressure caused by such factors as coughing, vomiting, hiccupping, and distension. Fascia regains about 10% of its tensile strength by the seventh postoperative day and reaches approximately 25% to 30% once the proliferation phase of healing is completed. By three months, 70% to 90% of the fascia's original strength is regained. Because it heals slowly, materials providing long-term wound support such as polyglyconate (Maxon) and polydioxanone (PDS II) have been shown to provide adequate wound support while minimizing the incidence of **fistula** formation and chronic scar pain associated with permanent sutures. The use of a continuous versus interrupted primary suture line evenly distributes wound tension along the length of the incision and reduces operating time by an average of 15 minutes. However, reliance on a single suture strand may result in **dehiscence** should the suture line fail. Studies cited by O'Dwyer and Courtney (2003)[2] contend that continuous closure with slow-absorbing monofilament suture is the most effective and efficient method overall. A recent study on abdominal wound **tensile strength** after midline laparotomy concluded that suture placement using the simple-interrupted technique should be approximately 4 to 6 mm from the edge of the wound (versus the conventional 10-mm placement) and that fascial closure should include the aponeurosis and exclude the rectus abdominis muscle. Several other trials are underway to determine the most effective and secure approach to fascial closure. Ultimately, the skill and preference of the surgeon, or if appropriate his assistant, will dictate the method used. Defects in the fascia may result in incisional hernia formation and are often buttressed with synthetic graft material to ensure consistency. During healing, a 40% return of tensile strength is achieved by the second postoperative month with maximum strength peaking around 1 year, although complete strength is never restored to preoperative levels.

Muscle

Because muscle does not tolerate suturing well, muscle-splitting or retracting incisions are the preferred method of entry into the abdominal cavity. When muscles are split along their fibers, only the fascia requires approximation. For midline laparotomy closure, rectus muscle approximation can be readily achieved via mass closure of the abdominal wall. In this approach, the peritoneum, posterior fascia, abdominal musculature, and anterior fascia are closed simultaneously using a running or interrupted primary suture line. Deitch (1997) recommends the Smead-Jones far-and-near technique (see Figure 11-1).[1]

This is a complex stitch in which a set of far-far sutures are placed through all layers of the abdominal wall below the subcutaneous tissue at 2 to 3 cm from the wound edges followed by 5-mm-wide near bites through the linea alba. Far and near bites are alternated along the length of the wound to provide both fascial coaption and superior wound strength.

Subcutaneous Adipose Tissue

Subcutaneous fat (adipose) presents a special challenge during wound closure. Like muscle, fat responds poorly to suture approximation due to its loose, watery composition. Many surgeons agree that suturing this layer is fruitless; however, others believe that some suturing is warranted to remove dead space. Because dead space is most common within the subcutaneous layer, careful approximation of the wound is critical. The use of a pressure dressing helps to minimize associated risks. When subcutaneous fat is sutured, absorbable materials that are broken down by hydrolysis are preferred.

Skin

Careful and meticulous closure of the skin is a very important step in the formation of a cosmetically acceptable scar and serves to significantly lower the risk of postoperative wound infection. Despite this fact, it is the most overlooked part of the operation. The following considerations will help the surgical assistant ensure that the goals of optimal cosmesis and infection prevention are met.

- The edges of the skin must be properly aligned and **everted** to ensure even coaptation. Misalignment can lead to the formation of dog ears or bunching of the skin at the ends of the incision.

- Epidermal sutures are in direct contact with the surface of the skin. Therefore, skin closure with multifilament materials can result in microbial wound contamination via wicking.

- Improper placement of the suture can cause dimpling or uneven wound edges that are unsightly when healed.

- Track marks may form on the skin during healing due to excessive tension on the suture line. Ischemia and skin necrosis may also develop.

- Excessive manipulation or pinching of the skin with tissue forceps can macerate wound edges.

- To facilitate closure, the tough layers of the skin are best sutured with the aid of a cutting needle.

When choosing a suture material, it is important to remember that the speed at which skin heals varies by location and the amount of tension applied to the wound edges.

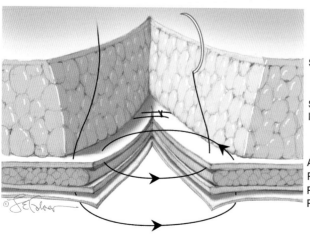

Skin

Subcutaneous layer

Anterior rectus sheath
Rectus abdominis m.
Posterior rectus sheath
Peritoneum

Figure 11-1 · Smead-Jones closure, near and far pattern. (Reproduced, with permission, from Yeomans ER, Hoffman BL, Gilstrap III LC, Cunningham FG, eds. *Cunningham and Gilstrap's Operative Obstetrics*. 3rd ed. New York, NY: McGraw Hill; 2017.)

Nonabsorbable monofilament sutures such as nylon and poly-propylene are typically preferred for epidermal approximation and are removed between the 3rd and 10th postoperative day. At this point, the skin has only had enough time to regain approximately 5% to 10% of its tensile strength. Although this seems like a premature period in which to remove the sutures, it is a necessary step in the prevention of suture tract epithelialization and wound infection. Removal is safe during this period as most wound tension is absorbed by the fascia. The use of fast-absorbing polyglactin 910 (Vicryl *Rapide*) eliminates the need for suture removal as the material is sloughed from the wound between the 7th and 10th postoperative day with complete absorption occurring by day 42.

As mentioned previously, the smallest diameter suture capable of holding the wound edges together should be used. The use of small sutures yields minimal tissue reactivity and enhances cosmesis. Size 5-0 to 6-0 sutures are recommended for the face, 4-0 to 5-0 for the hands, and 3-0 diameter sutures are usually ideal for closing incisions of the trunk and extremities.

ABDOMINAL WOUND CLOSURE TECHNIQUE

Given the considerations previously mentioned, Table 11-1 outlines common procedural steps in the closure of midline laparotomy. Variations in this technique may differ from surgeon to surgeon depending on their individual training and preferences. Physiologic patient characteristics may also dictate choice of wound closure method. Additional abdominal incisions may be closed using these same basic steps; although, wounds involving more than one fascial layer may require a multi-layered closure.

Needle holders are designed to grasp, hold, and facilitate the pushing of a curved surgical needle through body tissues. Most are ringed instruments with powerful jaws and ratchets. Because needle holders are designed to clamp metal, they may have inserts within the jaws that are made of ultra-hard tungsten carbide. Instruments with these inserts are readily identified by their gold rings. Other needle holders may have smooth jaws for fine needles or serrated jaws for heavy needles. Needle holders are available in a myriad of different widths, lengths, and styles. Ultimately, the type of needle holder chosen should be of the appropriate size and configuration for both the needle and anticipated procedural application.

BASIC SUTURING TECHNIQUES

While suturing, the surgical assistant should stand comfortably and in a position that optimizes forward movement of the hand and wrist. The elbows should be out and away from the sides of the body. The needle holder is held in the palm of the hand. The rings of the handle are typically occupied by

TABLE 11-1 • COMMON INTRAOPERATIVE STEPS IN THE CLOSURE OF MIDLINE VERTICAL LAPAROTOMY
Basic mass closure technique with running absorbable monofilament suture
1. Following anatomic replacement of the abdominal viscera and greater omentum, the wound is evaluated for the necessity of a drainage device. If a drain is needed, it is placed before suturing of the wound is initiated. Administration of a muscle-relaxing agent facilitates tension-free closure.
2. To prevent damage to the bowel and abdominal viscera, a metal ribbon retractor or Glassman visceral retainer (fish) may be placed under the posterior fascia.
3. The fascia is lifted at the superior end of the wound with heavy toothed forceps or Kocher clamps. Hand-held retractors may be needed for exposure.
4. Beginning a few millimeters superior to the apex of the incision, the first full-thickness suture pass is made 1 cm from each opposing edge of the wound.
5. The suture is knotted according to the type of suture material used. If using #1 polydioxanone, 5-6 square knot throws are indicated. Use of a double-loop strand is an ideal alternative for continuous closure because the absence of an anchoring knot increases the breaking strength of the suture and reduces the amount of foreign material left within the wound. Care should be taken when suturing the fascia to ensure that the tension is just enough to hold the wound edges in apposition without causing ischemia.
6. Running wound closure continues along the length of the incision with small bites of tissue taken no more than 1 cm apart from each other. The assistant follows the suture line by maintaining tension on the loose end of the strand. Clamps and hand-held retractors are repositioned as needed to expose the wound edges. The undersurface of the closure is palpated intermittently to ensure the absence of fascial gaps or inadvertently sutured viscera. Wide gaps in the facial closure can be approximated individually with an interrupted figure-of-eight stitch. The ribbon retractor or visceral retainer is removed prior to completion of the suture line.
7. The distal anchoring knot is securely seated and tied to prevent suture line disruption.
8. Once mass closure is completed, the subcutaneous tissues are irrigated and the skin is closed according to preference. The use of skin staples provides good cosmetic closure with minimal tissue reactivity.
9. A three-layer dressing is applied to the wound. If the presence of dead space is a concern postoperatively, a pressure dressing may be preferred.

Sources: Deitch EA, ed. *Tools of the Trade and Rules of the Road: A Surgical Guide*. Philadelphia, PA: Lippincott-Raven; 1997; Ellis H, Bucknall TE, Cox PJ. Abdominal incisions and their closure. *Curr Probl Surg*. 1985;22(4):1-51.

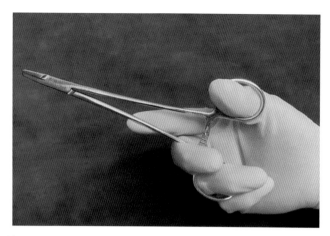

Figure 11-2 · Holding a needle driver.

the thumb and ring fingers. The index finger is placed along the shaft of the instrument for stability and security (see Figure 11-2). The needle should enter the skin at a right angle to the surface of the tissue or structure being sutured. To avoid bending the needle, it must be pushed along a circular axis following its curvature. Therefore, passage of the needle through tissue is accomplished by pronating the wrist. Some practitioners prefer to place their thumb outside the ring and manipulate the needle holder with the base of the thumb, about the area of the first metacarpophalangeal joint. Subtle movements of the proximal thumb are used to unlock the ratchet and open the jaws of the instrument. This method improves control and increases the degrees of rotational manipulation of the needle. If super pronation of the wrist is needed to facilitate proper placement of the needle, both the thumb and index fingers should be removed from the rings of the instrument.

To correctly place the needle within the jaws of the needle holder, it should be clamped along the body at approximately one-third the distance from the eye. Clamping the needle over the swage may weaken the needle and cause the suture to dislodge. When attempting to penetrate tough tissue, it may be necessary to reposition the jaws in the center of the needle body. Avoid placing excess pressure on the body of the needle. When clamped too tightly, needles may become warped or bent. Delicate handling of both needle and suture with the needle holder will help ensure their integrity and reduce tissue damage and the likelihood of suture line failure.

Once the needle passes through the tissues, it is withdrawn by grasping it with the hand in the pronated position. Rather than pulling the needle through the tissue, it is removed by gently rotating the wrist along the curvature of the needle in a small arc until the hand is in the supinated position. Clamping of the needlepoint must be avoided. If only the point is visible, the needle holder can be repositioned at the back of the needle to advance it further. The needle should be reset in the jaws of the needle holder during withdrawal, ideally before pulling the suture strand through the tissue. Doing so saves movement and time.

When assisting the surgeon during the placement of a continuous suture line, tension must be held on the loose strand until the next bite is taken. This is accomplished by following (grasping) the suture close to the wound yet out of the surgeon's line of sight. It is important to remember that excess tension can lead to ischemia and strangulation. The wound will swell with edema postoperatively, enhancing this effect. Therefore, just enough tension to hold the wound edges in apposition is sufficient.

COMMON SUTURE PATTERNS

Many options exist for the primary closure of surgical wounds. Primary suture lines are placed to hold the wound in approximation during first-intention healing. When additional wound support is needed to relieve excess tension on the primary suture line and eliminate dead space, use of a secondary suture line may be indicated. Examples of primary and secondary suture line techniques include the following.

Interrupted

Interrupted primary suture lines involve the placement of individually tied stitches along the length of the incision. Use of this technique is ideal for the closure of wounds under tension or in the presence of infection. Because interrupted sutures are not interconnected, they do not have the propensity to wick bacteria.

Simple Interrupted. The simple interrupted suture line (see Figure 11-3) is the most basic technique for approximating tissues within the body. For skin closure, the use of simple interrupted sutures provides a good cosmetic result when small

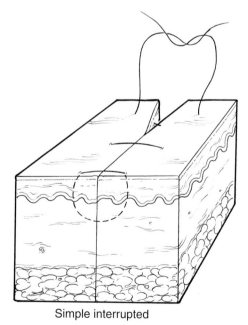

Simple interrupted

Figure 11-3 · Simple interrupted stitch. (Reproduced, with permission, from Minter RM, Doherty GM. *Current Procedures: Surgery.* New York, NY: McGraw Hill; 2010.)

bites of tissue are taken and when knot tying is snug and secure without over-tightening. Each stitch should be placed equidistant on either side of the incision and the stitches should be as far apart as they are wide. Because each stitch is independent, this method is considered the strongest and most secure of any suture pattern. If one stitch is compromised, disruption of the wound is localized, and the rest of the wound remains unaffected.

Subcuticular or Deep Buried. When used in the fascia or below the skin, the simple running or interrupted stitch may be placed so that the knot is tied underneath the tissue layers. This technique is known as the subcuticular or buried stitch. It provides an excellent cosmetic outcome and reduces tissue reactivity by burying the knot deep within the wound and is especially useful when placing large-diameter suture in thin patients.

Vertical Mattress. Vertical mattress sutures (see Figure 11-4) effectively approximate the epidermis with minimal tension by adding two epidermal-thickness bites to the simple interrupted technique. The technique involves placement of sutures at vertical right angles to the incision in a near-far pattern. The near component of the vertical mattress suture line provides coaptation of the skin, while the far component reduces the amount of tension on the wound. The far-far suture is placed 4 to 8 mm from the wound edge, somewhat deep in the wound below the dermis. The far-far passage of the needle is placed across both sides of the wound, and then the needle is positioned backwards in the needle driver. The near-near location is at a shallow depth and placed in the upper dermis. The near-near placement is placed 1 to 2 mm from the wound edge. Both

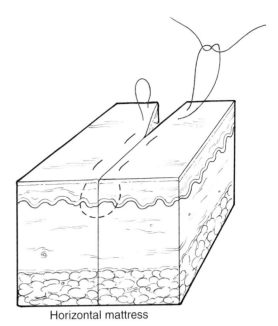

Horizontal mattress

Figure 11-5 · Horizontal stitch. (Reproduced, with permission, from Minter RM, Doherty GM. *Current Procedures: Surgery.* New York, NY: McGraw Hill; 2010.)

ends of the suture should be tied on one side of the wound. The stitch is tied so that the knot is on the side where the suture passage began.

Eversion of the skin results as the knots are secured and may lead to increased scarring. Despite this disadvantage, mattress sutures are ideal for use in the groin and extremities.

Horizontal Mattress. The horizontal mattress stitch (see Figure 11-5) is placed horizontally, axial to the wound edges, and in line with the incision. This technique everts the tissues and is commonly used in the skin and fascia.

The horizontal mattress stitch introduces the needle about 4 to 8 mm from the edge of the wound. The needle is passed through to the opposite side of the wound edge where it exits the skin. The needle is placed backwards in the needle driver, inserted into the skin parallel to the wound edge and passed from the far side of the wound back to the near side. The needle exits the skin about 4 to 8 mm down the original wound edge from the original insertion site. The suture is tied gently on the side of the wound where the suturing began.

Continuous

Continuous suture lines are created using a single suture strand that is anchored at one end of the wound, runs along the length of the incision to approximate the wound edges, and is anchored to the tissues at the opposite end. Primary suture lines of this type are typically used for the closure of long wounds. Because one strand is used, tension along the wound edges is evenly distributed. Use of this technique should be carefully considered because the entire wound may become jeopardized if any portion of the suture strand breaks or otherwise fails. Therefore, continuous suture lines are not recommended for

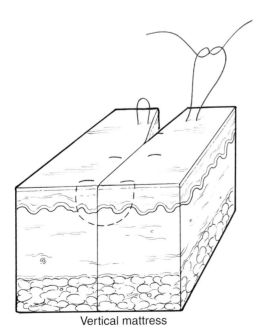

Vertical mattress

Figure 11-4 · Vertical mattress. (Reproduced, with permission, from Minter RM, Doherty GM. *Current Procedures: Surgery.* New York, NY: McGraw Hill; 2010.)

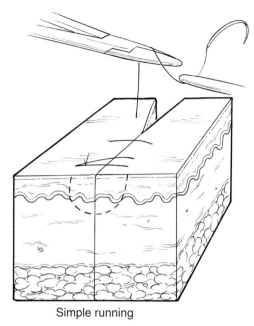

Simple running

Figure 11-6 · Continuous stitch. (Reproduced, with permission, from Minter RM, Doherty GM. *Current Procedures: Surgery*. New York, NY: McGraw Hill; 2010.)

wounds under excess tension, such as heart wall incisions. Options for continuous suture lines include simple and locking configurations.

Simple Continuous. Also known as a running stitch, the continuous suture line (see Figure 11-6) is commonly used throughout the body to close tissues such as the skin, peritoneum, and blood vessels. Because only two knots are typically required; continuous sutures can be placed in a fraction of the time needed for interrupted techniques. Simple continuous sutures are run obliquely over the incision and appear as solid lines that bridge the wound edges together. Each bite should be parallel to the wound and equally spaced. This technique may be utilized to approximate both internal and external wound layers. When used to close the skin, an acceptable cosmetic result is anticipated.

Continuous Locking. The continuous locking stitch (see Figure 11-7) is a modification of the simple continuous suture

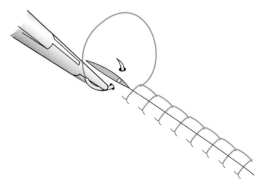

Figure 11-7 · Continuous locking stitch. (Reproduced, with permission, from Gomella LG, Haist SA. *Gomella and Haist's Clinician's Pocket Reference*. 12th ed. New York, NY: McGraw Hill; 2022.)

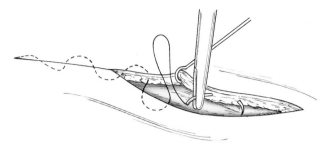

Figure 11-8 · Running subcuticular stitch. (Reproduced, with permission, from Minter RM, Doherty GM. *Current Procedures: Surgery*. New York, NY: McGraw Hill; 2010.)

line that provides excellent hemostasis and water resistance. It is placed by passing the needle through the loop made by the previous running stitch. Continuous locking sutures are especially useful for skin closure in patients with ascites or for the approximation of the myometrium following cesarean section.

Running Subcuticular. To further enhance cosmesis and minimize infection during the closure of Class I surgical wounds, skin edges can be held in approximation using a running subcuticular stitch (see Figure 11-8). This primary suture line technique involves the placement of either an absorbable or nonabsorbable suture within the dermis. The skin is gently everted with an Adson tissue forceps visualizing the dermal-epidermal section of the skin. The suture needle is placed at a 90° angle at the dermal-epidermal section; the wrist is pronated to take a deep horizontal bite that is parallel to the skin. Using the Adson forceps to stabilize the needle, it is advanced through the tissue, and then using the Adson forceps to hold the needle, it is repositioned in the needle driver for the next throw.

When absorbable material such as polyglycolic acid (Dexon, Dexon II) or poliglecaprone 25 (Monocryl) is used, the ends of the suture are anchored and knotted within the incisional apexes under the skin. Because nonabsorbable materials are eventually removed, these sutures are not knotted; rather, the tails of the suture line are left outside of the wound and pulled taught. Advantages of running subcuticular sutures include elimination of bacteria-wicking epidermal stitches, scarring from needle puncture sites, and track marks. Drawbacks include higher infection rates with clean-contaminated and contaminated wounds and increased operative time to place the suture line.

To achieve coaptation of the epidermis, the skin can be supported with adhesive tapes. Subcuticular closure is not recommended for large wounds or those under tension.

Pursestring. A purse string stitch is a continuous drawstring suture pattern that enables circular closure of a structure (see Figure 11-9). Common uses of this technique include closure of the cecum after removal of the vermiform appendix, the securing of drainage tubes within the urinary bladder, closure of the bowel around an intestinal stapler, and for the sealing of the aorta and right atrium around cardiopulmonary bypass cannulae.

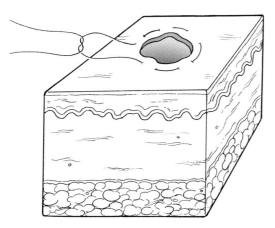

Figure 11-9 • Pursestring stitch. (Reproduced, with permission, from Minter RM, Doherty GM. *Current Procedures: Surgery*. New York, NY: McGraw Hill; 2010.)

Retention

When slow healing or disruption of the primary suture line is suspected or to support tissue healing by second intention, the wound can be reinforced with a secondary suture line in the form of **retention sutures** (see Figure 11-10). The use of a large nonabsorbable suture material placed through most (if not all) layers of the wound in an interrupted or figure-of-eight pattern lateral to the incision relieves tension on the wound edges and aids in the maintenance of coaptation during healing. A bumper may be slid over the exposed portion of the retention suture to relieve excess pressure and avoid suture cut through. The use of a suture bridge allows the tension of the suture line to be adjusted postoperatively. Retention sutures are most often used in patients suffering from immunocompromising conditions, and in the presence of wound stress due to increased intraabdominal pressure.

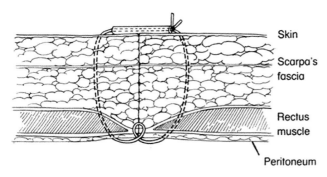

Figure 11-10 • Many surgeons use retention sutures bolsters or simple 2-in. sections of sterilized red rubber tubing in order to minimize the cutting of the suture into the skin during the inevitable postoperative swelling. Because of this swelling, the retention sutures should be tied loosely rather than snugly such that the surgeon can still pass his or her finger between the retention suture and the skin of the abdominal wall. (Reproduced with permission from Ellison E, Zollinger RM, eds. *Zollinger's Atlas of Surgical Operations*, 10e. New York: McGraw-Hill; 2016.)

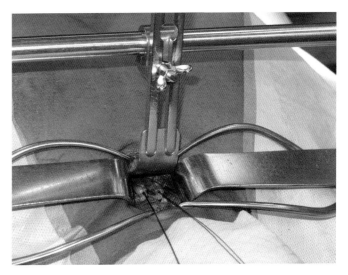

Figure 11-11 • Traction stitch. (Reproduced, with permission, from Sugarbaker DJ, Bueno R, Burt BM, et al. *Sugarbaker's Adult Chest Surgery*, 3rd ed. New York, NY: McGraw Hill; 2020.)

Traction

Traction sutures (see Figure 11-11) are used to retract tissues that are difficult to grasp or handle with conventional retracting instruments and position them away from the operative site. A nonabsorbable suture is placed through the structure and temporarily left in place.

The tails of the suture strand provide a mechanism for manipulation. In some instances, a clamp may be placed at the distal end of the tails to tag the suture or prevent it from being inadvertently pulled out. Once traction is no longer needed, the suture is removed. Examples of tissues commonly retracted in this manner include the sclera, myocardium, dura, and tongue.

KNOT TYING

Secure knots are needed to ensure that suture lines and vessel ligatures remain in place without slacking or disruption during the healing process. The goal of knot tying is to create well-seated and secure square knots. Square knots (also known as flat or reef knots) provide unparalleled security and are the preferred method of knot tying. Square knots are made by passing one suture strand over the other in a complete primary turn or throw (half knot), reversing the position of the strands, and placing a second half knot to secure the first. When additional security is needed, a second primary turn can be made on the first throw to prevent slippage. This modification is known as a surgeon's knot. It is necessary to note that a half knot is the first throw of a square knot; it is not to be confused with a half-hitch knot. Half-hitch knots are formed by looping one strand around the other and pulling the two strands taut into a slip knot. Half-hitch knots are often tied because of improper technique. Granny knots result from failure to reverse the strands between the half-knot throws of a square knot.

TABLE 11-2 • BASIC KNOT TYING PRINCIPLES
1. Hands should be placed equidistant from the location of the knot.
2. The length of the strands should be adequate to facilitate tying. Ideally, the tip of an outstretched finger should contact the knot.
3. The working strand should ideally be manipulated with the right hand, regardless of hand dominance.
4. Stand in a position that allows for comfortable tying and proper alignment of the knot.
5. Square knots provide the most security.
6. Avoid sawing or fraying of the strands.
7. Crossing of the strands or the hands should not occur on the first throw.
8. The position of the right and left hands should be reversed upon throw completion.
9. Throw directions should be alternated. Granny knots result from repetition of the same throw.
10. Apply sufficient tension to the knot to maintain apposition of the tissues, but avoid over tightening and ischemic strangulation.
11. The index finger should be used to seat the lower strand of the knot to avoid pulling up on the tissue or reversing the throw into a half-hitch knot.
12. Maintain equal tension on both strands when tying under tension to reduce knot slippage and formation of a half-hitch knot.
13. Practice makes perfect.

Sources: Caruthers B, May M, Ward-English L. *The Surgical Wound.* Englewood, CO: Association of Surgical Technologists; 1995; Wind GG, Rich NM. *Principles of Surgical Technique: The Art of Surgery.* 2nd ed. Baltimore, MD: Urban & Schwarzenberg; 1987.

Factors Affecting Knot Security

Factors that affect knot security include the friction coefficient of the suture material, the length of the suture ends following knotting and cutting, the type of knot method used, the configuration suture material (monofilament vs multifilament), and whether or not the suture strand is coated. Monofilament and coated multifilament suture materials require additional knots to reduce slippage.

It is important to remember that the integrity of the suture strand is weakened at the location of the knot. Poor knot tying decreases the strength of the suture even further and results in minimal knot tensile strength. Half-hitch (sliding) and granny knots only provide 20% of the security achieved by a well-seated square knot. As a surgical assistant, the ability to tie good knots is a skill that will be appreciated and recognized by the surgeon and reduce the risk of postoperative wound dehiscence, hemorrhage, and tissue strangulation. As with learning any skill, it takes many hours of repetitive practice to master. Table 11-2 lists the basic principles that must be followed in order to ensure proper technique. The three most common methods of knot tying are two-handed, one-handed, and instrument tying techniques.

Two-Handed Tying

The two-handed technique is the most meticulous approach to knot tying and, when performed well, provides the most security of any method. During tying, the left hand maintains constant, even tension on the long-fixed strand. The shorter free strand (working strand) is manipulated with the right hand by holding, releasing, and regrabbing the strand as needed.

One-Handed Tying

The one-handed tying technique (see Figure 11-12) differs from the two-handed method in that all the suture strand manipulation is performed using one hand while the opposite hand remains

perfectly still with constant tension on the fixed strand. This method increases the speed of tying and facilitates tying within deep cavities lacking sufficient space for the performance of the two-handed technique. Another advantage is that the needle holder does not have to be unclamped from the needle. The downside to one-handed tying is that it is difficult to achieve secure flat throws, limiting the security of the knots.

Instrument Tying

When closing the wound, knots may be secured using the instrument tying technique. To accomplish the first throw, the suture is pulled through the wound until a short tail is left protruding through the tissue. The needle holder is rolled over the long strand toward the short end. The short end is grasped in the jaws of the needle holder and the resulting knot is slid into the tissue and secured. The second throw is made by rolling the needle holder over the suture in the opposite direction.

CUTTING THE SUTURE

To cut the suture following placement of a secure knot, the tip of the scissors is used to follow the strand of the suture down to the knot. Once the knot is both felt with the tip of the instrument and visualized, the scissors are rotated 45° from the knot and the strands are evenly cut in one motion by opposing the blades of the scissors. Rotating the tips of the scissors helps avoid inadvertently cutting the knot. The tails of the suture must be cut short enough that irritation and inflammation of the tissues are minimized, yet long enough to ensure that the knot does not come unraveled. Additionally, long tails may get coiled in the next stitch. Uncoated multifilament sutures hold knots better than monofilament and coated materials and can be cut more closely. The tails of monofilament skin sutures should be left approximately 3 to 5 mm long.

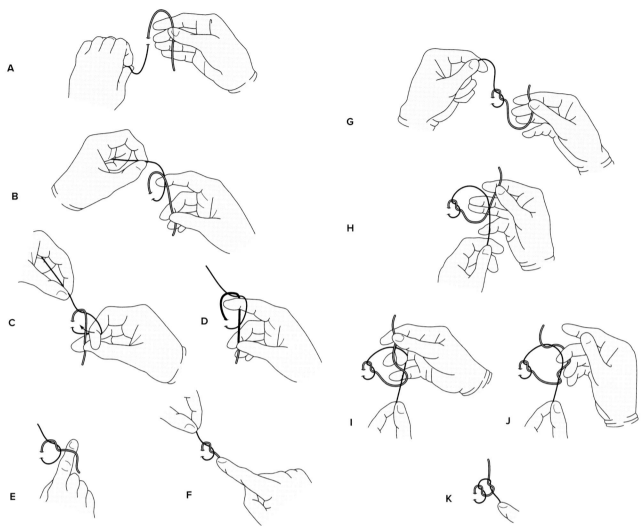

Figure 11-12 · One-handed knot tying. (Reproduced, with permission, from Gomella LG, Haist SA. *Gomella and Haist's Clinician's Pocket Reference*. 12th ed. New York, NY: McGraw Hill; 2022.)

POSSIBLE WOUND HEALING COMPLICATIONS

As with the surgical intervention itself, any number of complications can arise during wound healing. As previously noted, several factors that influence healing are inherent to the patient. However, those factors related to surgical site infection (SSI) and postoperative wound dehiscence are under the direct control of the surgical team members. A clear understanding of common complications, their risks, and the methods of preventing them are necessary to help ensure proper wound healing and patient recovery.

SURGICAL SITE INFECTION

SSI is one of the most acquired nosocomial infections. As infection ensues, the tissues are overcome by the presence of bacterial contamination, which may result in increased morbidity and mortality. The risk of SSI can be greatly increased depending upon factors such as the manner in which the

wound is approximated, the level of adherence to aseptic technique, how the tissues are handled intraoperatively, the removal and evacuation of blood and devitalized tissues, and the final classification of the wound. The administration of preoperative antibiotic prophylaxis may be indicated to reduce this risk.

In the prevention of SSI, there are several elements that must be considered. Because the degree of wound contamination is a key component of increased infection rates, strict adherence to sterile technique is paramount. Irrigation of the wound may also be indicated; however, there is debate over the effectiveness of this method in reducing SSI in clean wounds. If the wound presents with an elevated wound classification, debridement of nonviable tissue must be thorough and healing by second-intention granulation may be indicated. When employing primary tissue closure techniques, the wound edges must be adequately approximated and dead space must not be left between the tissue layers. This is especially relevant to adipose tissue layers. Overuse of suture material is contraindicated, and knots should be tied tightly enough to ensure approximation without

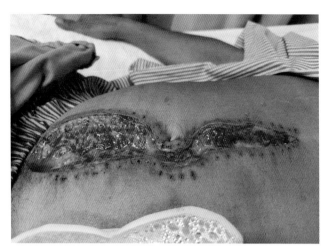

Figure 11-13 · Partial Revealed Wound Dehiscence Post Operatively. (Used with permission from Casa nayafana/Shutterstock)

strangulation and ischemia of the wound edges. The surgeon and surgical assistant must also consider the virulence of the microorganisms that may be present within the wound and the presence of undrained serum, blood, and foreign material. The use of a wound drain may be indicated in these instances.

DEHISCENCE

Dehiscence of the surgical wound (see Figure 11-13) is described as the separation of the fascial layer and usually occurs in the abdomen. According to Fischer, Fegelman, and Johannigman (1999), the incidence of postoperative wound dehiscence is approximately 2.6%.

Complete dehiscence of an abdominal wound may lead to protrusion of the viscera, a complication known as evisceration. Although several patient-related factors directly affect wound healing, correct wound closure technique, the proper selection of suture materials, and the maintenance of hemostasis can greatly reduce the likelihood of dehiscence. Surgical practitioners must also avoid the use of long, paramedian incisions whenever possible. Because dehiscence begins primarily in the fascial layer of the closed wound, the use of nonabsorbable, monofilament, interrupted sutures is indicated and may need to be accompanied by a secondary retention suture line. Other methods, such as the use of a pressure dressing, may also be utilized to reduce the presence of dead space and fluid accumulation that may separate the fascia.

HEMORRHAGE

Hemorrhage is typically evident early in the postoperative recovery of the surgical patient. Further surgery may be indicated for hematoma evacuation and to achieve hemostasis. Depending upon the amount of blood loss, shock may further complicate recovery. Meticulous attention to intraoperative hemostasis, careful tissue handling, and precise tissue approximation will serve to reduce the possibility of hemorrhage.

HERNIATION

Incomplete dehiscence of the surgical wound can lead to the **herniation** of body tissues or structures through defects in the fascia. The lower abdomen is the most common site of herniation. Hernias are typically diagnosed several months postoperatively, and complications such as bowel incarceration and tissue ischemia may also be present. In obese patients, the weight of body structures such as the panniculus adiposus can add additional stress to the surgical wound and result in incisional hernia formation. Proper and complete closure of the abdominal wound with an appropriate suture material can reduce this risk.

ADHESION

An **adhesion** is an abnormal attachment of two surfaces or structures that are normally separate. This attachment is created within the peritoneum due to the presence of fibrous tissue and is relatively common in patients with prior abdominal surgery. In patients with multiple abdominal surgeries, the incidence of adhesion formation is approximately 90%. Gynecologic surgery patients are especially at risk. Fibrous tissue growth is commonly extended beyond the specific surgical site and may include any number of nearby structures directly or indirectly impacted during surgery. Surgical team members can reduce the formation of tissue adhesions by using proper tissue handling techniques, keeping body tissues and structures moist by irrigating and minimizing blotting with dry sponges, maintaining sterile technique to reduce the risk of postoperative infection, and removing foreign material such as lint and powder granules from gloves.

SUTURE-SPECIFIC COMPLICATIONS

The selection of improper suture materials can also have an adverse effect on successful wound healing. Because body tissues react to any material implanted in the tissues, it is important for the surgeon and surgical assistant to have an in-depth working knowledge of the various options available for the closure of the surgical wound. Proper suture selection will vary from patient to patient and from tissue to tissue. Most adverse reactions to suture material are the result of improper absorption or tissue irritation due to sensitivity. Tissue reactions are most frequently attributed to the use of cotton or silk materials. Spitting of the suture from the wound, sinus tract creation, **edema,** and secondary scarring due to **ischemic necrosis** may result. Suture spitting can be prevented by burying the knot or running intracuticular knotless suture.

References

1. Deitch EA, ed. *Tools of the Trade and Rules of the Road: A Surgical Guide.* Philadelphia, PA: Lippincott-Raven; 1997.

2. O'Dwyer PJ, Courtney CA. Factors involved in abdominal wall closure and subsequent incisional hernia. *J R Coll Surg Edinb.* 2003;1(1):17-22.

Bibliography

Caruthers B, May M, Ward-English L. *The Surgical Wound.* Englewood, CO: Association of Surgical Technologists; 1995.

Cohen IK, Diegelmann RF, Yager DR, Wornum IL, Graham MF, Crossland MC. Wound care and wound healing. In: Schwartz SI, Shires GT, Spencer FC, Daly JM, Fischer JE, Galloway AC, eds. *Principles of surgery.* New York, NY: McGraw-Hill; 1999:263-295.

Columbia University Medical Center. Angiogenesis and wound healing, impaired angiogenesis in the elderly. 2011. http://www.columbiasurgery.org/cli/wound/impaired_angiogenesis.html. Accessed May 25, 2023.

Dattillo PP, King MW, Cassill NL, Leung JC. *Medical textiles: Application of an absorbable barbed bi-directional surgical suture.* Raleigh, NC: North Carolina State University. http://www.tx.ncsu.edu/jtatm/volume2issue2/articles/dattilo/dattilo%20full2.doc. Accessed May 26, 2023.

Dharmananda S. Abdominal adhesions: Prevention and treatment. 2003. http://www.itmonline.org/arts/adhesions.htm. Accessed May 26, 2023.

Doshi SJ. *A Complete Review of Wound Closure.* Cambridge, MA: Massachusetts Institute of Technology; 2002. http://dspace.mit.edu/bitstream/handle/1721.1/12833/27648464.pdf?sequence=1

Dunn DL, ed. *Wound Closure Manual.* Somerville, NJ: Ethicon, Inc; 2007.

Dunscombe AR. Sutures, needles, and instruments. In: Rothrock JC, McEwen DR, eds. *Alexander's Care of the Patient in Surgery.* 10th ed. St. Louis, MO: Mosby Elsevier; 2007:158-182.

Ellis H, Bucknall TE, Cox PJ. Abdominal incisions and their closure. *Curr Probl Surg.* 1985;22(4):4-51.

Fischer, JE, Fegelman, E, Johannigman, J. Surgical complications. In Schwartz SI, Shires GT, Spencer FC, Daly JM, Fischer JE, Galloway AC, eds. *Principles of surgery.* New York, NY: McGraw-Hill; 1999: 441-483.

Fuller JK. Sutures and wound healing. In: Fuller JK, Ness E, eds., *Surgical Technology Principles and Practice.* St. Louis, MO: Elsevier Saunders; 2005:321-346.

Howard RJ. Surgical infections. In: Schwartz SI, Shires GT, Spencer FC, Daly JM, Fischer JE, Galloway AC, eds. *Principles of Surgery.* New York, NY: McGraw-Hill; 1999:123-153.

Junge T, Price B, Ross T. Hemostasis and emergency situations. In: Frey KB, Ross T, eds. *Surgical Technology for the Surgical Technologist: A Positive Care Approach.* 3rd ed. Clifton Park, NY: Delmar Cengage Learning;2008:185-202.

Kudur MH, Pai SB, Sripathi H, Prabhu S. Sutures and suturing techniques in skin closure. *Indian J Dermatol Venereol Leprol.* 2009;75(4):425-434.

Lai SY, Becker DG, Edlich RF. Sutures and Needles. 2010. Retrieved from http://emedicine.medscape.com/article/884838-overview#aw2aab6b3. Accessed May 25, 2023.

Langenburg SE, Hanks JB. Principles of operative surgery. In: Sabiston, Jr DC, Lyerly HK, eds., *Sabiston Essentials of Surgery.* 2nd ed. Philadelphia, PA: Saunders; 1994: 98-103.

Nandi PL, Rajan SS, Mak KC, Chan S, So YP. Surgical wound infection. *Hong Kong M J.* 1999;5(1):82-86.

Niederhuber JE. Incisions, wound closure, & the healing process. In: Niederhuber JE, Dunwoody SL, eds. *Fundamentals of Surgery.* Stamford, CT: Appleton & Lange; 1998: 79-92.

Pieknik R. *Suture and Surgical Hemostasis: A Pocket Guide.* St. Louis, MO: Saunders Elsevier; 2006.

Price P, Smith C. Wound healing, sutures, needles, and stapling devices. In Frey KB, Ross T, eds. *Surgical Technology for the Surgical Technologist: A Positive Care Approach.* 3rd ed. Clifton Park, NY: Delmar Cengage Learning; 2008:278-303.

Retzlaff K, Agarwal S, Song D, Dorafshar A. *The four-step subcuticular suture technique. Plast Reconstr Surg.* 2010;126(1):p 50e-51e. doi: 10.1097/PRS.0b013e3181dab592

Venes D, Biderman A, Fenton B, et al., eds. *Taber's Cyclopedic Medical Dictionary.* 21st ed. Philadelphia, PA: F.A. Davis; 2009.

Wayne MA, Singer A. *Nine myths about wound care.* 2008. http://www.emedmag.com/html/pre/cov/covers/040110014.asp. Accessed May 26, 2023.

Weng R, Li Q, Zheng Y. Reduce suture complications by applying proper knot tying techniques. *Dermatol Surg.* 2010;36(8):1314-1318.

Why suture the peritoneum? The Lancet. 1987;329(8535):727.

Wind GG, Rich NM. *Principles of Surgical Technique: The Art of Surgery.* 2nd ed. Baltimore, MD: Urban & Schwarzenberg; 1987.

Zuber TJ. *The mattress sutures: vertical, horizontal and corner stitch. Am Fam Physician.* 2002;66(12):2231-2236.

12

Wound Dressings and Drains

Douglas J. Hughes and Rebecca Hall

Application of the dressing following surgery is a skill often delegated to the surgical assistant. It is important to have a strong working knowledge of the various types of dressing materials and their intended uses. The goals of dressing the wound are essentially to protect the wound, promote healing, control infection, facilitate debridement, provide compression, immobilize, and protect deep anatomic structures. There are many types of dressings available, ranging from the very simple to the very complex. Selection of the proper type and material is based on the following:

- Location, size, and type of wound
- Amount of exudate expected to drain from the wound
- Preference of the surgeon
- Size, age, and habitus of the patient
- Underlying patient medical conditions
- Condition of the skin around the wound
- Patient's comfort
- Cost of the materials

Once these considerations are made, the next step is to determine what the dressing is intended to do. The major actions or properties of dressings are adherence, absorption, and occlusion.

Adherence

At the point of contact with the wound, the dressing may be **adherent** or **nonadherent**. Adherent dressings cling to the wound and act as mechanical debriding agents when removed. During dressing changes, the adherent layer is ripped from the wound, taking necrotic tissue with it. This form of dressing may be used to debride wound healing by **second intention**. Most closed wounds (incisions) will be dressed with a nonadherent dressing. The contact layer of nonadherent dressings may be constructed from a material that resists clinging (such as Telfa) or may be impregnated with a petroleum-based lubricant (Adaptic, Xeroform) or other ointments.

Absorption

The ability of a dressing to absorb drainage is critical to the prevention of postoperative infection in wounds with expected **exudate**. As pus drains from the wound, it is trapped in the absorbent layer of the dressing. Gauze is an ideal absorbent material because it wicks bacteria away from the wound and into the dressing, where it is removed during dressing changes.

Occlusion

Fully **occlusive** dressings are used in the treatment of wounds such as abdominal evisceration and sucking pneumothorax; however, their usefulness is limited. Because occlusive dressings do not allow for evaporation and keep the skin airtight, they are prone to skin maceration, wound infection, and suture abscess formation. Some dressing materials, such as those impregnated with an emulsion (ie, Vaseline Gauze, Xeroform), are considered occlusive because they are resistant to drying and keep the skin moist; yet they are not impermeable because they facilitate the passage of secretions from the wound. Nonocclusive dressings (ie, Telfa, Adaptic) are widely used because they are permeable, promote evaporation, and limit the amount of bacterial growth within the wound by keeping the skin dry.

TYPES OF DRESSINGS

Once a determination of the overall goals and functions of the dressing has been made, one must decide which type of dressing will best suit the needs of the patient. Dressings should be large enough to cover the wound, tailored to its location, and specific to the nature of anticipated healing. Several options are available.

One-Layer Dressing

For small, clean incisions healing by first intention in which little or no exudate is expected, a one-layer dressing may be used. These dressings consist of a single layer of material that covers the wound, keeps it moist, protects it during initial healing, and supports epithelialization. Options include transparent, sterile polyurethane films (Opsite, Bioclusive), liquid collodion, aerosol adhesive sprays, foams, gels, hydrocolloids, and adhesive skin closure tapes (Steri-Strips). Dressings of this type are usually removed within 24 to 48 hours.

Three-Layer Dressing

Three-layer dressings are used when moderate to heavy exudate is expected and may be left in place longer than 48 hours. They consist of an inner contact layer, intermediate absorbent layer, and outer retention layer.

Contact Layer. The inner layer of a three-layer dressing is in direct contact with the surface of the wound. This layer should allow for the passage of secreted fluids into the middle layer. The contact layer should provide complete coverage of the wound and follow its anatomic contours. Depending on the nature of the wound, materials chosen for the contact layer may be adherent or nonadherent, occlusive, semi-occlusive, or nonocclusive. A wound for which normal, uncomplicated healing is expected can be dressed with a nonadherent, nonocclusive contact layer. Examples of common contact layers include nonadherent dressing materials (ie, Telfa, Adaptic), antibiotic ointments, and emulsion-impregnated gauze.

Absorbent Layer. The intermediate or absorbent layer is placed over the contact layer and is designed to absorb and wick fluids away from the wound. The thickness of this layer should be gauged by the amount of exudate expected to drain from the wound; however, if too much bulk is applied, compression of the wound may result in circulatory compromise. When moderate exudate is expected, gauze pads provide an ideal intermediate layer material. For heavy drainage, the use of fluff gauze (Kerlix), an ABD, or a combine dressing (Surgipad) will allow for greater absorbency.

Retention Layer. The outer layer of the three-layer dressing secures the contact and intermediate layers to the wound. Retaining materials may consist of tape, wrap (ie, Coban, Kling, Kerlix, Ace), stockinette, tube gauze, or **Montgomery straps** (see Figure 12-1). Montgomery straps are adhesive straps placed on the skin to secure the bandage and allow for frequent dressing changes without having to replace the tape each time.

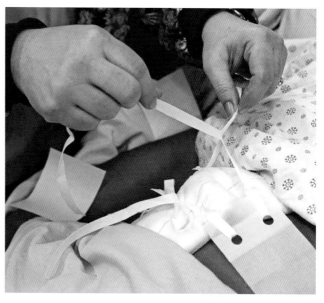

Figure 12-1 · Montgomery straps. (Reproduced, with permission, from Lynn PB. *Taylor's Clinical Nursing Skills: A Nursing Process Approach.* 5th ed. Philadelphia, PA: Wolters Kluwer; 2019.)

Pressure Dressing

When extensive surgery has been performed, use of a pressure dressing may be indicated to eliminate dead space, distribute pressure, absorb extensive drainage, influence wound tension, immobilize the wound, and provide the patient comfort. Pressure dressings are created by adding bulky material to the intermediate layer of a three-layer dressing.

Rigid Dressing

Casts and splints are examples of rigid dressings. They are commonly applied to traumatic wounds involving fractures for support and immobilization during healing. Plaster, fiberglass, or premanufactured (ie, finger split, knee brace) materials are available and their selection is largely based on availability and preference.

Bolster Dressing

To exert even pressure over an autografted wound such as a skin graft site and prevent the formation of hematomas or seromas under the graft, rolled gauze or other dressing materials may be sutured in place over the wound. This technique is known as a **bolster dressing** (see Figure 12-2).

Wet-to-Dry Dressing

The wet-to-dry dressing consists of dressing materials that are soaked in a sterile solution such as saline, antibiotic solution, or **Dakin's solution** and then applied over the wound and allowed to dry. As the dressing dries, it adheres to the wound. This process facilitates the removal of necrotic tissue from contaminated wounds during dressing changes. When healing by second intention, the wound should be repacked twice daily to facilitate thorough debridement. Because this method causes the patient a significant amount of pain and discomfort, dressing changes may be performed in the operating room under general anesthesia.

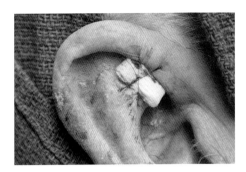

Figure 12-2 · Bolster dressing. (Reproduced, with permission, from Kantor J. *Atlas of Suturing Techniques: Approaches to Surgical Wound, Laceration, and Cosmetic Repair.* New York, NY: McGraw Hill; 2016.)

TABLE 12-1 • SKIN ADHESIVES	
Name	**Manufacturer**
Indermil Flexifuse®	Kendall
Dermabond Advanced®	Ethicon
Liquidband Flex®	Advanced Medical Solutions
Liquidband Optima®	Advanced Medical Solutions Limited
Derma + Flex®	Chemence Medical
Liquidband Exceed and Flow Control®	McKesson
SurgiSeal	Kebomed
SwiftSet™ Topical Skin Adhesive	Covidien
LiquiBand® Exceed™ XS Topical Skin Adhesive	Covidien

Wet-to-Wet Dressing

The wet-to-wet dressing is similar to the wet-to-dry dressing but differs in that the dressing is changed before it is totally dry. This method causes the patient less pain while providing a minimal amount of debridement.

Packing

The majority of surgical wounds are closed through first intention, but some are allowed to heal by secondary intention. This frequently involves packing and dressing of wound surfaces. Infected or necrotic wounds need in-depth surgical debridement, performed in the operating room. Such wounds are then often allowed to heal by secondary intention or delayed primary intention. They can be superficial or deep, and there can also be ever-changing sums of exudate, requiring frequent dressing changes.

Skin Glue

Cyanoacrylates were originally mass-produced in 1949. The first adhesives had an inflammatory effect on the tissues. In the 1970s, *N*-butyl-2-cyanoacrylate was developed and found to have insignificant tissue toxicity and good bonding strength, allowing for good cosmetic effects on the wound. *N*-butyl-2-cyanoacrylate has been used in Canada and other countries for the following situations:

- Cartilage and bone grafting
- Repair of damaged ossicles
- Embolization of gastrointestinal varices
- Covering corneal ulcers
- Covering canker sores
- Embolization in neurovascular surgery

There are several advantages to using skin glue, such as: it provides faster closure than stitches, provides a protective barrier from bacteria, eliminates the need for bandages, is waterproof, and there is no need for suture removal. The first widely used skin glue was Dermabond. Dermabond (2-octylcyanoacrylate) is the FDA-approved skin glue and has less toxicity and four times the strength of *N*-butyl-2-cyanoacrylate. It is more flexible, and the adhesive achieves maximum bonding strength within 2.5 minutes and is equal in strength to healed tissue at 7 days postopertively. DERMABOND PRINEO uses a liquid adhesive with self-adhering latex free mesh to close first intention wounds created from surgical incisions, trocar incisions from minimally invasive surgery and clean lacerations due to simple trauma. DERMABOND PRINEO is used in place of a subcuticular stitch or skin staples which penetrate skin tissue. Since Dermabond, there have been several skin adhesives that have come on the market. The SA should follow the manufacturer's instructions for application of their product (see Table 12-1).

DRESSING APPLICATION

Regardless of the type of material or technique used, application of the dressing follows the same basic concepts. The general process is as follows:

- Following closure of the wound and completion of a correct final count, the dressing materials are opened by the circulator and secured onto the field by the surgical technologist in the scrub role or scrub nurse.

- Using sterile technique, the wound is gently cleaned with a damp towel or sponge and patted dry.

- The contact layer of a three-layer dressing is applied over the entire wound with unsoiled gloves. If necessary, a skin adhesive (ie, tincture of benzoin, Mastisol) may be applied around the wound to secure the contact layer.

- If a drainage device is in place, the surgical wound is dressed separately from the stab wound incision. Slitted drain sponges are placed around the base of the drainage catheter. Emulsion-impregnated gauze may be used for occlusion around chest tubes.

- The contact layer is completely covered by the intermediate layer. This layer should be applied neatly and evenly.

- As the drapes are removed from the patient, the integrity and sterility of the dressing is maintained.

- Additional blood, body fluids, and skin prep solution are removed from the patient's skin.

- The retention layer is applied to secure the dressing. If a sterile retention layer is needed, it is applied prior to drape removal. The surgeon or surgical assistant is responsible for the application of rigid dressing materials as needed. If unsterile tape is used, this step may be performed by the circulating nurse.

- For closed nonchronic wounds, most dressings are changed using sterile technique within 48 hours.

CASTING / SPLINTING TECHNIQUE

Orthopedic injuries can include fractures, sprains, or postoperative immobilization. Swelling is often anticipated with these types of injuries. It is the body's natural reaction to injury. For this reason, splinting is often the optimal choice for the acute phase of the above-listed injuries. After the acute phase, a cast will be applied to further protect the injury during the repair phase. Splints are able to accommodate for the swelling in response to injury since it is not circumferential. If an accommodation is not made for the anticipated swelling of tissue, **compartment syndrome** may occur. Compartment syndrome compromises the neurovascular integrity of injured extremities. Symptoms of compartmental syndrome include pain, pressure, paresthesia, pulselessness, and swelling. If a patient experiences any of these symptoms, they should report to their physician or the emergency room for treatment. To diminish possible swelling of tissue, patients should apply the **RICE method** (Rest, Ice, Compression, Elevation) after a splint has immobilized the injury. Before applying any immobilization method, a preassessment should be completed. This assessment should include a neurovascular assessment, covering wounds with the appropriate dressing and secured with a rolled gauze, and acute fractures immobilized above and below the fracture when possible. All supplies should be gathered before the splint or cast is applied and the treatment should be explained to the patient.

Splinting

The size of the splint and cast padding is usually decided by the width of the patient's hand at the **MCP joint** for upper extremity and foot at the **MTP joint** for lower extremity. A 1- to 2-in cast padding and splint materials are usually appropriate for pediatric patients while a 3- to 4-in splint material is suitable for adults. If swelling is anticipated or already present, a stockinette is contraindicated due to compression issues and cast padding should be selected. Cast padding should start distally and proceed proximally. Wrap around the circumference completely twice to prevent slipping of the padding. Continuing from distal to proximal, overlap subsequent wraps at 50% to cover the extremity. The padding is wrapped at a slight angle to prevent gapping in the padding. The distal end should overlap 100% as well. Bony prominences such as radial styloid, olecranon, malleoli, calcaneus should be adequately padded to prevent pressure sores. Additional straps of padding can be applied to just these areas to assure proper padding. Room temperature or cool water

should be utilized, hot or warm water will hasten the exothermic reaction. A drape should be placed to keep the patient from getting wet during the process. Once a splint is placed, it is secured with a compression bandage or ace wrap, not too tightly, in case of possible swelling. It is important to leave a 1-in gap between the edges of the splint (see Figure 12-3). If the splint overlaps, it could become circumferential and will not allow for swelling. Patients should be instructed to avoid placing objects into the splint in order to scratch the skin, and should also prevent the splint from getting wet.

Casting

Casts are a circumferential form of immobilization and do not account for possible swelling. When cutting the stockinette, it should be longer than the cast to allow for the material to be flipped over the proximal and distal edges of the cast. The stockinette should be snug to the skin but not tight or binding. Any wrinkles should be smoothed out prior to the cast padding. Cast padding should be applied distally and proceed proximally. The first circumference of padding should be overlapped 100% for three times to ensure a comfortable cuff will be established when the stockinette is flipped over. All bone prominences should be assessed to ensure adequate padding. This extra step will prevent the formation of pressure sores within the cast. As with splinting, cool or room temperature water should be used for saturating fiberglass cast tapes. The Cooler water will slow the setting time allowing for proper molding prior to the exothermic reaction. To keep the strength of the cast uniform, the cast should be rolled evenly. The layers

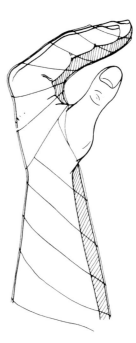

Figure 12-3 · Volar wrist and hand splint for immobilization of metacarpal shaft fractures and wrist injuries. (Reproduced, with permission, from Stone CK, Humphries RL, eds. *Current Diagnosis & Treatment: Emergency Medicine*. 8th ed. New York, NY: McGraw Hill; 2017.)

of the cast should be rubbed to seal the layers into a solid cast. This will give the cast strength, make it look good, and help prevent pressure sores by eliminating wrinkles. It is important to keep the cast narrow in the web space between the thumb and index finger and keep the palmar crease free to allow for movement of the fingers. The cast should be well molded to the body part. This allows for maximized strength and is accomplished by holding and molding the cast carefully using the palm and heel of your hands. A three-point fixation is often applied to mold displaced fractures in long bones to maintain fracture reduction. This can be accomplished by placing one hand on the apex of the fracture and the other on the opposite side distal to the apex and bringing them together to align the fracture fragments. After the initial layers of the cast or splint are applied, repeat the process on the setting plaster or fiberglass to mold the fracture fragments in place with the cast or splint (see Figure 12-4). This reduces the possibility of the fracture being displaced. Soft spots in casts can occur around the olecranon and calcaneus and are eliminated by applying an additional roll of cast tape over the area. Once the cast is set, it is imperative to evaluate the patient's neurovascular status.

The location and severity of the fracture will determine what type of cast will be applied. Options include:

- Short-arm casts for wrist fractures
- Long-arm casts to immobilize forearm or elbow fractures
- Long-leg casts, indicated for fractures that include the femur, tibia, or fibula, or complicated ankle fractures
- Short-leg casts work for ankle and foot fractures
- Hip spica casts, used for complete leg immobilization
- Body jacket casts for spinal immobilization

Cast Removal

Removal of a cast requires an electric cast saw or cutter. The blade is gently pushed into the cast as the blade oscillates back and forth. The saw blade is applied to the cast in an "up and down" motion along the cast in a straight line with a firm motion. The blade should never be pushed into the cast and pulled through the cast material. By firming but gently using the up and down motion, friction and heat can be avoided between the saw and cast material. Special precaution should be used when cutting over bony prominences, such as the styloid process or malleolus, to prevent cutting the skin. **Cast spreaders** will release the cast and allow it to be split into two halves. Use bandage scissors to cut the stockinette at each end of the cast. Pull the anterior half of the

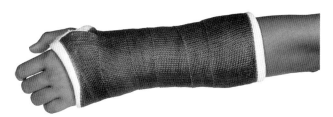

Figure 12-4 • Cast. (Used with permission from Stacy Nazelrod /Shutterstock.)

cast away from the posterior half and then cut the cast padding. Be mindful not to twist or rotate the remodeled bone.

Immobilization Devices

Slings. Injuries such as dislocations, partial rotator cuff injuries, small fractures, and tendon/ligament damage are treated with static shoulder orthoses (SOs) to protect the glenohumeral joint from subluxation. The most common device is a sling, which can be used along with a cast or a splint, or alone as an immobilization device.

Braces. Braces support, align, or hold a body part in the proper anatomical position. Braces are occasionally used after surgery is performed on an arm or a leg, or if an injury occurred. Braces generally have Velcro straps allowing for adjustments to the brace and easy removal. Braces offer less support and protection than a cast and may not be a recommended treatment option in all circumstances.

Collars. A cervical collar is indicated for post-surgery anterior cervical discectomy and fusion (ACDF). Post-surgical cervical collar use is thought to reduce post-operative pain, provide the patient with a sense of security to manage activities of daily living as well as reduce the incidences of non-fusion.

Traction. Immobilization may also be achieved through traction. Traction applies tension to correct the alignment of two structures (eg, two bones). The goal of traction is to guide the body part back into alignment and maintain the proper position. Traction may be used to:

- Stabilize and realign bone fractures, such as a broken arm or leg
- Help reduce the pain of a fracture before surgery
- Treat bone deformities caused by certain conditions, such as scoliosis
- Correct stiff and constricted muscles, joints, tendons, or skin
- Stretch the neck and prevent painful muscle spasms

DRAINS

Following surgery, body fluids and air accumulate within the wound naturally and may require drainage in order for proper wound healing to occur. Therefore, drains are often inserted prior to or during wound closure to aid in the prevention of dead space, seroma formation, or hematomas that can lead to infection and disruption of the wound. Other reasons to insert a drain include monitoring of drainage output, such as bile from the abdomen, or detecting anastomosis leaks. Chest tube drains are utilized in preventing pneumothorax or hemothorax.

When selecting and placing drainage devices, one must remember that drains are foreign bodies that may cause tissue reactivity, infection, or pressure necrosis. Although prophylactic infection prevention is a common indication for the use of drains, they communicate with the skin and provide a direct channel for the introduction of bacterial contamination.

Hence, drains should be used conservatively and cautiously, especially around joint spaces and near avascular planes created by synthetic grafts and other surgical implants.

To ensure proper placement, the straightest and most direct route to the skin should be used. A new stab wound is often created apart from the main surgical incision. The incidence of postoperative hernia formation may be increased if the drain is placed through the operative wound. The size of the stab incision will be indicated by the diameter of the drain, for example, a ¼-in Penrose drain will require the creation of a ¼-in stab incision. Once the incision is made, a hemostatic clamp is passed into the wound to create a tract or tunnel. The drain is then placed within the wound, grasped by the clamp at the end that will protrude from the skin, and pulled through the tract toward the outside of the body. The drain should be placed carefully and away from nerves, blood vessels, and sites of surgical anastomosis. To avoid dislodgment, drains are affixed to the skin using suture, adhesive tape, or another means as indicated by the type of drain used. It is imperative that proper sterile and aseptic technique is employed and that appropriate postoperative dressings are chosen.

There are several methods available to secure a drain.

- Roman garter technique by using silk suture, a common method for securing a drain
- Nylon suture
- Safety pin
- Drain clip
- Adhesive
- Tie-Lok™

After placement of the drain, two Tie-Lok™ components are placed around the body of the drain. The tail of the Tie-Lok™ is cut with scissors. A suture is then stitched to the skin and a separate loop of suture is placed through the hollow eye of the Tie-Lok component and is secured with a surgical knot.

Surgical dressing of a drain will be determined by surgeon preference or institutional practice. Common methods of dressing a drain include:

- A flat gauze sponge with a pre-cut T slit around the drain and secured with tape.
- Semi-occlusive dressing such as Tagaderm will decrease healing time and reduce patient discomfort.
- Chlorhexidine-impregnated disk is indicated for high-risk patients to prevent infection.

Removal of drains should be done as soon as clinically possible because the risk of infection is significantly increased if the drain is left in place longer than 3 to 4 days. Drains are classified into one of two groups, active or passive, based on their mechanism of action.

Passive Drains

Passive drainage devices are placed within the wound to allow a pathway for the removal of air and body fluids from an area of high pressure (within the wound) to an area of low pressure (outside the wound). To facilitate drainage, a gravity collection device may be connected to the drain. Examples of passive drains include the Penrose, Pezzer, Malecot, and T-tube drains.

Penrose. Penrose drains (see Figure 12-5) are one of the oldest and most commonly used passive drainage devices. These drains function by capillary action to move fluid away from the wound and consist of soft latex tubing that is available in several different diameters. Because they are soft, Penrose drains are easily manipulated and placed within the body and may be cut and shaped to fit around anatomic structures. To prevent retraction and slippage into the wound, the drain can be secured to the skin using a safety pin for transfixion. Significant drainage occurs within the first 24 to 48 hours following surgery, at which time fibrin begins to wall off the drain tract.

To counteract fibrin formation, the drain is withdrawn from the wound progressively, about 1 to 2 cm each day. Each time the drain is withdrawn, excess tubing is cut from its distal end and the safety pin is applied at the new location. To increase capillary action, some surgeons place rolled gauze within the lumen of the Penrose drain, a modification referred to as the cigarette drain.

Despite their advantages, Penrose drains are used by general surgeons with less and less frequency because they are inefficient when compared to more modern alternatives. Because of their reliance on capillary action, drainage of the wound only occurs when the pressure within the wound exceeds the resistance of the drain. Dressings must be changed frequently to avoid oversaturation that can reduce the capillarity of the drain tract.

Pezzer or Malecot. The Pezzer or Malecot catheter is often used to provide nephrostomy drainage if the normal flow of urine from the kidney to the bladder is blocked. Urine built up in the kidney can cause permanent kidney damage; therefore, any blockage must be addressed and treated. The self-retaining catheter is inserted through an incision in the abdominal wall into the renal pelvis.

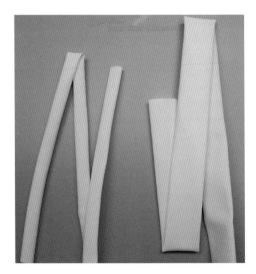

Figure 12-5 • Penrose drain. (From Cochran A, Braga R, eds. *Introduction to the Operating Room.* New York, NY: McGraw Hill; 2019. Used, with permission, from Ruth Braga, University of Utah.)

T-tube. T-tubes are inserted into the biliary system to drain bile away from the wound following biliary surgery or to aid in the operative correction of acute suppurative cholangitis. The top part of the tube, the "T," is placed in the common bile duct while the long bottom part of the tube is brought out of the abdomen through a small incision and connected to a bag. A gravity collection device known as a bile bag is attached to the drain to collect evacuated fluids. T-tubes are removed following normal results from a cholangiogram taken 24 hours postoperatively.

Active Drains

Drainage systems that use negative pressure to draw fluids and air from the wound are active drains. Negative pressure is created by attaching the drain to a pressurized manual collection device or mechanical vacuum pump. Active drainage system examples include the Hemovac, Jackson-Pratt, sump, and chest tube drains.

Hemovac. When moderate drainage is expected following orthopedic procedures, the Hemovac drain may be used. Hemovac drains consist of a drainage catheter attached to a sharp trocar that is passed through the layers of the cavity directly near the wound from inside to outside. Once inserted, the trocar point is removed with scissors and the drainage catheter tubing is cut to an appropriate length (see Figure 12-6).

The drain is attached to a collection device. Air is removed from the collection device manually by removing the stopper, squeezing the device, and replacing the stopper to create a negative pressure vacuum. The collection device will hold up to 450 mL of fluid. The drainage catheter size varies from 7 to 19 French or ¼, 1/8, 3/16, and 3/32 in.

Jackson-Pratt. The Jackson-Pratt drain is used following abdominal or soft tissue surgery to remove a moderate amount of fluid from the wound. Various diameters and configurations are available; the most common are 7- to 10-mm round and flat drains. Like the Hemovac drain, they consist of a drainage

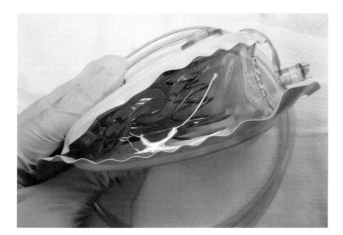

Figure 12-6 · Hemovac drain. (From Cochran A, Braga R, eds. *Introduction to the Operating Room.* New York, NY: McGraw Hill; 2019. Used with permission from Ruth Braga, University of Utah.)

catheter that is attached to a manual reservoir. Because they are composed of soft, pliable plastics they are useful for additional applications such as neurosurgery and breast procedures. Jackson-Pratt drains are secured to the skin using nonabsorbable suture.

Sump. In addition to drainage, the sump drainage system can also be used for irrigation of the wound and instillation of medications. Sump drains have large perforations on their lateral edge that reduce the likelihood of clogging. To create equalized negative pressure, they are attached to either in-wall or portable vacuum devices set between 80 and 120 mm Hg. Once fluid drainage slows and becomes negligible, the drain is removed completely from the wound.

Chest Tube. Chest tubes are used to remove fluid and maintain negative pressure within the pleural space following procedures or trauma of the thorax. When two ipsilateral tubes are inserted, one is placed superiorly to evacuate air, while the other is placed inferiorly to remove fluids that accumulate under gravitational force. Chest tubes may be straight or angled and are available in several diameters. A large nonabsorbable suture is placed through the skin and tied around the tube to prevent accidental removal. Because variances in pressure within the thoracic cavity can lead to collapsed lung, the tubes are connected to a special water seal drainage system. The chest tubes allow for drainage of air, blood, and other fluid from the intrapleural space. The chest tubes are connected to a drain system that uses three mechanisms to remove air and fluid from the pleural cavity, expiratory pressure, gravity, and suction. The first chamber collects the drainage from the pleural space, the second chamber provides a water seal, and the third chamber provides suction that is controlled by the level of water. It is essential the drainage system is lower than the chest to facilitate drainage and prevent backflow. For safety reasons, only **standard** suction devices should be used on any drain or device connected to the patient. The Neptune Suction System should never be hooked up to drains or chest tubes.

It is worthwhile noting that many hospitals currently use the Neptune® Waste Management System mobile unit for fluid waste and small debris from the surgical site during operative procedures. The Neptune® system is used with the Neptune® Docking station. The docking station waste disposal zone is commonly housed in an enclosed area in proximity to the operating rooms. The Neptune® System is a high flow, high suction system, and if not used with proper training can cause irreparable harm to the patient. The FDA reported that the Neptune 1 Silver and Neptune 2 Ultra Waste Management Systems were responsible for patient injuries, including:

- Hemorrhaging
- Soft tissue damage
- Muscle damage
- Vital organ damage
- Death

Bibliography

Abbott A, Halvorsen M, Dedering A. Is there a need for cervical collar usage post anterior cervical decompression and fusion using interbody cages? A Randomized Controlled Pilot Trial. *Physiother Theory Pract.* 2013;29(4):290-300. doi: 10.3109/09593985.2012.731627. Epub October 17; 2012. https://pubmed.ncbi.nlm.nih.gov/23074995/. Accessed May 26, 2023.

Bruns TB, Worthington JM. Using tissue adhesive for wound repair: a practical guide to dermabond. *Am Fam Physician.* 2000;61(5):1383-1388. https://www.aafp.org/afp/2000/0301/p1383.html. Accessed May 26, 2023.

FDA Issues Updated Safety Communication on Stryker Neptune Waste management Systems. March 27, 2013. https://www.infectioncontroltoday.com/operating-room/fda-issues-updated-safety-communication-stryker-neptune-waste-management-systems. Accessed May 26, 2023.

Hemovac Evacuators. https://www.zimmer.co.uk/medical-professionals/products/surgical-and-operating-room-solutions/hemovac-evacuators.html. Accessed May 26, 2023.

Immobilization. http://www.healthofchildren.com/I-K/Immobilization.html#ixzz6QIVu9IHH. Accessed May 26, 2023.

Kelishadi SS, Zeiderman M, Freeman DW, Tutela JP, Wilhelmi BJ, The Double Opposing Semiocclusive Drain Dressing. Published online September 7, 2015. https://www.ncbi.nlm.nih.gov/pmc/articles/PMC4714597/. Accessed May 26, 2023.

Shoulder brace. *Anesthesia Secrets.* 4th ed. 2011. https://www.sciencedirect.com/topics/nursing-and-health-professions/shoulder-brace. Accessed May 26, 2023.

Tarwari A, McFarlane J, Peters JL. A simple technique for securing drains. *Science Direct.* Elsevier, 2004;35(11):91-93. https://www.sciencedirect.com/science/article/pii/S1572346104000327. Accessed May 26, 2023.

13

Managing Perioperative Emergencies

Brenda K. Pointer

The ability to respond calmly in an emergency is one of the most valuable traits, which separates operating room personnel from other healthcare professionals. Despite preventive measures, a situation may arise in surgery, which calls for an emergent response. A surgical assistant must master the ability to identify warning signs and perform specific duties during an emergency. While emergencies are not commonplace, unless working in trauma, they can happen with any surgical procedure. The team must be educated and prepared to react quickly and efficiently. Emergencies in the operating room arise through three main causes: the first relating to the anesthetic, the second to the surgical procedure, and the third to a patient's health. In the event of respiratory or cardiac emergencies, the cause may be related to the anesthetic or surgical complications; however, there are cases where an emergent event is precipitated by the overall failing health of the patient. No matter the cause, the surgical assistant should have the ability to recognize an emergency as it unfolds and react accordingly to serve the needs of the team and patient, while assuring preventive measures are taken for the future.

ANESTHESIA EMERGENCIES

Anesthesia emergencies may include malignant hyperthermia, pseudocholinesterase deficiency, paralytic ileus, anaphylactic reactions, respiratory events, or cardiac events. While the anesthesia provider is the primary responder treating these complications through medication, the surgical team should be able to recognize the signs and symptoms and be available to assist in the team effort to resolve the emergency. Oftentimes, the sign or symptom will become evident in the amount of bleeding at the surgical site, the temperature of the body tissues, or the color of the skin and tissues. With the patient covered in drapes, it is the responsibility of the surgical team to bring awareness of changes identified to the anesthesia provider and surgeon.

Malignant Hyperthermia

Malignant hyperthermia, most commonly referred to as MH, is a genetically-transmitted syndrome that occurs in surgery when a patient is administered the muscle relaxant, succinylcholine, or an anesthetic agent such as halothane, enflurane, or isoflurane. The syndrome is seen mostly in males and may also be seen triggered outside the operating room by vigorous exercise. This emergency is one in which the whole team must respond to help save the life of the patient.

The first signs and symptoms of a MH crisis include tachycardia, tachypnea, and increased carbon dioxide levels. While a patient who is feeling pain or waking up might exhibit tachycardia and tachypnea, the carbon dioxide levels should indicate to anesthesia to explore the possibility of MH. These symptoms are followed by muscle rigidity, which may cause difficulty for the surgical assistant and surgeon in retraction. A later sign is the increase in core body temperature, which can go up to

107F degrees, and might be evident to anesthesia or the sterile team members when touching the skin or tissues of the patient.

Most facilities have a MH cart located in a common area for use in the operating rooms. Treatment for MH begins with discontinued use of the triggering agent and the administration of 100% oxygen to the patient. Medication administered is Dantrolene sodium (Dantrium) as a loading dose of 2.5 mg/kg and 1 mg/kg every 5 minutes thereafter up to 10 to 30 mg/kg. Intravenous fluids may be chilled to facilitate the cooling of the patient as well as utilizing chilled saline irrigation to any accessible body cavities except the bladder. Unsterile team members should pack the patient in ice at the axilla, base of the skull, and groin, if possible. Further interventions involve the placement of a Foley catheter with a urine meter to closely monitor urine output. Sodium bicarbonate is used to regulate acidosis while glucose is also needed for metabolism in the cells. Renal function and removal of waste is assisted utilizing mannitol, while heparin may be given to prevent clot formation in the blood.

Prevention of malignant hyperthermia can be difficult unless the patient has a family history of complications during surgery. In the event of a known history, a patient can be tested by undergoing a muscle biopsy using a local anesthetic. If confirmed, anesthesia providers would proceed with a general anesthetic avoiding triggering agents, or provide alternate modes of anesthesia, if appropriate. Additionally, if anesthesia has a suspicion of MH history, non-triggering anesthetic agents could be utilized prophylactically.

Pseudocholinestrase Deficiency

Pseudocholinesterase deficiency syndrome is a condition in which the patient has difficulty processing the choline ester medications used to paralyze the skeletal muscles in a patient during a general anesthetic, specifically succinylcholine and mivacurium. Typically, this syndrome is inherited; however, it may also result from malnutrition, kidney or liver disease, cancer, or major burns. Those affected by inheriting the gene obtained the gene from both parents. If the gene is inherited from only one parent, the person is a carrier and not affected. This syndrome is more commonly seen in Alaskan natives and patients of Persian Jewish descent and twice as often in women.

Unless a patient has been diagnosed with pseudocholinesterase deficiency syndrome from a previous surgery, this syndrome exists without symptoms. As a result, complications are often discovered at the end of a surgical procedure utilizing general anesthetic, when the anesthetist has minimal neurological response from the patient after discontinuing the paralytic agent. Once identified, the patient must be kept sedated, potentially for as long as 8 hours, until the paralytic wears off and the patient regains the ability to move and breathe without assistance.

Prevention is possible with full knowledge of patient and family history. If a patient has a family history of difficulty during anesthesia, they may undergo a blood test to identify pseudocholinesterase enzyme activity. Due to the potential for inheritance, family members should warn one another if they have difficulties processing and recovering from paralytics.

Anaphylactic Reaction

Anaphylaxis is the most extreme form of a Type I allergic reaction. This reaction occurs when a patient is exposed to a trigger, either a medication given by the surgeon or anesthesia provider or contact with a triggering substance such as latex. Muscle relaxants are the most common cause of anaphylaxis in the operating room followed by latex, antibiotics, and induction agents. Due to the lethality of an allergic reaction, patient allergies are included in the "time-out" at the beginning of every procedure to assure the operating room team members are cognizant of potential triggers. A person exposed to an allergen will initially respond with hives or wheezing; however, she may progress to difficulty breathing, tightening of the throat, rapid heartbeat, decreased blood pressure, or in extreme situations, cardiac arrest.

Rapid response to an allergic reaction is key in the treatment of the surgical patient. Administration of intravenous epinephrine, otherwise known as adrenaline, along with supplemental oxygen, is the primary treatment for a severe anaphylactic reaction to an allergen in the operating room during surgery. Additionally, anesthesia may provide an antihistamine, cortisone, or albuterol to improve respiration.

Prevention of anaphylaxis in the operating room begins with a thorough patient and family history with a focus on known allergies to medications or substances. In the event a medication, with a known sensitivity, must be administered during surgery, anesthesia may pre-treat the patient with antihistamines and corticosteroids. With respect to latex allergies, the focus rests on the patient's history and any previous exposures to latex. Patients with indwelling catheters, a history of multiple surgical procedures, allergy to bananas, or those who are healthcare workers are at a higher risk for an allergic response to latex. Providing a latex-free environment for all patients, whenever possible, reduces the risk of developing an allergy to latex through the reduction in exposure.

RESPIRATORY COMPLICATIONS

The most common respiratory complications in the operating room include aspiration, laryngospasm or bronchospasm, atelectasis, pneumothorax, and pulmonary embolism. These complications are often a result of preexisting respiratory conditions, smoking, chest wall deformities, obesity, or age; however, these may also be a result of the patient positioning necessary during surgery or the duration or severity of the procedure. Although the anesthesia provider monitors respirations, the entire surgical team is responsible to monitor patient responses to medications administered, changes in positioning, or effects of tissue manipulation and retraction especially when operating in the abdomen or thorax.

Aspiration

Aspiration occurs when the reflexes of the throat decrease, as a patient is rendered semi-conscious or unconscious, during the administration of anesthesia and gastric secretions enter the lungs. The acidic contents of the stomach cause chemical pneumonitis, which results in edema and collapse of alveoli and finally hypoxemia. Indications of aspiration include cyanosis, which is a bluish cast of lips and fingernail beds, dyspnea, and tachycardia. Treatment of aspiration begins with suctioning aspirate as well as lowering the head of the bed and tilting it to the right followed by oxygenation and positive pressure ventilation. If solid matter is aspirated, a bronchoscopy procedure may be necessary to remove the contents. Anesthesia will need to monitor blood-gas and acid-base determinations operatively and postoperatively for the proper treatment of the patient. Most often, patients are treated postoperatively with a broad-spectrum antibiotic.

Prevention of aspiration begins with a thorough patient history. If the patient has a known condition, such as gastroesophageal reflux disease (GERD), has ingested food or drink within 8 hours prior to surgery, or is potentially under the influence of drugs or alcohol, Sellick's maneuver or cricoid pressure during induction is indicated along with intubation using a cuffed tube. Preoperative medication should include Reglan, or a similar medication, to reduce the production of acid in the stomach and stimulate gut motility. Lastly, anesthesia may employ a technique called rapid sequence induction and intubation (RSII), which speeds up the intubation process, leaving the airway unprotected for a shorter amount of time than the normal induction and intubation process.

Laryngospasm and Bronchospasm

Laryngospasm and bronchospasm are respiratory complications commonly encountered in the operating room. While the laryngospasm occurs as a partial or complete closure of the vocal cords, bronchospasm is a narrowing of the bronchi caused by smooth muscle contraction. These two conditions are seen most often during the induction or emergence phases of anesthesia and commonly occur in patients with a history of smoking or asthma. Laryngospasm and bronchospasm are triggered by a spasm of the "gag" reflex due to excessive saliva, inadequate sedation, or airway inflammation. The most common characteristic of these conditions is a high-pitched wheezing or stridor prior to intubation or immediately following extubation. Treatment for spasm of the airway includes positive pressure ventilation followed by administration of a neuromuscular blocker, succinylcholine, to relax the muscular response. During extubation, anesthesia will often be forced to deepen the sedation or re-intubate the patient until oxygen levels return to normal and another attempt at extubation can safely occur.

In order to prevent these airway complications from occurring, knowledge of the patient's history is of the utmost importance. For patients with a known asthma or smoking history, an anticholinergic medication, such as Robinul, should be administered prior to surgery for a reduction in mucous secretion and saliva. An additional prevention measure is the utilization of aerosolized lidocaine to numb the throat and upper respiratory tract. Similarly, as in the prevention of aspiration, anesthesia personnel may utilize rapid sequence induction and intubation to swiftly secure and protect the airway.

Atelectasis

Atelectasis, a full or partial collapse of the lung, is more common postoperatively and has a potential to lead to bronchopneumonia. The increase in mucous production and shallow breathing due to pain or sedation following general anesthesia are contributing factors to the onset of atelectasis. Temperature, pulse, and respirations all increase with this condition while the patient will appear cyanotic having reduced breath sounds with faint crackling. Partial collapse will be evident on x-ray. Both treatment and prevention of atelectasis involve coughing and deep breathing, as well as early ambulation postoperatively.

Pneumothorax

While it is rare, pneumothorax is another potential surgical complication occasionally seen in the operating room, when entry is inadvertently made into the thoracic cavity. The patient will have shortness of breath and pain when breathing. In the event entry to the thoracic cavity is recognized during upper abdominal, breast, or renal surgery, the hole should be repaired with suture. If the lung fails to expand, treatment is a closed chest tube drainage system to enable the lung re-expansion. Prevention involves extreme care in identifying tissue and avoiding penetration into the thoracic cavity.

Pulmonary Embolism

Pulmonary embolism is a dangerous and significant cause of death in the operating room as well as postoperatively. This condition is caused by a blockage of the pulmonary artery by a blood clot, or fat, plaque, or air. Preexisting clotting or plaque conditions, the duration of the procedure, or pressure on major vessels of the venous return system may cause emboli. Venous stasis, or a slower blood flow, is contributing factor to deep vein thrombosis (DVT) and is more prevalent in patients with obesity, congestive heart failure, or dehydration. A patient in the operating room will present with a sudden increased heart and respiratory rate, while a postoperative presentation may include fever, dyspnea, chest pain, increased breathing, and elevated heart rate. Within 24 to 48 hours, the patient is at risk for acute respiratory distress syndrome (ARDS) often resulting in a high mortality rate.

As for prevention measures for any complication, knowledge of patient history is imperative to safely prepare a patient for surgery with risk factors for emboli. Prior to time-intensive surgical procedures or when a patient is at high risk for clotting, anti-embolism stockings are applied to the legs or the patient may be given pre- and postoperative heparin or warfarin to prevent clotting. Insertion of a Greenfield filter may be indicated if anticoagulants are unsuccessful in dissolving a preoperative clot. Surgery involving the manipulation of any major vessel increases the risk of plaque emboli. The surgical team should handle surrounding tissue gently, beginning with the prep of the area performed by the circulator or surgical assistant. In orthopedic procedures, care must be taken to suction all blood and body fluids prior to the manipulation of fractures or reaming of bone, as this may increase the risk for fat emboli.

CARDIAC COMPLICATIONS

While there are numerous cardiac complications, which may occur perioperatively, there are three main categories in which to focus as a surgical assistant. The changes in blood pressure during a surgical procedure often correlate with the control of operative site bleeding. Communicate any changes identified in the amount of bleeding at the site. Increases in bleeding may indicate an unexpected elevation in blood pressure, while a severe decrease in bleeding may indicate hypotension. Team members should be aware of the common arrhythmias occurring in the operative environment to assist anesthesia in awareness and management. Lastly, in the event of cardiac arrest in the operating room, a surgical assistant plays an important role in the treatment of an arresting patient.

Hypotension and Hypertension

Blood pressure is a significant factor in the management of the surgical patient. Whether the patient is hypotensive, with a low blood pressure, or hypertensive, with a high blood pressure, these conditions may affect the anesthetic administration as well as how the surgical team approaches a procedure. Dropping blood pressures during positioning leads the team to slow the positioning process or resume a neutral position to allow for stability of the pressure. During a procedure, low pressure may indicate the need to lighten anesthetics or it may suggest to the surgical team to assess for unidentified or excessive bleeding. Hypotension, if left untreated, could result in a deficit of blood to the brain and heart, eventually causing death. Other symptoms, which may accompany low blood pressure, include an elevation in pulse, elevated serum pH, decrease in urinary output, and reduced bleeding at the field. Treatment for a decrease in pressure depends on the cause. Anesthesia may need to lighten sedation, increase fluid volume, or it may be necessary to raise the patient's legs, if medications are unsuccessful in restoring a healthy pressure.

On the other hand, hypertension, often seen in arteriosclerotic patients, also must be brought under control in the perioperative setting. During a procedure, sudden hypertension might suggest an excessive replacement of fluid or the need for deepening of anesthetic. In the postoperative patient, it may occur due to poor pain control. Management of high blood pressure usually consists of oxygen, an antihypertensive beta-blocker, and a diuretic. Awareness of a patient's baseline blood pressure is key in assessing the patient throughout the perioperative process.

Arrhythmia

While there are a variety of arrhythmias, which may occur perioperative, atrial fibrillation is the most common seen in the surgical setting. Anticoagulation is often associated with the treatment of atrial fibrillation, thus presenting challenges with respect to the control of blood loss in patients with known A-Fib. Beta-blockers or calcium channel blockers are generally the best choice to control these arrhythmias. In the event the rhythm cannot be controlled, a patient may have to undergo cardioversion.

Premature ventricular contraction (PVC) is a condition where the myocardium is irritated and the heart beats prematurely. It is caused by caffeine or an imbalance of electrolytes, which may occur perioperative. This is generally treated with a lidocaine bolus, followed by a controlled drip. If untreated, this condition may lead to ventricular tachycardia (V-tach) which is evidenced by a rapid heart rate of over 100 bpm and as high as 220 bpm. V-tach must be treated immediately to prevent Ventricular fibrillation (V-fib), the most dangerous of arrhythmias.

In V-fib the heart beats rapidly and irregularly as the ventricles are not contracting properly and cardiac output eventually ceases. Cardiac defibrillation along with medications for myocardial stimulation and vasodilation are used to treat this deadly condition. A patient in V-fib is in danger of cardiac arrest, the most serious complication of arrhythmias.

Cardiac Arrest

In the event of cardiac arrest, the heart ceases with no electrical activity, which displays as a straight line on the ECG, asystole. Respiratory cessation will either precede or follow cardiac arrest. Most commonly, this occurs in patients with prior cardiac history or undergoing cardiac surgery. In an otherwise healthy patient, this may occur with major blood loss, respiratory obstruction, severe hypotension, sepsis, anesthetic overdose, or an underlying heart condition. The symptoms indicating cardiac arrest are the cessation of the heartbeat, fixed pupils, cyanosis, or dark blood at the surgical site.

Treatment begins with cardiopulmonary resuscitation (CPR) to restore oxygen to organs and defibrillate the heart to re-establish a rhythm. Anesthesia is responsible for breathing and respirations while a member of the surgical team, either the surgical technologist or the surgical assistant, is responsible for chest compressions. The start of CPR is accompanied by IV medications, such as epinephrine, vasopressin, and amiodarone, to aid in restoration of cardiac function.

For prevention measures, in a patient with a known heart condition, it is important to avoid stimulation during induction. The patient should be monitored closely with respect to ECG, arterial pressure, and oxygen saturation throughout the perioperative process. Early intervention, if issues arise, is key.

SHOCK

Shock occurs when there is a lack of the perfusion of blood to body tissues. This condition may occur for various reasons including complications with hypovolemia, sepsis, cardiogenic or neurogenic issues. While there are several causes of shock, hypovolemic and septic shock are the two most common in surgery. The symptoms of shock vary depending on the cause; however, most present with tachycardia, decrease in blood pressure and urine output, and vasoconstriction. This reaction is the body's way of preserving blood flow for essential organs to sustain life. Treatment of shock begins with a secure airway and an attempt to restore the circulatory function of the patient to normal levels. Each category of shock will use varied methods to restore blood pressure and profusion, depending on the cause.

Hypovolemic Shock

Assistance with visualization and control of bleeding are the most important tasks performed by the surgical assistant. Although some degree of blood loss is to be expected during surgery, uncontrolled hemorrhage is a life-threatening condition. This commonly occurs in patients with a congenital hemostatic defect such as hemophilia or Von Willebrand's disease as well as in patients taking blood-thinning medications such as Coumadin, heparin, or warfarin. There are numerous options to control bleeding in the surgical setting including chemical, thermal, and mechanical.

Topical chemical or biological control of bleeding occurs with milder incidences of bleeding or oozing of a generalized area. These medications come in many forms including sponges, powders, foam, or film. The chart gives examples of the various medicated products used to control minor bleeding by applying them to the area where bleeding occurs. Biological control involves the use of fibrin glue made up of calcium chloride and thrombin, which is mixed on the field and applied to the bleeding source.

The most common way to control bleeding in the operating room is the use of heat or thermal hemostasis. This is accomplished using an electrosurgical unit and grounding pad, bipolar cautery, lasers, or ultrasonic/harmonic scalpel. Heat has the ability to cut and coagulate tissues simultaneously, providing a bloodless field for the surgeon and assistant. Thermal hemostasis is most often utilized when bleeding is focused to a small- or medium-sized vessel. It may also be used in combination with mechanical techniques.

In the treatment of heavy bleeding or the necessity to divide a large vessel, there are several techniques for the mechanical control of blood loss. With unanticipated bleeding, direct pressure and patience are the first line of defense to gaining control. Assuring visualization prior to attempting a permanent solution for the bleeding is key. Once visualization is achieved and pressure has been applied to slow the bleeding, the use of clamps, hemostatic clips, or ligatures is employed to permanently stop the bleeding. In the event bleeding cannot be controlled and the estimated blood loss (EBL) exceeds safe limits, usually 1500 cc for the average adult; blood replacement is necessary.

In the event blood loss is anticipated in an elective procedure, patients may opt to give blood several months prior to surgery in order to receive their own autologous blood, if needed during the procedure. Blood may even be salvaged during a procedure by collecting lost blood into a cell saver, filtering it, and reinfusing it into the patient. In the absence of autologous blood, homologous, or donated, blood is used after typing and cross-matching to the patient. Figure 13-1 lists the four classifications of hemorrhage and symptoms associated at each level.

Providing careful dissection and clear visualization for the surgeon are ways the surgical assistant can help protect a patient from excessive blood loss. A keen awareness of the patient's medical history is imperative to the proper preparation and care for each individual. Swift access to life-saving

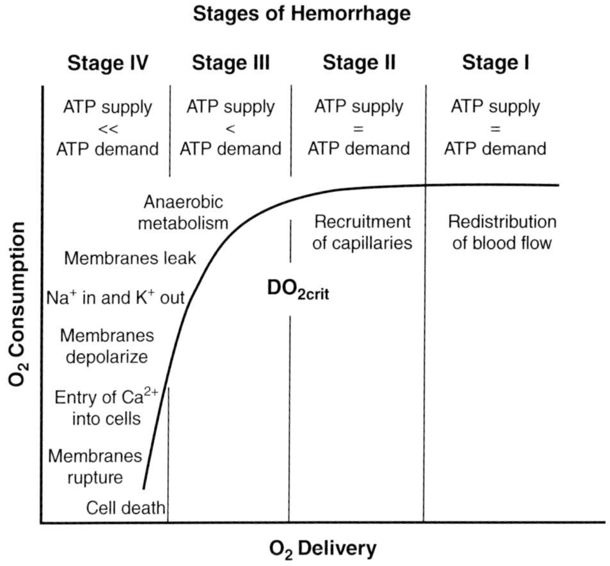

Figure 13-1 · Changes in oxygen consumption shown as a function of oxygen delivery. DO_{2crit}, critical oxygen delivery. (Reproduced, with permission, from Gutierrez G, Reines HD, Wulf-Gutierrez ME. Clinical review: hemorrhagic shock. *Crit Care.* 2004;8(5):373-381.)

medications and blood, especially with a known at-risk patient, is essential in providing safe patient care with respect to bleeding. In patients taking anticoagulants, the best prevention is to refrain from blood thinning medications for 5 to 7 days prior to surgery if possible.

Septic Shock

In patients with septic shock, the condition is caused by a severe infection, usually bacterial, when the body's response to fighting the infection eventually leads to severe vasodilation. Unfortunately, this condition has a 40% to 60% mortality rate and early diagnosis and treatment are key to survival. Treatment includes intubation to preserve oxygenation of tissues, fluids to increase circulatory volume, vasopressors, and most importantly, treatment of the infection through appropriate antibiotics and/or surgical debridement when indicated. A major complication of septic shock is disseminated intravascular coagulation (DIC), when blood clots form throughout the body in small vessels, thus inhibiting blood flow to all major organs and the peripheral vascular system. In a patient with DIC, complications may lead to acute respiratory distress syndrome (ARDS), where the blood oxygen levels are low due to the clots.

Cardiogenic Shock

Cardiogenic shock is associated with heart failure or myocardial ischemia, which leads to tissue hypoxia. An acute myocardial infarction is the primary cause of cardiogenic shock, which has a 50% to 80% mortality rate. Cardiogenic shock is diagnosed when other causes of shock and hypotension are ruled out, such as excessive bleeding, pulmonary embolism, or infection. In treatment, the source of the circulatory failure must be identified to determine appropriate measures.

Dysrhythmias or heart blocks are treated with medication for arrhythmia, a pacemaker, or cardioversion. When the cause lies with cardiac dysfunction, dopamine or epinephrine may be utilized, depending on the cardiac issue at hand.

Neurogenic Shock

The development of neurogenic shock occurs as a result of losing the impulse of vasoconstriction, most often associated with spinal cord injury in the high thoracic area. Once the patient's airway is stabilized, treatment involves administering fluids to increase volume and vasoconstrictors for preservation of the essential organs. The patient must be stabilized prior to considering surgery to repair the neurologic injury. Depending on the extent of the injury, repair has the potential to reverse the condition.

SURGICAL EMERGENCIES

Paralytic Ileus

Paralytic ileus, or pseudo-obstruction, is a condition in which the bowel is paralyzed and not permitting the passage of food through the digestive system. While it may be caused by gastroenteritis, infections of the abdomen, kidney or lung disease, hernias, adhesions, or low potassium levels, it may also be a result of abdominal surgery or the use of narcotics. This condition is one of the most common causes for intestinal obstructions in infants and children. Postsurgical patients experiencing abdominal swelling, pain and cramping, the inability to pass gas, and vomiting should undergo testing to rule out this condition.

Once an obstruction is identified through an abdominal CT scan, x-ray, barium enema, or an upper GI and small bowel series. The patient is treated using a nasal gastric tube or rectal tube to reduce the existing pressure followed by a clear liquid diet. Surgical intervention may be necessary if these treatments are not successful to relieve the obstruction.

Fire

The risk for fire or burns is a significant concern when working in an oxygen-rich environment such as the operating room. There are three types of fire extinguishers and it is important to use the one appropriate for the item on fire. Class A is for wood, paper, and textiles; class B for flammable liquids, oils, or gas; and class C for electrical or laser fires. In the event of a fire in the surgical suite, the operation of the fire extinguisher is through the acronym, PASS.

P=Pull the pin

A=Aim at the bottom of the fire

S=Squeeze the trigger

S=Sweep back and forth

When the fire occurs in the sterile field, it is the responsibility of the sterile team members to put out the fire. The first line of defense is often a wet towel or sponge to extinguish the

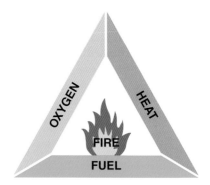

Figure 13-2 • Fire triangle.

fire. Burns can occur because of a light source laying directly on the patient's skin, an insufficient seal of the ET tube when using an ESU in a patient's mouth, or an accidental trigger of the ESU or laser when it is in contact with a nonsurgical area of the patient. Although most drapes are fire resistant, this does not mean high heat or sparks do not affect them. Often, they will melt and cause the underlying skin of the patient to suffer a burn.

Prevention of fires in the operating room depends on the risk components of the fire triangle in the operating room (Figure 13-2). When working with endoscopic equipment, the light source should remain on standby unless it is being utilized in the patient or stored safely on the mayo stand or a table. This will prevent the concentration of light from melting drapes or gowns and creating access to burn skin. As for burns using cautery, the ESU pencil should be stored in a holster or safely on the mayo stand or table. Laying the ESU on a patient may cause accidental activation of the handpiece and an unintentional burn. When utilizing the ESU in the mouth of a patient, a tight seal of the ET tube is imperative, as anesthesia gases are highly flammable if they come in contact with sparks generated by cautery.

ALL HAZARDS

All-hazards preparation is a term used to describe the desired response of a faction of the community during a crisis. In the case of the surgical assistant, this refers to the response of the healthcare community. As an allied health professional, the surgical assistant is a valuable part of the team when the medical community is activated for assistance. Hazards may include any natural disasters such as earthquakes, tsunamis, hurricanes, floods, tornados, or volcanos as well as man-made disasters such as accidents, infrastructure collapse, terrorism including biological or mechanical, explosions, or a pandemic. Each facility should have a plan for response in the event of a local disaster, especially ones prevalent in the area. Likewise, there are governmental agencies, local and state, responsible for planning and coordination in the event of an emergency.

At the Federal level, there are governmental and nongovernmental agencies that work together to coordinate a response depending on the nature of the disaster. The Protocol for disaster management falls under the Department of Homeland Security. The National Response Framework is the policy incorporated to ensure there is consistency throughout the country in any response.

- Federal Emergency Management Agency (FEMA)
  - Responsible for the coordination, management, and response for declared disasters.
- National Incident Management System (NIMS)
  - Responsible for implementation of FEMA guidelines
- National Response Framework (NRF)
  - Framework for disaster management
- National Disaster Medical System (NDMS)
  - Responsible for supporting state, local, tribal and territorial authorities by supplementing health and medical systems.
- Hospital Incident Command System (HICS)
  - Responsible for coordinating medical disasters with respective hospitals.
- Local Emergency Management Agency (LEMA)
  - Responsible for horizontal linkages with personnel in police, fire, emergency medical services, public works, and emergency management/homeland security departments.

The disaster cycle is comprised of the three phases including preparedness, mitigation, and response. Chief Resilience Officers facilitate the framework in which their communities handle community disaster root causes, vulnerability, mitigation, and/or recovery as part of their role.

- Comprehensive Emergency Management (CEM) plan
- Comprehensive Emergency Management (CEM) components

Through all the steps in the disaster cycle, the medical facilities must respond swiftly and efficiently to assure confidence from the community. In these situations, people primarily focus on health and safety, which places healthcare personnel at the forefront of any disaster, once food and shelter are secure.

Similar to Maslow's hierarchy of needs, the necessities of life should be a priority in any disaster situation. During the preparedness phase, plans are generated to respond using federal and state guidelines followed by assessment of the risk factors for the area for all types of disasters. Several agencies are involved in the planning such as police, fire, ambulance, mental health, public works, and many others. The next phase is mitigation, which may occur within preparedness or even within the response phase. In mitigation, the goal is to reduce the impact of the disaster when there is no way of preventing it from occurring. An example of mitigation might be a city that will be requiring houses to be built on stilts in a flood-prone area. The last phase is the response phase, when the disaster occurs, and plans go into action. Plans begin with evacuation, and progress to shelter, food, water, sanitation, and access to medical services. While the importance of shelter, food, and water is obvious, sanitation may not seem as critical until you examine the increase of infection in the absence of a sanitation system. Implementation of plans for regular and safe disposal of trash as well as medical waste is pertinent to the overall health of people sheltering in close proximity. Often, a point of distribution (POD) site is set up by the medical community to triage patients, or provide testing, medication, or vaccines in the most critically affected areas. In the case of many emergencies, especially a pandemic, the surgical assistant may be utilized on the "front lines" as screeners, due to the in-depth understanding and knowledge of cross-contamination. In addition, mental health and safety play critical roles in the management of a community during a disaster. Other agencies, such as police and fire, play an important role in the response process assuring safety needs are satisfied, thereby attaining the the second important step in Maslow's Hierarchy of Needs.

While things do not always go as planned, there should always be a framework for a response allowing for flexibility and adjustments along the way (see Table 13-1).

TABLE 13-1 • Primary Objectives of a Local Disaster Plan	
Objective	**Explanation**
Activation of emergency response personnel	Based on which organizations have been identified in the planning phase. The level of activation depends on the predetermined threshold or trigger.
Command post operations center	Responding personnel need a place to meet. This may correspond with the emergency operations center (EOP).
Public announcements, hazard, and service information	People in the community need to receive updated information about the emergency. The plan must include methods for information dissemination.
Management of resources	During a disaster, resources can be depleted or used inefficiently. The plan includes a resource management team that coordinates private and government sources of all types of resources.
Restoration of vital services	Critical services such as power, fuel, sewer, and roadways are essential to aiding victims and preventing additional emergency situations. A strategy for restoration of vital services is addressed at the planning stage.

Source: Reproduced with permission from Fuller JK, Fuller JR. *Surgical Technology, Principles and Practice,* 6th ed; Table 5-2.

SENTINEL EVENT AND INCIDENT REPORTS

Part of the profession of a surgical assistant is to assure the safety of our patients by minimizing the risks of harm or injury. While not all surgical cases will go as planned, any time there is harm, injury, or death, or the potential for either of these occurring as a result of an unplanned occurrence, documentation is necessary. This may pertain to issues such as a patient fall, burn, medication errors, or most severe, a patient death.

When a surgical assistant is involved in a procedure with an unplanned event causing potential harm to the patient, it is necessary to submit the appropriate report to risk management following the event. When filling out the form, it is imperative to include only facts and leave assumptions and opinions out of the report. Members of a risk management team will assess the event to assure proper protocol was followed and often implement new processes to prevent an event from reoccurrence. Procedures such as the "neutral zone" for sharps, time outs, and one-handed recapping of needles are direct results of assessing processes to improve safety of the patient and surgical team. The Safe Medical Device Act of 1990 is another process tracking medical equipment as well as implants which assures the safe operation and usage of these items.

Bibliography

American College of Allergy, Asthma, and Immunology. Anaphylaxis. 2018. https://acaai.org/allergies/anaphylaxis. Accessed August 6, 2019.

Association of Surgical Technologists. *Surgical Technology for the Surgical Technologist.* 5th ed. Boston; MA: Cengage Learning; 2017.

Brunicardi FC, Andersen DK, Billiar TR, et al. *Schwartz's Principles of Surgery.* New York, NY: McGraw-Hill Medical Publishing Division; 2005.

Gutierrez G, Reines HD, Wulf-Gutierrez ME. Clinical review: hemorrhagic shock. *Critical care (London, England),* 2004;8(5):373-381. https://doi.org/10.1186/cc2851. Accessed August 9, 2023.

Lieberman P. Anaphylactic reactions during surgical and medical procedures. *J Allergy Clin Immunol.* 2002;110(2 Suppl):S64-S69. doi:10.1067/mai.2002.124970

Jensen J, Kirkpatrick S. Local emergency management and comprehensive emergency management (CEM): A discussion prompted by interviews with Chief Resilience Officers. *ScienceDirect.* 2022. https://www.sciencedirect.com/science/article/abs/pii/S2212420922003557

Mayo Foundation for Medical Education and Research. Mayo Clinic Anaphylaxis. 2020. https://www.mayoclinic.org/diseases-conditions/anaphylaxis/diagnosis-treatment/drc-20351474. Accessed April 26, 2020.

Natal BL, Doty CI. Venous Air Embolism. 2017. https://emedicine.medscape.com/article/761367-overview#a7. Accessed September 21, 2020.

National Organization for Rare Disorders. Pseudocholinesterase Deficiency. 2005. https://rarediseases.org/rare-diseases/pseudocholinesterase-deficiency/. Accessed August 5, 2019.

National Organization for Rare Disorders. Malignant Hyperthermia. 2013. https://rarediseases.org/rare-diseases/malignant-hyperthermia/#affected-populations. Accessed September 16, 2020.

Phillips N. *Berry & Kohn's Operating Room Technique.* 11th ed. St. Louis, MO: Mosby Elsevier; 2017.

Ramkumar V. Preparation of the patient and the airway for awake intubation. *Indian J Anaesth.* 2011;55(5):442-447. https://doi.org/10.4103/0019-5049.89863. Accessed August 9, 2023.

Rothrock JC. *Alexander's Care of the Patient in Surgery.* 14th ed. St. Louis, MO: Elsevier; 2011.

Rothrock JC, Seifert PC. *Assisting in Surgery: Patient-Centered Care.* Competency and Credentialing Institute. 2009.

Snyder KC, Keegan C. *Pharmacology for the Surgical Technologist.* 4th ed. St. Louis, MO: Elsevier; 2017.

US National Library of Medicine. Shock. 2019. https://medlineplus.gov/ency/article/000039.html. Accessed August 4, 2019.

US National Library of Medicine. Pseudocholinesterase Deficiency. 2019. https://ghr.nlm.nih.gov/condition/pseudocholinesterase-deficiency. Accessed August 5, 2019.

US National Library of Medicine. Intestinal Obstruction and Ileus. 2018. https://medlineplus.gov/ency/article/000260.htm. Accessed August 6, 2019.

General Surgery

Jennifer Ickes, Shannon E. Smith, and Kerry R. Stanziano-Bradic

DISCUSSED IN THIS CHAPTER

1. Surgical anatomy and pathology
2. Perioperative Considerations for surgery
3. General Surgery Procedures
4. Role of the Surgical Assistant in general surgery

General surgery is a discipline focusing on surgical treatment of disease processes that are non-operative, elective, urgent, and emergent in nature. Broad knowledge and experience is required for diagnosis, preoperative, operative, and postoperative management of patients, including management of complications, in the following nine surgical components:

- Alimentary tract
- Abdomen and its contents
- Breast, skin, and soft tissue
- Head and neck, including vascular, trauma, endocrine, congenital and oncologic disorders—expressly tumors of the salivary glands, thyroid, parathyroid, oral cavity, and the skin
- Vascular system, excluding the heat and intracranial vessels
- Endocrine system, including thyroid, parathyroid, adrenal, and pancreas
- Surgical oncology, including multimodality coordinated management of the cancer patient by screening, surveillance, surgical adjunctive therapy, rehabilitation, and follow-up
- Comprehensive management of trauma to encompass musculoskeletal, hand, and head injuries. Responsibility for all phases of care for the injured patient—a key component of general surgery
- Absolute care of critically ill patients with underlying surgical conditions, in the emergency room, intensive care unit, and trauma/burn units

APPENDECTOMY

Appendectomy is the surgical removal of the appendix. Appendicitis is one of the most frequent indications for emergent abdominal surgery. Progression of acute appendicitis to perforation is unpredictable. Perforated appendicitis can be managed either operatively or non-operatively. Patients suspected of having sepsis require immediate surgical intervention; however, this is usually associated with higher complications, including abscesses and enterocutaneous fistulae, because of dense adhesions and inflammation. Due to their premorbid conditions, older patients present a higher risk for complications; therefore, definitive diagnostic studies should be obtained prior to surgical intervention.

Anatomy

Historically considered to be a vestigial organ, the function of the appendix has been a topic of debate and there has been no clear evidence for its function in humans. The appendix is credited with the development and preservation of a specific type of lymphoid tissue known as gut-associated lymphoid tissue (GALT), located in the lamina propria. The appendix produces immunoglobulins, bacteria-producing proteins, and is believed to be essential in maintaining the intestinal flora.

Located at the base of the cecum near the ileocecal valve, the vermiform appendix is a true diverticulum measuring 6 to 9 cm, on average. Unlike an acquired diverticulum, the appendix contains all the histologic colonic layers: mucosa, submucosa, circular and longitudinal muscularis, and serosa; however, the crypts have differences in irregularity. Although the appendiceal orifice is fixed in position and is consistent, the position of the tail is variable and may be found in various positions such as: retrocecal (but intraperitoneal), sub cecal, pre-ileal, post-ileal, pelvic, and may extend into the hepatorenal recess. Other factors such as posture, respiration, and adjacent bowel distention can influence the position of the appendix.

Blood supply is provided by the ileocecal artery's appendicular branch. Lymph drainage for the appendix and cecum occurs via the ileocolic lymph nodes and proceeds to the superior mesenteric nodes. Although drainage of the cecum occurs via several intermediate mesenteric lymph nodes, drainage for the appendix occurs via a singular intermediate node.

The superior mesenteric plexus (T10-L1) and Vagus nerves provide visceral innervation. Afferent sensory fibers from the appendix are carried via the sympathetic nerve fibers entering the spinal cord at T10 and corresponding to the umbilical dermatome. When the appendiceal wall becomes inflamed, the visceral afferent fibers are stimulated producing diffuse periumbilical pain. As the inflammation progresses, the nearby peritoneum becomes irritated stimulating somatic nerve fibers and producing more localized pain. The localization is dependent on the position of the appendiceal tail. The convergence of the taeniae coli is an important anatomical landmark and marks the area of the appendix. When followed anteriorly, the appendix can be located, identified, and resected.

Etiology

Acute appendicitis is primarily caused by luminal obstruction. In adult populations, it may be due to fecaliths, fibrosis, foreign bodies (food, calculi, parasites), or neoplasia. In pediatric populations, luminal obstruction may be caused by lymphoid hyperplasia. Early obstruction results in bacterial overgrowth of aerobic organisms in the early stages leading to mixed flora. Obstruction leads to referred visceral pain to the periumbilical region due to increased intraluminal pressure. This is believed to lead to impaired venous drainage, mucosal ischemia leading to bacteria translocation causing gangrene and intraperitoneal infection. The most common aerobic and anaerobic bacteria isolated in perforated appendicitis is *Escherichia coli* and *Bacteroides fragilis*.

Diagnostic Intervention / History & Physical Findings

Common presentation of acute appendicitis occurs in patients between the ages of 10 and 40 years. Upon presentation, approximately 75% of patients report pain with a duration of 24 hours or less. Subjective symptoms include nausea, vomiting, and anorexia. Presentation of anorexia and/or abdominal pain preceding vomiting is more consistent with acute appendicitis. The diagnosis of appendicitis is questionable when vomiting is the first symptom.

Physical exam findings consistent with the differential for appendicitis are dependent on the location of the appendix. Objective symptoms can be extremely variable depending on the location. A normal anterior location of the appendix will elicit a classic right lower quadrant (RLQ) tenderness over

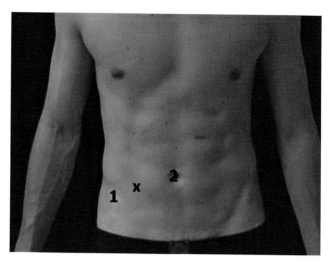

Figure 14-1 • McBurneys point. (Reproduced, with permission, from Brunicardi FC, Andersen DK, Billiar TR, et al, eds. *Schwartz's Principles of Surgery*. 11th ed. New York, NY: McGraw Hill; 2019.)

McBurney's point (see Figure 14-1). A positive Rovsing's sign (RLQ pain when left lower quandrant [LLQ] is pressed) may also be present with this location. A retrocecal location can elicit localized pain in the right flank and extension of the hip joint may cause pain due to stretching of the psoas muscle. When the inflamed appendix is located within the pelvis, the patient may have a positive obturator sign due to the obturator internus being stretched as the thigh is medially rotated and flexed. The patient may also experience irritation to the bladder and rectum such as suprapubic pain and pain with urination. The patient may feel the need to defecate. Post-ileal presentation may cause testicular pain and ureteral irritation in some males. In pregnant patients, the uterus may displace the appendix causing the patient to experience right upper quadrant (RUQ) pain. Patients with ruptured appendicitis and intra-abdominal sepsis usually present with diffuse peritonitis, tachycardia, and a temperature greater than 39°C.

Radiologic and laboratory studies may be utilized to compliment physical exam. A white blood count (WBC) and a C-reactive protein (CRP) are two common laboratory tests ordered in the initial workup for appendicitis. Patients presenting with acute appendicitis typically have leukocytosis of 10,000 cells/mm³. Patients with gangrenous or perforated appendicitis present with leukocytosis of approximately 17,000 cells/mm³. Pregnancy tests are essential for women of child-bearing age. A urinalysis may also be ordered to rule out pyelonephritis and nephrolithiasis. Liver function tests and serum chemistry studies including amylase and lipase are helpful in determining a diagnosis in patients with atypical presentation and physical exam findings.

In recent years, diagnostic imaging has moved to the forefront for diagnosing appendicitis. Computed Tomography (CT) with intravenous (IV) and enteral contrast have become the gold standard in evaluating appendicitis. Ultrasound remains a

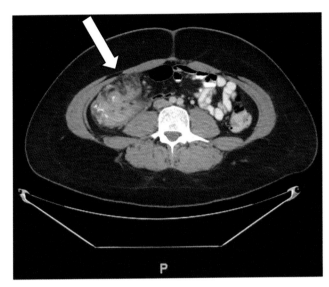

Figure 14-2 · Ultrasound of inflamed appendix. (Reproduced, with permission, from Elkbuli A, Diaz B, Polcz V, Hai S, McKenney M, Boneva D. Operative versus non-operative therapy for acute phlegmon of the appendix: Is it safer? A case report and review of the literature, Volume 50, 2018.)

relevant modality and is especially useful in evaluating pediatric patients and in early pregnancy (see Figure 14-2). Although ultrasound is more relatively available than CT scan and less expensive, the utility in obese patients is limited and it is user-dependent. Plain abdominal radiographs can be used in patients presenting with symptoms of diffuse peritonitis and intra-abdominal sepsis but should not be used to evaluate for appendicitis.

Preoperative Patient Preparation

Anesthesia. General anesthesia is administered to patient undergoing open approach or laparoscopic approach. Regional anesthesia may be used but is not common.

- Antibiotics should be given 30 to 60 minutes prior to skin incision.
  - Antibiotic choices for uncomplicated appendicitis: Cefoxitin, Ampicillin, and Cefazolin.
  - Antibiotic choices for patients with perforated appendicitis should cover gram-negative bacteria and anaerobes. These therapies include Piperacillin or combination of cephalosporin with metronidazole.

Positioning the Patient

- The patient is placed in the supine position.
  - Foley catheter may be ordered but is not routine for this approach.
- If laparoscopic approach is utilized, the patient will be placed in supine position and the arms may be tucked.
  - Foley catheter insertion is routine in this approach to decompress the bladder and lessen the risk of injury.

Draping the Patient

- The abdomen is prepped from xiphoid process to symphysis pubis and side to side as far laterally as possible.
- The patient is draped using four square towels and a transverse laparotomy drape.

Surgical Procedure (Open vs Laparoscopic Approach)

Metadata comparing laparoscopic and open approaches demonstrate relative comparisons between the two approaches with the laparoscopic approach resulting in a shorter length of stay (LOS), lower superficial infection rates, and faster return to work rates. The open appendectomy approach demonstrates lower intraoperative infection rates and shorter operative times. Cost analysis of the two procedures reveal they are relatively similar with the laparoscopic approach having an offset of cost due to the shorter LOS. Once the most common emergency general surgery performed in the Unites States, open appendectomy has given way to the laparoscopic approach as the gold standard for treating appendicitis. Although it is the preferred surgical approach, laparoscopic appendectomy is not always possible. Patients with a history of extensive abdominal and/or pelvic operations may require an open approach as well as pregnant patients; a gravid uterus may preclude laparoscopy.

In the open approach, the appendix is resected from the cecum and removed utilizing a McBurney incision, a muscle-splitting incision, in the right lower quadrant. Additionally, conversion from a laparoscopic approach to an open technique may be required based upon technical or anatomical reasons.

Open Approach Procedural Steps

- After the surgical prep and draping, a McBurney incision is made in an oblique fashion in the right lower quadrant.
- The patient is placed in Trendelenburg with the left-side down to facilitate exposure. **The surgical assistant (SA) should provide wound retraction utilizing handheld retractors such as a Richardson-Eastman or Goelet retractors**.
- The peritoneum is lifted with two Crile hemostats and incised using Metzenbaum scissors 15-blade scalpel.
- Once the peritoneum is incised, peritoneal fluid may be cultured using aerobic and anaerobic cultures. **The SA should provide suctioning using a Poole suction tip**.
- The appendix is readily identified. If there is difficulty in identifying the appendix, it can be located by tracing the anterior tinea of the cecum distally.
- Ligation of the mesentery may be needed to facilitate exposure.
- The appendix is grasped with a Babcock clamp. The base of the appendix is visualized and ligated.
- The appendiceal stump is imbricated using a 2-0 absorbable suture to perform a Z-stitch or purse string suture. **The SA will invert the appendiceal stump utilizing a Crile hemostat or DeBakey forceps**. This should be placed in a "dirty" container upon release.

- The wound is irrigated with normal saline and closed in a layered fashion. If significant contamination or abscess is present, the wound may be closed by secondary intention. A drain may or may not be placed.
- Dressings are applied.

Laparoscopic Procedural Steps

- After infiltration with local anesthetic, a periumbilical incision is made, and the peritoneal cavity is accessed using Hasson technique or optical trocar. If Hasson technique is utilized, stay sutures may be placed in the fascia using a suture such as a 0 Vicryl, UR-6.
- The abdomen is inflated with CO_2. The abdominal pressure should be ≤15 mm Hg.
- After infiltration with local anesthetic, 5-mm trocars are placed under direct visualization. One in the lower midline and one in the left lower quadrant, lateral to the epigastric vessels.
- The four quadrants are visualized and inspected for abnormal findings.
- The patient is placed in Trendelenburg position. The OR table may be tilted to the left to allow gravity to displace the small bowel and allow better visualization of the right lower quadrant.
- After clear visualization of the appendix and mesentery, the appendix is mobilized.
- The mesoappendix is splayed out by grasping the mesentery with an atraumatic grasping forceps. **Note: The inflamed tip of the appendix should not be grasped to avoid rupture**.
- Using a dissecting instrument, the mesentery is opened at the base of the appendix.
- Using an endoscopic vascular stapling instrument, the mesoappendix is divided through the Hasson port.
- Using an endoscopic cutting linear stapler, the base of the appendix is divided. The stapler should be rotated 180° to visualize the entire length and contents of the jaws. This maneuver should also be done during the division of the mesoappendix.
- If the appendix is minimally inflamed and small, it can be removed through the 10-mm Hasson trocar. If the appendix is large and/or suppurative, it may be placed in an endo-retriever bag for removal through the abdominal wall to lessen the chance of a surgical site infection. Removal of the appendix is directly visualize using the endoscope.
- The mesoappendix and staple line are visually inspected for bleeding and to ensure there is no leakage.
- The abdomen is adequately irrigated using the suction irrigator. The pelvis is inspected and irrigated as needed.
- The 5-mm ports are removed under direct visualization to ensure hemostasis of the abdominal wall.

- The abdomen is decompressed, and the periumbilical port is closed. If stay sutures were placed, the fascia can be closed by tying them together. If no stay sutures were used, the fascia can be closed using an absorbable suture such as a 0 Vicryl UR-6. The subcutaneous tissue is not closed. The skin is closed with an absorbable suture such as a 4-0 or 5-0 Vicryl or Monocryl.

Postop

- Dressings
  - Wound is dressed using steri strips and small, dry sterile dressings, or Dermabond.
- Orogastric tube
  - Removed prior to patient awakening
- Foley catheter
  - Removed at the end of the procedure
- Pain control
  - If a long-acting local anesthetic utilized, most patients can tolerate oral pain medications.
- Discharge
  - Most patients are discharged with 24 to 28 hours with oral pain medications.
  - Patients may be discharged with antibiotic therapy depending on operative findings.

BREAST PROCEDURES

Abstract

Breast procedures are performed for two reasons: to establish a diagnosis or to treat breast cancer. Tumors may occur because of hormone level changes from puberty that exist throughout a woman's natural life. These changes affect the breast tissue both physically and microscopically. Many impalpable breast lesions are now being detected as advances in breast cancer screening with mammography have continued to improve. Breast cancer is the most common cancer in women[1]; it accounts for nearly one of every three cancers diagnosed.

Anatomy and Physiology

The breasts are composed of two mammary glands located bilaterally on the pectoralis major fascia of the anterior wall of the chest. The mammary glands are surrounded by an adipose layer which is enclosed in a layer of skin. The breasts are located and extend from the second to the sixth rib and then extend horizontally from the lateral edge of the sternum to the axillary line (see Figure 14-3). The largest portion of the mammary gland lies on the connective tissue of the pectoralis major muscle and laterally on the serratus anterior. Cooper's ligaments also known as the suspensory ligaments of Cooper help maintain the breast structural integrity. A portion of mammary tissue extends laterally on the pectoralis major toward the axilla. This tissue is referred to as the *tail of Spence*.

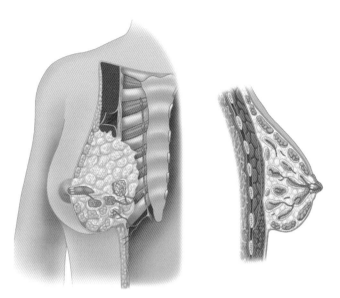

Figure 14-3 · Anatomy of the breast. (Reproduced, with permission, from Bland KI, Copeland EMI. *The Breast: Comprehensive Management of Benign and Malignant Diseases*. 4th ed. Philadelphia, PA: Elsevier/Saunders; 2009.)

Each breast contains 12 to 20 glandular lobes which are separated by connective tissue. Lactiferous ducts drain these lobes through a single lactiferous duct which opens on the nipple area. The nipple is located at the fourth intercostals space. The area surrounding the nipple is called the *areola*.

There are three major arterial systems that are responsible for blood supply to the breast. Two of the main sources include the branches of the internal mammary artery and the lateral branches of the anterior aortic intercostals. The pectoral branch serves as the third source which branches off a branch of the axillary artery.

The lymphatics drain into two main areas. The internal thoracic nodes are responsible for most of the lymph drainage deriving from the inner half of the breast (see Figure 14-4). This is why the lymph system can be a source for the spread and metastasis of disease to the chest wall or axillary area.

Core anatomical organ(s) affected are liver, lung, bone, and brain. Key landmarks and/or relevant associated structures include the breast that does not contain muscle tissue. It is composed of tissue that lies on top of the muscles that cover the chest wall.

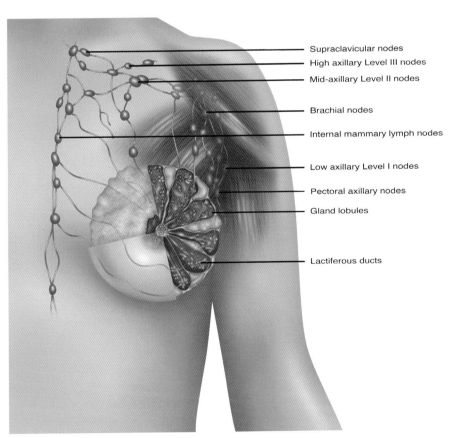

Figure 14-4 · Lymphatic pathways of the breast. (Used with permission from Gwen Shockey/Science Source)

Physiology. The primary function of the breasts is to produce milk for lactation. The breasts also drain lymphatics into lymph nodes located in the axilla and behind the sternum.

Etiology. Among the most complicated regarding cancers and considered to be unknown. Factors believed to be the cause include familial influences, environmental influences—exposure to ionizing radiation, dietary, endocrine disruptors, elevated estrogen exposure.

Diagnosis (modalities)

- **History:** affects primarily women but can occur in men
- **High risk:** women age 65 and older, genetic factors (inherited mutations of BRCA1 and BRCA2), family history (2 or more 1st degree relatives with breast cancer at a young age, history of previous breast cancer (risk for developing in opposite breast is five times greater), breast density
- **Moderate risk:** family history (1st degree relative with breast cancer), biopsy confirmed atypical hyperplasia, Ionizing radiation exposure, high estrogen levels
- **Low risk:** reproductive history (childless women or those giving birth the first time near age 30, menstrual history, oral contraceptives, hormone replacement therapy, obesity
- **Other risk factors:** alcohol, high socioeconomic status, Jewish heritage
- **Physical:** dimpling of the skin, changes in size and shape of breast, sudden nipple discharge, retraction of the nipple, swelling under the arm

Diagnostic Modalities Relevant to Condition/Procedure:

- Diagnostic laboratory exams: fine needle aspiration biopsy with cytologic examination of the aspirate
- Diagnostic imaging: mammography, ultrasonography, magnetic resonance imaging (MRI), molecular breast imaging, positron emission tomography
- Diagnostic procedures: breast biopsy

Procedural Considerations. Examples are nonsurgical treatment, surgical treatment, list of surgical approaches (open, laparoscopic, robotic, etc.). Patients that have large breasts may require an ESU (smoke evacuation system) and additional hemostatic clips due to increased bleeding.

Nonsurgical Treatment: Neoadjuvant treatment also known as pre-surgery treatment, ie, chemotherapy which can induce a (pCR) pathological complete response. Radiation therapy and hormonal therapy may also be used.

Usual Surgical Treatment and Options: Minimally invasive treatment options include breast biopsy, lumpectomy, wide excision of mass. Invasive treatment includes modified radical mastectomy (including lymph nodes with axillary dissection), possible salpingo-oophorectomy.

Surgical Approaches: Surgical approach is dependent on the size and location of the mass, cell characteristics, stage of cancer, and patient's choice. TNM (T=tumor, N=node, M=metastasis) is used to clinically stage the disease. These approaches may be accompanied by radiation therapy, chemotherapy, or hormonal therapy. A port insertion may also be performed for chemotherapy after the surgical procedure.

Preoperative Preparation: Additional labs/orders—If general anesthesia, patient would be Nil per os (NPO) after midnight. Patient is to bathe the night before, no perfumes, nail polish, deodorant, or lotions. Any requirements for procedure (no smoking, lose weight, psychological counseling, nutritional aspects, etc.) be followed.

Breast Conservation. Breast conservation surgery consists of resection of the primary breast cancer and a margin of normal looking breast tissue, adjunct radiation therapy, and evaluation of the regional lymph node status. For women diagnosed with stage I or stage II breast cancer, breast conserving therapy (BCT) is desired over a total mastectomy as BCT produces survival rates comparable to those after total mastectomy while conserving the breast. It also presents improved quality of life and aesthetic outcomes. Breast conservation surgery is considered the standard treatment for women with stage 0, I, or II invasive breast cancer.

Procedures

Breast Biopsy: Usual anesthesia considerations. Local anesthetic with IV moderate sedation, laryngeal mask airway, or general anesthetic with intubation.

Position: Patient is supine. Arms are positioned on arm boards with padding underneath.

Skin Prep: Specifics for surgical skin prep—surgeon preference. SA should include wire in prep and take special precaution so the wire is not dislodged. Betadine, Chloraprep, or Dynahex is generally used. Prep should start at center of breast, extend to patients' side and down to edge of table. Shoulder and upper arm should be prepped and should extend to unaffected breast side and include neck area.

Surgical Procedure: Procedure including the role of the assistant (SA, PA, resident).

- The radiologist places the wire prior to the patient entering the operating room. The surgeon makes the initial incision over the location of the lesion which is identified by placement of the wire.
- The SA provides counter traction as needed. Army Navy retractors or Goelet retractors are utilized as the surgeon dissects the tissue using the wire as the guide to the affected area.
- Specimen is manipulated with a Lahey tenaculum and bleeders are cauterized with electrocautery device. The surgeon may use a Metzenbaum or curved mayo scissor or electrocautery to dissect tissue containing the biopsy.
- The tissue is removed en bloc with the wire and sent to radiology for specimen mammography.

- The surgeon and SA utilize the bovie to cauterize bleeders. The field is kept sterile pending results of the biopsy. The SA waits until surgeon gets the report from radiology.
- Once specimen is confirmed, SA closes incision with 4-0 suture of surgeon's preference.

Postop Care: The patient should leave steri strips on the wound until they fall off, usually around 7 to 10 days. The patient will be instructed to not bathe for 1 to 2 days.

After a breast biopsy, there may be some bleeding, swelling, or bruising. The swelling will go down in time. The breast may be sore for several days and the patient may require pain medication. The patient should seek medical attention if there is any shortness of breath, chest pain, or signs of a blood clot in the leg.

Complications: Possible complications include:

- Fever higher than 101°F
- Chills
- Inflammation or unusual swelling around the area of the biopsy
- Bleeding, any drainage, or pus from the area of the biopsy
- Increased or worsening pain in the area
- The breast increasing in size

Lumpectomy

Anesthesia: Usual anesthesia considerations—anesthetic with IV moderate sedation, laryngeal mask airway, or general anesthetic with intubation.

Position: Patient is supine. Arms are positioned on arm boards with padding underneath.

Skin Prep: Specifics for surgical skin prep: Surgeon preference—Betadine, Chloraprep, or Dynahex is generally used.

Prep should start at center of breast, extend to patients' side and down to edge of table. Shoulder and upper arm should be prepped and should extend to unaffected breast side and include neck area.

Surgical Procedure: Procedure including the role of the assistant (SA, PA, resident). Steps highlighted, key landmarks, core nerves/arteries are to be identified.

- Incision is made in the direction of the skin lines or along border of areola above the tumor. A circumareolar incision may be used to give the patient a better cosmetic result. A radial incision will be used if the lesion is located extremely laterally or medially.
- The SA provides counter traction.
- The surgeon gently retracts the mass with an Allis clamp or Lahey tenaculum.
- The SA utilizes a Goelets or army navy retractor to provide exposure. Sharp dissection is used for removal of the mass with Metzenbaum scissors or scalpel with a #10 blade. Some surgeons may use an electrocautery device to maintain hemostasis while removing the mass.

- The SA should have a hemostat available to clamp any bleeders that cannot be cauterized.
- Once the mass is freed, the surgeon will mark the mass with a sterile marker or silk suture to provide its orientation in the breast. The specimen is sent to pathology fresh to perform a frozen examination.
- The team leaves the field sterile as they wait for pathology to confirm the mass contains the tumor and margins are clear.
- During this time, the surgeon and SA will cauterize or tie off any bleeding and irrigate the wound.
- When confirmation is given that the specimen contains the mass, the wound is closed with absorbable suture of 3-0 Chromic or surgeon's preference.
- The skin is then closed by the SA (surgeon's preference) usually with 4-0 Vicryl or 4-0 Monocryl running subcuticular stitch or staples.

Modifications/additional associated procedures commonly seen—the surgeon may utilize surgical clips and leave them in the operative site for the radiation oncologist to locate the exact site for radiation therapy.

Sentinel Lymph Node Localization

Anesthesia: General with laryngeal mask airway, or general anesthetic with intubation.

Position: Patient is supine. Arms are positioned on arm boards with padding underneath. Sequential wraps are placed on patient's legs.

Surgical Skin Prep: Surgeon preference—Betadine, Chloraprep, or Dynahex is generally used. Prep should start at center of breast, extend to patient's side and down to edge of table. Arm on affected side should be prepped including axilla area down to elbow circumferentially. Shoulder and upper arm should be prepped and should extend to unaffected breast side and include neck area.

Surgical Procedure: Procedure including the role of the assistant (SA, PA, resident). Steps highlighted, key landmarks, core nerves/arteries are to be identified. Patient is scheduled for Lumpectomy or Mastectomy. Prior to entering the operating room, the patient was injected with a labeling substance. This could be a radioactive tracer and/or blue dye. The surgeon utilizes a Geiger counter in order to determine where the nodes are located that would be positive for cancer. This can also be determined by visualizing where the blue dye has traveled.

- A sentinel node biopsy will pinpoint where the first several lymph nodes are located that the tumor has drained into. The sentinel nodes are where the cancer has first metastasized. If the sentinel node is positive, it is likely that a full axillary node dissection will need to be performed. If it is negative, the surgeon would only need to remove those sentinel nodes and an axillary node dissection would not need to be performed. The surgeon will make a small incision in the axilla (armpit).

- The SA will use Senn retractors or army navy retractors to expose the area being dissected.
- The surgeon will use Metzenbaum scissors and DeBakey forceps to carefully dissect the sentinel nodes away from the tissue. The nodes will be sent to pathology after removal to determine if they are positive or negative.
- An electrocautery device will be used to coagulate any bleeders.
- The SA will close the incision with suture of surgeon's preference of a 4-0 Vicryl or Monocryl is used.

Postop: Drains used/dressings—Mastisol, steri-strips, 4 by 4's, fluff gauze, and a surgical bra.

Prognosis with Treatment: If the cancer has not metastasized, prognosis is good. If the cancer is metastatic, 22% of patients have a survival rate of 5 years. The average rate of survival is approximately 3 years. It is dependent upon the length of time between initial diagnosis and metastasis, genetics, and other factors.

Potential Complications: Common to this procedure—hematoma, seroma, infection

Discharge Planning: Will feel mild discomfort for a few days. Bruising and mild swelling around incision are normal. Patient should rest the day of the surgery. Liquid diet and easy to digest foods and work up to normal diet. If general anesthesia, no alcohol or driving for 24 hours. Patient can take a shower, but not soak in a bathtub. Take pain meds as directed. Patient should always wear a snug bra. Return to normal activities in 24 hours. Keep wound dry for 48 hours.

Mastectomy and Axillary Dissection. A mastectomy is performed to surgically remove the entire breast. Typically, some of the skin and the nipple are also taken. There are several different types of mastectomies.

- Total or simple mastectomy, which is the removal of the entire breast.
- Modified radical mastectomy, is the removal of the entire breast and the axillary lymph nodes.
- Breast conserving surgery, the tumor and some healthy breast tissue is removed. Much of the breast remains.
- Skin sparing procedures may be utilized for a simple or modified radical mastectomy. The breast tissue is removed through a cut that is made around the areola.
- Radical mastectomy, which is the removal of the breast, chest muscles, and all the axillary lymph nodes under the arm. This surgery is not commonly performed anymore.

A mastectomy may be an option for many types of breast cancer, including:

- Ductal carcinoma in situ (DCIS), or noninvasive breast cancer
- Stages I and II (early-stage) breast cancer

- Stage III (locally advanced) breast cancer—after chemotherapy
- Inflammatory breast cancer—after chemotherapy
- Paget's disease of the breast
- Locally recurrent breast cancer

See Figure 14-5 for MRI examination revealing contralateral breast cancer.

The type of surgery you have depends on the following:

- Tumor size, type, and location
- Breast size
- Staging of the cancer
- If the cancer has spread to the lymph nodes
- If you have had radiation treatment
- Age and health
- A discussion between the patient and surgeon to determine best approach

Anesthesia: General anesthesia is utilized for the procedure.

Positioning & Prepping: Patient is positioned supine with arms on arm boards at less than a 90° angle. All bony prominences are padded.

Surgical Procedure:

- The surgeon will make a transverse elliptic incision with a knife. The SA will provide counter traction. The surgeon will utilize curved Metzenbaum scissors and the Bovie is utilized to free the skin edges from the fascia. The SA will utilize the Yankauer suction to evacuate any surgical plume from the field. The SA will also utilize sharp rakes or Freeman retractors to pull the skin up as it is being dissected off of the fascia.
- Bleeding vessels are coagulated using hemostats and ligated with either sutures or electrocautery device (bovie). The surgeon or SA will clamp the bleeders and tie with 3-0 Vicryl ties and cut with suture scissors.
- Surgeons may request warm, moist laparotomy sponges to protect the skin edges of the incision.
- The SA will grasp the breast tissue with Allis forceps as the surgeon dissects it free from the underlying pectoral fascia with Metzenbaum scissors.
- The tumor and all breast tissue are removed. Bleeding vessels are ligated by the surgeon and SA with a hemostat and the SA will tie the vessels with a 3-0 Vicryl. Suture is then cut with suture scissors.
- The surgeon will make a small incision and enter the wound with a hemostat. The SA will place the end of a Jackson Pratt drain into the jaw of the clamp and it will be tunneled to the outside of the incision. The SA will secure the drain to the skin with a silk suture and attach the grenade to the end for wound drainage.
- The SA will then apply a dressing of 4 by 4's, fluffs, and a surgical bra.

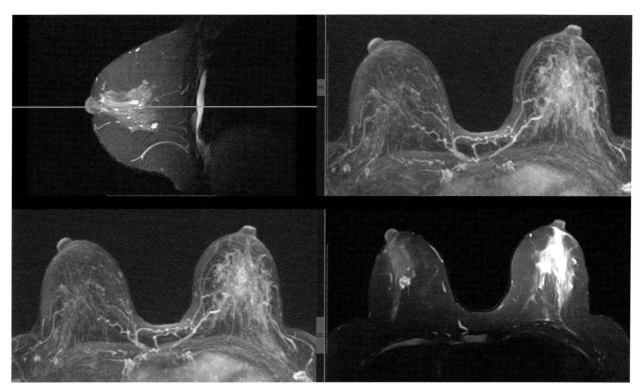

Figure 14-5 · X-ray Digital Mammogram or mammography is x-ray image of the breast in women for screening Breast cancer. (Used with permission from luckykdesignart/Shutterstock.)

Postop:

- Patients are taken to PACU to have vitals monitored.
- Patients can expect some pain, numbness, and a pinching sensation in the underarm area.
- Discharge instructions be given on how to care for the incision and drains, recognizing signs of infection, and understanding activity restrictions.
- Prescriptions for pain medication and possibly an antibiotic be given.

Complications:

- Bleeding
- Infection
- Pain
- Swelling (lymphedema) in your arm if you have an axillary node dissection
- Formation of hard scar tissue at the surgical site
- Shoulder pain and stiffness
- Numbness, particularly under your arm, from lymph node removal
- Buildup of blood in the surgical site (hematoma)

Modified Radical Mastectomy

Anesthesia: General anesthesia is utilized for the procedure.

Positioning & Prepping: Patient is positioned supine with operative arm on an arm board at less than a 90° angle. All bony prominences are padded. The specimen will be examined under a microscope to classify it (tumor size, type, grade, invasion, lymphocytic response, and clear margins).

Surgical Procedure:

- An oblique elliptic incision with lateral extension toward the axilla is made through the subcutaneous tissue including the nipple and areola.
- Bleeding is controlled with hemostats, ligatures, or electrosurgical pencil.
- A #3 knife handle with a #10 blade, Metzenbaum scissors, or electrosurgical pencil is utilized to undercut the skin creating skin flaps that are raised from the edges of the incision.
- The margins of the skin flaps should be covered with warm, moist lap sponges and retracted.
- Beginning near the clavicle and expanding down to the midsternum, the fascia and breast tissue is resected from the pectoralis muscle leaving the pectoralis major muscle unharmed.
- Intercostal arteries and veins are clamped and ligated.
- Dissection of the axilla is meticulously executed to prevent damage to the axillary vein and medical and lateral nerves of the pectoralis major muscle.

- Fascia is dissected off the lateral edge of the pectoralis muscle, ligated any vessels in the axilla. Fascia is dissected off the serratus anterior muscle.

- Thoracic and thoracodorsal nerves are preserved.

- Breast and axilla fascia is freed from the latissimus dorsi muscle and suspensory ligaments.

- Specimen is passed off the field.

- Hemostasis is checked; irrigation with normal saline will verify all bleeders have been coagulated.

- Jackson Pratt drains are inserted through a stab wound in the skin securing them with a non-absorbable suture.

- Absorbable suture is utilized to close subcutaneous tissue.

- Skin is often closed with running subcuticular absorbable suture.

Wound Dressings: Tape, antibiotic ointment, and a nonadherent wound dressing such as Adaptic will dress the wound. A simple gauze dressing or bulky absorbent dressing is secured by a surgical bra or ACE bandage.

Possible Complications:

- Excessive bleeding

- Infection in the surgical wound

- Depression

- Fluid accumulation under the skin (seroma)

- Excess blood or serum accumulation within the underlying skin of the surgical wound

- Reduced range of motion of the shoulder, due to nerve damage

- Obstruction of the lymphatic system (lymphedema)

- Loss of skin surrounding the site of the surgical procedure

Postop Care:

- Resume regular/daily activities slowly but as soon as possible.

- Warm compresses can be used to relieve pain at the incision site.

- Resume showering with unscented soap and keep the wound clean and dry. Avoid baths until the surgical wound is completely healed.

- To prevent blood clots and postop swelling, elevate legs during rest.

- Take stool softeners as needed to prevent constipation.

- Take any prescribed antibiotic medication.

- Avoid all activities that are physically strenuous for about 6 weeks after the procedure.

- Driving can be resumed after 2 weeks of being discharged.

- Avoid sex until healing is complete.

- Individuals should start with a clear liquid diet until the gastrointestinal tract resumes to function properly.

Axillary Node Dissection. Breast cancer will often spread first to lymph nodes located in the axilla next to the affected breast. The number of lymph nodes in the axilla fluctuates from person to person; the typical range is between 20 and 40. The first node that lymphatic fluid passes through is the sentinel lymph node. Sentinel lymph node biopsy is done by removing one to five Sentinel lymph node (SLNs) from the underarm. The lymph nodes are then examined to determine if they are positive for cancer.

ESOPHAGEAL PROCEDURES

The Esophagus, also spelled *oesophagus*, is the tubular structure that allows the passage of nutrition to the stomach where digestion and absorption of nutrients begin. When there is a disturbance with the esophagus the patient will have difficulty with consumption and surgical involvement may be necessary to allow continuity of the GI tract. The SA will perform several roles to the surgeon to achieve successful intervention.

Anatomy

The esophagus is the straight muscular tube which passes food from the pharynx to the stomach, located posterior to the cricoid cartilage and in front of the spinal column originating at the sixth cervical vertebra, the esophagus passes through the diaphragm at the esophageal hiatus, before entering the stomach at the gastroesophageal junction. Roughly 2 to 4 cm of the esophagus is normally located below the diaphragm.

The arterial supply to the esophagus begins with the upper portion supplied by the branches of the inferior thyroid arteries. Thoracic portion is delivered by the bronchial arteries and the esophageal branch that originates from the aorta. The diaphragm and abdominal section are distributed by the left inferior phrenic artery and esophageal branches of the left gastric arteries. Venous drainage is more complex. The upper and midpoint levels of the esophagus drain into hemiazygos and azygos veins. More importantly is the lower portion which drains into the esophageal branches of the coronary vein, a tributary of the portal vein.

Each end of the esophagus contains a muscular constriction named sphincters. The contractions of the structure, peristalsis, allows food to move down to the stomach. The sphincters maintain positive pressure and prevent the continuous entrance of air from the mouth and gastric content from the distal end. The upper esophageal sphincter (UES) is in a state of tonic contraction with a resting pressure of about 100 mm Hg. The UES prevents passage of air from the pharynx into the esophagus and reflux contents into the pharynx. The lower esophageal sphincter is 3 to 4 cm in length and is referred to the LES, its pressure ranges from 15 to 24 mm Hg. When swallowing the LES relaxes for 5 to 10 seconds to allow the food bonus to enter the stomach and then regain its resting tone. The LES is the most common problematic area with patients with reflux issues (see Figure 14-6).

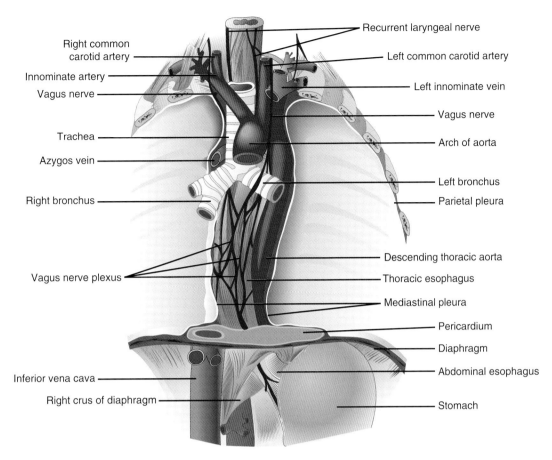

Figure 14-6 · Surrounding anatomical structures of the esophagus. (Reproduced, with permission, from Doherty GM, ed. *Current Diagnosis & Treatment: Surgery*. 15th ed. New York, NY: McGraw Hill; 2020.)

Diagnostics

Diagnosing esophageal malignancies and disruptions may be achieved using multiple imaging and tests, aside from symptomatic evaluation. Common diagnostic tests performed are gastroscopy, CT, MRI, PET imaging, and finally laparoscopy and thoracoscopy. An upper GI series will evaluate the esophagus, gastroesophageal junction, stomach, and duodenum whereas a Barium swallow will simply evaluate the esophagus and GE junction. Some patients require PH monitoring while diagnosing GERD and esophageal manometry which monitors the upper and lower esophageal sphincters. Depending on the chief complaint, the provider will determine which test will be of value in finding an accurate diagnosis.

Etiology

Common pathology associated with the esophagus can range from a stricture to cancer depending on location and severity. Beginning with the most common gastroesophageal reflux disease (GERD), some patients can be managed with medications, more chronic patients opt for surgical intervention. Complications of GERD may lead to esophagitis and Barrett's esophagus due to prolonged exposure of gastric acid. Zenker's diverticulum and tumors are structural defects

that may require surgical intervention (see Figure 14-7). Malignancies in the esophagus also require more in-depth surgical intervention and location will dictate which procedure is performed with any lymphatics that may also require removal.

Anesthesia

General anesthesia is preferred with esophageal procedures with airway maintained. Anesthesia may be required to insert and esophageal dilator such as a boujie to stent open the esophagus for certain procedures. Also, a nasogastric or oral gastric tube may be placed to deflate the stomach and evacuate any contents prior to beginning depending on the procedure.

Positioning and Prepping

Typical positioning for esophageal procedures is supine with arms extended no more than 90° on the operating room table. Reverse Trendelenburg is common for laparoscopic procedures to assist with retraction of anatomical structures that may interfere. Some patients that require a thoracic approach may be positioned in a lateral position. Depending on the incision site or port placement, the abdomen may be prepped with wide margins with facilities required prep solution.

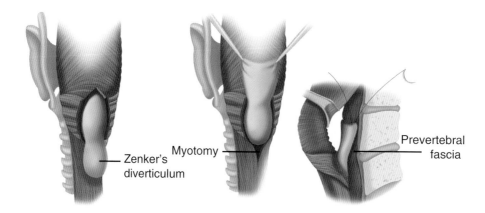

Figure 14-7 · Zenker's diverticulum. (Reproduced, with permission, from Brunicardi FC, Andersen DK, Billiar TR, et al, eds. *Schwartz's Principles of Surgery*. 11th ed. New York, NY: McGraw Hill; 2019.)

Surgical Procedure

Laparoscopic Nissen Fundoplication. The Nissen Fundoplication is anti-reflux procedure for patients with GERD to reinforce the incompetent Lower Esophageal Sphincter (LES). The top of the stomach is wrapped around the lower esophagus and reducing a hiatal hernia if present (see Figure 14-8). In the presence of a hiatal hernia, the LES migrates into the thoracic cavity and alters the normal pressure gradient between abdominal and thoracic cavity. The increase in pressure may alter the LES ability to prevent reflux. The Nissen will reinforce the LES making it less likely that acid will back up in the esophagus.

Indications for a Nissen Fundoplication include patients with GERD taking proton pump inhibitors that are incompletely responsive, esophageal manifestations of GERD, and complications of GERD (stricture, bleeding, aspiration, Barrett esophagus). There are few contraindications for the procedure,

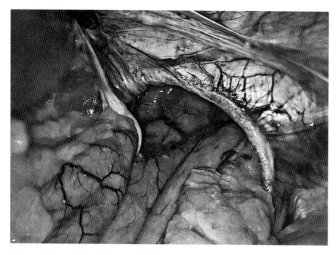

Figure 14-8 · Hiatal hernia defect. (Reproduced, with permission, from The Center of Weight Loss at Wood County Hospital, Bowling Green, Ohio.)

the morbidly obese patient with GERD may benefit from a gastric bypass surgery as opposed to Nissen Fundoplication.

Surgical steps are given in the following sections:

Incision and Trocar Placement

- Using #15 blade, trocars are strategically placed in the abdomen at different locations to accommodate the working instrumentation. The abdomen is inflated with carbon dioxide and a pneumoperitoneum is established to provide a space to work. The liver is retracted to provide exposure of the defect.

- The SA may place an assist port at this time. Note that if using a robotically assisted approach the SA will assist in the docking of the robot to the patient at this time. The SA will be responsible for exposure if using a laparoscope and maintain a clear visual of the field.

Mobilization

- The SA may be responsible for providing traction on the stomach as the surgeon begins dissecting the stomach free from the defect. Light traction may be necessary depending on the severity of the defect, the SA will use caution while retracting any tissue as to avoid injury to other nearby structures such as the spleen.

- The surgeon begins mobilization using the preferred ultrasonic device beginning with the cardia. With each section that is liberated the SA may retract the stomach in different directions as dictated by the surgeon.

- Next, the fundus and the upper portion of the greater curvature of the stomach are mobilized.

- Finally, the short gastric vessels between the fundus and the spleen are ligated and divided.

Nissen Formation

- Once the stomach has been mobilized, an atraumatic grasper is placed behind the esophagus and attaches to the fundus. The fundus is the pulled behind and around the esophagus, creating a 360° wrap.

- At this time anesthesia may insert an esophageal dilator of the surgeons choosing ranging from size 40-60 Fr to dilate and stent open the esophagus while the Nissen is sutured in place.
- The Nissen is sutured with non-absorbable sutures along with the Hiatal hernia defect (see Figure 14-9).
- Some hiatal defects are far larger than others and may require further repair than just sutures such as a biological graft or mesh.
- Some surgeons may choose to address the hiatal hernia defect before Nissen completion, this will be at surgeon's discretion (Figure 14-10).
- Upon completion the esophageal dilator is removed, and the field is inspected for any bleeding.

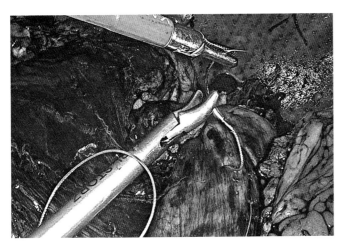

Figure 14-9 · Suturing of Nissen. (Reproduced, with permission, from The Center of Weight Loss at Wood County Hospital, Bowling Green, Ohio.)

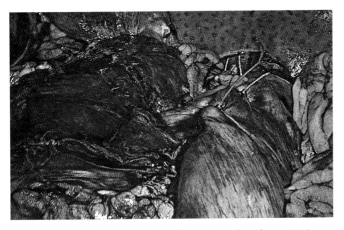

Figure 14-10 · Nissen completion. (Reproduced, with permission, from The Center of Weight Loss at Wood County Hospital, Bowling Green, Ohio.)

Wound Closure:

- Once the pneumoperitoneum is deflated and instrumentation removed, the SA will begin closure of the port sites using the surgeon preferred suture of choice. Small adhesive dressings are applied, and the patient is transferred to recovery.

Postop: Patients may have significant swelling in the operative area for the first 2 to 3 weeks postoperatively; therefore, patients must follow a strict diet during this time. Patients will be advised to take exceedingly small amounts of fluids at first 1 to 2 ounces and wait some time before taking any more such as 15 to 30 minutes. Fluids will be allowed, but not carbonated beverages or frozen drinks as this may lead to an esophageal spasm. Soft foods are only permissible at this time, patients will want to avoid food that is in chunks, patients will need to puree solids. The patient will be advised to sit upright while eating and remain in this position up to 60 minutes after eating. Patients will also be advised to prevent gas build up which may lead to pain by not using straws, slurp food, chew gum, and or suck on ice. Postoperative radiologic studies may be ordered and followed up by the surgeon.

Transoral Incisionless Fundoplication (TIF). Transoral Incisionless Fundoplication is considered another option to treat severe GERD and reduce a hiatal hernia defect by means of reconstructing the anti-reflux valve with no incision (see Figure 14-11). The procedure is an outpatient procedure under general anesthesia, using merely just a gastroscope and the TIF product of the surgeon's choice. The device itself creates a valve of 2-4 cm in length and creates a circumferential wrap greater than 270°. The SA will assist in the role of visualization with the gastroscope or potentially firing the TIF device, depending on surgeon preference.

Surgical procedure is mentioned in the following sections.

Introduction of Gastroscope

- The surgeon begins the procedure by advancing the gastroscope, while the preferred procedural equipment is opened and prepared. The device is then inserted over the endoscope and placed in the stomach.
- The SA may assist in the insertion of the device or provide visualization with the endoscope by holding it in place and maintaining air in the stomach to keep the stomach inflated. The scope is retroflexed to view the working field.

Advancement of Device

- As the device is advanced into the stomach, retraction of the tissue may be engaged at the esophageal gastro junction. The device begins with retracting this tissue into a molding mechanism.

Reduction of Hiatal Hernia: If hiatal hernia is present, it can be reduced and the esophagus lengthened by retracting the endoscope into the esophagus and using suction, can be repositioned below the diaphragm.

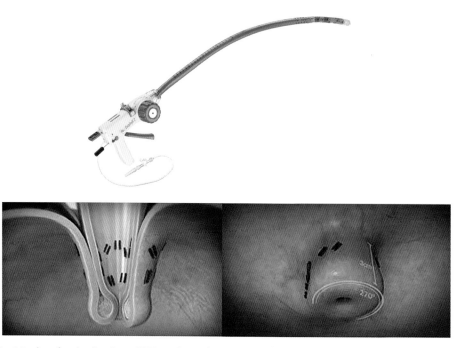

Figure 14-11 · Transoral incisionless fundoplication—TIF® 2.0 Procedure. (© 2018 from EndoGastric Solutions Inc., Redmond, WA.)

Valve Creation

- The device is repositioned and begins wrapping the fundus around the lesser curvature of the stomach. The device will then deploy a fastener that will hold the tissue in place and maintain the wrap.
- The wrap is tightened further with the device and the next fasteners placed 1 cm above the created line and repeated on the opposite side. The valve is extended creating a long 3 to 5 cm flap and secured with more fasteners.
- The device is removed and a final look with the gastroscope is completed.

Postop: The patient is the transported to recovery and typically a chest x-ray is completed before discharge. At time of discharge, the patient will go over diet instructions. The patient will be on a strict diet over the course of 4 weeks or as needed. The patient will be allowed to consume clear liquids for the first 24 hours, then progressing to full liquids for a week. Following that week, the patient will progress into soft foods leading into week 3, resuming a regular diet, but excluding meats and breads that week. Patient may also resume normal activity during this time.

Esophageal Gastrectomy. Esophageal Gastrectomy procedure is the resection of the distal esophagus and proximal stomach. Commonly performed to remove lesions and malignancies from the gastroesophageal junction and its associated lymphatics. The procedure itself is typically practiced in a minimally invasive laparoscopic technique but may also be performed as an open procedure depending on the patient and any of their comorbidities that may not allow the surgeon to

perform with the laparoscope. The SA will be responsible for exposure and assisting the surgeon in both scenarios.

Surgical steps are given in the following sections:

Incision

- Using #15 blade, trocars are strategically placed in the abdomen at different locations to accommodate the working instrumentation. The abdomen is inflated with carbon dioxide and a pneumoperitoneum is established to provide a space to work. The liver is retracted to provide exposure of the defect.
- The SA may place an assist port at this time. Note that if using a robotically assisted approach the SA will assist in the docking of the robot to the patient at this time. The SA will be responsible for exposure if using a laparoscope and maintain a clear visual of the field.

Mobilization

- The surgeon will begin by transecting the short gastric vessels using the heat source of choice. Once identifying the gastroepiploic artery, the surgeon will preserve the artery, as this will provide the blood supply to the gastric conduit.
- Next, the esophageal hiatus is released by the transection of the Freneau esophageal membrane and the GE junction is mobilized.
- The surgeon will then create a retroesophageal tunnel which will facilitate a Penrose drain which may be used to assist with retraction. Left gastric artery and vein are then identified and mobilized along with the associated lymphatic tissue. This tissue will also stay and be transported with the specimen to pathology.

Resection

- The surgeon may then begin resection using an endoscopic stapler containing a vascular size load and transect the left gastric vascular pedicle.

- The SA may be responsible for firing the stapler if procedure is robotic and surgeon prefers to not use a robotic stapler. In this case the SA will follow manufacture guidelines and the surgeon will direct the location of which the stapler will be deployed. If the SA is not holding any structure or deploying the stapler, the SA should have suction available at this time to maintain a clear field as the surgeon fires the stapler.

- With the distal esophagus now mobilized in the posterior mediastinum, the surgeon will begin to drain the lymphatic tissue between the aorta, pericardium, and right and left pleura which will also be included with the final specimen.

- The surgeon may perform an endoscopy to locate the exact site of the malignancy or tumor and mark the distal area of the location with cautery or marking of their choice. Typically, the lesser curvature stomach is chosen as a point of gastric transection. Lymphatics in this location are sent to pathology as well.

- The gastric conduit is then created using an endoscopic stapler with medium thickness loads. A stay suture may be placed on each side of the distal esophagus, and the esophagus is the next portion to be transected with the endoscopic stapler.

Specimen Removal

- The specimen is now liberated and will include distal esophagus, proximal stomach, and all associated lymphatics to be sent to pathology. The specimen may be placed in an endo retrieval bag and may be removed through an extended incision towards the end of the procedure.

Anastomosis

- The remaining esophagus is then opened, and the gastric conduit is sutured to the posterior aspect of the esophagus. The surgeon may overlap the esophagus and stomach in preparation for anastomosis.

- A gastrotomy is created and full thickness sutures are placed between the gastric conduit and the esophagus, incorporating the esophageal muscle and mucosa.

- The endo stapler is used to create the anastomosis between the two structures. The common channel is then closed in two layers using a running absorbable suture and an interrupted non absorbable suture as reinforcement. Any drain placement will occur at this time.

Wound Closure

- The specimen is removed, and the SA will begin closing the port sites, secure drain, and apply the preferred dressing of choice. The patient is then transported to recovery.

Postop: The patient may be NPO a few days after surgery, depending on the surgeon's preference. An upper GI series will be ordered to evaluate that the anastomosis is intact, and the emptying of the conduit is normal. Patient will then proceed to a clear liquid diet and be observed for any heart burn, reflux, and regurgitation. Postoperative day seven, the patient may return home if no complications are present with no restrictions.

Esophagectomy. An esophagectomy is a removal of a portion the esophagus, the approach to the procedure will depend on the location of the portion to be removed, the size of the tumor or malignancy, the extent of lymph node dissection to be performed. The methods to be discussed in this chapter will be the transhiatal and the transthoracic. Both procedures like the previously discussed, but with different approaches. The transhiatal will not only include the abdominal dissection but a neck dissection as well to assist with anastomosis. Thoracic will also begin with an abdominal approach and anastomose thoracically. Any of these procedures may be completed in an open approach with the same technique, only adjusted to accommodate the instrumentation. The SA will be responsible for maintaining clear visual of the field and completing any task such as retracting tissues, suctioning fluids, or deploying stapling devices at the surgeon's discretion.

Transhiatal Esophagectomy

Prepping and Positioning: This procedure will require and incision in the neck region as well. The patient will be placed supine, with neck hyperextended. Patient will be prepped from chin to pubis, using the preferred prep solution and proper dry time before placing drapes.

Surgical procedure is given in the following sections (see Figure 14-12):

Incision

- Using #15 blade, trocars are strategically placed in the abdomen at different locations to accommodate the working instrumentation. The abdomen is inflated with carbon dioxide and a pneumoperitoneum is established to provide a space to work. The liver is retracted to provide exposure of the defect.

- The SA may place an assist port at this time. Note that if using a robotically assisted approach the SA will assist in the docking of the robot to the patient at this time. The SA will be responsible for exposure if using a laparoscope and maintain a clear visual of the field.

Mobilization

- The surgeon begins mobilizing the greater curvature of the stomach using the preferred heat source. The surgeon then identifies and liberates the gastrohepatic ligament and then the right crus.

- The SA may retract the stomach as the surgeon is dissecting, the SA will use caution with the retraction as to not cause

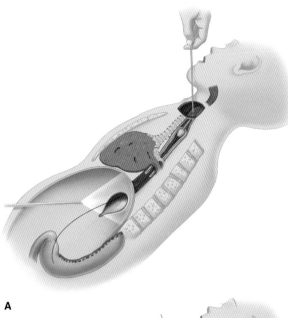

A

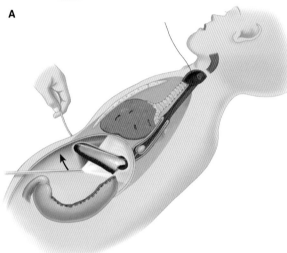

B

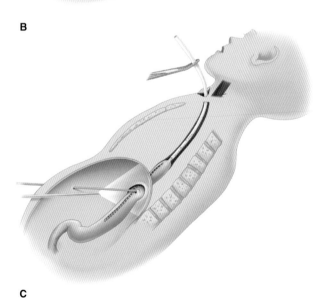

C

Figure 14-12 · Transhiatal esophagectomy. (Reproduced, with permission, from Brunicardi FC, Andersen DK, Billiar TR, et al, eds. *Schwartz's Principles of Surgery*. 11th ed. New York, NY: McGraw Hill; 2019.)

injury to nearby structures such as the spleen. Once the esophageal hiatus is exposed, the surgeon begins dissecting the mediastinum and mobilizing the thoracic esophagus.

- The surgeon will then move lower and begin taking down the gastrocolic omentum and the left gastric vessels at the origin. The surgeon will identify and preserve the gastro-epiploic vessel. To ensure a later tension free anastomosis, the Kocher maneuver may be performed at this time.

- The surgeon will then perform a pyloroplasty to widen and relax the pylorus.

Resection

- The proximal stomach is then divided using an endoscopic stapler. Again, the SA may be responsible for firing the stapler if procedure is robotic and surgeon prefers to not use a robotic stapler. In this case the SA will follow manufacture guidelines and the surgeon will direct the location of which the stapler will be deployed. If the SA is not holding any structure or deploying the stapler, the SA should have suction available at this time to maintain a clear field as the surgeon fires the stapler. After the proximal stomach is divided, the gastric conduit will be pulled into the mediastinum.

Neck Dissection

- Once resection is complete, the surgeon or another team will begin the dissection into the neck. The incision is typically made on the left side of the neck, to decrease the risk of injury to the recurrent laryngeal nerve, as it descends and recurs lower around the aortic arch rather than the subclavian artery on the right side.

- If the SA is holding retraction for this portion of the case, use caution while holding excessive lateral traction as to not injure any nearby structures.

- After the cervical esophagus is liberated and exposed, a Penrose drain may be used for retraction around the esophagus. The proximal esophagus is divided, and specimen will be pulled into the abdomen for removal through one of the port site.

Anastomosis

- If two teams present, surgeon working in the abdomen will then begin to anchor the stomach to the esophageal hiatus to reduce tension on the anastomosis. While the surgeon at the neck begins the anastomosis of the remaining esophagus to the gastric conduit.

Wound Closure

- Before closing, the surgeon may decide to put drains or a feeding jejunostomy tube at this time. Once drains are in place and specimen removed, the SA may begin closure of the incision sites and secure any drains at this time. Dressings are applied and the patient is transferred to recovery.

Postop: The patient may be NPO a few days after surgery, depending on the surgeon's preference. The patient will be encouraged to walk and increase activities as tolerated. Incentive spirometry will encourage the patient to expand their lungs. An upper GI series will be ordered to evaluate that the anastomosis is intact, and the emptying of the conduit is normal. Patient will then proceed to a clear liquid diet and be observed for any heart burn, reflux, and regurgitation. Postoperative day seven, the patient may return home if no complications are present with no restrictions. Patients typically make a full recovery between 6 and 8 weeks.

Transthoracic Esophagectomy. The transthoracic esophagectomy also known as the Ivor–Lewis technique, may be chosen by the surgeon and is performed in a two-stage technique. Beginning abdominally and performing the same mobilization techniques as a transhiatal, the patient is then repositioned on the left side for the thoracic. The anastomosis and specimen removal will be achieved thoracically.

Surgical procedure is mentioned in the following sections:

Incision

- Using #15 blade, trocars are strategically placed in the abdomen at different locations to accommodate the working instrumentation. The abdomen is inflated with carbon dioxide and a pneumoperitoneum is established to provide a space to work. The liver is retracted to provide exposure of the defect.

- The SA may place an assist port at this time. Note that if using a robotically assisted approach the SA will assist in the docking of the robot to the patient at this time. The SA will be responsible for exposure if using a laparoscope and maintain a clear visual of the field.

Mobilization

- Mobilization of gastric structure technique will remain the same as a transhiatal, see previous surgical steps for review.

Resection

- Once finished with mobilization, the transection of the proximal stomach may be initiated. The stapler is deployed across the lesser curve vessels toward incisura and then parallel with the greater curvature to avoid any spiralizing of the conduit (see Figure 14-13). The staple line is inspected for hemostasis and a suture is placed to mark 2 to 3 cm above the diameter change from the conduit. The suture will be the guide to stop retraction of the gastric conduit into the chest to avoid bringing the antrum too far into the thoracic space.

- The resected specimen may be reattached to the gastric conduit by placing a few sutures this technique can minimize bulk as the specimen and the gastric conduit are passed through the hiatus.

- Before the second stage of the procedure, some surgeons may choose to place a feeding jejunostomy tube at this time, as they will not have to enter the abdomen again as the last portion may be completed thoracically. The SA will begin closing all abdominal incisions and secure the feeding tube and apply dressings before repositioning patient for second portion.

Thoracoscopy

- The patient is repositioned in the lateral decubitus position for thoracic portion of case. The appropriate port sites are placed, and robot is reconnected if in use, the SA will assist with port insertion and visualization of the field with the scope. The patients are typically intubated with a double

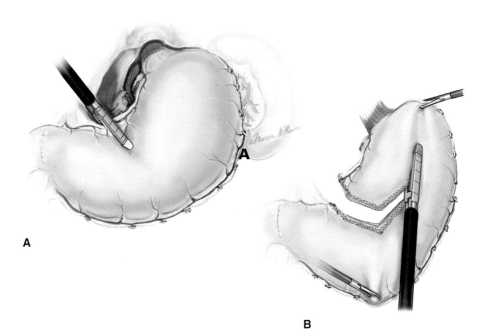

Figure 14-13 · Transection of the proximal stomach. (Reproduced, with permission, from Sugarbaker DJ, Bueno R, Burt BM, Groth SS, Loor G, Wolf AS, eds. *Sugarbaker's Adult Chest Surgery*. 3rd ed. New York, NY: McGraw Hill; 2020.)

lumen endotracheal tube and both lungs are inflated during the abdominal portion of the case. However, during the thoracic the right lung is isolated during thoracic dissection to provide better visualization and a larger working space.

Dissection

- Dissection will begin with the inferior pulmonary ligament, then the mediastinal pleura is dissected anteriorly between the esophagus and lung. The structure is then resected with the specimen up to the azygos vein. Subcarinal lymph nodes may be removed and taken with the specimen.

- The SA should use caution if using suction or manipulating any tissue to avoid injury to the posterior structures of the airway such as the right and left mainstem bronchi, the carina, and the trachea. The dissection is carried up to the azygos vein and the vein is then divided with and endoscopic stapler. The esophagus is mobilized and liberated from surrounding tissue, traction on the Vagus nerve is minimalized and the risk of recurrent nerve injury had decreased. The mediastinal pleura above the azygos recurrent nerve injury is decreased. The mediastinal pleura is preserved above the azygos vein and this will aid in maintaining the gastric conduit in the mediastinum and seal the surrounding tissue. This will also minimalize leakage of any cervical drainage into the chest.

- Once the specimen is mobilized the specimen and the gastric conduit are pulled into the field with gentle traction on the esophagus. The suture attaching the specimen and conduit are released. After the esophagus is completely mobilized, the proximal esophagus is divided, and the specimen is now liberated. The specimen will be removed from the posterior port incision that will be extended and placed with a wound protector.

Anastomosis

- The anastomosis of the remaining esophagus and the gastric conduit are achieved using an end-to-end anastomosis stapling device, the same device use in lower colon resections. The anvil of the stapler is placed with in the lumen of the esophagus and should be sized appropriately. The edges of the esophagus are then purse-string sutured around the anvil of the stapler. The gastric conduit is then brought up in the field and the proximal end is divided to open the conduit. The handle of the EEA stapler is then placed through the posterior port that was used earlier to remove the specimen, and into the open end of the conduit. The spiked end of the stapler is opened pushed out along the greater curvature at a site that is distal to the opening and well perfused. The anvil and spike are attached together, reapproximated, and deployed to from the anastomosis. The EEA stapler is carefully removed, and a nasogastric tube is inserted.

Wound Closure

- Once the NG tube is in place the open end of the conduit, used for the EEA stapler, may be divided by the endoscopic stapler, and removed from the chest cavity. The procedure now completed the cavity is irrigated, and chest tubes are

placed, as well as any drains at this time. The SA may begin wound closure and secure drains. Dressings are applied and the patient is transferred to recovery.

Postop: The patient may be NPO a few days after surgery, depending on the surgeon's preference. The patient will be encouraged to walk and increase activities as tolerated. Incentive spirometry will encourage the patient to expand their lungs. An upper GI series will be ordered to evaluate that the anastomosis is intact, and the emptying of the conduit is normal. Patient will then proceed to a clear liquid diet and be observed for any heart burn, reflux, and regurgitation. Postoperative day seven, the patient may return home if no complications are present with no restrictions. Patients typically make a full recovery between 6 and 8 weeks.

CHOLECYSTECTOMY

Procedure Identified: Cholecystectomy is the surgical removal of the gallbladder.

Abstract

There are more than 50 types of procedures to remove the gallbladder. These techniques have been improved over the years to increase lessened hospital stay and improve cosmetic results. Cholecystectomy is considered to be a low-risk surgery and in most cases the patient can go home the same day or the day after the procedure.

Anatomy and Physiology

The variation of the anatomy surrounding the gall bladder makes the procedure difficult in some cases. A surgeon's knowledge and awareness of the relevant anatomy is crucial to carrying out a successful operation. Anatomical variations or differences can cause damage to the biliary tract which can sometimes lead to morbidity if not corrected or treated immediately postoperatively.

The gall bladder is pear shaped and sits on the underside of the liver in an area known as the fossa. In certain cases, the liver is embedded in the parenchyma which is termed as an intrahepatic gallbladder. The surgeon must take care as to avoid tearing the liver to prevent bleeding and to avoid the large portal and hepatic venous branches.

The gall bladder consists of the fundus, the body, and the neck of the infundibulum. In the neck area is a region known as Hartman's pouch. When this area is distended it is usually indicative of gallstones. If Hartman's pouch is abnormally large, it can obstruct the surgeon's view of the cystic duct and the triangle of Calot. The triangle of Calot consists of the common hepatic duct (bile duct) located medially, the cystic duct located inferiorly, and the interior or underside of the liver located superiorly. The cystic duct connects the gall bladder to the bile duct and must be identified by the surgeon prior to ligation. It is normally 2 to 3 mm. in length. If the cystic duct contains stones, it can be slightly larger in diameter thus causing difficulty identifying it. The cystic artery is a branch of the right hepatic artery.

Core anatomical organ(s) affected: The gallbladder is a small, pear-shaped organ located on the underside of your liver. It stores bile made by the liver and sends it to the small intestine via the common bile duct (CBD) to aid in the digestion of fats. The CBD connects the liver, the gallbladder, and the pancreas to the small intestine. Gallstones blocking the CBD are the leading cause of cholecystitis. This blockage causes bile to build up in the gallbladder, and that buildup causes the gallbladder to become inflamed.

Gall stones in the bile duct are also the prominent cause of choledocholithiasis. If a stone becomes lodged in the duct, it can cause severe abdominal pain. Cholelithiasis can affect the stomach by causing bloating, gas pain, as well as nausea. The common bile duct connects the liver, gall bladder, and the pancreas to the small intestine and a blockage from a stone can also cause cholelithiasis.

Structures Identified Relative to Diagnosis-Liver

Location: The gall bladder is in a sulcus on the undersurface of the right lobe of the liver. It is located adjacent to the postero-inferior aspect of the liver, transverse colon, and superior part of the duodenum.

Arterial and venous supply: The arterial supply to the gallbladder is via the cystic artery—a branch of the right hepatic artery (which itself is derived from the common hepatic artery, one of the three major branches of the coeliac trunk). Venous drainage of the neck of the gallbladder is via the cystic veins, which drain directly into the portal vein. Venous drainage of the fundus and body of the gallbladder flows into the hepatic sinusoids.

Nerves: Vagus

Lymph nodes: Calot's node sometimes referred to as the sentinel lymph node of the gall bladder. It has also been referred to as Lund's node, or Mascagni's node. Calot's node will become inflamed in patients with Cholecystitis.

Key landmarks and/or relevant associated structures: The original definition of the triangle of Calot or Calot's triangle consisted of the 3 C's which included the common bile duct, the cystic duct, and the cystic artery. Most surgeons utilize the inferior border/surface of the liver as opposed to the cystic artery which was utilized in the original description by Calot.

Physiology (function or work of the organ[s]): The gall bladder's function is to store and concentrate bile. Bile is a yellow-brown digestive enzyme that is produced by the liver. The gall bladder is part of the biliary tract and is used as a reservoir that stores bile until it is needed in the body to aid in digestion.

Etiology: The major cause of gall bladder disease is due to gall stones which form due to a build-up of excessive cholesterol or bilirubin in the bile or incomplete emptying of the gall bladder. Gallstones can also form due to an excess of water that is removed from the bile by the gall bladder. There are two types of gall stones. The first type of gall stones are called cholesterol stones. These are the most common type. They are yellow green in color and make up about 80% of gallstones in patients with diseases of the gall bladder. The second type are called pigment stones and they are black in color and much smaller than cholesterol stones. They are made of bilirubin and are less common.

Diagnosis (Modalities)

History: family history of gall stones, female, over age 40, native American or Mexican descent, obese, pregnant, diabetic, taking birth control pills or hormone therapy treatment, have Crohn's disease, hemolytic anemia, or cirrhosis of the liver, or have lost a substantial amount of weight in a short time

Physical: upper right quadrant pain, right shoulder or back pain, epigastric pain, vomiting, indigestion, heartburn, gas, fever/chills, jaundice (yellow eyes or skin), dark urine, light colored stool (clay stool), anorexia, abdominal pain after eating

Diagnostic Modalities Relevant to Condition/Procedure

- Diagnostic laboratory exams: blood tests (check for signs of infection or blockage)
- Diagnostic imaging: ultrasound, CT scan, MRCP-Magnetic resonance cholangiopancreatography (see Figure 14-14)
- Diagnostic procedures: HIDA Scan, ERCP

Procedural Considerations

Examples are nonsurgical treatment, surgical treatment, list of surgical approaches (open, laparascopic, robotic, etc.).

- Nonsurgical treatment: combination of analgesics, anti-inflammatory drugs, antibiotic agents, and percutaneous drainage (usually a bridge to surgical treatment)
- Usual surgical treatment and options: Laparoscopic Cholecystectomy is the surgery of choice. In some cases, the procedure may have to be performed open or converted to an open procedure if the surgeon cannot initially identify crucial anatomical landmarks. This is essential for a safe laparoscopic approach.

Surgical Approaches

Cholecystectomy—Open approach: If a patient has been diagnosed with or is suspected to have cancer of the gallbladder, in their third trimester of pregnancy, suffers from cirrhosis with portal hypertension, or poor pulmonary reserve.[2] They may not be able to tolerate the pneumoperitoneum required for a laparoscopic approach.

Cholecystectomy-Laparoscopic approach: Patients that meet the criteria for the laparoscopic approach are informed prior to surgery that it may be necessary to convert the procedure to an open approach if necessary. The standard laparoscopy procedure uses four ports, but some surgeons have been able to modify the procedure and use less ports to decrease the chance of incisional hernias and for cosmetic reasons.

Preoperative Preparation. Additional labs/orders: abdominal ultrasound, HIDA scan, ERCP, bloodwork, chest x-ray, EKG. Any requirements for procedure (no smoking, lose weight, psychological counseling, nutritional aspects, etc.) as such not mentioned.

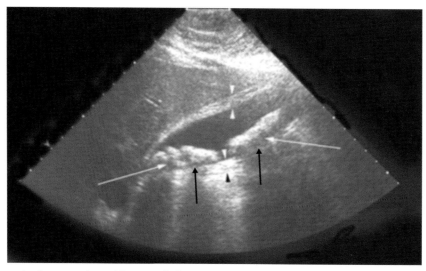

Figure 14-14 • Ultrasonography from a patient with acute cholecystitis. (Reproduced, with permission, from Brunicardi FC, Andersen DK, Billiar TR, et al, eds. *Schwartz's Principles of Surgery.* 11th ed. New York, NY: McGraw Hill; 2019.)

Anesthesia. Patients undergo a general anesthesia for open or laparoscopic cholecystectomy. Laparoscopic Cholecystectomy can cause problems related to cardiopulmonary effects of pneumoperitoneum, systemic carbon dioxide absorption, extraperitoneal gas insufflation, venous gas embolism and unintentional injuries to intra-abdominal structures especially in older patients.

Positioning and Prepping. Supine: Some surgeons will prefer that the right arm is tucked Specifics for surgical skin prep-An abdominal prep is performed for Laparoscopic and/or open procedure. Patient is in supine position with arms positioned on arm boards or the right arm may be tucked. Patient is prepped from nipple line to upper third of thighs down to right table line and left table line. Patient should be prepped in a circular motion using the aseptic solutions or one-step skin prep applicator noted on the surgeon's preference card.

Surgical Procedure

Procedure including the role of the assistant (SA, PA, resident). Steps highlighted, key landmarks, core nerves/arteries are to be identified.

Open Cholecystectomy

- The abdomen is opened through a right subcostal or upper midline incision usually with a #10 or #12 knife blade.
- The SA provides counter traction during initial incision.
- The surgeon and/or SA cauterizes capillary vessels with a bovie or electrocautery device. The second assistant will utilize the suction to evacuate surgical plume and take care to keep the bovie out of the vision of the surgeon and SA Larger vessels will be clamped, cut, and tied with suture (surgeon's preference) by the surgeon and/or SA.
- The second assistant will cut sutures as needed. Appropriate size retractors (army-navy, Goelets, or small Richardson) are placed as well as laparotomy packs for the surgeon to ex-

amine the abdominal cavity. It is the second assistant's duty to hold retractors in order to free up the SA' hands so he/she can assist the surgeon effectively.

- The common bile duct is palpated for evidence of stones and to determine pathological conditions. A Harrington or Deaver retractor is placed on the underside of the liver bed to provide exposure of the area. The retractor is held by the second assistant. Long tissue forceps (Debakey's) and suction are commonly used to manipulate the tissues.
- The SA will utilize moistened laparotomy packs, deep retractors and sometimes their hand to isolate surrounding organs from the gallbladder region. The other hand of the SA would utilize a Pean forceps on the body of the gall bladder to provide gentle traction.
- The peritoneal fold that overlies the junction of the cystic duct and common bile duct is incised by the surgeon with a #7 knife handle and a #15 blade, long Metzenbaum scissors, and forceps.
- The SA provides suction as the surgeon clamps, ligates, or electrocoagulates bleeding vessels.
- The surgeon will then utilize a sponge stick, peanut on a long Kelly clamp or tonsil clamp, and a blunt right-angled clamp to separate adhesions. Dissection continues in order to expose the neck of the gall bladder, the cystic duct, and the cystic artery. Lateral traction on the gall bladder neck provided by the second assistant provides access and visualization of the peritoneum that overlies the triangle of Calot. The surgeon can then incise the peritoneum.
- The surgeon then exposes the cystic artery where it enters the wall of the gallbladder. The cystic artery is clamped with ligating clips and then divided. On occasion, a patient may have multiple branches off the cystic artery, in which case it would be double ligated with silk or clamped with ligating

clips and divided. In some patients, abnormalities of the arterial and ductal anatomy are present.

- The surgeon and SA must be mindful of this and carefully identify these structures appropriately. The junction of the cystic duct and common bile duct are identified, and the cystic duct is dissected down to its junction with the hepatic duct. If stones are present in the cystic duct, the surgeon will utilize a right-angle clamp to milk the stones back into the gall bladder.
- The surgeon will then tie a suture around the proximal part of the cystic duct. A cholangiogram would now be performed if necessary. The surgeon will incise the cystic duct and insert the cholangiocatheter into the small incision. This will determine if the cystic duct has been identified properly. If it is not needed, the cystic duct is doubly ligated and divided. Some surgeons will opt to place an absorbable transfixation suture on the stump of the cystic duct.
- The gallbladder is then dissected off the liver bed with an electrocautery (bovie) and removed. Bleeding is controlled by electrocauterization or interrupted stitches. A drain is placed if necessary.
- The wound is closed in layers by the surgeon and SA. The first and second assistant will then apply the dressing.

Laparoscopic Cholecystectomy

- A small incision is made supraumbilically or infraumbilically with a #11 blade on a #7 knife handle by the surgeon. Pneumoperitoneum is created using the open or closed method depending on surgeon's preference.
- The surgeon then places an 11-mm trocar through the umbilical incision. The surgeon then inserts the laparoscope with the attached video camera through the port and views the peritoneal cavity. The surgeon is positioned on the left side of the patient and the SA is positioned on the right side. Each have monitors positioned on each side at eye level.
- Anesthesia then places the patient in reverse Trendelenburg position and tilts the bed slightly to the right. Three additional small incisions are made with a #15 blade by the surgeon and/or the SA The camera is held by either depending on who is making the incisions and inserting the trocars into the peritoneal cavity. These are inserted under direct visualization of the laparoscopic view.
- An atraumatic grasper or blunt grasper is inserted through the 5-mm port by the SA to grasp the gall bladder.
- The SA then retracts the gall bladder laterally to expose the triangle of Calot.
- The surgeon then identifies the junction of the gallbladder and the cystic duct. The surgeon inserts the endoscopic dissector, hook, and/or scissors through the port and partially dissects the base of the gall bladder from the liver bed.
- The SA will manipulate the gall bladder with the atraumatic grasper as needed. A suction/irrigator is also used to remove blood and smoke plume from the area being dissected.

- The surgeon then places hemoclips proximally and distally on the cystic artery and then uses endoscopic scissors to divide it. In most cases, a single use multi-clip applier is used. An intraoperative cholangiogram may be performed at this time.
- The surgeon will place a hemoclip proximally on the cystic duct and make a small incision on the anterior surface with an endoscopic scissor. The cholangiogram catheter is then inserted into one of the ports and inserted into the duct.
- The SA will place a sterile bag on to the C-Arm and the Radiology Technician performs the cholangiogram with the surgeon. After the cholangiogram is completed, two clips are placed distally on the cystic duct, and it is divided with the endoscopic scissors. A prettied loop ligature may also be used if the duct is too large.
- The surgeon then dissects the gallbladder out of its fossa. The surgeon inspects the area for hemostasis and proceeds to dissect the gallbladder from the underside of the liver. In most cases an endo-bag is used to contain the gall bladder.
- The surgeon inserts the endo-bag through the umbilical port and opens the bag.
- The SA places the gall bladder into the bag and releases the atraumatic grasper. The bag is then closed by the surgeon and removed through the umbilical port. The peritoneal cavity is decompressed.
- The surgeon places interrupted non-absorbable suture in the fascia of the umbilical port site incision.
- The SA then closes the remaining port incisions with 4-0 absorbable suture or staples. Dressings are applied (see Figure 14-15).

Modifications/additional associated procedures commonly seen are given in the following sections.

Open Common Bile Duct Exploration. This is rarely performed due to advances in technology. However, due to having a previous surgery it may be necessary.

- The surgeon makes a subcostal or midline incision. The gall bladder is removed. The surgeon identifies the common bile duct by using an aspirating syringe and fine gauge needle and then obtains a culture specimen. The common duct area is isolated with moistened laparotomy packs.
- The SA utilizes a narrow Deaver retractor to provide exposure. The surgeon places two traction sutures on the wall of the duct. (Below the entrance of the cystic duct) A #15 or #11 blade is used to make a longitudinal incision into the common duct. (Between the traction sutures).
- The incision is enlarged with Potts angled or Metzenbaum scissors. The surgeon removes visible stones with gallstone forceps. An isotonic solution is used in an Asepto syringe and a small-lumen catheter to remove remaining small stones and debris.
- The surgeon checks for patency of the common bile duct until it enters the duodenum. A choledochoscope may also be used to check for additional stones. Once the duct is clear

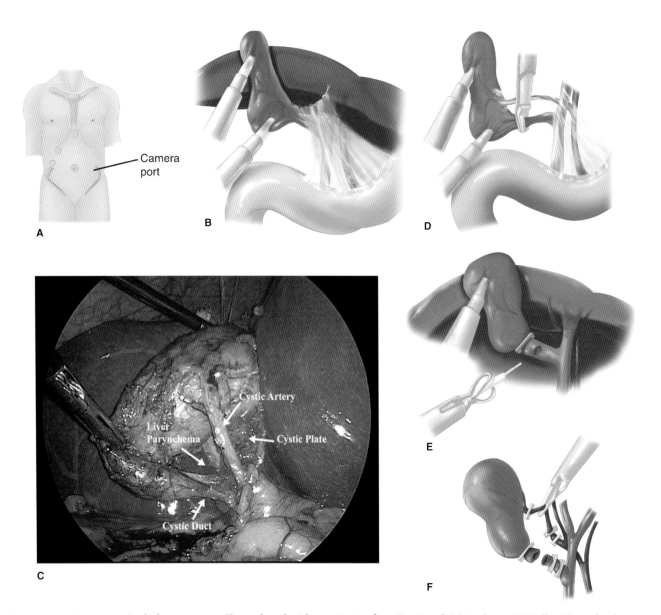

Figure 14-15 · Laparascopic cholecystectomy. (Reproduced, with permission, from Brunicardi FC, Andersen DK, Billiar TR, et al, eds. *Schwartz's Principles of Surgery*. 11th ed. New York, NY: McGraw Hill; 2019.)

of stones, the surgeon inserts a T-tube in the common bile duct and closes the duct ensuring that the tube is secure.

- The T-tube is then connected to a small drainage bag or container by the SA.

Conversion to Open Procedure. Once the surgeon enters the abdominal cavity with the laparoscope it may be evident that the patient has a porcelain gall bladder, or the gall bladder could perforate and will determine that the procedure will need to be converted to open. The surgeon may also not be able to identify the common bile duct with enough certainty to continue laparoscopically. Whatever the case may be, the table is already set up for an open cholecystectomy and the case would continue as described for an open case.

Choledochduodenostomy. The surgeon makes a midline incision. The SA provides counter-traction with a laparotomy sponge. The common bile duct and duodenum are identified and exposed. The surgeon utilizes Metzenbaum scissors and forceps to dissect the common duct free so it can be attached to the duodenum side-to-side or end-to-side. An intraluminal catheter is then inserted, and the incision is closed.

Choledochojejunostomy. The surgeon makes a midline incision. The SA provides counter traction with a laparotomy sponge. The jejunum is mobilized. After the surgeon identifies the common bile duct, the jejunum is transected. An anastomosis is performed between the common bile duct and the jejunum. A catheter is introduced. The surgeon then rejoins the jejunum. A drain may be placed, and the incision is closed.

Postop: Drains used/dressings: Open Cholecystectomy—open or closed drain if necessary. Surgeon's preference until drainage ceases. T-tube may be inserted if exploratory bile duct was performed. Dressings-4 by4's, abdominal pad, paper tape (surgeon's preference). Laparoscopic Cholecystectomy—open or closed drain if necessary. Surgeon's preference until drainage ceases. Dressings-Mastisol, steri-strips, band aids or small dressings and bioclusive (surgeon's preference).

Prognosis with Treatment: Example includes PT, radiation. Prognosis is excellent to very good if surgery was performed successfully.

Complications: Common to this procedure—Open Cholecystectomy and Laparoscopic Cholecystectomy—infection, bleeding, injury to common bile duct, injury to other organs, Incisional hernia.

Discharge Planning: Discharge planning is the same for both procedures; however, patients that undergo laparoscopic cholecystectomy will be discharged the next day in most cases. Open cholecystectomy patients within 2 to 3 days. Patient is not permitted to drive until pain medication is no longer needed. Normal diet is advised (some surgeons may order a low-fat diet). Gently wash area around incision with mild soap and water daily. Patient may take a shower. Bathtubs, pools, and hot tubs are not permitted until incision has closed/healed.

There may be several variations in the arterial supply to the gallbladder:

A. Cystic artery from right hepatic artery,

B. Cystic artery off the right hepatic artery arising from the superior mesenteric artery (accessory or replaced).

C. Two cystic arteries, one from the right hepatic, the other from the common hepatic artery.

D. Two cystic arteries, one from the right hepatic, the other from the left hepatic artery.

E. The cystic artery branching from the right hepatic artery and running anterior to the common hepatic duct.

F. Two cystic arteries arising from the right hepatic artery.

GASTRIC AND BOWEL RESECTION PROCEDURES

Introduction

The role of the gastrointestinal tracts is to transport, digest, and absorb nutrition. When there is a disturbance in any portion of the tract due to illness or abnormalities that can interfere with a patient's safety, surgical intervention may be an option to reestablish continuity of the tract. Surgical intervention will be determined by the surgeon and discussed with the patient. Procedures can range from traditional open to advanced laparoscopic, this may also include robotically assisted laparoscopy. The SA will play a key role in exposure in all the scenarios listed in procedure selection. The SA will also be beneficial in assisting with rerouting and anastomosis with the use of GI staplers and suturing.

Anatomy

The stomach is made up of four main regions: the cardia, the fundus, body, and pylorus (see Figure 14-16). The gastrophrenic ligament extends from the diaphragm to the cardia. The cardia is where the esophagus meets the stomach. To the left of the cardia is the fundus, below that is the body of the stomach which is the main portion of the stomach. The large fold in the body of the stomach where the mucosa and submucosa fall is called ruga. Moving distally, is the pylorus, which connects the stomach to the duodenum. The pyloric sphincter controls the stomach emptying into the duodenum. The arterial blood supply to the stomach include the left gastric artery; branches off the celiac artery, splenic artery, the left gastroepiploic and one branch of the left gastric artery and the gastroduodenal artery. Major nerves of the stomach include the anterior and posterior Vagus nerves and anterior and posterior nerve of Latarjet.

The stomach empties into the duodenum. The duodenum continues into the jejunum beginning at the ligament of Treitz. The small intestine is roughly 4 to 6 m long and connects with the large intestine at the cecum at the ileocecal junction. The colon is divided into seven sections (Figure 14-17). Beginning with the cecum transitioning into the ascending colon at the hepatic flexure. From the ascending colon around the hepatic flexure leads into the transverse colon. As the transverse colon leads to the splenic flexure, it then begins the descending colon, sigmoid, rectum, and anal canal. The colon has four layers: serosa, muscular, submucosa, and mucosa. Arterial supply faced during resection can include the right, middle and left colic arteries. Also, the inferior and superior mesenteric, and intercolic and sigmoid arteries. Lower arterial supply commonly encountered in lower anterior resections are the superior rectal artery.

The stomach obtains innervation from the autonomic nervous system. The parasympathetic nerve supply arises from the Vagus nerve. The sympathetic nerve supply arises from T6 to T9 and passes to the coeliac plexus via the greater splanchnic nerve. These also provide extrinsic innervation to the small intestine. The large intestine innervates from the mesenteric plexus. The distal anal canal receives somatic innervation from the pudendal nerve.

Diagnostic Procedures

Diagnostics in the gastrointestinal tract commonly use imaging to obtain a clear view of the tract and its functioning. Tests leading to the diagnosis of dysphagia and other malignancies include but are not limited to a Barium swallow study for the pharynx and esophagus, upper GI x-ray examination, endoscopy, ultrasound and CT scans of the abdomen may be ordered to visualize the areas in question in the stomach and bowel region.

Anesthesia

Anesthesia selected for gastrointestinal surgery typically is a general with the patient paralyzed and airway maintained.

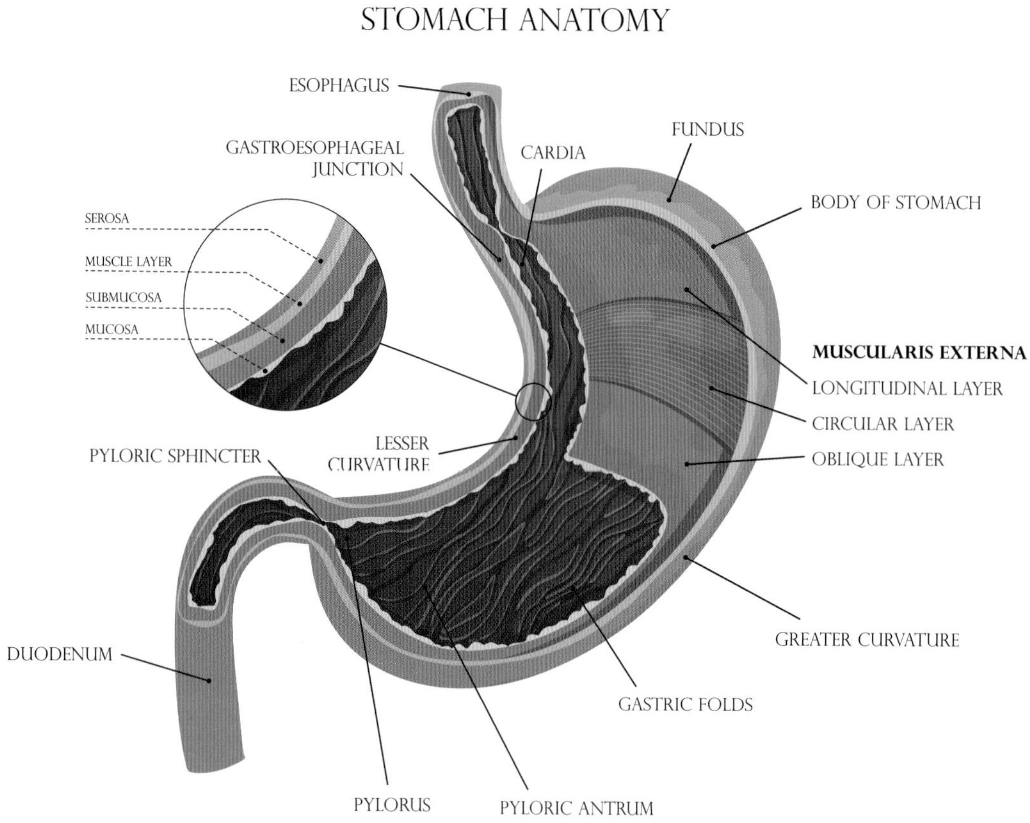

STOMACH ANATOMY

Figure 14-16 • Human stomach inside visualization with all layers and folds. Medical infographic, educational diagram. (Used with permission from Tatsiana Matusevich/Shutterstock.)

Nasal or Oral gastric tubes may be placed by anesthesia to deflate or drain fluids from the stomach and decompress the bowel in some cases. Pain control afterward has advanced from narcotics to using an epidural, spinal, or regional nerve block. Local anesthetic may be injected at portal sites for minimally invasive procedures, to promote analgesia to assist with postop pain.

Positioning

The SA may assist with positioning the patient on the operating room table. The patient, in most procedures, will be positioned supine with arms extended no more than 90° on the arm boards to protect the patient from nerve damage. Over extension of the arms may injure the brachial plexus. Depending on the procedure the patient may be placed in Trendelenburg or reverse Trendelenburg, the SA must take proper precautions to assure the patient will remain safe on the bed. Safety straps and foot boards may be used to prevent the patient from sliding on the bed when placed in another position. Lithotomy positioning may be used for resections on the lower portion of the colon. The most common injured nerve in lithotomy position is the peroneal nerve if positioning incorrectly. The SA must be mindful when positioning to not over flex the hips and knees of the patient while in stirrups to avoid over stretching and compressing the nerves such as the femoral nerve.

Prepping and Draping

An alcohol-based prep may be used to prep the abdomen. The SA must be conscious if using these types of preps, there may be a time needed to dry before applying the drapes to aid in the prevention of a fire in the operating room. Follow the manufacturer guidelines when using any prep solution.

Draping is based on the preference of the surgeon. Once the prep solution is dried, the site may be squared off with operating room towels and a large laparotomy or laparoscopic drape placed over the abdomen. Colorectal surgery may require the same type of draping for incision on the abdomen but lithotomy draping for the lower portion of the case.

Dressings

Dressings in Gastrointestinal surgery depend on the surgeon method of procedure. A large incision requires a larger absorbable dressing, while smaller puncture sites may only require a simple adhesive dressing such as band aids. The SA must be aware if the patient has any allergies that may affect choice in dressings.

Surgical Procedures

Gastrostomy. A Gastrostomy is a surgically created opening from the gastric mucosa to the skin. In most cases the gastrostomy will be used in providing nutrition to the patient. Other instances may be used to decompress or a drain for the

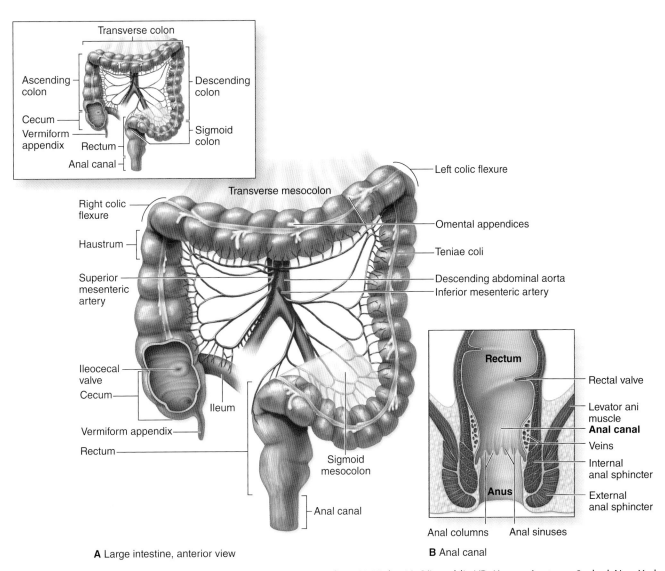

Figure 14-17 · Anatomy of the colon. (Reproduced, with permission, from McKinley M, O'Loughlin VD. *Human Anatomy*. 2nd ed. New York, NY: McGraw Hill; 2008.)

stomach. The procedure may be done endoscopically in an outpatient setting or inpatient at the bedside, using a gastroscope and a percutaneous gastrostomy tube equipment. The procedure may be accomplished laparoscopically as well in combination with other laparoscopic cases or if endoscopy is not an option for the patient.

Pathology: When the patient requires the insertion of a gastrostomy tube, this may be due to a finding that will no longer allow them to ingest their own nutrition. Malignancies may include tumors of the larynx, pharynx, esophagus, and proximal stomach. Dysphagia, difficulty swallowing, is potentially another reason for insertion of a gastrostomy tube. Esophageal stricture is another source for patients to have difficulty swallowing and therefore causing them to not consume food and fluids.

Surgical procedure is mentioned in the following sections.

Insertion of the Endoscope: The Patient will remain in the supine position for the duration of the procedure. Using a gastroscope the surgeon will inflate the stomach using air from the scope, providing a visual inspection of the mucosa. Then selecting the designated area for the tube insertion. An endoscopic looped snare is then threaded through the scope, used to capture the guidewire will be inserted. The SA may be used to provide visualization with the endoscope or assist with the tube insertion measures.

Percutaneous Insertion of Needle and Guide Wire: Once the area of insertion is prepped, a local anesthetic is injected at the site, then a trocar needle is inserted into the abdomen and visualized entering the stomach with the endoscope. A small stab incision is made with an #11 blade at the site of the trocar needle. An appropriately sized guide wire is inserted through the needle. Using the looped snare, the guidewire is captured and pulled out of the patient's mouth along with the endoscope, meanwhile the distal end of the guidewire remains threaded through the trocar needle.

Insertion of Gastrostomy Tube: After the retrieval of the guidewire and removal of the endoscope, the gastrostomy tube is lubricated and placed over the guidewire. The procedure is then reversed, pulling the gastrostomy tube down the esophagus into the stomach. The proximal end of the tube and guidewire is then pulled out through the needle insertion site, and guidewire removed. The endoscope may be reinserted to provide visual inspection of the gastrostomy tube. The SA may cut the end of the gastrostomy tube to proper length and insert sterile catheter plugs. Dressings are then applied, and the patient is then transferred to recovery.

Postop: Patients at discharge will be provided with care instructions for their gastrostomy tube such as proper handling and use, as well as cleaning and monitoring the tube site. The patient should contact physician if they contract a fever or if gastrostomy tube falls out with in the first 2 weeks of placement.

Gastrectomy. The surgical removal of the stomach and reconstitution of the alimentary tract. Partial gastrectomy may be achieved using the Billroth 1 and 2 procedures. Billroth 1 consists of removing the distal portion of the stomach and pylorus with an end-to-end anastomosis of the remaining stomach to the duodenum. Billroth 2 is nearly the same technique, but the divided ends of the duodenum are closed, and the jejunum is anastomosed to the stomach (gastrojejunostomy). Total removal of the stomach requires a Roux-en-Y, esophagojejunostomy.

Etiology: The most common reasons for a total gastrectomy are malignancy and uncontrollable bleeding using conservative measures.

Surgical procedure is given in the following sections:

Incision:

- Using a #10 blade, the surgeon will typically make an upper midline incision. Depending on preference a bilateral subcoastal (chevron) or thoracoabdominal may also be used.

- The SA will help in the assistance of exposure by retracting each tissue layer till visualization of the stomach is achieved, while also assisting with maintaining hemostasis of vessels.

Mobilization of the Lesser and Greater Curvature:

- The surgeon will then mobilize the greater and lesser curvature of the stomach using the preferred energy source for example: ultrasonic scalpel, vessel sealer, etc.

- The SA will maintain visualization by keeping the site clear with suctioning fluids and retraction of tissue. Any adhesions and peritoneal attachment to the pancreas will be released.

Division of the Duodenum:

- Once the stomach is mobilized, the duodenum is then divided using a surgical stapler.

- Next, the esophagus is transected with the reloaded stapler of choice and the stomach and duodenum are removed.

Anastomosis:

- A Roux-en-Y reconstruction will now begin, at least 45 cm of jejunum is recommended to be anastomosed to achieve a tension free loop to prevent any reflux that may occur.

- The SA will use proper bowel technique and control spillage using suction while anastomosing the esophagojejunal and end-to-end jejunal anastomosis (see Figure 14-18).

Wound Closure:

- The SA will then assist the surgeon with inspecting the anastomosis sites for any possible leakage and any hemostasis needed.

- The wound is then irrigated and closed. Beginning with the fascial layer using the surgeon's suture of choice, the SA will provide retraction as needed.

- The SA may close the subcutaneous tissue and skin to follow using the closing preference of the surgeon.

- After the wound is closed the SA will apply preferred dressings and patient is transferred to recovery.

Postop: The patient will be educated on proper diet and changes in bowel habits, as well as wound care for the incisions. Activities will be encouraged during hospital stay and increased as tolerated. Patients will be encouraged not to drive or lift over 10 to 20 lb until after postoperative appointment. Returning to work will be discussed and cleared at follow up visits with provider.

Bariatric Surgery. Bariatric surgery is the surgical treatment of obesity. Obesity is the second leading cause of preventable death behind smoking. Also known as "Weight loss" or "Weight reduction" surgery. Obesity is weight that is above what is considered healthy using the body mass index scale (BMI). BMI that is above 35 will qualify a patient for weight loss surgery.

Etiology: Obese patients may suffer from comorbidities that may perhaps be improved with weight loss surgery. These include but are not limited to cardiovascular disease, diabetes, hypertension, hyperlipidemia, sleep apnea, kidney, and arthritis. Weight reduction surgery may help with treatment, if not resolve these comorbidities as well as promote a healthy lifestyle.

Diagnostics: In addition to routine lab work and diagnostic imaging, patients will also be evaluated psychologically by a professional and meet with a nutritionist for education purposes.

Laparoscopic Sleeve Gastrectomy: The sleeve gastrectomy is a restrictive procedure that reduces the size of the stomach. This will limit the amount of food the patient will intake. The patient's appetite will reduce with the removal of the Ghrelin hunger hormone, therefore, decreasing food consumption and increasing weight loss.

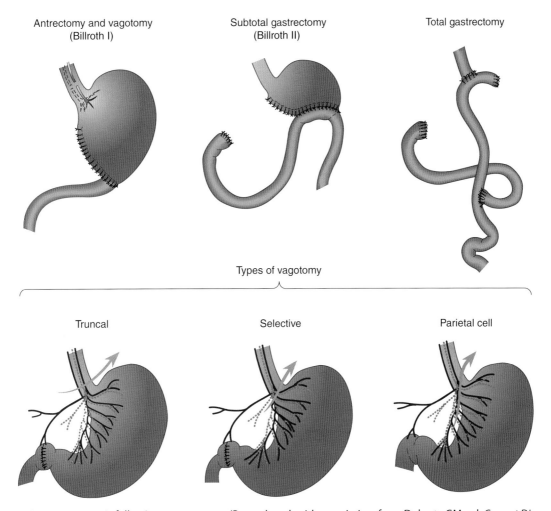

Figure 14-18 • Various anastomosis following gastrectomy. (Reproduced, with permission, from Doherty GM, ed. *Current Diagnosis & Treatment: Surgery.* 15th ed. New York: McGraw Hill; 2020.)

Surgical Procedure is given in the following section.

Incisions and Trocar Placement:

- Using a #15 knife blade, trocars are placed strategically in the abdomen at different locations to accommodate the working instruments.

- The abdomen is inflated with carbon dioxide and a pneumoperitoneum is established to provide space to work.

- The liver is then retracted to provide visualization of the stomach. The SA may assist in placing an assistant port on the section of the patient closest to them (note if the surgeon is using the robot, the SA will dock the manipulators of the robot to the appropriate port sites before beginning).

Gastric Mobilization:

- Once visualization of the stomach is achieved and the liver is retracted, using the preferred energy source, the surgeon will make a window into the omental bursa roughly 4 to 6 cm proximal to the pylorus. Then proceed superiorly and mobilizing the antrum.

- The SA will provide visualization of the site with the camera (if not robotically) and assist in the division of the omentum.

- Using atraumatic laparoscopic graspers, the SA may hold gentle traction of the omentum as the surgeon dissects each section.

- The stomach is then retracted, and the cardia is then mobilized. The SA must be mindful to surrounding structures that are in proximity while providing retraction of the stomach and omentum such as the spleen, as injury may easily occur (Figure 14-19).

Gastrectomy: Before the gastrectomy begins, a 32 French orogastric bougie is placed adjacent to the pylorus, this will reduce the risk of antral pouch dilation and will stent open the newly created stomach.

- Using the laparoscopic stapler containing a thicker load of no less than 60 mm, the surgeon will begin the gastrectomy. Beginning with the fundus and working superiorly to the cardia.

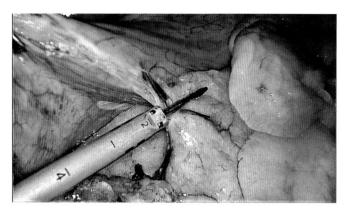

Figure 14-19 · Window being created into the omental bursa. (Reproduced, with permission, from The Center of Weight Loss at Wood County Hospital, Bowling Green, Ohio.)

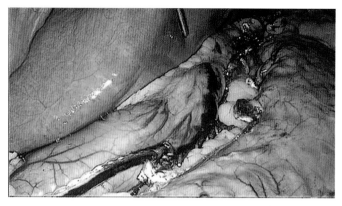

Figure 14-21 · Completion of gastrectomy sleeve. (Reproduced, with permission, from The Center of Weight Loss at Wood County Hospital, Bowling Green, Ohio.)

- Once the stomach is liberated, the staple line may be reinforced with suture unless using buttressing strips that can be attached to each staple load before stapling. The bougie is then removed and the staple line is inspected for bleeding (see Figures 14-20 and 14-21).

Omentopexy (Optional):

- Suturing of the divided edges of the omentum may provide additional reinforcement and gentle traction to prevent coiling of the stomach. Drains may potentially be placed at this time according to surgeon preference.

Wound Closure:

- The detached stomach is removed, and the puncture sites are closed with the surgeon preferred suture by the SA. Small adhesive dressings placed over the trocar sites by the SA and patient is transferred to recovery.

Laparoscopic Roux-en-Y Gastric Bypass. A largely restrictive and mildly malabsorption procedure that reroutes ingested food from the small pouch, created from the proximal stomach to segment of the proximal jejunum. Weight loss is achieved again by restricting the patient's intake and delaying of absorption.

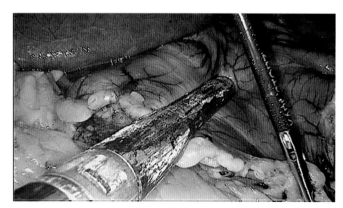

Figure 14-20 · Beginning staple of the gastrectomy. (Reproduced, with permission, from The Center of Weight Loss at Wood County Hospital, Bowling Green, Ohio.)

Surgery steps are given in the following section.

Incisions and Trocar Placement:

- Using a #15 knife blade, trocars are placed strategically in the abdomen at different locations to accommodate the working instrumentation on the stomach. The abdomen is inflated with carbon dioxide and a pneumoperitoneum is established.

- The SA may assist in placing an assistant port on the section of the patient closest to them (note if the surgeon is using the robot, the SA will dock the manipulators of the robot to the appropriate port sites before beginning).

Division of Jejunum:

- Once the abdomen is inflated, the liver is retracted, The SA will maintain exposure with the laparoscope. The omentum is then reflected and the ligament of Treitz is located. Counting 40-50 cm distal to the ligament of Treitz the jejunum is divided by an endoscopic surgical stapler.

Pouch Creation:

- The proximal portion of the stomach is divided, and the gastric pouch is created (see Figure 14-22). Leaving the proximal jejunum, the Roux limb is anastomosed to the gastric pouch, creating a gastrojejunal anastomosis.

- The surgeon may use traditional suturing techniques or use a circular end-to-end anastomosis stapler to complete the connection.

- The SA will maintain exposure by retracting any tissue that obstruct visualization, suctioning any fluid, and continue to maintain the laparoscope in position that provides the best view of the field.

Leak Testing:

- After the anastomosis is complete (see Figure 14-23), the pouch may be tested for leaks by instilling air or methylene blue. Endoscopy may also be used to inspect the anastomosis from inside the pouch. If no leaks are detected, the

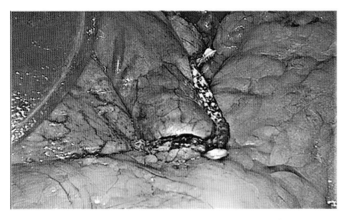

Figure 14-22 · Gastric pouch creation. (Reproduced, with permission, from The Center of Weight Loss at Wood County Hospital, Bowling Green, Ohio.)

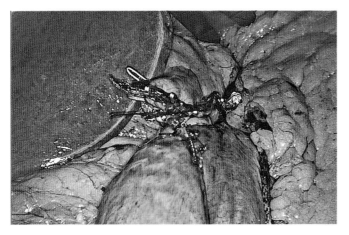

Figure 14-23 · Completion of gastrojejunal anastomosis. (Reproduced, with permission, from The Center of Weight Loss at Wood County Hospital, Bowling Green, Ohio.)

proximal jejunum is reconnected to the rest of the distal jejunum creating a three-way junction where delayed absorption occurs.

Inspection of the Abdomen:

- The abdomen is then inspected and irrigated, any drains to be used will be inserted at this time. Mesenteric defects requiring closure may be closed at this point in the procedure.

Wound Closure: The puncture sites are closed with the surgeon preferred suture by the SA. Small adhesive dressings placed over the puncture sites by the SA and patient is transferred to recovery.

Postop Bariatric Procedures: Activities for patients are highly encouraged after surgery, some patients are assisted with walking the day of surgery. Most bariatric programs have a strict diet schedule to be followed that have been discussed before surgery with a nutritionist. Typically, day 1, no food or drink are allowed, and an upper GI is scheduled to survey anastomosis and at the surgeon's discretion clear liquids may begin.

Patients are encouraged to not use a straw to drink fluids as this may increase gas and cause pain to increase. Week 1 of recovery will begin full liquids and protein drinks are frequently encouraged to increase nutrition. Weeks 2 and 3, the patient may begin to consume pureed food and still increasing protein. The next stage of the diet will be discussed at follow up appointment with provider and dietician to navigate the rest of the patient's success in the program. Again, each dietary restriction is based on the program at each facility.

Colon Resection. The surgical removal of a portion of or the entire large bowel. The resection may be an open procedure or a laparoscopic assisted, with both techniques achieving the same outcome. The resection may be completed with anastomosis of the colon back together, or creation of a stoma. The stoma may be permanent or temporary depending on the prognosis of the patient.

Etiology: Patients may possibly have a section of bowel that may be diseased, obstructed, and or necrotic and require removal. Common pathologies of the colon include Diverticular disease, Neoplasm (Polyps and Carcinoma), Ulcerative colitis, Crohn's disease, volvulus, intussusception, impaction, and obstruction.

Colon Resection with Colostomy: There are some instances that the colon may not be reestablished, a colostomy is then required. A colostomy involves bringing the proximal end of the divided colon or a loop of colon, through the anterior abdominal wall and suturing it to the skin. This creates a diversion for fecal matter, this may allow any infection to resolve or distal anastomosis to heal. A colostomy is only permanent if there is not enough colon to reconnect safely.

Surgical Procedure is given in the following section.

Incision:

- The surgeon will make a midline incision using a #10 knife blade and explore the abdominal cavity.
- The SA will maintain exposure by retracting tissue during dissection and assisting with hemostasis of vessels until self-retaining retractor is placed. If laparoscopically assisting the resection, the SA will help place trocars and maintain exposure with the camera.

Mobilization:

- Once adequate exposure is achieved, the surgeon will then identify the portion of the colon to be removed and begin mobilizing with the preferred energy source.
- The SA will assist with retracting any tissue that will interfere with visibility. The SA will be mindful of vascularity in the mesentery and notify if any bleeding is discovered.

Resection:

- After the colon is mobilized, the diseased section of colon will be resected using surgical staplers of the appropriate size no smaller than 75mm. The resected colon will be removed from the field, and stoma creation will begin.

Stoma Creation:

- The surgeon selects the ostomy site and makes a circular incision using electrosurgical cautery carrying all the way to the fascia.
- The SA will provide retraction with Army-Navy retractors and a cruciate incision is made into the fascia to assure room for the colon to be pulled to the skin surface with no tension. The colon is then pulled through the incision and sutured to the skin around the perimeter of the stoma (see Figure 14-24).

Wound Closure:

- Wound closure of the midline incision may occur before the suturing of the stoma perimeter to practice proper bowel technique, so long as the colon is secure. Each layer of the wound is closed using the surgeons preferred suture and closing technique.
- The SA will then apply the preferred dressings. The SA must ensure the skin around the stoma is clean and dry before placing the colostomy receptacle. The patient is then transferred to recovery.

Postop: Upon discharge patients will be given stoma care instructions and potentially meet with an ostomy nurse to answer any questions regarding special care of the stoma. Patients are encouraged not to lift over 5 lb and no driving until provider clears the patient at follow up visit. Activity increase should be gradual but is encouraged. These patients typically may return to work in 4 to 6 weeks with provider clearance.

Colon Resection without Colostomy:

Incision:

- The beginning steps will remain like the above procedure without the stoma creation. The surgeon will make a midline incision using a #10 knife blade and explore the abdominal cavity.

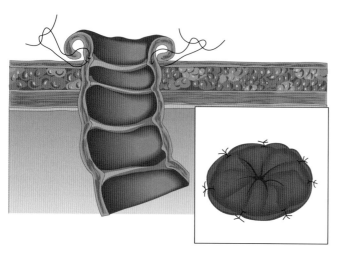

Figure 14-24 · Stoma creation through abdominal wall. (Reproduced, with permission, from Doherty GM, ed. *Current Diagnosis & Treatment: Surgery.* 15th ed. New York: McGraw Hill; 2020.)

- The SA will maintain exposure by retracting tissue during dissection and assisting with hemostasis of vessels until self-retaining retractor is placed. If laparoscopically assisting the resection, the SA will help place trocars and maintain exposure with the camera. The portion of colon to be resected will depend on the location of the pathology (see Figure 14-25).

Mobilization:

- The portion of bowel to be removed is identified and mobilized with the preferred energy source.
- The SA will assist with tissue retraction as well as notifying the surgeon of any bleeding vessels while releasing the bowel.

Resection:

- The surgeon will use a linear surgical stapler of choice to begin resecting the portion of bowel. The surgeon will make sure that there is enough bowel remaining to reconnect the GI tract.
- The mesentery is inspected to assure adequate blood flow to the remaining segments.

Anastomosis:

- There are a few bowel anastomoses options for the surgeon to choose to reconnect the bowel such as End-to-end, End-to-side, Side-to-Side, and Roux-en-Y. Depending on the anastomosis choice, certain shape and size staplers are available for each option.
- The SA may assist in the approximation of the segments and with firing the surgical staplers to be used.
- The two segments to be connected are placed together using the stapler of choice. Sutures may be placed to reinforce the staple line.
- The anastomosis is inspected for leaks and should be free of tension. Any mesenteric defects should be closed with preferred suture of the surgeon.

Wound closure:

- Once the wound has been irrigated, the surgeon will begin to close each layer with preferred closure method. The SA will then apply the preferred dressing and the patient will be transferred to recovery.

Postop: Activity such as walking will be encouraged during the patient's hospital stay and gradual increase as tolerated. Patients are typically on a low fiber diet for 6 to 8 weeks as the colon heals, the diet may advance as tolerated thereafter. Fluids are encouraged to keep the patient hydrated. The patient may experience loose stools and diarrhea for several months following surgery. The patients will not be allowed to lift over 20 lb, no vigorous exercising, and no driving until after postoperative appointment with provider. Depending on recovery, the provider will give clearance for return to work at follow up appointments.

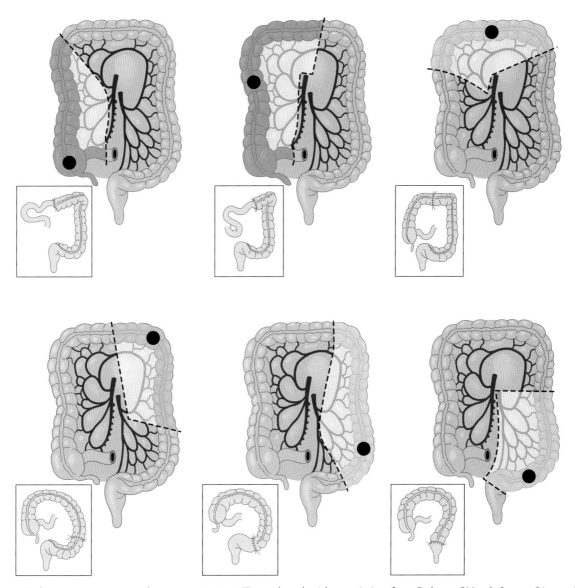

Figure 14-25 · Colectomy variations and anastomosis sites. (Reproduced, with permission, from Doherty GM, ed. *Current Diagnosis & Treatment: Surgery*. 15th ed. New York: McGraw Hill; 2020.)

Abdominoperineal Resection. Abdominoperineal resection is the complete excision of the sigmoid colon, rectum, and anus. This procedure will place the patient in supine or lithotomy for the abdominal portion. The perineal portion may require the patient in jackknife position. This procedure results in a permanent colostomy.

Pathology: APR is recommended for patients diagnosed with low rectal or anal malignancies, complications of Crohn's disease or ulcerative colitis, or even fecal incontinence.

Diagnostics: Colorectal diagnosis begins with history and physical examination, along with routine laboratory results reviewed. CT and MRI imaging may be completed prior to surgery. Colonoscopy may give a closer visual of the anus, rectum, and colon. Biopsies may be obtained during the endoscopic procedure.

Surgery steps are given in the following section.

Incision:

- Depending on the surgeon preference before the procedure begins, a purse-string may be used sew the rectum closed before perineal dissection.
- The surgeon will open the abdomen with a midline incision and explore the peritoneal cavity.
- The SA will continue to hold exposure until self-retaining retractor is placed.

Mobilization:

- The surgeon begins laterally dissecting the sigmoid colon along the peritoneal reflection, taking care to protect the left ureter and gonadal vessels as the pelvis is entered.

- Medial dissection to follow, again protecting the right ureter, and then developing the presacral space and releasing the rectum.

Resection:

- Using an articulating curved stapler, the rectum is resected. Then the proximal sigmoid is resected with a linear stapler.
- The surgeon will mobilize the proximal colon for permanent colostomy.

Stoma Creation:

- Using the same techniques from the colostomy procedure, the permanent stoma is created. The abdomen will then be closed, and the colostomy sutured to the skin.
- The appropriate dressings are placed by the SA, the team begins to prepare for the perineal dissection.

Perineal Dissection:

- The patient may be flipped to the prone position at this time if the perineal dissection requires jackknife position instead of lithotomy.
- The surgeon will make an incision around the anus, hemorrhoidal vessels are ligate and divided. Mobilization and removal of the sigmoid and rectal stump are through the perineal incision.
- The site is examined for bleeding and drains may be placed at this time.

Wound Closure:

- Perineal incision is closed, and the SA applies the dressing, and the colostomy receptacle and patient is transferred to recovery.

Postop: Upon patient discharge, the patient will be educated on stoma care and potentially meet with ostomy nurse, if facility provides it. The patient will be educated on proper diet as well as wound care for the incisions. Activities will be encouraged during hospital stay and increased as tolerated. Patients will be encouraged not to drive or lift over 10 to 20 lb until after postoperative appointment. Returning to work will be discussed and cleared at follow up visits with provider.

Splenectomy. There are multiple justifications for the removal of the spleen. Some diagnostics can lead to the prognosis of removal in a minimally invasive setting such as an elective laparoscopic case. In other instances, such as trauma, can lead to an open abdominal approach. The SA will play a key role in exposure in each setting and keeping the field clear for visualization.

Anatomy: The spleen (see Figure 14-26) located in the left upper quadrant, protected by ribs 10-12. Located below the diaphragm, the anterior medial surface of the spleen is near the cardiac end of the stomach. The splenic flexure is in proximity of the large colon. Supporting ligaments are formed from the peritoneum cover of the spleen (see Figure 14-27). Vascularity consists of the splenic artery and a branch of the celiac axis. The splenic vein drains into the portal system. The spleen defends the body by means of phagocytosis of microorganisms and damaged red blood cells. The spleen also performs as a blood reservoir.

Diagnostics: Preoperative imaging such as technetium or indium scanning, maybe used along with CT and MRI imaging to view the spleen. A gamma probe periop exam is sensitive to detecting an accessory spleen. Also, with general lab orders, prophylactic anticoagulation, and vaccine meningococcal,

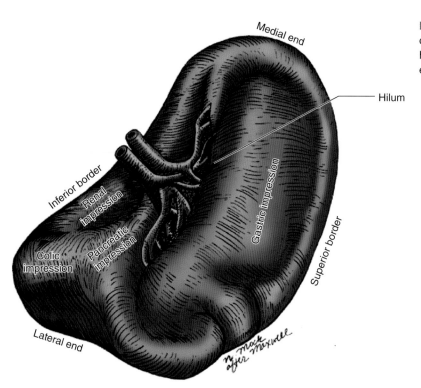

Figure 14-26 · Gross anatomy of the spleen. (Reproduced, with permission, from Zinner MJ, Ashley SW, Hines OJ, eds. *Maingot's Abdominal Operations.* 13th ed. New York, NY: McGraw Hill; 2019.)

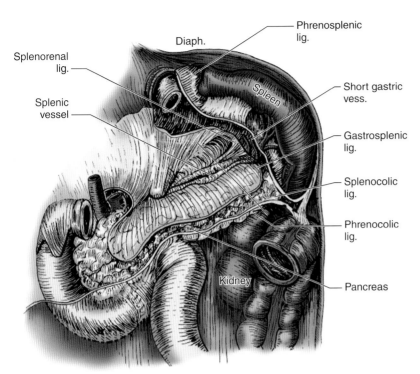

Figure 14-27 · Splenic ligaments. (Reproduced, with permission, from Zinner MJ, Ashley SW, Hines OJ, eds. *Maingot's Abdominal Operations*. 13th ed. New York, NY: McGraw Hill; 2019.)

pneumococcal, and haemophilus influenza type B are recommended before surgery. In some cases, a post op denatured RBC scintigraphy may be used to detect accessory spleen. Note that if accessory spleen is detected it is removed as well as it can maintain hyper splenic function (see Figure 14-28).

Etiology: Trauma, such as an injury during a vagotomy, to name just one of the urgent scenarios leading to an open splenectomy, but certain diagnosis may be more appropriate for an open abdominal approach such as portal hypertension, uncorrectable coagulopathy, severe ascites, and extreme splenomegaly.

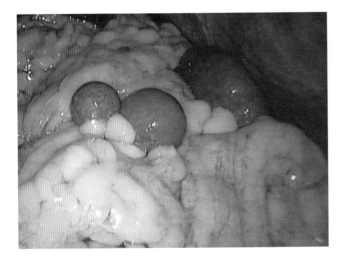

Figure 14-28 · Accessory spleen. (Reproduced, with permission, from Zinner MJ, Ashley SW, Hines OJ, eds. *Maingot's Abdominal Operations*. 13th ed. New York, NY: McGraw Hill; 2019.)

Other malignancies leading to the spleen removal include Hodgkin's and non-Hodgkin's lymphomas, chronic myelogenous leukemia, splenic anemia, ITP, tumors, cysts, and splenomegaly may be elective and use the laparoscopic approach.

Anesthesia: General anesthesia is commonly used with airway maintained. A nasal or oral gastric tube may be inserted to deflate the stomach prior to beginning to allow for better visualization. A regional block may be used for postoperative pain such as a spinal or epidural.

Positioning, Prepping, and Draping: In trauma cases, positioning may have to remain supine as time will be limited when getting access to the spleen. When preforming an elective laparoscopic case, the patient will be placed in the right lateral decubitus, with left side up at 45°. Positioning laterally, the SA will use the facilities equipment for lateral such as a bean bag. Gel pads and rolls may be used under bony prominences for protection and axillary roll in place to protect the associated nerves in that area. The operating room table may be flexed between the anterior superior iliac spine and the costal margin. During the procedure, the table will be placed in reverse Trendelenburg to assist with visualizing the field. The SA will prep the site with the appropriate solution provided by the facility and preferred draping sequence applied.

Surgical procedures are given in the following section:

Open Splenectomy:

Incision:

• The surgeon may use a midline abdominal incision or a subcostal approach, in some rare cases a thoracoabdominal tactic may be used.

- The SA will assist with retraction to provide exposure of the field as each layer is exposed of the abdomen.
- Once inside the abdomen, a self-retaining retractor may be placed if preferred by the surgeon.
- The SA will then assist with keeping the field clear of fluid with careful suctioning and moist lap sponges. Longer instrumentation will be required once dissection begins.

Dissection:

- The splenorenal, splenocolic, and gastrosplenic ligaments are clamped and divided. Any posterior adhesions to the spleen are released and the spleen is mobilized.
- The Short gastrics that are visible are ligated and detached from the spleen.
- Next, using fine dissection, the splenic vein and artery are clamped, divided, and ligated.
- The SA may assist with the removal of the clamps as the surgeon is ligating the vessels.

Removal:

- The spleen, now freed, is removed from the surgical field and passed off for pathology. Inspection of the cavity formally occupied by the spleen, for any bleeding vessels and are controlled.

Wound closure:

- Drains may be placed at this time. Then the SA may begin closing the wound in layers using the surgeon's preference of closure.
- The drain is secured, and dressings are applied.

Postop: Discharge instructions for patients after splenectomy include, not lifting anything over 10 lb, not overexerting to the point of fatigue, increase activity gradually, and climbing steps slowly and rest every few steps. Patients will be advised not to drive until first follow up appointment with provider, surgeon will decide when to resume normal activities. Patients will also need to keep current with vaccinations and notify other care providers of an absent spleen due to higher risk of infections.

Laparoscopic Splenectomy:

Incision:

- The Surgeon will begin by placing the first trocar, using preferred method of choice.
- The SA will provide visualization of the port site entries while holding the laparoscope.
- The SA may also assist in placing the ports if surgeon allows. If robotically assisted, the SA will assist in docking the Robot to the patient port sites.
- The surgeon will start visual inspection for an accessory spleen (Figure 14-28) mobilization begins.

Dissection:

- The left colon along the splenic flexure is mobilized first, this will mobilize the inferior pole and the SA to use an assist port that will allow retraction of the spleen.

- The SA must be cautious with the amount of traction as to not rupture the spleen.
- The lateral peritoneal attachment is incised using ultrasonic dissection and then the lesser sac is entered medially for dissection. As the spleen is mobilized even further, the SA will retract the spleen to allow access to the short gastrics and the main vascular pedicle.
- The short gastrics are then divided by the surgeon using the ultrasonic device, stapler, or clips.
- Robotically, the SA may be required to use these devices through the assist port.
- The splenic pedicle is carefully dissected from the medial and lateral aspects and divided.
- The artery and vein are finally divided using and endoscopic stapler and the spleen is then freed (see Figures 14-29 and 14-30).

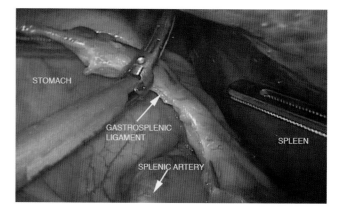

Figure 14-29 · Ligament mobilization. (Reproduced, with permission, from Zinner MJ, Ashley SW, Hines OJ, eds. *Maingot's Abdominal Operations.* 13th ed. New York, NY: McGraw Hill; 2019.)

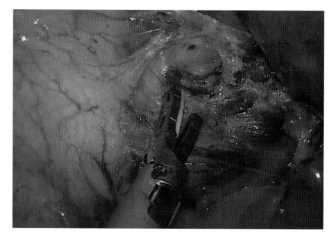

Figure 14-30 · Release of the short gastric vessels. (Reproduced, with permission, from Zinner MJ, Ashley SW, Hines OJ, eds. *Maingot's Abdominal Operations.* 13th ed. New York, NY: McGraw Hill; 2019.)

Removal:

- An endo bag may be placed to capture the spleen for removal. Before disconnecting the laparoscope, a visual inspection of the cavity for any bleeding, and a drain may be placed at this time.
- The laparoscopic or robotic equipment is removed from the field and the port incision containing the retrieval bag and spleen is extended and removed from patient.

Wound closure:

- The trocar sites and the incision are closed by the SA as to the preference of the surgeon. Drain is secured and dressings are applied.

Postop: Discharge instructions for patients after splenectomy include, not lifting anything over 10 lb, not overexerting to the point of fatigue, increase activity gradually, and climbing steps slowly and rest every few steps. Patients will be advised not to drive until first follow up appointment with provider, surgeon will decide when to resume normal activities. Patients will also need to keep current with vaccinations and notify other care providers of an absent spleen due to higher risk of infections.

HERNIAS

Procedure Identified: incisional/ventral hernia repair, umbilical hernia repair, inguinal hernia repair, femoral hernia repair

Abstract/introduction

A hernia is an abnormal protrusion of the peritoneum through the musculoaponeurosis. Hernias are caused by a weakness in the abdominal wall, congenital, or acquired. Hernias occur more often in males, but the most common hernia in both male and female patients is the indirect inguinal hernia. However, femoral hernias occur more often in women. A hernia repair is the most common surgical procedure performed and is considered the preferred treatment.

Anatomy and Physiology

A hernia can occur in several places in the abdominal wall. The abdominal wall consists of the external abdominal oblique muscles which are connected to the rectus sheath. Underneath the rectus sheath lies the rectus abdominis muscle which lies laterally to the right and left of the linea alba. The abdominal wall also contains internal abdominal oblique muscles.

Core anatomical organ(s) affected: A portion of the parietal peritoneum and sometimes a portion of the intestine may protrude through the defect. The most common places which are areas of weakness in the abdominal aponeurosis are the inguinal canals, femoral rings, and the umbilicus. Hernias can be reducible or non-reducible. If the contents of the hernia sac cannot be returned to the abdomen, it is referred to as an incarcerated hernia.

Incisional/Ventral Hernia

These most often occur postoperatively, especially when a T-shaped or vertical midline incision was used for a prior surgery.

Umbilical Hernia

Umbilical hernias are extraperitoneal and are basically tiny fascial defects on the underside of the umbilicus. Very common in children and repaired by re-approximating the fascia. In adults, the linea alba has a defect superior to the umbilicus. They are more common in obese patients and require surgical repair to prevent an incarcerated hernia. Surgical repair is indicated for an umbilical hernia even if the patient is asymptomatic.

Femoral Hernia

A femoral hernia will protrude beginning from the groin underneath the inguinal ligament and extend into the thigh. It consists of a tender mass and is inflamed. It is located below the inguinal ligament. They are often misdiagnosed and can often be mistaken for a lipoma, saphenous varix, enlarged inguinal lymph node, or a psoas muscle abscess. They have even been misdiagnosed as an inguinal hernia. Elective repair is always indicated for a femoral hernia.

Inguinal Hernia

There are several methods used to repair inguinal hernias. All of the surgical approaches that are used reestablish the integrity of the transversalis fascia while also reestablishing and strengthening the posterior inguinal floor. Most surgeons will opt to sew the transversalis fascia to the Poupart ligament in order to have a successful repair.

Organs Identified Relative to Diagnosis

Location – Femoral and Inguinal hernias are located in the groin. Umbilical hernia is located in the umbilicus region. Incisional hernias can be located anywhere on the abdomen where there is a weakness in the rectus abdominis muscle.

Arterial and venous supply-Saphenous vein

Nerves-Ileoinguinal Nerve

Lymph nodes-inguinal lymph nodes

Key landmarks and/or relevant associated structures: The external abdominal oblique muscles are attached to the rectus sheath. The linea alba extends superiorly and inferiorly from the xiphoid process to the pubis. The rectus abdominus muscles lie beneath the rectus sheath. The linea semilunaris lies lateral to the rectus abdominis. Originating from the seventh through twelfth costal cartilages, lumbar fascia, iliac crest, and inguinal ligament are the transversus abdominal muscles. They then insert on xiphoid process, linea alba and the pubic tubercle. The third and final layer of the abdominal wall includes the internal abdominal oblique muscles. These originate from the iliac crest, inguinal ligament and lumbar fascia and insert on the tenth to twelfth ribs and rectus sheath.

Etiology

Obese patients, patients that do heavy lifting or straining, previous surgery, steroid use, COPD, Hypoproteinemia

Diagnosis (Modalities): Upon Exam

History: common subjective symptoms and relevant family history-Previous surgeries related to the hernia area, relevant familial history, nutritional status

Physical: common objective symptoms-duration of symptoms, history of obesity, constipation, chronic cough, intra-abdominal pressure

Diagnostic modalities relevant to condition/procedure: Patient will present with nausea, vague abdominal pain, or epigastric pain.

Diagnostic laboratory exams: physical exam ultrasound, MRI

Diagnostic imaging: ultrasound, MRI, CT (see Figure 14-31)

Diagnostic procedures: physical exam

Procedural Considerations

Examples are nonsurgical treatment, surgical treatment, list of surgical approaches (open, laparascopic, robotic, etc.) Surgery is often the best choice and usually only choice for a hernia diagnosis. The following are types of hernias that require surgical repair. Hernia types are dependent upon where they are located. Incisional, Umbilical, Direct Inguinal, Indirect Inguinal, Epigastric and Femoral.

Nonsurgical Treatment. The patient must have a surgical repair or risk the chance of an incarcerated hernia or bowel obstruction. The hernia could also become strangulated where it would cut off the blood supply and the contents of the sac would be at risk for necrosis.

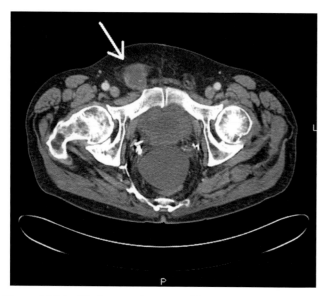

Figure 14-31 · CT of large right inguinal hernia. (Reproduced, with permission, from Brunicardi FC, Andersen DK, Billiar TR, et al, eds. *Schwartz's Principles of Surgery.* 11th ed. New York, NY: McGraw Hill; 2019.)

Usual Surgical Treatment and Options. Open, laparoscopic, or robotic surgical repair

Surgical Approaches. Femoral and Inguinal Hernias-Inguinal region or groin, umbilical hernias-supraumbilical, incisional-abdominal depending on where the hernia is located.

Preoperative Preparation:

- Additional labs/orders: routine blood work, stress test

- Any requirements for procedure: no smoking, lose weight may be recommended for obese patients, no heavy lifting prior to surgery.

- Usual anesthesia considerations: general, inguinal block, field block, spinal/epidural, regional with sedation, local with sedation

Position: Supine or dorsal recumbent with arms on padded arm boards less than 90°. Bony prominences are all padded.

Surgical Skin Prep: The SA will prep always following the surgeon's preference.

Inguinal/Femoral/Umbilical Hernia: The patient is prepped with an antimicrobial solution. A long cotton swab is used to clean the inside of the umbilicus. The patient is prepped from above the umbilicus to the mid-thigh on both sides. In males, the scrotal area is also prepped for inguinal hernias and a sterile drape is placed underneath.

Incisional Hernia: The SA will prep the entire abdomen from below the nipple line down to the groin area. If the patient has not been shaved in the preoperative area, the SA will shave and remove the hair prior to prepping.

Surgical procedure is given in the following sections:

Procedure Including the Role of the Assistant (SA, PA, resident):

Incisional hernia repair

- The SA will apply counter-traction as the surgeon makes the incision into the abdomen. The skin, scarpa's fascia, external oblique muscle and rectus sheath, and rectus abdominal muscle. Electrocautery will be utilized to coagulate bleeders. The scar tissue will be released.

- The SA will utilize a Richardson retractor to provide exposure. The hernia contents which are most often bowel and omentum will be returned to the abdomen. The muscle wall will be reinforced with suture.

- The SA will follow the suture for the surgeon as the muscle is re-approximated. The area of muscle weakness will be reinforced with a synthetic or biological mesh utilizing a suture of surgeon's preference. (Prolene is most often used.) The external oblique aponeurosis and Scarpa fascia are then closed.

- The SA will close the skin with a running 4-0 subcuticular stitch with suture of surgeon's preference or staples may be used.

Umbilical hernia repair

- The surgeon will make a peri-umbilical incision.

- The SA will provide counter-traction and cauterize any bleeding. The contents of the hernia will be exposed and dissected off of the fascia if necessary.

- The SA will utilize a small Richardson or army navy retractor to provide exposure. The contents, usually fat, omentum, and sometimes bowel will be returned to the abdominal cavity.

- The fascia will be re-approximated utilizing a 3-0 Prolene suture or surgeon's preference.

- The SA will follow the suture and cut when applicable. The fascia may be reinforced with a piece of synthetic or biological mesh utilizing a suture of surgeon's preference. (Prolene is most often used.)

- The SA will then close the skin with a 4-0 Vicryl or Monocryl suture. Staples may be used. (Surgeon's preference)

Femoral hernia repair

- The surgeon will make an inguinal incision, 1 cm above the medial half of the inguinal ligament. The SA will provide counter-traction.

- A plane will be created superficial to the external oblique aponeurosis. The surgeon will divide the rectus sheath along the linea semilunaris 4 cm above the inguinal ligament. This will preserve the inguinal canal while exposing the lateral border of the rectus abdominus muscle.

- The SA will retract the muscle medially with a small Richardson, Goelet, or Army Navy retractor. The surgeon will then divide the fascia transversalis and peritoneum. This will give access to the peritoneal cavity and compromised bowel.

- The bowel will be returned to the abdominal cavity and the fascia will be re-approximated utilizing a 3-0 Prolene suture or surgeon's preference.

- The SA will follow the suture and cut when applicable.

- The fascia may be reinforced with a piece of synthetic or biological mesh utilizing a suture of surgeon's preference. (Prolene is most often used.)

- The SA will then close the skin with a subcuticular running stitch or staples may be used. (Surgeon's preference).

- Examples of additional associated procedures commonly seen are Lotheissen repair, Lockwood repair.

Inguinal hernia repair—McVay/Cooper/ligament repair

- The SA will provide counter-traction for the transverse suprainguinal skinfold incision or oblique incision. The incision will extend through the Scarpa's fascia and extend to the external oblique aponeurosis (see Figure 14-32). The SA and surgeon will clamp bleeders with a hemostat and ties or utilize the electrocautery device.

- The surgeon will then open the external oblique aponeurosis by making a small incision over the inguinal canal. The aponeurotic flaps are reflected back along with the iliohypogastric and ilioinguinal nerves with mosquito or small hemostat clamps.

- The SA will utilize army navy or Goelets retractors or a Weitlaner may be used for traction to expose the area. The nerves are identified to prevent injury. The ilioinguinal nerve is a sensory nerve which innervates the medial thigh and the scrotum. The cremaster muscles are opened, and the cord is exposed. The conjoined tendon is a medial fibrous portion of the internal oblique. The cord and attached structures are dissected away from the canal.

- The SA will utilize a DeBakey forceps to assist the surgeon during this step. The SA will then pass a penrose drain through the hole and the two ends will be clamped with a hemostat for gentle traction of the vessels and vas deferens. The cord is examined to determine if it is an indirect hernia. Indirect hernias are defined by the sac being located adjacent to the cord. The sac originates from the internal ring lateral to the epigastric vessels and is attached to the cord. If it is indirect, the sac is dissected away from the cord and freed from the neck of the hernia.

- The sac is opened with Metzenbaum scissors, and the SA and surgeon will place hemostats on the edges of the sac. The abdominal contents (omentum/bowel) will be returned to the peritoneal cavity.

- The surgeon will place a purse string suture around the neck of the sac. The SA will follow the suture and ensure it does not get tangled. The excess peritoneum of the hernia is excised with Metzenbaum scissors.

- The SA will hand the specimen to the Surgical Tech or Scrub Nurse. The ligated stump will retract back into the peritoneal cavity.

- The surgeon will then determine if a direct hernia is present in the inguinal floor. A piece of mesh may be used to reconnect the transversalis fascia.

- The SA will now follow the suture as the surgeon begins at the pubic tubercle and continues laterally to the internal ring. The superior portion may be sutured to Coopers Ligament if the inferior transversalis fascia is weak or nonexistent. The repair is then carried laterally, and the transversalis fascia is connected to the inguinal ligament. If there is too much tension, a piece of synthetic surgical mesh will be attached to the shelving edge of the inguinal ligament. The cephalad edge will be attached to the conjoined tendon and the lateral edge will be split to make room for the spermatic cord.

- The SA will utilize DeBakey forceps to help place the mesh and cut suture with suture scissors when indicated. Once the integrity of the posterior inguinal floor is restored, the cremaster muscles are reapproximated around the cord. The external oblique aponeurosis and Scarpa fascia are then closed.

- The SA will close the skin with a running 4-0 subcuticular stitch with suture of surgeon's preference or staples may be used.

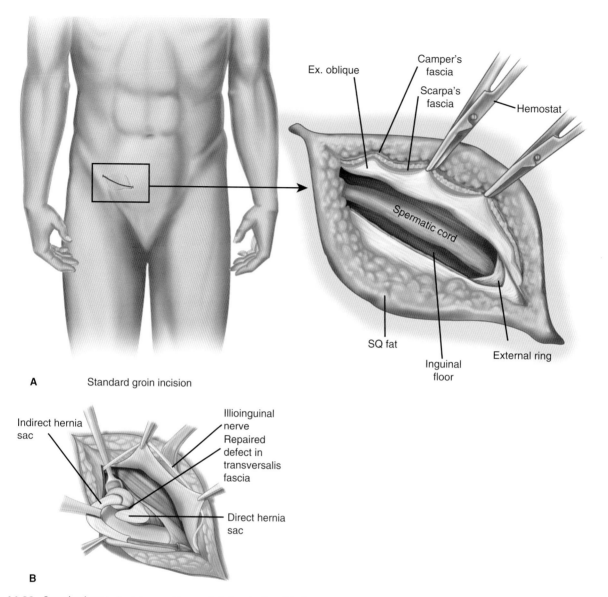

A   Standard groin incision

B

Figure 14-32 · Standard groin incision and layer of abdominal wall in hernia repair. (Reproduced, with permission, from Brunicardi FC, Andersen DK, Billiar TR, et al, eds. *Schwartz's Principles of Surgery.* 11th ed. New York, NY: McGraw Hill; 2019.)

Additional associated procedures commonly seen are the Shouldice Repair, Mesh-Plug Repair, Shouldice repair which was introduced in 1887 and is still used by some surgeons but has been replaced with newer techniques. The Bassini Repair was introduced in 1940.

Postop: Drains used/dressings: The SA will place Mastisol, steri-strips, 4 by 4 gauze and tape over the incision

- Prognosis with treatment, eg, PT, radiation: Patient will schedule follow-up exam with surgeon 2 weeks postop. Patient can resume normal routine after follow-up exam if no complications

- Potential complications common to this procedure: Wound Infection, Mesh reaction, Bleeding, Recurrence, painful Scar, urinary retention, seroma/hematoma, postoperative neuralgia, constipation

- Discharge planning: Patient will be discharged same day, no lifting or straining, normal diet, patient can usually return to normal activity 2 weeks postoperatively.

LIVER

Anatomy

The liver lies in the upper right quadrant of the abdominal cavity, just beneath the diaphragm and situated on top of the stomach, right kidney, and intestines. It is the largest organ, cone shaped, reddish-brown in color and weighs about 3 lb. The external covering is comprised of dense connective tissue and is identified as Glisson's capsule. The main blood supplies to the liver included the hepatic artery and the hepatic portal vein.

The liver holds about 13% of the body's blood supply and is comprised of four lobes, the larger right lobe and left lobe, the smaller caudate lobe and quadrate lobe. The anatomic right and left lobes of the liver are divided by the ligamentum teres and umbilical fissure. However, the middle hepatic vein is the functional dividing line between the right and left liver. The left liver is further divided by the falciform ligament into a medial and lateral segment.

Segments of the liver: Left lateral segment is further divided into superior (segment II) and inferior (segment III) and left medial segment (segment IV). The right liver is divided into anterior (segments V & VIII), posterior segments (Segments VI & VII).

Both lobes divide into eight segments that contain thousands of lobules. The lobules are the functional unit of the liver. Each lobule contains a hepatic duct, a hepatic portal vein branch and a branch of the hepatic artery, nerves, and lymphatics. A central vein in the center of each lobule presents venous drainage into the hepatic veins. The hepatic veins drain into the inferior vena cava (IVC). The lobules also contain hepatic cords, hepatic sinusoids, and bile canaliculi. The sinusoids have a delicate epithelial padding made of Kupffer cells (phagocytic cells that consume bacteria and toxins). The sinusoids drain into the central vein. The lobules are connected to small ducts that connect with larger ducts forming the common hepatic duct. The common hepatic duct carries bile to the gall bladder and duodenum by way of the common bile duct. The common bile duct opens into the duodenum in an area called the ampulla of Vater.

Functions of the Liver

The liver is vital in the metabolism of carbohydrates, proteins, and fats. It metabolizes nutrients into glycogen which helps regulate blood glucose levels and serves as energy sources for the brain and body functions. All the blood leaving the stomach and intestines passes through the liver. The liver processes this blood and breaks down, balances, and creates the nutrients and metabolizes drugs into structures that are easier to use for the rest of the body or making them nontoxic. More than 500 crucial functions have been identified with the liver. Some of the more well-known functions include the following:

- Production of albumin, a protein that keeps fluids in the bloodstream from leaking into surrounding tissue.
- Production of bile, to carry away waste and aids in the absorption of fats in the small intestine during digestion
- Production of specific proteins for blood plasma
- Production of cholesterol and special proteins to help carry fats through the body
- The liver stores substantial amounts of vitamins A, D, E, K, and B12, as well as iron and copper.
- The liver removes excess glucose (sugar) from the bloodstream and stores it as glycogen
- Regulation of amino acids
- Filters blood removing toxins, byproducts, and other harmful substances
- Conversion of poisonous ammonia to urea

- Clearing the blood of drugs and other poisonous substances
- Resisting infections by making immune factors and removing bacteria from the bloodstream
- Clearance of bilirubin, also from red blood cells

Hepatic Resection

A liver resection is usually performed to address primary tumors, benign conditions such as hepatolithiasis and metastatic tumors. There are three common approaches to a liver resection.

- Anatomic approach is indicated when evidence points to malignant cells are distributed along the portal venous segmental supply.
- Enucleation approach addresses benign lesions can be removed due to a limited chance of local invasion.
- Nonanatomic approach is utilized to include resections appropriate for a pathologic process and a tumor debulking.

Types of Hepatectomy

Right hepatectomy	Also called a hemi-hepatectomy, this surgical procedure is the re-sectioning of the liver on the right side of Cantlie's line.
Left hepatectomy	Consisting of three parts: hilar dissection of the left portal pedicle, mobilization of the left liver, and parenchymal dissection.
Left lateral hepatectomy	Also identified as left lateral liver sectionectomy, this surgical procedure in when the left lobe of the liver is removed. This involves all the liver tissue left of the falciform ligament.
Extended right hepatectomy	Recognized as trisegmentectomy, this surgical procedure becomes needed when malignant tumors dominate a large section of the right lobe with extension into the medial segment of the left lobe.
External left hepatectomy	This approach is used when large, left-sided, and central hepatic lesions expand to involve the right anterior sectoral portal pedicular structures.
Segmental hepatectomy	This surgical procedure includes the resection of one or more anatomic segments of the liver, with the most common anatomic segments are the right posterior sectionectomy and left lateral sectionectomy and caudate lobe resection.

Etiology

Patients with liver cancer (Hepatocellular Cancer or HCC) who have one or two small tumors will be eligible for liver resection surgery.

A liver resection will be undertaken to treat benign hepatic neoplasms such as:

- Hepatocellular adenoma
- Hepatic hemangioma

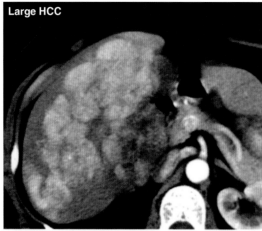

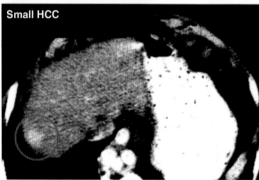

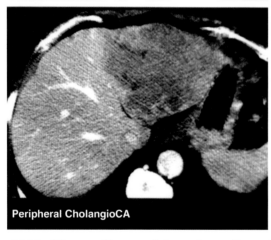

Figure 14-33 · CT image of hepatocellular carcinoma. (Reproduced, with permission, from Brunicardi FC, Andersen DK, Billiar TR, et al, eds. *Schwartz's Principles of Surgery*. 11th ed. New York, NY: McGraw Hill; 2019.)

- Focal nodular hyperplasia
- Metastases that arise from colorectal cancer
- Hepatocellular carcinoma
- Intrahepatic gallstones
- Parasitic cysts

Diagnosis

Several tests will be performed to determine the necessity for a hepatic resection. These tests will determine if there is cancer and if it has spread outside the liver (see Figure 14-33).

- Physical examination
- Blood tests
- CT scan
- Ultrasound tests
- MRI
- Angiograms
- Biopsy
- Esophagogastroduodenoscopy (EGD)

Devices Used for Dividing Liver Parenchyma and Achieving Hemostasis

Blunt fracture and clips
Monopolar cautery (Bovie)
Bipolar cautery
Argon beam coagulator
CUSA ultrasonic dissector
Hydro-Jet water jet dissector
Harmonic Scalpel, AutoSonix ultrasonic transector-coagulator
LigaSure tissue fusion system
SurgRx EnSeal tissue sealing and transection system
Gyrus PK cutting forceps
Endovascular staplers
TissueLink sealing devises
Habib 4× Laparoscopic sealer
InLine bipolar linear coagulator

Procedural Considerations

Slight Trendelenburg may be requested to facilitate the procedure. Many surgeons will use a right subcostal incision. If a median sternotomy or right thoracotomy incision is used, then chest instruments will be required.

Positioning, Prepping, and Draping

The patient is positioned supine with arms on padded arm boards less than 90°. The patient will receive a Foley catheter. The abdomen is prepped from nipple line to mid-thigh.

Anesthesia

The patient will be under general anesthesia. A Nasogastric tube may be inserted after the patient has been intubated.

Surgical Procedure

- The surgeon will make a right subcostal incision opening the abdomen with the possibility of a partial or complete left subcostal extension across the midline. The SA will assist in hemostasis using suction or sponging in between cauterizing vessels, keeping the field clear and dry for visualization.

- The liver is examined to determine the pathology and resection course. Anatomic resections usually involve two or more hepatic segments, while non-anatomic resection

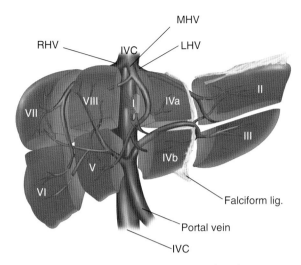

Figure 14-34 • Hepatic anatomy. (Reproduced, with permission, from Brunicardi FC, Andersen DK, Billiar TR, et al, eds. *Schwartz's Principles of Surgery*. 11th ed. New York, NY: McGraw Hill; 2019.)

involves resection of the metastases with a margin of uninvolved tissue (segmentectomy) (see Figure 14-34).

- A self-retaining retractor such as the Bookwalter is placed in the abdomen, and the abdomen is packed with moist lap sponges. The SA will assist in the assembly of the self-retaining retractor, making sure all segments are attached appropriately and securely to the OR bed frame, and not directly resting on the patient's body.
- Intraoperative sonography is performed to evaluate all segments of the liver. Ultrasound guided digital intraparenchymal isolation of vessels is utilized during the resection.
- The liver vascular inflow & outflow should be controlled before parenchymal division.
- The liver parenchyma is delicately resected using the CUSA.
- Take down the round and falciform ligaments and uncover the anterior surface of the hepatic veins.
- If performing a left hepatectomy, divide the left triangular ligament.
- If performing a right hepatectomy, mobilize the right lobe from the right coronary and triangular ligaments.
- Open the gastrohepatic ligament, palpate the porta hepatis, checking lymph nodes to determine extrahepatic metastasis.
- Once the liver is resected, the remaining liver is assessed for bleeding and bile leakage. The SA will also assist with inspecting for bleeding and spillage and notify surgeon if any is visible.
- The remaining liver may be sutured with 2-0 or 3-0 absorbable suture, or an intended layer of eschar developed using an electrosurgical pencil or the argon beam coagulator.
- Abdominal drains may be placed along the liver bed and secured externally with non-absorbable suture. The SA may be responsible for suturing the drain in place, to the patient's skin without damaging the preferred drain of choice.

- The abdominal wound is closed in layers and dressings applied. The SA may close the abdominal layers using the surgeon preferred suture and method.

Postop

- Gastrointestinal upset that could include gas, diarrhea, constipation, and nausea
- Tiredness
- Headache
- Low grade fever

Complications

- Bleeding
- Biliary fistula
- Atelectasis
- Pleural effusion
- Infections are comparatively rare but not uncommon.

Liver Transplantation

A liver transplantation is performed to replace a liver that is no longer functioning properly, (liver failure). The liver can be replaced with a healthy liver from a deceased donor or a portion of a healthy liver from a living donor. Liver transplantation is proposed for patients with chronic hepatocellular disease, chronic cholestatic disease, metabolic liver disease, primary hepatic cancer, acute fulminant liver disease.

Signs and Symptoms of Liver Disease

- **Gastrointestinal bleeding:** Portal hypertension causes alternative routes for blood to return to the heart. Small veins throughout the abdomen, outside the liver, become enlarged and thin walled due to the abnormally high amount of blood flow due to increased pressure. Bleeding in the intestinal tract can be life threatening.
- **Fluid retention:** Liver failure results in low albumin levels force fluid out of the bloodstream, which cannot be reabsorbed. Fluid will accumulate in tissues the abdomen (ascites). Fluid retention is treated first by limitation of dietary salt intake, second with diuretics and intermittent drainage through needle aspiration.
- **Encephalopathy**: Failure of the liver to clear ammonia and other toxins from the blood will allow the substances to accumulate.
- **Jaundice**: Bilirubin is not cleared from the body and bilirubin levels increase in the blood in liver failure. The skin and all tissues of the body will then take up a yellow color.

Causes of Chronic Liver Disease in the United States

- Viral Hepatitis
  - Hepatitis B: Hep B infections account for 5% of all liver transplants
  - Hepatitis C: Accounts for 50% of all liver transplant recipients

- Alcoholic Liver Disease
  - Liver failure due to alcoholism is the second most common indication for liver transplants.
- Metabolic Liver Disease
  - Non-alcoholic steatohepatitis (NASH) is the deposition of fat within liver cells which results in inflammation that injures and scars the liver.
- Autoimmune Liver Disease
- Genetic Liver Disease
- Budd-Chiari syndrome
- Hepatocellular Carcinoma

Diagnostics. A scoring system, called MELD (Model for end stage Liver disease), is utilized to determine how sick a person is from his or her liver disease. The MELD scoring system is highly predictive of the risk of death caused by chronic liver disease.

The MELD score is determined by the results of three objective and readily available laboratory tests:

1. Total bilirubin
2. Prothrombin time
3. Creatinine that measures kidney function

As a patient becomes more ill as their liver function deteriorates, the MELD score will move a patient to a higher position on the waitlist. The list is also organized by blood type.

Anesthesia. The patient is intubated under general anesthesia. Extensive blood loss is a possibility so anesthesia should work with the circulator to confirm blood products will be available as needed. Ten units of packed red blood cells (RBCs) and fresh frozen plasma (FFP) and one unit of pooled donor platelets should be available for the procedure. Cell saver may also be utilized to offer autotransfusion.

As many as 50 intraoperative labs may be drawn throughout the procedure and are taken immediately to the lab for timely feedback to the surgeon.

Positioning, Prepping, and Draping. The patient is placed supine with arms on padded arm boards less than 90° on a gel pad or pressure reducing OR table pad. Knees are slightly flexed and padded. A Foley catheter is placed after anesthesia. Heal protectors are used and SCD's are placed and turned on prior to anesthesia induction. The safety strap is placed over the lower thighs. A Bair Hugger is applied over the upper body, neck, and head to aid in maintaining normothermia.

The patient is prepped from the neck to the mid-thigh, bedline to bedline and draped for a laparotomy procedure.

Surgical Procedure

- Bilateral subcostal incisions with a midline incision extended toward the umbilicus. The xiphoid can be removed if needed and the right side of the chest entered if necessary.

- Peritoneum is entered through a cutdown incision and hemostasis achieved with cautery and suture ligatures as necessary.
- The hilar structures are isolated, and the lobes of the liver mobilized.
- The retro hepatic vena cava is isolated and identified, along with the hepatic artery, portal vein, common bile duct, and inferior vena cava.
- Once isolated the above vessels are transected and the diseased liver is removed.
- The donor liver is situated in the right upper abdomen and an end-to-end anastomosis to the vena cava and portal vein is performed using double armed Prolene suture.
- Any venous clamps are removed, and blood flow is reestablished to the vena cava and portal vein.
- Anastomosis sites are checked for leaks.
- The donor liver is monitored for a color change from dusky to pink.
- Arterial flow is re-established by suturing the donor's and recipient's hepatic arteries.
- Finally, biliary drainage is accomplished by suturing the donor's and recipient's common bile ducts.
- If biliary atresia was the indication for liver disease, a choledochoenterostomy into a Roux-en-Y of jejunum is performed.
- Arterial anastomoses are checked for leaks.
- Drains are placed in front and behind the liver.
- The abdomen is closed in layers and dressed in a three-layer dressing.

Complications

- Primary non-function or poor function of the newly transplanted liver
- Hepatic artery thrombosis
- Portal vein thrombosis
- Biliary leaks or stricture
- Bleeding
- Infections

Immunosuppression. The goal of the immune system is to identify anything foreign inside the body and that includes any transplanted organs. Liver transplant recipients will need to take certain drugs to keep their body from rejecting the newly transplanted liver. Common drugs used to prevent organ rejection include:

- Corticosteroids (methylprednisolone is given intravenously; prednisone is given orally) – steroids prevent activation of lymphocytes
- Calcineurin inhibitors (cyclosporine, tacrolimus) – they block the function of calcineurin, a molecule that signals the lymphocyte pathway and the production of multiple cytokines

- Mycophenolate mofetil – (Cellept®, Myfortic®) converts to mycophenolic acid in the body and inhibits the ability of the lymphocytes to replicate DNA

- mTOR inhibitors (sirolimus; everolimus): mTOR stands for mammalian Target Of Rapamycin. mTOR belongs to a family of enzymes known as kinases and is involved in checkpoint regulation of the cell cycle, DNA repair, and cell death. Inhibition of mTOR stops T cells from progressing

- Antibodies that target the lL-2 receptor – a signaling molecule that amplifies the immune response

- Antibodies that remove T cells from circulation (Thymoglobulin®, OKT-3®)

Outcomes. Outcomes for liver transplantation are very good but can fluctuate substantially depending on the reason for the liver transplant as well as considerations related to the donor. Presently, the overall patient survival 1 year after liver transplant is 88%. Patient survival 5 years after liver transplant is 73%.

Acute cellular rejection occurs in 25% to 50% of all liver transplant recipients within the first year after transplantation with the highest risk period within the first 4 to 6 weeks of transplantation. Injury to the liver is typically facilitated by immune cells, T cells or T lymphocytes. The first sign is generally unusually elevated liver lab test results. When rejection is suspected, a liver biopsy is performed.

PANCREAS

Pancreaticoduodenectomy (Whipple Procedure)

Pancreatic cancer is the fourth common cause of death due to cancer and a 5-year survival rate is only around 12%. The pancreaticoduodenectomy or Whipple procedure, is the surgical procedure of choice for pancreatic ductal adenocarcinomas. The first pancreaticoduodenectomy was performed by Dr. Allessandro Codivilla in 1898 and later modifed by Dr. Walter Kausch in 1912. Dr. Allen Whipple improved the Whipple into a one stage procedure in 1940 (see Figure 14-35).

Anatomy and Physiology. The pancreas is a retroperitoneal organ and located between the spleen and duodenum. The pancreas is an elongated organ that's approximately 15 cm long and has a tapered shape. It is divided into the head, uncinate process, neck, body, and tail. The head of the pancreas and the uncinate process are supplied by superior and inferior pancreaticoduodenal arteries, branches from the gastroduodenal artery and middle colic artery. The neck, body and tail receive their blood supply from the splenic artery through the dorsal pancreatic artery, greater pancreatic artery, and transverse pancreatic artery. The head of the pancreas is drained by the four pancreaticoduodenal veins, which drain into the superior mesenteric vein (SMV) or portal vein (PV). The venous drainage for the neck, body and tail of the pancreas is the splenic vein. The main duct (Wirsung) begins in the tail, extends the entire length of the pancreas, and connects with the bile duct in the head of the pancreas to form the ampulla of Vater, which opens into the duodenum. Movement of bile is regulated by the sphincter of Oddi.

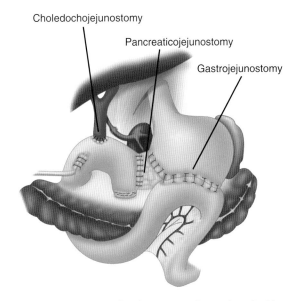

Choledochojejunostomy
Pancreaticojejunostomy
Gastrojejunostomy

Figure 14-35 · Pancreaticoduodenectomy. (Reproduced with permission from Gaw JU, Andersen DK. Pancreatic surgery. In: Wu GY, Aziz K, Whalen GF, eds. *An Internist's Illustrated Guide to Gastrointestinal Surgery*. Totowa: Humana Press; 2003.)

The pancreas is considered both an exocrine and endocrine gland. Over 80% of the organ is comprised of exocrine pancreatic tissue, which is a bulk of specialized cells called pancreatic acini. These produce enzymes that blend with bile to assist in digestion. The remaining cells are endocrine cells responsible for the portion of the pancreas called "islets of Langerhans;" a cluster of small slightly granular endocrine cells that produce and secrete insulin and glucagon to maintain the balance of sugar (glucose) and salt in the body.

Etiology

- Cancer located at the head of the pancreas
- Pancreatic neuroendocrine tumors (PNETs)
- Intraductal papillary mucinous neoplasms (IPMN)
- Bile duct cancer
- Adenocarcinoma of the ampulla of Vater
- Duodenal adenocarcinoma
- Chronic pancreatitis
- Pancreatic trauma

Diagnostics. There are several diagnostics that will help the physician determine whether someone has pancreatic cancer. They include Ultrasound, computerized tomography (CT) scans, magnetic resonance imaging (MRI) and, sometimes, positron emission tomography (PET) scans, and a tissue biopsy. The CA19-9 is a blood test that measures the amount of a protein called CA19-9 in the blood. CA19-9 is a tumor marker made by cancer cells or the response of normal cells to cancer in the body. The CA19-9 may clarify how the cancer responds to treatment.

Pancreatic cancer is rarely detected at its early stages when it's most treatable. This is because it regularly doesn't cause symptoms until after it has spread to other organs. Pancreatic cancer treatment options are decided based on the scope of the cancer. Options may consist of surgery, chemotherapy, radiation therapy or a combination of these. The stages of pancreatic cancer are indicated by Roman numerals ranging from 0 to IV. The lowest stages indicate that the cancer is confined to the pancreas. By stage IV, the cancer has spread to other parts of the body.

Procedural Considerations. Due to the complexity of a Whipple procedure, pancreatic cancer is treated through a multidisciplinary team approach that includes surgeons, gastroenterologists, oncologists, radiologists, nurses, and nutritionists. Most tumors begin in the head of the pancreas of the exocrine gland. They often obstruct the bile duct and may extend to the duodenum, intestines, even the spine. A Whipple can be performed through an open approach, laparoscopic or robotic. This is a joint decision between the patient and surgeon as to what approach is best.

Position, Prepping, and Draping. The patient will be positioned supine with arms on padded arm boards less than 90°. Additional padding for any pressure points as the procedure could last 5 to 6 hours. SCDs are applied and started prior to anesthesia and a Bair Hugger will be applied to maintain normothermia. A Foley catheter is placed once the patient is unconscious. The patient is prepped from the nipple line to mid-thigh and bedline to bedline.

Anesthesia. The patient is placed under general anesthesia and a NG tube placed after intubation. The patient should be typed and crossed for anticipation of the administration of blood products.

Surgical Procedure

- The abdomen is incised through an upper transverse, a bilateral subcostal or long paramedian incision. The SA will assist in hemostasis using suction or sponging in between cauterizing vessels, keeping the field clear and dry for visualization.

- A cut down is completed through peritoneum and the abdomen is packed with lap sponges and a self-retaining retractor to visualize and protect vital viscera, the SA will maintain exposure of the field and assist with the placement of the self-retaining retractor, assuring the proper assembly and that it is not resting on the patient's body.

- The parietal and visceral peritoneal surfaces, the ligament of Treitz, the omentum, and the entire small and large intestine are examined for the presence of metastasis. The celiac axis is inspected for lymph node involvement. Questionable looking lymph nodes outside the proposed area of dissection are sent for frozen section. A pancreaticoduodenectomy (PD) is not completed if the biopsy is positive for metastatic cancer.

- The duodenum is mobilized using the Kocher maneuver with Metzenbaum scissors and blunt dissection.

- Mobilization of the duodenum continues and loose connective tissue is separated from the duodenum with an ESU and bleeding vessels are ligated with silk suture, the SA may assist with the ligation of vessels depending on the comfort level of SA and surgeon.

- The gallbladder dissected from the liver, and the distal common hepatic duct is divided close to the level of the cystic duct entry site. The proximal bile duct is left without a clamp to avoid crush injury, and the distal bile duct is clamped or sutured to prevent the spillage of the bile and tumor cells. The bile duct is retracted caudally, and portal dissection continued at the anterior aspect of the portal vein, the SA will assist with inspecting the field and notifying the surgeon if any bleeding or bile spillage has occurred.

- The gastrocolic ligament and gastrohepatic omentum are divided using curved forceps and are ligated or transfixed.

- The division of the gastroduodenal artery facilitates uncovering the anterior surface of the portal vein and enables the dissection of the portal vein behind the pancreatic neck. The portal vein is identified above the neck of the pancreas and SMV inferior to the neck of the pancreas. Blunt dissection downwards along the portal vein is designed to create a plane in front of the portal vein and behind the neck of the pancreas.

- The prepyloric area of the stomach is mobilized.

- The operative field is prepared for anastomosis.

- Two long Allen or Payr clamps are placed near the midportion of the stomach to complete the transection.

- The duodenum is exposed, the common duct is divided, and the hepatic end is tagged for later anastomosis.

- The jejunum is clamped with two Allen forceps and the duodenojejunal flexure is divided.

- The pancreas is divided and the duct isolated.

- The SA will continue to provide exposure by keeping the field clear of any fluid for surgeon to maintain visualization.

- Mobilization of the duodenum continues, and the inferior pancreaticoduodenal artery is divided.

- The specimen is removed.

- Standard reconstruction consists of the pancreatic anastomosis (PA) first, followed by the bile duct, and finally, the duodenum to establish the GI continuity.

- For the pancreatojejunostomy, the duct to mucosa anastomosis is created sandwiched between the end of the pancreatic duct remnant and side of jejunum in a retrocolic fashion.

- The reconstruction is followed by end-to-side hepaticojejunostomy with interrupted single layer synthetic absorbable suture.

- The third anastomosis performed is the gastrojejunostomy in patients who have had a classic pancreaticoduodenectomy with distal gastrectomy or duodenojejunostomy.

- Drains are placed and the abdomen is closed in layers.

- The SA may be responsible for suturing the drain in place, to the patient's skin without damaging the preferred drain of choice.
- Abdominal three-layer dressing is applied. The SA may close the abdominal layers using the surgeon preferred suture and method.

Postop. Postoperative management includes keeping the patient NPO for the first day and progressing slowly with clear liquids and later a low-fat diet in frequent small meals. The stomach is decompressed overnight after surgery with a naso-gastric tube, which is typically removed the next morning if there are not any issues. The drains are removed slowly once the output is minimal, there is no evidence of pancreatic fistula, and the patient is tolerating a normal diet.

Complications

- Delayed gastric emptying
- Pancreatic fistula
- Post pancreatectomy hemorrhage
- Wound infection
- Intra-abdominal abscess

HEMORRHOIDECTOMY

Hemorrhoids are swollen veins in your anus and lower rectum. Hemorrhoids can grow inside the or under the skin around the anus. A hemorrhoidectomy is an out-patient surgical procedure performed to remove internal or external hemorrhoids when nonsurgical treatments fail.

Causes

The veins around your anus stretch and can bulge or swell when under pressure. Hemorrhoids can develop from:

- Straining during bowel movements
- Sitting for long periods of time on the toilet
- Having chronic diarrhea or constipation
- Being obese
- Being pregnant
- Having anal intercourse
- Eating a low-fiber diet
- Regular heavy lifting

Procedural Considerations

Many surgeons will perform a proctoscopy to rule out rectal disease before surgery. Preoperative anal dilation will aid to expose the vessels and contribute to patient comfort. Spinal, caudal epidural, local and general anesthesia are options to discuss with your surgeon and anesthesia provider. The patient is positioned jack knife with the buttocks taped open. A rectal instrument tray is needed.

Surgical Procedure

- The surgeon will insert an anal retractor to expose the hemorrhoids
- The hemorrhoid is grasped with an Allis or Babcock clamp
- An absorbable suture I placed around the apex of the hemorrhoid
- The hemorrhoid is excised through sharp dissection

Types of Hemorrhoidectomies	
Closed	Excision of hemorrhoidal tissue uses a sharp dissection with a scalpel, scissors, electrocautery, or even laser followed by complete wound closure with absorbable suture., usually chromic suture.
	Postoperative care includes frequent sitz baths, mild analgesics, and avoidance of constipation. Closed hemorrhoidectomy is successful 95% of the time.
	Possible complications consist of pain, delayed bleeding, urinary retention/urinary tract infection, or fecal impaction
Open	Hemorrhoidal tissue is removed in the same manner as in a closed procedure, but the incision is left open.
	Surgeons select an open hemorrhoidectomy when the location or amount of diseased tissue makes wound closure problematic, or the likelihood of postoperative infection is high.
Stapled	Stapled hemorrhoidectomy is primarily used in patients with grade III and IV hemorrhoids.
	During stapled hemorrhoidectomy, a circular stapling device is used to excise a circumferential ring of excess hemorrhoid tissue, thereby lifting hemorrhoids back to their normal position within the anal canal.
	Stapling additionally interrupts hemorrhoid blood supply. Studies have indicated that stapled hemorrhoidectomy results in less postoperative pain and shorter recovery.
Rubber band ligation	A rubber band is positioned around the base of the hemorrhoid within the rectum. The band cuts off circulation, and the hemorrhoid shrivels away in a few days.
Lateral internal sphincterotomy	Lateral internal sphincterotomy or opening of the inner anal sphincter muscle is sometimes performed during hemorrhoidectomy in patients with high resting sphincter pressures.

- Care is taken to avoid the rectal sphincter
- The anal mucosa is closed with a 2-0 absorbable suture
- A petroleum gauze dressing is placed over the wound

ANAL FISSURE

An anal fissure is a small tear in the mucosa that lines the anus. An anal fissure may develop when you pass hard or large stools during a bowel movement. Anal fissures usually cause pain and bleeding with bowel movements. You may well experience spasms in the anal sphincter.

Causes

- Passing large or hard stools
- Constipation and straining during bowel movements
- Chronic diarrhea
- Anal intercourse
- Childbirth

Less Common Causes of Anal Fissures

- Crohn's disease or another inflammatory bowel disease
- Anal cancer
- HIV
- Tuberculosis
- Syphilis

Procedural Considerations

Some diagnostic tests may be recommended to rule out other diagnosis. These include an anoscopy, flexible sigmoidoscopy or colonoscopy. Nonsurgical treatments include increasing your intake of fiber and fluids, soaking in warm water after bowel movements to relax the anal sphincter and promote healing. Your physician may prescribe: Externally applied nitroglycerin (Rectiv) to help increase blood flow to the fissure and promote healing of the sphincter. Topical anesthetic creams such a lidocaine may help with pain relief. Botox injection will paralyze the anal sphincter muscle and relax spasms. Blood pressure medications such as Procardia or Cardizem can help relax the anal sphincter.

A chronic anal fissure that is resistant to other treatments may require surgery. Surgeons typically perform a procedure called lateral internal sphincterotomy (LIS), which entails cutting a small portion of the anal sphincter muscle to reduce spasm and pain, and promote healing.

Bibliography

Abdel-Misih SR, Bloomston M. Liver anatomy. *Surg. Clin. North Am.* 2010; 90(4):643–653. https://doi.org/10.1016/j.suc.2010.04.017. Accessed June 1, 2023.

American College of Surgeons. Section III: Surgical Specialties. n.d. https://www.facs.org/education/resources/residency-search/specialties/general. Accessed June 1, 2023.

Anal Fissures. https://www.mayoclinic.org/diseases-conditions/anal-fissure/symptoms-causes/syc-20351424. Accessed June 1, 2023.

An Overview of the Pancreas—Understanding Insulin and Diabetes. https://www.endocrineweb.com/author/1072/sargis. Accessed June 1, 2023.

Aragon RJ, Solomon NL. Techniques of hepatic resection. *J Gastrointest Oncol.* 2012;3(1):28–40. https://doi.org/10.3978/j.issn.2078-6891.2012.006. Accessed June 1, 2023.

Baylor Medicine. Healthcare: Breast Cancer. Mastectomy | Baylor Medicine (bcm.edu). Accessed June 1, 2023.

Chari RS, Shah SA. Chapter 54: Sabiston Textbook of Surgery. In: Townsend CM, Jr., Beauchamp RD, Evers BM, Mattox KL, eds. *Biliary system.* 18th ed. Sec X. St. Louis, MO: WB Saunders; 2008:54, 1474-1414.

Dahdaleh FS, Heidt D, Turaga KK. The appendix. In: Brunicardi F, Andersen DK, Billiar TR, et al, eds. Schwartz's Principles of Surgery, 11th ed. McGraw-Hill. https://accesssurgery.mhmedical.com/content.aspx?bookid=2576&sectionid=216215350. Accessed September 21, 2020.

D'Cruz JR, Misra S, Shamsudeen S. Pancreaticoduodenectomy. In: StatPearls [Internet]. Treasure Island, FL: StatPearls Publishing; 2021. https://www.ncbi.nlm.nih.gov/books/NBK560747/. Accessed June 1, 2023.

Ellison E, Zollinger RM, Jr., eds. *Zollinger's Atlas of Surgical Operations.* 10th ed. McGraw-Hill. https://accesssurgery.mhmedical.com/content.aspx?bookid=1755&sectionid=119128923. Accessed September 21, 2020.

Haisley KR, Hunter JG. Gallbladder and the extrahepatic biliary system. In: Brunicardi F, Andersen DK, Billiar TR, et al., eds. *Schwartz's Principles of Surgery. 11th ed.* McGraw-Hill; 2021. https://accesssurgery.mhmedical.com/content.aspx?bookid=2576&sectionid=216215815. Accessed June 1, 2023.

Hemorrhoids. https://www.mayoclinic.org/diseases-conditions/hemorrhoids/symptoms-causes/syc-20360268. Accessed June 1, 2023.

Hodge BD. Anatomy, Abdomen and Pelvis, Appendix. 2019. https://www.ncbi.nlm.nih.gov/books/NBK459205/#article-32438.s4. Accessed June 1, 2023.

Hunter JG, Spight DH. *Atlas of Minimally Invasive Operations.* https://accesssurgery.mhmedical.com. New York, NY: McGraw-Hill Education; 2018.

Liver: Anatomy and Functions. Johns Hopkins Medicine. https://www.hopkinsmedicine.org/health/conditions-and-diseases/liver-anatomy-and-functions. Accessed June 1, 2023.

Markman M. Liver Resection. CTCA. cancercenter.com. Accessed June 1, 2023.

Mastectomy. Mayo Clinic. Mastectomy - Mayo Clinic. Accessed June 1, 2023.

Moyer A, Naglieri C. *Current Diagnosis and Treatment: Surgery.* 15th ed. New York, NY: McGraw Hill Education; 2020. http://accesssurgery.mhmedical.com. Accessed June 1, 2023.

Moyer A, Naglieri C. *Maingot's Abdominal Operations.* 13th ed. New York, NY: McGraw Hill Education; 2019. http://accesssurgery.mhmedical.com. Accessed June 1, 2023.

Mulholland MW, Albo D, Dalman RL, Hawn MT, Hughes SJ, Sabel MS. *Operative techniques in surgery.* Philadelphia, PA: Wolters Kluwer Health; 2015.

Pancreatic Cancer. Mayo Clinic. https://www.mayoclinic.org/diseases-conditions/pancreatic-cancer/diagnosis-treatment/drc-20355427. Accessed June 1, 2023.

Perry B, Connaughton JC. Abdominoperineal resection: how is it done and what are the results? *Clin Colon Rectal Surg.* 2007;20(3) 213-220. https://www.ncbi.nlm.nih.gov/pmc/articles/PMC2789508/. Accessed June 1, 2023.

Rothrock JC, McEwen DR. *Alexanders Care of the Patient in Surgery.* St. Louis, MO: Elsevier Mosby; 2015.

Sentinel Lymph Node Biopsy. NIH. National Cancer Institute. Sentinel Lymph Node Biopsy - National Cancer Institute. Accessed June 1, 2023.

Sissons B. What to know about recovering after a breast biopsy. Medically reviewed by Selchick F. 2021. https://www.medicalnewstoday.com/articles/breastbiopsy-recovery. Accessed June 1, 2023.

Sugarbaker D. *Sugarbaker's Adult Chest Surgery.* 3rd ed. New York, NY: McGraw Hill Education. http://accesssurgery.mhmedical.com. Accessed June 1, 2023.

Tangella K. Modified Radical Mastectomy. Updated March 28, 2019. Modified Radical Mastectomy (dovemed.com). Accessed June 1, 2023.

University of California San Francisco, Department of Surgery. Henorrhoidectomy. ucsf.edu. Accessed June 1, 2023.

USFC. Transplant Surgery. Department of Surgery. Liver Transplant. ucsf.edu. Accessed June 1, 2023.

Weaver V; UCSF Helen Diller Family Comprehensive Cancer Center. A Biophysical-Computational Perspective of Breast Cancer Pathogenesis and Treatment Response (researchgate.net). 2009. https://www.researchgate.net/publication/235105561_A_Biophysical-Computational_Perspective_of_Breast_Cancer_Pathogenesis_and_Treatment_Response. Accessed June 23, 2023.

Zinner M, Ashley S. *Maingot's Abdominal Operations.* 13th ed. https://accesssurgery.mhmedical.com. New York, NY: McGraw-Hill Education; 2019.

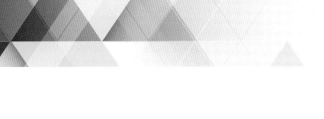

15

Obstetric and Gynecologic Surgery

Kathleen Duffy and Sara Adams

DISCUSSED IN THIS CHAPTER

1. Surgical anatomy and pathology
2. Perioperative considerations of surgery
3. Surgical procedures
4. Role of the surgical assistant in GYN and Obstetric cases

SURGICAL ANATOMY

The female reproductive system is made of both external (Figure 15-1) and internal (Figure15-2) components. Externally, gynecologic anatomy begins with the mons pubis. Anterior to the pubic symphysis, the mons pubis consists of adipose tissue, and is more prominent in females than in males. As a whole, external genitalia is collectively known as the vulva. The labia majora, the most lateral components of the vulva, span from the mons pubis to the perineum. Positioned just medially from the labia majora is the labia minora, which surrounds the clitoris from above and below. The clitoris is located superior to the urethral opening and houses the urethral meatus and Bartholin's glands. Bartholin's glands, which are paired, secrete a mucous-based lubricant for the vagina. The vagina is the tubular cavity spanning between the exterior opening and the uterine cervix. Its blood supply comes from the pudendal arteries.

Internally lies the uterus, a pear-shaped organ located between the bladder and rectum. This organ consists of the cervix, body, fundus, and cornua. The cervix forms the inferior portion of the uterus, the body is the midsection, and the fundus is the superior portion. The cornua, located superiorly and laterally, form the entry point of the fallopian tubes.

The uterus is held in place in the pelvis by a series of suspension ligaments. Cardinal ligaments are located anteriorly, pubic ligaments are posteriorly, and sacral are inferiorly. The broad ligament is formed by a fold of peritoneal tissue, and contains fallopian tubes, round and ovarian ligaments, blood vessels, and nerves.

The fallopian tubes extend bilaterally from the cornua of the uterus. Ovaries are located distally to the fallopian tubes at the lateral pelvic wall. Not only do they release eggs for fertilization, but they are also responsible for releasing estrogen and progesterone.

Blood supply to the uterus is accomplished by uterine branches of the internal iliac arteries. Fallopian tubes receive vascularity from uterine and ovarian branches. The ovarian arteries come directly from the abdominal aorta. Hypogastric arteries also play a major role, giving rise to the obturator, pudendal, and uterine arteries.

Uterine lymph nodes drain from the utero-ovarian pedicle to the external iliac area. Nodes tend to be larger in size during pregnancy. Lymph drainage from the fallopian tubes begins at the broad ligament and meets up with drainage from the uterus and ovaries, to periaortic and lumbar nodes.

Sciatic, obturator, and femoral nerves are present in the pelvis. The vagina receives innervation from the vaginal plexus and pudendal nerves. Nerves associated with the uterus include ovarian and hypogastric plexuses, and second through fourth spinal roots. Sympathetic nerve fibers of the fallopian tubes are located in lumbar plexuses, parasympathetic fibers are from the ovarian plexus, and second to fourth sacral nerves. Innervation of the ovaries comes from sympathetic, parasympathetic, and autonomic fibers of the ovarian plexus. Ilioinguinal, iliohypogastric, and genitofemoral nerves are also present in the pelvis, and should be considered during any pelvic procedures.

POSITIONING THE GYN PATIENT

Sequential compression devices, DVT prophylaxis, are placed on the patient prior to anesthesia induction. If the patient has any joint issues or range of motion issues, the patient should

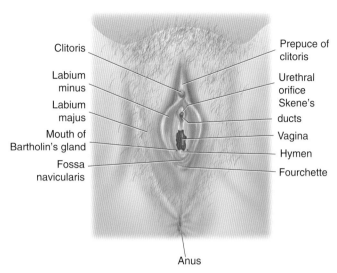

Figure 15-1 · External anatomy. (From Brunicardi FC, Andersen DK, Billiar TR, et al, eds. *Schwartz's Principles of Surgery*. 11th ed. New York, NY: McGraw Hill; 2019.)

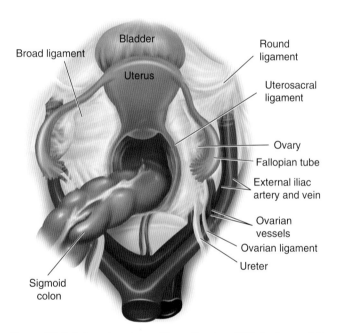

Figure 15-2 · Internal anatomy. (From Brunicardi FC, Andersen DK, Billiar TR, et al, eds. *Schwartz's Principles of Surgery*. 11th ed. New York, NY: McGraw Hill; 2019.)

be positioned while awake. Arms are positioned so as to not extend the arms more than 90° to prevent brachial plexus injuries. Padding the arms will prevent radial and ulnar nerve injury.

Lithotomy position is often utilized for vaginal procedures. Stirrups, once attached to the bed, should be equal in height. The patient's legs are placed in the stirrups at the same time. Failure to do so may cause hip hyperflexion or lumbosacral nerve damage. Make sure the patient's heels are seated as deep as possible into the boot of the stirrup, and the angle of the boot is such that the pressure is on the heel, and

not the patient's calf or the medial/lateral aspect of the knee before securing the straps. It is important that the buttocks do not sit too far beyond the cutout in the mattress. Poor positioning may put excess pressure on the sacrum. Make sure the knees are aligned with the opposing shoulder. The knees should not be too far abducted, and after removing the bottom of the bed, always test the movement of the stirrup to be sure that the knees don't adduct when the stirrups are simultaneously lowered into "laparoscopic position." Ensure that sequential compression hoses are not compromising the secured legs; patient comfort and avoidance of pressure points are key.

Arms are either placed on arm boards or tucked at the sides, depending on the procedure. For any procedure requiring a supine position, the arms should be on padded arm boards making sure that the arms and hands are well padded. Arms should not exceed angles greater than 90°. For laparoscopic or robotic procedures, arms should be tucked to avoid injury either by the robot or any other laparoscopic equipment. Make sure pressure points are well-padded and reposition and pad any intravenous lines or monitor cords to keep them from pressing against the arms. Fingers and hands should also be protected from the break in the operating table. Digits are at a risk for being crushed when the foot of the bed is raised at the end of a procedure.

Trendelenburg is often required to provide better visualization. The patient must be properly secured or laid on special foam padding to prevent sliding during the procedure. It's always a good idea to move the patient into steep Trendelenburg before continuing to be sure that there will be no movement during the surgery.

PREPPING THE GYN PATIENT

For cases performed in supine position, an abdominal prep is used. Prepping starts at the origin of the incision, moving in a circular motion, outward and from bedside to bedside. The umbilicus, considered the dirtiest area, is prepped last.

For vaginal preps, betadine or gentle cleansing soap is used, along with three prepping sponges. Each sponge begins at the lower abdomen, extending downward over the pubis. Inner thighs are cleaned next, moving from the genital area outward to the mid-thigh. The vagina is prepped last, followed by buttocks and anus. Once a sponge has made contact with the contaminated areas, it is discarded.

Any hair that is exposed and included in the sterile field is clipped. If a procedure requires both abdominal and vaginal preps, two separate sets of sponges are needed.

SURGICAL PROCEDURES

Cervical Cerclage (Shirodkar Procedure)

Overview: Cervical cerclage repairs or reinforces a weakened cervix and prevents miscarriage. This procedure may be performed in a clinical setting or operating room and does not require a surgical assistant (SA).

Anesthesia: Regional block or general anesthesia

Positioning: Lithotomy with arms out on arm boards

Prepping: Vaginal prep. Be careful, as the patient is pregnant.

Draping: Lithotomy drape

Procedure:

- The vaginal mucosa is incised with a 15 blade, anterior and posterior to the cervix.
- The bladder is gently retracted and held out of the way to prevent injury.
- A thin tape of synthetic material is passed through both incisions, surrounding the cervix.
- Once in position, the tape is tightened and sutured to remain in place.
- The anterior and posterior incisions are sutured and closed.
- Note: Cerclage may also be achieved with the McDonald procedure, in which a purse string suture is placed through cervical tissue instead of a synthetic tape.

Postoperative complications: Although there are no common postop complications to these procedures, there are risks associated with performing a Cervical Cerclage which include:

- Infection
- Bleeding
- Premature contractions
- Rupture of membranes (water breaking)
- Miscarriage or preterm delivery if the stitch fails

Caesarian Section

Overview: Caesarian section is performed when labor fails to progress, a baby is breech, or if there are any other threatening situations. Patients with past multiple pregnancies, and especially prior C-sections, are also candidates for the procedure. The SA role should focus mainly on placing retractors for exposure, using suction to keep blood and fluid out of the field, and applying fundal pressure on the uterus to remove the baby.

Anesthesia: Epidural, or General anesthesia if the baby is in fetal distress.

Positioning: Supine with arms out on arm boards. A bump may be placed under the patient's right hip, to minimize pressure on the vena cava caused by the uterus.

Prepping: A Foley catheter is inserted to drain the bladder and monitor urine output. An abdominal prep is performed, from nipples to mid-thighs, and from bedside to bedside.

Draping: Block towels around abdomen, then laparotomy drape. A special C-section drape may be used, equipped with side pockets.

Procedure:

- An abdominal incision is made with a 10 blade, either Pfannensticl or vertical, long enough to accommodate the size of the infant. Electrocoagulation may be used at this point to stop bleeding especially if the patient is awake and under regional anesthesia.
- Rectus muscles are separated at the midline to expose the transversalis facia and peritoneum. Once visualized, the peritoneum is opened, taking care not to injure any abdominal organs. Handheld retractors are used for exposure.
- A self-retaining retractor may be placed at this point to hold the incision open.
- The uterus is quickly but carefully palpated to determine the size and presenting part of the fetus as well as the direction and degree of rotation of the uterus.
- A bladder flap is gently created by sharp and blunt dissection at the reflection of the peritoneum above the upper margin of the bladder and overlying the anterior lower uterine segment. The bladder flap is retracted with a bladder retractor.
- The surgeon will inspect the uterus for adhesions or uterine windows from prior C-Sections or surgeries. The uterus is opened approximately 2 cm above the bladder flap. The Uterine incision can be extended laterally using large bandage scissors or using lateral pressure.
- The presenting membranes are incised, and amniotic fluid is suctioned out.
- All retractors are removed. The fetal head is gently elevated, either manually or by use of obstetric forceps, through the incision, aided by transabdominal fundal pressure to help expel the fetus.
- As soon as the head is delivered, a bulb syringe or aspirator tip is used to aspirate the exposed areas and mouth to minimize aspiration of amniotic fluid and its contents.
- Once cleared, the shoulders are delivered taking care not to cause shoulder dystocia.
- Once the infant is delivered, the neonatologist will time the blood flow through the placenta to the baby, and when advised the umbilical cord is clamped and divided, and the baby is then passed to a separate neonatal team for evaluation. Cord blood samples are taken from the placental side of the umbilical cord. Oxytocin is then administered by the anesthesia provider to contract the uterus.
- The placenta is delivered by gently massaging the uterus, or by manual removal. Any remnants of placenta should be removed using a wet lap and wiping the myometrium. It is critical to make sure that there is no placental tissue left inside the uterus, which could cause excessive bleeding and possible return to the OR for retained placenta.
- The edges of the uterine incision are clamped using T-Clamps or Sponge Sticks, and the uterus is sutured back together typically in two layers, locking the first layer, and imbricating the second.
- The surgical area is then inspected for bleeding. Additional figure-of-eight sutures are placed, if necessary. Bi-lateral abdominal cavities (Gutters) are then cleaned and irrigated, ovaries, fallopian tubes, and uterine vessels are inspected.

- Attention is then turned to closing the surgical site. Peritoneum may or may not be closed, depending on surgeon preference. The facia is closed using heavy suture. The subcutaneous layer is closed with a fast-absorbing suture and skin is approximated with either staples or subcuticular sutures.
- After the wound is closed, fundal pressure is applied expressing any clots from the vagina.
- Abdominal dressings and peri-pad are applied.

Note: Should this be an emergency, the patient is intubated using rapid sequence induction. The Foley has already been in place and no bump is placed under the patient. The baby needs to be removed as quickly as possible.

Postoperative complications:

- Post-surgery infection or fever
- Too much blood loss
- Injury to organs
- Emergency hysterectomy
- Blood clots
- Reaction to medication or anesthesia
- Emotional difficulties
- Scar tissue and difficulty with future deliveries
- Death of the mother
- Harm to the baby

Risks and complications for the baby:

- Premature birth
- Breathing problems
- Low APGAR scores
- Fetal injury

Endometrial Ablation

Overview: Ablation is used to treat heavy menstrual periods, abnormal bleeding, or anemia. The process affects endometrial tissue and may stop bleeding completely. The procedure is quick and requires little recovery time. This procedure does not require an SA.

Anesthesia: Regional block or general anesthesia using an Laryngeal mask airway (LMA) if done in the operating room

Positioning: Lithotomy with arms out on arm boards

Prepping: Vaginal prep

Draping: Under buttocks drape, lithotomy sheet

Procedure:

- The cervix is dilated to accommodate the size of the ablation device to be used.
- A diagnostic hysteroscopy is performed to visualize the uterine cavity.
- There are several different ways to ablate endometrial tissue—a resectoscope with a roller ball attachment, cryotherapy, thermal heat, or radiofrequency.
- After ablation, the device and hysteroscope are removed, and a peri-pad is applied.

Postoperative complications: Complications of endometrial ablation are rare and can include:

- Pain, bleeding, or infection
- Heat or cold damage to nearby organs
- A puncture injury of the uterine wall from surgical instruments

Pregnancy can occur after the procedure, but it is a high risk to mother and baby. Once the lining of the uterus is altered, the risk increases for an ectopic pregnancy.

Total Abdominal Hysterectomy

Overview: The uterus and cervix are removed through an abdominal approach.

Anesthesia: General anesthesia using an endotracheal tube

Positioning: Supine with arms out on arm boards. The patient will also be placed in slight Trendelenburg.

The SA role should focus on placing retractors and other duties to aid in surgeon visualization.

Prepping: An abdominal prep is performed, from nipples to pubis, and from bedside to bedside. A vaginal prep is also performed, and a Foley catheter is placed to drain the bladder and monitor urine output.

Draping: Block towels around abdomen, laparotomy drape

Procedure:

- An incision is made with a 10 blade, either Pfannenstiel or vertical midline.
- Bleeders are cauterized and the incision is developed down to the facia. The facia is exposed using a handheld retractor and the facia is opened either by Electrocautery or Metzenbaum scissors, depending on the incision. The muscle is split using blunt dissection and then the peritoneum entered taking care to prevent bowel injury.
- A self-retaining retractor is placed for optimal visualization and protection of any abdominal contents.
- The patient is placed in Trendelenburg, and moist laparotomy sponges are used to pack away bowel, preventing injury.
- A visual inspection of the pelvis is performed. The uterus is grasped with a tenaculum and retracted cephalad. It is important to keep the uterus in its normal anatomical position.
- Once the round ligaments are located, they are clamped with a Heaney clamp, divided with scissors, sutured, and tagged with hemostats laterally.
- The anterior layer of the broad ligament is separated on each side, transected, and the bladder is separated from the anterior cervix using a wet lap sponge.

- Ureters are identified and avoided to prevent injury.
- Broad ligaments are clamped with Heaney clamps, divided with scissors and sutured, or they are divided using a thermal device such as the Ligasure or ENSEAL.
- Uterosacral ligaments are clamped with straight Heaney clamps divided and sutured bilaterally down the length of the cervix, followed by the cardinal ligaments. This step is repeated on the other side.
- Curved Heaney clamps grasp below the cervix bilaterally and a circumferential incision is made above the clamps freeing the specimen, and it is removed. The vagina is then closed using heavy suture taking care not to suture the bladder into the vaginal cuff.
- Stumps from the uterosacral and round ligaments are anchored to the closed vagina.
- The abdominal cavity is inspected for hemostasis.
- Moist laparotomy sponges are removed from the cavity and counted, and the self-retaining retractor is taken out.
- Attention is then turned to closing the surgical site. Peritoneum may or may not be closed, depending on surgeon preference. The facia is closed using heavy suture. Depending on surgeon preference, the surgeon closes one side, the SA closes the other and the two suture lines meet in the middle. The subcutaneous layer is closed with a fast-absorbing suture and skin is approximated with either staples or subcuticular sutures.
- Abdominal dressings are applied, and an abdominal binder may be used.
- A peri-pad is also placed in case of any vaginal drainage (see Figure 15-3).

Total Abdominal Hysterectomy with Bilateral Salpingo-Oopherectomy

Overview: The uterus, cervix, fallopian tubes, and ovaries are removed through an abdominal approach.

The procedure is as listed above for a total abdominal hysterectomy. The procedural changes are that of removing both ovaries and associated fallopian tubes.

Operative procedure:

- The abdominal cavity is opened, as described for total abdominal hysterectomy.
- After the round ligament is ligated, a window is developed through the broad ligament and the tube, ovary and the infundibulopelvic ligament is clamped with a Kelly clamp, cut and ligated.
- The anterior layer of the broad ligament is separated on each side, transected and the bladder is separated from the anterior cervix using a wet lap or raytex.
- The procedure is as described for the total abdominal hysterectomy, the wound is closed, and dressings are applied.

Vaginal Hysterectomy

Overview: If there is adequate space, the patient may be a candidate for vaginal hysterectomy.

Anesthesia: General anesthesia; in some cases, a regional block may be used.

Positioning: Lithotomy with arms out on arm boards. The patient will also be placed in Trendelenburg.

Prepping: Vaginal prep

Draping: One towel across the abdomen, under buttocks drape, lithotomy sheet

Procedure:

- A Foley catheter is inserted to drain the bladder and monitor urine output.
- The cervix is grasped with a tenaculum.
- Local containing epinephrine is used to control bleeding and aid in tissue dissection.
- An incision is made circumferentially around the cervix.
- Scissors are used to enter the posterior cul-de-sac, and a long-weighted speculum is inserted, providing a barrier and protecting the rectum from injury.
- The anterior cul-de-sac is entered next, and scissors are used to dissect the anterior cervix away from the bladder. A small Deaver or similar retractor may be inserted to protect the bladder.
- Uterosacral ligaments are identified, clamped, divided, and tied. Once the most lateral ends are tied, they are tagged to make for an easier closure.
- Uterine vessels and parametrial structures are identified, clamped, divided, and tied.
- At the cornua of the uterus, round and utero-ovarian ligaments are divided to free the fallopian tubes and ovaries.
- Once the specimen is freed, it is removed.
- Interrupted sutures are used to close the vagina.
- A cystoscopy may be performed to check for any potential injury to the bladder and ureters.
- Vaginal packing may be inserted, and a peri-pad is placed (see Figure 15-4).

Laparoscopic Assisted Vaginal Hysterectomy

Overview: An alternative to abdominal hysterectomy, LAVH provides a less invasive approach.

Anesthesia: General anesthesia

Positioning: Lithotomy with arms padded and tucked at the sides. Patient will be placed in steep Trendelenburg.

Prepping: Abdominal prep, from nipples to pubis, and bedside to bedside. A vaginal prep is also needed.

Draping: Block towels around abdomen, under buttocks drape, and lithotomy sheet

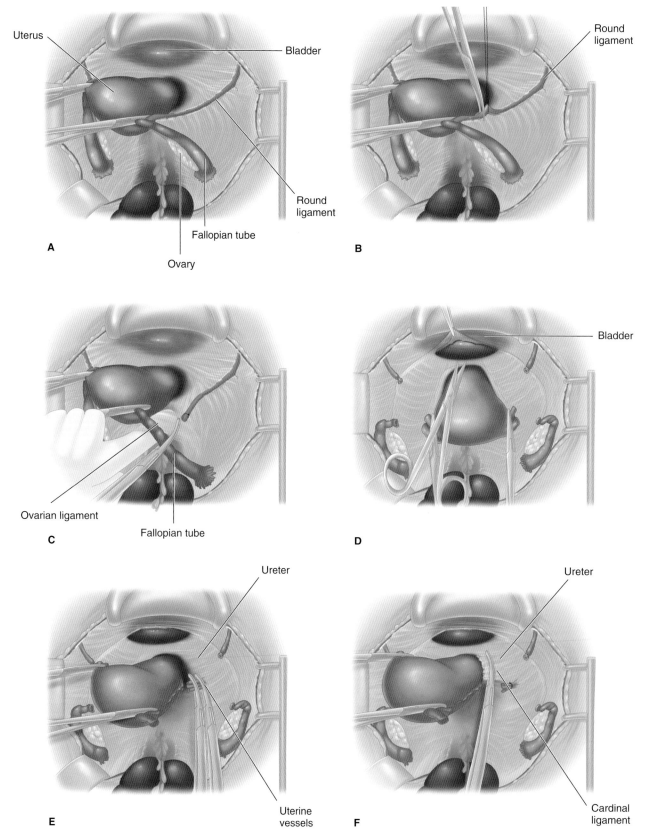

Figure 15-3 · Abdominal hysterectomy. (From Brunicardi FC, Andersen DK, Billiar TR, et al, eds. *Schwartz's Principles of Surgery*. 11th ed. New York, NY: McGraw Hill; 2019.)

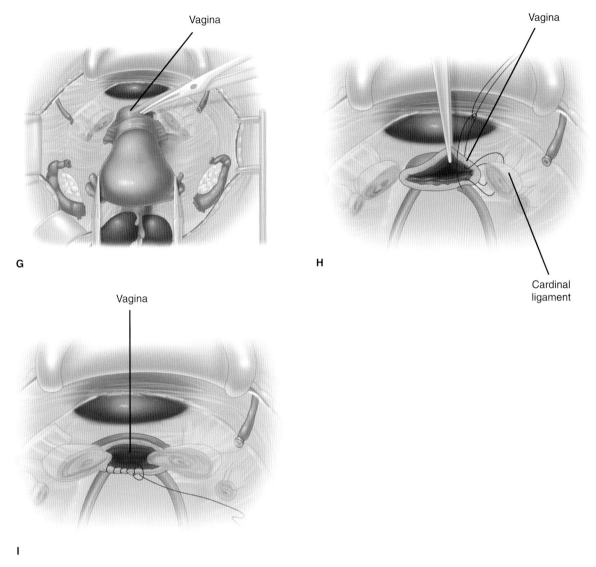

Figure 15-3 (*Continued*)

Procedure:

- A Foley catheter is inserted to drain the bladder and monitor urine output.
- While the surgeon dilates the cervix and places the uterine manipulator, the SA passes laparoscopic cords off the surgical field.
- After placing the uterine manipulator, the surgeon changes their gloves and begins entry into the abdominal cavity.
- Using towel clips to support the skin, a small incision is made through the umbilicus and a Veress needle is introduced into the abdominal cavity. Saline is pushed through the Veress needle to determine that it has passed through all three layers into the abdominal cavity. This will avoid any subcutaneous air that may occur if the Veress needle is not inserted deep enough. The Insufflation tubing is attached, and Insufflation is started.

- Once the intra-abdominal pressure reaches 15 mm the Veress needle is removed, and the camera port is placed. The camera is inserted to inspect the abdominal cavity for any anomalies and pathology.
- Two more ports are placed laterally on both sides of the camera port under direct visualization to avoid injury to the inferior epigastric artery. The SA may be asked to place ports on his or her side.
- The abdomen is visually inspected, and pictures may be captured.
- Bowel graspers, Maryland dissectors, laparoscopic needle drivers and an energy dissector are used for the procedure.
- The ureters are identified and avoided to prevent injury.
- The fallopian tubes are grasped and retracted to expose the infundibulopelvic and round ligaments, which are divided with the energy dissector.

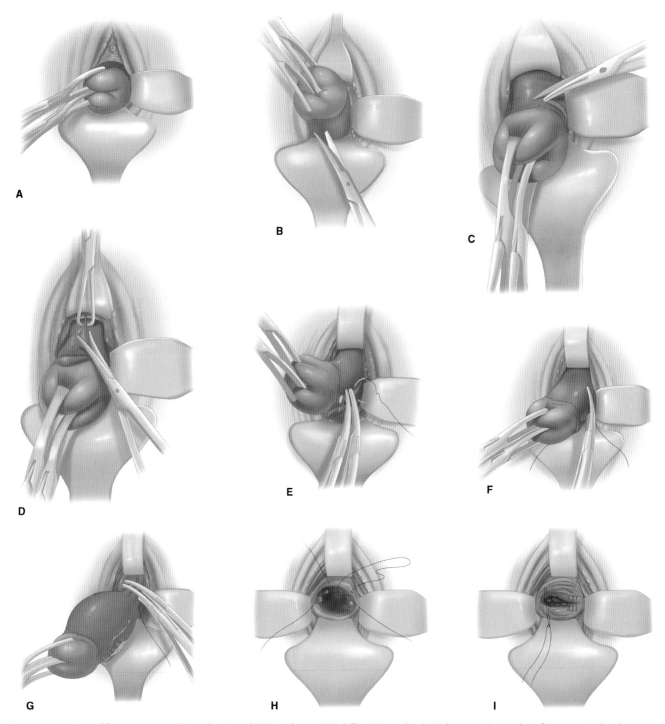

Figure 15-4 · Vaginal hysterectomy. (From Brunicardi FC, Andersen DK, Billiar TR, et al, eds. *Schwartz's Principles of Surgery*. 11th ed. New York, NY: McGraw Hill; 2019.)

- The bladder is dissected away from the anterior cervix.
- Uterine vessels are sealed and divided, and tissue is dissected circumferentially around the cervix.
- A colpotomy exposes the ring of the uterine manipulator allowing for removal of the specimen.
- The specimen is removed through the vagina. A vaginal occluding device is placed after removal to prevent gas from leaking out of the body and to keep the abdominal cavity inflated for suturing the cuff.
- Hemostasis is achieved, and the vaginal cuff is closed intracorporeally with a running or interrupted suture.
- The abdomen is irrigated with saline and all fluid is suctioned out.

- Instruments are removed, trocars are opened to deflate the abdomen and then pulled out.
- Port sites are closed, and dressings are applied. A peri-pad is placed, and an abdominal binder may be used.

For extracorporeal vaginal cuff closure:
- A three-quarter sheet is draped over the sterile field, the bed height is raised, and stirrups are readjusted to prepare for the vaginal portion of the procedure.
- Interrupted sutures are used to close the vagina.
- A cystoscopy may be performed to check for any potential injury to the bladder and ureters.
- Vaginal packing may be necessary, and a peri-pad is placed.

Robotic Hysterectomy

Overview: Another minimally invasive alternative to abdominal hysterectomy, this procedure allows for more meticulous dissection, and better angles. The SA plays a large role in robotic surgery. Once the ports have been placed, the surgeon breaks scrub to operate from the console across the room, leaving the SA in control over the sterile field. Using laparoscopic graspers to provide counter traction is key, as well as using suction and irrigation.

Anesthesia: General anesthesia with oral-gastric tube placed to prevent injury to the stomach.

Positioning: Lithotomy with both arms padded and tucked. Patient will also be placed in Trendelenburg.

Prepping: Abdominal prep from nipples to pubis, and bedside to bedside. A vaginal prep is performed also.

Draping: Block towels around the abdomen, under buttocks drape, lithotomy sheet.

Procedure:
- A Foley catheter is inserted to drain the bladder and monitor urine output.
- While the surgeon dilates the cervix and inserts a uterine manipulator, the SA passes off laparoscopic and robotic tubing and cords.
- After placing the uterine manipulator, the surgeon changes their gloves and begins entry into the abdominal cavity.
- Using towel clips to support the skin, a small incision is made through the umbilicus and a Veress needle is introduced into the abdominal cavity. Saline is pushed through the Veress needle to determine that it has passed through all 3 layers into the abdominal cavity. This will avoid any subcutaneous air that may occur if the Veress needle is not inserted deep enough. The Insufflation tubing is attached, and Insufflation is started.
- Once the intraabdominal pressure reaches 15 mm the Veress needle is removed, and the camera port is placed. The camera is inserted to inspect the abdominal cavity for any anomalies and pathology.

- Two more robotic ports are placed laterally on both sides of the camera port under direct visualization to avoid injury to the inferior epigastric artery. An assistant port is placed between the camera and lateral port under direct visualization, just below the ribs. The SA may be asked to place ports on his or her side.
- The abdomen is inspected, and pictures may be captured.
- With help from the circulator, the robot is moved into position and robot is docked.
- The camera is inserted into the camera port and the pathology is targeted. Once successful targeting has occurred, all other arms are docked.
- Robotic instruments on hand include a grasper, Maryland dissector or fenestrated bipolar forceps, vessel sealer, monopolar scissors, and monopolar spatula. The robotic instruments of choice are inserted into the proper ports, attached to the robotic arm, and inserted into the abdominal cavity under direct visualization to avoid injury to the patient. Any laparoscopic instrumentation used by the SA is introduced through the assistant port.
- Using both monopolar and bipolar instrumentation, the vessels are sealed and transected. For a bilateral salpingectomy, the utero-ovarian ligament is divided, and the fallopian tube is removed. For bilateral salpingo-oophorectomy, the infundibular pelvic ligament is dissected along with the broad ligaments down to the cervix.
- The bladder is dissected away from the anterior cervix.
- Uterine vessels are sealed and divided, and tissue is dissected circumferentially around the cervix.
- A colpotomy exposes the ring of the uterine manipulator allowing for removal of the specimen.
- The specimen is removed through the vagina. A vaginal occluding device is placed after removal to prevent gas from leaking out of the body and to keep the abdominal cavity inflated for suturing the cuff.
- Hemostasis is achieved, and the vaginal cuff is closed with a running or interrupted suture.
- The abdomen is irrigated with saline and all fluid is suctioned out.
- Robotic instruments are removed, the robot is undocked, and trocars are removed.
- Port sites are closed, and dressings are applied. A peri-pad is placed, and an abdominal binder may be used.

Supracervical Hysterectomy

A modification of a simple hysterectomy, supracervical hysterectomy (or subtotal) refers to amputating the uterus at the internal os of the cervix, leaving the cervix behind. Supracervical hysterectomies may be performed laparoscopically or robotically, avoiding abdominal or vaginal incisions. The fundus of the uterus is freed, bagged, and morcellated through an extended umbilical port site. One risk to consider for this procedure is the possibility of cancer developing within the cervical stump.

Robotic Supracervical Hysterectomy with Sacral Colpopexy

Overview: Another minimally invasive alternative to abdominal sacral colpopexy, this procedure allows for more meticulous dissection, and better angles. The SA plays a large role in robotic surgery. Once the ports have been placed, the surgeon breaks scrub to operate from the console across the room, leaving the SA in control over the sterile field. Using laparoscopic graspers to provide counter traction is key, as well as using suction and irrigation.

Anesthesia: General anesthesia with oral-gastric tube placed to prevent injury to the stomach.

Positioning: Lithotomy with both arms padded and tucked. Patient will also be placed in Trendelenburg.

Prepping: Abdominal prep from nipples to pubis, and bedside to bedside. A vaginal prep is performed also.

Draping: Block towels from xiphoid process, laterally on both sides, and across symphysis pubis. Under buttocks drape, leggings and major abdominal drape is placed. Hint: Place the major abdominal drape on the patient upside down. This will allow for the longer end of the drape to go toward the anesthesia provider and give the assistant more room. Hint: Using small strips of Ioban to secure the towels to the patient ensures that the major abdominal drape sticks and will not move during the surgery.

Procedure:

- A Foley catheter is inserted to drain the bladder and monitor urine output.

- The SA passes off laparoscopic and robotic tubing and cords.

- Using towel clips to support the skin, a small incision is made through the umbilicus and a Veress needle is introduced into the abdominal cavity. Saline is pushed through the Veress needle to determine that it has passed through all three layers into the abdominal cavity. This will avoid any subcutaneous air that may occur if the Veress needle is not inserted deep enough. Alternate to the Veress needle, the surgeon may choose to use a Mini Gel point. This requires a cut-down entry through the umbilicus into the abdominal cavity. The ring is placed making sure there are no loops of bowel pinched by the internal ring. The gel cover is placed, and the Insufflation tubing is attached, and Insufflation is started.

- Once the intraabdominal pressure reaches 15 mm the Veress needle is removed, and the camera port is placed. If the Mini Gel point is used, the camera trocar is placed through the Gel point self-sealing cover. The camera is inserted to inspect the abdominal cavity for any anomalies and pathology.

- Three more robotic ports are placed, two laterally on the left side of the patient and one laterally on the right side of the patient under direct visualization to avoid injury to the inferior epigastric artery. An assistant port is placed between the camera and lateral port under direct visualization, just below the ribs. The SA may be asked to place ports on his or her side.

- The abdomen is inspected, and pictures may be captured.

- The patient is placed in steep Trendelenburg to allow for any bowel in the pelvis to shift toward the head. This will expose the sacrum. Then the patient is moved slightly out of Trendelenburg.

- With help from the circulator, the robot is moved into position and robot is docked.

- The camera is inserted into the camera port and the pathology is targeted. Once successful targeting has occurred, all other arms are docked.

- Robotic instruments on hand include a tenaculum, Maryland dissector or fenestrated bipolar forceps, vessel sealer, monopolar scissors, and monopolar spatula. The robotic instruments of choice are inserted into the proper ports, attached to the robotic arm and inserted into the abdominal cavity under direct visualization to avoid injury to the patient. Any laparoscopic instrumentation used by the SA is introduced through the assistant port.

- From the console, the surgeon will grasp and manipulate the uterus with a robotic tenaculum.

- Using both monopolar and bipolar instrumentation, the vessels are sealed and transected. For a bilateral salpingectomy, the utero-ovarian ligament is divided, and the fallopian tube is removed. For bilateral salpingo-oophorectomy, the infundibular pelvic ligament is dissected along with the broad ligaments down to the cervix.

- The bladder is dissected away from the anterior cervix.

- Uterine vessels are sealed and divided, and tissue is dissected circumferentially around the cervix.

- The cervix is transected, and the uterus is placed either in a bag or upper left quadrant to be removed before closing.

- Hemostasis is achieved and the endocervical canal is burned.

- Attention is then turned to the sacral colpopexy.

- Using the robotic monopolar scissors and bipolar graspers of choice, the surgeon will locate the sacrum and incise the peritoneum to expose the sacral promontory.

- The surgeon grasps the cervical stump with the tenaculum. The surgeon will manipulate the cervical stump to accommodate the dissection of the bladder and the rectum from the vagina.

- Bladder dissection is carried into the vesicovaginal space to the level of the trigone, and the rectovaginal space to the level of the perineal body.

- Using laparoscopic graspers, the SA will be asked to grasp the bladder and to pull it cephalad, being careful not to injure the bladder. This will allow the surgeon access down the anterior and posterior vaginal wall respectively.

- Peritoneum overlying the sacral promontory is tented up and entered sharply. Dissection is carried inferiorly to meet the dissection from below in the cul-de-sac.

The anterior longitudinal ligament and the presacral vessels are identified.

- Either the surgeon, or the SA will sterilely prepare the Y mesh. Typically, one side of the Y is folded back toward the tail and attached to the tail of the mesh using a vicryl suture, leaving long suture tails. This will be grasped by the SA and introduced into the patient through the assistant port knot side up. This allows for proper placement of the mesh over the cervical stump.

- The mesh is placed with the crotch of the Y directly over the endocervical canal along the posterior vagina. If necessary, the length is trimmed, and the excess removed through the assistant port so there will be no discomfort for the patient.

- The mesh is tacked to the posterior vagina using Gore-Tex suture.

- Once the surgeon places the sutures, the tenaculum is moved to grasp and secure both the mesh and the cervical stump.

- Attention is then turned to the anterior vagina and bladder.

- Using the robotic tenaculum, the surgeon will pull the cervix down toward the sacrum to expose the anterior vagina. The SA will grasp the bladder in the same manner taking care not to injure the bladder.

- The surgeon will then place the opposing side of the Y mesh deep into the area between the vagina and bladder, assuring that there are no folds, and trimming the mesh if necessary, and attach the mesh to the vaginal wall using Gore-Tex or another non-absorbable, soft suture.

Attention is then turned to the sacrum:

- EEA sizers or a similar instrument is placed into the vagina against the cervix. This will push the cervical stump into the pelvis.

- Simultaneously, the surgeon will manipulate the cervix cephalad using the tenaculum, and the tail of the mesh is pulled toward the sacrum. This will pull the cervical stump cephalad, along with the bladder, basically removing the cystocele.

- If necessary, the tail of the mesh will be trimmed and attached to the anterior longitudinal ligament using Ethibond suture or another strong non-absorbable soft suture.

- The mesh is then attached to the sacrum using Ethibond suture.

- The whole area of mesh is reperitonealized utilizing 0 Monocryl securing both ends with lapra-ty suture clips. No mesh should be exposed so there is no injury to bowel.

- The robotic instruments are removed the robot is undocked and the surgeon joins the assistant at the field. The uterus is placed in an endo-catch bag and is drawn out through the Gelport in the umbilicus. Morcellation may be required.

- The facial defect in the umbilicus is closed.

- If possible, the SA will suction any excess gas from the belly.

- Trocars are removed.

- Port sites are closed, and dressings are applied. A peri-pad is placed.

Radical Hysterectomy

A radical hysterectomy may be performed robotically or through an open abdominal incision. In addition to a simple hysterectomy, pelvic and periaortic lymph nodes are dissected and removed. Parametrial tissue is also separated from the pelvis and removed as part of the specimen, along with Omentum. The complex and more thorough tissue dissection raises the risk of injury to the bowel and rectum, ureters, bladder, nerves, and major blood vessels. It is important for the SA to have a knowledge of the anatomy and basic vascular surgery, just in case of vessel injury and significant blood loss.

Postoperative complications of a hysterectomy:

- Bleeding
- Damage to ureters, bladder, or bowel
- Infection
- Blood clots
- Early menopause if ovaries are removed
- Vaginal problems such as prolapse

Pelvic Exenteration (Wertheim Procedure)

Overview: If a patient has recurring localized cervical cancer, and has received a maximum amount of radiation, a pelvic exenteration may be necessary. This surgery may also be considered for certain rectal cancers. A hysterectomy with bilateral salpingo-oophorectomy is a large part of the procedure; however, it also incorporates steps from other surgical specialties. If cancer has spread to areas outside the pelvis, the operation is aborted. If completed, exenteration includes removal of the distal colon and rectum, bladder, creation of a urinary diversion, and creation of a permanent colostomy.

Anesthesia: General anesthesia

Positioning: Lithotomy with arms out on arm boards. Patient is also placed in Trendelenburg.

Prepping: A generous abdominal prep, from nipples to midthighs, and bedside to bedside. A vaginal and perineal prep is also performed.

Draping: Block towels around abdomen, under buttocks drape, and laparotomy sheet, cut to expose the perineal area.

Procedure:

- A large midline incision is made with a 10 blade.
- Once the abdomen is opened, the cavity is examined for any evidence of metastasis. Suspicious areas are biopsied and sent to pathology for a frozen section.
- A self-retaining retractor is placed for optimal exposure, and moist laparotomy sponges are used to pack bowel and avoid injury.
- A hysterectomy with bilateral salpingo-oophorectomy is performed.
- Pelvic lymph nodes are removed, being careful not to cut or damage iliac vessels.

- The rectum is dissected and mobilized.
- A cystectomy is performed, along with the creation of a urinary diversion.
- The distal colon, rectum, and anus are removed (abdominoperineal resection).
- Posterior vaginal tissue may undergo reconstruction later.
- The perineum is closed.

Hemostasis is achieved, and all moist laparotomy sponges are removed from the abdomen and counted.

- A permanent colostomy is created.
- The peritoneum is closed, followed by the fascia, and skin is approximated.
- Dressings and stomal appliances are put in place. Perineal dressings are also applied (see Figure 15-5).

Postoperative complications:

- Fever
- Sepsis
- Thromboembolic events
- Acute kidney injury (AKI)
- Superficial wound separation
- Dehiscence and evisceration
- Necrotizing fasciitis
- Bowel relation complications

Myomectomy

Overview: Myomectomy is performed to remove uterine fibroid tumors, which can cause abnormal bleeding and infertility. Uterine leiomyomas can be excised with a laparotomy or robotic procedure, or with a hysteroscopy if they are growing within the uterine cavity. Approximate size, number, and location of fibroids can be mapped out with the help of an MRI. During an open myomectomy, the SA should focus on placing retractors, suctioning, and providing adequate exposure. Robotic-assisted myomectomy has some advantages over an open method. It lowers the risk of complications allowing for

a shorter hospital stay and faster recovery. The surgery also allows for removal of difficult-to-remove fibroids. If the procedure is done robotically, the SA will be responsible for injecting Vasopressin around the fibroids to prevent massive blood loss from the uterus, using a tenaculum to hold the fibroid as it is removed, suctioning, passing suture and supporting the surgeon by holding the suture as the surgeon closes the uterus and applying any hemostatic agents to the uterus.

Anesthesia: General anesthesia

Positioning: Lithotomy with arms out on arm boards (or tucked if laparoscopic or robotic procedure)

Prepping: Abdominal prep, from nipples to pubis, and from bedside to bedside. A vaginal prep is also performed.

Draping: Block towels around the abdomen, under buttocks drape, lithotomy drape

Open procedure:

- A Foley catheter is inserted to decompress the bladder and monitor urine output.
- If fibroids exist within the uterine cavity, a diagnostic hysteroscopy is performed, and a Myosure or similar device is used to remove them.
- A Pfannenstiel incision is made with a 10 blade.
- As the SA uses a retractor to maintain exposure, the abdomen is opened.
- Once the peritoneum is incised and opened, a self-retaining retractor is placed, and ringed moist laparotomy sponges are packed into the abdomen to retract bowel and avoid injury.
- A visual inspection of the uterus, fallopian tubes, and ovaries is performed.
- When a fibroid is located, Vasopressin may be injected. This helps to minimize blood loss, and to separate tissue planes for optimal dissection.
- An incision is made over the fibroid. Note that multiple fibroids may be accessed through the same incision sites.
- A tenaculum, or even a towel clip, may be used to grasp the fibroid and manipulate while uterine tissue is dissected. Electrocautery or a knife blade is used to remove the tumor.
- Once hemostasis is achieved, the uterine incision is closed with absorbable suture.
- All moist laparotomy sponges are removed from the abdomen and counted.
- The self-retaining retractor is removed.
- The peritoneum is closed, followed by the fascia, and the skin is approximated.
- Abdominal dressings are applied, and an abdominal binder may be used.

Robotic Myomectomy

- A Foley catheter is inserted to drain the bladder and monitor urine output.

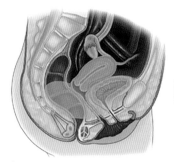
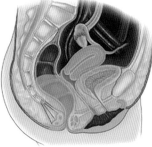

A   B

Figure 15-5 · Pelvic exenteration. (From Brunicardi FC, Andersen DK, Billiar TR, et al, eds. *Schwartz's Principles of Surgery.* 11th ed. New York, NY: McGraw Hill; 2019.)

- While the surgeon dilates the cervix and inserts a uterine manipulator, the SA passes off laparoscopic and robotic tubing and cords.

- After placing the uterine manipulator, the surgeon changes their gloves and begins entry into the abdominal cavity.

- Using towel clips to support the skin, a small incision is made through the umbilicus and a Veress needle is introduced into the abdominal cavity. Saline is pushed through the Veress needle to determine that it has passed through all three layers into the abdominal cavity. This will avoid any subcutaneous air that may occur if the Veress needle is not inserted deep enough. The Insufflation tubing is attached, and Insufflation is started.

- Once the intraabdominal pressure reaches 15 mm the Veress needle is removed, and the camera port is placed. The camera is inserted to inspect the abdominal cavity for any anomalies and pathology.

- Two more robotic ports are placed laterally on both sides of the camera port under direct visualization to avoid injury to the inferior epigastric artery. An assistant port is placed between the camera and lateral port under direct visualization, just below the ribs. The SA may be asked to place ports on his or her side.

- The abdomen is visually inspected, and pictures may be captured.

- With help from the circulator, the robot is moved into position and robot is docked.

- The camera is inserted into the camera port and the pathology is targeted. Once successful targeting has occurred, all other arms are docked.

- Robotic instruments on hand include a grasper, Maryland dissector or fenestrated bipolar forceps, monopolar scissors, and monopolar spatula. The robotic instruments of choice are inserted into the proper ports, attached to the robotic arm and inserted into the abdominal cavity under direct visualization to avoid injury to the patient. Any laparoscopic instrumentation used by the SA is introduced through the assistant port.

- The SA will be instructed to inject vasopressin around the fibroids using an injection cannula placed through the assistant port. Vasopressin should be diluted with injectable saline. Note: the SA must aspirate the syringe after inserting the needle into the uterus to verify it won't be injected directly into a blood vessel. This will aid in developing the tissue planes for dissection.

- From the console, the surgeon will incise and dissect the uterus until the fibroid cavity is developed.

- The SA will grab the fibroid using a laparoscopic tenaculum, being aware of surrounding tissues and organs. The surgeon will continue to dissect the fibroid from the uterus assisted by the SA.

- Once the fibroid is removed from the uterus it must be placed in an endo-catch bag. An accurate count of the number of fibroids removed from the uterus is imperative. The bag should be closed completely to avoid any fibroids from falling out, and the string end tagged with a hemostat on the outside of the assistant port.

- The uterus is inspected for bleeding.

- At this time, the robotic instrumentation is changed to the needle drivers of choice and the suture is passed either through the assistant port, or the robotic port before the needle driver is placed into the robotic arm.

- The surgeon closes the uterus in layers with the SA following and keeping the suture from knotting.

- After closing, the uterus is inspected for bleeding, the abdomen irrigated, suctioned and inspected for bleeding, and hemostatic agents are applied.

- All instruments are removed from the trocars, the camera is removed, and the insufflation is turned off. Using the suction irrigator, the remaining gas is suctioned from the belly to aid in the patient having less postop shoulder pain.

- The robot is undocked, and the trocars are removed.

- The surgeon will scrub back into the case. Depending on the number and size of the fibroid, either the assistant port incision is extended to accommodate morcellation, or a mini-laparotomy may be performed to remove/morcellate the fibroids.

- Large facial defects are closed with heavy suture and the skin is approximated with subcuticular sutures or staples.

- Dressings are applied.

Postoperative complications:

- Excessive blood loss
- Scar tissue
- Pregnancy or childbirth complications
- Rare incidence of hysterectomy
- Rare chance of spreading malignant tumor
- Blockage of fallopian tubes
- Intestine looping

Fallopian Tubes / Ectopic Pregnancy

Overview: A pregnancy is ectopic when it is located in any area other than within the uterus. Although most ectopic pregnancies occur within the fallopian tubes, they may also be found in the ovaries, cervix, pelvis, and omentum. This occurrence can be fatal if not addressed right away, as a major complication is rupture and hemorrhaging. An ectopic pregnancy can't progress as normal. The fertilized egg can't survive, and the developing is a real imminent danger to the mother.

If an ectopic pregnancy is detected early enough, the patient may receive an injection of methotrexate for treatment. A transvaginal ultrasound is performed to confirm the exact location of the pregnancy. Laparoscopic surgery is the most common method of management, involving a salpingectomy with use of a vessel sealer to divide and ligate. For patients at a higher risk, or for emergencies, a laparotomy is performed.

Anesthesia: General anesthesia

Positioning: Supine with arms out on arm boards. Patient will be placed in Trendelenburg.

Prepping: Abdominal prep, from nipples to pubis, and bedside to bedside.

Draping: Block towels around abdomen, laparoscopy drape

Procedure:

- A Foley catheter is inserted to drain the bladder and monitor urine output.
- The SA passes off laparoscopic tubing and cords.
- A camera port is placed, and the abdomen is inflated.
- Additional working ports are placed. The SA may be asked to place ports on his or her side.
- The abdomen is visually inspected, and pictures may be captured.
- Once the affected side is identified, the fallopian tube is grasped with a Babcock or non-traumatic instruments.
- Cautery is used to incise the fallopian tube at the location of the ectopic pregnancy.
- The tissue is removed from within, and the tube is left open.
- Hemostasis is achieved, the camera is removed, and ports are opened to deflate the abdomen and then pulled.
- Port sites are closed, and dressings are applied.

Postoperative complications:

- Rupture of the fallopian tube with internal bleeding which may lead to hypovolemic shock

EXTERNAL GENETALIA PROCEDURES

Vaginal repair is done to correct a cystocele or a rectocele and to reestablish the support of the anterior and posterior vaginal walls restoring the bladder and rectum to their normal positions.

A cystocele is a herniation of the bladder that causes the anterior vaginal wall to bulge downward. A rectocele is formed by a protrusion of the posterior vaginal wall into the vagina.

Vaginal retractors or a Lonestar retractor are used for exposure. The labia may be sewn back of exposure is inadequate.

Cystocele Repair

- The bladder is drained to prevent injury.
- Local containing epinephrine is used to control bleeding and aid in tissue dissection.
- Tissue between the bladder and vagina is exposed and the tissue distal to the urethral meatus grasped with an Allis Clamp, and another Allis clamp is placed a few centimeters proximal to this. An incision is made between Allis clamps.
- Vaginal epithelium is separated from vaginal muscularis as laterally as possible on each side using Metzenbaum scissors and blunt dissection with a ray tec sponge.

- The arcus tendinous fascia pelvis was then identified on each side and completely cleaned off.
- The lateral aspect of the vesicovaginal fascia is then attached to the arcus tendinous fascia pelvis on each side with interrupted 2-0 vicryl sutures.
- Excess vaginal epithelium is excised, and vaginal epithelium is reapproximated using 2-0 vicryl running suture.

Rectocele Repair

- Local anesthetic containing epinephrine is used to control bleeding and aid in tissue dissection.
- Two Allis clamps are placed on skin and perineal body and posterior fourchette.
- A diamond-shaped incision is made between the allis clamps.
- Vaginal epithelium is trimmed from vaginal muscularis superiorly and dorsally.
- Allis clamps are placed on both sides of the incision and dissection is continued up to the posterior vaginal fornix and laterally.
- The rectovaginal fascia is reapproximated using a 2-0 vicryl interrupted suture.
- Excess vaginal epithelium is excised, and vaginal skin is approximated using 2-0 Vicryl running suture.
- Crown perineorrhaphy is performed with 2-0 and 3-0 Vicryl.
- The vagina may be packed with 2-in vaginal packing to which antibiotic or antifungal cream may be added.

Postoperative complications of cystocele/rectocele:

- Anesthesia complications
- Infection
- Bleeding
- Injury to pelvic structures
- Dyspareunia
- Recurrent prolapse
- Failure to correct the defect

Read more: https://www.surgeryencyclopedia.com/Ce-Fi/Cystocele-Repair.html#ixzz7CCxKyyQk

Tubal Ligation

Overview: Tubal ligation for sterilization is typically performed after delivery, within 24 to 36 hours. If a patient undergoes Caesarian section, ligation is often performed then; if the patient delivers vaginally, a laparoscopy or mini-laparotomy may be suggested.

Anesthesia: General Anesthesia or regional block

Positioning: Arms tucked for laparoscopy, or on arm boards post C-section

Prepping: Abdominal prep from nipples to pubis, and bedside to bedside.

Draping: Block towels around abdomen, laparotomy sheet

Procedure:

- Depending on the approach, a 10 blade is used to make a mini incision in the abdomen, or ports are placed for laparoscopic surgery. If performed after a C-section, the procedure is done prior to closure of the abdomen.

- The uterus, fallopian tubes, and ovaries are inspected. The tubes are identified.

- Each tube is grasped with a Babcock or non-traumatic grasper.

- Electrocautery is more commonly used to burn the tubes. A portion of the tube may be excised, or a small clip may be placed across the tube to achieve sterilization.

- Hemostasis is achieved.

- The abdomen is closed, and dressings are applied.

Postoperative complications:

- Bleeding
- Postoperative pain
- Infection
- Organ damage
- Anesthesia complications
- Ectopic pregnancy
- Failure to close the fallopian tube

Vesicourethral Suspension (Marshall-Marchetti-Kranz)

Marshall Marchetti Kranz suspension is performed for the correction of stress incontinence caused by an abnormal urethrovesical angle. The intent of the Marshall Marchetti Kranz operation is to bring the bladder and urethra into the pelvis by suturing para-urethral vaginal tissue to the back of the symphysis pubis. A modification of this technique is the Birch procedure. The approach mimics the Marshall Marchetti Kranz until placement of the buttressing sutures. Instead of attempting difficult periosteal sutures, the surgeon places non-absorbable size 0 suture into the Cooper ligament from each side of the bladder neck. The Birch is technically easier, and long-term results are equivalent.

Procedural considerations: The patient is usually placed in a moderate Trendelenburg position, frog-legged, with supports under each knee to allow for inter-operative vaginal manipulation. Abdominal and vaginal preps are required. A Foley catheter is inserted into the urethra at the beginning of surgery. This procedure is combined with an abdominal hysterectomy. Surgeon and assistant double glove for vaginal manipulation. The patient will commonly have a vaginal pack and a urethral catheter with or without a super pubic catheter and possibly a wandering postoperatively

Operative procedure:

1. A Foley catheter is inserted into the bladder through the urethra.

2. A suprapubic transverse incision is made to expose the pre-vesicle space of Retzius.

3. The bladder retractor is positioned with small moist laparotomy pads in place.

4. The bladder and urethra are freed from the posterior surface of the rectus muscle and symphysis pubis by gentle blunt manipulation.

5. The assistant places two fingers into the vagina lifting the urethra upward against the symphysis pubis to facilitate ease of repair of the periurethral musculofascial structure.

6. A heavy non-absorbable atraumatic suture on a Heaney needle holder is placed to the supporting fascia of the vaginal wall on each side of the urethra. The suture is passed through the symphysis pubis providing support to the urethra and bladder neck. A row of three sutures are placed on each side.

7. The area is drained, and the wound is closed in layers and dressed.

8. Vagina may be packed with 2-in packing which should be removed after 24 to 36 hours.

Transvaginal Bladder Suspension

Vesical neck suspensions have distinct advantages over traditional open retropubic urethrovesical suspensions. The incision is superficial, the bladder and bladder neck are not dissected, and the para urethral tissues that suspend the bus circle neck or buttressed vaginally

- The labia minora may be sutured laterally to expose the vaginal introitus.

- The weighted speculum is placed into the vagina.

- A super pubic catheter is generally placed through a stab wound in the usual manner.

- A Foley catheter is placed intra-urethrally and the bladder is drained.

- With a gentle traction on the intraurethral Foley, the anterior vaginal wall is palpated to locate the bladder neck.

- Often a local anesthetic and vasopressin are injected into the anterior vaginal wall for bleeding and pain management into aid and tissue dissection.

- An inverted U incision is made with the legs of the U distal to the bladder neck and the base of the U midway between the bladder neck in the external urethral meatus. The vaginal tissue is dissecting laterally from the legs of the U toward the pubic bone of the periurethral fascia.

- Using sharp dissection with scissors the surgeon opens the retropubic space. All adhesions within the space and along the original length are released with blunt figure dissection.

- Bilaterally, helical stitches of heavy non-absorbable monofilament suture material on a mayo needle our place faster way to incorporate the urethropelvic fascia at the medial edge of the retropubic space with the pubocervical facia and anterior vaginal wall.

Postoperative complications:

- Inability to urinate
- Infection
- Overactive bladder
- Anesthesia complications

FETAL SURGERY

Fetal surgery also known as **fetal reconstructive surgery**, **antenatal surgery**, **prenatal surgery**, is a growing branch of maternal fetal medicine (MFM) that covers any of a broad range of surgical techniques that are used to treat birth defects in fetuses who are still in utero.

There are three main types: open fetal surgery, which involves completely opening the uterus to operate on the fetus minimally invasive fetoscopic surgery, which uses small incisions and is guided by fetoscopy and sonography; and percutaneous fetal therapy, which involves placing a catheter under continuous ultrasound guidance.

Fetal intervention is relatively new. Advancing technologies allow earlier and more accurate diagnosis of diseases and congenital problems in a fetus.

It often involves training in obstetrics, pediatrics, and mastery of both invasive and non-invasive surgery, meaning it takes several years of residency, and at least one fellowship (usually more than 1 year), to be able to become proficient. It is possible in the United States to become trained in this approach whether one started in obstetrics, pediatrics, or surgery. Because of the very high risk and high complexity of these cases, they are usually performed at Level I trauma centers in large cities at academic medical centers, offering the full spectrum of maternal and newborn care, including a high-level neonatal intensive care unit (Level IV is the highest) and suitable operating theaters and equipment, and a high number of surgeons and physicians, nurse specialists, therapists, and a social work and counseling team. The cases can be referred from multiple levels of hospitals from many miles, sometimes across state and provincial lines. In continents other than North America and Europe, these centers are not as numerous, though the techniques are spreading.

Postoperative complications:

- Rupture of the uterus
- Fetal death
- Operative complications
- Early labor
- Potential failure to treat the birth defect

Bibliography

Allen G, Caruthers B. Obstetric and Gynecological Surgery. In: Frey KB, Junge TL, eds. *Surgical Technology for the Surgical Technologist: A Positive Care Approach*. 2nd ed. Boston, MA: Delmar Cengage Learning; 2004:477-552.

C-Section Complications. American Pregnancy Association. https://americanpregnancy.org/healthy-pregnancy/labor-and-birth/c-section-complications/. Accessed June 7, 2023.

Complications of a Hysterectomy. NHS. www.nhs.uk. Accessed June 7, 2023.

Complications of Myomectomy. https://www.mayoclinic.org/tests-procedures/myomectomy/about/pac-20384710. Accessed June 7, 2023.

Cornforth T. Possible Complications After a Tubal Ligation. 2020. verywellhealth.com. Accessed June 7, 2023.

Duska L, Gregory T, Kohn E, Temkin S. Gynecology. In: Brunicardi FC, Andersen DK, Billiar TK, ed. *Schwartz's Principles of Surgery*. 11th ed. New York, NY: McGraw-Hill; 2019. https://accesssurgery.mhmedical.com/content.aspx?bookid=2576&sectionid=216211905. Accessed.

Ectopic Pregnancy. The Mayo Clinic. https://www.mayoclinic.org/diseases-conditions/ectopic-pregnancy/symptoms-causes/syc-20372088. Accessed June 7, 2023.

Endometrial ablation. Mayo Clinic. https://www.mayoclinic.org/tests-procedures/endometrial-ablation/about/pac-20393932. Accessed June 7, 2023.

Fetal Surgery. https://www.mayoclinic.org/tests-procedures/fetal-surgery/about/pac-20384571. Accessed June 7, 2023.

Goldman MA. Gynecologic and obstetric surgery. *Pocket Guide to the Operating Room*. 2nd ed. Philadelphia, PA: F. A. Davis Company; 1996.

Llamas M. Bladder Sling complications. Drugwatch. https://www.hopkinsmedicine.org/health/treatment-tests-and-therapies/roboticassisted-myomectomy. Accessed June 7, 2023.

Moore RD, Miklos JR. Vaginal repair of cystocele with anterior wall mesh via transobturator route: efficacy and complications with up to 3-year follow-up. *Advances in Urology*. 2009;2009(743831):8. https://doi.org/10.1155/2009/743831. Accessed June 7, 2023.

Ramirez PT, Salvo G. *Complications of Pelvic Exenteration*. In Principles of Gynecologic Oncology Surgery, 2018. Elsevier Publishers. Science Direct.

Robotic Assisted Myomectomy. Johns Hopkins Medicine. https://www.hopkinsmedicine.org/health/treatment-tests-and-therapies/roboticassisted-myomectomy. Accessed June 7, 2023.

Rothrock J, Smith D, McEwen D. Gynecologic surgery and cesarean birth. *Alexander's Care of the Patient in Surgery*. 12th ed. St Louis, MO: Mosby, Inc.; 2003:455-517.

Valle M, Federici O, Ialongo P, Graziano F, Garofalo A. Prevention of complications following pelvic exenteration with the use of mammary implants in the pelvic cavity: Technique and results of 28 cases. *J Surg Oncol*. 2011;103(1):34-38. doi: 10.1002/jso.21716.

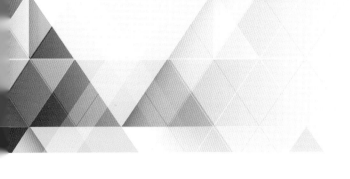

16

Genitourinary Surgery

Sandra Freymuth

DISCUSSED IN THIS CHAPTER

1. Anatomy and pathology of the genitourinary system
2. Pre- and postop surgical considerations
3. Surgical procedures

ANATOMY OF THE GENITOURINARY SYSTEM

The urinary system consists of the kidneys, ureters, bladder, and urethra. Urologists also typically treat conditions of the adrenal glands and male reproductive organs—phallus, testis, epididymis, scrotum, and prostate. The urinary system filters blood and creates urine as a waste byproduct. It also plays a role in regulating blood pressure and volume, electrolytes, metabolism, and blood pH (see Figure 16-1).

The adrenal glands cap each one of the kidneys and are encased in Gerota's fascia and produce hormones and steroids including cortisol, aldosterone, adrenaline, norepinephrine, Dehydroepiandrosterone (DHEA), and androgenic steroids. Oxygenated blood comes to the kidneys via three arteries stemming from the inferior phrenic artery (superior adrenal artery), the aorta (middle adrenal artery), and the renal artery (inferior renal artery). The venous return is via a short vein directly into the vena cava from the right kidney and adrenal gland.

The capsule is the outer connective tissue layer of the adrenal gland. The cortex is derived from embryonic mesoderm and secretes corticosteroids and androgen hormones. It is divided into an additional three layers (from external to internal): the zona glomerulosa which produces aldosterone, the zona fasciculata which secretes cortisol, and the zona reticularis which produces androgens. The medulla is the center of the adrenal gland containing chromaffin cells which secrete adrenaline including epinephrine and norepinephrine and enkephalins which function in pain control (see Figure 16-2).

Disorders of the adrenal glands can lead to adrenal insufficiency also known as Addison's disease, Cushing syndrome, adrenal hyperplasia, overactive adrenal glands, hyperaldosteronism also known as Conn's syndrome, pheochromocytomas, and rarely cancer. Additionally, adrenal "incidentalomas" are unsuspected adrenal masses detected while ongoing cross-sectional imaging for an unrelated condition and represent the most common presentation of all adrenal masses. The differential for these tumors is quite broad and includes benign non-functioning adenomas, adrenal myelolipomas, functional tumors, and metastasis.

The kidneys are bean-shaped organs that filter waste and produce urine as a byproduct. They balance electrolytes and pH and serve to contribute to fluid homeostasis. They have a superior and inferior pole, and the medial surface features the renal hilum where the blood supply and ureters are found. The kidneys lie in the retroperitoneum along the psoas muscles. The right kidney is lower than the left because it is displaced by the liver. There is typically one renal artery and vein that attach to the aorta and vena cava directly, but duplications are common. The kidneys are covered by Gerota's fascia and bind them to the abdominal wall. Under the renal fascia lies the renal capsule and cortex. The inner renal parenchyma, consisting of about a million urine-producing nephrons, extends into columns that project toward the renal sinus and divide into 6 to 10 pyramids. The papilla, or "tip" of each renal pyramid, rests against the minor calyx which collects all urine and converges to form a major calyx. Multiple major calyces then join together like a funnel to form the renal pelvis which connects to the ureter to drain urine from the kidney to the urinary bladder. Kidney innervation consists of both afferent and efferent nerves. These nerves make up the renal plexus and receive

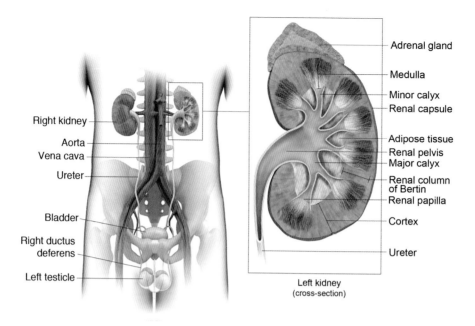

Figure 16-1 · Genitourinary system. (Reproduced, with permission, from Elsayes KM, Oldham SAA, eds. *Introduction to Diagnostic Radiology.* New York, NY: McGraw Hill; 2014.)

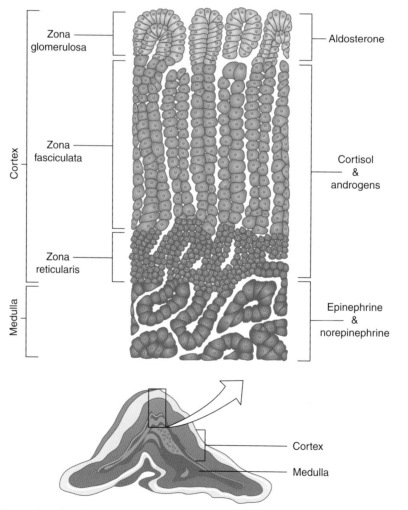

Figure 16-2 · Adrenal gland. (Reproduced, with permission, from Molina PE, ed. *Endocrine Physiology.* 5th ed. New York, NY: McGraw Hill; 2018.)

inputs from the celiac and aorticorenal plexuses, as well as the least splanchnic nerves.

There are many disorders of the kidneys ranging from stones, cysts, tumors, and functional disorders. Because the kidneys are responsible for filtering and removing waste products, excess water, toxins, and other impurities from the body, when renal function is compromised, medical intervention is necessary. The kidneys also regulate pH, salt, and potassium levels, and produce hormones that control blood pressure and the production of red blood cells. End-stage renal disease is treated with dialysis or kidney transplantation and is caused when the nephrons are damaged from diabetes, hypertension, other chronic medical conditions, or from chronic obstructive uropathy. Other conditions that affect the kidneys include kidney stones, glomerulonephritis, polycystic kidney disease, infections, malignancies, and obstructions that lead to hydronephrosis.

The ureters extend from the renal hilum and travel along the psoas muscle to the base of the bladder. They drain urine collected in the renal calices from the renal pelvis by way of peristalsis. Obstructions of the ureters caused by stones or strictures can produce hydronephrosis of the kidney. The ureters can be stented to facilitate the flow of urine and stones and strictures can be managed surgically by several different methods.

The urinary bladder is a muscular, hollow organ that acts as a reservoir for urine. Physiologically, it stores urine at a low pressure to protect the kidneys from damage and completely expels urine at a socially convenient time. The urinary bladder is positioned in the pelvis inferior to the peritoneum and behind the pubic symphysis. Extending from the dome of the bladder toward the umbilicus is the median umbilical ligament which represents the obliterated urachus leftover from embryonic development. The ureters enter the bladder posteroinferiorly and the ureteral orifices and urethra mark the borders of the trigone on the bladder floor. The orifices are approximately 2.5 cm apart. The bladder neck is formed by thickened fibers of the detrusor muscle and acts as a sphincter.

Conditions that affect the bladder include cystitis, urinary incontinence, overactive bladder, stones, and cancer. Physicians often perform urinalysis, KUB imaging, and cystoscopy to diagnose bladder problems.

The prostate is a gland that surrounds the urethra and ejaculatory ducts in males. It is positioned in the pelvis immediately anterior to the rectum and can be palpated through the rectal wall by a digital rectal exam. The prostate produces a thin, milky secretion consisting of calcium, citrate, phosphate ions, clotting enzymes, and most notably, a protein-hydrolyzing enzyme known as prostate-specific antigen or PSA. These secretions make up approximately 30% of the semen. Sixty percent of semen is derived from fluid produced by the seminal vesicles. Each of the two seminal vesicles is associated with its corresponding ductus (vas) deferens and are also removed during a radical prostatectomy for prostate cancer. Benign prostate hyperplasia, also known as an enlarged prostate, is present to some degree in approximately 90% of men by the age of 70 and can obstruct the flow of urine.

The urethra is a channel that connects the urinary bladder to the external urinary meatus and allows for the expulsion of urine from the body. It passes through the prostate and penis in males and is bound to the anterior vaginal wall in females and differs dramatically in length between the two sexes. The female urethra is 3 to 4 cm long whereas the male's is 18 cm on average. A thickened portion of the detrusor (bladder) muscle forms the internal urethral sphincter which constricts the urethra and allows for retention of urine in the bladder. The external urethral sphincter, located deep in the pelvic floor and inferior to the prostate in males, is made of skeletal muscle innervated by the pudendal nerve which allows for voluntary control over voiding.

The male testes, situated within the scrotum, are combined endocrine and exocrine glands that produce sperm and androgens, mainly testosterone. The thick, white capsule covering the testicle is called the tunica albuginea. Within the testes, there are hundreds of lobules containing seminiferous tubules—tiny, coiled ducts where the sperm are produced. The sperm travel from the tubules to the rete testis, efferent ducts, and epididymis where they mature. The tail of the epididymis turns into the vas deferens which passes through the spermatic cord and inguinal canal and ends at the terminal ampula uniting with the seminal vesicle where the sperm are stored as part of semen until they are expelled during ejaculation.

The penis and the scrotum make up the external male genitalia. The scrotum, a pendulous dual-chambered sac of muscle and skin, contains the testes, epididymis, and spermatic cord which incorporates the vas deferens, testicular vessels, and associated lymphatic channels. The two compartments are separated by a septum called the scrotal raphe. The scrotum regulates the temperature of the testes by relaxing and contracting accomplished by the cremaster and dartos fascia. Dartos fascia is a connective tissue found in the penile shaft, foreskin, and scrotum.

The penis is the male sex organ and serves as a conduit for urine and semen to leave the body. It is made up of the corpus cavernosum erectile bodies and corpus spongiosum with the urethra passing through it. Covering the glans, if it is not surgically removed via circumcision, is the foreskin. A ventral fold of skin called the frenulum attaches the foreskin to the head of the penis. Running dorsally along the sides of the penis is the corpus cavernosum, two cylindrical columns of tissue that fill with blood and cause the penis to become erect. The corpus spongiosum, a single column of erectile tissue, passes along the ventral side of the penis and fills with blood during an erection holding the urethra open (see Figure 16-3).

There are multiple conditions affecting the scrotum and testes including hydroceles, testicular torsion, and testicular cancer. Penile cancer is rare and typically starts in the skin cells of the penis, but other conditions are more common. Priapism is a persistent, painful erection typically lasting longer than 4 hours. Peyronie's disease is a buildup of plaque or scar tissue within the penis which causes it to curve and sometimes causes pain. And phimosis is a condition where the foreskin cannot be retracted back off the glans of the penis. Paraphimosis is

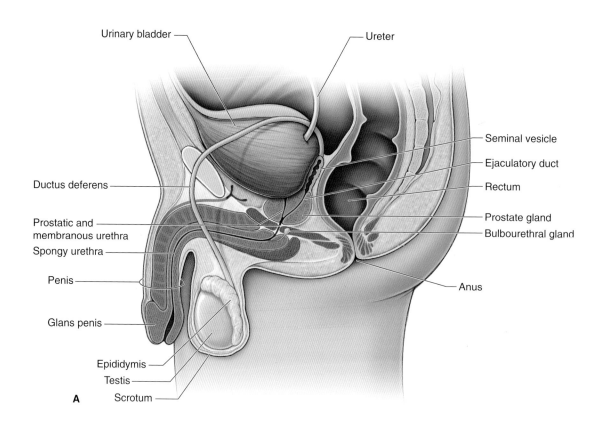

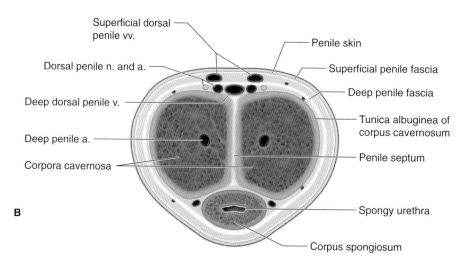

Figure 16-3 · Male reproductive anatomy. (Reproduced, with permission, from Morton DA, Foreman KB, Albertine KH. *The Big Picture: Gross Anatomy*. New York, NY: McGraw Hill; 2011.)

when the foreskin gets stuck behind the head which can cause obstruction of blood flow leading to ischemia and even necrosis if not treated immediately.

Anesthesia

Due to the various types of urologic surgical procedures, a range of anesthesia options are utilized. General anesthesia is always used for major operations but spinal anesthesia or monitored anesthesia care with intravenous sedation may be used for certain minor procedures such as cystoscopy. General anesthesia with endotracheal tube can allow for paralysis in major surgeries while general anesthesia with laryngeal mask airway (LMA) is easier to perform and decreases cardiovascular instability related to reduced anesthetic requirements. Cystoscopy can also be performed in the office with local lidocaine gel or even without anesthesia. Local anesthesia can be used for regional blocks, circumcisions, and vasectomies.

Fluid loss increases during surgery, so it is important that the anesthetists provide sufficient fluid replacement. Some surgeons like to restrict the amount of fluids given during certain

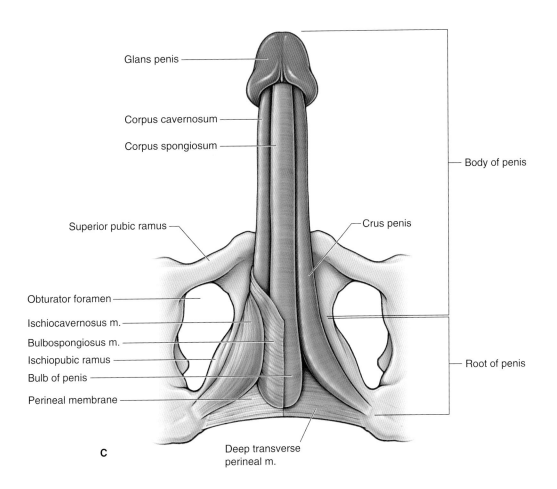

Glans penis

Corpus cavernosum

Corpus spongiosum

Body of penis

Superior pubic ramus

Crus penis

Obturator foramen

Ischiocavernosus m.

Bulbospongiosus m.

Ischiopubic ramus

Bulb of penis

Perineal membrane

Root of penis

C

Deep transverse
perineal m.

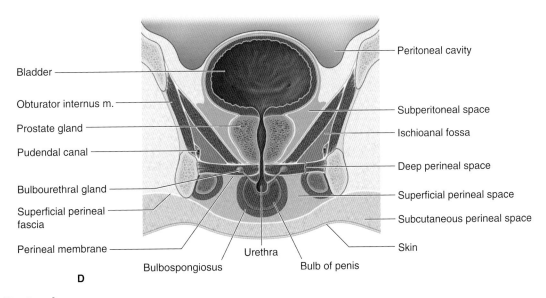

Peritoneal cavity

Bladder

Obturator internus m.

Subperitoneal space

Prostate gland

Ischioanal fossa

Pudendal canal

Deep perineal space

Bulbourethral gland

Superficial perineal space

Superficial perineal
fascia

Subcutaneous perineal space

Perineal membrane

Skin

Bulbospongiosus

Urethra

Bulb of penis

D

Figure 16-3 ▪ (*Continued*)

procedures, namely prostatectomies, to prevent obscuring the surgical field with excessive urine once the bladder is incised and to help minimize edema from the steep Trendelenburg position. It is also noteworthy that there is significantly less fluid loss in laparoscopic and robotic cases when compared to open abdominal surgeries.

Some urologic cases present unique challenges to the anesthesia provider. Adrenal tumors such as pheochromocytomas can cause hypertension and arrhythmias and extra care is taken while monitoring these patients under anesthesia. Arterial lines and Swan-Ganz catheters are frequently utilized. Communication between the surgeon and the anesthesia provider is essential, especially when ligating the venous drainage for the tumor as this maneuver can cause sudden and profound hypotension in the normally hypertensive patient.

Certain medications are also frequently administered by the anesthetist in urologic procedures. Lasix (furosemide) is given to increase urine output. Methylene Blue, Indigo Carmine, or fluorescein may be administered to visualize the ureteral orifices. Mannitol is sometimes used for partial nephrectomies to increase renal blood flow and decrease ischemia-related injuries due to its antioxidant/free radical scavenging properties.

Preparing the Patient for Surgery

Techniques employed are dependent upon the operation being performed. When the groin must be accessed during the procedure, the patient is usually placed in stirrups in the dorsal lithotomy position. Care is taken to prevent overflexion of the hips, injury to the peroneal, femoral, and lumbosacral nerves, and finger/hand injury when the arms are tucked while in the lithotomy position.

Many patients are placed in extreme Trendelenburg positions in order to provide improved access to the pelvic anatomy (the bowels are then displaced cephalad). Newer foam/padded positioning systems are available to prevent the patient from sliding on the bed when it is tilted but utilizing sufficient straps, shoulder braces, and/or padding is vital to patient safety. Trendelenburg allows for excellent visualization of the pelvis, but lung volume may be compromised, especially during laparoscopic procedures. Communication with the anesthesia provider is important.

Patients undergoing nephrectomy are typically placed in a lateral decubitus position with or without the use of the kidney rest with the affected side positioned upwards. The operating table is often flexed just above the iliac crest (at the level of the umbilicus) to provide extra space between the rib cage and the anterior superior iliac spine. An axillary roll is utilized to relieve pressure and prevent brachial plexus nerve injury. The bottom leg is padded and bent and pillows are placed between the legs. The lower arm is placed on a padded arm board and the upper arm may be positioned above it using pillows, blankets, or a padded positioning device. Tape and/or safety straps assure the patient will not slide on the bed if it is tilted during the operation (see Figure 16-4).

The solution utilized for preoperative skin preparation is typically dependent on surgeon preference, but a general rule is to not use alcohol-based formulas in or on a mucous membrane such as the vagina. Towels and fenestrated drapes are often utilized for abdominal procedures and leggings are used when the patient is in lithotomy positioning.

Drains and Catheters

Surgical drains are often placed whenever the urinary tract is opened to provide drainage for potential postoperative urinary leakage. The drain is placed in the abdomen or pelvis adjacent to the surgical site and is often removed 1 to 3 days postoperatively at which time the output has tapered off or is demonstrated not to contain urine.

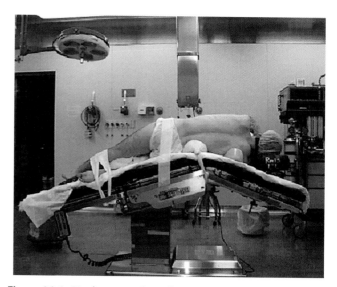

Figure 16-4 • Nephrectomy lateral position. (Reproduced, with permission, from Yokoyama M, Ueda W, Hirakawa M. Haemodynamic effects of the lateral decubitus position and the kidney rest lateral decubitus position during anaesthesia. *Br J Anaesth*. 2000;84(6):753-757.)

Urinary catheters are inserted pre- or peri-operatively to empty the bladder but can also be used to fill the bladder during certain procedures. In prostatectomies, they are used to help identify the urethra and bladder neck during vesicourethral anastomosis. Suprapubic catheterization is utilized in specific situations after operations on the bladder or urethra or where the urethra is compromised or obstructed.

SURGICAL PROCEDURES

Adrenal Gland

Adrenalectomy. An adrenalectomy is the removal of the adrenal gland that caps the kidney. It is usually performed in cases of cancer or functional tumors that are producing excess hormones. Adrenocortical carcinoma and other malignant adrenal tumors are rare. More common are functional tumors and "incidentalomas" which are found by chance on imaging during workup for an unrelated condition.

Pathology: Adrenalectomies are performed for a number of different diseases and disorders. Cushing's syndrome can be caused by excess glucocorticoid production in an adrenal tumor in about 20% to 25% of cases. Primary hyperaldosteronism (also known as Conn's syndrome) is caused by a functional tumor of the adrenal gland and is three times more frequent on the left side than the right. Pheochromocytomas are catecholamine producers (epinephrine, norepinephrine, metanephrine, and normetanephrine) and lead to significant hypertension poorly controlled by medications, headache, diaphoresis, and palpitations.

Diagnostic Procedures: Diagnosis of adrenal tumors depends on the type. In Cushing's Disease, a pituitary tumor must be ruled out and diurnal serum cortisol levels are measured.

In Cushing's syndrome, a dexamethasone suppression test is conducted to confirm adrenal pathology as the cause of elevated cortisol production. A tumor is suspected if no depression of the steroid level occurs. Adrenocorticotropic hormones are measured, and CT scans are performed to help locate the tumor. Hyperaldosteronism is suspected if serum potassium is low and a tumor can be diagnosed following a series of blood tests measuring plasma renin and aldosterone levels at different intervals. Meta-iodobenzylguanidine (MIBG) scintigraphy nuclear scan, CT scans, and/or MRIs may be performed. These tests are also commonly used to diagnose pheochromocytomas in addition to plasma-free metanephrine blood testing and oral clonidine suppression tests.

Procedural sequence:

- Patient is positioned either supine or lateral depending on the preferred approach. If a lateral incision is being utilized, the affected side is positioned up. From here, the steps will depend on whether an open or a minimally invasive approach is used. For open adrenalectomy, access to the abdomen is gained through either a flank supracostal or thoracic abdominal incision. For a minimally invasive approach, access is through the placement of multiple trocars that are typically placed in the midclavicular line in a trans-peritoneal fashion.

- In a left adrenalectomy, the colon is mobilized first which includes taking down the splenorenal and splenocolic ligaments. The surgical assistant (SA) will help maintain exposure with suction and retraction. In a right adrenalectomy, the liver may be lifted and retracted by the assistant before mobilizing the hepatic flexure of the colon and duodenum (Kocher maneuver) and opening Gerota's fascia.

- Any crossing vessels along the plane of dissection are cauterized or ligated medially toward the renal hilum until the renal vein is identified.

- The kidney is gently retracted downwards to bring the adrenal gland into view. Excess traction can cause bleeding from small vessel attachments from the liver or spleen, so caution is needed.

- The gland is mobilized along its lateral border and adipose tissue surrounding the adrenal is gently teased away.

- The blood supply varies from the left and right sides. The arterial supply usually consists of multiple small branches, but the venous anatomy is more consistent, draining into the vena cava on the right and the renal vein on the left. Regardless of the side, the adrenal vein is dissected out and ligated usually with clips placed by the surgeon or assistant. In cases of pheochromocytoma, ligation of the vein should be done as early as possible. This is imperative as manipulation of the tumor can release excess catecholamines into the vascular system leading to hypertensive crisis.

- Once the blood supply is ligated and the rest of the adrenal gland isolated and freed, the wound bed is inspected for bleeding and Gerota's fascia is closed.

Kidney

Kidney Stone Surgery: Nephrolithotomy involves removing a stone from the kidney. It is usually accomplished minimally invasively through extracorporeal shockwave lithotripsy (ESWL) treatment. Fluoroscopy is used to locate the kidney stone and shockwaves are used to break up the stone. Occasionally, in cases of a very large or hard stone, a percutaneous nephrolithotomy can be performed. For percutaneous nephrolithotomy, an interventional radiologist or urologist first gains access to the kidney through the flank. A wire is placed from outside the patient's flank, through the kidney and down the ureter to the bladder using fluoroscopy. The tract is then dilated and a nephroscope is directed into the kidney, at which time the stone is fragmented using ultrasonic, pneumatic, and/or laser treatment. Smaller kidney stones are often treated with ureteroscopy and laser lithotripsy via a retrograde approach from the urethra. Because of the success of these minimally invasive procedures, an open or laparoscopic anatrophic nephrolithotomy procedure is rarely required, usually in cases of large staghorn renal calculi.

Pathology: Renal calculi form as a buildup of certain waste products in the kidneys such as calcium oxalate and other mineral and salt deposits. Stones can cause flank pain, infection, fever, hematuria, and hydronephrosis.

Diagnostic Procedures: Calculi are usually diagnosed with typical radiological scans such as plain abdominal x-rays and urograms. A CT scan can be used to identify weakly radiolucent stones. Urine cultures are often positive for UTI with large staghorn stones. It is imperative to treat positive urine cultures prior to surgical intervention to avoid preventable cases of urosepsis.

Anatrophic nephrolithotomy surgery—steps highlighted:

- Patient is placed in a lateral position and entry into the abdominal cavity is gained.

- Depending on which side is affected, the anatomy is different so the colon or the duodenum is mobilized to provide visualization of the renal hilum. Retraction of the liver is provided by the assistant if needed.

- The renal vein and artery are skeletonized.

- Gerota's fascia is incised and the renal capsule is exposed.

- The avascular plane of the kidney (Brodel line) is usually identified by gently clamping the posterior segmental artery and having the anesthesia provider inject methylene blue and mannitol.

- The renal artery is then usually occluded with an atraumatic bulldog-type clamp. In a robotic procedure, this clamp is usually applied laparoscopically by the assistant. The vein may also be similarly clamped. Some surgeons may choose not to occlude the blood supply at all and rely solely on the proper dissection of the kidney through Brodel's line which is supposed to be avascular. However, limiting the blood by clamping the renal artery is very common.

- Renal hypothermia is sometimes utilized to reduce ischemic damage to the kidney. If the surgeon chooses this approach, a dam is placed around the kidney with the help of the assistant and ice is packed within the barrier. The kidney is cooled for 10 to 20 minutes before the renal capsule is incised.

- The renal capsule is then sharply incised, and the stone is exposed. The parenchyma is bluntly separated, and the stone is gently elevated from the kidney. Radiographs are helpful to identify potential stones in adjacent calyces.

- The pelvis is closed around a catheter or double J stent and then the capsule is closed in two layers. Deep absorbable stitches are utilized followed by interrupted, usually buttressed with a clip bolster or fat pad.

Nephrectomy. Nephrectomy is the removal of a kidney. Since the anatomy of the kidney differs between left and right, it is important to understand these variations when operating. The right kidney is lower than the left because of displacement by the liver. Due to the position of the inferior vena cava and aorta, the right renal artery is usually longer than the left and the left renal vein is longer than the right. The left renal vein also commonly receives tributaries from the phrenic, adrenal, gonadal, and lumbar veins. Abnormalities in renal vasculature are present in up to 75% of patients and supernumerary arteries are very common.

Pathology: Nephrectomy is performed for a number of both malignant and benign reasons including renal tumor or mass, severe polycystic kidney syndrome, medically untreatable or recurrent infections, renal abscess nonfunctioning kidney associated with hypertension or nephrolithiasis, or irreparable trauma. A "simple nephrectomy" (named so because it does not include the removal of Gerota's fascia, not because the procedure itself is easy) is typically performed for some pathology. Otherwise, a total radical nephrectomy is indicated. Renal cell carcinoma (RCC) is the most common malignancy of the kidney, and radical nephrectomy is the primary treatment since RCC is relatively refractory to chemotherapy and radiation therapy. RCC has a relatively unique biology in that the tumor can extend into the renal vein and even inferior vena cava. Intracaval tumors are often dealt with a multidisciplinary approach that involves a vascular surgeon or even cardiac surgeon as these tumors can sometimes extend all the way up the inferior vena cava and into the right atrium.

Diagnostic Procedures: Nonfunctioning kidneys can be diagnosed by an excretory urogram, diuretic nuclear renal scan, or CT scan. Occasionally, stents or urostomy tubes are placed to confirm that lack of function documented by contrast studies isn't caused by an obstruction. Renal ultrasound, pyelography, CT scans, and MRI are often used to diagnose and confirm a renal mass. Up to 80% of solid renal masses are renal cell carcinomas and are easily visualized on a CT scan. They can be biopsied before surgery depending upon the imaging appearance of the tumor. Surgery can be avoided for biopsy-confirmed oncocytoma which are known to be benign. Angiomyolipomas often show signs of macroscopic fat on CT scan and can be monitored when small because of their benign nature. However, as angiomyolipomas grow to greater than 4 cm, they are at risk for hemorrhage and surgical intervention may be warranted.

Procedural sequence in total nephrectomy:

- Patient is positioned laterally with the affected side facing up. Access to the abdomen is gained through either a flank or thoracic-abdominal incision or through the placement of multiple trocars in the midclavicular line for laparoscopic transperitoneal surgery. Large tumors and those with IVC tumor thrombus are often performed via subcostal or chevron incision in the supine position.

- In a left nephrectomy, the colon is mobilized first. In a right nephrectomy, the liver may be lifted and retracted by the SA before mobilizing the colon and duodenum (Kocher maneuver) and opening Gerota's fascia.

- The gonadal vein and ureter are identified just below the lower pole of the kidney and the ureterogonadal dissection is continued up toward the hilum. Any crossing vessels along the plane of dissection are cauterized or ligated.

- For a right nephrectomy, a plane is created between the gonadal and the IVC to identify the psoas muscle which the kidney rests upon and on the left, the ureter and gonadal are lifted similarly to visualize the psoas.

- The renal vein and artery are identified and skeletonized to facilitate adequate clipping or stapling which is often carried out by the SA in robotic cases.

- The adrenal vein is then identified and either spared or included in the resection depending on whether or not there is indication for excision of the adrenal gland in addition to the kidney. This depends upon the location and extent of the renal tumor.

- The renal artery is always ligated first followed by the renal vein. Hem-o-lok clips or a vascular stapler are typically utilized for this step in laparoscopic/robotic surgery. In robotic surgery, the SA is vital during this step. They must have a steady hand and be well-versed in the operation of the clip or stapler of choice to avoid accidentally tearing the vessels. In open cases, the vessels are often controlled with 0 silk-free ties or suture ligatures.

- The ureter is then clipped by the surgeon or assistant and transected at the level of the iliac crossing.

- The kidney is separated from its lateral attachments. Any remaining attachments to the liver or spleen are taken down and the kidney is freed off the psoas.

- Hemostasis is confirmed, and the specimen extracted from the wound. If minimally invasive, it is bagged by the assistant and removed through an extended port site incision either midline or through a muscle-splitting Gibson incision.

- Retroperitoneal lymph node dissection is often indicated for large renal masses and urothelial carcinoma. The borders of dissection on the right side are as follows: the renal vasculature cephalad, the ureter laterally, the aorta medially, the bifurcation of the iliac vessels caudally, and the anterior spinous ligament posteriorly. The borders of dissection on the left side are as follows: the renal vasculature cephalad, the ureter laterally, the vena cava medially, the bifurcation of the iliac vessels caudally, and the anterior spinous ligament posteriorly (see Figure 16-5). Care must be taken to achieve adequate hemostasis and lymphostasis with clips and bipolar electrocautery. Patients are at risk for postoperative chylous ascites and should maintain a low-fat diet.

Procedural sequence in partial nephrectomy:

- The steps for a partial nephrectomy are the same as a total until after the dissection of the hilum. For a partial nephrectomy, the renal artery and vein are temporarily clamped rather than ligated. The renal vein can be clamped for very large and centrally located tumors but otherwise is left patent to allow for some retrograde blood flow and renal perfusion.

- Gerota's fascia is peeled off the kidney to expose the tumor and its borders are marked with cautery using the ultrasonic probe as a guide.

- Once the renal vein and artery are identified, the tumor is located using a sterile ultrasound probe. Recently, with the introduction of special robotic cameras and equipment, indocyanine green (ICG) dye has been utilized to help identify at least partially exophytic kidney tumors. The kidney will glow green under the fluorescent lighting, but the tumor will remain dark. ICG can alternatively be given to better characterize the renal vasculature.

- The renal artery and often the vein are then gently occluded using a bulldog-type clamp. In a robotic procedure, these are often placed by the SA. The artery is always clamped first. The start of ischemic time is noted as soon as the artery is clamped. Maximal preparation before clamping is mandatory to ensure renal warm ischemia time is kept to a minimum.

- If using ice to induce renal hypothermia, a barrier made of laps and/or an isolation bag is introduced and filled with ice-slush. The kidney is allowed to cool for 10 to 20 minutes before the tumor excision begins.

- The tumor is then sharply dissected free from the normal kidney parenchyma. The SA utilizes suction to maintain the visual field.

- After the tumor is excised, the kidney defect is closed in two layers. An absorbable suture, commonly a 3-0 Monocryl, is used to close the deep layer and collecting system if it was entered. Larger absorbable interrupted Vicryl stitches with bolsters are used for the second layer to reapproximate the cortical edges. In a robotic procedure, the assistant places the bolsters, usually in the form of large or extra-large hemolok clips, and secures the end of the sutures with lapra-ty's.

- The bulldog clamps are removed from the renal artery and vein and total ischemic time is noted.

- The kidney is examined for hemostasis and additional sutures may be placed or tightened with Hem-o-lok clips or Lapra-ty's.

- Gerotas is sewn back over the defect and a drain is often placed.

- The specimen is bagged and removed from the wound and the wound is closed in layers.

Procedural sequence in nephroureterectomy:

- The steps for a nephroureterectomy are the same as a total nephrectomy until the clipping and transection of the ureter.

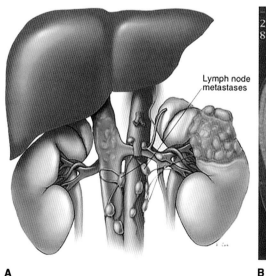
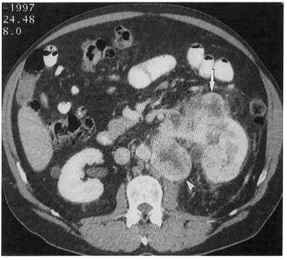

Figure 16-5 · Retroperitoneal lymph node dissection. (Reproduced, with permission, from Sheth S, Scatarige JC, Horton KM, Corl FM, Fishman EK. Current concepts in the diagnosis and management of renal cell carcinoma: Role of multidetector CT and three-dimensional CT. *Radiographics.* 2001;21:Spec No:S237-S254.)

- After the renal vein and artery are transected and the kidney freed from all of its attachments, the ureter is identified and dissected out all the way down to the bladder. Gentle traction on the ureter helps facilitate this.

- To ensure that the entire ureter and a small cuff of bladder is removed, a cystoscopy is sometimes performed just prior to the nephrectomy and the ureteral orifice is partially disarticulated from the bladder using a resectoscope loop or Collin's knife. Alternatively, the bladder may be backfilled with saline by the assistant or a nurse to identify the ureterovesical junction.

- At this point, the ureter may be clipped before it is excised along with a bladder margin. The aim is to minimize spillage and tumor seeding. If done robotically, the SA is responsible for all clipping.

- The bladder is closed in two layers and a drain is left according to surgeon preference. The drain is typically placed adjacent to the bladder closure.

- The kidney and ureter are extracted through an extended incision and the wound is closed in the typical fashion.

- Retroperitoneal lymph node dissection is often indicated for large renal masses and urothelial carcinoma. The borders of dissection on the right side are as follows: the renal vasculature cephalad, the ureter laterally, the aorta medially, the bifurcation of the iliac vessels caudally, and the anterior spinous ligament posteriorly. The borders of dissection on the left side are as follows: the renal vasculature cephalad, the ureter laterally, the vena cava medially, the bifurcation of the iliac vessels caudally, and the anterior spinous ligament posteriorly. Care must be taken to achieve adequate hemostasis and lymphostasis with clips and bipolar electrocautery. Lumbar vessels can be particularly perilous. Patients are at risk for postoperative chylous ascites and should maintain a low-fat diet.

Procedural sequence in pyelolithtomy: Pyelolithotomy is performed for a retained stone in the renal pelvis and is becoming uncommon with less invasive treatments readily available. Failing a percutaneous nephrolithotomy or ESWL may indicate the need for a pyelolithomy for removal of renal calculi (see Figure 16-6).

Surgery—steps highlighted:

- Oftentimes, cystoscopy with ureteral stent placement is performed at the beginning of the procedure. Patient is then placed in a lateral position and entry into the abdominal cavity is gained.

- The intestines are reflected to obtain visualization of the renal pelvis and ureter.

- Gerota's fascia is incised and perirenal fat dissected away so that the ureteropelvic junction is clearly defined.

- A longitudinal incision is made into the renal pelvis and the stone or stones are carefully extracted. The incision may be extended for larger calculi.

- The renal pelvis is then closed with 4-0 absorbable suture in a running fashion and a drain is placed and secured.

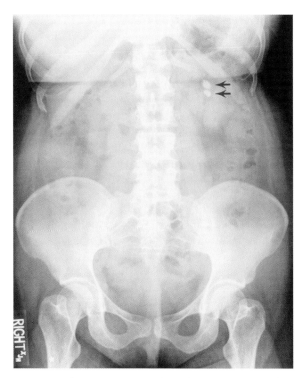

Figure 16-6 • Kidney stone. (Reproduced, with permission, from Chen MYM, Pope TL, Ott DJ. *Basic Radiology*. 2nd ed. New York, NY: McGraw Hill; 2011.)

Ureter

Ureteroscopy. Ureteroscopy is performed to visualize the ureter and insides of the kidney—renal pelvis and calyces. A ureteroscope is placed through the urethra and bladder into the ureter. A biopsy and/or images can then be taken of suspicious tissue, or a stone can be broken up and removed. Laser lithotripsy of ureteral stones is facilitated by passing a small laser fiber through the ureteroscope. Snares or baskets can then be used to remove the fragments. Typically, this is done without the use of an SA. Ureteroscopy is always performed with fluoroscopy and a safety wire. A temporary ureteral stent is often left at the conclusion of the procedure.

Ureterotomy. Ureterotomy is the surgical incision into a ureter. It is performed to remove a stone or as a procedural step in part of a larger procedure such as a pyeloplasty, pyelolithotomy, ureteral reimplantation, cystectomy, or other operation that involves the ureters. Most of those procedures are covered separately in this chapter.

Ureteral Reconstruction. The ureter may need to be reconstructed for several reasons such as cancer, stricture, obstruction, or trauma, or as part of a larger procedure such as a cystectomy. Sometimes, such as the case with trauma or ureteral injury, the ureter can simply be re-anastomosed. If the injury or stricture is low enough, the ureter can be reimplanted directly into the bladder. In cases where a larger part of the ureter needs to be removed, it can be replaced and reconstructed with a portion of bladder (Boari flap procedure) or bowel. When the lower portion of the ureter is removed, it is often necessary to perform a psoas hitch procedure where the bladder is mobilized cephalad to allow the shortened ureter to be reimplanted. Ureteral reconstruction options are dictated by the underlying pathology and remaining ureteral length. For proximal ureteral issues that cannot be immediately re-anastomosed (uretero-ureterostomy), surgical options are replacement with ileal interposition, boari bladder flap, transuretero-ureterostomy, or auto-transplantation down to the pelvis. While transuretero-ureterostomy seems like a good idea, it is fraught with potential issues as both kidneys are now tied to one outflow tract. This has obvious risks when stone disease and malignancy are part of the underlying disease so both kidneys are subject to one stone or cancer recurrence. For mid-ureter pathology, boari bladder flap and psoas hitch reconstructions are ideal. For distal ureteral pathology, ureteroneocystostomy or ureteral reimplant is the best option.

Pyeloplasty. Open (or laparoscopic) pyeloplasty is the surgical reconstruction of the renal pelvis and the gold standard for treatment of a ureteropelvic junction obstruction (UPJO) usually from a crossing vessel or acquired stricture. Ureteroscopy with laser endo-ureterotomy and stenting is a minimally invasive procedure that has good efficacy with stricture but will simply not address UPJ obstruction secondary to crossing vessel or high insertion of the ureter into the renal pelvis.

Pathology: UPJ obstruction can be either congenital or acquired. It impairs the flow of urine from the kidney to the bladder and often causes flank pain, progressive renal insufficiency, and hydronephrosis. Congenital causes of UPJ obstruction include intrinsic narrowing of the ureteropelvic junction, high insertion of the ureter into the renal pelvis, or compression of the ureter by a band of tissue or renal vessel (up to 50% of cases). Acquired obstruction is often caused by trauma or strictures but also by tumor or stones.

Diagnostic Procedures: Intravenous pyelogram, renal scan with furosemide washout, and retrograde pyelograms are used to diagnose UPJ obstructions and CT scans, and ultrasound has also been found to be helpful.

Surgery—steps highlighted:

- If a stent has not already been placed in the affected ureter, it is done so at the beginning of the procedure.
- After stent placement, the patient is placed in a lateral position with the affected side up.
- The abdominal cavity is safely entered, and the retrospective colonic flexure is mobilized and the bowel reflected. Adequate retraction and suction are provided by the SA.
- The proximal ureter is identified, and the ureteral stent should be able to be palpated.
- The renal pelvis can then be identified by following the ureter cephalad.

- At this point, a crossing vessel or stricture is encountered and the pelvis and ureter are dissected free around it and the adjacent structures.
- If a crossing vessel is the cause of the obstruction, the blood supply is spared by transecting the ureter and repositioning it to the other side of the vessel so that it is no longer being compressed.
- If the obstruction is caused by a stricture, the damaged section of ureter is cut out and removed.
- The proximal ureter is then spatulated and anastomosed with 4-0 absorbable suture in a running fashion around the stent to the renal pelvis.
- A drain is placed, and the wound is closed in layers.

Bladder

Cystoscopy. Cystoscopy is used to visualize the inside of the bladder for a number of diagnostic and therapeutic reasons. This can be done in conjunction with a larger procedure or by itself. Cystoscopy is sometimes also performed during difficult urinary catheter placement.

A cystoscope is passed through the urethra into the urinary bladder which is then filled with a saline solution or sterile water so that the inside of the bladder can be visualized. From here, the bladder wall and the ureteral orifices can be inspected, biopsies taken, tumor resected, bladder stones removed, and additional procedures performed. There is usually no need for an SA for these cases.

Cystectomy. Cystectomy is the total or partial removal of the urinary bladder and is usually performed because of cancer. A partial cystectomy is reserved for smaller lesions that cannot be removed successfully by transurethral resection of bladder tumor (TURBT). Tumors amenable to partial cystectomy are solitary muscle-invasive lesions in both time and space. A requirement for partial cystectomy is also the ability to have sufficient margin circumferentially and ample distance from the trigone. Simple cystectomy is rarely performed and is the removal of the entire bladder while leaving adjacent structures intact and without a lymph node dissection. Indications for simple cystectomy include benign conditions such as neurogenic bladder or pain. Radical cystectomy, however, is a major operation involving multiple organs and sometimes even multiple surgical specialties. In males, radical cystectomy involves the removal of not only the urinary bladder but also the prostate, and seminal vesicles. In women, the urethra, uterus, broad ligaments, and part of the vaginal wall are also excised in addition to the bladder. An extensive lymphadenectomy is performed in both sexes.

Reconstruction after removal of the bladder often involves the use of the small bowel or colon for urinary diversion where a piece of bowel is used to create a urinary diversion. There are many different approaches to replacing a diseased bladder. These include cutaneous fistulas such as nephrostomies and ureterostomies, implantation of the ureters directly into the sigmoid colon, and implantation into pouches made of isolated sections of bowel most commonly distal ileum. In addition to

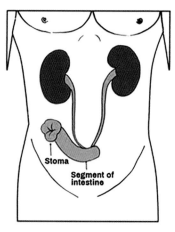
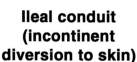

Ileal conduit (incontinent diversion to skin)

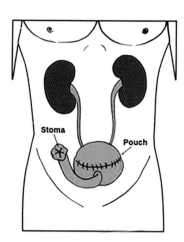

Continent cutaneous reservoir (continent diversion to skin)

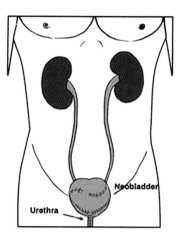

Orthotopic neobladder (continent diversion to urethra)

Figure 16-7 · Cystectomy. (Reproduced, with permission, from Pardalidis P, Nikolaos Andriopoulos N, Pardalidis N. Robotic orthotopic neobladder: The two chimney technique. In: Ziglioli F, Maestroni U, eds. *Modern Approach to Diagnosis and Treatment of Bladder Cancer.* IntechOpen; 2021. doi: 10.5772/intechopen.91525 [www.intechopen.com/chapters/78553])

bowel conduits that are connected to a urostomy bag, there are also continent catheterizable reservoirs and orthotopic neobladder reconstructions (see Figure 16-7).

Pathology: High-grade muscle-invasive urothelial carcinoma (formerly known as transitional cell carcinoma) is an indication for radical cystectomy. The procedure is carried out for high tumor grade, infiltration of the muscle, visceral fat, or adjacent organs, and cancers that have failed TURBT and chemo/immunotherapy. Patients often undergo neoadjuvant chemotherapy prior to radical cystectomy.

Diagnostic Procedures: Diagnosis is usually made through TURBT and staged with CT scans of the abdomen and pelvis. PET scans can be used to evaluate for metastasis to the bone in patients with symptoms or elevated serum calcium or alkaline phosphatase levels.

Procedural sequence in radical cystectomy in men: Step order differs depending on whether an open or minimally invasive procedure is being performed. In an open procedure, the anterior bladder and prostatic attachments are taken down first whereas they are left for later in a laparoscopic or robotic procedure.

- Patient is placed in Trendelenburg in either a supine or lithotomy position depending on whether or not urethrectomy is planned at the time of the initial surgery and a catheter is placed in the bladder.

- Entry into the abdomen is obtained laparoscopically or through a lower midline incision.

- Often, adhesions to the colon must be taken down. Adequate suction and retraction are provided by the SA.

- The ureters are identified where they cross the common iliac vessel and are dissected free down to the level of the bladder where they are ligated and divided, and the distal ends are tagged and brought out of the pelvis and safely tucked away until later. If doing a laparoscopic/robotic procedure, a short piece of suture can be tied to a hemo-lok clip before it is used to ligate the ureter making it easier to locate and manipulate later.

- The pouch of Douglas and Denonvilliers fascia is identified, and a plane is developed in a blunt fashion between the rectum and the bladder. The peritoneal incision made for the ureteral dissection can be continued to help identify this plane.

- The dissection continues caudally to the seminal vesicles and Denonvielliers fascia to the apex of the prostate.

- An extended bilateral pelvic lymphadenectomy is performed and incorporates the internal, external, obturator and common iliac lymph node packets. The borders of dissection are the inguinal ligament caudally, the common iliac vessels cephalad, the genitofemoral nerve anteriorly, the pelvic side wall laterally, the bladder medially, and the internal iliac vessels posteriorly. Hemostasis and lymphostasis are achieved with bipolar electrocautery and clips. In a robotic procedure, these clips are placed by the SA.

- The pedicles of the bladder and prostate should now be easily visualized. The anterior division of the internal iliac artery, which branches into the inferior and superior vesical artery, is ligated and divided.

- The endopelvic fascia surrounding the prostate is then opened and the levator muscle attachments are cleared away exposing the prostate and apex.

- At this time, a nerve-sparing prostatectomy may be performed if indicated. The neurovascular bundles posterior and lateral to the prostate are spared using a combination of sharp and blunt dissection. In robotic procedures, the perforating vessels are clipped by the SA and divided by the surgeon with minimal use of cautery.

- The space of Retzius is bluntly opened and the dissection is extended laterally until the ventral surface of the bladder and the prostate are exposed.

- The vas deferens are encountered laterally, dissected free, and divided.

- The anterior dissection of the bladder and prostate can now be completed. The urachal remnant by the umbilicus is dissected free from its attachment and the bladder is mobilized down to the level of the endopelvic fascia and puboprostatic ligaments.

- The dorsal venous complex is secured with 0 or 2-0 absorbable suture. It is then incised proximal to the suture and the urethra is transected exposing the Foley catheter.

- The prostatic dissection is then completed, and any remaining prostatic attachments and pedicles are clipped, often by the assistant, and divided by the surgeon with cold scissors up to and beyond the apex.

- The Foley catheter is clipped to avoid urine spillage and divided. It is placed in an endobag by the assistant along with the prostate and bladder and removed from the patient.

- The urinary diversion of choice is then performed. The most common is an ileal conduit using a section of the terminal ileum. The most distal 10 to 15 cm of terminal ileum is spared to allow for adequate Vitamin B12 absorption.

- An incision into an avascular section of the mesentery is made between the ileocolic and right colic arteries which is approximately 10 to 15 cm from the ileocecal valve and the bowel divided with Endo GIA stapler. This can either be done by the surgeon using an open, laparoscopic, or robotic stapler or by the SA.

- Making sure there are enough mesenteric vascular arcades to supply the chosen segment of bowel, the surgeon selects a point on the proximal ileum to divide it. The isolated loop of bowel should be about 15 cm long.

- Ileal re-anastomosis is performed cephalad to the conduit in a side-to-side fashion using Endo GIA and TA staplers. The mesenteric window is closed to avoid internal herniation of the bowel.

- This isolated segment of the bowel will act as the new urinary reservoir. Open-ended single J stents are inserted bilaterally, and the terminal ends of the ureters are spatulated and anastomosed to the proximal end of the conduit using one of several techniques. Absorbable sutures are used and can be placed in a running or interrupted fashion.

- A stoma is then created with the distal end of the conduit by the surgeon and assistant. A circular plug of subcutaneous fat and skin is excised from the chosen stoma site on the abdomen. The fascia is incised and muscle split to allow entry into the abdominal cavity. The distal conduit is brought up through the defect taking care not to twist the mesentery and compromise the blood flow. The conduit can be gently sutured to the posterior fascia to prevent parastomal hernia. The stoma is matured, and its edges everted using interrupted absorbable sutures per the Brooke technique.

- With the urinary diversion complete, the bladder and prostate can be bagged and removed en bloc (if not done so already), drains may be placed, and the wound is closed in the usual fashion.

Procedural sequence in radical cystectomy in women: Step order differs depending on whether an open or minimally invasive procedure is being performed. In an open procedure, the anterior bladder is taken down first whereas it is left for later in a laparoscopic or robotic procedure.

- Patient is placed in Trendelenburg and in the lithotomy position, a catheter is placed in the bladder, and a sponge stick is placed in the vagina.

- Entry into the abdomen is obtained laparoscopically or through a lower midline incision.

- Often, adhesions to the colon must be taken down. Suction and retraction are provided by the SA.

- A total radical hysterectomy with bilateral salpingo-oophorectomy is performed first. The broad and round ligaments are dissected, ligated, and divided as well as the other lateral structures and attachments until the uterus, tubes, and ovaries are fully mobilized. The assistant will often help by positioning the uterus with a uterine manipulator or the sponge stick that was placed vaginally at the beginning of the case.

- The ureters are identified where they cross the common iliac vessel and are dissected free down to the level of the bladder.

- Just lateral to the medial umbilical ligaments, the peritoneum is opened, and the dissection is extended laterally on either side of the bladder.

- The ureters are ligated and divided at the bladder insertion and the distal ends are tagged and brought out of the pelvis and safely tucked away until later. If doing a laparoscopic/robotic procedure, a short piece of suture can be tied to a hemo-lok clip by the assistant before it is used to ligate the ureter making it easier to locate and manipulate later.

- The pedicles of the bladder are identified and the anterior division of the internal iliac artery, which branches into the inferior and superior vesical artery, is ligated, and divided.

- The posterior fornix of the vagina is easily visualized because of the previously inserted sponge stick and is incised.

- The incision is carried along the lateral wall of the vagina and is continued distally until reaching the urethra.

- The bladder can then be taken down anteriorly. The peritoneum is incised and the space of Retizus is developed, and the bladder is fully mobilized.

- The urethrectomy can be performed intracorporeally or through the vagina. In either case, an inverted U-shaped incision is made around the urethra, and it is mobilized anteriorly and laterally followed by the posterolateral dissection.
- The entire specimen is removed en bloc.
- The posterior aspect of the vagina is then mobilized, and strong, absorbable sutures are used to close the vaginal defect.
- An extended bilateral pelvic lymphadenectomy is performed and incorporates the internal, external, obturator, and common iliac lymph node packets. The borders of dissection are the inguinal ligament caudally, the common iliac vessels cephalad, the genitofemoral nerve anteriorly, the pelvic side wall laterally, the bladder medially, and the internal iliac vessels posteriorly. Hemostasis and lymphostasis are achieved with bipolar electrocautery and clips.
- The urinary diversion of choice is then completed.
- Drains are placed, and the wound closed in the usual fashion.

Bladder Neck Suspension/Vaginal Wall Sling. Bladder suspension is performed for urinary incontinence in women. Incontinence is common in older women and following vaginal delivery. It occurs often alongside prolapse because of denervation and weakening of the pelvic floor muscles but may also be caused by detrusor (bladder) muscle instability. It is important to differentiate stress incontinence from urge-related incontinence as the former is treated surgically and the latter is treated with behavioral modification and medications. Both are quite common in the aging woman. Repair with an anterior vaginal wall sling is appropriate for treatment of incontinence caused by intrinsic sphincter dysfunction or bladder-neck hypermobility. Modifications of the procedure are also utilized to treat patients with low-grade cystoceles. The most common procedure used today to treat urinary stress incontinence is the mid-urethral sling.

Diagnostic Procedures: Diagnosis of urinary incontinence is usually made by a clinical history and examination. The patient may be asked to cough with a full bladder to observe the effects. A cystoscopy may be performed, or more in-depth urodynamic testing may be warranted.

Surgery—steps highlighted:

- Patient is placed in a lithotomy position and draped to expose the vagina and suprapubic region with the anus covered for sterility.
- A weighted vaginal speculum is inserted, and silk sutures are often used to retract the labia for better exposure.
- A Foley catheter is placed and the bladder is drained.
- The vaginal wall is grasped with an allis clamp halfway from meatus to bladder neck and 10cc of saline or local anesthetic is injected just under the anterior vaginal wall beneath the proposed incision site. This has a dual purpose of pain control and hydro-dissection of the vaginal epithelium from the underlying connective tissue.
- A midline anterior vaginal wall incision is made at the level of the mid-urethra.
- A pocket is developed between the vaginal wall and underlying urethral and paraurethral tissue and extended laterally.
- Being careful not to puncture the bladder, a special percutaneous needle carrier/vaginal trocar is then passed through the vaginal wall and the retropubic space to exit above the pubic symphysis approximately 2.5 cm lateral to the midline. Small puncture incisions can be made in the suprapubic region over the exit sites to facilitate the passage of the trocars. This describes the transvaginal tape or sling procedure, also known as TVT. Another approach is to pass the trocars through the obturator foramen and out laterally in the groin region. This is known as the TOT procedure.
- The suspending sutures of the mesh are then threaded into the trocar with the ligature carrier and retrieved at the abdominal skin site.
- Cystoscopy is performed to confirm that the bladder was not injured.
- After passing the ends of the mesh bilaterally, it is tensioned appropriately around the urethra to stabilize it.
- Once correctly positioned, the tails of the mesh protruding from the abdominal wall are cut off just below the skin.
- The wounds are irrigated, Foley replaced, and vaginal packing inserted.

Prostate

TURP. Transurethral resection of the prostate (TURP) is performed in cases of benign prostatic hyperplasia (BPH) otherwise known as an enlarged prostate. A cystoscopy is performed and the prostatic urethra is visualized. The enlarged prostate is then removed endoscopically with a resectoscope cautery loop or laser. Larger prostatic adenomas can be treated with an open or laparoscopic surgery called a simple prostatectomy. Indications for surgical intervention for BPH include voiding dysfunction from the enlarged prostate, persistent gross hematuria, obstructive uropathy, recurrent urinary tract infection, bladder calculi, and urinary retention. Other more minimally invasive procedures include greenlight laser prostatectomy, transurethral microwave therapy, uro-lift procedure, among others.

Prostatectomy. Radical prostatectomy is performed for malignancy of the prostate. A less aggressive simple prostatectomy is reserved for extremely large benign prostatic adenomas in cases of BPH. For years, open retropubic radical prostatectomy has been the gold standard for treatment of prostate cancer that requires surgical intervention. Recently, however, robotic-assisted prostatectomies have arguably replaced open surgery as the treatment of choice and the new gold standard. The DaVinci robot allows for excellent visualization and nerve sparing which may decrease erectile and urinary continence complications postoperatively. It also can significantly reduce blood loss. The prostate can also be removed through a perineal approach. There are also less invasive options for prostate cancer including brachytherapy, external beam radiation therapy, and focal ablation techniques such as cryotherapy and high-intensity focused ultrasound therapy (HIFU).

Pathology: Up to 90% of prostate cancers are adenocarcinomas and many arise simultaneously in multiple zones of the prostate. The cancer may spread to the bladder neck, ejaculatory ducts, and/or seminal vesicles. Distant metastasis is usually to the bone. Prostate cancer is graded by Gleason score and not all cases of prostate cancer need to be treated. Some patients have slow-growing carcinomas that can be monitored for years and sometimes indefinitely. Patients with a higher Gleason score of greater than or equal to 7 usually benefit from surgical removal or other treatment. Older men are at higher risk; it is less common in men under 50 years of age but can be more aggressive in younger patients.[9]

Diagnostic Procedures: Prostate cancer is initially diagnosed with a PSA (prostate-specific antigen) blood test, DRE (digital rectal exam), and finally confirmed with a biopsy. MRI fusion biopsy is rapidly becoming a diagnostic tool employed by centers of excellence. BPH is diagnosed based on patient history and symptoms, digital rectal exam, and urinalysis.

Procedural sequence in radical prostatectomy:

- Patient is placed in a supine or lithotomy position in deep Trendelenburg, draped appropriately with the penis prepped into the field, and a Foley catheter is placed.

- Entry into the abdominal cavity is gained.

- Often, adhesions to the colon must be taken down. Suction and retraction are provided by the SA to maintain the visual field.

- Steps may differ based on surgeon preference, but many choose to dissect out the seminal vesicles first (known as a posterior approach) while others begin by taking down the bladder from the anterior abdominal wall.

- If the seminal vesicles and vas are dissected out first, the peritoneum is incised just above the rectovesical junction.

- The vas deferens are transected and the seminal vesicles are freed from their attachments. The seminal vesical arteries are clipped by the assistant prior to being divided. Minimal cautery is used around the tips of the seminal vesicles because the erectile nerves are in this area. Denonvilliers fascia and vas deferens are identified in the midline and a plane is developed between the rectum and the bladder (see Figure 16-8).

- The anterior dissection of the bladder begins by identifying and incising the peritoneum just lateral to the medial umbilical ligaments. The urachal remnant is cauterized prior to being divided because remnant vessels can still be patent. Space of Retzius is mobilized with sharp and blunt dissection as the bladder is dropped to the level of the endopelvic fascia and puboprostatic ligaments. The prostate is defatted.

- The endopelvic fascia surrounding the prostate is then opened and the dorsal venous complex is exposed. Puboprostatic ligaments are taken down sharply.

- The dorsal venous complex is carefully secured with 0 or 2-0 absorbable suture to minimize bleeding. It is important for the assistant to check and make sure the Foley catheter moves freely and was not inadvertently sutured during this process.

- The catheter is gently manipulated by the assistant to help delineate the junction between the prostate and the bladder.

- An incision is made at that junction with every effort made to spare the bladder neck depending on the extent of the malignancy. Once the bladder is entered, the ureteral orifices are inspected, and the assistant uses the Foley to retract the prostate upwards to facilitate the posterior bladder neck dissection.

- The surgeon divides the posterior portion of the bladder neck to expose the vas and seminal vesicles. The prostate is lifted anterior by the seminal vesicles to continue the posterior and lateral dissection. Often, the SA will help with exposure by lifting one of the seminal vesicles while the surgeon retracts the other.

- At this time, a nerve-sparing prostatectomy may be performed if indicated. The neurovascular bundles posterior and lateral to the prostate are spared using a combination of sharp and blunt dissection. Perforating vessels are clipped by the SA and divided by the surgeon with minimal use of cautery. The pedicles on either side of the prostate are clipped and ligated and the dissection continues up toward the apex.

- When the dissection is completed, the dorsal venous complex and urethra are divided and the prostate is placed in an endobag for later retrieval.

- A bilateral pelvic lymphadenectomy of the internal, external, and obturator lymph node packets is performed. The borders of dissection are the inguinal ligament caudally, the bifurcation of the iliac vessels cephalad, the external iliac vein anteriorly, the pelvic side wall laterally, the bladder medially, and the internal iliac vessels posteriorly. Hemostasis and lymphostasis are achieved with bipolar electrocautery and clips.

- The bladder neck is inspected to determine if it needs reconstruction which may be accomplished by tailoring it with a 2-0 or 3-0 Vicryl suture.

- Before the anastomosis of the bladder to the urethral stump, a special "Rocco" stitch, usually an absorbable 3-0 Monocryl or V-loc suture, may be placed to reapproximate the posterior layer of the rhabdosphincter to the remnant Denonvilliers fascia and posterior surface of the bladder. This takes the tension off of the anastomosis.

- The vesicourethral anastomosis is created with a running doubled-armed absorbable suture. The Foley is passed in and out by the assistant during each throw of the needle to help with visualization. The stitch is usually started by placing one needle at the 6 o'clock position and the other at the 5 o'clock position on the posterolateral aspect of the bladder. They are passed through the bladder outside-in and then through the urethra inside-out at the same

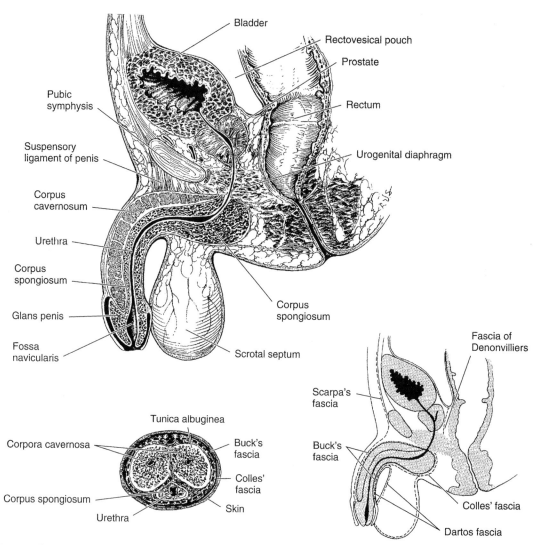

Figure 16-8 · Denonvilliers fascia. (Reproduced, with permission, from McAninch JW, Lue TF, eds. *Smith & Tanagho's General Urology*. 19th ed. New York, NY: McGraw Hill; 2020.)

position and run toward the top of the urethra. When both stitches meet, they are tightened and tied, completing the anastomosis.

- A new Foley catheter is placed and the bladder by the assistant and is filled to check for leaks.

- A drain may be placed at this time.

- The specimen is extracted, and the wound closed in the appropriate fashion.

Procedural sequence in simple/suprapubic prostatectomy:

- Patient is placed in a supine or lithotomy position in deep Trendelenburg, draped appropriately with the penis prepped into the field, and a Foley catheter is placed.

- Entry into the abdominal cavity is gained.

- A Foley is placed by the assistant so that the bladder may be filled and adequately distended.

- A longitudinal incision is made into the posterior bladder wall proximal to the bladder neck.

- Retraction sutures may be placed to help hold the bladder

open for better visualization.

- The ureteral orifices are identified.

- The bladder urothelium/mucosa is incised circumferentially over the prostate taking care to preserve the ureteral orifices. The adenoma is freed from the peripheral zone of the prostate in the avascular plane using a combination of blunt and sharp dissection.

- Hemostasis is achieved with electrocautery and the bladder neck mucosa in the enucleation site is reapproximated with 2-0 or 3-0 absorbable suture.

- The bladder is closed in two layers with 2-0 Vicryl or absorbable v-loc suture.

- The assistant places a large three-way Foley and the balloon is inflated to approximately 20cc. The bladder is filled to test the closure.

- The Foley is hooked up to CBI (continuous bladder irrigation), a drain placed, the specimen extracted, and the wound closed in layers.

Penile

Penile Implant. Penile implants are primarily used for men with erectile dysfunction only after other forms of treatment have failed. They come in either semi-rigid or inflatable forms. The inflatable prosthetics have a reservoir filled with saline that is pumped into the penile implant to create an erection. The malleable implants maintain a constant semi-rigid state and are easy to use but can be uncomfortable for some patients (see Figure 16-9).

Surgery—steps highlighted:

- The patient is placed in a supine position and prepped and draped in a regular fashion.
- A Foley catheter is inserted into the urethra and the bladder is emptied.
- A Lone Star or Wilson self-retaining ring retractor is placed by the surgeon and assistant to help facilitate exposure and the penis is put on traction to expose the penoscrotal junction.
- A transverse skin incision is made at the penoscrotal junction, dartos fascia is exposed and incised, and skin hooks are placed.
- The tunica albuginea of both corporas are exposed and stay sutures are placed.
- An incision is made with a scalpel into each corpora and, using Metzenbaum scissors, extended vertically.

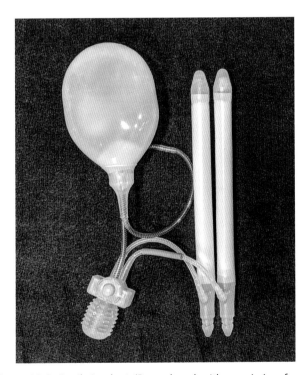

Figure 16-9 · Penile implant. (Reproduced, with permission, from Brunicardi FC et al, eds. Schwartz's Principles of Surgery. 11th ed. New York, NY: McGraw Hill; 2019.)

- The corporal space is dilated with Brook's or Hegar dilators both proximally and distally making sure both cylinders are symmetric.
- The length of the dilated corporal cylinders is measured to determine the proper implant size.
- The corporal spaces are irrigated with antibiotic solution.
- The device and reservoir are prepared, making sure the tubing is free of air bubbles, and the connecting tubes are clamped with rubber-shods.
- The proximal part of the cylinder is inserted into the corporal space.
- Then, the Furlow instrument is inserted and used to pass a Keith needle at the tip on each side to facilitate the distal placement of the cylinders.
- After it is placed correctly, the corporotomies are closed using the previously placed stay sutures.
- A subdartos pouch is made for the pump in the middle of the scrotum using a nasal speculum or ring forceps to create the space.
- The pump is inserted into the pouch, ensuring that the deflation button is positioned anteriorly.
- The pump's tubing is passed through stab incisions to emerge from the posterior side of the pouch.
- The opening of the top part of the pouch is closed with 2-0 nonabsorbable suture.
- The pump is then connected to the cylinders and tested.
- The external ring is identified using a small Deaver retractor and the spermatic cord is pushed aside medially to protect it.
- The transversalis fascia is punctured to access the retropubic space, and a pocket is created with blunt dissection.
- Either a Deaver or a nasal speculum is placed in the pocket and opened, and the reservoir is inserted.
- The reservoir is then filled with normal saline and tested.
- The final connection between the pump and the reservoir is completed.
- The wound is closed in two layers. The dartos fascia is closed with 2-0 absorbable suture and the skin is closed with 3-0 absorbable suture.

Testicular

Hydrocelectomy. A hydrocele is an accumulation of fluid between the tissue layers in the scrotum. They can be congenital or acquired and although it is a benign condition in and of itself, it can sometimes cause pain or social embarrassment necessitating surgical correction.

Diagnostic Procedures: Diagnosis of hydrocele is usually easily made with a physical exam. It must be distinguished from an inguinal hernia by confirming the swelling is confined to the scrotum. A scrotal ultrasound can also be performed.

Surgery—steps highlighted:

- Patient is placed in a supine position and the scrotum is shaved and prepped.

- An incision is typically made transversely in between any obvious blood vessels which can be visualized by grasping the hydrocele and pressing it anteriorly against the skin.

- The incision is carried down through dartos fascia to the surface of the tunica vaginalis layer using cautery to maintain hemostasis.

- The hydrocele is freed from Dartos with blunt dissection before the sac is opened and excised. The remaining sac is inverted and then oversewn with absorbable suture making sure to preserve adequate aperture around the spermatic cord. A penrose drain is often placed via a dependent incision in the scrotum.

- Dartos is closed with running Vicryl suture.

- The scrotum is then closed with absorbable suture and dressed in the usual fashion.

Orchiectomy. Orchiectomy is performed for a number of reasons including tumor, hormonal therapy for advanced prostate cancer, or certain benign intrascrotal processes such as an injury, necrosis from torsion, or chronic epididymo-orchitis. Radical orchiectomy for malignancy is performed via inguinal approach because of lymphatic drainage. Simple orchiectomy for prostate cancer or benign etiologies is performed via scrotal incision.

Pathology: Although testicular tumors are rare, the majority are germ-cell tumors and many are correlated to a history of cryptorchidism (undescended testicles).

In patients with advanced prostate cancer, bilateral orchiectomy has been shown to be beneficial by decreasing testosterone production and slowing the progression of the cancer.

Diagnostic Procedures: The majority of testicular tumors can be palpation during examination. Ultrasound can be utilized to rule out other conditions and elevated tumor markers can help confirm the diagnosis but normal levels cannot be used to rule out cancer.

Surgery—steps highlighted:

- Patient is placed in a supine position and the lower abdomen and groin are shaved, prepped, and draped appropriately.

- An oblique incision is made just above the inguinal ligament as would be made for an inguinal hernia repair. (The operation can also be done trans-scrotally for some benign disease).

- The external ring is identified and the external oblique aponeurosis is incised taking care not to damage the underlying ilioinguinal nerve.

- The spermatic cord is dissected circumferentially, elevated with a Penrose drain, and tourniqueted with the Penrose.

- The testes are then mobilized from the scrotum and passed up through the internal ring into the surgical field where it is freed from its gubernacular attachments using electrocautery.

- Cremasteric muscle fibers are dissected off of the spermatic cord which should now be free up to the internal inguinal ring.

- The vas deferens is ligated and divided. The remainder of the spermatic cord including the testicular vessels is controlled with silk suture ligature. The suture is left long in case the remainder of the spermatic cord is needed to be removed as part of retroperitoneal lymph node dissection at a later date. After the spermatic cord is doubly ligated, it is divided and allowed to retract into the retroperitoneum.

- The wound is inspected, irrigated, and checked for hemostasis before it is closed. The external oblique aponeurosis is re-approximated with Vicryl suture, taking care to preserve the ilioinguinal nerve.

- The external oblique and skin are closed, and a pressure dressing is applied.

Vasovasostomy. Vasectomy reversal is estimated to have around a 50% success rate. Sperm production is usually maintained after vasectomy, but complications can occur from the anastomosis, obstructions caused by infections or changes to the epididymis, and even immunologic reactions to the spermatozoa (see Figure 16-10).

Procedural Sequence:

- The patient is placed supine and enough room is made around the bed for the microscope to be brought in.

- An incision is made in the scrotum over the side of the previous vasectomy if it can be located and the testicals are delivered into the field.

- The vas is grasped above and below the vasectomy defect with Babcock clamps or vessel loops and fully mobilized from its surrounding adhesions.

- A small incision is in the inferior end of the vas and the epididymis is squeezed to express fluid from the vas.

- The superior end is then incised, and the lumen is identified with a small probe.

- The two ends are overlapped and joined together with a side-to-side anastomosis using 6-0 prolene suture. An end-to-end anastomosis could also be used. Fibrin glue may be placed to ensure the repair is completely free of any leaks.

- If there is still an obstruction, a vasoepididymostomy or alternative anastomosis may need to be performed.

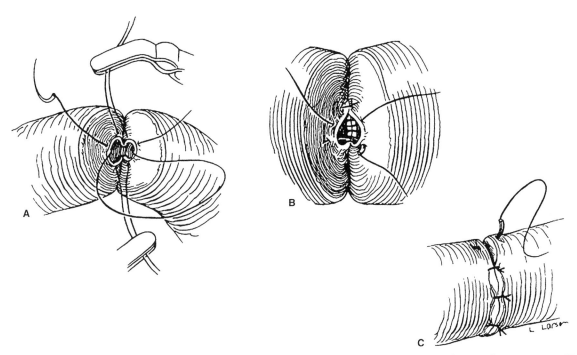

Figure 16-10 Vasovasostomy. (Reproduced, with permission, from McClure RD. Microsurgery of the male reproductive system. *World J Urol.* 1986;4(2):105-114.)

• Once satisfied with the anastomosis, the adventitial tissue is approximated and the dartos layer is closed. The skin is closed with a subcutaneous suture and a dry, bulky dressing is applied to the scrotum.

Bibliography

Asakura C, Iwasaki H, Sato I, Izumi Y, Kunisawa T. *Effect of Fluid Restriction During Robotic-Assisted Laparoscopic Prostatectomy on Postoperative Renal Function*, October 2016. www.asaabstracts.com/strands/asaabstracts/abstract.htm?ycar=2016&index-=4&absnum=3643. Accessed June 9, 2023.

Bemelmans BLH, Chapple CR. Are slings now the gold standard treatment for the management of female urinary stress incontinence and if so which technique? Curr Opin Urol. 2003;13(4):301-307. https://pubmed.ncbi.nlm.nih.gov/12811294/. Accessed June 9, 2023.

Chopra S, Srivastava A, Tewari A. Robotic radical prostatectomy: The new gold standard. *Arab J Urol.* 2012;10(1):23-31.

Graham SD, Jr., Keane TE. Pheochromocytoma. In: *Glenn's Urologic Surgery,* 8th ed. Lippincott Williams & Wilkins (LWW).

Lugo-Baruqui JA, Ayyathurai R, Sriram A, Pragatheeswar KD. Use of mannitol for ischemia reperfusion injury in kidney transplant and partial nephrectomies-review of literature. *Current Urology Reports,* Springer US, January 2019. link.springer.com/article/10.1007/s11934-019-0868-6. Accessed June 9, 2023.

Phillips NM, Hornacky A. *Intra*operative patient care / positioning the patient. In: *Berry & Kohn's Operating Room Technique.* Elsevier; 2021:494-499.

Preparation and approaches to adrenal excision. In: Smith JA, Preminger GM, Howards S. *Hinman's Atlas of Urologic Surgery.* Elsevier; 2019:1058-1059.

Surgical basics/operative management. In: Smith JA, Preminger GM, Howards S. *Hinman's Atlas of Urologic Surgery.* Elsevier; 2019: 12-14.

Tracy CR. *Prostate Cancer.* 2023 https://emedicine.medscape.com/article/1967731-overview#a1. Accessed June 9, 2023.

Ophthalmic Surgery

Terry Herring

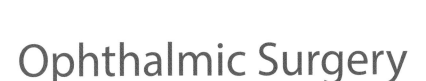

DISCUSSED IN THIS CHAPTER

1. Ocular anatomy and physiology
2. Diagnostics and indications for surgeries of the eye
3. Pharmacology for ophthalmic surgery
4. Role of the surgical assistant in eye surgery

EYE ANATOMY

The eye includes the eyeball and its appendages. The eyeball is very nearly the same size in all persons; the apparent difference in the size of the eyes is due to a difference in the distance between the angles of the eyelids from end to end of the visible portion of the eyeball.

The eye socket (orbit) is a cavity filled with muscles that move the eyeball, blood vessels to supply nourishment, nerves, and cushions of fat. The eyeball rotates in the socket, pulled about by suitable muscles. The eye is protected in the front by eyelids, of which the upper lid is the more movable, being able to cover the entire eyeball in front. The inner sides of the eyelids are covered by the conjunctiva (mucous membrane), which also covers the front of the eyeball. The edges of the eyelids are lined with eyelashes which help to keep out flying particles, such as dust. Wherever there are hairs, there are sebaceous glands, which secrete a fatty substance to soften and lubricate the hair and skin; the edges of the eyelids are equipped with such glands. When the secretion is excessive, the yellowish matter occurs along the eyelids after a night's sleep, sometimes even being abundant enough to stick the lids together momentarily (see Figure 17-1).

The lacrimal or tear-producing apparatus is in the eye. This system supplies moisture, which keeps the eyeball wet. Under emotional stress, when one cries, the tears are produced in abnormal quantity and sometimes overflowing down the cheeks. However, the tears are often carried off by the lacrimal canals, which open by a pore into the inner corner of each eye. Tears eventually drain into the nasal cavity and the pharynx and are swallowed. The act of blinking keeps the moisture from the lacrimal glands evenly distributed over the eyeball, eliminating any accumulated particles, and washing it clean several times a minute.

The muscles of the eye, attached to the back of the eyeball in the orbit, are so arranged that they can move the eyes from side to side, or up and down, or obliquely, or rotate them, at will. These movements, which are controlled by six muscles attached to the sclera, increase the range of vision, which is further amplified by turning the head. These muscles working in a coordinating fashion include six extraocular muscles (EOMs) and two oblique muscles. The EOMs include four rectus muscles, the superior, inferior, lateral, and medial muscles. The two oblique muscles include the superior and inferior muscles. These muscles help keep the two eyes aligned, moving simultaneously with a gentle adjustment of muscles and nerves. If this adjustment of muscle coordination is impaired, a condition known as strabismus occurs (see Figure 17-2).

The eye itself is the shape of a globe and is nearly spherical in its central part. Three coats of tissue protect the eyeball: the outer is the sclera, which is the thick, fibrous part enclosing about three-fourths of the eyeball. The second coat includes the iris, which is the visible colored portion of the eye; its center is the aperture through which light rays enter and allows us to see. A ring of muscle within the iris permits the contracting or narrowing of the pupil; the pupil is smaller in bright light than in diffused light.

The color of the eyes is due to the melanin pigment in the iris. This pigment is always of lighter or darker yellow color, forming what we ordinarily call black eyes, brown eyes, or gray eyes, depending on its intensity. Blue eyes occur when this

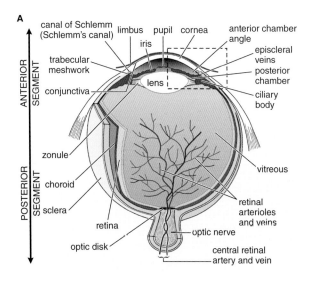

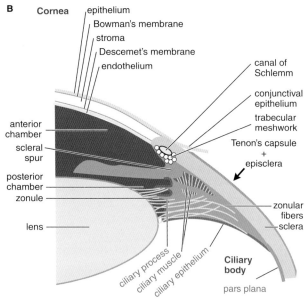

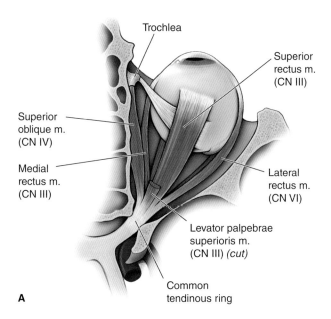

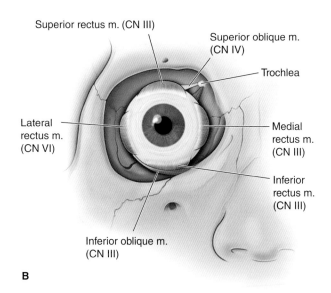

Figure 17-1 • Anatomy of the eye. (Reproduced, with permission, from Brunton LL, Hilal-Dandan R, Knollmann BC, eds. *Goodman & Gilman's the Pharmacological Basis of Therapeutics.* 13th ed. New York, NY: McGraw Hill; 2018.)

Figure 17-2 • Muscles of the eye. (Reproduced, with permission, from Morton DA, Foreman KB, Albertine KH. *The Big Picture: Gross Anatomy.* 2nd ed. New York, NY: McGraw Hill; 2019.)

same pigment is more deeply embedded; the absorption of light forms the blue color in the outer portions of the iris.

The third coat of the eye is on the inner and rear of the eyeball; it is called the retina. Its complex structure of blood vessels and nerve cells in the apparatus receives the stimuli of light rays entering the eyeball through the cornea and transmits the nerve impulses to the brain. For the most part, the eye is constructed like a small camera, having a lens that can be automatically adjusted for nearer and farther distances. In front of the crystalline lens is a space filled with transparent aqueous humor (water-like); behind it is the inner globe on the eye, filled with vitreous humor (jelly-like) which is also transparent. The lens acts somewhat like an artificial glass lens to focus on the sensitive retina and retains the rays of light passing through the cornea and pupil.

The anterior portion of the eye is divided into two different chambers, the anterior and posterior chambers. The anterior chamber is located in front of the iris, while the posterior chamber is located behind the iris. A clear, watery fluid referred to as the aqueous humor is produced by the ciliary body and drains from the eye through an angle formed by the junction of the cornea and the sclera, exiting the eye through the canal of Schlemm. If the fluid does not drain and continues to build up in the eye, an increase in the intraocular pressure (IOP) will occur. If goes undetached, it can lead to the loss of vision and a condition referred to as Glaucoma.

PREOPERATIVE PROCEDURES

Positioning the Patient for Ophthalmic Surgery

Most ophthalmic surgical procedures are performed with the patient in the supine position. The head is stabilized in a supportive headrest or doughnut. Some ophthalmologists like to use a wrist rest; this will allow additional support of the surgeon's hands during the ophthalmic procedure. Regardless of the type of headrest that may be utilized, the patient's head must be level with the top of the bed.

Before the case, it is essential to make sure the patient is as comfortable as possible. Most ophthalmic patients are older and have lower back problems. Placing a pillow under the patient's knees will help take some of the pressure off the lower back to decrease the discomfort. Many facilities utilize a unique stretcher to minimize having to move these patients, which may increase their IOP; these unique stretches can be converted into a chair in the postoperative area.

Anesthesia

As with any surgical procedure, adequate anesthesia is vital to the success of the surgery. With ophthalmic surgical procedures, local anesthesia (topical or regional) with monitored sedation has become the safer standard. Usually, patients that are good candidates for local include those that are calm, cooperative, and able to follow verbal commands.

Local anesthesia can be performed in the pre-operative area or within the operating room (OR) suite. Regardless of the location for the anesthesia, a dedicated setup is necessary, which includes a finger-control syringe and infiltration needles (25-27 gauge), and the local anesthetic. Based on the surgeon's preference, the infiltration may include lidocaine 1% or 2%. Lidocaine has a rapid onset and usually diffuses well into the surrounding tissue. For longer or complicated procedures, the surgeon may include a Marcaine solution (0.25-0.75%) combined with the lidocaine solution. Also, to reduce bleeding and prolong the local anesthetic, epinephrine (1:50,000 to 1:200,000) may be added. Based on the fact, epinephrine is a vasoconstrictor, it should be used with caution, especially with patients that are hypertensive, diabetic, or have a history of cardiovascular disease. In addition to the local anesthetic, hyaluronidase (hyalase) may be added. If utilized, the hyaluronidase will enable the anesthetic agent to spread, producing wider anesthesia.

Retrobulbar injections, used less frequently, may be utilized to temporarily paralyze the EOMs. These injections usually are performed about 10 to 15 minutes before the procedure. Based on the surgeon's choice of anesthetic agent(s), the solution is injected behind the globe of the eye, blocking the ciliary ganglion and nerves.

For procedures that involve the eyelids, a facial nerve or peribulbar block can be performed. These blocks prevent the patient from being able to squeeze the eyelids during the procedure.

For anterior segment surgical procedures, a new technique, intracameral anesthesia, may be utilized. This technique anesthetizes the iris, which is innervated with nerves, which make it very sensitive. After applying a topical anesthetic, about 0.25 to 0.50 ml of 1% lidocaine is administered through a small paracentesis incision in the corneal. If this technique is utilized, unpreserved lidocaine (MPF) must be used. If inadequate blocking of the iris occurs, the patient may experience discomfort with any iris manipulation. Otherwise, this technique allows the patient to be more aware of the intraoperative phase of the surgery.

General anesthesia is mostly used with selective cases, including pediatric patients and cases that may last a long duration, and provide control over the intraoperative phase of surgery.

Prepping and Draping

After the patient has been anesthetized, the operative eye(s) needs to be cleaned with an antiseptic solution. If the patient does not have an iodine allergy, most facilities utilize the standard 5% betadine solution. Before starting the prep, a small cotton ball may be placed in the ear to keep the prepping solution from pooling in the ear. Also, if the procedure is being performed under topical, the operative eye(s) may involve the instillation of drops. The prep area includes the eyelid, starting at the inner aspect and extending outward, including the inner aspect at the nose, forehead, and outer aspect toward the ear, usually ending at the chin. Often the eyelashes are cleaned with a cotton-tip applicator; it is essential not to come into contact with the cornea, which may cause a corneal abrasion.

Eye Dressings

To perform the necessary function, eye dressings must be appropriately applied. After the procedure and the instillation of any eye drops or ointment, the eyelid needs to be immobilized by applying pressure. The proper technique involves applying an eye pad doubled in half, followed by a second eye pad over the folded pad. If bleeding is a major concern, double pads may be utilized. After confirming no tape allergic, a small ½ inch of adhesive tape in an overlapping fashion is applied.

Some procedures may only require the application of an eye shield. Unlike the pad, the shield is to protect the eye from physical injury. Patients may be instructed to apply the shield at night time to prevent accidental rubbing of the eye.

Ophthalmic Pharmacology in Surgery

Ophthalmic surgery requires the use of several different types of medications, which are administered preoperative, intraoperative, and postoperative. The surgical assistant (SA) is primarily concerned with the medication that is used during the intraoperative period and the various classifications of ophthalmic drugs and their action. These intraoperative medications can be administered to the patient through different methods or routes. The most common routes include solutions, suspension, ointments, and gels. Despite the route of admission, ophthalmic medication delivery can be challenging based on the complex nature and structure of the eye.

Ophthalmic surgery, as with all surgical specialties, requires adequate anesthesia. In today's ophthalmic surgeries, local anesthesia (topical or regional) has become safer and the standard of care. Successful surgery under topical requires constant communication with the patient. Patients that are able to follow verbal commands are the best candidates for this type of anesthesia.

Intracameral anesthesia has grown in popularity. This type of anesthesia is instilled into the anterior segment of the eye. This technique anesthetizes the iris. The iris consists of muscles and nerves. The intracameral administration of local anesthesia helps to eliminate pain and allows the patient to be more cooperative during the surgical procedure. Despite the benefits of intracameral anesthesia, there is a risk of toxic anterior segment syndrome. This inflammatory reaction can be a result of improper concentration and exposure to preservatives. If intracameral anesthesia is used, the SA needs to be aware of the potential for corneal toxicity caused by medication that might be used intracamerally. Also, improper concentration and preservatives can cause endothelial damage.

Most often, ophthalmic medication is given in combination. The combination of ophthalmic agents provides an effective method to address different conditions that can occur. For example, an antibiotic, steroid, and nonsteroidal anti-inflammatory drug (NSAID) may be prescribed. Combining these agents helps keep the ocular surface lubricated to minimize postoperative complications.

Table 17-1 lists the most common ophthalmic medications and their usage.

TABLE 17-1 • MOST COMMON OPHTHALMIC MEDICATIONS AND THEIR USAGE		
Generic Name	**Brand Name**	**Usage**
Anesthesia (Topical)		
Tetracaine ophthalmic	Pontocaine	Provides surface anesthesia of the cornea, comes in drops or ointment
Proparacaine ophthalmic	Ophthaine	
Lidocaine ophthalmic	Akten	
Anesthesia (Local)		
Lidocaine hydrochloride	Xylocaine	Administered via infiltration or via regional block (retrobulbar or facial nerve block) to provide adequate pain control
Bupivacaine hydrochloride	Marcaine	
Antibiotics		
Azithromycin	Azasite	Treat ocular infections
Besifloxacin	Besivance	
Bacitracin	AK-Tracin	
Bacitracin-neomycin-polymixin B	AK-Spore	
Ciprofloxacin	Ciloxan	
Gentamicin	Gentasol/Gentak	
Erythromycin	Erythromycin	
Ofloxacin	Ocuflox	
Gatifloxacin	Zymar; Zymaxid	
Tobramycin	Tobramycin	
Levofloxacin	Levofloxacin	
Corticosteroids		
Prednisolone	Prelone	Inhibit inflammatory response Unlike steroids, NSAIDs cause little, if any, rise in IOP
Prednisolone acetate	Pred Forte	
Dexamethasone	Decadron	
Triamcinolone acetonide	Kenalog	
Loteprednol etabonate	Lotemax	

(Continued)

TABLE 17-1 • *(Continued)*

Cycloplegics (Dilation)

Tropicamide	Mydriacyl	Dilates pupil
Cyclopentolate	Cyclogyl	
Atropine sulfate	Atropisol	

Dyes

Fluorescein sodium	Fluress	Corneal or vessel abnormalities
Trypan blue	VisionBlue	Stain anterior capsule

Hyperosmotic Agents

Mannitol	Osmitrol	IV osmotic diuretic used to reduce IOP

Irrigants

BSS	Endosol	Used to keep the cornea moist, can be used in anterior or posterior segments
BSS enriched with bicarbonate, dextrose, and glutathione	BSS Plus	

Miotics (Parasympathetic Constriction)

Pilocarpine HCl	Pilocar	Constricts pupil
Acetylcholine HCl	Miochol-E	
Carbochol	Miostat	

Mydriatics (Dilation)

Phenylephrine HCl	Neo-Synephrine	Dilates pupil but permits focusing

NSAIDs

Ketorolac tromethamine	Acular	Prevent and relieve pain and inflammation
Nepafenac	Nevanac	
Flurbiprofen	Ocufen	
Ketorolac	Acular	
Diclofenac	Voltaren	
Bromofenac	Xibrom	

Steroids

Betamethasone sodium phosphate and betamethasone acetate	Celestone	Treat inflammation and relieve symptoms such as swelling, pain, redness, or irritation
Desamethasone	Decadron	
Prednisolone acetate	Pred Forte	
Fluorometholone acetate	Flarex	

Viscoelastics

Sodium hyaluronate Chondroitin sulfate	Healon Amvis Provisc Viscoat DuoVisc	Protect the corneal endothelium

SURGICAL PROCEDURES

Dacryocystorhinostomy

A dacryocystorhinostomy is best understood by reviewing the anatomy of the lacrimal system. The lacrimal system, which consists of glands, provides a drainage system for tears. The system consists of the puncta, canaliculi, lacrimal sac, and nasolacrimal duct (see Figure 17-3).

- Puncta: The puncta are openings within the eyelids through which tear fluid drains from the eyes. These openings are located at the medial canthus of the eye.
- Canaliculi: The canaliculi, located in the medial aspect of the eyelid, provide an opening for the tears to drain onto the outer surface of the conjunctiva. These small channels may also be referred to as the lacrimal canals or lacrimal ducts.
- Lacrimal sac: The lacrimal sac, which provides storage for the overflow of tears, connects the superior and inferior canaliculi. The system drains the tears from the surface of the eye into the nasal cavity.
- Nasolacrimal duct: The nasolacrimal duct, also known as the tear duct, is a canal through which tear fluid drains from the lacrimal sac into the inferior nasal meatus. The canal opens within the eye socket between the maxillary and lacrimal bones.

These tears consist of a watery solution compound that contains a bactericidal enzyme called lysozyme. The primary function of these enzymes is to clean, lubricate, and keep the eye moistened.

Pathology. When the tear ducts become blocked, the lacrimal sac becomes infected. Dacryocystitis is an inflammation of the lacrimal sac. The usual signs of inflammation can be noted within the medial canthus, which includes pain, redness, and swelling. Dacryocystitis can lead to complete blockage of the lacrimal system.

Diagnostic Procedures. Diagnosis of dacryocystitis can be determined relatively by merely accessing the eye for any visible signs of dacryocystitis, including pain, redness, and swelling. During the routine examination, the physician may place pressure on the lacrimal sac to see if any visible pus or mucoid material can be expressed from the punctum (openings in the eyelid).

Surgery—Steps Highlighted. The following are the steps involved in the surgery:

- **Incision is made in the medial canthus**
  Using a #15 blade, the surgeon makes an incision into the medial canthus exposing the nasal bone. The SA needs to keep the incisional site clear of blood, using Frazier suction or cotton-tip applicators.
- **Osteotomy is performed in the lacrimal bone**
  Before the osteotomy is performed, the surgeon removes the periosteum from the nasal bone using a small Freer or periosteal elevator. To enlarge the opening, the surgeon may use a Kerrison rongeur or a small dental drill. If the Kerrison is used, the SA needs to keep the tip of the rongeur cleaned. This is often performed by using a moisten 4 × 4 sponge.
- **Incision is made into the lacrimal sac**
  Before the incision, a Bowman lacrimal probe is used to identify the blockage. Using a #11 blade, the surgeon makes an incision into the lacrimal sac. The SA needs to have the Frazier suction ready to remove any of the contents that may be located within the lacrimal sac. Also, a similar incision is made into the nasal mucosa.
- **Lacrimal duct intubation**
  The SA passes the surgeon the Silastic lacrimal duct intubation set for placement into the inferior and superior puncta. Afterward, the silastic tubing is passed through the osteotomy site into the nasal cavity. The SA needs to have a straight hemostat available to retrieve the end of the tubing. The tubing will be cut short enough to allow it to retract into the nostrils, making it invisible.
- **Anastomoses of the lacrimal sac and the nasal mucosa**
  The surgeon uses a vicryl suture (4-0 to 6-0) to close the lacrimal flap with the nasal mucosa.

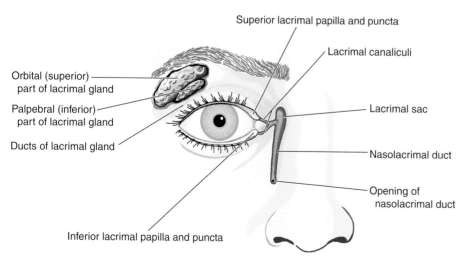

Figure 17-3 · Lacrimal system. (Reproduced, with permission, from Brunton LL, Hilal-Dandan R, Knollmann BC, eds. *Goodman & Gilman's the Pharmacological Basis of Therapeutics.* 13th ed. New York, NY: McGraw Hill; 2018.)

Superior lacrimal papilla and puncta

Lacrimal canaliculi

Orbital (superior) part of lacrimal gland

Palpebral (inferior) part of lacrimal gland

Ducts of lacrimal gland

Lacrimal sac

Nasolacrimal duct

Opening of nasolacrimal duct

Inferior lacrimal papilla and puncta

- **Wound closure**

  The wound is closed according to the surgeon's preference. The SA applies antibiotic ointment to the wound. An ophthalmic ointment is usually allied to the lower cul de sac. The patient may be instructed to apply continuous ice packs to help with postoperative swelling.

Enucleation

Enucleation involves the removal of the entire globe.

Pathology. Enucleation usually involves pathology relating to tumors, injury, or severe pain with a dysfunctional eye.

Diagnostic Procedures. The ophthalmologist may perform any of the following diagnostic tests to determine if an enucleation is indicated.

- Dilated retinal exam
- Ultrasound imaging
- Optical coherence tomography
- Magnetic resonance imaging (MRI)
- Fine needle biopsy
- Pupil reflex tests
- Fundus photography and angiography
- Fundus autofluorescence and echography
- Surgical biopsy called an orbitotomy (anterior or lateral)

Surgery—Steps Highlighted. The following are the steps involved in the surgery:

- **Incision is made into the conjunctiva**

  The SA prepares the eye by placing a speculum for exposure of the globe. The surgeon makes a 360° conjunctiva incision around the limbus of the globe of the eye, using a #15 blade or Westcott scissors.

- **Identification of the four rectus muscles**

  Using a muscle hook, the four rectus muscles are identified. The SA holds the muscle hook while the surgeon places the preferred suture in a double-locked fashion at the insertion site of each muscle. After placement of the sutures, the surgeon will excise each muscle from the globe.

- **The optic nerve is severed**

  Once all the muscles are excised, the SA will pull the globe anteriorly (forward), exposing the optic nerve. The surgeon will clamp the optic nerve, leaving the clamp attached to the nerve for 30 to 60 seconds. Afterward, the surgeon will use the enucleation scissors to sever the optic nerve. A monopolar cautery is used to cauterize the stump of the optic nerve.

- **Implant is inserted**

  After the socket has been cleared, irrigated, and hemostasis has been achieved, the surgeon will insert the implant using a sphere introducer. It is crucial to have a variety of sizes available; adult sizes can range from 14 to 18 mm.

- **Wound closure**

  Once the implant and conformer are in place, the rectus muscles are sutured over the sphere, using a 4-0 or 5-0 absorbable suture. The tendon capsule and conjunctiva are closed, using a 5-0 absorbable suture. Before the dressing, the SA applies antibiotic ointment followed by a pressure eye dressing.

Repair of Orbital Fractures

Not every orbital or blowout fracture requires surgery. If surgery is needed, the repair involves an open reduction and internal fixation (ORIF) of the orbital bones, which consist of seven bones, which includes the frontal, zygomatic, maxillary, sphenoid, ethmoid, palatine, and lacrimal bones (see Figure 17-4). Based on the anatomical location, infections may be a major consideration.

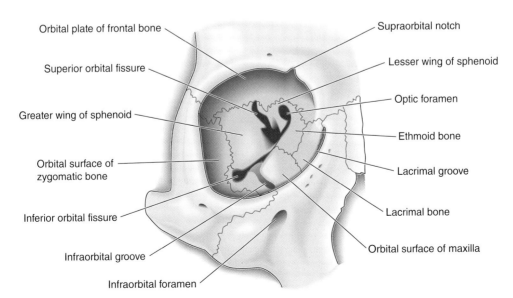

Figure 17-4 · Bony anatomy of the orbit. (Reproduced, with permission, from Riordan-Eva P, Augsburger JJ, eds. *Vaughan & Asbury's General Ophthalmology.* 19th ed. New York, NY: McGraw Hill; 2018.)

Pathology. Orbital fractures are usually a result of high-speed blunt trauma to the globe and may involve the entrapment of the EOMs. If the muscles are entrapped, the patient may experience diplopia (double vision).

Diagnostic Procedures. Computed tomography (CT) is a useful diagnostic tool for detecting orbital fractures. However, the CT scan may not reveal that a muscle is entrapped, so a clinical examination is often needed. If the patient has herniation of the inferior rectus into the maxillary sinus, this can be noted on the CT scan.

Surgery—Steps Highlighted. The following are the steps involved in the surgery:

- An incision is made into the lower eyelid using a #15 blade. The SA needs to keep the incisional area clear of blood, using cotton tip applicators or weck-cell sponges or suction.

- To provide exposure, the surgeon will place a traction stitch between the lower eyelashes and the incision. The SA may need to provide additional exposure using blunt-tip retractors.

- Using tenotomy scissors, the surgeon will dissect the tissue to expose the infraorbital rim. After exposure to the rim, the surgeon will use a Freer elevator to dissect the periosteum.

- To prevent eye injuries, the SA needs to retract the eye superiorly, using a moistened orbital retractor. Care should be taken not to put too much pressure on the eye.

Keratoplasty

Keratoplasty or corneal transplant involves the removal of the damaged corneal tissue and its replacement with donor corneal tissue. The cornea is the transparent front part of the eye, which can become damaged when injured or an infection occurs. The only way to restore vision is to replace the cornea.

Keratoplasty may be either lamellar or partial penetrating procedure, in which a half thickness of the cornea is used to transfer from the donor to the recipient. This procedure does not involve the anterior chamber of the eye. However, the penetrating or full-thickness does involve the anterior chamber. Since the anterior chamber is involved, viscoelastic is used to minimize the damage to the endothelial cells.

Both partial penetrating and full-thickness corneal transplants require the use of a cutting trephine. A trephine is used to remove the affected cornea, creating a smooth round cut.

Pathology. The cornea, which is the transparent front part of the eye, helps focus light so that vision is clear. The cornea is avascular and consists of five layers: epithelium, Bowman's membrane, stroma, Descemet's membrane, and endothelium. Injury, inherited conditions, or keratoconus are conditions that may cause scarring and cloudy of the cornea.

Diagnostic Procedure. Several diagnostic tests may be performed to determine corneal damage and provide crucial information during the preoperative phase. Corneal topography is a standard test performed to diagnose the early stages of keratoconus and thinning of the corneal surface. This diagnostic test will note any corneal steepening and asymmetry.

Keratometry is the measurement of corneal curvature by the use of a keratometer. During this diagnostic test, a circle of light is reflected on the cornea to determine the basic shape of the cornea. The cornea's surface is measured in diopters, and the keratometry reading is referred to as *k* readings.

Specular microscopy or endothelial cell count (ECC) is performed to examine the endothelium of the cornea, which is a single inner layer of cells in contact with the aqueous humor. The average endothelium cell count can range from 1800 to 4000 cells/mm^2; the average count is around 2800 cells/mm^2. Unfortunately, endothelial cells do not regenerate. So, it is vital during any anterior intraocular surgery that the endothelium is protected. For example, during cataract extraction, the use of phacoemulsification may damage these cells. This damage can be minimized with the use of a viscoelastic substance and by keeping the phacoemulsification power and usage time to a minimum.

Surgery—Steps Highlighted. The following are the steps involved in the surgery:

- Preparing the donor cornea: The SA assists the surgeon in the preparation of the donor cornea, which is often prepared in a container with OptiSol storage solution. Also, the SA needs to note the color of the OptiSol solution. A pink color indicates a normal pH.

  After the surgeon has determined the size of the graft, which is often 0.2 to 0.5 mm larger than the recipient measurements, a trephine will be utilized to cut the donor cornea. Once the cornea has been cut, the SA needs to make sure the graft does not dry out. The residual tissue from the cornea needs to be sent to the laboratory for culture and sensitivity (C&S) testing.

- Preparing the recipient cornea: A suction trephination system, such as the Hanna, is used to excise the cornea tissue. After the surgeon has determined the area and applied the trephine, the SA applies suction. After a 90% corneal depth has been achieved, the suction is released. The surgeon may use Westcott or Vannas scissors to trim the edges of Descemet's membrane.

- In preparation for the graft, the surgeon may use a viscoelastic agent to protect the iris and minimize damage to the donor endothelium. Also, to provide support, the surgeon may suture a scleral support ring to the cornea.

- To strategically place the interrupted sutures, the surgeon may use a calibrated marker. A 10-0 Nylon suture is used to suture the graft in place. Once placed, the surgeon or the SA will cut the suture using Vannas scissors. After the placement of the sutures, the knots are buried into the recipient tissue.

- Replacement of the anterior chamber: Once the graft is secured into place, the surgeon will reform the eye with balanced salt solution (BSS) or sodium hyaluronate. It is vital to make sure the wound is secured and watertight. However, it is critical that the sutures not be placed too tight; this could create a "doughnut effect" on the donor graft.

- To minimize infections, the surgeon may inject antibiotics and steroids, subconjunctivally. The SA covers the eye with the selected dressing.

Scleral Buckle

Retinal detachment involves a separation of the retina from the choroid (see Figure 17-5). This separation can occur anywhere in the retina and requires some surgical correction, like a scleral buckle. Often, the detachment is a result of traction of the vitreous body, inflammation, or an injury that may cause vitreous shrinkage.

Pathology. A tear or rhegmatogenous detachment is when the vitreous becomes detached from the retina, allowing fluid to collect underneath. The accumulation of the fluid may continue and create a tear (see Figure 17-6). The tear can create symptoms that include flashes of light, halos around lights, and floaters. Some patients may describe a curtain-like shadow across their field of vision. Often these symptoms are accommodated by a painless loss of vision.

Diagnostic Procedures. A retinal tear or detachment can be diagnosed during a routine eye examination but will often require that the patient's pupils be dilated. The dilation provides a better view of the posterior portion of the eye and the retina.

Treatment. The extent of the tear and the degree of detachment will determine which method of treatment is needed. The most common treatment methods include scleral buckle, pneumatic retinopexy, and vitrectomy with intraocular gas or oil tamponade.

The scleral buckle (described below) involves the placement of a circumferential band (see Figure 17-7), which causes the sclera to indent so that the choroid will be pushed back against the retina, closing the hole.

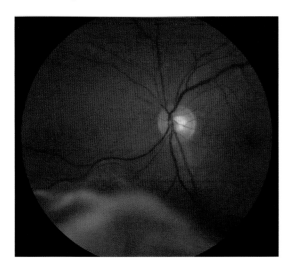

Figure 17-5 · Retinal detachment. (Reproduced, with permission, from Loscalzo J, Fauci AS, Kasper DL, Hauser SL, Longo DL, Jameson JL, eds. *Harrison's Principles of Internal Medicine.* 21st ed. New York, NY: McGraw Hill; 2022.)

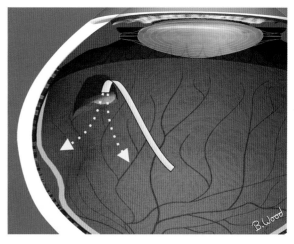

Figure 17-6 · Retinal tear. (Reproduced, with permission, from Riordan-Eva P, Augsburger JJ, eds. *Vaughan & Asbury's General Ophthalmology.* 19th ed. New York, NY: McGraw Hill; 2018.)

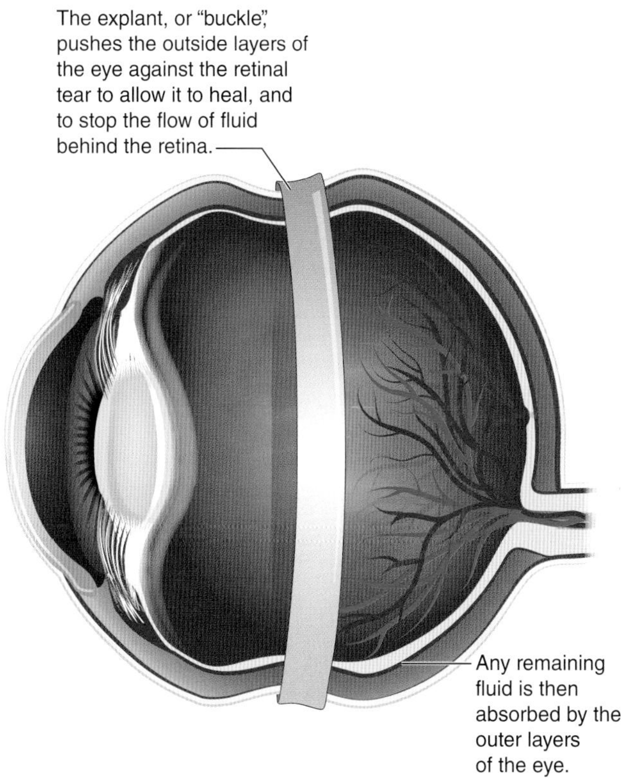

The explant, or "buckle", pushes the outside layers of the eye against the retinal tear to allow it to heal, and to stop the flow of fluid behind the retina.

Any remaining fluid is then absorbed by the outer layers of the eye.

Figure 17-7 · Scleral buckle.

Pneumatic retinopexy, a less invasive procedure, involves injecting expandable gas into the vitreous cavity, creating a closure of the hole.

Vitrectomy involves removing the vitreous gel or preretinal membranes that are causing traction and tearing on the retina. The vitreous gel is replaced with a gas or oil, creating a tamponade effect to close the hole and repair the tear.

Surgery—Steps Highlighted. The following are the steps involved in the surgery:

- The SA prepares the eye by placing a speculum for exposure of the globe. The surgeon makes a 360° peritomy using Westcott scissors. Using conjunctival scissors, the surgeon bluntly dissects the conjunctiva.

- **Isolation of the rectus muscles**
  Using a muscle hook as a sling, the rectus muscles are identified, and a traction suture is placed using a 2-0 or 4-0 Silk suture. The SA tags the traction suture, which will provide access to the posterolateral section.

- **Inspection of the retina**
  The circulation nurse places the indirect ophthalmoscope on the surgeon's head. The SA supplies the surgeon with a 20-diopter indirect lens. Once the holes or tears are identified, they are marked with the diathermy.

- **Placement of circumferential buckle**
  The surgeon places a horizontal mattress suture in the sclera, which will be used to hold the Silastic band in place. Before tying the sutures, the surgeon drains the subretinal fluid via a scleral incision, which is made down through the choroid.

- **Intravitral sulfahexafluoride (SF-6) gas may be injected**
  With the use of indirect ophthalmoscopy, any holes or tears which were not closed by the Silastic band may be treated with the use of gas. This gas will expand and keep the hole or tear closed against the buckle.

- To minimize infections, the surgeon may inject antibiotics and steroids, subconjunctivally. The SA covers the eye with the selected dressing.

Adjunctive Chemotherapy

For patients that have had previous surgery for retinal detachment, silicone oil may be used. The oil acts as a type of vitreous substitute, pushing the retina back against the wall of the eye. After 3 to 4 months, the silicone oil is often surgically removed.

Trabeculectomy

Glaucoma is the result of increased IOP within the eye. In order to drain the aqueous humor from the anterior chamber, a small channel, known as a trabeculectomy, is performed.

Pathology. Glaucoma is a disease process that impacts the optic nerve and creates visual loss. Patients develop increased IOP based on the fact that there is an obstruction of the outflow of aqueous humor. If the IOP is left untreated, then permanent vision loss may occur. Contrary to what people believe, IOP has no direct correlation with a patient's blood pressure. A normal IOP range is between 12 and 22 mm Hg.

Diagnostic Procedures. Patients are often asymptomatic until the disease is in the advantageous stages. Patients are encouraged to undergo routine eye exams, to screen for elevated IOPs. Patients that present with elevated IOPs undergo additional diagnostic tests.

Several diagnostic tests may be utilized to detect glaucoma. More popular tests include the use of the tonometer to measure the pressure, pachymetry mapping, which measures the central corneal thickness (CCT), and visual field test to measure the extent of damage to the optic nerve from elevated IOPs.

Treatment. The degree of glaucoma will determine the treatment to be performed. Glaucoma can be treated with eyedrop medications. These drops can reduce the amount of aqueous fluid or reduce the pressure by helping the fluid drain. Also, glaucoma can be treated with laser surgery. The two most popular laser surgeries to treat glaucoma are trabeculoplasty and iridotomy. Trabeculoplasty is for patients that have open-angle glaucoma; these patients have a decreased function of cells in the trabecular meshwork. For patients with angle-closure glaucoma, an iridotomy is performed. When angle closure occurs, the iris is pushing against the lens and angle. The aqueous production continues to occur; however, the fluid is not drained, causing an increase in the IOP.

If surgery is needed to create a new drainage channel for the aqueous humor, a trabeculectomy (described below) or implanting glaucoma devices might be needed.

Surgery—Steps Highlighted. The following are the steps involved in the surgery:

- The SA prepares the eye by placing a speculum for exposure of the globe. The surgeon may place a bridle suture within the superior rectus muscle. Using beaver blade and forceps, the surgeon makes an incision into the conjunctiva. Afterward, to create a conjunctival flap, the surgeon uses Westcott scissors to separate the Tenon capsule from the sclera. The SA needs to irrigate with BSS while the surgeon uses the Wetfield cautery for hemostasis.

- **Creation of a scleral flap**
  Using a beaver blade or crescent knife, the surgeon creates a scleral thickness flap with a 4-mm limbal base. If the surgeon suspects a risk of failure, chemotherapeutic agents such as 5-fluorouracil (5-FU) or Mitomycin C may be utilized. Using a soaked weck-cell sponge, the agent is placed on top of the outlined scleral flap. The agent remains in place for 3 minutes; afterward, the area is irrigated well with BSS.

  Note: Based on the fact that these are chemotherapy drugs, hospital policy needs to be followed for disposal and instrument decontamination.

- **Trabecular meshwork is excised**
  Using a 15°-stab blade, the surgeon makes a stab wound to enter the anterior chamber along the base of the sclera flap. Using non-tooth forceps, the SA will need to hold the scleral flap. Care must be taken not to pull the tissue away from the base. The surgeon will use Descemet's punch or the Vannas scissors to create a peripheral iridectomy.

- **Incision closed**
  The surgeon closes the scleral flap using a 10-0 nylon suture. To reform the anterior chamber, the surgeon will inject BSS through a paracentesis incision. Closure of the Tenon's and conjunctival incisions is performed using an absorbable suture. At this point, the surgeon will use a weck-cell to ensure watertight closure.

TABLE 17-2 • MUSCLES, NERVE, FUNCTION, AND TESTING

Muscle	Nerve	Function	Testing
MR	3rd	Nasal	Look to Nose
LR	6th	Temporal	Look Away
SR	3rd	Elevate, Intorts, Adducts	Up and Out
IR	3rd	Depress, Extorts, Adduct	Down and Out
Superior Oblique	4th	Intorts, Depress, Abducts	Look Down and In
Inferior Oblique	3rd	Extorts, Elevates, Abducts	Look Up and In

IR, inferior rectus; LR, lateral rectus; MR, medial rectus; SR, superior rectus

Vitrectomy

In order to provide a better assessment of the retina, a vitrectomy may be performed. The vitreous is removed through the pars plana. Afterward, gas or oil may be used to replace the vitreous.

Pathology. Retinal tears can damage blood vessels, causing a vitreous hemorrhage. Also, patients that develop scar tissue formation after injuries require a vitrectomy to remove the scar tissue within the vitreous cavity. If the scar tissue is not removed, this may place traction on the vitreous humor, which can create a retinal detachment.

Diagnostic Procedures. When looking into the eye with an ophthalmoscope, the physician is able to view the retina. The retina should be lying against the chorodial layer of the eye. However, during a retinal detachment, this layer becomes separated from the choroid.

If additional diagnosis examination is needed to view the posterior portion, ultrasound may be utilized. The same technology that is utilized during pregnancy to view the fetus can be used to view the posterior segment of the eye.

Surgery—Steps Highlighted. The following are the steps involved in the surgery:

- With Westcott scissors and pick-ups with teeth, incisions are performed superotemporally, superonasally, and inferotemporally into the conjunctiva and Tenon's capsule.
- Using the wet field cautery, hemostasis is achieved. During this phase, the SA needs to irrigate with BSS.
- Using a caliper, the surgeon measures 3.5 mm to 4 mm from the limbus; this will be utilized as the entry point of the ora serrata. Based on the surgeon's preference, a nylon suture may be placed to hold the infusion cannula.
- Using a microvitreoretinal knife, the surgeon will create one or more sclerotomies at the upper border of the lateral muscle and the medial side. The sclerotomies will be the entry point for the infusing cannula and the vitrectomy handpiece. The SA needs to make sure the cornea remains moistened with BSS; otherwise, the cornea may dry out, making visibility very difficult.
- Surgeon closes sclerotomies with an 8-0 vicryl or any suture of choice. Closure of the conjunctiva and Tenon's capsule

incisions are performed using an absorbable suture. To minimize infections, the surgeon may inject antibiotic and steroid medications. The SA applies selected antibiotic ointment and covers the eye with the selected eye dressing.

Strabismus

Strabismus is the inability of the two eyes to focus on the same object (Table 17-2). The most common form of strabismus is esotropia, which is the turning in of the eyes. Other types of strabismus include exotropia, in which one eye turns out or away from the direction of sight; hypertropia, in which one eye turns up; and hypotropia, in which one eye turns down. Because of ocular misalignment, images are projected to noncorresponding parts of the retina. Vision will be impaired since the fovea is getting information from different fields of view. Because it is not possible to focus on two images at one accurately, the brain will tune out input from the deviated eye and use the aligned eye to focus. This process will avoid double vision and lead to amblyopia, in which the brain does not learn to see through the affected eye. If left untreated, the weaker eye may regress to the level of partial blindness. Strabismus mainly involves children; however, it can occur in adults. In adults, strabismus is usually the result of trauma or stroke.

Pathology. The six EOMs control the position of the eyes (Figure 17-8). If a problem with the muscles or the nerves controlling the EOMs occurs, it can cause paralytic strabismus. Cranial nerves III, IV, and VI control the EOMs. An injury to cranial nerve III causes the associated eye to deviate down and out. An injury to cranial nerve IV, which can be congenital, will cause the eye to drift up and perhaps slightly inward. An injury to cranial nerve VI causes the eyes to deviate inward. It may be caused by several factors based on the relatively long path of the nerve. At any given time, only one eye (fixating eye) can focus on the target of interest while the other eye deviates.

Diagnostic Procedures. An eye examination is required to diagnose strabismus; special attention needs to be given to ocular motility. Ocular motility refers to the movements of the eye in all directions. Strabismus is the failure of the eyes to direct their gaze at the same object, often resulting from muscular imbalance. Ocular misalignment may be comitant or incomitant (Table 17-3, Figure 17-9).

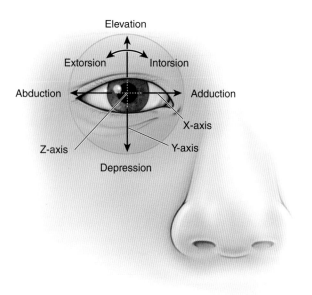

Figure 17-8 · Six extraocular muscles. (Reproduced, with permission, from Morton DA, Foreman KB, Albertine KH. *The Big Picture: Gross Anatomy.* 2nd ed. New York, NY: McGraw Hill; 2019.)

TABLE 17-3 • CLASSIFICATIONS OF STRABISMUS

Comitant Strabismus	Incomitant Strabismus
Deviation angle measures same in all fields of gaze	Deviation angle measures differently in fields of gaze
Both eyes move together well with no restriction or paresis	Characterized by limitation of ocular rotations due to ocular restriction or paresis
Usually not secondary to neurological involvement	Paresis always one of lateral rectus muscles, usually resulting from palsy of abducens nerve (CN VI)
Includes most types of congenital and childhood strabismus	Diplopia present when eyes turned in direction of paralyzed muscle

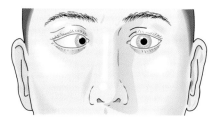

Primary position: right esotropia

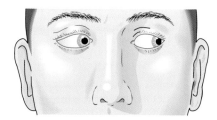

Left gaze: no deviation

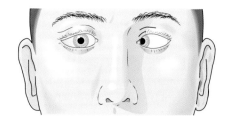

Right gaze: left esotropia

Figure 17-9 · Strabismus. (Reproduced, with permission, from Riordan-Eva P, Augsburger JJ, eds. *Vaughan & Asbury's General Ophthalmology.* 19th ed. New York, NY: McGraw Hill; 2018.)

Surgery—Steps Highlighted. The following are the steps involved in the surgery.

Note: Narrative describes correction with a recession. It is intended to illustrate basic surgical principles of strabismus surgery, which can be applied to other techniques.

- The SA prepares the eye by placing a speculum for exposure of the globe. The surgeon may place a bridle suture (0 silk) through the sclera at the 12 o'clock position (Figure 17-10).

- **Isolating the muscle**
The surgeon uses 0.5-mm toothed forceps to grasp the limbus in the intranasal quadrant and rotate superotemporally. The SA passes the Westcott scissors, and a buttonhole incision is made in the conjunctiva. Bleeding is controlled with cautery. While the surgeon is using the cautery, the SA irrigates with BSS. Once bleeding is controlled, the SA passes muscle hooks to the surgeon. Utilizing a two-muscle hook technique, the muscle is isolated

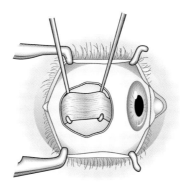

Exposure of lateral rectus

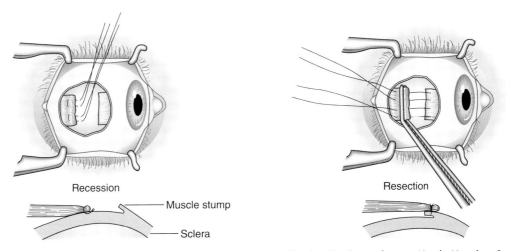

Recession   Resection

Muscle stump

Sclera

Figure 17-10 · Strabismus correction. (Reproduced, with permission, from Riordan-Eva P, Augsburger JJ, eds. *Vaughan & Asbury's General Ophthalmology*. 19th ed. New York, NY: McGraw Hill; 2018.)

on the muscle hook. (If SA holds muscle hooks, it is important not to tug on the muscle during surgery. This can create an oculocardiac reflex). The SA passes a 6-0 vicryl to the surgeon for suture placement, just posterior to the insertion. Also, the surgeon will place two locking sutures at the superior and inferior aspects of the muscle.

- **Muscle excised**
  The SA passes the Westcott scissors to the surgeon to disinsert the muscle from the sclera. The sutures support the remaining ends of the muscle.

- **Muscle attachment**
  The caliper is used to mark the location of the new insertion point. The surgeon attaches the muscle back to the scribe mark made by the caliper and secures it with a suture.

- **Closing the conjunctiva**
  The conjunctival incision is closed with a 5-0 or 6-0 absorbable suture. Alternatively, some surgeons may close the incision with cautery or tissue glue. The SA applies ophthalmic drops or ointment. Because no intraocular surgery has been performed, a patch is not needed.

Bibliography

Frey KB. *Surgical Technology for the Surgical Technologist: A Positive Care Approach*. 5th ed. Boston, MA: Delmar Cengage Learning; 2018.

Fuller JK. *Surgical Technology: Principles and Practice*. 7th ed. St. Louis, MO: Elsevier; 2018

Jordan DR, Anderson RL, Mawn L, American Academy of Ophthalmology. *Surgical Anatomy of the Ocular Adnexa: A Clinical Approach*. 2nd ed. New York, NY: Oxford University Press; 2012.

Stein HA, Stein RM, Freeman MI. *The Ophthalmic Assistant: A Text for Allied and Associated Ophthalmic Personnel*. 9th ed. St. Louis, MO: Elsevier Saunders; 2013.

Sturm RA, Larsson M. Genetics of human iris colour and patterns. *Pigment Cell Melanoma Res*. 2009; 22(5), 544-562.

18

Otorhinolaryngology

Jennifer Consorte and Rebecca Hall

DISCUSSED IN THIS CHAPTER

1. Anatomy of the ear, nose and throat
2. Diagnostics and indications for surgery
3. Surgical procedures related to ENT
4. Role of the surgical assistant in ENT

The word "otorhinolaryngology" or its shorter form, "ENT," is derived from the Greek root words: otos (ear), rhino (nose), laryngo (windpipe), and logos (science). Otolaryngologists train in medical and surgical remedies for hearing loss, ear infections, balance disorders (vertigo), ringing ears (tinnitus), and some cranial nerve disorders (Table 18-1). They also handle hereditary auditory situations.

Otolaryngology, or the ENT field of medicine, can be traced to the 19th century when physicians recognized that the head and neck consisted of many interrelated structures. Physicians established procedures and instruments for assessing and treating pathologies of the head and neck, ultimately establishing a medical specialty. According to the American Academy of Otolaryngology, it is the oldest medical specialty in the United States.

EAR ANATOMY

The ear is a sensory organ of hearing and equilibrium consisting of the external, middle, and inner ear. The external ear gathers sound pressure waves and guides them in the direction of the tympanic membrane (TM). The external ear consists of the auricle or pinna and the external auditory canal (**EAC**) (see Figure 18-1). The pinna is comprised of elastic cartilage with overlying skin. The shape of the pinna affects each sound amplification of incoming sounds uniquely, assisting in the vertical localization of sound. The external auditory canal is a curved tubal structure directly posterior to the temporomandibular joint. It is comprised of 1/3 cartilaginous tissue laterally and bone in the medial 2/3 of the structure. The **tragus** demarcates the anterior canal and sits directly behind the parotid gland.

The facial nerve leaves the **stylomastoid foramen** 1 cm deep to the tip of the tragus. The **fissures of Santorini** create small fenestrations through the anterior and inferior portions of the ear canal. The cartilaginous contains hair follicles, sebaceous glands, and ceruminous glands that generate cerumen, or ear wax. The mastoid bone is part of the temporal bone and lies behind the ear canal. It can be palpated behind the ear where the bone of the skull ends, and the muscles of the neck begin. The outer cortex of the mastoid bone is solid, although it is mainly composed of trabeculae. The trabeculae form a complex network of air-containing passages that form the antrum, or bony cavity, that opens into the middle ear.

The space of the middle ear is air-filled, narrow, and is divided into an upper and lower chamber. The middle ear space is rectangular in shape and can be divided into three regions: the upper epitympanum, the middle mesotympanum, and the lower hypotympanum. The outer or lateral wall of the middle ear space is created by the **TM**, (see Figure 18-2). The ceiling is a thin plate of bone, called the tegmen, that divides the middle ear cavity from the cranial cavity and brain above. The floor is comprised of a thin bony plate that separates the middle ear cavity from the jugular vein and the carotid artery. The posterior wall communicates with the mastoid air cells and mastoid antrum through the aditus. The anterior wall is the opening of the eustachian tube and unites the middle ear with the nasopharynx. The middle ear contains a mucous membrane that is uninterrupted with the pharynx and mastoid cells, allowing for possible infection to travel to the middle ear such as otitis media or mastoiditis. Aeration of the air-filled spaces of the temporal bone is accomplished via the eustachian tube. The **eustachian tube** also equalizes pressure in the middle ear with

TABLE 18-1 • TYPES OF HEARING LOSS			
Category	Description	Causes	Symptoms
Sensorineural	The most common type of hearing loss. A permanent hearing loss develops when there is damage to either the tiny hair-like cells of the inner ear or the auditory nerve itself. This prevents or weakens the transfer of nerve signals to the brain.	Meniere's disease A side effect of medications Trauma Exposure to loud noises Presbycusis Heart disease Diabetes Congenital hearing loss Tumors Strokes	Speech of others is heard but hard to understand Difficulty following a conversation with multiple people Tinnitus Difficulty listening in noisy surroundings Difficulty hearing high-pitched sounds Noises seem too loud or quiet A feeling of vertigo
Conductive	A less common type of hearing loss. It occurs when there is an obstruction or damage to the outer or middle ear that prevents sound from being conducted to the inner ear. It may be temporary or permanent.	Stenosis or a narrowing of the ear canal Wax impaction Exostoses Otitis externa Obstructions caused by foreign bodies inserted into the ear Microtia Fluid in the middle ear Otosclerosis Otitis media	Easier time hearing out of one ear than the other Pain in one or both ears Sensation of pressure in one or both ears Difficulty or frustration with telephone conversations A foul odor emanating from the ear canal A feeling that one's own voice sounds louder or different
Mixed	Loss of hearing acuity resulting from a combination of conductive and sensorineural factors	Mixed hearing loss generally occurs when the ear sustains some type of trauma. It also can happen gradually over time when one type of hearing loss is combined with another	The symptoms of mixed hearing loss will be some combination of those listed above for the other two types of hearing loss

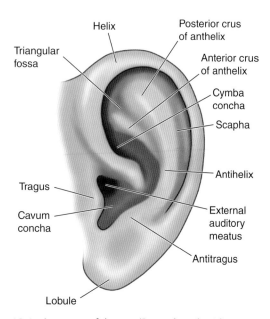

Figure 18-1 • Anatomy of the ear. (Reproduced, with permission, from Lalwani AK, ed. *Current Diagnosis & Treatment in Otolaryngology—Head & Neck Surgery*. 4th ed. New York, NY: McGraw Hill; 2020.)

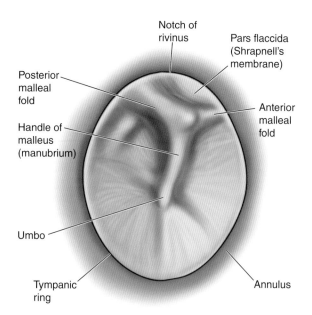

Figure 18-2 • Tympanic membrane. (Reproduced, with permission, from Lalwani AK, ed. *Current Diagnosis & Treatment in Otolaryngology—Head & Neck Surgery*. 4th ed. New York, NY: McGraw Hill; 2020.)

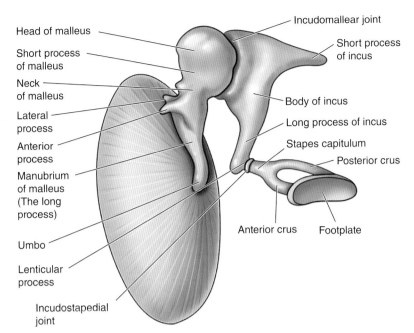

Figure 18-3 Ossicles of the ear. (Reproduced, with permission, from Lalwani AK, ed. *Current Diagnosis & Treatment in Otolaryngology—Head & Neck Surgery.* 4th ed. New York, NY: McGraw Hill; 2020.)

atmospheric pressure. Another element of the middle ear is the articulated **ossicular chain**, comprising the malleus, incus, and stapes (see Figure 18-3). The ossicular chain expands across the middle ear space and conducts vibrations (airborne sound waves) from the TM across the middle ear into the **oval window** and the fluid-filled inner ear. The branches of the internal and external carotid artery supply blood to the middle ear.

The inner ear is a membranous, curved space located in the pyramid-shaped medial area of the temporal bone. It contains hair cell receptors that provide us with both hearing and balance and is protected from loud noise by the tensor tympani and stapedius muscle which are connected to the ossicles and provide attenuation of otherwise damaging sound waves. The inner ear consists of a bony labyrinth filled with a watery fluid (**perilymph**) that encircles and infuses a membranous labyrinth filled with endolymph. The inner ear has two main parts: the **cochlea**, the hearing portion, and the **vestibular labyrinth,** the balance portion.

The cochlea is snail shaped and is separated into three compartments: the scala vestibuli which relates to the oval window, the scala tympani which relates to the round window, and the cochlear duct. The scala vestibuli and scala tympani are lined with perilymph while the cochlear duct contains endolymph. The **organ of Corti** is the neural organ for hearing and can be found on the basilar membrane of the cochlear. Thousands of hair cells are set in motion by vibrations passing through the ossicles and oval window to the perilymph. The vestibular labyrinth is comprised of the utricle, the saccule, and the three semi-circular canals. The utricle and saccule utilize bidirectional coding as there are hair cells oriented in both directions across their surface. Because of this, a single macule can produce both excitatory and inhibitory signals with an alteration of the head position.

The semi-circular canals are little canals lined up at right angles (90°) to each other. This enables the brain to recognize which direction the head is moving. Each of the canals is positioned to respond in distinct planes of movement. The semi-circular canals are filled with fluid and contain small calcium crystals (**cristae**) embedded in the lining.

CRANIAL NERVES

The trigeminal (fifth cranial) delivers sensory innervation to the face, oral cavity, nose, nasal cavity, and maxillary sinuses. It gives motor innervation to the muscles of mastication. The eighth cranial nerve, or the auditory nerve originates from the inner ear and terminates in the brain. This nerve conveys both balance and hearing information to the brain. Along with the eighth cranial nerve runs the seventh cranial nerve. The seventh cranial nerve, or facial nerve, is a bone-covered structure that runs through the temporal bone and controls the muscles of facial expression, and functions in the transmission of taste sensations from the anterior two-thirds of the tongue.

LYMPHATIC SYSTEM OF THE HEAD AND NECK

The head and neck comprise an intricate lymphatic network of more than 300 superficial and deep nodes. The lymphatic system provides immunologic and circulatory functions by draining tissue fluid, plasma proteins, and other cellular debris into the bloodstream. As the lymph nodes trap foreign matter, like bacteria, viruses, or tumor cells, the nodes become enlarged or infected. Lymphadenopathy is a considerable clinical discovery related to acute infection, granulomatous disease, autoimmune disease, and malignancy. The enlargement of certain nodal groups is a marker of pathologically affected organs and tissues, specifically regarding malignancy. Detailed knowledge of the anatomic relationship of the lymphatic system and the structures they drain is crucial in providing proper treatment in patients with cancers of the head and neck.

Superficial nodes that drain into the deep cervical nodes that lie along the internal jugular vein are:

- Occipital, retro auricular, and parotid nodes drain lymph from the scalp, auricle, and middle ear.
- Submandibular nodes drain lymph from the face, sinuses, mouth, and tongue.
- Retropharyngeal nodes drain lymph from deeper structures of the cranium and superior section of the pharynx.

Deep cervical nodes drain into the thoracic duct or right lymphatic duct. The thoracic duct empties into the intersection of the left internal jugular vein and the left subclavian vein. The right lymphatic duct drains into a parallel site on the right side at the root of the neck (see Figure 18-4). The nasal cavity, the paranasal sinuses, and the pharynx drain into the retropharyngeal nodes. The submandibular nodes drain the mouth, lips, and external nose. The tip of the tongue drains into the submental nodes, and the lymph nodes of the posterior tongue drain into the cervical nodes.

ETIOLOGY

Chronic suppurative otitis media (CSOM), illustrated by frequent or lengthy episodes of acute otitis media lasting for more than 12 weeks, may produce damage to the TM, causing a non-healing perforation. The TM is divided into two membranes, the pars tensa and the pars flaccida. The pars flaccida, also called Shrapnell's membrane, is the triangular flaccid portion of the TM. It is situated above the malleolar folds connected to the bone at the notch of Rivinus. The pars tensa is the tense portion of the TM and is considered the main portion of the TM. The periphery of the pars tensa forms the fibrocartilaginous ring called Gerlach's ligament. TM perforations (TMPs) can appear in the pars tensa or the pars flaccida. Upper respiratory tract infection, malnutrition, eustachian tube dysfunction, and poor hygiene are factors that may lead to CSOM. The history of tympanoplasty began in the 1950s when Wullstein and Zollner popularized the technique of using overlay graft to reconstruct the perforated TM and restore the sound conduction apparatus of the middle ear.

Diseases of the mastoid are the most common reason to perform a mastoidectomy. Mastoiditis and cholesteatoma are both common causes of chronic ear drainage and may lead to a mastoidectomy. Mastoiditis is a bacterial infection of the

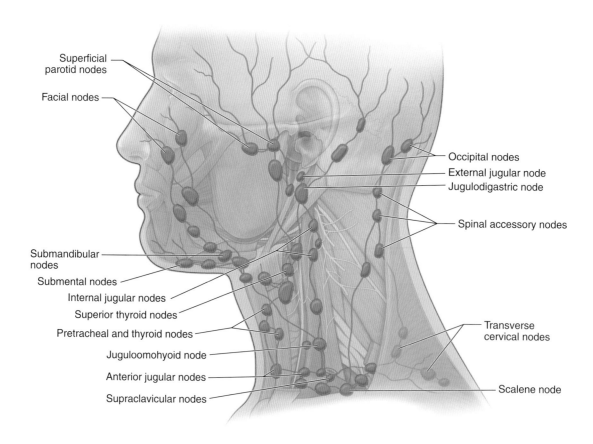

Figure 18-4 · Lymphatic system of the head and neck. (Reproduced, with permission, from Lalwani AK, ed. *Current Diagnosis & Treatment in Otolaryngology—Head & Neck Surgery*. 4th ed. New York, NY: McGraw Hill; 2020.)

mastoid air cells surrounding the inner and middle ear. The mastoid bone, which is part of the temporal bone of the skull, is comprised of these air cells. The mastoid air cells are designed to shield the delicate structures of the ear, regulate ear pressure, and safeguard the temporal bone during trauma.

When the mastoid cells become infected or inflamed, due to unresolved otitis media, mastoiditis may occur. Acute mastoiditis usually involves children, but adults can also be affected.

A **cholesteatoma** is an atypical, noncancerous skin growth that can grow in the middle section of your ear, at the back of the eardrum. It may be a birth defect, but generally caused by recurrent middle ear infections. A cholesteatoma often builds as a cyst, or sac, that sheds layers of old skin. A cholesteatoma can cause bone damage, dizziness, infection, or even abscesses. The signs and symptoms of cholesteatoma consist of foul-smelling **otorrhoea,** hearing loss, TMP, and possible attic retraction. Sizeable invasive cholesteatomas may necessitate a mastoidectomy as well as reconstruction of the TM and ossicular chain.

Cochlear implant surgery is usually accompanied by a mastoidectomy to reach the appropriate anatomical landmark. It allows for good visualization and insertion of the cochlear implants at the proper angle. Acoustic neuromas or facial nerve tumors are often removed through a mastoid approach or translabyrinthine approach where the bony and membranous labyrinth are removed as well.

CONDITIONS OF THE EXTERNAL EAR

Infective and Inflammatory Disorders of the External Ear

- Impetigo encompasses the epidermis of the auricle and is frequently triggered by *Staphylococcus aureus* or *Staphylococcus epidermidis*. It will display as red papules, which can evolve into vesicles, or open crusting sores. Treatment entails antibiotics and local wound care.

- Erysipelas comprises the dermis of the ear and is frequently caused by group-A hemolytic streptococcus. The patient experiences pain, erythema, and edema of the auricle. The affected area is delineated from uninvolved skin and can be treated with oral antimicrobials. Intravenous antibiotics are suggested if rapid reduction of the erythema and edema is not seen within 48 hours.

- Relapsing perichondritis is an autoimmune disease that can mimic the above infections. Relapsing perichondritis will involve only the skin adherent to the ear cartilage, while erysipelas involves the entire auricle, including the lobule.

Trauma

- Trauma is classified as blunt or penetrating. Blunt trauma to the pinna can be caused by a range of events, such as boxing, wrestling, self-mutilation, or deliberate force with a blunt object.

- Blunt trauma can lead to hematomas or seromas with separation of the perichondrium and underlying cartilage that disrupts the nutritional support of the auricular. To prevent harmful repercussions, fluid collections should be treated quickly through an irrigation and debridement (I & D) procedure. Dressing should include cotton bolsters sutured close to the incision to prevent fluid re-accumulation. Failure to treat this condition in a timely manner leads to a condition known as *cauliflower ear*. Penetrating trauma includes lacerations to avulsion of the auricle. Treatment of lacerations encompasses wound approximation from one to three layers depending on cartilage and pinna involvement.

Tumors

- The most common skin cancer of the auricle is basal cell carcinoma and is addressed through a local excision. If the lesion is recurrent, a Mohs procedure may be necessary.

- Squamous cell is less common than basal cell and is treated through local excision if the lesion is small. Resection of the auricle may be indicated for large invasive lesions.

- If malignant melanoma involves the auricle, a wide local excision is indicated. Extensive lesions may include a parotidectomy or regional neck dissection.

CONDITIONS OF THE EXTERNAL EAR CANAL

- *Pseudomonas aeruginosa* is the leading cause of the inflammatory condition otitis externa. It can be caused by trauma to the canal through the misuse of cotton swabs in the ears or water trapped in the ear canal known as *swimmer's ear*. Treatment typically involves ototopical fluoroquinolones, but other ototopical antibiotics are available as well.

- Most external ear canal infections are bacterial, although *Aspergillus niger* and *Candida albicans* will cause fungal infections that require the use of antifungal agents to treat.

- A herpes zoster infection is the source of Ramsay Hunt syndrome causing external otitis. It will present as vesicles containing the epithelium of the external canal. Hearing loss, facial nerve paralysis, and vertigo are associated with Ramsay Hunt syndrome. Treatment includes antivirals such as acyclovir or valacyclovir, as well as steroids for cranial nerve pathology.

DIAGNOSTIC MODALITIES

Audiometry

Patients who have a hearing loss, whether it is damage to the organs of hearing, or a tumor in or around the ear, should have an audiogram performed. An audiometry assessment is a noninvasive hearing test that measures a person's ability to hear different sounds, pitches, or frequencies. While wearing earphones, the patient has a range of sounds directed to one ear at a time.

The loudness of sound is measured in decibels (dB).

- A whisper is about 20 dB.
- Loud music ranges from 80 to 120 dB.
- Sound from a jet engine is about 120 to 140 dB.

The tone of sound is measured in frequencies (Hz).

- Low bass tones range from 50 to 60 Hz.
- High-pitched tones range 10,000 Hz or higher.
- Normal hearing range is from 250 to 8,000 Hz at 25 dB or lower.

Word Recognition

Patients may also be given a word recognition test. This test will assess a person's ability to distinguish between different sounds that sound similar. A poor word recognition score can mean the patient will do poorly with a traditional hearing aid and may be a candidate for a cochlear implant.

Tympanometry

A tympanometry test can help identify perforated eardrum, ossicle bone damage, or tumors of the middle ear. The middle and inner ears are comprised of bony structures, soft tissue structures, and fluid-filled spaces.

Tuning Fork

A tuning fork will test bone conduction and sensorineural hearing function of the cochlea.

Brainstem Evoked Response Test

The brainstem evoked response (BSER), brainstem auditory evoked response (BAER) test, and automated auditory brainstem response (AABR) test are a 60-minute exams to obtain more information about the hearing nerve. While you relax, a computer will measure how your hearing nerve responds to sounds.

Distortion Product Otoacoustic Emission Testing

A distortion test checks outer hair cell function. It helps to determine the part of the ear that may be damaged. It is also a nonparticipatory test useful in young children who cannot have a regular audiogram.

Electronystagmography

Electronystagmography is a test performed to assess the functioning of the inner ear and nerves that connect the brain, ears, and eyes. It is helpful in diagnosing vestibular abnormalities.

Facial Electromyography

Facial electromyography is a test to record electrical activity in facial muscles and can determine the prognosis of a facial paralysis or weakness.

Auditory Brainstem Response Test (ABR)

An auditory brainstem response (ABR) test is used to test the response of the brainstem to electrical stimuli. It provides physicians with information about potential hearing loss.

Computed Tomography / Magnetic Resonance Imaging

Using a high-resolution magnetic resonance imaging (MRI) allows for optimized and accurate images of the auditory and vestibular system. Computed tomography (CT) scans are radiographic findings that offer visualization of bone, soft tissue, and intracranial and extracranial pathologic disorders. High-resolution CT scanning is needed to adequately visualize the delicate structures of the middle and inner ears. The MRI should consist of a three-dimensional reconstructed images. MRIs use magnetic and radiofrequency waves to reproduce cross-sectional images without ionizing radiation. An MRI will capture fat and fluid highlighting them as bright areas. A combination of a CT and MRI can aid in accurately predicting disease location and the extent of the damage for a variety of conditions of the head and neck, as well as tumors in the oral cavity, and pathologic conditions of the external auditory canal, middle ear, and the mastoid.

Tympanoplasty

Tympanoplasty is performed to repair a perforated TM, as well as possible reconstruction of the ossicles, with the goal of restoring hearing and preventing recurrent infections. Historically, Horst Ludwig Wullstein and Fritz Zöllner established the tympanoplasty using split-thickness and full-thickness skin grafts to reconstruct the perforated TM and reestablish the sound conduction apparatus of the middle ear. The current approach uses temporalis fascia grafts for reconstruction. Risks of performing a tympanoplasty include pain, bleeding, infection, failure of the graft, recurrence, further surgery, worsening hearing loss or deafness, dizziness, and facial nerve injury resulting in facial palsy or to the chorda tympani nerve resulting in taste disturbances.

Diagnostic Tests to Determine TMPs

- Radiography and MRI are not utilized unless the surgeon suspects ossicular destruction and/or cholesteatoma. Most TMPs are diagnosed using routine otoscopy.
- Small perforations may necessitate otomicroscopy.
- Middle ear impedance testing.
- Audiometry for initial TMP diagnosis and again before surgery.
- Preoperative and postoperative audiography.

The most common grafts used to repair the eardrum include:

- Temporalis fascia
- Tragal or conchal cartilage
- Periosteum
- Canal skin
- Alloplastic grafts

Temporalis fascia is the most common graft utilized. Cartilage can be harvested from either the tragus or the conchal if a postauricular approach is being used. Tragal cartilage is harvested with perichondrium connected through a small incision at the internal surface of the tragus.

Temporalis fascia is available through the same postauricular incision that is used for the tympanoplasty; otherwise, a separate incision is made in or beyond the postauricular hairline if a transcanal or endaural procedure is used. A benign amount of donor site morbidity ensues, with postoperative pain over the temporalis muscle the most common symptom patients' experience.

- The postauricular incision is marked and injected with lidocaine with epinephrine.
- Dissection is carried down to the fascia.
- The graft is harvested.
- Muscle is removed from the fascia graft, and the graft is located to the back table for future use (see Figure 18-5).

Preparation of the Patient

General Anesthesia: Supine position with the head rotated approximately 30 to 45 ° away from the surgeon. After induction, the patient is often rotated 180°. The head of the patient is often positioned at the foot of the bed to allow the surgeon to place their legs under the operating room (OR) table while sitting.

Arms may be tucked with all bony prominences padded. A pillow under the knees to relieve lower back pressure. The patient will be secured to the bed with straps at the level of the chest and hips to allow for rotation of the OR table. Check with the surgeon if using N_2O during the maintenance phase of anesthesia. N_2O should be turned off prior to graft placement as it can cause an increase in ear pressure pushing on the new graft.

Skin Prep: If hair removal is necessary, surgical clippers should be used. Hair should be about 1 to 2 cm away from a postauricular and endaural incision site. Using betadine swabs or a povidone-iodine 10% solution poured on 4 × 4s, the area is prepped around the back of the ear, down the neck and hairline, and portion of the cheek. The ear canal is also swabbed or prepped ensuring there is no pooling of solution in the ear.

Draping: May be towels around the head (turban) head wrap in addition to a drape to cover the patient's body.

Microscopic Approach. The postauricular approach and transcanal approach are commonly utilized when using the microscope. The Lempert endaural approach is rarely used today. The patient is injected postaurically and in the ear canal using xylocaine with epi and a 27-gauge needle.

- The surgeon will make canal incisions to form a tympanomeatal flap.
- An incision is made about 1 cm posterior to the auricle skin fold. The surgical assistant (SA) will retract the ear anteriorly.
- The periosteum over the mastoid is reflected anteriorly using a periosteal elevator until the underside of the canal skin is exposed.
- The incision is carried down through the musculoperiosteum to create a flap which is elevated toward the ear canal entering the bony canal.
- Skin along the posterior aspect of the bony canal is elevated until the surgeon reaches the tympanomeatal flap incisions.
- The flap is raised, and the middle ear is entered.
- The ossicular chain is repaired at this stage if needed.
- The limbus is undermined; the TM is lifted; and the perforation is covered with a graft medially.
- The graft should cover the TM and be anchored to the ear canal.
- Care is taken to avoid the chorda tympani in the posterior region.

Endoscopic Approach. A less invasive approach to repairing TMPs can be accomplished through an endoscopic approach. It offers a wider view of the middle ear anatomy, eliminating external incisions thereby reducing operative and recovery time.

Endoscopic tympanoplasty is accomplished using a transcanal approach. Deepithelization will be performed as needed. The incision in the ear canal may be endaural, lateral, circumferential, or swing door. This will allow the creation of the tympanomeatal flap and annulus to be elevated giving access to the middle ear. The malleus is peeled off the TM and repair of the ossicular chain (ossiculoplasty) is completed if necessary.

The prepared graft is put in place medially to the TM and lateral to the malleus. Gel foam sponges are placed in the middle and outer ear canals. Studies show tympanoplasty to be 93% successful in patients, especially when the temporalis fascia graft is utilized.

Massive middle ear cholesteatoma that involves the mastoid, presence of obstruction, and exostosis in the external ear canal will prevent an endoscopic approach.

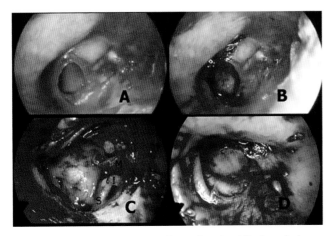

Figure 18-5 · Endoscopic views of a perforation (A), denuded edge of the perforation (B), elevated tympanomeatal flap and middle ear cavity (C), graft placed lateral to the malleus and medial (over-underlay) to the membrane remnant (D). M, malleus; I, incus; S, stapes. (Reproduced, with permission, from Akyigit A, Sakallioglu O, Karlidag T. Endoscopic tympanoplasty. *J Otol.* 2017 Jun;12:62-67.)

Butterfly Myringoplasty. The butterfly myringoplasty can be performed for nonmarginal perforations. The ossicular chain should be intact. The procedure will use a cartilage graft. Under general anesthesia, the perforation is evaluated by a 0° rigid scope of either 2.7 or 4 mm in diameter. The edge of the perforation is deepithelized. The conditions of the middle ear and ossicles are examined. The size of the perforation is determined using an angled pick. The cartilage graft is prepared leaving perichondrium on both sides. The graft should be 0.5 mm wider than the actual perforation. The graft is positioned medial to the TM with the use of an endoscope and verified with a pick. Gelfoam is placed at the borders of the graft and TM.

General Complications. The general complications of tympanoplasty include:

- Infection
- Graft failure
- Chondritis
- Injury to the nerve (chorda tympani)
- Sensorineural hearing loss (SNHL) and vertigo
- Increased conductive hearing loss
- External auditory canal stenosis

Mastoidectomy

The mastoid receives air from the eustachian tube, and any blockage will lead to mastoiditis. Mastoiditis will present with drainage from the affected ear, ear pain, fever, headache and possible hearing loss, redness, swelling and tenderness behind the affected ear. Tests to confirm mastoiditis include:

- A white blood cell count to confirm the presence of an infection
- CT scan
- MRI
- X ray of skull
- Possible spinal tap to determine if the infection spread to the spinal column

Nonsurgical treatment will involve hospitalization with an antibiotic regimen. Oral antibiotics will be prescribed for home treatment. If the antibiotics are unsuccessful, a mastoidectomy is indicated.

Preoperative. The preoperative procedures include:

- History and physical (H&P)
- Diagnostic lab reports
- CT scan
- MRI
- Signed consent form

Approaches. **Simple mastoidectomy** involves opening the mastoid bone, removing the infected air cells, and draining the middle ear.

Complete or canal wall up mastoidectomy removes all the mastoid air cells along the tegmen, sigmoid sinus, pre-sigmoid dural plate, and posterior wall of the external auditory canal. The posterior wall of the external auditory canal is maintained.

Canal wall down mastoidectomy involves a complete mastoidectomy including the removal of the posterior and superior osseous external auditory canal. The TM is remodeled to separate the middle ear space from the mastoid cavity and ear canal.

Radical mastoidectomy will remove mastoid air cells, eardrum, most of the middle ear structures, and ear canal. The eustachian tube is often eliminated with soft tissue to reduce the risk of a chronic otorrhea. A skin graft can be placed in the middle ear to reduce the risk of fluid discharge.

Modified radical mastoidectomy is a less severe form of radical mastoidectomy and allows for saving some of the middle ear structures including the TM.

Preparation of the Patient

General Anesthesia: Supine position with the head rotated approximately 30 to 45° away from the surgeon. After induction, the patient is often rotated 180°. The head of the patient is often positioned at the foot of the bed to allow the surgeon to place their legs under the OR table while sitting.

Arms may be tucked with all bony prominences padded. A pillow under the knees to relieve lower back pressure. The patient will be secured to the bed with straps at the level of the chest and hips to allow for rotation of the OR table.

Surgical Procedure. The incision area is often injected with lidocaine or marcaine with diluted epinephrine from the region of the mastoid tip to include the linea temporalis.

A curvilinear postauricular incision is made 5 to 10 mm to the postauricular sulcus. Skin and subcutaneous tissue is elevated off the mastoid periosteum and temporalis fascia by way of sharp dissection. The skin flap is elevated, and a T- or 7-shaped incision is made with the top of the T at the linea temporalis from the zygomatic root to the occipital mastoid suture. Hemostasis is maintained with a monopolar cautery. The periosteum is elevated to expose the spine of Henle and the ear canal. See Figure 18-6. The SA will place a Weitlaner retractor to hold the auricle forward.

Using a drill, a cutting burr is utilized to mark the tegmen superiorly, the sigmoid sinus posteriorly, the posterior bony external ear canal anteriorly, and the digastric ridge inferiorly. The drill is used to remove the mastoid bone. The semicircular canal offers a landmark to recognize the dissection has reached the depth of the facial nerve. The antrum is identified at the deepest and the most anterior part of the dissection. The open antrum provides air circulation between the mastoid and the middle ear. A cholesteatoma can extend from the middle ear to the mastoid as well as to the antrum area. The diseased mastoid lining and any cholesteatoma are removed with a high-speed drill from the mastoid cavity.

The wound is usually closed with absorbable deep sutures to bring the periosteum back together. Buried interrupted sutures are placed in the deep dermal layer. The epidermis is closed

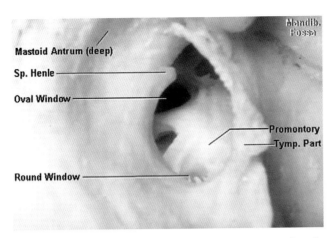

Figure 18-6 · Spine of Henle. (Reproduced from Cohen-Gadol A. *The Neurosurgical Atlas*. https://www.neurosurgicalatlas.com/; https://assets.neurosurgicalatlas.com/eyJidWNrZXQiOiJuc2F0bGGFzLWFFzc2V-0cyIsImtleSI6Im5IdXJvYW5hdG9teVwvUmhvdG9uX1B1YnNcL1JQM-jZfMTEuanBnIiwiZWRpdHMiOnsicmVzaXplIjp7ImZpdC6lmNvdm-Vyliwid2lkdGgiOjEyMDB9LCJqcGVnIjp7InF1YWxpdHkiOjY1fX19.)

with a running stitch or by tissue adhesive. Mastisol and steri strips are used to dress the wound if a running stitch is applied. Complications include:

- Facial nerve injury
- Hearing loss
- Vertigo
- Taste disturbance
- Cerebrospinal fluid leak
- Need for revision
- Postoperative infection
- Postoperative bleeding

Patients will remain for several hours in recovery, then discharged home. They can expect mild pain which can be controlled with pain medications. Recovery can take up to 6 weeks and hearing evaluations will be performed after recovery. Patients should not blow their noses for 4 weeks. Ear drops may be prescribed. Instructions will include: no bending, lifting, straining aerobic exercise, heavy work, or traveling without surgeon approval. Ibuprofen and aspirin should be discontinued 2 weeks prior to surgery and 1 week after surgery.

NASAL ANATOMY

The nose is an olfactory and respiratory organ located in the middle of the face. The internal part of the nose, the nasal cavity, lies above the roof of the mouth. There are four functions associated with the nasal cavity:

- Responsible for the sense of smell
- Drains and clears the paranasal sinuses and lacrimal ducts
- Warms and humidifies inspired air
- Removes and traps pathogens and particulate matter from the inspired air

The nose consists of:

- **External meatus.** Triangular-shaped projection in the center of the face.
- **External nostrils.** Two chambers divided by the septum.
- **Septum.** Made up primarily of cartilage and bone and covered by mucous membranes. The cartilage also gives shape and support to the outer part of the nose.
- **Nasal passages.** Passages that are lined with mucous membranes and tiny hairs (cilia) that help to filter the air.
- **Sinuses.** Four pairs of air-filled cavities, also lined with mucous membranes. The sinuses are cavities, or air-filled pockets, near the nasal passage. There are four different types of sinuses:
- **Ethmoid sinus.** The ethmoid sinuses are located in the spongy ethmoid bone near the bridge of the nose and form air cells between the eyes. They are present at birth and grow until the age of 12. Blood supply to the ethmoid sinuses arises from the anterior and posterior ethmoidal arteries from the ophthalmic artery and the sphenopalatine artery from the terminal branches of the internal maxillary artery.
- **Maxillary sinus.** This bilateral sinus is the largest of all the sinuses. They are located lateral to the nasal cavity and beneath the orbits. The maxillary sinus decreases skull weight, generates mucus, and affects the tone quality of a person's voice. The blood supply to the maxillary sinus is provided by the superior, anterior, middle, and posterior alveolar arteries, the infraorbital artery, and the greater palatine artery. The maxillary sinus has six borders that are comprised of:
  - the medial wall: nasal surface of the maxilla;
  - the lateral wall: zygomatic process of the maxilla;
  - the inferior wall: alveolar process and a section of the palatine process;
  - the superior wall: orbital surface of the maxilla and forms the floor of the orbit;
  - the anterior wall: anterior surface of the maxilla; and
  - the posterior wall: infratemporal surface of the maxilla.
- **Frontal sinus.** The frontal sinus is an air-filled, triangular-shaped cavity located superior to all other paranasal sinuses, positioned within the frontal bone. It does not develop until around 7 years of age. The blood vessels supporting the frontal sinus include the supraorbital and anterior ethmoidal arteries.
- **Sphenoid sinus.** This sinus is located deep in the face, posterior to the upper part of the nose. It does not typically develop until adolescence. The sphenoidal sinuses vary in shape and size from person to person. The blood supply to the sphenoid sinus is carried out by the posterior ethmoidal branches of the ophthalmic arteries and nasal branches of the sphenopalatine arteries (see Figure 18-7).

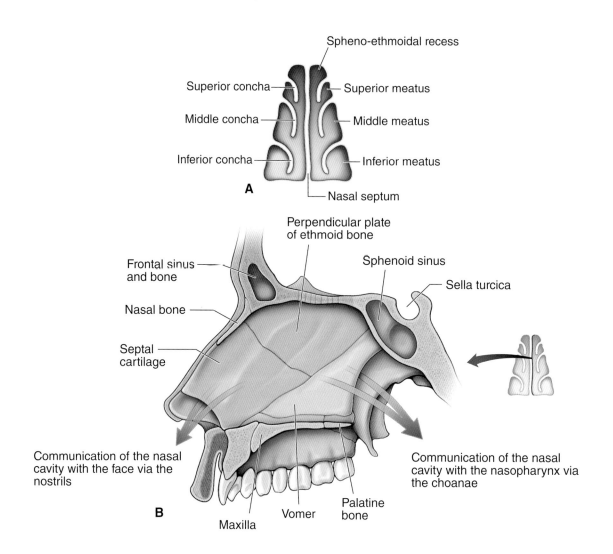

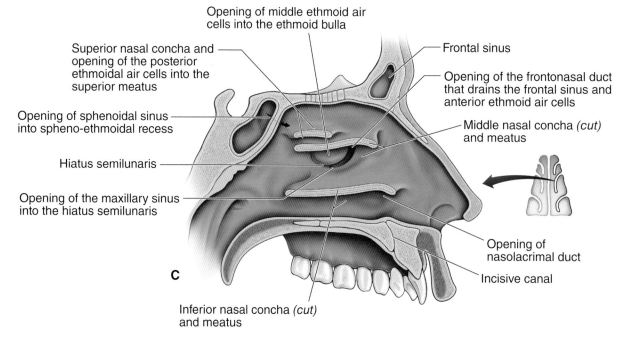

Figure 18-7 · Anatomy of the nose. (Reproduced, with permission, from Morton DA, Foreman KB, Albertine KH. *The Big Picture: Gross Anatomy.* 2nd ed. New York, NY: McGraw Hill; 2019.)

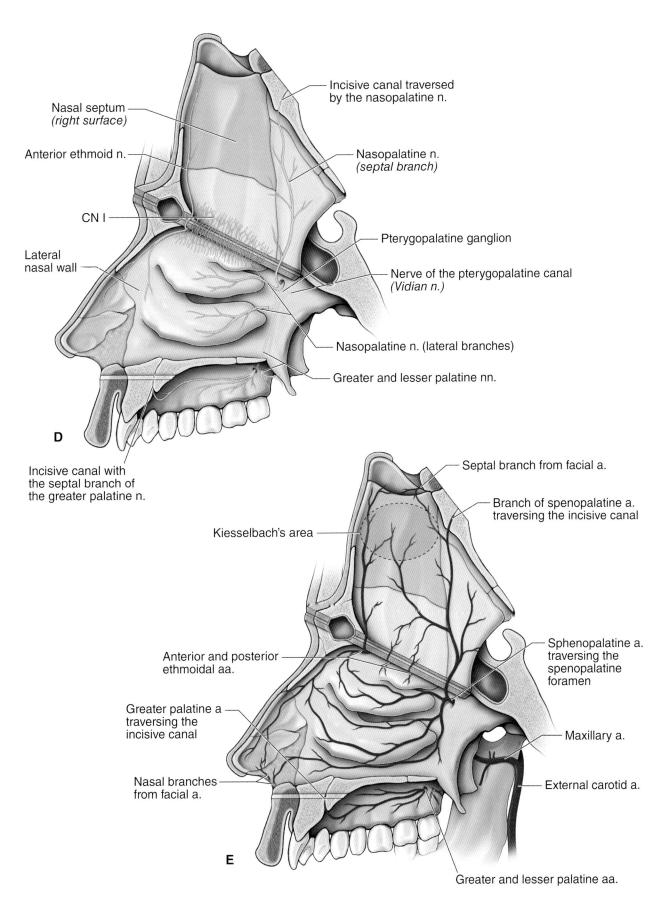

D

Nasal septum
(right surface)

Anterior ethmoid n.

CN I

Lateral
nasal wall

Incisive canal traversed
by the nasopalatine n.

Nasopalatine n.
(septal branch)

Pterygopalatine ganglion

Nerve of the pterygopalatine canal
(Vidian n.)

Nasopalatine n. (lateral branches)

Greater and lesser palatine nn.

Incisive canal with
the septal branch of
the greater palatine n.

E

Septal branch from facial a.

Branch of spenopalatine a.
traversing the incisive canal

Kiesselbach's area

Anterior and posterior
ethmoidal aa.

Greater palatine a
traversing the
incisive canal

Nasal branches
from facial a.

Sphenopalatine a.
traversing the
spenopalatine
foramen

Maxillary a.

External carotid a.

Greater and lesser palatine aa.

Figure 18-7 · *(Continued)*

DIAGNOSTIC AND TREATMENT MODALITIES

Sinus Surgery

Ethmoidectomy. May be performed to open the ethmoid sinus cavity to improve drainage into the nasal airway.

Maxillary Antrostomy. The maxillary sinus will be opened, clearing the blockage to allow fluid from the maxillary sinus to drain more efficiently, as well as reducing the reccurrence of sinus infections.

FESS and Septoplasty. These types of cases will usually have a "set up tray" on a separate prep/small table or mayo. It is considered a "clean procedure." It will include a nasal speculum, smooth bayonet forceps, medicine cups labeled with local and topical anesthesia, controlled syringes with needles, and cottonoids. The doctor will usually inject local anesthesia and pack the nose with two cottonoids per nostril or may use cotton balls.

Functional Endoscopic Sinus Surgery (FESS)

Patient Position and Prep: The patient is positioned supine, and the OR table may be reversed or rotated 90° with the patient's head at the foot of the table to give the surgeon access. Some surgeons prefer a gel headrest or shoulder roll to slightly hyperextend the neck for easier access. The patient's bony prominences are well padded, and arms are tucked. A nasal 0°, 45°, or 30° endoscope is used to visualize the sinuses.

Anesthesia: FESS procedures are performed under general anesthesia.

Surgical Procedure

- Anti-fog or (FRED) should be available.
- Depending on the disease or blockage, tissue can be removed by a variety of biting forceps, biopsy forceps (Blakesley), Kerrison rongeur, tru-cut forceps, scissors, curette, sickle knife, or mushroom punch forceps.
- A FESS may include excision of the ethmoid tissue and partial or total resection of the middle turbinate.
- If performing a total sphenoethmoidectomy or sphenoidotomy, a micro-debrider is used.
- Specimens will be sent separately as left and right.

A **FESS** may use *image-guided surgery* as well.

Once dissection or resection is complete, hemostasis is achieved by nasal packing soaked in topical anesthetic, or Meropack, which is a bioresorbable nasal packing that is left in and resorbed in about 2 weeks. Another hemostatic agent used is MeroGel, which can be injected to help with adhesions as well as hemostasis. A dressing may be optional which could be sinus packing, Gelfilm, or no packing/dressing at all.

An SA should become familiar with sinus instruments, as well as all equipment used in sinus surgery.

Postoperative Complications: The patient will be monitored in post-anesthesia care unit (PACU). The patient should have the head of the bed elevated, vitals monitored, any bleeding addressed and have an ice pack available to help with swell or bruising. Possible complications include orbital trauma and cerebral spinal fluid (CSF) leak.

Nasal Cavity Procedures

Septorhinoplasty: Congenital anomalies or trauma can lead to deformities of the external nose and nasal septum. A septorhinoplasty addresses a deviated septum or enlarged turbinates that can make it hard to breathe normally and increases the risk of sinus infections due to poor drainage. The procedure also improves the appearance of the external nose.

Indications for Surgery

- Polyps
- Chronic/recurrent sinusitis
- Deviated septum
- Abnormal growth/cancer
- Enlarged turbinates
- Cosmetic
- Obstructive sleep apnea (OSA)

A septorhinoplasty can be performed as an outpatient or inpatient procedure, under general anesthesia, or local as well. The SA should be familiar with both approaches and their role in each. They may be required to function in a dual role as the surgical tech and SA.

Preoperative

- H&P
- Diagnostic lab reports/CT scan images
- Cardiac clearance if needed
- Signed consent form

Surgical Positioning: The OR bed is turned 180° to allow for right-handed surgeons to work on the patient's right side. The patient is supine with the right arm tucked. The bed may be placed in reverse Trendelenburg greater than 45° to minimize intraoperative bleeding.

Skin Prep: These procedures are considered clean contaminated procedures and there will be no prep.

Draping: May be towels around the head (turban) head wrap with a drape to cover the patient's body.

Surgical Procedure

Septoplasty

- The nostril on the affected side is opened with a nasal speculum and an incision is made with a #15 blade in the mucous membrane and perichondrium
- It is divided with a freer elevator or a Cottle elevator.
- Cartilage is incised with a round knife or Ballenger swivel knife and is removed with a Takahashi forceps.
- If a bony spur is to be removed, have available a nasal osteotome, chisel, and mallet.

- Hemostasis is achieved by using hemostatic agents or electrosurgical pencil (Bovie) or suction cautery.
- Incision is sutured with plain gut or chromic (3-0) or (4-0) suture on a small taper needle.
- The SA should have external splints according to the surgeon's preference. Splints may need to be cut to fit patient and have "mustache" dressing.
- Secretions are removed from pharynx to reduce the risk of aspiration. Have ice packs ready in PACU.

Rhinoplasty: The procedure will change the external appearance of the nose by reshaping the underlying framework. The surgeon may use a rasp for dorsal hump reduction, partial excision of lateral and alar cartilages, shortening of the septum, and osteotomy of nasal bones.

Postoperative Complications: Have head elevated, bleeding, bruising/swelling around eyes, and CSF leak.

Caldwell-Luc

In late 1897, three surgeons working autonomously—George Caldwell of the USA, Scanes Spicer of England, and Henri Luc of France—explained the concept of an anterior antral window for surgical excision of diseased sinus mucosa, to be used in combination with an inferior meatal antrostomy.

The **Caldwell-Luc** procedure is an approach for surgical treatment of the severely diseased maxillary sinus, or more commonly known for the removal of maxillary tumors. A middle meatal antrostomy will ensure adequate drainage and aeration of the sinus and allow for removal of diseased tissues in the sinuses under direct vision.

The Caldwell-Luc operation is reserved for selected patients with an extensive maxillary disease, particularly those with massive polyposis or fungal disease. Failure to clear the maxillary mucosa completely could result in early postoperative recurrence of disease. The anterior and inferior regions of the maxillary antrum are especially difficult to access endoscopically.

Indications

- Complicated acute or chronic rhinosinusitis, usually as an adjunct to endoscopic sinus surgery (ESS)
- Pterygomaxillary space surgery
- Maxillary floor fractures
- Foreign body retrieval
- Benign tumor removal
- Combined with ESS: orbital decompression and inverting papilloma removal

Technique

- With the patient under general anesthesia, lidocaine-epinephrine solution is injected into gingivobuccal sulcus, and cottonoids that are soaked in a vasoconstrictor are placed in nasal cavity.
- A gingivobuccal sulcus incision is created above canine fossa.
- Incision continued through periosteum laterally to the level of the first molar.
- The periosteum is elevated superiorly by the SA, identifying the infraorbital nerve.
- The maxillary antrum is opened with an osteotome.
- The infraorbital nerve and anterior superior alveolar nerve should be protected.
- Punch forceps can be used to enlarge window.
- An antrostomy is created by passing a curved hemostat under the inferior nasal concha.
- Cysts and tumors are removed.
- Gingival incision is then closed with absorbable sutures.
- Prognosis is good.

Endoscopic Approach

- To begin the procedure, the middle turbinate is moved medially to provide access.
- A large maxillary antrostomy is produced using conventional endoscopic techniques.
- The medial maxillary sinus wall is resected and continues posteriorly to the junction of the medial and posterior sinus walls.
- A 70° endoscope, angled forceps will aid in the removal of the mucosa from the posterior maxillary sinus wall.
- The surgeon may change to a 120° endoscope to allow for full visualization of the anterior maxillary sinus.
- Coakley curettes are utilized to remove diseased mucosa until all bony maxillary sinus walls are exposed.
- An angle-tipped burr is applied to drill down the remaining bony abnormalities.

Postoperative Complications

- Facial edema
- Infection
- Bleeding
- Hematoma
- Negative reaction to anesthesia
- Damage to nasal passages
- Numbness in the infraorbital and anterior superior alveolar nerves
- Dacryocystitis
- Constant epiphora due to damage to the lacrimal duct
- Devitalized teeth
- Oroantral fistulae
- Facial hypoesthesia
- Mucoceles

ANATOMY OF THE ORAL CAVITY

Hard palate. This separates the nose from the mouth.

Soft palate. The back of the roof of the mouth.

Epiglottis. This helps keep food and liquids out of the trachea when you swallow.

Larynx (voice box). This makes sound used for speaking.

Eustachian tube. The tube that connects the throat to the ear.

Nasopharynx. The area at the top of the throat behind the nose.

Oropharynx. The area at the middle of the throat behind the mouth.

Hypopharynx. The area at the lower part of the throat.

Esophagus. The tube that carries food and liquids from the throat to the stomach.

Trachea. The tube that carries air between the throat and the lungs.

Lymph nodes. Bean-shaped organs that help the body fight infections.

What Is the Throat?

The throat is a ring-like muscular tube that acts as the passageway for air, food, and liquid. The throat also helps in forming speech. The throat consists of:

- **Larynx (also known as the voice box).** The larynx is a cylindrical grouping of cartilage, muscles, and soft tissue that contains the vocal cords. The vocal cords are the upper opening into the windpipe (trachea), the passageway to the lungs.
- **Epiglottis.** A flap of soft tissue that is located just above the vocal cords. The epiglottis folds down over the vocal cords to help prevent food and irritants from entering the lungs.
- **Tonsils and adenoids.** They are made up of lymph tissue and are located at the back and the sides of the mouth. They protect against infection, but generally have little purpose beyond childhood.

DIAGNOSTIC, AND TREATMENT MODALITIES

Procedures of the Oral Cavity

Adenotonsillectomy

Indication for Surgery

- Recurrent tonsilitis
- Nasopharyngeal obstruction/adenoids
- Enlarged tonsils
- Halitosis
- OSA

Preoperative

- H&P
- Diagnostic lab reports/images
- Diagnostic sleep study
- Cardiac clearance if needed
- Signed consent form

Prepping and Positioning: The patient is positioned supine with the bed rotated 90° to facilitate the surgeon access with head of patient at top/edge of the bed.

A shoulder roll is utilized to extend the neck.

A pillow is placed under the knees.

One note, the base of the OR table may be turned to give surgeon room as well as the mayo for better position. If doing tonsil abscess, the position would be semi-Fowlers with arms placed on the patient's lap with a pillow and secured with pads and padded footboard that supports the feet.

Anesthesia: General Anesthesia.

Skin Prep: These procedures are considered a "clean" procedure and there is no skin prep.

Draping: May be towels around the head (turban) head wrap with a drape to cover the patient's body.

Supplies that the SA needs to be familiar with are the bovie extender, coblator sizes and tubing, as well as the coblator generator. The SA should be familiar with all the supplies and medications that may be on the field (Table 18-2) and work closely with your surgical technologist on making sure the preference card is updated and all equipment is in the room and available.

Uvulopalatopharyngoplasty (UPPP)

The purpose of this procedure is to increase the size of the pharyngeal airway as well as for intractable snoring and OSA that has not responded to nonsurgical treatments. This procedure will involve the uvula, portions of the soft palate, tonsils, unnecessary pharyngeal mucous membranes, and depending on obstruction site portions of the hard palate, palatoglossus muscles, and even base of the tongue (see Figure 18-8).

Surgical Procedure

- A mouth gag is placed, and is tissue excised depending on the severity of the soft palate, muscles, tonsils, and hard palate.
- They can be removed by using bovie pencil, or special instrumentation (laser, coblation, or #15 blade).
- Suture (vicryl or chromic stitch on small taper needle) may be used or clips to control hemostasis.
- Once wounds are closed the area is cleansed of clots, mouth gag is removed and the patient is extubated and transferred to PACU.

Postoperative Complications. Excessive bleeding, airway obstruction, swelling.

Parotidectomy

The most common reasons to perform a parotidectomy are to address benign and malignant tumors of major salivary glands. The parotid glands develop at about 6 to 7 weeks of gestation.

TABLE 18-2 • MEDICATIONS COMMONLY USED IN OTORHINOLARYNGOLOGIC SURGERY

Category	Dose/Route	Purpose/Action	Adverse Reactions
Local Anesthetics			
Lidocaine, 0.5% or 1%	Local injection	Inhibits pain and temperature fibers, used to dilute epinephrine	Cardiovascular, hypotension, confusion, dizziness, headache, nausea, vomiting, tremor, weakness, injection site pain, cardiac arrest, cardiac dysrhythmia, seizure, methemoglobinemia
Tetracaine (Pontocaine)	Topical; 0.25%-0.5% by nebulization or direct application	Inhibits pain, represses gag reflex	Pain, redness, urticaria, hypotension, severe burning, stinging, swelling, chills, dizziness, nausea, vomiting, slow, fast, or irregular heartbeats
Benzocaine/Tetracaine/ Cetacaine	Topical: available in gel, liquid, and spray	Inhibits pain, represses gag reflex; local anesthetic	Dry mouth, dizziness, hives, irritation, erythema, local oozing, localized vesiculation, pruritus), eschar, xeroderma
Benzocaine	Topical; available in 20% gel and 20% spray	Inhibits pain, represses gag reflex	Dry mouth, dizziness, localized erythema, localized rash, urticaria, methemoglobinemia
Topical Lidocaine Hydrochloride	2% viscous solution, 4% solution	Local anesthetic	High doses may cause cardiac dysrhythmias, minor burning and stinging of mouth and throat on initial contact
Cocaine Hydrochloride	4% topical, packing instilled not cavity or spray	Local anesthetic	CNS depression, CNS stimulation, hypertension, tachycardia, anxiety, drug abuse, drug dependence, nervousness, tonic-clonic epilepsy
Vasoconstrictors			
Oxymetazoline Hydrochloride (Afrin Nasal Spray, Neo-Synephrine, Nasacon)	0.05% nasal spray	Nasal decongestant used for vasoconstriction	Headache, insomnia, nervousness, dry nose, nasal congestion (rebound; chronic use), nasal mucosa irritation (temporary), sneezing, nasal stinging/burning, cardiac dysrhythmia, hypertension, tachydysrhythmia
Epinephrine	1:100,000 to 1:200,000	Used for vasoconstriction	Palpitations, tachydysrhythmia, paleness and sweating, nausea and vomiting, asthenia, dizziness, headache, tremor, pain in eye, anxiety, apprehension, nervousness, dyspnea, cardiac dysrhythmia, hypertensive crisis, pulmonary edema
Antibiotics			
Mupirocin (Nasal Bactroban)	2% topical	Antibacterial and lubricant for nasal packing, applied topically to skin incisions	Dermatologic, local pain, disorder of taste, headache, nausea, dysgeusia
Bacitracin	Topic ointment	Antibacterial, antibiotic	Swelling, contact dermatitis, pruritus, anaphylaxis
Steroids			
Triamcinolone Acetonide (Aristocort, Kenalog)	Topical	Used topically to lubricate packs or expand packing	Acneiform eruption, allergic contact dermatitis, atrophic striae, desquamation, folliculitis, hypertrichosis, hypopigmentation, local dryness, maceration of the skin, miliaria, perioral dermatitis, skin atrophy, skin blister
Cortisporin Otic Suspension (Neomycin and Polymyxin B Sulfates/Hydrocortisone)	Topical	Used after otologic surgery as an anti-inflammatory/ antibiotic agent	Itching, pain, stinging, burning, ototoxicity, drug-induced hypersensitivity (sensitization to kanamycin, paromomycin, streptomycin, and gentamicin)

Sources: https://www.rxlist.com/consumer_lidocaine_lidopen/drugs-condition.htm; https://www.drugs.com/mtm/tetracaine-topical.html

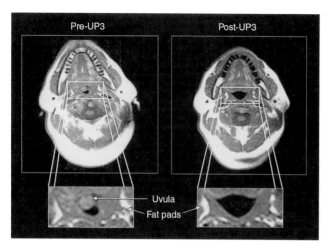

Figure 18-8 · Uvulopalatopharyngoplasty. (Reproduced, with permission, from Lalwani AK, ed. *Current Diagnosis & Treatment in Otolaryngology—Head & Neck Surgery.* 4th ed. New York, NY: McGraw Hill; 2020. Image contributed by Schwab RJ, et al. University of Pennsylvania Health System, Philadelphia.)

They form two lobes that lie in front of the ears. The blood supply of the parotid gland is supplied by the external carotid artery.

The parotid gland is the largest of the salivary glands, and is approximately the size of a walnut. It lies inferior to the zygomatic arch extending from the mastoid process of the temporal bone across the outer surface of the masseter muscle. It is bordered by the anteromedial aspect of the sternocleidomastoid muscle inferiorly, and mandibular canal posteriorly. It is covered in a layer of connective tissue, yellowish in appearance and irregularly shaped. Fatty tissue and the facial nerve separate the two lobes of the parotid gland, which opens in the mouth near the second maxillary molar. The opening is called the parotid duct or Stensen's duct.

The parotid gland has lymph nodes in the superficial and deep lobes. The superficial group drains the pinna, scalp, eyelids, and lacrimal glands. The deep group drains the gland, middle ear, nasopharynx, and soft palate.

The primary function of the parotid gland is the creation of saliva. Saliva is a hypotonic solution that contains electrolytes, macromolecules, and enzymes. Saliva is responsible for many important roles:

- Delivers lubrication for the mouth
- Helps in mastication (chewing)
- Assists in swallowing, speaking, and digesting
- Helps break down food for digestion
- Inhibits infection in the mouth and throat
- Assists in preventing tooth decay

Etiology

- Chronic parotitis is a nonspecific sialadenitis that is often diagnosed in the dental office. The patient will present with decreased salivation, stasis, and an ascending retrograde duct infection.

- Sialadenitis is triggered by multiple bacteria or viruses or various obstructions. A decrease in saliva can lead to increased infection, pain, and swelling. Sialadenitis can be treated with oral hydration, warm compresses, antibiotics, and medications that increase saliva.
- Sialolithiasis arises when a stone or other small particle becomes embedded in Stensen's duct. It is the most common cause of salivary gland disease and disorders. The patient presents with painful swelling often during and after eating. Surgery is often required to remove the stone.

Indications for Surgery

- Inflammatory conditions
- Infectious processes
- Congenital malformations
- Benign or malignant neoplasms

Preoperative

- H&P
- Biopsy to collect cells from the parotid gland
- Diagnostic lab reports
- MRI or CT scans
- Cardiac clearance if needed
- Signed consent form
- The TNM staging system is used for parotid gland tumors

Prep and Positioning. The patient is positioned supine, neck slightly extended, with the affected side of the face up. The entire operative side of the face, mouth and outer canthus of the eye, the ear, and the forehead are prepped.

Anesthesia. The procedure is accomplished under general anesthesia with the endotracheal tube fixed to the contralateral side. Muscle relaxants are avoided so facial nerve function can be monitored.

Surgical Approaches. Extracapsular dissection. The facial nerve is not identified. The tumor is resected utilizing facial nerve monitoring and is suggested for benign lesions that are not pleomorphic adenoma.

Partial/Superficial: The tumor is resected with a cuff of parotid tissue, utilized for benign lesions and lymph node metastasis into the superficial lobe.

Total Parotidectomy: The entire gland is removed, applied for aggressive malignant tumors, deep lobe tumors, sentinel lymph node excision if located in the deep lobe, vascular malformations, or large tumors.

Radical Parotidectomy: The entire gland and facial nerve are removed. Utilized commonly when preoperative facial paralysis is already present, or when the malignant tumor has involved the nerve. Nerve grafting may be considered.

Surgical Procedure

- A modified Blair incision is used starting in the preauricular skin crease, around the ear lobe posteriorly and extending inferiorly into a cervical skin crease below the body of the mandible. Bleeding vessels are attended to with the ESU.
- After the dermis and platysma muscle is incised, the skin is raised between the superficial musculoaponeurotic system (SMAS) and fascia of the parotid.
- With fine-toothed pickups and dissecting scissors, the skin flap is elevated and retracted applying silk sutures fastened to hemostats.
- The upper portion of the sternocleidomastoid (SCM) is retracted by the SA. The auricular nerve is identified, and the lower part of the parotid gland is elevated with curved hemostats. Often, the auricular nerve is sacrificed, however, the posterior branch can be preserved.

The assistant plays an important role by monitoring the face for muscle contraction during the procedure.

- Using blunt dissection, the superficial temporal artery, vein, and the external jugular vein are exposed.
- The tail of the parotid is dissected from the anterior edge of the SCM muscle, and the digastric muscle is identified. The external jugular vein may be divided and ligated, although it is possible to conserve the vein to decrease bleeding during the procedure or provide a source for anastomosis during a reconstructive flap.
- The temporal, zygomatic, mandibular, and cervical branches of the facial nerve are exposed and protected.
- The diseased portion of the parotid gland is removed. If the diseased portion is superficial, the parotid gland with the tumor is removed with ligation and separation of the parotid duct. If the diseased portion is deep, the facial nerve is lightly retracted by the SA, and the parotid tissue is taken from beneath the nerve. Kocher retractors are used by the SA to retract the mandible. The external carotid artery is exposed. The internal maxillary and superficial temporal arteries may be sacrificed.
- Before closure, the integrity of the facial nerve is checked, and function is assessed with a nerve stimulator.
- The wound layers are closed using absorbable suture. A small drain is inserted, the skin is sutured by the SA with nonabsorbable suture and a pressure dressing is utilized.

Postoperation. Facial nerve function should be assessed as soon as possible once the patient is in recovery.

Complications

- Hematoma
- Facial paralysis
- Seroma
- Surgical site infection
- Frey's syndrome
- First bite syndrome
- Loss of sensation around the ear
- Surgical site depression
- Salivary fistula

ANATOMY OF THE NECK

- Important structures that are contained in or pass through the neck include the seven cervical vertebrae, spinal cord, the jugular veins and carotid arteries, part of the esophagus, the larynx and vocal cords, and the sternocleidomastoid and hyoid muscles in front and the trapezius. Other important muscles include:

- Sternohyoid
- Omohyoid
- Platysma
- SCM
- Trapezius

There are important structures related to the head and neck surgery. This brief overview of muscles, veins, arteries, and nerves is just a brief summary. It is important the SA has knowledge and training in advanced anatomy and physiology (A&P) to become efficient in assisting during these procedures.

The platysma muscle is located in the superior thorax between cartilage of second rib and acromion of the scapula; it is a flat thin broad muscle covering the sides of the neck. It covers superior portions of the pectoralis muscle as well as anterior length of the clavicle. It covers the external jugular vein and innervated by a branch of the facial nerve. The SCM is a long muscle on both sides of the neck that will be exposed/retracted and divided during neck dissection.

Infrahyoid muscles are a group of muscles that start inferior to the hyoid bone. They consist of the omohyoid muscle and the sternohyoid muscle, which is straplike, a narrow ribbon-like muscle band, that arises from the inner portion of the clavicle and sternum. It extends to the lower portion of the hyoid bone. Deep to the sternohyoid is the sternothyroid muscle, which inserts on the thyroid cartilage. These "straplike" muscles will be retracted when a thyroidectomy is being performed.

The head and neck receive majority of the blood supply from the carotid and vertebral arteries. The neck is supplied by arteries other than the carotid that will be discussed as an overview. They include right and left subclavian arteries, thyrocervical trunk, inferior thyroid artery, ascending thyroid artery, and transverse cervical artery.

The right common carotid artery comes from the bifurcation of the brachiocephalic trunk. The subclavian artery is the other branch of the carotid. The left common carotid artery comes from the arch of the aorta. The right and left common carotid arteries ascend up the neck, lateral to the trachea.

Near the superior margin of the thyroid cartilage the carotid arteries split into the external and internal carotid.

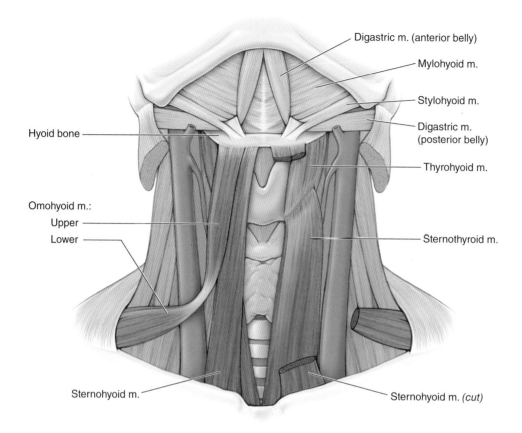

Figure 18-9 · Anatomy of the neck. (Reproduced, with permission, from Morton DA, Foreman KB, Albertine KH. *The Big Picture: Gross Anatomy*. 2nd ed. New York, NY: McGraw Hill; 2019.)

The external carotid arteries supply blood to the head and neck. These arteries travel up the neck and posteriorly to the mandibular neck and end up within the parotid gland where it then divides into the superficial temporal artery and maxillary artery. The internal carotid artery supplies blood to the brain and eyes.

The neck is supplied by arteries other than the carotids that the SA should be familiar with when assisting on head and neck surgical procedures. The right and left subclavian arteries provide the thyrocervical trunk. This trunk has several vessels that supply the neck.

The inferior thyroid artery is the first branch off the thyrocervical trunk and it supplies the thyroid gland.

The ascending cervical artery comes off the inferior thyroid artery, medially in the neck. It provides blood vessels to the posterior prevertebral muscles.

The transverse cervical artery is another branch off the trunk and provides blood supply to the trapezius and rhomboids.

The recurrent laryngeal nerve is an important structure that is identified and protected during surgery. The recurrent laryngeal nerve contains motor and sensory fibers that innervate the vocal cord and the sensory fibers supply sensation to the larynx. It the nerve is damaged, injured or cut during surgery hoarseness can happen or if cut the vocal cord may cause the airway to become obstructed and the patient may require a tracheotomy (see Figure 18-9).

DIAGNOSTIC AND TREATMENT MODALITIES OF THE NECK

Thyroidectomy

Indications for Thyroid Surgery

Thyroid nodule

- Hyperthyroidism
- Hypothyroidism
- Cancer
- Trauma

Preoperative

- H&P
- Diagnostic lab reports: images, cardiac clearance (if needed or required)
- Diagnostic test reports: needle biopsy or previous biopsy if indicated
- Surgical permit consent form

Preparation of the Patient (May Vary Depending on Doctor Preference)

General anesthesia. Foley catheter based on doctor preference.

Supine with arms tucked or extended on padded armboards.

Table may be flexed with pillow under knees to avoid back muscle strain. Another position may be reverse Trendelenburg with padded footboard secured on table.

Skin Prep: May vary from procedure, including anterior neck to the level of the infra-auricular border and the lower lip to above the nipple. For a laryngectomy, the prep will also include the axilla and down the sides of the neck and shoulder. Depending on the class of the neck dissection prep may include face up the hairline.

Draping for Neck Surgery: May include "crunched-up towels" on either side of the neck to prevent "pooling," followed by four squared towels. Followed by a split sheet, head drape, or thyroid drape.

Draping for radical neck dissection head drape (drape sheet with two folded towels around the head "clamped"): The neck is draped with towels secured by suture or staples and patient is covered with a fenestrated sheet of doctor's choice.

As the SA you will need to be familiar with instruments and retractors utilized to retract muscles and other structures during surgery, being aware of the major arteries, veins, and nerves. Some commonly used hand-held retractors are army/navy, skin hooks, and green retractors.

Surgical Procedure

- A transverse incision is made through skin, fascia, and platysma muscle, 2 cm above sternoclavicular junction.
- Platysma muscle is retracted by the SA with a hand-held or self-retainer retractor the midline fascia is incised between the strap muscles.
- Bleeding vessels are ligated with ties, hemoclips, or suture ligature (nonabsorbable) while preserving anterior jugular veins. The SCM muscle is usually not divided but if large gland or tumor is involved, it may have to be divided for additional exposure.
- The inferior and middle thyroid veins are ligated and divided.
- The superior thyroid artery is identified and ligated. Care of the superior laryngeal nerve is taken and identifying the upper parathyroid gland is taken.
- The inferior thyroid artery and the inferior parathyroid are identified and only branches of the artery that supply the thyroid are ligated.
- The thyroid lobe and isthmus are dissected, while protecting the recurrent laryngeal nerve. Any bleeding vessels are clamped and ligated. If parathyroid glands were removed, they would be re-implanted.
- If strap muscles were divided, they would be reapproximated with fine interrupted absorbable or nonabsorbable suture. A drain may be used, and hemostasis is controlled, and closure of wound is facilitated utilizing surgeon's preference for a careful closure. The SA should be prepared for a cosmetic closure with a subcutaneous fine absorbable suture.
- Dressing may consist of steri-strips, surgical glue, or small gauze with minimal tape.

- If performing a parathyroid, only vessels that supply the parathyroid are ligated and thyroid gland is preserved.

Postoperation. Depending on the SA role, you may have written instructions for all patients that will include postoperative care. For in-patients, you may follow up on rounds with doctor. If out patient, care of dressing, drain care, pain control, and diet (soft foods, avoid hot food or drink) are mentioned, and postoperative doctor's appointment is made.

Potential Complication. Swelling, bleeding, hoarseness that does not improve, fever, neuropathy (nerve injury or damage) numbness, tingling, muscle weakness.

If skin graft or skin/muscle flaps were perfomed, the SA should be cognizant in regards to the condition and the survival of flaps, observing any (dead skin, redness, inflammation, warm/hot skin around graft/flap site).

Laryngectomy

Laryngectomy is the process of removal of larynx. Cancer of the larynx is classified:

- ***Supraglottic:*** From epiglottis and include false cords
- ***Glottic:*** Floor of the ventricle to below the glottis and vocal cords
- ***Infraglottic***: Below true vocal cords to cricoid cartilage.
- ***Transglottic***: Lesions from the ventricle to true and false cords and subglottically.

This procedure is usually performed for malignancy. Nonsurgical treatment can include radiation, laser, or palliative care. Surgery can be performed as: hemi laryngectomy, partial or total with a radical neck dissection.

Laryngectomy: This involves the removal of hyoid bone, cricoid cartilage, two or three rings of the trachea, and the larynx (consist of epiglottis, false cords and true cords). Postoperative considerations include loss of voice, breathing through a trach, no swallowing problems observed.

Supraglottic Laryngectomy: Hyoid bone, epiglottis, and false vocal cords are removed. **Postoperative considerations**: normal voice, may aspirate when introduced to liquids and should have normal airway because trachea is not removed.

Hemi-Laryngectomy: It is the removal of one true vocal cord, one false cord, arytenoid cartilage, which is the superior border of the cricoid cartilage, and half of the thyroid cartilage. **Postoperative considerations**: hoarseness in voice, normal airway, and no problem swallowing.

Partial Laryngectomy: It is the removal of one vocal cord. **Postoperative considerations**: Hoarseness may occur but also may have almost normal voice, normal airway, and normal swallowing.

Total Laryngectomy Procedure

- The procedure begins with a midline incision from the suprasternal notch just above the hyoid bone.
- The strap muscles are divided as well as isthmus.

- The hypoglossal nerves are preserved. The laryngeal nerves are exposed and ligated when performing a total laryngectomy.

- Vessels are clamped and ligated. Trachea may be divided between second and third rings and the endotracheal tube is replaced (trach tube) or repositioned from tumor.

- The larynx is freed from cervical esophagus. The blunt dissection will continue to pharynx and cervical esophagus well away from tumor.

- The tumor is removed, and nasogastric tube is placed into esophagus and the defect is closed with a running absorbable suture (3-0 Vicryl).

- The nasogastric tube is guided down to pharyngeal suture line. The tracheostomy will stay in place till swelling goes down, stoma is matured so patient will have stoma after trach is removed.

- A drain is placed and secured with drain stitch and closure of deep cervical fascia and muscles (strap/platysma).

- Skin closure by staples.

- Dressing is optional depending on doctor preference choice of a moderate pressure dressing to no dressing and just ointment covering stapes.

As the SA you should be knowledgeable of the neck anatomy and work on closing with your surgeon.

Glossectomy

A glossectomy is the surgical removal of all or part of the tongue. It is accomplished to inhibit malignant growth such as oral cancer. Usually, only a portion of the tongue is removed through procedures such as a hemiglossectomy (half of the tongue) or a subtotal glossectomy (more than half the tongue, but less than the entire tongue) or a total glossectomy (tongue excision) may be performed.

Anatomy

The tongue is a unique organ located in the oral cavity and plays a vital role in mastication, deglutition, taste, speech, and articulation. It is divided into anterior and posterior sections. The anterior portion is called the oral or presulcal part of the tongue. The posterior portion is referred to as the pharyngeal or postsulcal part of the tongue. The base of the tongue refers to the postsulcal part that forms the ventral wall of the oropharynx, while the root of the tongue refers to the presulcal section of tongue that is attached to the floor of the mouth. The tongue is split into halves by an avascular midline raphe and lined with keratinized and nonkeratinized stratified squamous epithelium. The sensory mucosa is responsible for taste perception.

Anteriorly and laterally the tongue is surrounded by the upper and lower rows of teeth. Superiorly, it is bordered by the hard and soft palates. Inferiorly the root of the tongue is continuous with the mucosa of the floor of the mouth, with sublingual salivary glands and vascular bundles located below the mucosa of the floor of the mouth. The palatoglossal and palatopharyngeal arches and the palatine tonsils are associated laterally to the posterior third of the tongue. The dorsal surface of the epiglottis and posterior wall of the oropharynx is posterior to the base of the tongue.

The eight paired muscles of the tongue are named for the direction in which they run: superior and inferior longitudinal, transverse, and vertical muscles. The intrinsic muscles are confined to the body of the tongue. Four extrinsic muscles, the genioglossus, styloglossus, hyoglossus, and palatoglossus originate outside the tongue and insert into the body of the tongue.

Motor innervation to the tongue is from the hypoglossal nerve. In the neck, the nerve crosses anterior to the internal and external carotid arteries and can be found inferior to the digastric muscle which needs to be identified and protected as it is at high risk for injury during neck dissections.

The external carotid artery gives arterial supply to the tongue through the lingual artery and tonsillar branch of the facial artery. Venous drainage is through tributaries to the lingual vein. Lymphatic drainage includes the submental and submandibular lymph node basins along with the upper jugular chain neck lymphatics. The lymphatic drainage is important to understand when treating squamous cell carcinoma of the tongue where there is a risk of cervical lymph node metastases.

Etiology

- Tobacco
- Alcohol
- Diet and nutrition
- Viruses
- Radiation
- Ethnicity
- Familial and genetic predisposition
- Oral thrush
- Immunosuppression
- Use of mouthwash
- Syphilis
- Dental factors
- Occupational risks

Diagnostics

- Physical examination
- Visual inspection and palpation of the tumor
- Flexible laryngoscopy
- Imaging
- Panendoscopy

Preparation. A thorough medical history should be taken at the preliminary clinical consult. The patient should share information about prior oncologic treatments, any chemotherapy or radiation to the head and neck, prior neck surgeries, vascular surgeries, airway procedures, and trauma to the area.

Anesthesia. It will be important for anesthesia to know if there is a history of difficult intubation from prior surgery, subglottic stenosis, and history of tracheostomy as they will affect the airway plan. Awake nasal fiberoptic intubation may be advised if good airway landmarks are present. Awake tracheostomy may be ideal if airway landmarks are destroyed or if the surgeon feels it is the safest option.

Skin Prep and Positioning. Transoral glossectomy without neck dissection is often considered a "clean-contaminated." If a neck dissection and reconstruction is to be performed, the patient is prepped and draped for a sterile procedure.

Cancer Staging System

The TNM system is applied for staging head and neck cancers. TNM is scored based on attributes of the tumor (T), cervical lymph node involvement (N), and distant metastasis (M). The Tumor (T) stage is scored as follows:

- Tis: Carcinoma in situ.
- T1: Tumor is less than or equal to 2 cm with a depth of invasion (DOI) less than or equal to 5 mm.
- T2: Tumor is less than or equal to 2 cm with DOI greater than 5 mm, or tumor is 2 to 4 cm with DOI less than or equal to 10 mm.
- T3: Tumor is greater than 4 cm, or DOI > 10 mm.
- T4: Advanced local disease and invasion into surrounding structures.

Contraindications. Contraindications include comorbidities that may make surgery unachievable or unresectable disease regarding the malignancy that includes total carotid artery encasement, skull base extension, and invasion into the paraspinal musculature.

Surgical Approach. There are three common approaches for a glossectomy: transoral glossectomy, glossectomy via lip-split mandibulotomy, and glossectomy via transcervical pull-through. The transoral is the removal of the tongue tissue through the mouth. It does have limited access and exposure to the posterior region. The lip-split offers the widest exposure; however, it is very time consuming with risks of complications. The lip-split procedure utilizes a sagittal osteotomy to open the mandible to permit inferior transposition of the tongue for a transoral-transcervical exposure of the tongue and pharynx. The transcervical pull-through releases the tongue into the neck through the floor of the mouth. This approach does not require a mandibular reconstruction.

Transoral Procedure

- Self-retaining retractors and mouth gags are utilized to obtain transoral exposure.
  - Molt, Fergusson, or Jennings mouth gags are often used.
- Traction is applied to the tongue by placing traction sutures or a Backhaus towel clamp on the tongue.
- Mucosal and muscle incisions are made with cautery, laser, or a knife.

- Mucosal margin incisions of 1 to 2 cm are made down to the muscle.
- A second traction suture on the specimen will add another direction of counter traction.
- Muscular incisions are made to procure normal tissue onto the deep margin.
- Prudent hemostasis and ample margins are key during the muscular dissection.
- Ventral margins may reach onto the floor of the mouth.
- Margins of 1 cm should be achieved when there is a malignancy.
- Mucosal and deep muscle margins are sent for margin assessment.
- The tongue can be closed primarily, left to heal by secondary intention, or reconstructed.

Glossectomy via Lip-Split Mandibulotomy

- Neck dissection midline through the lip with a 1-cm mucosal lip incision anterior to the gingiva.
- A median mandibulotomy is created between the central incisors by extending the incision along the mucosal lip through the vermillion border.
- The labial artery is usually clipped or cauterized.
- Muscular cuts are done through the orbicularis oris, mentalis, and the lip depressors, onto the periosteum of the mandible.
- A 15 blade is used to make gingival cuts between the central incisors.
- Mandible flaps are elevated by the SA to expose the bone.
- Subperiosteal dissection is accomplished to provide exposure to secure a fixation plate across the osteotomy.
- A reconstruction plate is contoured and positioned on the inferior border of the mandible.
- A sagittal osteotomy is executed.
- The mandible is spread open, and the mylohyoid muscle is observed.
- A glossectomy is accomplished.
- Specimen is sent to check for clear margins.
- The facial nerve should be identified and safely retracted by the SA.
- Any soft tissue over osteotomies is ablated down to cortical bone.
- Bone cuts are made and will allow for additional exposure.
- Soft tissue and mandibular reconstruction is required at this point.
- Resected bone is reconstructed with a free bone graft or vascularized osseous free tissue transfer.
- Reductions and internal fixation is realized with mandibular plates or lag screws.
- The lip split incision requires closure of the gingiva and mucosal lip using chromic or monocryl.

- The muscle layers of the chin and neck are reapproximated followed with closure of the muscles by the surgeon and the skin by the SA.

Glossectomy via Transcervical Pull-Through

- The transcervical approach is accomplished through a neck dissection.
- The subplatysmal flaps are elevated.
- The cervical lymph node dissection of the submandibular triangle is accomplished.
- The anterior transoral glossectomy is performed.
- Mucosal cuts are created on the anterior tongue along the dorsal and ventral surfaces.
- The floor of the mouth is released through mucosal cuts along the floor of the mouth.
- Lingual mucosa of the alveolus is incised for tumors that involve the floor of the mouth.
- The periosteum is elevated off the lingual cortex of the mandible.
- Reconstruction is supported by tooth extraction, alveoloplasty, and circum-dental inset sutures.
- Once the tumor is removed from the tongue, the mylohyoid, and anterior digastric muscles are released from the mandible.
- Specimen is removed and margins are checked.
- Reconstruction is accomplished and the incisions are closed by the surgeon and SA.

Postoperative Complications. Prior head and neck radiation may affect wound healing. Other conditions that could affect a good outcome include malnutrition, hypothyroidism, chronic steroid use, autoimmune conditions, and smoking. Pain, bleeding, infection, chyle leak, fistula, nerve damage, sequelae of healing, and risks of anesthesia will also interfere with a good outcome.

Mandibulectomy

The mandible is a singular bone that has a unique horse-shoe shape and is identical on both sides. The mandible is the moving part of the jaw and all muscles of mastication attach to it.

The ramus is the second largest component of the mandible after the body, and it extends from the gonial angle of the mandible. The masseter muscles attach to the ramus laterally, and the pterygoid muscle and sphenomandibular ligament attach to the medial walls of the ramus. The ramus divides into two processes at the most superior point.

The coronoid process sits anteriorly, and the condylar process sits posteriorly and articulates with the temporal bone. The coronoid process is attached to the temporalis muscle, which aids in mastication. It also aids in opening and closing the jaw. The bony extrusion behind the coronoid process is the condylar process which forms the bony component of the temporomandibular joint, along with the temporal bone.

The body of the mandible contains the most anatomical landmarks of the mandible and is rectangular in shape.

The most important part of the mandible is the alveolar process as it holds the teeth through a joint known as gomphosis. Gomphoses line the upper and lower jaw in each tooth socket. Teeth are responsible for biting, chewing, cutting, and grinding, as well as speech and pronunciation along with facial tissue support.

The medial side of the ramus holds the mandibular foramen, which encapsulates the inferior alveolar nerve and its branches. The lateral body of the mandible includes the mental foramen anteriorly, which is home to the mental nerve and its corresponding vessels.

The external oblique line can be seen on the lateral side. On the medial side of the mandible there are seven major structures, including the superior and inferior genial tubercles and the digastric fossa, which are observed in the midline, and includes the mylohyoid line, whose posterior border allows for the attachment of the pterygomandibular raphe. The mylohyoid line divides the submandibular and the sublingual fossae.

Etiology

- Infectious etiologies
- Osteomyelitis
- Osteoradionecrosis
- Malignant squamous cell carcinoma
- Severe maxillofacial trauma

The occurrence of bisphosphonate-related necrosis of the mandible has increased lately, triggering the need to perform a mandibulectomy to remove the impacted portion of the mandible. There are two types of a mandibulectomy:

- Marginal mandibulectomy: Just the area with cancer is removed. A great deal of the jawbone is retained to avoid reconstructive surgery.
- Segmental mandibulectomy: The complete jawbone is taken and then reconstructed.

Contraindications to mandibulectomy are often related to cardiovascular hemodynamic instability or metabolic comorbidities. Patients who undergo a mandibulectomy will often also require a neck dissection.

Airway management is an important aspect of the treatment process. Some patients may require a tracheotomy, others may require nasotracheal tube intubation and overnight ventilatory support. A patient whose disease involvement is limited to the mandible and whose airway is easily visualized may undergo the procedure with a nasotracheal intubation and not a tracheotomy. This includes patients who receive immediate mandibular reconstruction with free-tissue transfers. They are kept overnight with a nasotracheal tube in the ICU, followed by extubation the next day.

In patients who present with large mandibular tumors that have destroyed the outer cortex of the mandible; a computer-generated pre-bent plate of the affected mandible may be necessary. A plastic model is constructed to be used as the base to create a template for the mandibular plate post resection. An internal fixation system allows stabilization of the fragments once the affected portion of the mandibular model is resected.

The model is made to the exact scale of the patient. This allows the reconstruction bar to be bent to the perfect contour on the patient's mandibular model and the plate is sterilized for use during the procedure.

Anesthesia. A mandibulectomy is performed under general anesthesia. The endotracheal tube is positioned so it does not impede access to the anatomical structures. For patients with lesions limited to only the mandible, the endotracheal tube is placed as a nasotracheal in most cases. If the lesion is lateralized and the patient does not require intermaxillary mandibular fixation, the endotracheal tube can be placed transorally and secured to the contralateral side of the mouth. A transoral resection that involves adjacent soft tissue may require a tracheotomy to control the airway. Cases with a free flap will dictate an arterial line. The use of vasopressors can affect free flap survival, so anesthesia should be made aware of this approach.

Position. The patient is positioned supine and rotated 180° away from anesthesia with the patient's feet adjacent to the anesthesia provider. A donut is used for the head and a shoulder roll will aid in placing the shoulders in a moderate degree of extension and tucking the arms. The surgeon will need access to the patient's head and neck and potential free flap donor sites. Patients scheduled for a free flap will require an arterial line for monitoring.

Prep. The face, neck, and chest are prepped with povidone-iodine scrub and paint and the patient is draped for a head and neck procedure.

Procedure

- A mandibulectomy can be approached transcervically or transorally. It all depends on the disease process as to which approach will be applied.

- A benign growth that involves the mandible or small to medium malignant tumors, the resection can be achieved transorally in many patients.

- In a transoral approach, the mucosal incision is made close to the teeth that will be resected or close to the alveolar ridge in patients who are edentulous.

- A periosteal elevator is used to elevate the soft tissues off the mandible. Once exposure is complete, the appropriate bone cuts can be determined pre-resection.

- For patients with extensive malignant disease requiring a wide resection, the transcervical approach utilizing lip splitting or visor flap incisions is deemed more appropriate.

- Complete excision of the tumor with clear margins can render the patient disease free of oral cavity carcinoma.

Postoperative Considerations. The patient will have a Foley catheter during and after surgery. The catheter will be removed when the patient is out of the ICU and up walking around. Patients who have undergone free flap construction are checked using a Doppler, capillary refill, color, and turgor pressure. An implanted Doppler probe is placed during surgery around the vessel of concern and is removed once the flap is deemed "viable." This allows continual assessment of the vascular supply to the flap.

Patients will have a Dobhoff tube (nasogastric tube) or a peg tube. The Dobhoff tube is only temporary and used for nutrition and medications while the incision site heals. The Dobhoff tube is usually in place for 2 to 4 weeks.

If a bilateral procedure was performed, a patient will have a tracheotomy that lasts for about 3 weeks to 3 months. A mandibulectomy may have a pectoralis, fibula, iliac crest, rib, or a reconstruction plate used to reconstruct the mandibular bone that was removed during surgery.

Most patients are seen between 7 and 14 days after discharge for suture removal and dressing changes. This is followed up by consistent visits every 1 to 2 months for the first year.

Neck Dissection

Position. Supine with head on padded foam, gel donut, or other head support with the face turned to the contralateral side. A shoulder roll may be used to slightly hyperextend the neck. General anesthesia, SCD (compression hose device) on patient's legs and hooked up to machine. The arm of the operative side is padded and tucked, and other arm is placed on padded arm board and secured. If the surgeon is going to get a skin graft, then the thigh area is prepped as well and draped in preparation for skin graft if necessary. A Foley catheter is inserted. A pillow may be placed under knees.

Skin Prep. Surgeon's choice. The prep will begin from (may need to place sterile cotton ball in ear) the neck and will extend from hairline to nipples and down to table at the sides. If going perform a skin graft. and second prep will be needed

Procedure

- There are several incision types that are used but it depends on the tumor and which structures will be removed. The Y-shaped or H-shaped incisions are very common. The structures to be identified include the platysma, external jugular vein, SCM, carotid artery (which is identified and preserved), and the vagus nerve (identified and preserved) (see Figure 18-10).

- The other vessels/arteries during this procedure will be divided and ligated. The procedure of the tumor will be removed, and cervical lymph nodes as well will be sent.

- Depending on the procedure, a mandibulectomy may need to be performed as well as a tracheostomy.

- The field is examined for hemostasis, drains are placed, and the incision closed.

- A small needle absorbable suture is used for closure and drains are secured and staples or sutures for skin.

Dressing. Surgeon's preference Usually ointment applied to staples and drain sites.

Postoperation. Excessive bleeding from site as well as drains. This should be monitored due to the highly vascular areas.

Reconstruction. The key functional elements of reconstruction are that the flap has enough bulk to create a convex floor of mouth to avoid pooling of secretions and to facilitate articulation, and that the hyoid be suspended from the mandibular

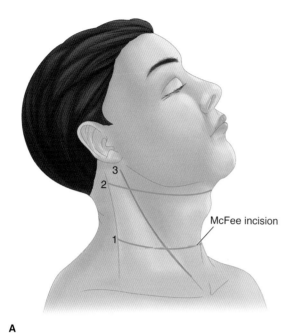

A

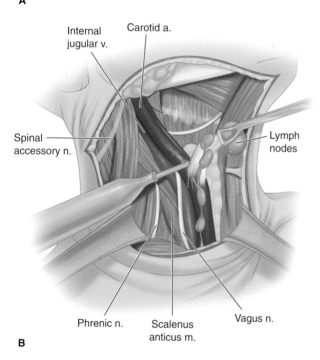

B

Figure 18-10 · Neck dissection. (Reproduced, with permission, from Brunicardi FC et al, eds. *Schwartz's Principles of Surgery.* 11th ed. New York, NY: McGraw Hill; 2019.)

arch to facilitate breathing and swallowing. A range of flaps will provide adequate tissue volume, that is, pectoralis major, latissimus dorsi, anterolateral free thigh, or rectus abdominis free flaps. Radial-free forearm flaps should not be used as they have inadequate bulk and result in a concave floor of mouth and a sump that interferes with deglutition and causes pooling and spillage of saliva and food. Mandibulectomy may necessitate free fibula flap reconstruction.

Tracheostomy

Anatomy. The trachea is cartilaginous and somewhat cylindrical but is compressed posteriorly. It is approximately 11 cm long and less than one inch in diameter. The trachea starts from the inferior part of the larynx (cricoid cartilage) in the neck and runs inferiorly behind the sternum where it divides at the carina into the right and left main stem bronchi. (See Figure 18-11.)

The trachea is surrounded by many vital structures in the neck and chest. In the neck, the esophagus lies posterior to the trachea and the heart and travels downward through the mediastinum and the hiatus of the diaphragm. The thyroid gland is positioned anterior and lateral to the trachea from the point of the cricoid cartilage to the second or third tracheal rings. The thyroid isthmus is at the midline and each thyroid lobe attaches laterally onto the trachea wrapping around the cricoid cartilage and tracheal rings. These two structures share a common blood supply from the inferior thyroid artery. The thoracic trachea and carina attain blood from the bronchial arteries that arise from the aorta.

A tracheostomy is performed when there is a need for an alternative airway. A cannula is inserted in the trachea through a midline incision placed below the cricoid cartilage. It can be temporary or permanent. It is performed as an emergency procedure if there is upper respiratory tract obstruction. Cuffed tracheostomy tubes are recommended for patients at risk for aspiration or pneumocephalus or patients receiving positive-pressure ventilation. Reasons to perform a tracheostomy include:

- Anaphylaxis
- Birth defects of the airway
- Burns of the airway
- Cancer in the neck
- Chronic lung disease
- Diaphragm dysfunction
- Injury to the larynx or laryngectomy
- Need for prolonged respiratory or ventilator support
- Obstruction of the airway by a foreign body
- OSA
- Subglottic stenosis
- Severe neck or mouth injuries
- Tumors
- Vocal cord paralysis

Anesthesia. A scheduled tracheostomy is performed under general anesthesia. Emergencies are done under local anesthesia.

Positioning. The patient is placed in supine position with a roll to raise the shoulders and hyperextend the neck and head. The neck is prepped, and sterile drapes are applied. An additional tracheostomy tube and obturator should be always kept with the patient in case the tube becomes dislodged or plugged with secretions.

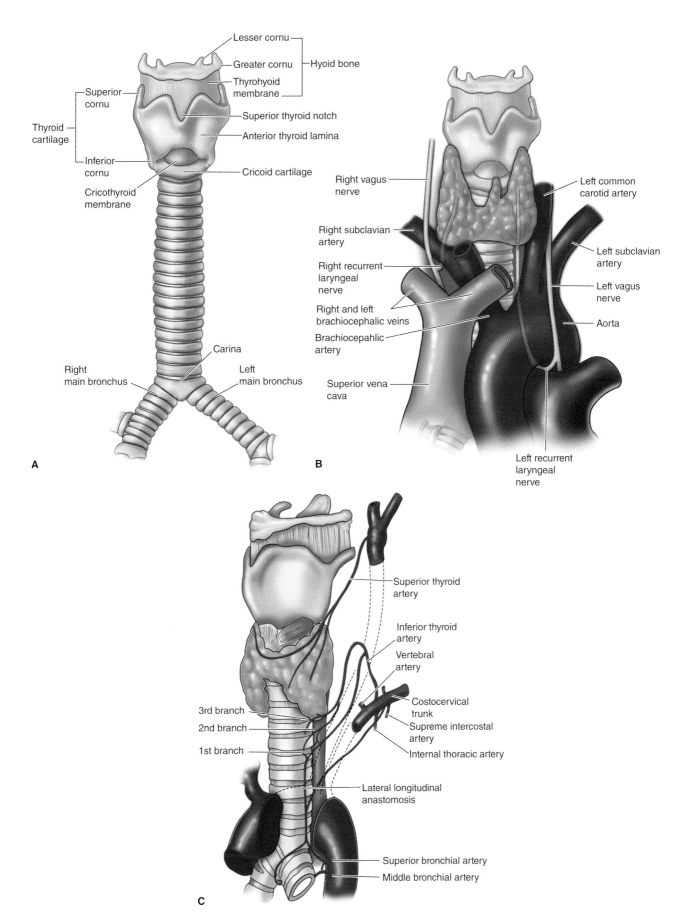

A

Lesser cornu
Greater cornu — Hyoid bone
Thyrohyoid membrane
Superior cornu
Thyroid cartilage
Inferior cornu
Cricothyroid membrane
Superior thyroid notch
Anterior thyroid lamina
Cricoid cartilage
Carina
Right main bronchus
Left main bronchus

B

Right vagus nerve
Right subclavian artery
Right recurrent laryngeal nerve
Right and left brachiocephalic veins
Brachiocepahlic artery
Superior vena cava
Left common carotid artery
Left subclavian artery
Left vagus nerve
Aorta
Left recurrent laryngeal nerve

C

Superior thyroid artery
Inferior thyroid artery
Vertebral artery
3rd branch
2nd branch
1st branch
Costocervical trunk
Supreme intercostal artery
Internal thoracic artery
Lateral longitudinal anastomosis
Superior bronchial artery
Middle bronchial artery

Figure 18-11 · Trachea. (Reproduced, with permission, from Lalwani AK, ed. *Current Diagnosis & Treatment in Otolaryngology—Head & Neck Surgery*. 4th ed. New York, NY: McGraw Hill; 2020.)

Operative Steps

- Surgeon will inject lidocaine with epi into the subcutaneous tissue.
- Incision is made along Langer's lines just below the Cricoid cartilage (Adam's apple).
- Soft tissues and the platysma and strap muscles are divided.
- Thyroid gland is identified, and isthmus is retracted or divided as necessary with the help of the SA.
- The plane between the isthmus and the trachea is separated with a blunt hemostat exposing the thyroid gland and displaying the underlying trachea rings (second and third).
- The isthmus may be transected with the aid of two curved clamps.
- The transected ends of the isthmus are oversewn, or ligated with absorbable sutures.
- A #11 blade is used to make a horizontal incision through the second and third tracheal rings.
- Tube is inserted into the trachea and secured with two 2-0 silk sutures sewn into the trachea.
- Suture is secured with air knots which will be cut during the first tracheostomy change in about 5 to 7 days.
- It may be attached to a ventilator if additional support is needed.
- The tube is secured with a band around the neck.

Postoperative Care. A nurse will help the patient in learning to adapt and speak with a tracheostomy.

Risks

- Damage to the thyroid gland
- Lung collapse
- Scar tissue in the trachea

TRANSORAL ROBOTIC SURGERY (TORS)

Transoral robotic surgery utilizes a surgical robot with arms to remove cancer from hard-to-reach areas of the throat and mouth. The camera attached to the robot gives a three-dimensional image for the surgeon at the console. The surgeon guides instruments placed on the robot arms to remove the cancer.

The DaVinci surgical system is most often used for robotic surgery. You can use the SI, XI, and SP. TORS aids in robotic assisted en-bloc resection of oral pharyngeal, hypo pharyngeal, and laryngeal T1 and T2 tumors, as well as resection of base of tongue tumors.

Benefits

- Quicker return to normal activity.
- Shorter hospitalization.
- Reduced risk of long-term swallowing problems that are more commonly seen with chemo, radiation, or traditional open surgery.
- Fewer complications than open surgery.
- Less scarring than traditional surgery.
- Less risk of infection.
- Less risk of blood transfusion one compared to open surgery.
- No routine use of tracheostomy during surgery compared to routine use for open surgery.

Complications

- Bleeding that may be life threatening.
- Difficulty swallowing.
- Tracheotomy possible.
- Loss of feeling in tongue.
- Changes of taste or loss of taste.

TORS Applications

- Tonsil
- Tongue base
- Palate
- Pharyngeal wall
- Parapharyngeal space
- Supraglottic
- Glottis
- Pyriform sinus

Patient Selection, Docking, and Positioning

- Early stage tonsillar, base of tongue, and supraglottic lesions

Contraindications

- Standard contraindications for head and neck surgery

Specific Contraindications for TORS

- Fixation of tumor to preverbal fascia
- Inability to adequately open mouth
- Retropharyngeal location of carotid arteries
- Limited neck mobility
- Mandibular invasion
- Carotid artery involvement
- 50% or more of tongue base

OR Configuration

This is the same for all TORS procedures. If using DaVinci Si or DaVinci Xi, use arms 1, 2, 3, and not arm 4.

Robot should be brought in at a 30° angle to the patient's bed.

The SA works at the head of the patient, seated, and has direct access to the surgical site. The SA performs these important functions during the case:

- Suction
- Retraction
- Application of hemoclips as well as instrument changes

TABLE 18-3 • TABLE OF RETRACTORS USED IN TRANSORAL ROBOTIC SURGERY

Retractor	Features	Limitations
Crow-Davis	Easily accessible, familiar to staff	Limited for base of tongue, hypopharynx, and larynx exposure
McIvor	Easily accessible, familiar to staff	Limited for base of tongue, hypopharynx, and larynx exposure, closed frame
Dingman	Large frame, cheek retractors, tie down points, accessible	Limited base of tongue, hypopharynx, and larynx exposure, closed frame
FK/FK-O	Large frame, a variety of blades created for exposure of certain areas, integrated suction, modified for TORS (FK-WO)	Closed frame, expensive
LARS	Intended for laryngeal procedures, curved frame, variety of blades, vertically adjustable blades, instrument attachment	Closed frame, expensive
Medrobotics Flex	Devised for TORS, curved frame assorted blades, blade modification in various planes, incorporated suction	Closed frame, expensive

Patient Positioning

- Patient in supine position
- Intubation with laser tube
- 2-0 silk stich is placed through the tongue and pulled out of mouth for positioning of mouth gag and teeth protectors. There is an assortment of mouth gags available including the FK–FKO, which is often used. A Crow-Davis is also commonly used. (See Table 18-3).

Camera Arm and Instrument Docking

- The camera arm is positioned in a vertical line over the patient's chest. Insertion angle should be perpendicular to the angle of the mouth gag. The SA will fine tune this angle according to patient's size.
- Camera cannula tip is placed at the level of the mouth gag. It is very important that the bedside SA ensures that the endoscope is not resting on any teeth during this procedure.
- The camera endoscope must be lower than the instrument arms.
- Right instrument arm is brought in and positioned at the level of the mouth gag, keeping distance between camera arm and right instrument arm to avoid external collisions.
- Insertion angle should be adjusted so that the instrument when inserted can be seen just past the tip.
- Left arm is brought in and is positioned the same as the right arm.
- Instrumentation for cautery and other is surgeon preference.

This set-up is the same for all TORS procedures.

Postoperation

- Intubated patients to ICU
- Antibiotic prophylaxis is mandatory
- Oximetry around the clock

Bibliography

Akyigit A, Sakallıoglu O, Karlidag T. Endoscopic tympanoplasty. *J Otol.* 2017; 2(2):62-67. https://doi.org/10.1016/j.joto.2017.04.004; https://www.ncbi.nlm.nih.gov/pmc/articles/PMC5963455/

Bigcas JLM, Okuyemi OT. Glossectomy. [Updated 2021 Jul 30]. In: StatPearls [Internet]. Treasure Island (FL): StatPearls Publishing; 2021 Jan. https://www.ncbi.nlm.nih.gov/books/NBK560636/

Brar S, Watters C, Winters R. Tympanoplasty. https://www.ncbi.nlm.nih.gov/books/NBK565863/. Updated June 24, 2021.

Burke D. *Mastoiditis.* Medically reviewed by Alana Biggers. https://www.healthline.com/health/mastoiditis. Updated on December 6, 2017.

Department of Otolaryngology, University of Pittsburgh. *Hearing Assessments and Diagnostic testing.* http://www.otolaryngology.pitt.edu/centers-excellence/center-audiology-and-hearing-aids/hearing-assessments-and-diagnostic-testing

Department of Otorhinolaryngology—Head & Neck Surgery, McGovern Medical School. Ear Anatomy – Inner Ear. UTH Health. https://med.uth.edu/orl/online-ear-disease-photo-book/chapter-3-ear-anatomy/ear-anatomy-inner-ear/

Dhillon N. Anatomy. In Lalwani AK (ed.), *Current Diagnosis & Treatment Otolaryngology—Head and Neck Surgery,* 4e. New York, NY: McGraw-Hill; 2020. https://accesssurgery.mhmedical.com/content.aspx?bookid=2744&sectionid=229669207

Ear Institute of Chicago. *Mastoidectomy.* https://www.chicagoear.com/our-services/ear-surgery/mastoidectomy/

El Sayed Ahmad Y, Winters R. *Parotidectomy.* https://www.ncbi.nlm.nih.gov/books/NBK557651/. Last Update: July 31, 2021.

Fagen J. Total glossectomy for tongue cancer. Open access atlas of otolaryngology, head & neck operative surgery. Total glossectomy for tongue cancer (uct.ac.za)

Frontal Sinus. Wikipedia. https://en.wikipedia.org/wiki/Frontal_sinus. Accessed July 19, 2023.

Funk E, Baker A, Goldenberg D, Goyal N. An Overview of Retractor Systems Used in Transoral Robotic Surgery. Penn State College of Medicine. https://www.otopa.org/uploads/1/0/3/7/103751734/baker_aaron_-_an_overview_of_retractor_systems.pdf

Glick Y, Hacking C. Caldwell-Luc Operation. https://radiopaedia.org/articles/51780. Accessed on September 29, 2021.

Goel A, Hacking C, Gajera J, et al. Sphenoid sinus. Radiopaedia.org. https://doi.org/10.53347/rID-24668; https://radiopaedia.org/articles/24668. Accessed on July 13, 2023.

Grujičić R. Paranasal Sinuses. Ken Hub. https://www.kenhub.com/en/library/anatomy/the-paranasal-sinuses. Accessed July 19, 2023.

Grujičić R. Maxillary Sinus. Ken Hub. https://www.kenhub.com/en/library/anatomy/maxillary-sinus. Accessed July 19, 2023.

Hayes K. The Anatomy and Function of the Nasal Cavity. Very WellHealth. https://www.verywellhealth.com/nasal-cavity-anatomy-5097506. Accessed July 19, 2023.

Hawkins J. Human Ear Anatomy. https://www.britannica.com/science/ear/Tympanic-membrane-and-middle-ear. https://www.intercoastalmedical.com/2018/03/30/what-exactly-does-an-otorhinolaryngologist-treat/

Isaacson B. *Mastoidectomy*. Edited by Meyers DA. https://emedicine.medscape.com/article/1890933-overview#a3. Updated October 1, 2019.

James MB, Arthur FS. *Essentials of Surgery*. Saunders/Elsevier Publishers.

Kennedy KL, Lin JW. Mastoidectomy. https://www.ncbi.nlm.nih.gov/books/NBK559153/. Updated June 10, 2021.

Koroulakis A, Jamal Z, Agarwal M. Anatomy, Head, Neck, Lymph Nodes. https://www.ncbi.nlm.nih.gov/books/NBK513317/

Krans B. *Tracheostomy*. Medically reviewed by Gerhard Whitworth RN. https://www.healthline.com/health/tracheostomy#uses. Updated on December 6, 2018.

Kumar M, Nanavati R, Modi TG, Dobariya C. Oral cancer: etiology and risk factors: a review. *J Cancer Res Ther*. 2016 Apr-Jun;12(2):458-63. doi: 10.4103/0973-1482.186696. PMID: 27461593.

Lindman JP. Tracheostomy. Edited by Soo Hoo GW. https://www.medscape.com/answers/865068-32759/what-is-the-anatomy-of-the-trachea

Louis Mandel DDS, Erin Leighwitek BS. Chronic parotitis: diagnosis and treatment. *J Am Dent Assoc*. Dec 2001;132(12):1707-1711. https://www.sciencedirect.com/science/journal/00028177

Martini N. *Fundamentals of Anatomy & Physiology*. 11th ed. In P. J. Frederic H. Martini, *Fund*. New York: Pearson; 2018: 838-843.

Mastoiditis. Medically reviewed by Minesh Khatri, on July 31, 2019. https://www.webmd.com/cold-and-flu/ear-infection/mastoiditis-symptoms-causes-treatments

Mayfield Brain and Spine. Audiometry Test. https://mayfieldclinic.com/pe-hearing.htm

Mroz M. Types of Hearing Loss. https://www.healthyhearing.com/help/hearing-loss/types. Last reviewed on May 4, 2020.

Nose. Cleveland Clinic. https://my.clevelandclinic.org/health/body/21778-nose. Accessed July 19, 2023.

Oghalai JS, Brownell WE. Anatomy and physiology of the ear. In Lalwani AK (ed.), *Current Diagnosis & Treatment Otolaryngology—Head and Neck Surgery*, 4e. New York, NY: McGraw-Hill; 2020. https://accesssurgery.mhmedical.com/content.aspx?bookid=2744&sectionid=229676006

Phillips N. *What Is a Mastoidectomy?* Medically reviewed by Judith Marcin. https://www.healthline.com/health/mastoidectomy. Updated on June 6, 2017.

Reilly BK. Tympanoplasty Technique. Edited by Meyers AD. https://emedicine.medscape.com/article/2051819 technique. Updated on March 02, 2016.

Rothrock JC. Rothrock JC, *Alexander's Care of the Patient in Surgery*, 14th ed. St. Louis: Elsevier; 2011:566-585 & 657-707.

Russell PT, Becker SS. Caldwell–Luc Surgery. https://entokey.com/caldwell-luc-surgery/

Saxby AJ, Jufas N, Kong JHK, Newey A, Pitman AG, Patel NP. Novel radiologic approaches for cholesteatoma detection: implications for endoscopic ear surgery. *Otolaryngol Clin North Am*. 2021 Feb;54(1):89-109. doi: 10.1016/j.otc.2020.09.011. Epub 2020 Nov 2. PMID: 33153729.

Seemann MD, Beltle J, Heuschmid M, Löwenheim H, Graf H, Claussen CD. Image fusion of CT and MRI for the visualization of the auditory and vestibular system. *Eur J Med Res*. 2005 Feb 28;10(2):47-55. https://pubmed.ncbi.nlm.nih.gov/15817422/

Sphenoid Sinus Anatomy. Healthline Medical Network. https://www.healthline.com/human-body-maps/sphenoid-sinus#1. Accessed July 19, 2023.

Trachea. Cleveland Clinic. https://my.clevelandclinic.org/health/body/21828-trachea. Accessed July 19, 2023.

Varvares MA, Walen SG. Mandibulectomy. Medscape. https://emedicine.medscape.com/article/1890889-overview. Updated on September 24, 2019.

What Exactly Does an Otorhinolaryngologist Treat? Intercostal Medical Group; March 30, 2018.

What Is Otolaryngology? Columbia University; Department of Otolaryngology Head and Neck Surgery. https://www.entcolumbia.org/about-us/what-otolaryngology

Whyte A, Boeddinghaus R. The maxillary sinus: physiology, development and imaging anatomy. *Dentomaxillofac Radiol*. 2019 Dec;48(8):20190205. doi: 10.1259/dmfr.20190205. Epub 2019 Aug 13. Erratum in: *Dentomaxillofac Radiol*. 2019 Sep 10;20190205c. PMID: 31386556; PMCID: PMC6951102.

Zimlich R. The Anatomy of the Parotid Gland. VeryWell Health. December 25, 2020. Parotid Gland: Anatomy, Location, and Function (verywellhealth.com)

19

Orthopedic Surgery

David Magaster, Jennifer Paling, Cynthia Kreps, and Jessica Wilhelm

DISCUSSED IN THIS CHAPTER

1. Fracture management
2. Skeletal anatomy and physiology
3. Diagnostics and surgeries of the skeletal system
4. Role of the surgical assistant in orthopedic surgery

INTRODUCTION

Orthopedic surgery, a branch of orthopedics, is a medical specialty that focuses on the diagnosis, treatment, and prevention of conditions or injuries that affect the musculoskeletal system. This includes bones, muscles, joints, tendons, ligaments, and other connective tissues that support and move the body.

The field of orthopedics includes several subspecialties that include trauma, sports medicine, reconstructive surgery, spine, pediatric orthopedics, and musculoskeletal oncology.

According to the CDC, accidents are the fourth leading cause of death in the US today. Musculoskeletal injuries are very common and often require treatment or surgery. The surgical assistant (SA) is a valuable team member during surgery and should be well versed in all aspects of orthopedics.

FRACTURE MANAGEMENT

Orthopedic surgeons manage most fractures internally with the use of plates. Plates come in many designs based on the bone in which it is designed to fix too. Some plates come with the ability to only compress fractures, whereas others are designed for both compression and buttressing of a fracture. Some plates are also capable of being contoured to match a patient's specific anatomic shape and others are manufactured already with the appropriate contouring for that bone. Plates also come in a variety of lengths and screw hold combinations. Depending on the surgeon's desired effect of the plate on the fracture, the plates have screw holes with threads for locking the screw into the plate or smooth holes for compression screws. Ultimately, the goal of a plate is to provide an internal structural support for the bone to stabilize the fracture and to support bone healing.

The screws utilized to fixate the plate to the bone come in many varieties. When the surgeon wants to use the plate as a buttress, locking screws are utilized in the threaded holes of the plate. Locking screws have threads in the head of the screw, which interlocks with the plate. The screws locking into the plate prevent the screw head from compressing the plate onto the bone. The locking screws and shaft threads are small since the locking screw will be placed through each cortex of the bone. It is important when placing locking screws that the bone is not overdrilled since the locking mechanism prevents the surgeon from realizing that the screw has not engaged the cortex. Locking screws are usually placed only after the fracture has been confirmed reduced.

If the surgeon needs to compress the fracture, the surgeon will use cortical screws in the smooth holes of the plate. Cortical screws have smooth and wide heads which allows the screw to slide along the plate's screw hole. This movement allows the screw head to compress the plate downward onto the bone, which will compress the fracture segments together. The cortical screws also have fine threads along the shaft to engage in the cortices of bone. Typically, only two cortical compression screws are used when plating a fracture. One screw engaged on each side of the fracture moves the fracture pieces toward each other. Compression of the fracture can also occur without a plate when utilizing a cortical screw.

To compress a fracture without a plate, a lag screw technique can be utilized. For the lag screw technique to work, the screw must lie perpendicularly to the fracture plane. To complete the lag screw technique, the near cortex is drilled to the same size as the outer diameter of the screw being placed. Using a centering drill guide, the far cortex is now drilled to the size of the inner diameter of the screw without the threads. A counter sink is used to allow the screw head to sit further into the bone. This prevents the screw head from interfering with the fibular plate and/or applying excess pressure on the skin. A depth gauge is used to determine the screw length, and the screw is inserted with a manual screwdriver. Since the near cortex is drilled to the same size as the screw, the screw threads will not be able to purchase into the bone. However, the far cortex is under-drilled enough to allow the screw threads to purchase in the bone, moving the far fracture piece toward the near fracture piece. This compresses the fracture. Not all fractures qualify for a lag screw technique, but it is a great mechanism to hold fractures together.

When compressing a fracture that occurs in metaphyseal bone, cancellous screws are used. The threads are coarse and widely spaced, which allow the screw to capture more of the spongy medullary bone for fixation and not rely on the cortical bone for fixation. Cancellous screws also have smooth head to engage in the smooth holes of the plates. These screws can also come partially threaded, which allow it to be utilized as a lag screw. Washers are used often with cancellous screws since these screws are placed in thinner cortical regions of the bone. The washers prevent the screw head from sinking farther into the cortex then it is supposed to.

Screws come in a wide range of diameters and lengths. Plate and screw manufacturing companies have specialized trays for each type of fracture seen in the operating room (OR). These trays contain the most used lengths and diameters for that specific fracture type. These manufacturer trays also contain the drill bits, drill guides, K-wires, and even specialty instruments needed to complete the procedure.

If internal fixation of a fracture is not possible, then the surgeon will place an external fixator to stabilize the fracture. External fixation is used often for severely comminuted fractures, open fractures with high risk of infection, malunions, or hemodynamically unstable patients. The complexity and size of the external fixator all depends on the location of the fracture. However, the basic application principles remain the same. Two pins are placed in the bones on either side of the fracture then clamps are placed on the pins. These clamps allow multiple rods to be attached to the pins across the fracture. With the rod to clamp connections loose, the fracture site is mobile and reduceable. The surgeon will externally reduce the fracture, then have the SA tighten the rod to clamp connections. When the rods are tightened to the clamps, the fracture is no longer mobile which provides the stability necessary for the bone healing process to begin. Placing an external fixator requires the use of intraoperative fluoroscopy to confirm the placement of the pins as well as the reduction of the fracture. This is considered a minimally invasive technique since no large incisions are created to visualize the fracture reduction. External fixation is the secondary plan for all internal fixation procedures, so having a tray available is important to prevent excessive delays during the surgery.

SHOULDER

Anatomy

The shoulder is one of the largest and highly intricate joints in the body. It offers more mobility than any other joint in the human body. The ball and socket joint of the shoulder is formed where the humerus fits into the scapula. Even with the variety of activity, the humeral head remains precisely centered in the glenoid. The acromion is the bony ridge off the scapula. The clavicle meets the acromion in the acromioclavicular joint. The coracoid process is a hook-shaped bony construct that projects from the scapula (see Figure 19-1). The rotator cuff is the collection of muscles and tendons that surround the shoulder to give it support and permits for the wide range of motion. The bursa is the small sac of fluid that cushions and protects the tendons of the rotator cuff and the labrum forms a cup for the head of the humerus to reside. The superior glenohumeral ligament (SGHL), middle glenohumeral ligament (MGHL), inferior glenohumeral ligament (IGHL), and coracohumeral ligament helps to stabilize the shoulder.

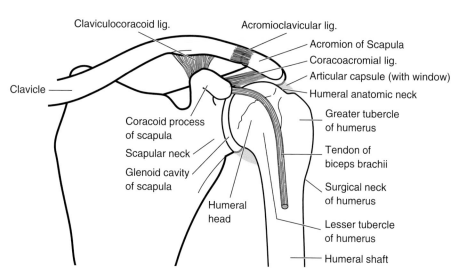

Figure 19-1 · Shoulder anatomy. (Reproduced, with permission, from Suneja M, Szot JF, LeBlond RF, Brown DD. *DeGowin's Diagnostic Examination.* 11th ed. New York, NY: McGraw Hill; 2020.)

Signs and Symptoms

- **Frozen shoulder:** Inflammation that develops in the shoulder and causes pain and stiffness.
- **Osteoarthritis:** Although wear and tear arthritis is common with aging, the shoulder is less often affected by osteoarthritis than the knee.
- **Rheumatoid arthritis:** A type of arthritis when the immune system attacks the joints, causing inflammation and pain.
- **Gout:** A form of arthritis in which crystals form in the joints, causing inflammation and pain.
- **Rotator cuff tear:** A tear in one of the muscles or tendons surrounding the top of the humerus.
- **Shoulder impingement:** The acromion (edge of the scapula) presses on the rotator cuff as the arm is lifted.
- **Shoulder dislocation:** The humerus or one of the other bones in the shoulder slips out of position.
- **Shoulder tendonitis:** Inflammation of one of the tendons in the shoulder's rotator cuff.
- **Shoulder bursitis:** Inflammation of the bursa, the small sac of fluid that rests over the rotator cuff tendons.
- **Labral tear:** Overuse or trauma can cause a tear in the labrum, which is the cuff of cartilage that helps stabilize the shoulder joint.

Rotator Cuff Repair

Anatomy. The shoulder contains several bursae that reduce friction where the muscles and tendons transverse across the capsule. These bursae include the subacromial, subcoracoid, subdeltoid, and subscapular. Inflammation of any of these bursae is called bursitis. Subacromial bursitis is the most common.

The supraspinatus tendon is separated from the deltoid, acromion, and coracoacromial by the subacromial bursae. Issues created in this area are called impingement.

Four articulations make up the shoulder joint: sternoclavicular, acromioclavicular, glenohumeral, and scapulothoracic. To maintain correct anatomic function, all these work in tandem. The supraspinatus and the infraspinatus pull the humeral head into the glenoid, which counteracts the forces of the deltoid muscle. The deltoid muscle forces the head of the humerus upward, causing impingement of the supraspinatus and the infraspinatus loses function from an injury. This impingement can be surgically repaired via acromioplasty.

The rotator cuff consists of four muscles located around the scapula. The supraspinatus muscle sits on the top of the scapula and is the most common rotator cuff muscle torn. The infraspinatus and teres minor muscles are located posteriorly on the wing of the scapula. The subscapularis is located anteriorly on the wing of the scapula (see Figure 19-2). The tendons of all the rotator cuff muscles fuse and connect to the humeral head. The function of the rotator cuff is to keep the humeral head against the glenoid fossa, which creates the shoulder joint. The insertion sites of the cuff to the humeral head: supraspinatous, infraspinatus, teres minor insert on greater tubercle of humerus and subscapularis inserts on lesser tubercle of the humerus.

Etiology. Rotator cuff tears tend to occur from chronic wear and tear of the tendons; however, an acute tear can occur from heavy lifting or trauma. When the tendon of a rotator cuff pulls away from the humeral head, pain and loss of motion can occur. A partial rotator cuff tear has damage to the soft tissue, but the tendon is not completely transected. A full thickness rotator cuff tear has a completely transected tendon that is usually torn off the humeral head (see figure 19-3). Occasionally,

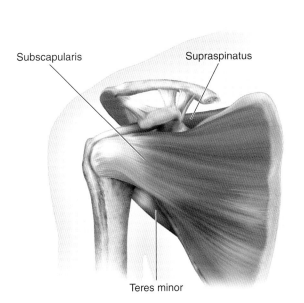
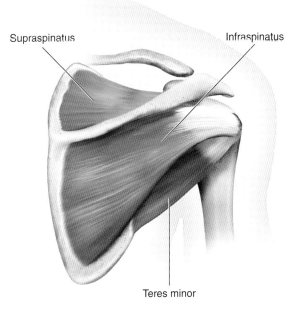

Figure 19-2 · Rotator cuff muscles, showing anterior (A) and posterior (B) views. (Reproduced, with permission, from Parks EH. Practical Office Orthopedics. New York, NY: McGraw Hill; 2017.)

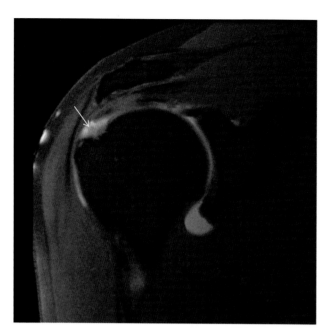

Figure 19-3 · Rotator cuff tear. (Reproduced, with permission, from Brunicardi FC et al, eds. *Schwartz's Principles of Surgery*. 11th ed. New York, NY: McGraw Hill; 2019.)

a bone defect in the humeral head is seen where the tendon has detached. Mild tears can be medically managed; however, larger tears need to be treated surgically.

Nonsurgical Treatment

- Rest
- Ice
- Physical therapy
- Steroid injections
- Analgesics such as Ibuprofen or Acetaminophen

Diagnostics. The physician will perform a physical exam to confirm an injury to the rotator cuff. The patient may also have x-rays, ultrasound, or a magnetic resonance imaging (MRI) to validate soft tissue injuries.

Positioning and Prepping. Shoulder procedures can be accomplished with the patient in either the lateral decubitus position (LDP) or the beach chair position (BCP).

Anesthesia. Surgically, rotator cuff tears are repaired using either the arthroscopic or open technique. The technique chosen is based on surgeon's training and size of rotator cuff tear. Severely torn rotator cuffs are repaired open, while more manageable tears are repaired arthroscopically.

For a rotator cuff repair, general anesthesia is utilized to ensure complete relaxation of the patient throughout the procedure. The endotracheal tube is taped to the opposite side of the operative arm to prevent dislodgment during the procedure. Injury to the eyes during this procedure is a major concern due to the sterile personnel's proximity to the face. Taping extra foam padding to the face and/or placing padded goggles over the patient's eyes will aide in protecting the patient's face from

injury. If the patient chooses to receive one, an interscalene nerve block aides in postoperative pain relief for about 24 to 48 hours post-surgery. Most facilities perform the block in the preoperative holding area, so be aware that the patient will not have control over their operative arm while maneuvering over to the OR bed.

Open Technique

Positioning, Prepping, and Draping. Following induction, the patient is positioned in the BCP. A Schlein shoulder positioner or a beanbag positioner is utilized to secure that patient in this position. The operative arm is prepped circumferentially from wrist to lateral neck, then a sterile large drape is placed under the operative arm and across the patient's body. An impervious stockinette is placed over the hand and extended to the mid-humerus. A Coban is wrapped around the arm to hold the stockinette in place. While the arm is still held in the air, an impervious U-drape is placed under the arm at the axilla. One limb of the drape is wrapped anteriorly around the shoulder at the level of the clavicle and the other limb of the drape is wrapped posteriorly around the shoulder at the spine of the scapula. A second impervious U-drape is placed at the base of the lateral neck and the limbs of the drape follow the same path as the other U-drape. To complete the sterile field, a re-inforced split sheet is placed underneath the operative arm as close to the axilla as possible. The limbs of the split sheet follow the same path as the impervious U-drape. A second reinforced split sheet is placed at the base of the lateral neck and each limb is unfolded following the same path as the impervious U-drape. An incise drape covers the exposed skin of the shoulder prior to incision.

Surgical Procedure

- An approximately 4-cm skin incision is made parallel to the lateral border of the acromion and dissection through the subcutaneous tissue continues to the deltoid muscle. The deltoid is dissected off the insertion point at the acromion ensuring that a small cuff of deltoid is left to reattach the muscle to.

- At this point an acromioplasty can be performed to remove any bone spurs that have formed beneath the acromion. The acromioplasty is performed with a power drill and a small burr. The SA is responsible for irrigating the bone during the acromioplasty to prevent the bone from overheating.

- The bursa surrounding the shoulder joint is dissected to gain access to the humeral head. With the humeral head exposed, the rotator cuff tear is visible.

- The SA is providing retraction of the soft tissues using small Eastman retractors or Army Navy retractors.

- The surgeon may also place Weitlaner retractors to provide self-retaining retraction during the procedure. Once the rotator cuff is adequately identified, the tendon is repaired using a size 0 permanent braided polyester suture. The figure of eight suture technique is utilized to ensure a strong hold for the tendon repair.

- Once the rotator cuff is repaired, closure begins. The deltoid muscle is reattached to the acromion the size zero permanent braided suture.

- The dermis is closed with a 3-0 absorbable braided suture then the skin incision is closed using 4-0 absorbable monofilament suture.

Dressing. Prineo® is applied to the skin incision and 4 × 4s are applied after the Prineo® has time to dry. Abdominal pads can also be added for extra pressure. Cotton-based tape is used to hold the gauze or pads onto the patient. A shoulder immobilizer is placed almost immediately following surgery. The patient must wear the immobilizer for around 6 weeks to allow the tendons time to heal. An ice pack is placed on the shoulder for postoperative swelling management and pain relief.

Arthroscopic Technique

Positioning, Prepping, and Draping. Positioning for the arthroscopic technique varies based on surgeon's preference. Surgeons may choose the BCP or LDP. When using the LDP, a Vac-Pac is used to maintain the lateral position. Placing the nonoperative arm out on an arm board and an axillary roll is placed in the axilla. All boney prominences are padded, and the operative arm is prepared to be placed in traction. A padded sleeve is placed over the arm to the elbow and Coban is used to secure the sleeve to the patient's arm. The sleeve has a loop that is hooked onto a shoulder traction holder that is attached directly to the end of the operative bed. The shoulder holder has a pulley system that allows weights to be placed on the opposite end to pull traction on the arm. This traction opens the joint space for exposure during the procedure.

The operative arm is prepped circumferentially from elbow to lateral neck with care taken to prep the entire axillary region. A sterile large drape is placed under the operative arm and across the patient's body. A sterile towel is wrapped from the elbow to hand and a Coban is wrapped around the arm to hold the towels in place. An impervious U drape is placed under the arm at the axilla. One limb of the drape is wrapped anteriorly toward the chest, and the other limb of the drape is wrapped posteriorly around the base of the scapula. A second impervious U-drape is placed at the base of the lateral neck and the limbs of the drape follow the same path as the other U-drape. To complete the sterile field, a reinforced split sheet is placed underneath the operative arm as close to the axilla as possible. The limbs of the split sheet follow the same path as the impervious U-drape. A second reinforced split sheet is placed at the base of the lateral neck and each limb is unfolded following the same path as the impervious U-drape. Strips of incise drape is used to secure the edges of the drape around the surgical field.

Surgical Procedure

- After the time-out is performed, the arthroscopy trocars are placed. A total of six trocars in varying combinations can be placed around the shoulder joint depending on the severity of the rotator cuff tear. An anterior trocar is located about one inch in front of the acromioclavicular joint. Two lateral trocars are placed at 1 inch and 3 inches laterally to the acromion. A posterior trocar is placed in the soft spot of the shoulder joint about two inches from the posterior border of the acromion. An anterior and/or posterior accessory trocar can be placed 1 inch away from the superior lateral trocar if additional access points are needed.

- A 4-mm 30° lens is placed in the posterior trocar to examine the glenohumeral joint. This allows the surgeon to review the rotator cuff tear from the inferior surface of the tendon as well as to evaluate the labrum and articular surfaces.

- Through the lower lateral trocar, the surgeon inserts soft tissue shaver to remove any bursal adhesions and release the coracoacromial and coracohumeral ligament.

- The lens is switched into the lower lateral trocar and the soft tissue shaver is placed in the posterior trocar. This gives the surgeon a view of the posterior cuff for release. The rotator cuff tear is now exposed and ready for repair. Throughout this portion of the procedure, the SA is aiding the surgeon by holding the camera and managing the cords.

- Anchors are placed into the humeral head in varying configurations based on the size of the rotator cuff tear. A small crescent tear utilizes a single triple anchor. A moderate crescent tear uses two-anchor double row suture bridge, and a large U-shaped rotator cuff tear uses a four-anchor double row suture bridge. The anchors are either self-tapping or require the bone to be tapped prior to insertion and are also made of either metal or biodegradable plastic. The anchors all have a braided ultra-high-molecular-weight polyethylene suture of different colors attached to them.

- Regardless of the repair technique chosen, the anchors are placed medially in the humeral head avoiding the articular surface. Utilizing the horizontal mattress technique, a suture passer retrieves one of the sutures and passes it through the supraspinatus tendon. Arthroscopic graspers aide in the retrieval of the suture and gauging the mobility of the tear during repair.

- After the sutures are passed through the tendon, the ends are passed through a trocar closest to the repair and extracorporeal knots are thrown. The knots are pushed into place using a knot pusher.

- Anchor systems are available that utilize knotless techniques for anchoring the rotator cuff repair. Some anchors also have holes to pass suture through from other anchors to attach the tendon to the humeral head. During the anchoring process, the SA helps organize the suture and holds the camera while the surgeon ties the knots.

- After the rotator cuff is securely anchored to the bone, the trocars are removed, and the skin incisions are closed. Surgeon's preference dictates if the skin incisions are closed with absorbable or nonabsorbable suture. A deep buried suture technique is used with an absorbable suture and a simple interrupted or horizontal mattress suture technique is used with nonabsorbable suture.

Dressings. Because the incisions are only 5 mm, surgeons may choose to only use steri-strips to close the incision. Each incision is covered with a 2 × 2 gauze and small Tegaderm™. A shoulder immobilizer is immediately placed, and an ice pack is placed on the shoulder for postoperative relief.

Arthroscopic rotator cuff repairs are still limited for larger tears; however, innovations in the anchor technology are enabling surgeons to use this minimally invasive technique more often. Arthroscopic repairs decrease infection and wound complications compared to the open repair. The patient's postoperative pain control and recovery is also easier with the arthroscopic repair due to the smaller incision size and lack of muscle dissection.

Postop Complications. Complications included shoulder stiffness, failure of healing, infection, reflex sympathetic dystrophy, deep venous thrombosis, and death.

Bankart Repair

The Bankart lesion is named after Arthur Sydney Blundell Bankart (1879–1951), a British orthopedic surgeon. In his initial report, Bankart described an avulsion injury of the fibrocartilaginous soft tissues along the anteroinferior glenohumeral joint occurring in correlation with anterior shoulder dislocation.

Etiology. Trauma is the most common cause that leads to shoulder instability including shoulder dislocation. The glenoid labrum and ligaments can tear when the arm is forced backwards, letting the humeral head to dislocate from the glenoid. Failure of the ligaments to heal results in an unstable shoulder where the ball of the joint can slip from its center placement of the glenoid with minimal force. Younger patients are more susceptible to repeat dislocations than older patients.

The most common form of ligament injury is the Bankart lesion, which is when the ligaments are torn from the front of the socket. Glenohumeral dislocations are primarily triggered by an abduction, extension, and external rotation movement. The repair requires the torn tissue be sutured back to the rim of the socket.

There are two types of Bankart lesions:

- A soft tissue is an anteroinferior labrum avulsion damage of the glenoid rim. The posterior capsule may be stretched and the IGHL is torn.
- A bony Bankart lesion highlights a fracture of the anterior inferior glenoid rim along with the soft tissue injury.

Symptoms

- Pain when reaching overhead
- A sense of instability in the shoulder
- Catching, locking, popping, or grinding in the shoulder
- Occasional night pain or pain with daily activities
- Decreased range of motion
- Loss of strength

Diagnostics

- MRI: The MRI can also measure the related medial displacements of the IGHL underneath the glenoid.
- A soft tissue lesion can be seen on arthroscopy and an MR arthrography.
- Radiographs will identify a bony Bankart lesion.

Nonsurgical Treatment. Older people and people who are not real active may benefit from immobilization with a sling for a few weeks. The arm is placed in front of the body in internal rotation with a small pillow under the armpit to abduct the arm slightly. This is followed by intensive physical therapy to regain some strength, stability, and mobility of the shoulder itself.

Other nonsurgical treatments include analgesics, muscle relaxants, or lidocaine to help with the pain and allow for a closed reduction.

Patient Positioning and Prepping. The patient is placed in a supine position or semi-Fowler's with a sandbag or folded sheet under the shoulder. The arm is prepped with dura prep and draped free and wrapped in a sterile arm sleeve connected to 10 to 15 pounds of traction. The ideal position is forward flexion of 20°-20° and abduction of 30° to allow for better exposure for the anterior repair.

Anesthesia

- General anesthesia is preferred, although the procedure can be performed with a scalene block as well.

Surgical Procedure

- A posterior arthroscopic portal is created, and a diagnostic arthroscopy is completed to confirm the Bankart lesion. Diagnostic arthroscopy should include evaluation of the labrum, capsular tissue, rotator cuff and biceps tendons, and humeral head.
- An anterior-superior access is established, medial to the anterolateral corner of the acromion. A spinal needle is used to confirm correct position and a cannula is inserted.
- An anterior portal is created above the subscapularis tendon, positioned lateral to the tip of the coracoid process.
- The drill guide is positioned on the anterior rim at a 45°e angle and a 7-mm cannula is inserted.
- The anterior glenoid rim is prepared through the anterior ports by removing fibrous tissue from the rim down to the bony bed.
- The capsuloligamentous structures are mobilized with the use of an elevator.
- A shaver is used to remove the tissue between the glenoid and the labrum.
- Mobilization of the Bankart lesion is accomplished.
- It is important that the ligamentous-labral tissues are returned to their anatomic position on top of the articular cartilage anteriorly.
- An arthroscopic grasper is used to verify the reduction before proceeding.

- The drill guide is inserted through an anterior portal, so the suture anchor can be placed at the 5 o'clock position around the anteroinferior capsulolabral tissue.

- The subscapularis is tented, and a sharp trocar is pushed into the glenohumeral joint.

- The trocar is removed, and the drill guide is positioned on the anterior rim at the 5 o'clock position.

- The arthroscope is placed in the anterior-superior portal for inserting the suture anchors and suturing the anterior ligamentous-labral complex.

- A 2.8-mm suture anchor is drilled into the anterior rim at the 5 o'clock position.

- A 2.8-mm Fastak anchor is a one-step anchor that is screwed into the bone with power (see Figure 19-4).

- The wound is irrigated, and trocar incisions are closed according to surgeon's preference.

- The shoulder is placed in an immobilizer.

Risks and Complications. The risks of surgery for shoulder instability include but are not limited to the following:

- Infection
- Injury to nerves and blood vessels
- Inability to carry out the planned repair
- Stiffness of the joint
- Tear of the rotator cuff

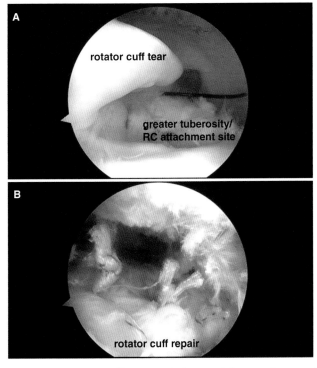

Figure 19-4 · Rotator cuff repair. A. Arthroscopic image of supraspinatus tendon tear. B. Completion of the repair using suture anchors embedded in the greater tuberosity of the humerus. (Reproduced, with permission, from Brunicardi FC et al, eds. *Schwartz's Principles of Surgery*. 11th ed. New York, NY: McGraw Hill; 2019.)

- Pain
- Persistent instability
- The need for additional surgeries

Slap Repair

The term "SLAP" stands for "Superior Labrum Anterior to Posterior" and is applied to define a tear or detachment of the labrum that begins at the anchor site for the biceps (anterior) and extends backward (posterior) from this point. A "SLAP tear" basically means that the labrum is being stripped away from the underlying bone. The labrum is an attachment site for several ligaments and tendons that include the long head of the biceps muscle, which is attached to the superior edge of the labrum.

Etiology. SLAP tears occur at the front of the upper arm where the biceps tendon connects to the shoulder. Trauma is responsible for approximately a third of all SLAP tears. Some tears arise more over time from repetitive strain, particularly in older adults whose cartilage becomes more brittle with age. SLAP injuries are frequent in athletes, particularly those who have repetitive actions such as throwing. A SLAP repair will use suture anchors to reattach the torn labrum to the glenoid.

Surgical Procedure

- The SLAP tear is identified, and excess/damaged tissue is removed.

- A small hole is drilled into the bone where the labrum has torn away from the socket.

- An anchor is placed into this hole; attached to the anchor is a strong suture.

- The suture is used to tie the torn labrum snuggly against the bone.

- Additional anchors are placed as needed to secure to the torn labrum.

Postop. The shoulder will be kept in a sling for 3 to 4 weeks. Physical therapy will include passive range of motion exercises. Once the sling is removed, strength training can begin. Athletes can start sports specific exercises after 12 weeks. It takes 6 months before the shoulder is fully healed.

Shoulder Arthroscopy

The word arthroscopy comes from two Greek words, "arthro" (joint) and "skopein" (to look). The word indicates "to look within the joint." Shoulder arthroscopy is a diagnostic tool that helps diagnose shoulder conditions.

Etiology. A standard arthroscopy is often performed to confirm a diagnosis and basic procedures such as, removal of loose bodies; lysis of adhesions, synovial biopsy; synovectomy; and bursectomy. It is often the surgical approach for the stabilization of dislocations, correction of glenoid labrum, biceps tendon, rotator cuff repairs, and relief of impingement syndrome.

Position and Prepping. The patient is placed in a lateral or semi-Fowler's. Lateral position requires use of the vacuum beanbag device and semi-Fowler's requires a 'beach chair' positioner. The affected extremity is placed in a shoulder suspension system and an immobilizer is applied to the forearm to provide distraction to the glenohumeral joint. The extremity is abducted at 40° to 60° and forward flexed at 10° to 20° with 5- to 15-pound weights placed on a pulley system to distract the joint. The shoulder is prepped and draped free to allow full range of motion throughout the procedure.

Anesthesia. A shoulder arthroscopy is often performed under general anesthesia. There are other options, such as the interscalene brachial plexus block (ISB) as it is one of the most effective anesthesia techniques offered for arthroscopic shoulder surgery. The posterior suprascapular block is also used during a shoulder arthroscopy.

Surgical Procedure

- An 18-gauge spinal needle is introduced through the posterior soft spot and guided anteriorly toward the coracoid process.
- The glenohumeral joint is distended with normal saline or lactated Ringers solution.
- The surgeon will inject 0.25% bupivacaine with epinephrine 1:200,000 at the needle spot to minimize bleeding.
- A stab incision with a #11 blade is made over the needle site.
- A sharp trocar and cannula is placed through the posterior joint capsule.
- After penetration of the capsule, the sharp trocar is replaced with a blunt obturator.
- An arthroscope connected to the camera and light source is introduced into the space and inflow and outflow tubing is connected to the obturator.
- Operative instruments are placed through an anterior portal that is established laterally to the coracoid process.
- A third portal may be established near the anterior portal or the supraspinous fossa portal.
- A switching stick will aid in changing the scope port.
- The joint is visualized by moving and rotating the arm.
- Glenoid tears are often repaired with absorbable fixation tacks.
- The joint is irrigated and injected with postop pain medication into the portal.
- Trocar incisions are closed and dressed with a 4 × 4.
- The arm is placed in a soft sling.

Postop. The sling is worn for up to 6 weeks. Ice helps with the swelling and can help to decrease pain after surgery. The patient is prescribed postoperative pain medication.

Shoulder Arthroplasty

The most common indication for an arthroplasty procedure is pain that has not responded to conservative management or a severe fracture. The first recorded procedure of shoulder arthroplasty was performed in 1894 by the French surgeon, Jean Pean. The original implant was comprised of a platinum and rubber implant for the glenohumeral joint. Charles Neer is recognized as leading the advancement of modern total shoulder arthroplasty (TSA), developing more modern prostheses for surgical procedures beginning in the 1950s. There are three main approaches to shoulder reconstruction surgery: hemiarthroplasty, TSA, and reverse total shoulder arthroplasty (rTSA). The indications for a TSA include:

- Osteoarthritis
- Rotator cuff injuries
- Fractures
- Rheumatoid arthritis and other inflammatory disorders
- Osteonecrosis

Hemiarthroplasty. A hemiarthroplasty of the shoulder is also called a partial replacement. During the procedure, the humerus is replaced with a prosthetic while the glenoid is left intact. Shoulder hemiarthroplasty is indicated in severe condition of osteoarthritis when only the humeral head is damaged, or a fracture affects only the proximal humerus. An optional procedure is a resurfacing hemiarthroplasty which does not require a stem component, instead the humeral head is resurfaced with a prosthetic component. This procedure is indicated for managing arthritic conditions of the shoulder and preferred for young, athletic patients.

Total Shoulder Arthroplasty. Total shoulder replacement arthroplasty is a well-recognized surgery for eliminating pain and restoring function to the arthritic shoulder. The arthritic ball is replaced by a smooth metal ball fixed to the humerus with a stem. The arthritic glenoid is resurfaced with high-density polyethylene prosthesis. These prothesis become fixated by allowing bony ingrowth through the porous ends of the components.

Reverse Total Shoulder Arthroplasty. This procedure is indicated for patients suffering from osteoarthritis or compound fractures of the humerus, in conjunction with a deficiency of the rotator cuff complex. Recently, however, recommendations have expanded to include etiology that were hard to treat with traditional anatomical shoulder arthroplasty, such as acute proximal humerus fracture, chronic locked dislocation, chronic pseudo paralysis caused by irreparable rotator cuff without arthritis, glenohumeral arthritis with severe glenoid bone loss, immunological arthritis, malunited/nonunited proximal humerus fracture, failed shoulder arthroplasty and tumors. An rTSA refers to a procedure where the prosthetic ball and socket that make up the joint are reversed.

Positioning and Prepping. The patient is placed in a 45° semi-Fowler's position with the nonoperative arm on a padded arm board. The affected shoulder is positioned a little off the edge of the OR bed to provide full access to the shoulder. A pillow under the knees will support the lower back and heels are padded. Head and neck alignment should be in neutral alignment. Male patients' genitalia should be free of any pressure from the semi-Fowler's position. A safety strap is positioned across the patient on the OR bed. The operative arm is placed on a padded surface or in a hydraulic positioner which allows for full extension and external rotation of the arm. The operative arm is prepped circumferentially with an alcohol-based prep solution from chin to waist, posterior shoulder, and axilla. The shoulder is draped with shoulder arthroplasty drapes.

Anesthesia. A TSA is performed under general anesthesia and a nerve block.

Surgical Procedure

- A 6-inch incision is made between the deltoid and pectoralis major muscles from the coracoid process of the scapula to the humerus. A surgical landmark is the cephalic vein found lying in the deltoid pectoralis groove.
- Dissection continues to the deltoid and the cephalic vein is identified and mobilized. Branches of the cephalic vein may be ligated with the ESU.
- The pectoralis tendon is exposed, and the cephalic vein is retracted laterally along with the deltoid.
- The SA will retract the deltoid laterally and the pectoralis major medially.
- The superior pectoralis tendon is released 1 cm using the ESU and the conjoined tendon is visualized.
- The clavipectoral fascia is separated parallel to the conjoined ligament from the distal pectoralis major to the coracoacromial ligament proximally.
- The arm is abducted and internally rotated to visualize the subacromial space.
- Dissection continues under the coracoacromial ligament, and the SA will place a retractor in the subacromial space.
- Attention is given to freeing adhesions from the subacromial and subdeltoid spaces.
- The axillary and musculocutaneous nerves are identified, and the SA will retract the conjoined tendons avoiding these structures.
- The arm is externally rotated, and anterior humeral circumflex vessels are exposed and coagulated near the inferior subscapularis.
- The biceps tendon is exposed.
- The superior portion of the subscapularis is mobilized.
- The capsular insertion onto the humerus is released along the medial neck avoiding the axillary nerve.
- Once the humerus is freed, the surgeon dislocates the humeral head.
- Osteophytes are removed from the humeral neck and the humeral head is removed.
- The humerus is prepared and a trial stem and humeral head are selected.
- The SA will expose the glenoid with shoulder retractors placed in the posterior and inferior glenoid.
- The inferior aspect of the subscapularis is released.
- The anterior capsule is incised with a knife from the coracoid to the inferior scapularis and the SA will expose the glenoid.

- The labrum and remaining cartilage are excised.
- The glenoid is prepared by reaming, drilling, and using sizers from the trial system.
- The glenoid is trialed for proper fit with the humeral trial head.
- The trial is removed, the glenoid is irrigated, and the cement is prepared.
- Cement is placed into the cancellous bone in the glenoid and an impactor helps seat the components into place.
- Excess cement is removed with a freer elevator.
- The humerus and stem are trialed.
- The implants are implanted with the aid of the impactor.
- The shoulder is reduced and irrigated.
- The subscapularis is sutured with Ethibond.
- Morphine or Demerol is injected for postop pain control.
- The SA will close superficial layers with absorbable suture.
- The wound is dressed with Kerlix fluffs and abdominal pad.
- A shoulder brace offers stability of the shoulder.

Postop. The patient is given tylenol with codeine and will remain in the hospital on the second or third day. Rehabilitation begins the same day of surgery by encouraging the patient to ambulate. They should avoid lifting anything heavy, pushing or pulling for up to 6 weeks after surgery. Driving is delayed until the patient has the necessary motion and strength.

Complications

- Infection
- Instability
- Periprosthetic fractures
- Glenoid complications

HUMERUS

Anatomy

The humerus is one of three bones that comprise the elbow joint. The *radius* and the *ulna* are the other two bones. The elbow is a hinged joint.

The distal end of the humerus has two articulating surfaces. The capitellum on the lateral side articulates with the proximal radius, specifically the radial (lesser sigmoid) notch on the anterior surface. The trochlea is located on the long axis of the humerus and articulates with the ulna on the medial side, specifically the trochlear (greater sigmoid) notch.

Common flexor muscles that originate from the medial epicondyle (superior to the trochlea) are pronator teres, flexor carpi radialis (FCR), palmaris longus, flexor digitorum superficialis (FDS), and flexor carpi ulnaris (FCU).

Common extensors originating from the lateral epicondyle are the anconeus, extensor digitorum communis (EDC), extensor carpis radialis longus (ECRL), extensor carpis radialis brevis (ECRB), and extensor digiti minimi (EDM).

The humerus shaft is cylindrical but distally becomes triangular. The *brachialis, triceps, brachioradialis, pectoralis major, deltoid,* and *coracobrachialis* muscles are responsible for movement. The *radial* nerve innervates these muscles and courses along the spiral groove.

Five muscles comprise the proximal humerus structure. The *pectoralis major* displaces the humerus anteriorly and medially. The *supraspinatus, infraspinatus,* and the *teres minor* externally rotate the greater tuberosity and the *subscapularis* internally rotates the lesser tuberosity. The supraspinatus, infraspinatus, teres minor, and subscapularis (SITS) are the muscles that form the rotator cuff.

Proximal humerus fractures are the third most common fracture, especially in the elderly (>65 year-old) population. Females are twice as likely as males to suffer from this fracture as a result of a ground-level fall on an outstretched arm. As the age increases in this population, there is a higher percentage of more complex fractures.

Open Reduction Internal Fixation (ORIF) of Dual Bone Forearm Fracture

Procedural Considerations. Confirm that preop x-rays are available in the room along with the C-arm. The patient will be supine with a hand table. The C-arm will come 90° perpendicular to the hand table. Confirm the appropriate plate system is in the room according to the surgeon's preference. A tourniquet is applied to the upper arm per the surgeon's preference.

Positioning and Prepping

• Confirm a beach-chair, beanbag, or lateral pegboard.

Anesthesia. An ORIF of a forearm fracture is performed under general anesthesia.

Surgical Procedure

• The incision is made at the *deltopectoral* groove or just below the coracoid process if the patient is obese and the grove cannot be identified. Dissection provides identification of the *deltopectoral* fascia near the *cephalic* vein.

• The *cephalic* vein is retracted either medially or laterally, while the deltoid is retracted laterally, and the pectoralis retracted medially. Avoid damage to the terminal branches of the axillary nerve when placing retractors.

• The SA should abduct the arm to relax the deltoid muscle for better visualization and for placing Steinman pins posterior to the deltoid to retract the said muscle. Identification and retraction of the short-head biceps and coracobrachialis medially with tension sutures provides visualization of the fracture.

• The fracture is reduced with appropriate large bone clamps. Again, the SA will rotate the arm to allow the surgeon to confirm proper alignment with the head, greater tuberosity, and the shaft. Placement of the plate is accomplished via a drilled outer cortex to provide placement of a "non-locking" plate to the bone.

• Drill, measure, and screw the bi-cortical screws in the humeral shaft and unicortical screws in the humeral head.

• Perform irrigation with copious amounts of normal saline.

• The capsule is closed with the tension sutures previously used for retraction of the short-head biceps and coracobrachialis.

The fascia, sub-q, and skin are closed per the surgeon's preference.

• Dress with bulky dressing, apply sling for comfort.

Humerus Shaft Fractures

Etiology. Humeral shaft fractures occur in two populations: young patients with high energy trauma and elderly patients with low energy injuries (see Figure 19-5).

Anatomy. The humerus shaft is cylindrical but distally becomes triangular. The *brachialis, triceps, brachioradialis, pectoralis major, deltoid,* and *coracobrachialis* muscles are responsible for movement. The *radial* nerve innervates these muscles and courses along the spiral groove.

Procedural Considerations. Nonoperative treatment is a splint providing that there is no major soft tissue loss or a vascular injury requiring surgical intervention. Operatively, there are two choices: open reduction internal fixation (ORIF) or intramedullary nailing (IMN).

Diagnostic. The physician will do an examination and take orthogonal radiographs, which may include an AP and lateral view as well as a transthoracic lateral view.

Positioning and Prepping. Hand table attachment or beanbag for positioning the patient in a supine position.

Depending on where the fracture is located on the shaft, a tourniquet may or may not be used. If it is utilized, a sterile tourniquet should be applied.

Anesthesia. Depending on the severity of the humeral fracture, the procedure may be done with a local under sedation or a general anesthesia.

Surgical Procedure. A posterior or anterolateral surgical approach will depend on the mechanism of injury and the best way to place plates to facilitate bone repair. Both approaches will be discussed below as different anatomical landmarks will be noted.

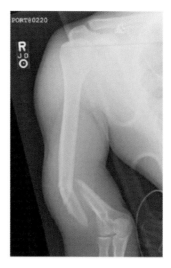

Figure 19-5 · Humerus fracture. (Reproduced, with permission, from McMahon PJ, Skinner HB. *Current Diagnosis & Treatment in Orthopedics.* 6th ed. New York, NY: McGraw Hill; 2021.)

Posterior Approach

- An incision along the posterior aspect of the midline is extended to the olecranon fossa. Identify the long and lateral heads of the *triceps* muscle laterally.

- Identify the biceps and the brachialis through blunt dissection and then retract the long head medially and the lateral head laterally. Identify and retract (to protect) the radial nerve proximal to the medial head of the triceps in the spiral groove. Bluntly dissect the medial head of the triceps to expose the fracture site.

- Gentle traction and rotation provided by the SA will allow the surgeon to reduce the fracture and maintain fixation with bone clamp(s). Establish the appropriate plate to facilitate fixation through six cortices above and below the break. A 4.5-mm Dynamic compression plate (DCP) should be used if fixation is on a large bone and a 4.5-mm Locking compression plate (LCP) if the bone is smaller.

- The surgeon's preference will dictate the suture used for fascia, subcutaneous tissue, and skin closure. Along with types of dressings. A sling should be used for support.

Anterolateral Approach

- An incision is made from the proximal deltoid tuberosity to just above the antecubital crease. At the distal aspect of the incision, the lateral antebrachial cutaneous nerve should be identified and protected.

- Use a finger for blunt dissection of the biceps and brachialis. Identify the musculocutaneous nerve under the biceps muscle. Follow the nerve distally to the terminal branch of lateral antebrachial cutaneous and isolate to protect the nerve branch. Dissect the brachialis and the brachioradialis muscles to expose the radial nerve. Isolate the radial nerve so the nerve could be readily observed at any time during the procedure. Expose the fracture between the radial nerve medially and the musculocutaneous nerve laterally.

- Gentle traction and rotation provided by the SA will allow the surgeon to reduce the fracture and maintain fixation with bone clamp(s). Establish the appropriate plate to facilitate fixation through six cortices above and below the break. A 4.5-mm DCP plate should be used if fixation is on a large bone and a 4.5-mm LCP plate if the bone is smaller.

- The surgeon's preference will dictate the suture used for fascia, subcutaneous tissue, and skin closure. Along with types of dressings. A sling should be used for support.

- Intramedullary nailing can be performed either antegrade or retrograde.

Distal Humerus Fractures

A break of the lower distal part of the *humerus* occurs in 30% of all orthopedic fractures, most commonly in young males and elderly females.

Procedural Considerations. First, a fracture of the elbow joint can complicate mobility if not properly repaired. Nonoperatively, cast immobilization can be utilized with nondisplaced fractures.

Operatively, closed reduction and percutaneous pinning (CRPP) for displaced fractures. ORIF for supracondylar and intercondylar/bi-columnar fractures and a total elbow arthroplasty (TEA) for distal bi-columnar fractures in elderly patients.

Positioning and Prepping. Before the patient enters the OR, confirm beanbag or lateral pegboard is available for positioning the patient in an LDP.

Confirm that preop x-rays are available in the room along with the C-arm. The C-arm will be perpendicular to the patient.

Anesthesia. The procedure will be performed with the patient under general anesthesia.

Surgical Procedure

- A direct posterior approach starts with an incision proximal to the olecranon at the midline of the posterior distal humerus. Curve laterally to the tip of the olecranon along the lateral aspect of the olecranon process. Continue to curve medially over the middle posterior aspect of the subcutaneous ulna.

- Fully dissect the ulna nerve and mark it with a vessel loop or a Penrose. Continue to dissect the deep posterior fascia and bluntly split the triceps fascia.

- Lift the triceps muscle from the humerus to expose the olecranon fragment proximately. Further, identify the sensory branch of the radial nerve laterally and follow proximately to identify the complete nerve route. Elevate the anconeus muscle on the lateral side to expose the joint laterally.

- At this point, debridement of clots and debris should be performed. Determine if the entire articular surface is present.

- Use 2.0-mm wires to medial and lateral condyles to hold the fracture in place.

- Place plate over K-wire to enable placement of cortical screws and leave screws loose to allow for adjustments Place two screws proximately, both medially and laterally.

- Replace K-wires with additional two cortical screws.

- Obtain compression of the fracture with the use of two compression screws. Place remaining screws.

- Perform range of motion tests.

- Perform irrigation with copious amounts of normal saline. Release the tourniquet and address any bleeding.

- Close per surgeon's preferences for deep layer, sub-q, and skin.

- Dress with bulky dressing, apply long arm split splint with the arm in extension.

- Sling for comfort.

FOREARM

Olecranon Fractures

Most olecranon fractures are sustained by the usual subjects. High-energy injuries in the young and falls by the elderly (see Figure 19-6).

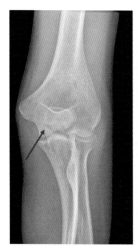
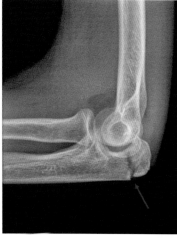

Figure 19-6 · Olecranon fracture. (Reproduced with permission from Hospital for Sick Children, Toronto, Canada, 2018.)

Anatomy. Muscles involved in olecranon fractures are the triceps muscle, that inserts onto the proximal, posterior ulna. The anconeus muscle inserts on the lateral aspect of the olecranon. Both muscles are innervated by the radial nerve. Additional anatomy is in the previous section, Distal Humerus Fractures.

Diagnostic. A fracture of the olecranon is diagnosed by a physical examination along with frontal and lateral view x-rays.

Procedural Considerations. Tension bands and intramedullary fixation are indicated in non-comminuted fractures.

ORIF is indicated with comminuted fractures, fractures with dislocation, and oblique fractures that extend distally to the coronoid.

Radiologic studies need to be performed to determine whether the repair is a simple traverse fracture to be repaired with a tension band technique, or an oblique and communicated fracture to be using plates and screws.

Positioning and Prepping. A supine position is used with the patient moved to the edge of the table and the arm draped over the chest. A lateral position using a beanbag to support the patient could also be used. A tourniquet should be placed and after exsanguination, engage the tourniquet at 200 to 250 mmHg.

Anesthesia. An olecranon fracture may be performed using local with sedation or general anesthesia.

Surgical Procedure

- The surgeon will perform subcutaneous dissection above the fracture and along the margin of the ulna.
- The incision should extend proximately from the ulna, around the olecranon laterally, and along the side of the distal humerus. A Weitlaner retractor should be placed distally and proximately.
- Debride the fracture site.
- Elevate periosteum with key elevator.

- Reduce fracture with the use of K-wire and bone clamps placed both above and below the fracture site while reducing the fracture through the extension of the arm.
- Check alignment of the plate and use lag bolts for any oblique fractures. Triceps should be bluntly dissected proximately to expose the tip of the olecranon.
- Drill pilot with 2.5-bit gauge and screw. Place the first non-locking screw on the proximal ulna. Then use a combination of locking and non-locking screws from the distal humerus to the proximal ulna.
- Obtain x-rays to confirm good alignment.
- Perform irrigation with copious amounts of normal saline.
- Release the tourniquet and address any bleeding or finish closure and then release the tourniquet. Close as per surgeon's preferences for deep layer, subcutaneous, and skin.
- Dress with bulky dressing, apply long arm posterior splint with 70° to 80° flexion of the arm.
- Sling for comfort.

Posterior Approach to the Radius. Identify Lister's tubercle on the dorsal side of the distal radius and the lateral epicondyle as prominent features and locate the fracture via the c-arm. The incision should be over the center of the fracture. Blunt dissection between the Extensor Carpi Radialis brevis (ECRB) and extensor digitorum communis (EDC) and extending proximately will help to expose the posterior interosseous nerve (PIN) within the supinator muscle. This will assist in exposing the radius for plate placement. Pronation of the arm will prevent impingement of PIN.

Posterior Approach to the Ulna. Identify the olecranon and the ulnar head. Make an incision over the fracture and then dissect through the extensor carpi ulnaris (ECU) and flexor carpi ulnaris (FCU) distally and the FCU and anconeus proximally.

Debride the hematoma and fracture fragments on the radius. Use bone clamps at either end of the fractures to approximate the correct alignment. Apply longitudinal traction and rotation to facilitate fixation. Use a bone clamp to provide temporary stabilization until the plate provides permanent stabilization. The same debridement, approximation and temporary stabilization should be provided for the ulna.

Place plate(s) and screw with two bi-cortical screws closest to the fracture first and then place the remaining screws in the plate.

Obtain x-rays to confirm good alignment.

Perform irrigation with copious amounts of normal saline.

Perform closure per surgeon's preferences for deep layer, subcutaneous, and skin, then release the tourniquet.

Dress with bulky dressing, apply sling for comfort.

ORIF Distal Radius

Etiology. An ORIF of the distal radius procedure repairs a fracture of distal radius that can include the articular surface.

These fractures are very common, making up 44% of all hand and wrist emergency room visits in the United States. Distal radial fractures occur across gender and age ranges; however, the mechanism of injury changes as the patient ages. The younger population have distal radial fractures from high-energy trauma. The older population have distal radial fracture more commonly from falls on an outstretched hand.

The direction in which the fracture occurs also determines the type of fracture. A Colle's fracture, first described in 1814 by Dr. Abraham Colles, occurs from an impact of an outstretched hand. The palmar force creates a fracture of the radius that tilts upward. Less common is a Smith fracture, which occurs from a fall or impact to a bent wrist. In 1847, Dr. Robert Smith described this distal radius fracture variation where the radius tilts downward. The surgical repair is the same for both fracture variation; however, the reduction technique is modified based on the direction of the radius.

Anatomy. The distal radius is one of the bones that create the wrist joint along with the scaphoid and lunate carpal bones. The distal radius as a lateral projection called the styloid process and a notch that the ulna articulates with. Ligaments connect these bones together to form the wrist joint. The palmar radiocarpal ligament attaches the distal radius to multiple carpal bones and the radial collateral ligament connects the radial styloid process to the scaphoid. Multiple tendons of the forearm muscle travel along the forearm to connect to the wrist and hand. Superficially, the muscles of the anterior forearm are the FCU, palmaris longus, and FCR. Below these muscles is the Flexor digitorum superficialis Extensor Carpi Radialis brevis (ECRB) muscle. In the deep anterior compartment, the flexor pollicis longus, flexor digitorum profundus, and pronator quadratus muscles are located. The ulnar artery and nerve run deep along the ulna and branches into the hand. The radial artery is located superficially running along the radius and is at risk from injury during this procedure. The median nerve runs medially between the flexor digitorum profundus and FDS muscles and transverses the wrist through the carpal tunnel.

Anesthesia. The procedure is performed under general anesthesia.

Positioning, Prepping, and Draping. The patient is placed supine on the OR table with the operative arm outstretched on floating hand table. A floating hand table is recommended since it does not have a leg that interferes with C-arm positioning. General anesthesia is primarily used; however, an axillary nerve block can be utilized for intraoperative regional anesthesia and/or postoperative pain relief. After induction, the OR bed is turned 90° away from anesthesia, with the operative arm outward. The tourniquet is now placed high on the patient's arm and set to 250 mmHG.

Once positioning is completed, the surgeon may want to take initial x-rays prior to prepping. This is to test the reduction of the fracture and ensure that the operative plan is still appropriate. Once the surgeon is satisfied, the operative arm is prepped circumferentially with an alcohol-based prep solution from fingers to tourniquet. After the surgical prep is completed, the surgical team is now able to sterilely drape the operative arm. A sterile large drape is laid on top of the hand table underneath the raised operative arm. A sterile blue towel is placed securely around the operative arm at the base of the tourniquet. A towel clip is used to secure the ends of the blue towel together. Next, a sterile impervious stockinette is placed over the hand. This is utilized only during the draping procedure to cover the fingers of the patient. Most surgeons will remove the stockinette when finished draping to have access to the thumb for pulling traction. Next, an upper extremity drape placed on the patient. The hole of the extremity drape is passed over the hand up to the operative arm's elbow. A rolled towel is placed in the dorsum of the hand to mimic a fist, then the operative arm is exsanguinated with an Esmarch®. After exsanguination, the tourniquet is inflated.

Surgical Procedure

- Once the tourniquet is inflated, the open reduction and internal fixation of the distal radius begins. A sterile hand immobilizer may be used to keep the patient's wrist in the pronated supinated position on the hand table; however, some surgeons may choose to have their SA hold the hand in the correct position.

- A linear skin incision is made down the radial border of the FCR tendon.

- The SA retracts the tendon toward the ulna with a Senn retractor, which allows the surgeon to continue the dissection downward toward the radius.

- The radial artery needs to be identified and protected with a Senn retractor during the tissue dissection.

- The median nerve should also be identified and protected if near the incision site. The surgeon may also utilize two dull Weitlaner retractors as the dissection continues deeper.

- The flexor pollicis longus muscle is retracted medially to expose the pronator quadratus muscle. The pronator quadratus muscle is incised leaving a small cuff to repair the muscle attachment later.

- The muscle is dissected off the radius and the Weitlaner retractor is adjusted to hold the muscle belly away. The distal radial fracture is now exposed.

- With the distal radius exposed, the fracture site is cleared of debris and clots to allow for appropriate reduction.

- Traction is applied by holding the hand and pulling longitudinally away from the patient's body while holding the arm above the wrist in place.

- While the SA holds the traction, K-wires are placed across the fracture fragments to hold the fracture reduction. One K-wire is passed through the radial styloid into the radial cortex beyond the fracture. An addition K-wire may be placed perpendicularly to the first K-wires to hold any other large fracture pieces in place.

- Intraoperative fluoroscopy is utilized to ensure accurate reduction with the K-wires before proceeding with the plate and screw process.

- The plating system for a distal radial fracture has a shaft with locking and compression screw holes, as well as a wider distal end that is anatomically like the distal radius.

- The distal end of the plate only has locking screw holes since distal radial fractures tend to be more comminuted and difficult to compress so close to the wrist joint. It is important that the plate sits as high on the distal radius as possible without it or the screws interfering with the joint surface.

- On the proximal side of the plate, a 1.8-mm drill bit is used to drill a compression screw hole in the oblong hole. The oblong hole allows the plate to slide and compress the plate to the bone farther.

- A depth gauge measures the needed length of 2.4-mm cortical screw, and the screw is now screwed into the compression hole.

- A power screwdriver is utilized first then a hand screwdriver is used to hand tighten the screw. If more compression is needed, a second cortical screw can be inserted into a different plate hole.

- Intraoperative fluoroscopy checks the reduction of the fracture and placement of the plate.

- After the cortical screw is placed in the shaft, the distal locking screws are placed. Utilizing a threaded drill guide, a 1.8-mm drill bit creates the holes. The number of locking holes utilized in the distal end depend on the fracture pattern since you cannot place a screw into unstable bone.

- Care also is taken not to drill into the articular surface of the distal radius. A depth gauge is now used to measure the length of screw needed, and a 2.4-mm locking screw is inserted into the threaded hole.

- A power screwdriver with a torque limiter is used for the screw insertion. All holes that a screw is usable in are utilized in the distal end of the plate. The K-wires can be removed after at least three proximal locking screws are placed.

- Intraoperative fluoroscopy confirms the articular surface has not been breached by any of the screws and that the fracture reduction is still intact.

- Finally, the proximal locking screws are inserted into the shaft of the plate. A 1.8-mm drill bit creates the hole then a depth gauge measures the needed length.

- Using a power screwdriver with a torque limiter, the locking screw is inserted. At least two locking screws are inserted into the plate depending on the length of plate utilized.

- Final intraoperative x-rays are taken to confirm the appropriate placement of all screws and that fracture reduction is intact before closure begins.

- To cover the plate, the pronator quadratus muscle is reattached to the radius using a 2-0 absorbable braided suture.

- Reattachment is sometimes not possible due to the muscle being too small. The patient will not experience any loss of function if the pronator quadratus is not reattached.

- Placing as many tissue layers as possible between the plate and the outside incision is important to slow any potential infection spread to the plate.

- The dermis is closed with a 3-0 absorbable braided suture and the skin is closed with an intracuticular 4-0 absorbable monofilament suture.

Dressings. After final closure, the dressings are placed on the incision. Dermabond® is used to seal the incision and given time to dry. A 4 × 4 gauze is placed over the incision and a 4-inch cotton roll is used from hand to elbow. A volar plaster splint stabilizes the wrist until the incision heals, and a 3-inch ace is wrapped from hand to elbow to hold the splint in place. Some surgeons will choose to use a carpal tunnel splint instead of creating a plaster splint.

Postop Complications. The most common complication following ORIF of a distal radial fracture is malunion. To prevent extensive loss of wrist range of motion, revision surgery to correct the malunion is essential. Usually, an external fixator will be placed to correct the malunion. Surgeons will monitor the patient for infection with patient's more at risk for infection when a K-wire is left through the skin to be removed later.

Transposition of Nerve

The second most common peripheral nerve entrapment is the cubital tunnel syndrome. It is often the cause of pain and disability for many. There are conservative and operative options for treatment once it is correctly diagnosed.

Anatomy. The cubital tunnel is established by the cubital tunnel retinaculum. It spans across a gap of about 4 mm between the medial epicondyle and the olecranon. The floor of the tunnel is created by the capsule and posterior band of the medial collateral ligament of the elbow joint and contains the ulnar nerve among other structures. The ulnar nerve is the terminal branch of the medial cord of the brachial plexus. It descends the arm anterior to the medial intermuscular septum and later penetrates the septum at the terminal third of its length. The ulnar nerve progresses under the septum and next to the triceps muscle and crosses the cubital tunnel to enter the forearm where it passes between the two heads of the FCU muscle.

Etiology. The precise cause of cubital tunnel syndrome is unknown. However, there are several instances excessive pressure is applied to the ulnar nerve:

- The ulnar nerve frequently slides back and forth from the medial epicondyle, triggering irritation

- Pressure applied on the elbow for long periods of time

- Inflammation on the elbow joint

- Bumping your "funny bone" inside of your elbow, that produces an electric shock sensation and loss of feeling in your little and ring fingers

- Prior fracture or dislocations of the elbow

- Bone spurs/arthritis of the elbow

- Cysts close to the elbow joint
- Repetition in movements while the elbow is bent or flexed

Symptoms. The symptoms of cubital tunnel syndrome can resemble other conditions such as medial epicondylitis.

- Numbness and tingling in the hand and/or ring and little finger, especially when the elbow is bent
- Hand pain
- Weak grip and clumsiness due to muscle weakness in the affected arm and hand
- Aching pain on the inside of the elbow

Diagnostics. The physician will do a complete history and physical examination along with several tests:

- **Nerve conduction test.** A test that demonstrates how fast signals travel down a nerve to find a compression or constriction of the nerve.
- **Electromyogram (EMG).** An EMG will test the forearm muscles controlled by the ulnar nerve. If the muscles are not working correctly, it may be a sign that there is trouble with the ulnar nerve.
- **X-ray.** An x-ray will rule out arthritis or bone spurs in your elbow.

Nonsurgical Treatments

- **Rest.** Avoid actions where the elbow is bent for prolonged periods of time. Keep the elbow straight and do not apply pressure to it.
- **NSAIDs.** Nonsteroidal anti-inflammatory drug (NSAIDs) will help diminish swelling around the nerve.
- **Braces or splints.** A padded brace or splint will keep your elbow in a straight position at night.
- **Physical therapy.** Nerve gliding exercises help the ulnar nerve slide through the cubital tunnel at the elbow and the Guyon's canal at the wrist, which can help with symptoms and also reduce stiffness in the arm and wrist.

Surgical Treatment

- **Ulnar Nerve Anterior Transposition.** This procedure is indicated when the nerve has slid out from behind the bony ridge of the medical epicondyle. The nerve is moved to one of three positions: on top of the muscle (subcutaneous transposition), within the muscle (intramuscular transposition), or under the muscle (submuscular transposition).
- **Cubital Tunnel Release.** The cubital tunnel is opened to release the pressure the nerve because the nerve does not slide out of position when the elbow is bent. As the tunnel heals, new tissue will grow making the tunnel larger.
- **Medial Epicondylectomy.** This procedure eliminates part of the medial epicondyle. It facilitates the release of the nerve when the elbow is bent.

Anesthesia. This procedure is accomplished under general or regional anesthesia using a sterile tourniquet.

Patient Position and Prep. The patient is positioned supine with affected arm placed on a hand table externally rotated and flexed slightly so that the posteromedial aspect of the elbow is exposed. A tourniquet is placed prior to the prep. The arm is prepped circumferentially from the axillary to the wrist. The medical epicondyle is palpated to locate the ulnar nerve. The location of the ulnar nerve posterior to the medial epicondyle is marked extending 6 to 10 cm in both proximal and distal directions with a skin marker.

Surgical Procedure

Ulnar Nerve Transposition

- The tourniquet is inflated, and a 10- to 12-cm incision is made on the lateral aspect of the elbow near the epicondyle.
- The SA provides visualization with retractors.
- The fascia and FCU muscle are divided.
- The ulnar nerve is freed, and the medial intermuscular septum is dissected.
- The nerve is pulled anteriorly and placed deep into the brachialis flexor muscle origin.
- A fascial flap is created from the superficial fascia of the medial epicondyle muscles to prevent nerve slippage.
- The flexion and extension of the elbow is checked to verify that the nerve is released and no new deformity at the flap had been created.
- The SA will irrigate the wound.
- The subcutaneous layer is closed with 3-0 absorbable suture.
- The SA will close skin with 3-0 Ethilon interrupted suture.

Postop. A plaster cast or splint is applied to the elbow in a 90° angle. This position is maintained for a period of 2 to 4 weeks. This allows the skin incision to heal and the ulnar nerve to get used to the new location.

HIP

Anatomy

The hip joint consists of a ball and socket joint, where the ball is the femoral head, and the socket is the acetabulum of the pelvis (see figure 19-7). The femoral head is attached to the femoral shaft by the femoral neck. The acetabulum has a fibrocartilaginous extension called the labrum. The labrum attaches to edge of the acetabulum and provides joint stability and lubrication. The acetabulum and femur are held together by multiple capsular ligaments. The iliofemoral ligament is located anteriorly from just below the anterior inferior iliac spine to the femur. The pubofemoral ligament is located anteroinferior to the hip joint. It attaches from the iliopubic prominence and obturator membrane to the femur. The ischiofemoral ligament attaches posteriorly from the ischium to the base of the greater trochanter. The ligamentum teres is located intracapsular and attaches the femoral head to the acetabulum. This ligament contains the foveal artery which is the vascular supply

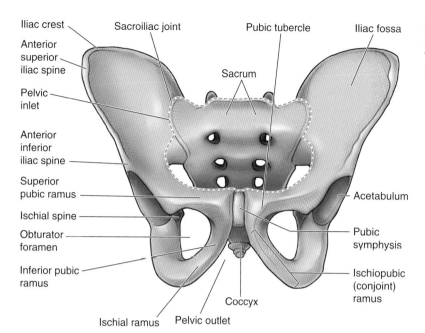

Iliac crest
Anterior superior iliac spine
Pelvic inlet
Anterior inferior iliac spine
Superior pubic ramus
Ischial spine
Obturator foramen
Inferior pubic ramus
Ischial ramus
Pelvic outlet
Coccyx
Sacroiliac joint
Pubic tubercle
Sacrum
Iliac fossa
Acetabulum
Pubic symphysis
Ischiopubic (conjoint) ramus

Figure 19-7 · Hip anatomy. (Reproduced, with permission, from Morton DA, Foreman KB, Albertine KH. The Big Picture: Gross Anatomy. 2nd ed. New York, NY: McGraw Hill; 2019.)

to the femoral head and injuries to this ligament may lead to avascular necrosis of the femoral head. The hip joint is also supplied by the medial and lateral circumflex femoral arteries which are branches for the profunda femoris artery. Considering the hip joint is responsible for numerous actions of the lower limb, there are many muscle groups associated with this joint. The hip flexor muscles located anteriorly are the psaos major and minor, the iliacus, and the pectineus and rectus femoris muscle. Posteriorly, the extensor muscles are the gluteus maximus, semitendinosus, semimembranosus, and biceps femoris muscles. Medially are the hip adductor muscles, adductor magnus, adductor longus, adductor brevis, gracilis, and pectineus muscles. Laterally, the gluteus medius and tensor fascia latae muscles are responsible for abduction of the hip joint. The deep hip internal rotator muscles are the tensor fascia latae and gluteus minimus muscles. Lastly, the external rotators of the hip joint are the gemellus superior and inferior, Obturator externus and internus, quadratus femoris and piriformis muscles. The piriformis muscle tendon is an important landmark to locate the hip joint during a total hip arthroplasty. The nerves responsible of innervating the muscles of the hip joint include the femoral, obturator and superior gluteal nerves. The sciatic nerve runs posteriorly to the hip joint and needs to be identified and protected during the procedure.

Total Hip Arthroplasty

The idea of replacing the hip joint began in the last 1800s and continued to evolve well into the mid-1900s. Sir John Charnley is seen as the father of the modern total hip arthroplasty with his low friction arthroplasty design. His design that he developed in the early 1960s consisted of a metal femoral stem, a polyethylene acetabular component and bone cement. While many variations have been developed over the last 50 years, Charnley's design is embraced in all total hip arthroplasties. Total hip arthroplasty is considered one of the most successful

orthopedic procedures with over 450,000 procedures performed in the United States each year.

The implant options for total hip arthroplasty vary by manufacturing company; however, there are four types of total hip arthroplasty devices that are available in the United States. The most common option is the metal on polyethylene type. With this type, the acetabular component is metal but has a polyethylene liner, and the femoral stem and head components are metal. The ceramic on polyethylene device option has a metal acetabular component with a polyethylene liner, but the femoral head component is ceramic. There is also the option of ceramic on ceramic as well as ceramic on metal, where the acetabulum component is metal, and the femoral head component is ceramic. The surgeon's preference will dictate which device option and manufacturer is used for the total hip arthroplasty. A manufacturer representative is available for every procedure to ensure a successful case with their device. With these devices, the surgeons have options about how to fixate the implants to the bone. Commonly, the implants are cemented in using a methyl methacrylate cement, which allows the implant to adhere better to the raw boney surface. Cementless also known as press fit techniques have been developed to replace using bone cement. The surface of these implants has a special coating that allows for bone ingrowth allowing for the purchase to the raw boney surface.

Etiology. A patient qualifies for a total hip arthroplasty due to severe hip joint pain that is not treatable with less invasive procedures. The most common cause of hip joint pain is arthritis, caused from either osteoarthritis, rheumatoid arthritis, or posttraumatic arthritis. Occasionally, a patient may develop avascular necrosis of the femoral head due to a hip injury. The injury decreases the blood flow to the femoral head which results in the surface of the bone to breakdown. Also, congenital hip defects may cause an increased chance of arthritis and patients will need hip replacements at a younger age. Proximal femoral shaft and neck fracture may also require a hip replacement to repair the fracture. This could mean a total hip replacement or just a partial hip replacement, where just the femoral head and neck are replaced.

Anesthesia. General anesthesia is the most common method of anesthesia used for a total hip arthroplasty. The surgeons may also choose spinal anesthesia for their patients instead of general anesthesia. Spinal blocks decrease the patient's postoperative nausea and vomiting as well as the time to discharge from the post-anesthesia care unit. All in all, the goal is to have a smooth transition from the OR to rehabilitation for an optimal patient outcome. The surgeon's preference also dictates whether a patient receives a Foley catheter. Length of surgery as well as if a patient has a spinal block are determining factors for the need of a Foley catheter. Not placing a Foley catheter is becoming more common to decrease the risk of catheter-associated urinary tract infections and increase ambulation postoperatively.

Positioning, Prepping, and Draping. Given the complexity of the hip joint, surgeons have developed multiple approaches to the total hip arthroplasty. One approach is the posterior approach, where the patient is placed in the LDP. The patient is held in the LDP with either a beanbag, pegboard, or a Wilson frame. The key is to choose lateral positioners that will keep the patient's hip stable during the procedure. Like the posterior approach, the direct lateral approach can be performed lateral or supine position and it access the hip joint through dissecting the gluteus medius muscle. Finally, the direct anterior approach is performed in the supine position while the patient is placed on a specialized traction bed, such as a Hanna table. The patient may also be on a standard OR bed; however, the specialized traction bed is preferred by most surgeons. Exposure is more difficult with this approach; however, due to the decreased dislocation risk, it has become increasingly popular with the surgeons.

Posterior Approach. For the posterior approach, the patient is placed on the OR bed in the supine position with the surgeon's preferred lateral positioners in place. After anesthesia induction, the patient is placed in the lateral position, and care is taken to protect the lower arm's brachial plexus with an axillary roll and pad the nonoperative lower leg. The operative leg is prepped circumferentially from the toes to the anterior superior iliac spine (ASIS). A team member will hold the operative leg in the air while the sterile team begins to sterilely drape the patient. A large drape is placed over the nonoperative leg covering the end of the OR bed. Next, four sterile blue towels are placed at the base of the hip, at the ASIS, at the midline covering the genitalia, and above the natal cleft. Towel clips or staples are used to hold the towels in place. An impervious split sheet is placed at the ASIS and is wrapped medially along the edge of the genitalia and laterally above the natal cleft. A second impervious split sheet is placed under the raised operative leg at the base of the hip and wrapped along the same regions as the first split sheet. An impervious stockinette is placed over the toes and unwrapped to the tibial tuberosity.

A Coban is used to secure the stockinette to the leg. The second assistant or surgical technologist will continue to hold the leg up, so the final layer of drapes can be placed. A reinforced split sheet is placed under the operative leg at the base of the hip and the limbs extended along the edge of the genitalia and just above the natal cleft. At the ASIS, an orthopedic bar drape or a reinforced split sheet is used to cover the distal portion of the sterile field. An isolation drape impregnated with iodine or plain is used to cover the exposed skin after the draping is completed.

Surgical Procedure

- After the sterile field is established, an incision is made with a 10 blade with the greater trochanter as the midpoint. From the greater trochanter, the incision extends no more than 5 cm proximally and distally.

- Surgeons may choose to decrease the size of the incision to help postoperative healing; however, that does limit the exposure of the hip joint.

- Once the skin and subcutaneous tissue is dissected, an incision is made in the tensor fasciae latae and a Charnley retractor is placed to provide exposure.

- Dissection continues through the tissue to locate the short external rotators of the hip.

- The SA slowly internally rotates the hip by lifting the foot and dropping the knee to expose the posterior portion of the hip joint.

- The short external rotator muscle tendons are tagged with a size zero braided absorbable suture then excised to expose the hip joint.

- A hemostat is placed on the end of the suture and hung under the Charnley retractor. This allows for easy identification of the tendons later for repairing.

- A capsulectomy is performed to expose the femoral head and acetabulum.

- With the bony structures of the hip exposed, the SA is now able to dislocate the femoral head either anteriorly or posteriorly. For an anterior dislocation, the femoral head is placed under traction with the knee flexed and abducted. Then the femoral head is externally rotated away from the acetabulum. An anterior dislocation requires an additional sterile bag drape to be attached to the edge of the OR bed for the foot to be placed in.

- For a posterior dislocation the femoral head is placed under traction with the knee flexed and adducted. Next, the femoral head is internally rotated away from the acetabulum. This leaves the foot in the upward direction, so care must be taken to not contaminate it with your head. Using a sterile hood during a total hip arthroplasty is highly recommended.

- The SA will need to stabilize the leg throughout the procedure.

- Since the femoral head and neck are now exposed, a femoral neck osteotomy is performed to remove the femoral head.

- A large oscillating saw blade is used to complete the osteotomy, and the SA uses Bennett retractors or Hohmann retractors to protect the soft tissue around the femoral neck while the osteotomy is performed. Without the femoral head, the acetabulum is readily accessible for reaming.

- The SA will use a combination of Cobra retractors, Bennett retractors, and Hibbs retractors around the acetabulum for exposure and protecting soft tissue during the reaming process. Be aware of the sciatic nerve when retracting posteriorly.

- The acetabulum is reamed until all the cartilaginous surface of the acetabulum is removed then a trial prosthesis is placed into the reamed acetabulum. Next, the femoral canal is prepared for reaming.

- The SA places the leg centrally on their abdomen to provide support during the reaming process as well as pushing the knee forward which places the femur into a better position for reaming.

- A Cobra retractor is placed also under the end of the femur to lift the femur out of incision for better exposure. The femoral canal is reamed to the appropriate size based on the canal's diameter.

- While the surgeon reams the canal, the SA must maintain exposure and stability of the operative leg. A trial femoral stem component as well as femoral head is placed, and the hip is reduced.

- To reduce the hip, the SA places traction on leg then completes the opposite rotation from the dislocation. Once the hip is reduced, the surgeon completes range of motion exercises to test the functionality and stability of the trial components.

- Any changes that need to be made to the type and sizing of the components are decided at this point.

- When the surgeon is satisfied with the size and type of component choices, the hip is dislocated again.

- All the trial components are removed, and the surgical site is flushed with pulse lavage.

- The manufacturing company's representative will confirm the permanent implant size with the surgeon and the circulating nurse will open implants onto the field.

- If the surgeon chooses to cement fixate the femoral stem, then cement will be mixed at this time.

- The permanent acetabular components are placed first, so the SA needs to place the Cobra retractors and Bennett retractors again to fully expose the acetabulum. Depending on the manufacturer of the implant, the acetabular component is either press fitted or attached via screws.

- Next, the femoral stem component is placed, and the SA must repeat the same exposure as before of the femur. The femoral stem can be press fit or cemented in. The femoral stem has a peg at the end that allows the femoral head to be snapped on, so the replaced joint will still have the same ball and socket joint functionality.

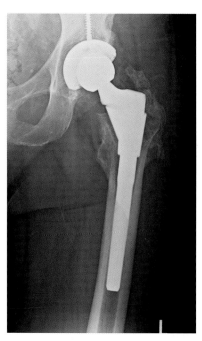

Figure 19-8 ∙ Hip replacement. (Reproduced, with permission, from McMahon PJ, Skinner HB. *Current Diagnosis & Treatment in Orthopedics*. 6th ed. New York, NY: McGraw Hill; 2021.)

- After the final prosthesis is placed, the hip is reduced as the cement is given time to fully harden (see Figure 19-8).

- Any excess cement is removed at this time to prevent loose bodies in the joint space. Another round of pulse lavage irrigation is used to aide in the removal of errant bacteria and debris, then closure can begin.

- The tagged short external rotator muscle tendons are reattached to the hip joint using a size zero braided absorbable or nonabsorbable suture.

- The tensor fasciae latae is closed using a number one absorbable suture, utilizing either interrupted sutures or running a barbed suture.

- If the subcutaneous layers are thick, then a few interrupted absorbable sutures are used to assist in closing the dead space.

- The dermis is then closed with a 2-0 absorbable suture, either utilizing interrupted sutures or running a barbed suture.

- Skin is closed with either staples or a buried running 3-0 absorbable barbed suture.

Direct Anterior Approach.   For the direct anterior approach, the patient is positioned on a specialized traction OR bed with both feet secured into the boots attached to the lever arms. The traction placed on the operative leg allows for additional retraction of the femur and dislocation of the femoral head. The operative leg is prepped from mid abdomen to the top of the boot with an alcohol based surgical solution. After the appropriate dry time, four sterile blue towels are placed around the surgical site. One blue towel just above the ASIS, and one blue towel placed at the knee. Another blue towel placed over the perineal post, and the last blue towel is placed lateral at the edge of gluteus maximus. A stapler is used to hold the towels in place. Two split sheet drapes are used to complete the sterile field by following the borders created by the blue towels. An incise drape that is either impregnated with iodine or plain is placed over the entirety of the surgical site.

Surgical Procedure

- The incision for the direct anterior approach is approximately 10 cm long and runs lateral to the ASIS distally on the anterior thigh.
- The tensor fascia latea is then incised, but care is taken to protect the lateral femoral cutaneous nerve.
- The nerve is dissected and moved medially with a Charnley retractor holding it and the subcutaneous tissue back.
- The surgeon will continue to dissect toward the plain between the rectus femoris and gluteus medius. Once that plain is developed, the Charnley retractor is moved deeper to adequately expose the anterior hip joint.
- A capsulectomy is performed to expose the acetabulum and femoral neck.
- Slight traction is placed on the operative leg to pull the femoral head slightly away from acctabulum. Hohmann retractors or Mueller retractors are placed around the femoral neck to protect the soft tissue during the femoral neck osteotomy.
- After the osteotomy is completed, the femoral head is removed from acetabulum using a corkscrew. Traction is now released from the operative leg.
- To access the acetabulum, the operative leg is externally rotated using the lever arms of the traction bed.
- The acetabulum is reamed to the depth required to remove all cartilaginous surface. Because exposure is limited due to the incision location, intraoperative fluoroscopy is utilized to ensure the appropriate angle of reaming.
- The SA is continuing to retract the soft tissue away from the acetabulum for protection and exposure.
- The trial acetabular component is placed then the femoral preparation can begin. Much like the acetabulum, exposure of the proximal femur is difficult so a sterile bone hook that is attached to the OR bed is inserted on the posterior side of the femur.
- The bone hook is controlled by a foot pedal attached to the OR bed and the hook can lift the proximal femur anteriorly.
- Along with utilizing the lever arms to place the operative leg in extension, adduction and external rotation, the proximal femur becomes adequately exposed for reaming.
- The SA will use Hohmann retractors to protect the soft tissue during the reaming process. A trial femoral stem and femoral head prosthesis is placed, and the hip is reduced utilizing the lever arms.
- With all traction released, the surgeon can complete the range of motion exercises to check the stability and functionality of the hip joint.

- If the surgeon is satisfied, the hip is dislocated, the trial prostheses are removed, and the permanent acetabular and femoral components are implanted. The permanent components can be press-fit or cemented onto the bone.
- The lever arms are used to reduce the hip and intraoperative fluoroscopy can also be used to check for appropriate positioning of the implants.
- If cement is used, it is vital that all excess cement is removed to prevent irritation of the hip joint.
- After the implants are set, pulse lavage is used to wash out the surgical site and wound closure can begin.
- The tensor fasciae latae is closed using a number one absorbable suture, utilizing either interrupted sutures or running a barbed suture.
- If the subcutaneous layers are thick, then a few interrupted absorbable sutures are used to assist in closing the dead space.
- The dermis is then closed with a 2-0 absorbable suture, either utilizing interrupted sutures or running a barbed suture.
- Skin is closed with either staples or a buried running 3-0 absorbable barbed suture.

Dressings. Dressings vary by surgeon's preference, but more surgeons are using dressings that seal the incision to prevent microbial contamination. For a suture closure, Prineo® is used to seal the incision for up to 6 weeks. If staples are used, then a nonadherent dressing like Telfa® is used to cover the incision. Next, 4 × 4 gauze and/or abdominal pads cover the incision, and a cloth surgical tape is used to secure the dressings. Another common option is to use an Opsite Post-op Visible® or Aquacel® AG surgical dressing to cover the incision. These dressings are not removed for multiple days and have antimicrobial properties to help prevent surgical site infections. The surgeon may choose to use an abduction pillow to prevent the patient from dislocating their hip directly following surgery.

Postop Complications. Following total hip arthroplasty, the patient is monitored for deep vein thrombosis and the goal is to being physical therapy by day two of surgery. Early ambulation helps prevent deep vein thrombosis and helps speed recovery. Risk of dislocation is high with the posterior approach due to the incision and repair of the short external rotator muscles; however, the direct anterior approach also has a dislocation risk. Dislocation of the total hip requires additional surgeries to reduce the hip joint with the potential needs for revision surgery if dislocation continuously happens. Nerve injury is another complication following a total hip arthroplasty. The superior gluteal, femoral, and sciatic nerves are all at risk from aggressive retraction of the soft tissue, leg lengthening or component placement.

Revisions

The are several reasons that revision surgery would not involve the hip components. A revision arthroplasty for wound closure, psoas release, heterotopic bone excision, and periprosthetic fracture.

Revisions affecting modular components could be for a poly (polyethylene) exchange or a titanium sleeve. A nonmodular component would be an acetabular exchange. This would be the most common reason for a revision. Sometimes both components are replaced with new components, an antibiotic spacer(s) or a girdlestone is performed.

Diagnostics. AP pelvis radiographs along with full-length femur x-rays.

Revision Synopsis

Closing is per the surgeon's preference, but #5 Ethibond is often used for the capsule, #1 PDS to reinforce the capsule and approximate the adipose tissue, and #2 PDS for interrupted subcuticular stitches. Depending on the condition of the patient's skin, we can use staples or #2-0 nylon interrupted suture. The dressing is Xeroform, sponges, ABD, and Medipore tape. An abduction pillow is a must since patients are not compliant.

A revision hip arthroplasty can be as simple as a poly swap or as difficult as removing failed components and placing antibiotic spacers. If you are replacing components, the old components need to be removed and the acetabulum or the femoral canal must be re-prepped. Take out the component, clean the cement out with a Moreland set. The set has some big curettes, pituitary forceps, and various types of osteotomes to scrape old cement out, especially if there is infection. More times than not, a Midas Rex with an AM-1 bit is used to debride the cement from the intramedullary walls, without putting a hole in the bone. Broach again because the canal is wider. Trial the head and stem and then cement in the real thing. Close in the usual fashion but sometimes the repairs need modifications to cover some bone or hardware, so the patient is not coming in next week for additional skin closure.

Congenital Hip Dislocation

Congenital hip disorders (CHDs) arise when a child is born with or suddenly develops an abnormality in the hip joint. Developmental dysplasia of the hip (DDH) and congenital dislocation of the hip (CDH) are the most common CHDs. In hip dislocation, the ball is not located in the socket, and that distinguishes it from DDH (see Figure 19-9).

Symptoms. Symptoms vary depending on the type and severity of the disorder, but may include:

- Legs that turn outward or appear to be different leg lengths
- Limited, excessive, or abnormal range of motion of the hips
- Delayed gross motor development

Diagnosis. The most common way to diagnose CHD is through a physical exam. The physician will maneuver the patient's hips and legs while listening for clicking or clunking sounds that may suggest a dislocation.

The exam includes two tests: the Ortolani test where the physician will apply upward force while they abduct the hip and the Barlow test where the physician applies downward force while moving the hip in adduction.

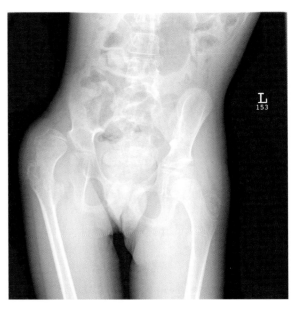

Figure 19-9 · Congenital hip displacement. (Reproduced, with permission, from Maitin IB, ed. *Current Diagnosis & Treatment Physical Medicine & Rehabilitation.* New York, NY: McGraw Hill; 2015.)

Treatment. If a child is less than 6 months of age and diagnosed with CHD, they will be fitted for a Pavlik harness. The harness presses their hip joints into the sockets. It abducts the hip bones by securing their legs in a froglike position. The harness is worn for 6 to 12 weeks depending on the severity of the diagnosis.

If the harness is unsuccessful, there are several options for surgical treatment. The surgeon may perform a closed reduction, or a tendon lengthening procedure and physically position the hips through an open reduction. After an open reduction, the patient's hips and legs will remain in a cast for at least 12 weeks. If the patient is 18 months or older and treatment has been unsuccessful, the surgeon may perform femoral or pelvic osteotomies to reconstruct the hip.

LOWER EXTREMITY

Pelvic Ring Fractures

The mechanism of injury is typically high-energy blunt trauma as in motor vehicle accident (MVA) or as vehicle versus pedestrian. Mortality for closed fractures is as high as 15% and 50/50 survival rate for open fractures. Hemorrhage is the leading cause of death. Increased comorbidities are age >60 years, increased Trauma Score, need for more than four transfusions, and an APC III score. That is an anterior-posterior compression (APC) injury with a disruption of the anterior and posterior SI ligaments. This creates a substantial vascular injury.

Other orthopedic injuries could include chest injury (63%), long bone fractures (50%), and spinal fractures (25%). Other surgical specialties such as urology, general, and neurology would be simultaneously involved with this type of patient.

Anatomy. The ring structure (or pelvic girdle) is comprised of the sacrum and two innominate (Latin, nameless or not named bones). The innominate bones consist of three bones: ischium, pubis, and ilium. The innominate bones fuse into the acetabulum.

There is a multifaceted group of ligaments that provide stability to the pelvic ring. These ligaments resist external rotation, flexion, AP translation. and cephalad-caudad displacement. The strongest ligaments in the body are the posterior sacroiliac complex.

Vascularly, the common iliac system begins near the L_4 bifurcation of the abdominal aorta. The venous plexus in the posterior pelvis accounts for 90% of the hemorrhage damage with this type of trauma.

Procedural Considerations. Open fracture principles dictate the following trauma management steps for this type of injury: (1) initial evaluation; (2) exclusion of life-threatening injuries; (3) prevent infection; (4) healing of the fracture; and (5) restoration of function. The use of a pelvic binder is the usual initial trauma management step. But a binder can sometimes mask injuries by creating erroneous false-negative x-rays and poor CT images. External fixation can help to alleviate negative outcomes due to ongoing blood loss. If the injuries include an external rotation component, the case supersedes an emergent laparotomy.

Inform the following specialties: urology for possible posterior urethral tear and bladder rupture; have an available suprapubic catheter for placement; general surgery for abdominal issues; and neurology for spinal cord or head trauma.

Diagnostics. Injuries are evaluated by a physical exam, x-rays to evaluate the severity of the broken pelvic bone and a CT to aid in a treatment plan and surgical approach.

Treatment Options. Any pelvic binding should be centered over the greater trochanters to effect indirection reduction.

External fixation works by decreasing pelvic volume. A single pin, bilaterally in the column of the supracetabular bone from the anterior inferior iliac spine (AIIS) toward the posterior superior iliac spine (PSIS), could provide stabilization. Multiple half pins in the superior iliac crest have also been employed as an external fixation method.

Anterior ring stabilization can be obtained via a single superior plate. The surgical approach would be through a Pfannenstiel incision and can be performed with any laparotomy or genitourinary (GU) procedures. Posterior ring stabilization can be accomplished with anterior sacroiliac (SI) plating.

KNEE

Knee Arthroscopy

Anatomy. The knee joint is part of the lower extremity. It is the connection of the thigh and the leg and is considered a hinge joint. Three bones that come together at the knee joint include the tibia, femur, and the patella. The fibula is located next to the tibia and knee joint. The tibia, femur, and patella are all covered with a smooth layer of cartilage where they contact each other at the knee joint. A sesamoid bone, the fabella sits behind the knee joint. Articular cartilage is the smooth lining that covers the end of the bones. The meniscus sits between the femur and tibia and acts as a shock absorber. There are four major ligaments that connect the bones: anterior cruciate and posterior cruciate ligaments in the center of the joint and they cross each other. The medial ligament resides on the inner side and the lateral collateral ligament on the outer side of the knee joint. The quadriceps muscle group provides strength with knee extension. The hamstring muscles allow for strength in flexion. The patellar tendon that resides on the front of the knee is part of the quadriceps structure. The synovium lines the joint space and produces synovial fluid within the joint. A bursa resides in front of the knee and underneath the skin.

Etiology

- Loose bone fragments
- Damaged or torn cartilage
- Inflamed joint linings
- Torn ligaments
- Scarring within joints

Indications for Knee Arthroscopy

- Diagnose injuries
- Repair injured soft tissues and bones
- Remove damaged or inflamed tissue

Patient Position and Prep. The patient is placed on the OR bed in a supine position. A tourniquet is placed over cotton webbing on the operative leg. The nonoperative leg is placed in a cushioned leg holder. The operative leg may be placed in a circumferential leg holder, or the leg is positioned approximately 5 cm superior to the proximal patella using a lateral post. The leg is prepped from mid-thigh to mid-ankle. The foot of the table is lowered.

Surgical draping for a knee arthroscopy is completed in layers. An impervious stockinette is placed over the leg and secured with Coban. An impervious split drape is placed around the leg distal to the tourniquet. A second split drape may be placed around the leg in an opposite fashion. An arthroscopic extremity drape is applied.

Anesthesia. There are many options for anesthesia during a knee arthroscopy which include a saphenous nerve block, peripheral, nerve block, spinal, monitored anesthesia care (MAC), or a general.

Surgical Procedure

- The tourniquet pressure is set to 350 mmHg for a normal adult.
- A stab incision is made with a #11 knife blade.
- The irrigation cannula and trocar are inserted into the lateral suprapatellar pouch near the superior pole of the patella.
- Lactated Ringers or normal saline is the medium used for visualization and distending the knee joint.

- The surgeon will place an additional stab incision anterolaterally or anteromedially 2 to 3 mm above the tibial plateau or patella tendon at the joint line.
- A sharp trocar and sheath are inserted through the capsule.
- A blunt trocar is used to pass the sheath into the knee joint.
- A 30° scope is inserted for visualization.
- A spinal needle is inserted to determine the angle for instruments.
- The cruciate ligaments and menisci are probed to determine any damage.
- The scope is moved to the opposite portal for examination of the entire knee joint.
- Continuous irrigation helps keep the operative field clear.
- The SA will inject Bupivacaine with epinephrine to minimize bleeding and provide postop pain control.
- The SA will close portal incisions with nylon or vicryl and steri-strips.
- Gauze sponges, Army battle dressing or abdominal pad (ABD), and elastic bandages are applied to the leg.

Postop Complications

- Nerve injury
- Infection
- Deep vein thrombosis
- Allergic reaction

Arthroscopic Anterior Cruciate Ligament Reconstruction

Anatomy. The anterior cruciate ligament (ACL) is a two bundled ligament found in the knee joint that is responsible for the prevention of extreme medial and lateral rotation as well as anterior translation. The ACL originates from the posterior corner of the lateral femoral condyle within the intercondylar notch. The ACL inserts medially on the anterior surface of the tibia. The ACL merges with the anterior horn of the medial meniscus. Its blood supply is provided by the middle and inferior geniculate artery; however, the ACL has areas of poor vascularity. This lack of consistent blood supply greatly effects the healing potential of ACL tears.

ACL tears are one of the most common orthopedic injuries, and around 200,000 reconstructions are performed each year. ACL tears occur following a sudden change in direction while pivoting or landing from a jump. ACL tears can also occur from high energy implants to the knee. These tears are seen most often in athletes though anyone is at risk for an ACL rupture. Women are three times more likely to rupture their ACL then men, and approximately half of all patients will develop osteoarthritis of the knee in the coming decades following the ACL tear. The ACL tear is classified as either a partial or complete rupture of the ligament with the occasional bone avulsion or bruising (see Figure 19-10).

Procedural Considerations. ACL tears are repaired by reconstructing the torn ligament with a new grafted ligament. There are two different types of grafts that can be used for an ACL reconstruction. Autografts are most used for the ACL reconstruction since this technique utilizes the patient's own ligament. The surgeon will harvest the graft from either the patellar tendon or the semitendinosus tendon of the ipsilateral leg. Patellar tendon is believed the "gold standard" for ACL repair autografts due to its ease of harvest; however, long term studies show the semitendinosus grafts fair similarly. Disadvantages of an autograft include donor site pain and weakening of remaining tendon. An alternative to autograft is the allograft. An allograft is taken from a cadaver tendon, either the patellar, Achilles or tibialis tendon. Some advantages of using an allograft are decreased surgical times and no donor site complications; however, allografts have a higher failure rate then autografts and come at a higher cost. Ultimately, the surgeon will choose which type of graft is best for the patient's ACL reconstruction, but it is

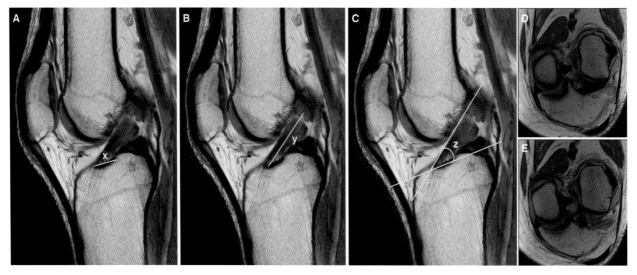

Figure 19-10 · Magnetic resonance imaging of a torn anterior cruciate ligament (ACL). (Reproduced, with permission, from Brunicardi FC et al, eds. *Schwartz's Principles of Surgery.* 11th ed. New York, NY: McGraw Hill; 2019.)

important to communicate prior to the surgical time to ensure all grafts and supplies are available. The reconstruction can be performed via an arthrotomy (open technique) or arthroscopic (minimally invasive). The arthroscopic technique is the most widely used since the patient has less post operative pain and infection risk.

Patient Position and Prep. The patient is placed supine on the OR bed and prepared for anesthesia.

When choosing positioners for an ACL reconstruction, the goal is to allow full flexion of the knee during the procedure. Using a lateral thigh post-positioned at the tourniquet and a foot support positioned to allow maximum flexion is common for an ACL reconstruction. Surgeons may also choose to use a leg holder at the level of the tourniquet and drop the foot of the bed. This allows gravity to rest the leg at flexion.

The operative leg is now prepped circumferentially from toes to tourniquet. Most orthopedic surgeons are using alcohol-based prep solutions for its increased efficacy as a skin antiseptic over non-alcohol-based prep solutions. Utilizing two personnel to prep the operative leg helps prevent contamination of the leg during the prepping process. One person holds the leg off the operative bed while the other preps the leg circumferentially. Once the leg is prepped, a sterile large drape is laid on top of the operative bed beneath the raised operative leg. This covers the nonoperative leg as well. A sterile blue towel is placed securely around the operative thigh at the base of the tourniquet. A towel clip is used to secure the ends of the blue towel together. Next, a sterile impervious stockinette is placed over the foot and passed up the leg to mid-tibia. An arthroscopy drape is placed over the foot and placed at the mid-thigh. The end of the built-in bag is pulled below the knee to catch the excess irrigation from the fluid management system.

Anesthesia. General anesthesia is mostly used for an ACL reconstruction to ensure complete relaxation. The patient may receive a femoral nerve or adductor canal block for postoperative pain relief. A Foley catheter is placed since the procedure is usually longer than 3 hours. A tourniquet is also placed high on the operative thigh to be used in case of excessive bleeding during the reconstruction. Routine inflation of the tourniquet is not common during an ACL reconstruction.

Surgical Procedure

- The ACL reconstruction begins with placing three trocars. Using an 11 blade, two trocars are placed beneath the patella, one medially and one laterally to the patellar tendon. An additional trocar is placed laterally beneath the other medial trocar.

- With the trocars in place, the surgeon uses a 30° arthroscope and a soft tissue shaver to resect the ligamentum mucosum. This exposes the intercondylar notch that the ACL is located. Examination of the torn ACL is completed at this time to determine if the rupture was complete or if there are intact ligament fibers left. The surgeon can now determine the length and thickness of graft needed.

- If the surgeon is using an allograft, the harvesting step is not needed; however, if using an autograft, the surgeon must take the time to harvest the needed tendon for the ACL reconstruction.

- When harvesting the semitendinosus tendon, a 3-cm incision is made from the lateral articular line and the tibial tuberosity.

- When the tendon is observed, a tendon stripper is used to complete the harvest.

- The harvested tendon is debrided of any muscle fibers and is folded directly in half. The graft is placed on a tensioner and the two limbs are sutured together.

- A size zero ultra-high-molecular-weight polyethylene suture is used to complete the running lock stitch on the graft.

- After tensioning and suturing, the graft length should be no more than 7.5 cm and the diameter should be around 1 cm. For harvesting the patellar tendon, an 8-cm incision is made from the inferior border of the patella to just beyond the tibial tubercule.

- The borders of the patellar tendon are dissected to give an adequate measurement for the graft. From the middle of the patellar tendon, a 1-cm width graft is measured and incised longitudinally using a scalpel.

- At each end of patellar graft, a bone plug is created using a small oscillating saw. A 1-cm wide by 2-cm long bone plug is removed from the patella, and a 1-cm wide by 2.5-cm-long bone plug is removed from the tibial tubercle. Once the graft is completely removed, careful planning of the size of the bone plugs are needed to ensure a proper fit during implantation.

- The bone plug needs to be able to easily pass through 1-cm sizer.

- Also, the femoral plug can be no longer than 2 cm, whereas the tibial plug can be no longer than 2.5 cm. Autografts will need to be prepared in a similar fashion depending on which type of tendon graft is given.

- The SA can prepare the graft while the surgeon returns to the arthroscopic preparation of the knee joint.

- The ruptured ACL is removed using the soft tissue shaver, and care is taken to leave any intact fibers behind.

- The femoral and tibial attachment sites are carefully marked and planned to ensure the best attachment trajectory of the graft. The femoral tunnel is created next through the accessory trocar.

- Under intraoperative fluoroscopy, a 1-cm-wide reamer is used to create the femoral tunnel. The tunnel is created slowly to ensure the proper trajectory and placement.

- Passing sutures are placed through an eyelet pin left in the femoral tunnel and pulled through the knee laterally. It is important that the looped end of passing suture stays in the femoral tunnel.

- Place a hemostat on the end of the suture to prevent it from being removed. The tibial tunnel is created by drilling a guide pin from approximately 2 cm medially to the tibial tubercle into the tibial joint surface.

- The trajectory of the tibial guide pin is confirmed utilizing intraoperative fluoroscopy. A cannulated drill bit, which is the size of the measured ACL graft, is placed over the guide pin. The tibial tunnel is slowly reamed in the desired direction while utilizing intraoperative fluoroscopy to monitor the trajectory.

- The tunnel is cleared of any soft tissue using a radio ablation probe and soft tissue shaver. The looped suture is grasped and passed through the tibial tunnel.

- During the reaming of the tunnels, the SA holds the camera and assists with the suture passing once the graft preparation is completed.

- With the tunnels created, the ACL graft can be placed into the knee joint via the tibial tunnel. The suture on the graft is passed through the looped sutured located through the tibial tunnel. The graft is then pulled into the knee joint by pulling on the passing suture that is located on the outside of the lateral knee. This pulls the ACL graft into the femoral tunnel. Before passing the ACL graft through the tunnels, double check the diameter sizing to ensure that the graft is still 1 cm in diameter. This will prevent the graft from getting stuck through either of the tunnels.

- With the knee is flexion, the ACL graft is now fixated to the femur with either a titanium or bioresorbable interference screw.

- The ACL graft is placed under as much tension as possible by pulling on the suture ends out of the tibial tunnel; then the knee is moved in flexion and extension approximately 20 times to remove any slack from the ACL graft.

- Placing the knee in extension, the surgeon pulls tension on the graft sutures and places an interference screw.

- The SA will retract the incision with Senn retractors to aide in visualizing the outer portion of the tibial tunnel.

- With the ACL graft fixated to the femur and tibia, the surgeon assesses the knee's stability and range of motion.

- With the ACL graft reconstruction complete, the closure begins. If the patellar allograft was used, the paratendon and the remaining patellar tendon are closed with a size zero absorbable braided suture using the buried interrupted technique.

- The dermis of the donor site incision is closed with a 2-0 absorbable braided suture, and the skin of all the incisions are closed with a 3-0 absorbable monofilament suture using the intracuticular technique.

- The incisions are covered with steri-strips and 4 × 4 gauze.

- The leg is wrapped from toes to thigh with an ace bandage before a hinged knee brace locked in extension is placed.

- An ice pack is placed on the knee for postoperative swelling and pain relief.

Postop Care. For 4 weeks postoperatively, the patient is partial weight bearing while locked in extension. From weeks 4 through 6, the knee brace is slowly opened to flexion and may be able to resume normal function by four months postoperatively.

Postop Complications. Postoperatively, the patient is monitored for complications. Patients need to be monitored for signs of deep vein thrombosis and infection postoperatively. For the patellar tendon donor site, anterior knee pain, patellar fracture, and patellar tendon tears are all risks. Knee stiffness is common with ACL reconstruction; however, physical therapy helps correct this complication. The key to preventing the stiffness is early movement after surgery. Even though the success rate of ACL reconstruction is around 85%, complications may arise that need to be addressed.

Total Knee Arthroplasty

The concept of replacing the articular surfaces of the knee joint has been around since the late 1800s; however, the first modern total knee replacement was performed in 1968 by Frank Gunston. He developed a polycentric total knee arthroplasty that combined metal and polyethene on the weight bearing surface of the knee joint. Over the decades, new technological advancements have made the total knee arthroplasty more patient specific and successful. Computer- or robotic-assisted surgery and patient specific instrumentation have utilized three-dimensional imaging to improve the patient outcomes after total knee arthroplasty. Understanding how the knee joint works has allowed for these advancements, which has made the total knee arthroplasty the most common orthopedic procedure performed in the United States. Over a half of a million total knee arthroplasties are performed annually.

Etiology. A patient qualifies for a total knee arthroplasty primarily due to cartilage damage on the articular surface. Osteoarthritis comprises 95% of all total knee arthroplasties; however, other arthritic conditions like rheumatoid arthritis or posttraumatic degenerative arthritis are also indications for total knee arthroplasty. A patient's tibiofemoral alignment may also make them a candidate for total knee arthroplasty. When the tibia turns inward from the femur, it puts more strain and pressure on the lateral condyles. This condition is called genu varum and the leg is "bow-legged." When the tibia turns outward from the femur, it puts more strain and pressure on the medial condyles. This condition is called genu valgum and the leg is "knock-kneed." The excess strain and pressure on the condyles cause pain and increase cartilaginous wear, which may eventually require a total knee arthroplasty (see Figure 19-11). Unstable fractures that involve the joint surface may also require a total knee arthroplasty.

Regardless, nonsurgical, or minimally invasive treatments will be exhausted before a patient is worked up for a total knee arthroplasty. These treatments include weight loss, nonsteroidal anti-inflammatory medication, corticoid steroid injections, and/or arthroscopic debridement. If these less invasive treatments have failed, the patient's quality of life must be drastically diminished for a surgeon to decide to perform the total knee arthroplasty.

choose to leave the cruciate ligaments intact, which requires the design of the implant to adapt to the patient's native ligaments. These cruciate-retaining implants are designed to allow the posterior and/or the ACL to stay in place and function accordingly. Another implant design component of the total knee is the bearing type. If the implant is a fixed-bearing implant, the polyethylene tibial component is securely attached to the metal tibial component. This allows the femoral component to roll on the polyethylene component. If the implant is a mobile-bearing implant, the polyethylene is placed on a rotating platform. This allows the knee to rotate medially and laterally a few more degrees than a fixed-bearing design.

Along with implant design choice, the surgeon has multiple options for fixating the implant to the bone. The most common option for implant fixation is using a polymethylmethacrylate bone cement. A relatively newer option is to utilize cementless fixation, where the implants are press-fit onto the bone. The implants are made of material that encourages the bone to grow into the surface of the implant. Lastly, some implants offer the option of hybrid fixation, where the surgeon can use cement fixation for one component and press-fit for the other component.

Positioning. When the patient enters the OR, they are placed supine on a standard OR bed. The arms are placed on arm boards at slightly less than 90°.

Anesthesia. General anesthesia is the most common method of anesthesia used for a total knee arthroplasty. A femoral nerve block may also be used in conjunction with general anesthesia for postoperative pain relief. The nerve block is performed in the preoperative holding area by an anesthesiologist, and it gives the patient excellent postoperative pain relief without the excessive use of opioids. Surgeons may also choose spinal anesthesia for their patients instead of general anesthesia. Spinal blocks decrease the patient's postoperative nausea and vomiting as well as time to discharge from the post-anesthesia care unit. All in all, the goal is to have a smooth transition from the OR to rehabilitation for an optimal patient outcome. Surgeon's preference also dictates whether a patient receives a Foley catheter. Length of surgery as well as if a patient has a spinal block are determining factors for the need of a Foley catheter. Not placing a Foley catheter is becoming more common to decrease the risk of catheter-associated urinary tract infections and increase ambulation postoperatively.

Prepping and Draping. Once induction is completed, the patient is prepped and draped for surgery. At this time the Foley catheter is placed per the surgeon's request. A tourniquet may also be placed at this time, but the use of tourniquets during total knee arthroplasties are a surgeon's preference. More surgeons are beginning to not utilize tourniquets due to the increased wound healing complications associated with tourniquet use. Ultimately, if the surgeon chooses to use a tourniquet, it must be placed high on the thigh to prevent any encroachment into the sterile field. The operative leg is now prepped circumferentially from toes to tourniquet or the hip. Most orthopedic surgeons are using alcohol-based prep

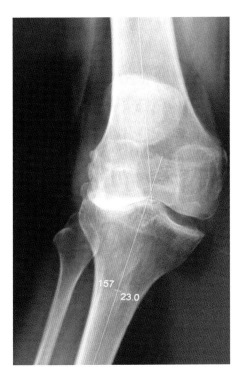

Figure 19-11 · Valgus deformity. (Reproduced, with permission, from Brunicardi FC et al, eds. *Schwartz's Principles of Surgery*. 11th ed. New York, NY: McGraw Hill; 2019.)

Anatomy. The knee joint is composed of three boney structures that are connected with various ligaments to perform the hinge motion. These boney structures are the distal femur, proximal tibia, and patella. These bones have a cartilaginous articular surface which allows for smooth motion. In the knee joint, the meniscus is found which is a wedge-shaped cartilaginous structure. The meniscus cushions and stabilizes the knee joint. The femur and tibia are joined with the medial and lateral collateral ligaments on the outside of the knee joint. On the inside of the knee joint, the anterior and posterior cruciate ligament attached the femur to the tibia. The collateral ligaments control the side-to-side motion of the knee joint, and the cruciate ligaments control the back-and-forth motion of the knee joint. The patella is held in place by two tendons. On the proximal side, the quadriceps tendon is attached to the patella and the quadriceps muscles. On the distal side, the patellar tendon attaches the patella to the tibial tuberosity. The neurovascular bundle for the knee joint runs posteriorly through the popliteal fossa. The neurovascular bundle consists of the popliteal artery, popliteal vein, and tibial nerve. The common fibular nerve also runs posteriorly; however, it exits the popliteal fossa and wraps around the fibular head laterally.

With over 150 different designs of total knee implants from various manufacturers to choose from, the studies have shown that not one implant type is superior to the other. The choice of implant remains with surgeon's preference as well as what a patient's specific anatomy requires. One design option is a posterior stabilized implant. With these implants, the cruciate ligaments are removed, and the tibial component is designed to act like the posterior cruciate ligament. Some surgeons may solutions for its increased efficacy as a skin antiseptic over non-alcohol-based prep solutions. Utilizing two personnel to prep the operative leg helps prevent contamination of the leg during the prepping process. One person holds the leg off the operative bed while the other preps the leg circumferentially. Once the leg is prepped, a sterile large drape is laid on top of the operative bed beneath the raised operative leg. This covers the nonoperative leg as well. A sterile blue towel is placed securely around the operative thigh at the base of the tourniquet or high on the thigh if a tourniquet is not placed. A towel clip is used to secure the ends of the blue towel together. Next, a sterile impervious stockinette is placed over the foot and passed up the leg. Surgeon's preference will dictate if the stockinette stops at mid-tibia or is rolled up to the patient's mid-thigh. If the surgeon requests the stockinette goes above the knee, then a whole will be cut at the knee after the final drapes are placed. Next, either a lower extremity drape or two split drapes are place on the operative leg. A lower extremity drape has a hole cut into it that requires the drape to be passed from the toes up to the operative leg's mid-thigh. The split sheets have a U cut out, which allows the SA to place the drape at the base of the operative site and pass the two limbs of the drape around the knee. The surgeon chooses which final drape they prefer to use. The final step of draping the operative leg for a total knee arthroplasty is placing an incise drape around the knee. The incise drape comes impregnant with iodine for increased antisepsis or plain. Again, the use of the incise drape will be at the surgeon's discretion.

Surgical Procedure

- After the draping is completed, the knee is placed in flexion and an approximately 10-cm skin incision is made medially over the patella using a ten blade.

- The skin incision begins 2 cm proximal to the patella, and then extends distally to the anterior tibial tuberosity.

- A fascial incision can now be created in the deep fascia surrounding the knee.

- A small Eastman retractor is utilized at the proximal apex of the skin incision to extend the fascial incision into the vastus medius muscle fascia.

- The fascial incision curves around the patella and extends distally along the patellar tendon with care being made to not fully transect the patellar tendon. A quadriceps sparing technique can be utilized which involves leaving the vastus fascia intact, essentially creating a smaller fascial incision which decreases a patient's postoperative pain.

- The order in which a surgeon completes a total knee arthroplasty depends on the surgeon's training and system they are using. The boney components can be resurfaced in any order deemed by the surgeon's preference. All total knee replacement systems have unique cutting guides and equipment that is used to complete the total knee arthroplasty. A manufacturing company representative is usually present for all total knee arthroplasties to assist the surgical team with the manufacturer's tray.

- Once the fascial incision is created, the patella is reflected to expose the femur and tibia. Osteophytes and meniscus are removed from all boney surfaces utilizing a rongeur.

- The femoral cutting guide is used to excise the correct depth of bone. The depth of cuts is kept as minimal as possible to preserve as much bone as possible. The goal of the cuts is to only remove the cartilaginous surface of the bone and correct any varus or valgus deformity.

- The SA is retracting the skin edges back and protecting the medial and lateral collateral ligaments from the saw blade.

- Typical instruments used to achieve femoral exposure are Eastman retractors and Hohmann retractors.

- A femoral component trial is placed to check for the correct sizing of the implant.

- Next, the tibial articular bone is resurfacing utilizing the manufacturing company's specific cutting guides.

- The SA will continue to protect the medial and lateral collateral ligaments with Hohmann retractors or Z retractors.

- The femur also needs to be retracted away from the tibia to expose the entire articular surface. A PCL retractor or bent Hohmann is used for femoral retraction.

- The tibial implant component has a small stem that extends to the boney canal, so the tibial canal will be reamed based on the manufacturer's recommendations.

- The tibial component trial is now placed with the temporary polyurethane spacer.

- With the trial femoral and tibial components intact, the knee is placed in extension to assess joint stability.

- When the surgeon is satisfied with the size implants chosen, the patellar osteotomy is performed.

- The SA will hold the cutting guide to hold the patella steady during the sawing. Three pilot holes are drilled into the patella to allow the patella component to sit easier in the patella.

- The patella component trial is placed, and the knee is worked in various range of motion exercises to test stability and functionality.

- When the surgeon is satisfied with the component trials fit, the permanent implants are opened onto the field to be implanted.

- If the surgeon chooses a cement fixation, the cement is now mixed and placed in a cement gun to deliver it onto the bone and implants. The permanent femoral component is fixated first, then the tibial components and lastly the patellar component (see figure 19-12).

- The SA is retracting the soft tissues away from the boney structures to give the best exposure when placing the permanent implants.

- With all the permanent implants impacted into place, the surgeon and SA thoroughly removes any excess cement before it hardens.

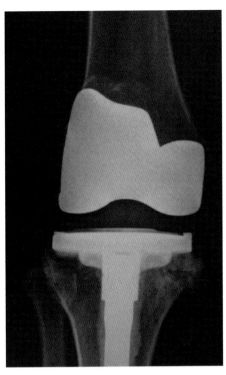

Figure 19-12 · Right total knee replacement. (Reproduced, with permission, from Brunicardi FC et al, eds. *Schwartz's Principles of Surgery.* 11th ed. New York, NY: McGraw Hill; 2019.)

- It is vital the cement not located underneath the implants are removed to prevent any floating bodies in the knee joint.

- While the team is waiting for the cement to harden, the tourniquet (if used) is released, and hemostasis is achieved. After around 5 to 10 minutes of cement curing time, the surgeon will extend the knee and complete range of motion exercises to confirm the permanent implant's fit and functionality of the knee.

- Closure techniques vary between surgeons, but the deep fascia is closed with a number one or zero absorbable suture.

- Many surgeons have switched to closing the layers with a running barbed suture, which decreases closure time as well as decreases knot spitting from multiple interrupted sutures.

- If the surgeon chooses, a suction drain may be placed in the intraarticular space to prevent hematoma formation. The drain is removed after no more than 48 hours.

- The dermal layer is closed with a zero or 2-0 absorbable suture, typically using a running barbed suture.

- The skin layer is closed with staples or a 3-0 absorbable barbed suture.

Dressings. Dressings also vary by surgeon's preference, but more surgeons are using dressings that seal the incision to prevent microbial contamination. For a suture closure, Prineo® is used to seal the incision for up to 6 weeks. If staples are used, then a nonadherent dressing like Telfa® is used to cover the incision. Next, 4 × 4 gauze and/or abdominal pads are used with a lightly wrapped 4-inch kerlix around the knee joint.

Compression is achieved for the leg by wrapping from the toes with a 4-inch ace wrap to the mid-thigh with a 6-inch ace wrap. Care is taken when taking the drapes off as well as wrapping the leg that the drain is not accidentally removed. An ice pack is wrapped around the knee joint to help with postoperative pain and swelling. The drain is secured to the ace wrap to prevent tugging.

Postop Complications. Following total knee arthroplasty, the patient will be monitored for deep vein thrombosis and hematoma. The goal is to ambulate and being physical therapy within 24 hours of surgery to decrease recovery times. Postoperative complications to be aware of are periprosthetic joint infections, aseptic loosening, and peroneal nerve palsy. A periprosthetic joint infection can be devastating to the patient, requiring additional operations, weeks of intravenous antibiotic therapy, and potentially a revision of the implanted components. It is vital that the surgical team executes impeccable sterile technique during the procedure to help prevent a periprosthetic joint infection to occur. Utilizing a pulse lavage device to irrigate the joint multiple times throughout the procedure also aides in preventing bacteria and debris from settling in the joint.

Above-the-Knee Amputation (AKA)

Etiology. The main causes of limb loss and the need for surgical amputation are vascular disease (54%), which includes diabetes and peripheral arterial disease (PAD), and trauma (45%). Trauma is a common occurrence resulting in upper extremity amputation, while vascular disease is the major reason for lower extremity amputation. Infection, tumor, or congenital abnormalities are indications for amputations.

African Americans are up to four times more likely to have an amputation than white Americans.

Nearly half of the individuals who have an amputation due to vascular disease will die within 5 years postop. This is a higher 5-year mortality rate than for breast, colon, or prostate cancers.

Fifty-five percent of diabetic patients who have a lower leg amputation will require amputation of the second leg within 2 to 3 years.

Anatomy. The thigh is composed of three compartments: anterior, medial, and posterior. These compartments surround the only bone in the thigh, the femur.

The anterior compartment contains the four muscles that delineate the quadriceps: the rectus femoris, vastus lateralis, vastus intermedius, and vastus medius. This musculature is innervated by branches of the femoral nerve. The saphenous nerve branches from the femoral nerve to innervate the medial skin of the thigh and leg. The IT (iliotibial) band traverses the lateral border of the thigh and is superficial to the vastus lateralis. The sartorius is the longest muscle in the body and runs obliquely from the ASIS on the lateral edge of the hip bone, traversing medially and inferiorly toward the medial edge of the knee.

The medial compartment contains the adductor magnus, adductor longus, adductor brevis, and the gracilis. These muscles are innervated by the obturator nerve. The adductor magnus is also innervated by the sciatic nerve. The femoral artery and vein also reside in the medial compartment.

Positioning, Prepping, and Draping. The usual equipment needed for an AKA is an orthopedic set with retractors, clamps and possibly an amputation knife. An oscillating or Gigli saw and drill. Sutures and ties according to the surgeon's preference. Sterile tourniquet if the amputation is going to be higher than mid-thigh.

Patient Position and Drape. The patient is placed on the OR table in a supine position. After the patient receives general anesthesia, place a bump under the buttocks on the operative side, shave the thigh, and apply the tourniquet if not using a sterile one, 1015 drape, and Bovie grounding. The patient is prepped and draped in a sterile fashion with bottom sheets under the leg and thorax. Impervious U-drapes are employed, ending with an extremity sheet or double U-drapes.

Surgical Procedure

- The leg is marked for incisions just above the knee. Usually, with an anterior/posterior flap configuration with a longer anterior flap.
- A circumferential incision along the marked lines is continued through sub-q tissue into the fascial plane.
- Anterior compartment muscles are dissected down to the femur with cautery used extensively to control bleeding. Muscle groups should be transected 1 to 2 inches longer than the planned femoral bone cut to allow the muscle to cover the bone, which will add cushioning for better prosthetic use postop.
- The quadriceps are transected with more cautery.
- Femoral vessels are identified and isolated. The femoral artery and veins are individually clamped, transected with each proximal segment ligated with 2-0 silk suture.
- The posterior muscle groups are transected; the sciatic and saphenous nerves are isolated, sharply transected (to prevent the formation of a neuroma), and tied off with a 2-0 vicryl tie and allowed to retract. This is done to any other branching nerves that are encountered.
- The femur is cleaned with a periosteal elevator.
- An oscillating saw is used to cut the femur and bone wax is applied to bleeding from the bone marrow.
- A rasp is used to smooth the edges of the bone.
- Drill holes are placed laterally and posteriorly of the femur.
- The adductor magnus tendon is attached to the lateral aspect of the femur with a nonabsorbable suture with the leg held with a 5° to 10° of adduction.
- The quadriceps muscle is attached over the distal femur to the posterior aspect of the adductor magnus tendon, again with a nonabsorbable suture, while holding the hip in full extension.
- The fascia lata is attached to the medial fascia.

- Per the surgeon's preference, a drain is placed deep to the fascial layers to reduce hematoma.
- The fascia, subcutaneous tissue, and skin are closed in a layered fashion.
- The skin closure should not be overtightened to prevent necrosis of the stump.

Sterile soft dressings are applied, along with a compression dressing.

Postop Complications. AKA complications include muscle atrophy, wound site infections, wound dehiscence, and prosthetic wear wounds. Abduction and flexion contractures may also occur. An abduction contracture can be prevented by confirming that the IT band is affixed to the femur. Posttraumatic stress disorder (PTSD), phantom pain, and depression are known psychological complications of amputations.

Femur

Femur Fracture Management. Approximately 300,000 femur fractures occur annually in the United States. The causes of these femur fractures vary between high energy traumas like a motor vehicle accident or a low energy trauma like a fall out of bed. The age demographic also varies as well. The average age of a femur fracture patient is 80 years old. Younger adults with femur fractures were typically caused by a high energy trauma, whereas the older patients, especially women, are osteoporotic and a short fall can cause the femur fracture. Femur fractures also vary in their location along the bone: proximal, shaft and distal. A proximal femur fracture occurs anywhere from the femoral head and 5 cm below the lesser trochanter. These can be further categorized into femoral neck fractures, intertrochanteric, or subtrochanteric fractures. Femoral neck fractures are classified using the Garden's classification system. Type 1 and 2 are nondisplaced and type 3 and 4 are displaced. This classification allows for better management of the fracture. A femoral shaft fracture occurs anywhere along the long portion of the bone before it widens at the condyles. Femoral shaft fractures occur in different patterns. These fracture patterns are transverse, spiral, oblique, segmental and comminuted. A distal femur fracture occurs from the distal metaphyseal-diaphyseal junction to the articular surface of the femoral condyles. The location of the femur fracture as well as the fracture pattern determine the surgical technique required to femur fixation.

Anatomy. The femur is the longest bone in the body. The proximal femur consists of the femoral head, femoral neck, and the greater and lesser trochanters. The femoral head articulates with the acetabulum to form the hip joint, and the femoral neck is angled at approximately 130° to the femoral shaft. The greater trochanter is large tuberosity located laterally to the femoral neck to which the short external rotators of the hip attach. The lesser trochanter is located on the posteromedial side of the femur below the femoral neck. The iliopsoas attaches to the lesser trochanter. On the anterior side of the femur, the intertrochanteric line connects the greater and lesser trochanter and is the attachment point for the hip joint capsule and iliofemoral ligament. On the posterior side, the greater and lesser trochanter are connected by the intertrochanteric crest, where the quadratus femoris muscle attaches. The medial circumflex femoral artery supplies the proximal femur, and injury to this vessel may cause avascular necrosis of the femoral head. The femoral shaft extends distally with a slight medial bowing. This bowing allows the knee to be closer to the body's center of gravity which increases stability. Anteriorly, the quadriceps muscles are found along the femoral shaft and posteriorly the hamstring muscles are found. The femoral shaft narrows at the midshaft and widens again distally at the epicondyles. The distal femur consists of the medial and lateral epicondyles as well as the medial and lateral condyles. These structures including the intercondylar fossa created the femoral component of the knee joint. The epicondyles are raised prominences on the medial and lateral side of the distal femur. The medial and lateral collateral ligaments originate here. The adductor tubercle is located on the superior aspect of the medial epicondyle in which the adductor magnus muscles attaches. The medial and lateral condyles articulate with the tibia, patella, and menisci of the knee joint. Posteriorly between the two condyles, the intercondylar fossa serves as an attachment point for the anterior and posterior cruciate ligament.

Patient Positioning. Depending on the location and choice of surgical fixation, the position of the patient varies; however, the table chosen must allow for fluoroscopy to access the leg from pelvis to knee. If the surgeon needs traction throughout the procedure, then a fracture or Hana® table may be used. The patient stays supine on these tables and the operative foot is placed in a traction boot, which aligns the fracture site using mechanical traction on the femur. A flat top Jackson table can also be utilized if the surgeon needs to position the patient laterally or the surgeon prefers using manual traction versus mechanical traction from the fracture or Hana® table. The SA is tasked with applying the traction when a flat top Jackson table is used. For the lateral position, a beanbag or pegboard positioner is utilized.

Surgical Considerations. The surgical technique chosen for femoral neck fractures depends on the blood supply being intact. A displaced femoral neck fracture has a higher risk of avascular necrosis, so the standard surgical technique is a hemiarthroplasty. For nondisplaced femoral neck fractures where the vasculature typically is intact, percutaneous hip pinning is utilized. After induction, the patient's operative leg is placed in traction using a fracture or Hana® table. This allows for the reduction of the femoral neck fracture to stay stabilized throughout the procedure.

Draping. The operative leg is draped using either two split sheets from the ASIS to just below the knee joint or a vertical isolation drape that adheres to the operative site and drapes over the entire field. Fluoroscopy is vital during this procedure and will also need to be draped.

Surgical Procedure

- Incision is made laterally over the greater trochanter and the tensor fascia lata is incised to allow the aiming arm to sit flush against the bone.
- With the aiming arm sitting below the greater trochanter, guidewires are inserted through the aiming arm holes. The goal is to have two to three parallel placed guidewires inserted through the femoral neck into the femoral head.
- Fluoroscopy is used throughout the guidewire placement to ensure the screws will stay parallel within the bone.
- A depth gauge is slide onto the end of the guidewire to determine the length of screw required for fixation. This technique recommends subtracting 5 mm from the length measured on the depth gauge.
- A 3.6-mm cannulated drill bit is used over the guidewire to drill the bone. The 7.0-mm cannulated cancellous screws are inserted over the wires completing the fixation. If the bone is too soft, a washer can be placed over the screw to prevent the screw head from plunging into the outer cortex.
- Final fluoroscopy is taken to confirm proper fixation and screw length. The tensor fascia lata is repaired using size 0 absorbable braided suture with a figure of eight suture technique. The dermis is closed next with a 2-0 absorbable braided suture using a buried interrupted suture technique.
- Finally, the skin is closed using a 4-0 absorbable monofilament using an intracuticular suture technique. Some surgeons may request a stapled skin closure. Placing a waterproof and antimicrobial impregnated dressing over the incision decreases the risk of wound infection for these fracture patients.

Surgical Considerations for Lower Extremity. For intertrochanteric and subtrochanteric femur fractures as well as proximal femoral shaft fractures, fixation is achieved through antegrade IMN (see Figure 19-13).

Patient Position and Draping. The patient is typically positioned on the fracture or Hana® table; however, the surgeon may choose the lateral approach. A beanbag vacuum positioner is commonly used for the lateral approach. The patient's operative leg is draped as described above and fluoroscopy is also draped and needed for the entirety of this procedure.

Surgical Procedure Antegrade Approach

- For the antegrade approach, incision is made 3 cm above the greater trochanter staying in line with the femur.
- Continue to use the 10 blade to dissect through the tensor fascia lata then bluntly sweep the tissues to feel for the top of the greater trochanter.
- Using fluoroscopy for guidance, the guide wire is inserted starting medially on the tip of the greater trochanter staying in line with the canal. Stop the advancement of the guide wire at the level of the lesser trochanter. It is important that biplanar fluoroscopy images are taken to ensure the guide wire is inserted in the correct space.

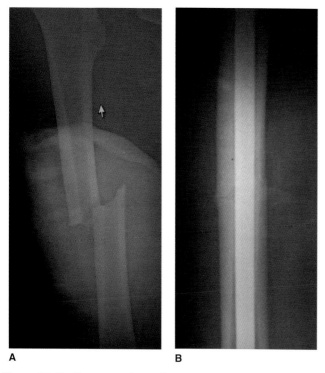

A   **B**

Figure 19-13 · Transverse femur fracture and intramedullary nail. (Reproduced, with permission, from Brunicardi FC et al, eds. *Schwartz's Principles of Surgery*. 11th ed. New York, NY: McGraw Hill; 2019.)

- With a soft tissue protector placed over the guide wire, an entry reamer is used to broach the medullary canal. The guide wire is removed, and a long ball-tip reaming rod is placed down the femoral canal passed the fracture site until it hits the distal end.

- If it was not done prior to incision, the intramedullary nail length and diameter is measured using the radiolucent ruler provided at this time. Before the nail is placed on the sterile field, laterality is confirmed because the nail has a side specific bow throughout the implant.

- With the ball-tip reaming rod in place, the surgeon can ream the intramedullary canal. Beginning with a 9-mm reamer, the surgeon will continue to size up by 0.5 or 1.0 mm until chatter is heard from the reamer.

- When the reamer is being removed, the SA will use the rod pusher sometimes referred to as the gear shift to prevent the ball-tip reaming rod from being removed passed the fracture line.

- The surgeon may choose to not ream the canal on elderly patients because the bone is already soft enough.

- The intramedullary nail is attached to the insertion handle and aiming arm, ensuring that all the targeting guides line up with the holes in the nail.

- The intramedullary nail is placed over the ball tip guidewire and slowly advanced down the canal until the nail is completely inserted into the bone. For longer nails, a mallet may be required to complete the advancement, but be sure

to place the hammer guide to be on the insertion handle for a point of contact for the mallet.

- Once the nail has crossed the fracture line, the ball-tip reaming rod is removed.

- To compress the inter/subtrochanteric femoral neck fracture, a helical blade is inserted through the intramedullary nail into the femoral head.

- A guide sleeve is inserted into the 130° aiming arm and an incision is made where the guide sleeve hits the skin.

- Turning the compression nut on the guide sleeve compresses the sleeve against the femur to ensure the proper length of helical blade is measured. Fluoroscopy is utilized to confirm the placement of the guide sleeve.

- Under fluoroscopic guidance, a 3.2-mm guide pin is inserted through the guide sleeve passing through the femur into the femoral head. Biplanar images are taken at the hip to confirm the guide pin is centrally located in the femoral neck and head as well as stopping at approximately 5 mm away from the far cortex.

- The helical blade's length is measured, and the cannulated drill bit's depth is set equal to the helical blade's length.

- Once the bone is drilled, the helical blade is inserted by hand and the final millimeters inserted using a mallet. The helical blade is locked into the intramedullary nail by tightening the preassembled locking mechanism through the top of the nail.

- A flexible hexagonal screwdriver is passed through the top of the insertion handle until it is engaged in the locking mechanism and turned until tightened.

- Next, the distal locking screws (1-2) are inserted. Surgeons can use the guide sleeves through the aiming arm to ensure a direct path for the screws or the surgeons will free hand the technique.

- If the surgeon free hands the distal screw insertion, fluoroscopy will position in the lateral view to give the surgeon perfect circle view of the screw holes in the intramedullary nail.

- A small stab incision is made over the location of the screw hole in the intramedullary nail. The 4.0-mm drill bit drills through prefabricated hole in the nail penetrating both cortices.

- Biplanar fluoroscopy confirms the correct trajectory of the drill bit.

- A depth gauge is used to measure the length of the screw, and the screw is inserted by hand through the nail. For femoral shaft fractures, compression of the fracture site is achieved by back slapping on the intramedullary nail before inserting the proximal locking screws.

- With the distal locking screws in place, an extension device is attached to the insertion handle and a slotted mallet slides back against the extension device pulling the nail distally.

- Then the proximal locking screws are placed instead of a helical blade.

- The insertion handle and aiming arm are removed and an end cap can be inserted if needed. The end caps are cannulated to pass over a 3.2-mm guidewire placed through the top of the intramedullary nail.

- Final biplanar fluoroscopy images are taken at the hip and the knee to ensure proper placement of the intramedullary nail and screws.

- In the two larger incisions, the tensor fascia lata is repaired using size 0 absorbable braided suture with a figure of eight suture technique.

- The dermis is closed next with a 2-0 absorbable braided suture using a buried interrupted suture technique.

- Finally, the skin is closed using a 4-0 absorbable monofilament using an intracuticular suture technique. Some surgeons may request a stapled skin closure.

- Placing a waterproof and antimicrobial impregnated dressing over the incisions decrease the risk of wound infection for these fracture patients.

Distal Femur. For fractures located in the distal third of the femur, a retrograde intramedullary femoral nailing surgical technique is utilized for fixation. It is important to note that the fracture must be 4 cm away from the articular surface to allow proper fixation.

Patient Position and Drape. The patient is positioned supine on a radiolucent table like the flat top Jackson table. Fluoroscopy needs to have access to both the knee and the hip. The operative leg is prepped from toes the level of the umbilicus. A sterile stockinette is placed over the foot to the mid-tibia and sterile split sheets are used to drape the operative field. The operative field runs from the mid-tibia to the ASIS. Sterile knee positioning triangles are used intraoperatively to flex the knee approximately 90°.

Surgical Procedure

- A longitudinal skin incision is made just below the patella over the patellar tendon.

- The patellar tendon is retracted laterally using an army navy retractor to gain access to the articular surface of the femur.

- Under biplanar fluoroscopy guidance, a guide wire is placed centrally on the intercondylar notch and advanced approximately 15 cm into the medullary canal. Ensuring the guide wire is centrally located in the canal is critical for the successful insertion of the retrograde intramedullary nail.

- Care is also taken not to plunge posteriorly to avoid injuring the structures in the popliteal fossa.

- A soft tissue protection sleeve is passed over the guide wire and a 13.0-mm drill bit opens the medullary canal.

- The guide wire is removed, and a long ball-tip reaming rod is placed down the femoral canal passed the fracture site until it hits the distal end.

- If it was not done prior to incision, the intramedullary nail length and diameter is measured using the radiolucent ruler provided at this time.

- Before the nail is placed on the sterile field, laterality is confirmed because the nail has a side specific bow throughout the implant.

- With the ball-tip reaming rod in place, the surgeon can ream the intramedullary canal. Beginning with a 9-mm reamer, the surgeon will continue to size up by 0.5 or 1.0 mm until chatter is heard from the reamer.

- When the reamer is being removed, the SA will use the rod pusher sometimes referred to as the gear shift to prevent the ball-tip reaming rod from being removed passed the fracture line.

- The surgeon may choose to not ream the canal on elderly patients because the bone is already soft enough.

- The intramedullary nail is attached to the insertion handle and aiming arm, ensuring that all the targeting guides line up with the holes in the nail.

- The intramedullary nail is placed over the ball tip guidewire and slowly advanced down the canal until the nail is completely inserted into the bone. For longer nails, a mallet may be required to complete the advancement, but be sure to place the hammer guide to be on the insertion handle for a point of contact for the mallet.

- Once the nail has crossed the fracture line, the ball-tip reaming rod is removed. The distal locking screws are now placed utilizing a guide sleeve and a 4.2-mm drill bit.

- A stab incision is made directly in line with the guide sleeve and fluoroscopy ensures that the drill bit passed through the nail and both cortices of the femur.

- A depth gauge measures the required length of the distal locking screw before placement. Typically, two distal locking screws are placed. The two proximal locking screws can now be placed.

- Fluoroscopy will position in the lateral view to give the surgeon a perfect circle view of the screw holes in the intramedullary nail.

- A small stab incision is made over the location of the screw hole in the intramedullary nail. The 4.2-mm drill bit drills through prefabricated hole in the nail penetrating both cortices. Biplanar fluoroscopy confirms the correct trajectory of the drill bit.

- A depth gauge is used to measure the length of the screw, and the screw is inserted by hand through the nail.

- The insertion handle and aiming arm are removed and an end cap can be inserted if needed. The end caps are cannulated to pass over a 3.2-mm guidewire placed through the end of the intramedullary nail.

- Final biplanar fluoroscopy images are taken at the hip and the knee to ensure proper placement of the intramedullary nail and screws.

- For wound closure, the dermis is closed with a 2-0 absorbable braided suture using the deep buried interrupted suture technique and the skin is closed with a 4-0 absorbable monofilament suture using the intracuticular technique.

- The surgeon may want a stapled skin closure.
- Placing a waterproof and antimicrobial impregnated dressing over the incisions decrease the risk of wound infection for these fracture patients.

For 24 hours following fracture fixation, the femoral compartment pressures are monitored, and a postoperative x-ray confirms placement of implants and fracture reduction. As tolerated, the patient may begin physical therapy on postoperative day one and released from the hospital after a few days. Full weight bearing using crutches, or a walker can occur as soon as the patient's pain allows. The patient will follow up with the surgeons for the next 12 weeks to ensure proper fracture healing.

Distal Condylar Femur Fracture. For distal condylar femur fractures, an open reduction and internal fixation is the standard surgical approach.

Patient Position and Drape. The patient is positioned supine or lateral on a radiolucent table like the flat top Jackson table. Fluoroscopy needs to have access to both the knee and the hip. The operative leg is prepped from toes the ASIS. A sterile stockinette is placed over the foot to the mid tibia and sterile split sheets are used to drape the operative field. The operative field runs from the mid tibia to the hip. A sterile tourniquet may be placed high on the thigh from intraoperative bleeding control. If the patient is in the supine position, sterile knee positioning triangles are used intraoperatively to allow for knee flexion.

Surgical Procedure

- A lateral skin incision is created from Gerdy's tubercle curving downward to align with the femoral shaft. The incision ending depends on the fracture location.
- Some surgeons may choose to do a minimally invasive technique which utilizes stab incisions to insert the screws versus one large incision.
- The tensor fascia lata is incised in line with the skin incision which exposes the vastus lateralis muscle.
- The muscle is released from intermuscular septum and retracted anteriorly to expose the fracture site.
- Weitlaners hold the femoral exposure open, though SA may need to use an army navy retractor to retract any soft tissue is not contained by the Weitlaners.
- The fracture site is irrigated and cleaned of any debris before reduction.
- Reduction of the fracture site is achieved using pointed reduction clamps or K-wires. The length of the plate is determined by the fracture pattern.
- There needs to be at least four screw holes proximal to the fracture site for proper fixation. Plate placement against the femur is critical to ensure the distal screws are parallel to the knee joint and will not penetrate the articular surface.
- Guide wires are placed through the plate into the femoral condyles to secure the placement prior to screw fixation, and lateral fluoroscopic images confirm the plate placement.

- With the plate in the proper position, a combination of 5.0-mm and 7.3-mm screws are used for distal plate fixation. A 5.0-mm drill bit is used for 7.3-mm screws and a 4.3-mm drill bit is used for the 5.0-mm screws.
- If desired, a compression screw is used first to compress the plate to the femur, then the rest of the screws inserted are locking screws.
- Fluoroscopy confirms proper screw trajectory and length. For the proximal screw insertion, a plate holding forceps holds the plate down to the femoral shaft to ensure proper plate placement.
- For compression of the proximal plate, 4.5-mm cortical screws are drilled using a 3.2-mm drill bit.
- A depth gauge is utilized to measure the correct length of screw before insertion. Typically, one to two cortical screws are placed, and then the rest of the proximal screws placed are 5.0-mm locking screws. A 4.3-mm drill bit is used for the 5.0-mm screws. Final biplanar fluoroscopy confirms fracture reduction and fixation before closure begins.
- The wound is irrigated and the vastus lateralis muscle is tacked over the plate with a 0 absorbable braided suture.
- The tensor fascia lata fascia is closed using the 0 absorbable braided suture utilizing the buried interrupted suture technique.
- Dermis is closed with a 2-0 absorbable braided suture utilizing the buried interrupted suture and the skin is stapled closed.
- Placing a waterproof and antimicrobial impregnated dressing over the incisions decrease the risk of wound infection for these fracture patients, and a knee immobilizer is placed on the operative leg.

TIBIA/FIBULA

Tibial Plateau Fractures

Etiology. As a high energy, patients are primarily males in their 40s, whereas the low energy injuries are by elderly females in their 70s from falls.

The lateral tibia plateau is convex while the medial plateau is concave. The muscle structure that attaches to the anterolateral tibia is the anterior compartment musculature. The pes anserine muscle attaches to the anteromedial tibia. It is the medial tibia plateau that bears 60% of the knee's load.

ExFix/Ilizarov is suited for severe open fractures with an elevated chance of contamination.

ORIF is recommended for medial and bicondylar fractures. Postop infection is increased if the patient has any of the following factors: male, smoker, pulmonary disease, bicondylar fracture patterns, and intraoperative time exceeding 3 hours.

External fixation is accomplished with two 5-mm half-pins in the distal femur and two in the distal tibia. The fixator is locked in slight flexion. This treatment allows the soft tissue swelling to subside. The ExFix usually remains in place for 2 to 4 months.

In an ORIF, the lateral incision is most common. A straight or hockey-stick incision anterolaterally from just proximal to the joint line to just lateral to the tibial tubercle. Restore the joint surface with either direct or indirect reduction techniques. Large bone clamps should be used to maintain joint reduction. Screws can be used alone for simple split fractures or depression fractures that need to be elevated percutaneously. Non-locking plates are indicated for simple partial articular fractures. Locking plates for fixed angle constructs and where less compression is needed on or near the periosteum and the soft tissue.

Drill, measure, screw, and repeat. Close with 0-vicryl if tissue allows closure. Use 3-0 Vicryl for subcuticular stitch and interrupted nylon for skin closure. Soft dressing followed by ACE bandage to assist with the swelling.

Tibial Shaft Fractures

Tibial shaft fractures are the most common long bone fracture. It accounts for 4% of all fractures seen in the Medicare population. This fracture is a result of both high energy trauma and low energy trauma. For the former injury, it is caused by direct forces from an MVA or sports encounter, usually young males. With a high-energy injury, the fibula is fractured at the same level. The later injury, low energy, is the elderly and often, an osteoporotic female falling. The low-energy fracture is a torsional injury, and the fibula is broken at a different level than the tibia.

The tibia is a triangular bone. It has a wide metaphyseal region and is narrow distally. Muscles that tend to be deforming forces on the bone are patellar tendon, gastrocnemius, the pes anserinus, and anterior compartment musculature. If the injury is extensive there can be a neurovascular compromise of the following nerves: deep and superficial peroneal, sural, tibial, saphenous, and posterior tibial.

Closed low-energy injuries can utilize closed reduction and cast immobilization. This is ideal for patients that may be nonambulatory or unfit for surgery. Use a long leg cast and convert to a patella tendon bearing brace 4 weeks out.

External fixation can be useful for proximal or distal metaphyseal fractures. This solution has a higher incidence of malalignment.

Intramedullary fixation is valuable and appropriate for the majority of tibial fractures. It is well-suited for mid diaphysis fractures. If severe bacterial contamination or infection is present, nailing may spread infection through the medullary canal and should be avoided. External fixator pins are a common source of contamination. If such pins appear to be infected or have been present for more than 2 to 3 weeks, preliminary pin removal, debridement, and antibiotics may be advisable before nailing.

A tibial IMN system, triangle, large bone clamps (preferably sharp periarticular), and step stool. Move the lights to avoid contamination of the guidewire. C-arm. Small bump under ipsilateral hip.

The most common approach is the medial parapatellar. Flex the knee over the triangle and mark your operative site. Landmarks should be the inferior pole of the patella, borders of the patella tendon, joint line, and the tibial tubercle. The incision is the inferior patella pole distally toward the tibial tubercle. The SA can retract the patellar tendon laterally and place a Gelpi to maintain access. The starting point for the *guide pin* is just medial to the lateral tibial spine. Use the cannulated starting point reamer to open the canal.

The SA can prep the ball-tip guidewire with a slight bend in the tip of the wire. Provide a soft tissue guide over the wire before the surgeon starts the wire. With imagining, push the ball-tip guidewire with a T-handle to the distal end of the fracture site. Reduce the fraction by pulling traction over the triangle. Once reduced, manually push guidewire past fracture site. Use X-ray to confirm placement both from AP and laterally.

Start reaming with a size 9-mm reamer and increment by 0.5 to 1.0 mm. Use the step stool for a better angle of reaming. Reaming has to be 1.0 full size above the implant (ream 10-mm for 11-mm nail). Attach proximal targeting guide, mark the skin for 2 or 3 static holes. Make an incision and with a hemostat and spread the soft tissue to the bone. Place the trocar on the bone and remove the inner sleeve and drill through the first cortex and nail. Measure when hitting the second cortex (the second cortex adds 2 to 5 mm). Continue drilling through the second cortex. Insert the screw and repeat the process for a second or third screw.

Bring knee to full extension and place on a sterile bump. Acquire perfect circles for the distal interlocking screw. Cut, spread, drill, measure, and screw as before with the proximal interlocking screws.

Irrigate with copious amounts of saline and cauterize anything bleeding. Close the patella tendon with 0-vicryl. Sub-q with layered 3-0 vicryl. Staples or interrupted suture for the skin. Soft dressing and ACE from distal thigh to the toes to prevent edema.

Tibial Pilon Fractures

This is a more common injury with males and an average age of 35 to 40 years. This is usually a result of an MVA or a fall from height. Seventy-five percent of these fractures have an associated fibula fracture. This fracture involves the weight-bearing surface of the ankle joint.

The distal tibia forms the inferior quadrilateral surface and pyramid-shaped medial malleolus. It articulates with the talus and fibula laterally via the fibula notch. Vascularization is via the anterior tibial artery, posterior tibial artery, and peroneal artery. The tibial nerve passes deep to the soleus and the posterior aspect of the medial malleolus. The common peroneal nerve bifurcates to the superficial and deep peroneal nerves. The saphenous nerve is a continuation of the femoral nerve from the thigh. The sural nerve innervates the lateral aspect of the leg and foot.

Immobilization is only indicated if there are stable fracture patterns without articular surface displacement, the patient is critically ill, or nonambulatory. A long leg cast for 6 weeks is followed by a fracture brace and ROM exercises.

ORIF is indicated as a definitive fixation for the majority of pilon fractures.

Both the large frag and small frag sets. Large bone holding clamps. Extra batteries. And do not forget the surgeon's lead with the C-arm.

The approach for an ORIF is via multiple small incisions that can include a direct anterior approach to the ankle, anterolateral approach to the ankle, anteromedial approach to the ankle, and a medial approach. After the fracture is exposed, reduce and use bone clamps on the fibula to establish the lateral column length. Reduce the articular surface. Plating can be an anterior, anterolateral, anteromedial, medial, or posterior technique for the tibia. Although the fibula is not weight-bearing, it may need ORIF placement also. The closure may be needed on both the medial and lateral sides. This is where the SA can cut down patient anesthesia time by closing one side with a 0-vicryl. Subcuticular with 3-0 vicryl and interrupted nylon for the skin. Soft dressing with ACE from knee to ankle to relieve some postop swelling.

External Fixation.   Indications for the use of external fixation in tibial shaft fractures include open fractures with extensive soft tissue devitalization and contamination, the stabilization of closed fractures with high grade soft tissue injury, or compartment syndrome. External fixation is preferred when the fracture configuration extends into the metaphyseal/diaphyseal junction of the joint making other modalities problematic. Circular and hybrid techniques have provided definitive treatment of complex periarticular injuries such as tibial plateau and distal tibial pilon fractures. Hexapod fixators can provide gradual reductions of the tibial shaft or periarticular injuries and in cases where acute distraction and reduction could compromise neurovascular aspects.

Etiology. Acute trauma applications will more commonly use monoliteral frame configurations. For diaphyseal injuries, the monoliteral frame is used with large pins for skeletal stabilization.

- Simple monoliteral fixators allow individual pins to be placed at different angles and varying angles when they connect to the bar. This is beneficial when adjusting the pin position to avoid areas of soft tissue compromise.
- Monotube-type fixators have pin placement predetermined by the multipin clamps. Universal articulations between the body and clamps allow for easy manipulation when reducing a fracture.

High energy fractures usually involve the metaphyseal regions and call for small tensioned wires to provide better mechanical stability and longevity.

- Small tensioned wire circular frames or hybrid frames can be beneficial in patients with severe tibial metaphyseal injuries that are combined with soft tissue compromise, compartment syndrome, or patients with multiple injuries.
- Hexapod fixators consist of six distractors and 12 ball joints with allow for 6° of freedom of bone fragment displacement. This permits for gradual three-dimensional correction or acute reduction with a simple frame.

Open tibial diaphyseal fractures are often treated with closed intramedullary nailing; however, there may be circumstances that indicate external fixation.

- Significant contamination and severe soft tissue injury
- A fracture that extends into the metaphyseal-diaphyseal junction of the joint

External Fixation Considerations

- A severely comminuted fracture will require a more complex frame to control motion
- Weight bearing
- The ability to bridge the joint to provide stability for both hard and soft tissues
- The frame must allow for multiple debridement and possible soft tissue reconstruction

Physical Considerations

- The neurovascular status with notation of the presence or absence of the anterior and posterior tibial pulses
  - A weak or absent pulse may indicate subsequent vascular injury or compartment syndrome and should further be evaluated with ankle-brachial index or arteriogram
- Soft tissue evaluation and formal grading of the open fracture which will help determine pin placement and fixator configuration (see Figure 19-14).

ANKLE & FOOT

ORIF of Ankle

Etiology. Ankle fractures occur because of extreme bending forces on the ankle. The exaggerative inversion or eversion stresses on the ankle joint, which causes ligaments to tear and potentially the malleoli to fracture. Compression trauma to the ankle from a fall or motor vehicle accident can also cause ankle fractures. The incidences of ankle fractures are on the rise due to the increase activity in the older demographics, though this fracture is seen often across age groups and genders. Stable ankle fractures only need immobilization without surgery. If the ankle joint is unstable due to the fracture, then surgery is required to prevent any mobility issues.

Anatomy. The ankle joint is formed from the distal tibia, distal fibular and the talus. The most distal portion of the tibia and fibula are referred to as the malleoli and extended medially and laterally along the talus. These bones are held together at the joint by multiple ligaments. On the lateral side, the ligaments consist of the anterior talofibular ligament, the calcaneofibular ligament and the posterior talofibular ligaments. On the medial side of the ankle, the deltoid ligament holds the medial malleolus to the talus. Multiple tendons also travel along the retinaculum of the ankle joint. Laterally, the personal brevis and long tendons travel just posteriorly to the lateral malleolus of the fibula. Medially, the posterior tibial tendon and flexor digitorum longus tendon travel just posteriorly to the medial malleolus of the tibia, and the anterior tibial tendon run just anteriorly.

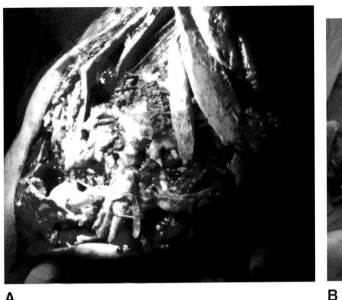
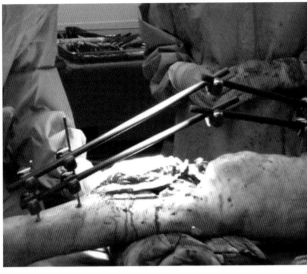

A   **B**

Figure 19-14 · Comminuted tibia-fibula fracture and external fixator temporarily stabilizes fracture. (Reproduced, with permission, from Brunicardi FC et al, eds. *Schwartz's Principles of Surgery*. 10th ed. New York, NY: McGraw Hill; 2015.)

Superficially, the long saphenous vein and saphenous nerve run along the tibia anterior to the medial malleolus. The posterior tibial vein, artery and nerve run deep to the flexor longus digitorum tendon. The anterior tibial artery travels on the anterior surface of the tibia across the ankle joint. On the fibular side of the ankle, branches of the fibular artery feed the lateral portion of the ankle. The sural nerve runs along the fibular artery posteriorly to the lateral malleolus, and the superficial peroneal nerve runs anteriorly along the fibula across the ankle joint.

An open reduction and internal fixation of the ankle consists of the repair of a malleolar fracture of the tibia and/or fibula. Occasionally, the distal portion of the fibular shaft may also be involved in the fracture. If the fracture only involves the lateral malleolus and medial malleolus then the fracture is a bimalleolar fracture. If the fracture also involves the posterior malleolus of the tibia, then the fracture is a trimalleolar fracture. The timing of the fracture repair depends on whether the fracture is open or closed. An open fracture is considered an emergency and is repaired within a few hours of the injury. This is key to preventing an infection from the break in the skin. A closed fracture is splinted in the emergency room and is scheduled for outpatient surgery a few days to 2 weeks later depending on the soft tissue swelling. The patient must stay non-weight bearing to prevent any further damage to the bone.

Positioning. The patient is placed in the supine position on a standard OR bed to prepare for induction.

Anesthesia. General anesthesia is the most common choice when performing an open reduction and internal fixation of the ankle. This allows for adequate relaxation and pain management during the repair. For postoperative pain relief, a popliteal block can be given which usually lasts around 24 hours. Though not commonly needed, spinal nerve block or femoral nerve block can be used in place of general anesthesia for high-risk patients. Because of the fracture, it is important that the patient stays relaxed to help with the reduction of the fractures.

Positioning and Draping. After induction, the patient positioning is finalized. A large bump is placed under the operative hip to correct the external rotation of the leg. This allows the lateral malleolus to be accessed easier. Another positioner option if available is the Bone Foam® ramp. This ramp elevates the operative leg on a stable surface while being radiolucent. The Bone Foam® ramp prevents the contralateral leg from interfering with the lateral x-ray images. Because this procedure requires intraoperative fluoroscopy, the standard OR bed must be turned so the long portion of the bed does not interfere with the C-arm extending under the bed. Placing the removal head piece at the distal end of the bed is not recommended as the large metal hinge pieces may interfere with the anterior to posterior fluoroscopy images. A nonsterile tourniquet is placed around the thigh for control of any intraoperative bleeding due to the bone fracture. The tourniquet is placed far from the incision site in case the incisions need to be extending more proximally to repair the fractures.

Once patient positioning is complete, the operative leg is prepped circumferentially from toes to knee. Commonly, an alcohol-based prep solution is used for this procedure, and care must be taken to not disrupt the fracture too much during the prep process. Two personnel may be needed to carefully prep the operative leg. After the surgical prep is completed, the surgical team is now able to sterilely drape the operative leg. A sterile large drape is laid on top of the operative bed beneath the raised operative leg. This covers the nonoperative leg as well. A sterile blue towel is placed securely around the operative thigh at the base of the tourniquet. A towel clip is used to secure the ends of the blue towel together. Next, a sterile impervious stockinette is placed over the entire foot. This is utilized only during the draping procedure to cover the toes of the patient. Most surgeons will remove the stockinette at the completion of the draping and cover the toes with an extra sterile glove or wrap the toes with Coban®. Next, a lower extremity drape placed on the patient. The hole of the extremity drape is passed over the toes up to the operative leg's knee. Because intraoperative fluoroscopy is utilized during this procedure, a large drape or C-Armor® drape is attached on the operative leg side of the bed to maintain sterility of the field when the C-arm is taking lateral x-rays. The operative leg is exsanguinated from toes to thigh using an Esmarch, and then the tourniquet is inflated to 350 mmHg.

Surgical Procedure

- To repair the lateral malleolus, an approximately 7-cm incision is made directly over the lateral malleolus extending proximally along the fibula. The incision may need to be extended longer depending on the fracture pattern into the fibular shaft.

- The SA should stand at the patient's foot or on the operative side next to the surgeon. This allows the SA to visualize the surgical field and assist more appropriately.

- As the surgeon dissects through the soft tissue, the SA retracts using Senn retractors and then two Weitlaners are placed to expose the fracture site and free up the SA's hands. Care is taken to not damage the peroneal tendons. The soft tissue needs to be dissected away from the fibula to allow the plate to lay flat against both the proximal and distal ends of the fibular fracture. It is key however to not over dissect the tissue away, which decreases the blood supply to the fibula.

- Once the fracture site is identified, the fracture is clean out of blood clots and debris. Bone fragments may also be found inside the fracture and need to be removed to facilitate the fracture reduction. The key to a successful fracture reduction is ensuring nothing is trapped between the two ends of the fracture.

- Irrigation and a Frazier suction tip as well as a Penfield number four dissector help clean out the fracture. Usually, if the fracture is not reducing cleanly enough, then more debris or clot can be found inside the fracture blocking its reduction.

- The fibular fracture reduction is held in place with a bone tenaculum or a lobster claw forceps. When using these bone holding clamps, be sure to position them so the clamp does not block where the plate will lay.

- A lag screw can be used to compress the fracture which will allow the bone-holding clamps to be removed before plating occurs.

- After the fracture is fully reduced, the fibular plate and screws are placed. Intraoperative fluoroscopy is utilized in both the anterior and lateral planes to ensure the screws are the correct size and the fracture stays reduced.

- A plate is chosen that allows at least three screw holes above and below the fracture line. Screws are placed through the

plate to fixate the plate to the fibula. Various combinations of locking and/or compression screws are placed using power to achieve maximum support for the fracture reduction. The screws need to be bicortical, but not extending into the ankle joint or too far into the interosseous membrane.

- To help with exposure, the SA can use Senn retractors or small Bennett retractors to hold the soft tissue away from the plate and screws. While the screws are being placed into the plate, soft tissue may get spun into the threads which effects its purchase into the plate.

- With these fracture patterns, a disruption in the syndesmosis is likely. The syndesmosis is located just above the ankle joint where the tibia overlaps the fibular posteriorly. When the ankle is stressed with extreme rotation, the ligaments that hold the syndesmosis together become stretched or torn.

- Repairing the syndesmosis is critical to the stability and movement of the ankle joint. Under fluoroscopy, the surgeon will stress the patient's syndesmosis by externally rotating the ankle. The fluoroscopy image will show if the syndesmosis separates. If it does separate, then a fibulotibial positioning screw is used.

- Through one of the distal fibular plate screw holes, a 2.5-mm drill bit is used to drill across the fibula into the tibia. The SA holds the foot at a 90° angle to ensure proper anatomic position of the ankle and parallel placement of the screw to the ankle joint. It is also critical to stabilize the leg to prevent shifting of the bones during drilling.

- The drill needs to be angled from posterior to anterior since the fibula sits posteriorly to the tibia. A depth gauge measures the needed screw length, and a 4.5-mm screw of that desired length is placed across at least three cortices of bone.

- Intraoperative fluoroscopy confirms the repair of the syndesmosis. If unsure, the contralateral leg's syndesmosis can be imaged intraoperatively for comparison.

- With the syndesmosis stabilized, the medial malleolus fracture can now be repaired. A 2-cm incision is created distally from the tip of the medial malleolus and curved upward toward the tibia. Be aware of the long saphenous vein and nerve while making the incision to prevent injury. Once identified, the long saphenous vein and nerve can be protected behind a dull Weitlaner or Senn retractor.

- The fracture site is exposed and clean out of all debris and clot. A small bone tenaculum is used to reduce the fracture; then a 1.6-mm K-wire is drilled perpendicularly to the fracture from the tip of the medial malleolus into the tibial medullary canal.

- A second 1.6-mm K-wire is placed in the same plane to temporarily hold the fracture, ensuring that one K-wire is placed anteriorly, and the other is placed posteriorly. This allows for enough room to place the screws through the malleolus.

- Intraoperative fluoroscopy confirms the placement of the K-wires. With the K-wires in the appropriate positions, a

2.5-mm cannulated drill with a drill sleeve is placed over the K-wire, and the bone is drilled to the end of the K-wire.

- Care is taken to avoid drilling into the ankle joint or past the far cortex of the tibial shaft. The bone is drilled over each K-wire, while using fluoroscopy to confirm the fracture maintains reduction.

- A depth gauge that fits over the K-wire is used to measure the needed length for each screw site. Occasionally, a washer may be needed under the screw head if the medial malleolar bone is weakened. The washer prevents the screw head from penetrating too far into the bone.

- A cannulated 4.0-mm cancellous screw of the required length is placed over one of the K-wires and inserted into the bone with a manual screwdriver. This step is repeated with the other K-wire. Care is given to not overtighten the screw to prevent damage to the tip of the medial malleolus.

- Intraoperative fluoroscopy will confirm the placement of the screws and ensure the proper anatomic alignment of the ankle joint.

- After final x-rays confirm the fixation of the fractures, closure can begin. Using a size 0 absorbable braided suture, soft tissue and/or any fascia is closed over the plates and screws. The goal is to cover the plates and screws with as many layers between it and the outside skin. The more layers between the metal implants and the outside of the body means decreased chance that any superficial infections would reach the implants.

- If a surgical site with an implant becomes infected to deeply into the tissue, then that implant must be removed to treat the infection. This has potentially devastating consequences for the patient's mobility.

- The dermis is now closed using a size 2-0 absorbable braided suture then the skin is closed with either staples or a 4-0 absorbable monofilament intracuticular suture. Skin closure depends on surgeon's preference, and the patient's limb swelling.

Dressings. For a stapled incision, the dressings include a petroleum impregnated gauze and 4 × 4 gauze. For an intracuticular sutured incision, steri-strips are placed over the incision with or without the use of Dermabond® first to seal the incision. Then, 4 × 4 gauze is placed over the steri-strips. Now, regardless of incision closure, the ankle needs to be wrapped for compression. Kerlix® roll gauze is used from below the toes to mid-tibia to hold the 4 × 4 gauze intact. Then, a 4-in ace wrap is wrapped from just below the toes to mid-tibia. The ace wrap needs to be wrap snuggly but not so tight that it inhibits the leg's circulation. While the incision is healing, the limb needs to be immobilized in a fracture boot or posterior splint. Place a pillow under the operative leg for postoperative comfort and elevation.

Postop Complications. The most common postoperative complication following an open reduction and internal fixation of the ankle is wound healing issues. Because of the thinner tissues over the malleoli, these incisions are the most difficult to heal. Wound healing issues may lead to infection and loss of soft tissue. Both could potentially require multiple reoperations. Malunion of the fracture is also a postoperative complication that requires reoperation. If the fracture does not heal properly, the patient will have pain and decrease ankle mobility. To best avoid these complications, the SA must approximate the tissues well and avoid extensive retracting on the skin.

Achilles Tendon Repair

Anatomy. The Achilles tendon is the thickest and strongest tendon in the human body. The origin is near the middle of the calf, and merges with the gastrocnemius muscle proximally. The gastrocnemius is a fusiform muscle created by two heads, medial and lateral; each one separately crosses the knee joint. The medial and lateral heads of the fusiform muscle fuses in a single muscle belly occupying the posterior superficial compartment of the lower leg. The soleus is deep to the gastrocnemius and with the gastrocnemius, the soleus forms the three-headed triceps surae, which allows plantarflex of the ankle joint via the Achilles tendon. The plantaris is a small and thin vestigial muscle that originates from the popliteal surface of the femur. The Achilles tendon has three vascular areas: the peroneal artery that supplies the midsection and the posterior tibial artery that supplies the proximal and distal sections. The mid-section of the tendon has poor vascularization. The average length of the Achilles tendon is 15 cm, although it can range from 11 to 26 cm. The gastrocnemius, soleus, and plantaris muscles act as ankle flexors. The gastrocnemius is involved in walking, jumping, and running and the soleus muscle is a stabilizer of the foot while standing.

Etiology. Achilles tendon rupture is most often caused by a sudden, forceful motion that stresses the calf muscle. This can happen during an intense athletic activity or even during simple running or jumping. Middle-aged adults are especially likely to get this kind of injury.

Contraindications to an Achilles Repair. There is much debate in the literature about treatment for Achilles tendon rupture with the two options comprising of a conservative or surgical approach. Many studies have shown that the re-rupture rates are higher in cases of nonoperative management. More recently studies have demonstrated equivalent or improved rates of re-rupture compared with surgical intervention. However, many people continue to be treated with surgical repair and physiotherapists will continue to see them for postoperative rehabilitation

Diagnostics. Clinically they present with a palpable gap on palpation, increased passive dorsiflexion, lack of heel raise, and a positive Thompson test. A Thompson test is performed to determine if the Achilles tendon is ruptured. This is done by squeezing the calf muscles while the patient is kneeling or lying face down with feet hanging unsupported. An MRI may be ordered.

Equipment. Instrumentation includes ortho soft tissue and tendon strippers.

Positioning and Prepping. After induction, a nonsterile tourniquet is placed around the thigh for control of any intraoperative bleeding. The patient is then turned into the prone position over chest rolls.

Once patient positioning is complete, the operative leg is prepped surgically and circumferentially from toes to knee. Commonly, an alcohol-based prep solution is used for this procedure. Two personnel may be needed to carefully prep the operative leg. After the surgical prep is completed, the surgical team is now able to sterilely drape the operative leg. A sterile large drape is laid on top of the operative bed beneath the raised operative leg. This covers the nonoperative leg as well. A sterile blue towel is placed securely around the operative knee. A towel clip is used to secure the ends of the blue towel together. Next, a sterile impervious stockinette is placed over the entire foot. This is utilized only during the draping procedure to cover the toes of the patient. Most surgeons will remove the stockinette at the completion of the draping and cover the toes with an extra sterile glove or wrap the toes with Coban®. Next, a lower extremity drape placed on the patient. The hole of the extremity drape is passed over the toes up to the operative leg's knee. The operative leg is exsanguinated from toes to thigh using an Esmarch, and then the tourniquet is inflated to 350 mmHg.

Anesthesia. General anesthesia is the most common choice when performing an Achilles tendon repair. This allows for adequate relaxation and pain management during the repair. For postoperative pain relief, a popliteal block can be given which usually lasts around 24 hours. Though not commonly needed, spinal nerve block or femoral nerve block can be used in place of general anesthesia for high-risk patients.

Indications for Surgery

- Achilles' tendinosis
- Achilles' tendon tear
- Foot defects or deformities
- Plantar fasciitis

Approaches to Surgical treatment

- Gastrocnemius recession or lengthening the calf muscles will reduce stress on the Achilles tendon.
- Debridement and repair if the tendon is intact.
- Debridement with tendon transfer if the tendon is damaged.
- Achilles tendon rupture surgery to reattach the torn ends of the tendon with suture.

Surgical Procedure

- A posteromedial longitudinal incision 10 to 12 cm long is made with a #10 blade. The incision is approximately 1 cm medial to the tendon and is deepened to the paratenon.
- The SA will maintain the foot in equinus position during surgery.

- The ends of the ruptured tendon are identified. The Achilles tendon is always under some degree of tension and may have retracted proximal along the gastrocnemius muscle.
- A tendon grasping forceps may be needed to retrieve the tendon. Once both ends of the tendon are secured with a traumatic clamp the length of the tendon is evaluated.
- One popular type of repair is the Krachow whipstitch (see Figure 19-15).
- Suture used for the repair is usually a nonabsorbable suture ranging in size from 2-0 to #5.

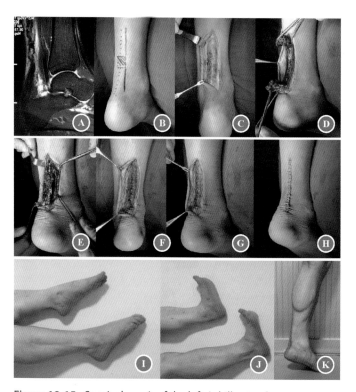

Figure 19-15 · Surgical repair of the left Achilles tendon rupture using the Krackow and tendon-bundle techniques. (A) Disruption of the Achilles tendon continuity as observed during MRI. (B) A longitudinal incision 1 cm off the posterior median tibial side of the Achilles tendon. (C) The flap was lifted superficially from the peritendinous sheath canal of the Achilles tendon to both sides to reveal the edges of the Achilles tendon on both sides. (D) A longitudinal incision of the peritendinous sheath canal of the Achilles tendon in the posterior median line revealed Achilles tendon rupture, which appears as horsetail-shaped irregular severed ends. (E) Krackow continuous locking edge sutures were performed on both sides of the Achilles tendon with a No. 2 Ethibond suture. (F) A 4-0 PDS suture was used to close the peritendinous sheath of the Achilles tendon. (G) After closing the peritendinous sheath, the taut Achilles tendon was pressed against the posterior tibial border. (H) Suture of the closed incision. (I–J) Active plantar flexion and dorsiflexion of the ankle at the final follow-up. (K) Unipedal standing heel lift. (Reproduced, with permission, from YANG Y, WEI Q, LI Z, et al. Management of Acute Achilles Tendon Rupture Using the Krackow and Tendon-Bundle Techniques. *Chin J of Plast and Reconstr Surg.* 2021;3(1):5-10; Figure 1.)

- As surgeon is approximating the ends of the tendon, the SA will place the foot in flexion.
- Layers are closed by the SA.
- Dressings are placed and a posterior short leg splint is applied with the foot in gravity equinus position.

Complications of Achilles Tendon Surgery

- Swelling
- Complications with healing
- Loss of strength in the calf muscle
- Scarring of the tendon
- Constant pain after surgery
- Another tear

Lapidus Bunionectomy

A lapidus bunionectomy is a procedure in which the first metatarsal bone is fixated to the medial cuneiform bone with a plate and screws to stabilize and correct a moderate to severe bunion. The procedure involves removing a small wedge of bone at the base of the metatarsal to allow for reduction of the bunion. Fusing the joint at the base of the metatarsal helps prevent any possible return of the deformity.

Anatomy. Bones of the foot include the 7 tarsals, 5 metatarsals, and 14 phalanges. The tarsus posterior hindfoot and proximal midfoot include seven bones which are talus, calcaneus, cuboid, navicular, and three cuneiforms.

The talus is the only bone of the foot that articulates with the tibia and is gripped by the malleoli, transferring body weight and dividing it between the calcaneus and the forefoot or hammock. The hammock spring ligament is suspended across a gap between the calcaneus and the navicular bone.

The talus has a groove for which the tendon of the flexor hallucis longus follows is flanked by a lateral and medial tubercle. The calcaneus is the largest and strongest bone in the foot. On the lateral surface is the fibular trochlea where longus and brevis tendons lie.

The navicular bone is located between the talus and the three cuneiforms anteriorly. The navicular tuberosity is the site for tendon attachments forming the medial longitudinal arch of the foot.

The cuboid bone is lateral in the distal row off the tarsus. Within the tuberosity of the cuboid is a groove for the fibularis tendon. The three cuneiform bones are the medial, intermediate, and lateral. They articulate with the navicular posteriorly.

Metatarsus is the forefoot and consists of five metatarsals that are numbered from the medial side. The base of the metatarsals has large tuberosity that provides tendon attachments.

On the planter side of the first metatarsal is a medial and lateral sesamoid bone. Fourteen phalanges make up the digits. The great toe has two phalanges and the other four digits have three phalanges each: proximal, middle, and distal. Each phalanx has a base, shaft, and head. All of these tuberosities and prominences can be palpated on examination.

Foot Fascia and Muscles. Deep fascia of the dorsum of the foot is thin and communicate with the inferior extensor retinaculum and laterally is continuous with the plantar fascia. The thick central part of the plantar fascia forms the strong plantar aponeurosis. The plantar fascia holds the longitudinal arches of the foot. The plantar fascia divides into five bands that hold the fibrous digital sheaths that enclose the flexor tendons.

In the midfoot and forefoot, there are three compartments of the sole: the medial compartment is covered by the thin medial plantar fascia and contains adductor and flexor tendons, plantar nerve, and vessels.

The central compartment is coved by the dense plantar aponeurosis and contains adductor and flexor tendons, lateral plantar nerve, and vessels. The lateral compartment is coved by thin lateral plantar fascia and contains adductor and flexor tendons.

The forefoot has a fourth compartment that contains the metatarsals, muscles, and vessels.

The fifth compartment is the dorsal compartment of the foot that contains muscles and neurovascular structures of the dorsum of the foot.

Blood Supply and Nerve Supply. Arteries of the foot are the terminal branches of the anterior and posterior tibial arteries.

The dorsalis pedis artery is a major blood supply to the foot. After passing the first interosseous space, it becomes the first dorsal metatarsal artery that supplies the great toe and a deep planter artery. The deep planter artery passes deep into the sole of the foot joining the lateral planter artery to form the deep planter arch.

The lateral tarsal artery, a branch of the dorsalis pedis artery, runs lateral to supply the tarsal and joints.

The arcuate artery runs across the bases of the four lateral metatarsals, anastomosing with the lateral tarsal artery to form an arterial loop. Branches of the arcuate artery supply the second, third, and fourth dorsal metatarsals.

Cutaneous innervation of the foot is supplied medially by the saphenous nerve that comes off the femoral nerve ending on the medial side of the foot and the head of the first metatarsal. The medial and the intermediate dorsal cutaneous nerve supply most of the dorsum of the foot. The deep fibular nerve supplies the anterior compartment muscles and then finally emerges as a cutaneous nerve that supplies the webbing between the first and second toe, as the first common dorsal digital nerve. Both the deep and the superficial originate from the common fibular nerve.

Coming off the larger and smaller branch of the tibial nerve is the medial and lateral planter nerves. The medial is distal to the foot and supplies skin to the side of the sole and the first three digits. The lateral planter nerve passes lateral to the foot supplies several muscles and the skin lateral of the sole and the fourth digit.

The sural nerve is formed by the union of branches off the tibial and fibular nerves. It passes inferior to the lateral malleolus and supplies the lateral aspect of the hindfoot and midfoot. The calcaneal nerve comes from the tibial and sural nerve passing from the posterior aspect of the leg to the heel, supplying the skin of the heel.

Etiology. Lapidus bunionectomy should only be considered when conservative treatment modalities have been depleted. The primary objectives are to eradicate pain, fix primary deformities, and reestablish a stable platform for ambulation. The major indications for the surgery are:

- Rheumatoid arthritis
- Degenerative joint disease
- Posttraumatic arthritis
- Chronic pain
- Joint instability
- Neuromuscular disease

Contraindications to the triple arthrodesis include:

- Active infection
- Short first metatarsal
- Adolescent patients with active growth plates
- Uncontrolled comorbidities
- Gross arthritis

Diagnostics. Indication for a lapidus bunionectomy will begin with a physical examination of the great toe. Radiographs will include medial, oblique, and lateral views to assess joint quality and joint positioning.

Equipment. Equipment include a standard foot ortho set, small fragment set of plates and screws, power equipment, and C-arm needed for confirmation of joint positioning.

Positioning and Prepping. The patient is supine with bony prominences padded and arms placed on arm boards less than 90°. A tourniquet is placed around the upper calf, depending on surgeon's preference. The foot and leg are prepped in a circumferential manner to themed calf or knee. The foot is draped according to surgeon's preference using a lower extremity drape.

Anesthesia. The patient is placed in general anesthesia.

Surgical Procedure

- A medial incision is made over the metatarsal beginning at the neck of the proximal phalanx.
- Using sharp dissection, the joint capsule is exposed and opened using a flap technique. Seaburger retractors are placed by the SA. Metatarsal head is exposed.
- All soft tissue attachments are released using a McGlamory.
- The proximal third of the metatarsal is removed, depending on which repair is warranted, with the micro saw.
- Proper alignment is done with K-wires by placing in the medullary canal.
- Depending on technique plates and screws or just screws can be used for alignment.
- The SA will irrigate and then close the layers.
- Joint capsule is closed.
- The skin is sutured closed.
- The SA will apply the dressing.

- The foot is placed in a splint and the patient is non-weight bearing.

Complications

- Non-weight bearing for 6 to 8 weeks
- Nonunion of realignment
- Hardware failure
- Infection

Triple Arthrodesis

The triple arthrodesis is an effective procedure in various pedal conditions and gait disorders. The term "triple" arthrodesis is a fusion procedure of three joints of the hindfoot: the subtalar joint (talus and calcaneus), the talonavicular joint, and the calcaneocuboid joint.

Anatomy. The bony structures consist of the talus, calcaneus, cuboid, and the navicular. The talus and calcaneus make up the subtalar joint. The anterior articular portion of the calcaneus and cuboid make up the CC joint. This is the first joint resected during a triple arthrodesis. Other important structures consist of: the artery of the tarsal sinus and venous that supply to the extensor digitorum brevis, the sural and intermediate dorsal cutaneous nerves, as well as the peroneal tendons, the extensor digitorum brevis muscle belly, and the peroneus tertius tendon. The posterior tibial tendon is encountered medially, and possibly the deltoid artery and tarsal canal artery along with the great saphenous vein and its tributaries.

Etiology. Triple arthrodesis should only be considered when conservative treatment modalities have been depleted. The primary objectives are to eradicate pain, fix primary deformities, and reestablish a stable platform for ambulation. The major indications for the surgery are:

- Valgus foot deformities that cannot be adequately braced
- Collapsing pes planovalgus deformity (flat foot)
- Advanced tibialis posterior tendon dysfunction
- Tarsal coalition
- Rheumatoid arthritis
- Degenerative joint disease
- Posttraumatic arthritis
- Chronic pain
- Varus foot deformities that cannot be adequately braced
- Cavus and cavovarus (elevation of the longitudinal plantar arch of the foot)
- Talipes equinovarus or clubfoot
- Joint instability
- Neuromuscular disease

Contraindications to the triple arthrodesis include:

- Active infection
- Acute charcot arthropathy (loss of sensation, in the foot and ankle)

- Arterial insufficiency
- Uncontrolled comorbidities
- arthritis

Diagnostics. Indication for a triple arthrodesis will begin with a gait analysis and also with the knee, ankle, and foot positions assessed. Radiographs will include weight-bearing dorsoplantar, medical oblique, and lateral views to assess joint quality and joint positioning. A calcaneal axial view can assess the degree of correction needed in relation to calcaneal valgus or varus. A CT verifies the integrity of the subtalar joint. Weight-bearing CT scans may be carried out in office. An MRI will evaluate soft tissue structures and a DEXA scan assesses osteoporosis. A scanogram is useful in the evaluation of any limb length deformities.

Equipment. Equipment for the triple arthrodesis includes a standard foot ortho set, screws sized from 6.5 to 8 mm for the subtalar joint, 4.5-mm screws to fixate the midtarsal joints, plates, and staples along with a laminar spreader, various osteotomes, curettes, saw, drill, K-wires, and burrs. Fluoroscopy will be needed for confirmation of joint positioning.

Positioning and Prepping. The patient is supine with bony prominences padded and arms placed on arm boards less than 90°. A tourniquet is placed around the upper thigh. The foot and leg are prepped in a circumferential manner to the knee. The foot is draped according to surgeon's preference. The iliac crest will be prepped if a bone graft is anticipated.

Anesthesia. The patient is placed in general anesthesia.

Surgical Procedure

- The lateral incision is made between the sural nerve and the superficial peroneal nerve using a #15 blade. The surgeon will use the electrosurgery unit (ESU) to coagulate any bleeders.
- The incision is continued deep reaching the fascia that covers the extensor digitorum brevis muscle.
- The SA will place retractors for visualization.
- The extensor digitorum brevis muscle is dissected off its origination site on the sinus tarsi.
- Fibrofatty tissue in the sinus tarsi is removed to expose the subtalar joint.
- All subtalar joint attachments are released including the interosseous ligament exposing the anterior and middle facets.
- The incision is followed distally exposing the calcaneal cuboid joint and the dorsal ligaments are released.
- The medial incision is made in the medial gutter of the ankle and lengthened to the inferior aspect of the navicular.
- The SA will retract the saphenous vein superiorly.
- The capsular tissue of the talonavicular joint is incised along the same line with the incision.
- A cobb elevator may be used to expose the joint.

- The talonavicular joint is resected.
- Curettes or osteotomes may be utilized for cartilage resection and exposure of the subchondral bone.
- Adequate resection of cartilage and fenestration of the bone ensures an adequate osseous union.
- Curettes or osteotomes, or even a sagittal saw, is used to remove articular surfaces of the calcaneocuboid joint.
- The SA will cut the bone into small pieces, and it will be saved for the fusion.
- The subtalar joint is prepped for the arthrodesis using a burr to provide sufficient subchondral bone exposure.
- The talonavicular joint is manually manipulation and either K-wires or Steinmann pins provide internal temporary fixation.
- The subtalar joint and calcaneocuboid are also fixated with K-wires or Steinmann pins.
- Once the foot is set in the optimal position for the fusion, the subtalar joint is permanently fixated utilizing screws.
- The talonavicular joint along with the calcaneocuboid joint are also permanently fixated
- The foot is placed in position with the heel in neutral to slight eversion and the midtarsal joint is placed in slight valgus.
- The SA will irrigate, and the layers are closed.
- The skin is sutured closed.
- A drain may be placed to prevent hematomas.
- The foot is placed in a splint and the patient is non-weight bearing.

Complications. Complications after a triple arthrodesis include:

- Wound dehiscence
- Nonunion of arthrodesis
- Hardware failure
- Infection
- Vascular disruption to the talus due to arterial insult during dissection
- Early osteoarthritis of the ankle joint due to the improper final position of the arthrodesis sites

HAND SURGERY

Carpometacarpal (CMC) Joint Arthroplasty

Etiology. Thumb arthritis is common with aging and occurs when cartilage wears away from the ends of the bones that form the joint at the base of your thumb—also known as the carpometacarpal (CMC) joint.

Anatomy. The wrist and hand consist of three parts: (1) the carpals, or wrist bones; (2) the metacarpals, or bones of the palm; and (3) the phalanges, or bones of the digits. The wrist is comprised of eight bones arranged in two rows. The proximal row contains the scaphoid, lunate, triquetrum, and pisiform. The distal row includes the trapezium, trapezoid, capitate, and hamate. There are five metacarpal bones, whose head forms the knuckles. The phalanges encompass 14 bones in each hand. There are three bones in each finger and two in each thumb. Patterns of injury result from the distinctive anatomy of the hand.

Cartilage. The primary function of hyaline articular cartilage is to provide a cushion between opposing joint surfaces. Articular cartilage is avascular, aneural, and does not replicate. The thinnest articular surfaces in the body can be found in the interphalangeal joints of the fingers. Fractures of the articular surface that involve subchondral bone appear to heal without an intermediate stage of fibrocartilage when compression screws are used to stabilize them.

Ligaments. Ligaments are flexible bands of fibrous connective tissue that link the bones of the skeleton. They permit full function while preserving joint integrity and stability thereby preventing dislocation. Ligaments of the hand may be intracapsular or capsular. Collateral ligaments of the interphalangeal joints are considered intracapsular as they are identified within the synovial membrane. Accessory collateral ligaments are considered capsular and are closely bound to the capsule making it hard to identify them as separate structures.

Tendons. The tendons of the fingers and thumbs are enclosed in a protective layer called a tendon sheath. Tendons serve as the physical connection between muscle and bone.

They remove the need for muscle to extend the entire length between the origin and the insertion point. They transmit the force of the muscle contraction and allow the muscle to be located at a distance from the joint on which it acts upon. Pulleys are bands attached to the bones at intervals along the tendon sheath. Tendons consist of three regions: the origin at the musculotendinous junction, the tendon proper, and the insertion into bone. As tendons advance from origin to insertion, they pass through specific connective tissue sheaths.

Fascia, Muscle, and Compartment of the Palm. The fibrous digital sheaths are ligament tubes that enclose the synovial sheaths and the superficial and deep flexor tendons. Several septums and compartments separate muscles, tendons, vessels, and nerves. The compartments include: hypothenar, thenar, interosseous, adductor, central compartments, and medial and lateral fibrous septums.

Between the flexor tendons and the fascia are two potential spaces, the thenar and the mid-palmer space.

These compartments, spaces and septums, will contain infections from spreading to other parts of the hand.

The intrinsic muscles of the hand are in these five compartments: the thenar muscles include the abductor pollicis brevis, flexor pollicis brevis, and the opponens pollicis. These muscles are mainly for the opposition of the thumb.

The hypothenar muscles include the abductor digiti minimi, flexor digiti minimi brevis, and opponens digiti minimi which move the little finger. The palmais brevis is a small muscle in the subcutianous tissues by the hypothenar but not in the compartment.

The short muscles of the hand are the lumbricals and the interossei.

Nerve Supply of the Hand. Nerves may contain both motor and sensory fibers or either one. The basic unit ofthe nerve is the neuron and its supporting elements. Sensibility is one of the most important functions of the hand. A hand that lacks sensibility is poorly used even though the tendons and joints might present as normal.

Four main nerves provide motor and sensory function to the hand: the median, radial, musculocutaneous, and ulnar nerves. These nerves are considered peripheralbranches of the brachial plexus. The four nerves enter the forearm through various muscle and fascial planes. These pathways are potential sources of entrapment.

Vascular Supply of the Hand. Radial and ulnar arteries are the main arteries to the hand. Superficial and deep venous palmer arches, associated with the superficial and deep palmer arteries, drain into the deep veins of the forearm. Dorsal digital veins unite to form the dorsal venous network.

Superficial to the metacarpals on the lateral side is the cephalic vein and on the medial side.

The basilica vein arises from the dorsal venous network.

Anesthesia

- General anesthesia is preferred, although the procedure can be performed with an axillary nerve block as well.

Symptoms

- Pain when grasping
- Catching, locking, popping, or grinding in the CMC joint
- Pain with daily activities
- Decreased range of motion
- Loss of strength

Diagnostics. X-rays will show diminished space between joint surfaces and joint subluxation.

Nonsurgical Treatment. Immobilization with a wrist wrap during activities. Other nonsurgical treatments include nonsteroidal to help with the pain.

Positioning, Prepping, and Draping. The patient is placed supine on the OR table with the operative arm outstretched on floating hand table. A floating hand table is recommended since it does not have a leg that interferes with C-arm positioning. General anesthesia is primarily used; however, an axillary nerve block can be utilized for intraoperative regional anesthesia and/or postoperative pain relief. After induction, the OR bed is turned 90° away from anesthesia, with the operative arm outward. The tourniquet is now placed high on the patient's arm and set to 250 mmHG.

Once positioning is completed, the operative arm is prepped circumferentially with an alcohol-based prep solution from fingers to tourniquet. After the surgical prep is completed, the surgical team is now able to sterilely drape the operative arm. A sterile large drape is laid on top of the hand table underneath the raised operative arm. A sterile blue towel is placed securely around the operative arm at the base of the tourniquet. A towel clip is used to secure the ends of the blue towel together. Next, a sterile impervious stockinette is placed over the hand. This is utilized only during the draping procedure to cover the fingers of the patient. Most surgeons will remove the stockinette when finished draping to have access to the thumb for pulling traction. Next, an upper extremity drape is placed on the patient. The hole of the extremity drape is passed over the hand up to the operative arm's elbow. A rolled towel is placed in the dorsum of the hand to mimic a fist, then the operative arm is exsanguinated with an Esmarch®. After exsanguination, the tourniquet is inflated.

Surgical Procedure

- With a 15 blade an incision is made on the radial side at the base of the thumb over the trapezium.

- The SA can use a double skin hook or a set of Ragnell retractors to hold back the skin.

- With a pair of Stevens tenotomy scissors, a blunt dissection is carried out; be careful to identify and safeguard the dorsal radial sensory nerve. This can then be retracted back with the skin. It is important to identify the radial artery.

- The joint capsule is opened, and the trapezium is dissected out. Drill holes can be placed in the bone to make it easier to rongeur out (see Figure 19-16).

- A 0.62 K-wire can be driven in with a pin driver to use as a joystick and a 6900 Beaver blade may be used to dissect the trapezium out.

- At the base of the cavity, you should be able to identify the FCR tendon. It needs to be identified and followed up the arm.

- Tiny horizontal incisions can be made, one just proximal to the wrist joint and one midway up the arm in the skin, just above the FCR.

- A hemostat may be used to dig into the incision and pull out the tendon, resting it on the tines of the hemostat.

- Once the FCR is identified it is cut at the midpoint of the palmar side of the arm. The hemostats are then used to strip the FCR attachments down to the incision over the CMC joint.

- The FCP is brought into the CMC joint.

- A hole is drilled at a 35° to 45° angle in the base of the metacarpal from the proximal base into the shaft on the opposite side of the bone. This is to allow the FCR tendon to be passed into and then back out of the bone. This is done to stabilize the joint and prevent the joint from collapse.

- It is then attached to itself to prevent it from going back through the tunnel.

- The use of a running (sewing) stich is utilized to weave in and out up the length of the tendon. You should be able to identify the radial artery in the cavity before filling the space, as not to put compression on it.

- Pull the tendon down on itself to accordion what is left and push it into the cavity, effectively filling the space.

- The wound is then copiously irrigated.

- The capsule is then closed, careful not to damage the radial nerve when closing the capsule and skin.

Dressings. After final closure, the SA will apply the dressings. Dermabond® is used to seal the incision and given time to dry. A 4 × 4 gauze is placed over the incision and a 4-inch cotton roll is used from hand to elbow. A thumb Spica splint or cast is applied, and a 3-inch ace is wrapped from hand to elbow to

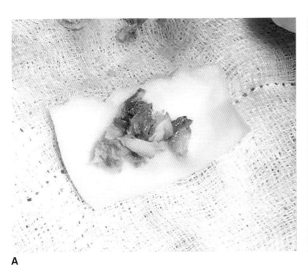
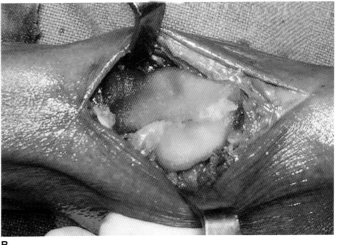

A   **B**

Figure 19-16 · Arthroplasty operative technique. (A) Trapezium crushed and put inside a sponge covering. (B) Trapezium graft put inside the cavity created after trapeziectomy. (Reproduced, with permission, from Kapoor C, Kansagra A, Jhaveri M, et al. First carpo-metacarpal joint arthritis: Interpositional arthroplasty using trapezium. *Cureus.* 2016;8(11):e861.)

hold the splint in place. Some surgeons will choose to use a carpal tunnel splint instead of creating a plaster splint.

Postop Complications. Surgical complications include infections and nerve damage.

Fasciotomy

Anatomic compartments organize the muscles, arteries, nerves, and veins of the extremities. These compartments are separated by thick fascia, which inhibits expansion when swelling occurs. If extensive swelling occurs in a compartment, the pressure builds which leads to the compression of the vessels. This compression is called compartment syndrome. Compartment syndrome is categorized as acute or chronic. Acute compartment syndrome occurs following a crush injury, high impact trauma, fracture, or reperfusion after ischemia. Chronic compartment syndrome develops after overuse of the muscles in the extremities, so body builders, runners and the military are at risk. When the compartment syndrome continues without relief, the ischemia leads to muscle and nerve necrosis and potential amputation. To relieve the pressure, incisions are made in the surrounding fascia which allows for the expansion of the muscle. This is called a fasciotomy and is considered an emergency procedure.

Anatomy. The upper extremity is divided into three sections: the upper arm, the forearm, and the hand. The upper arm contains two compartments: the anterior and the posterior compartments. The anterior compartment contains the biceps brachii, coracobrachialis, and brachialis muscles. These are innervated by the musculocutaneous nerve and supplied by branches of the brachial artery. The posterior compartment contains the triceps brachii muscle, radial nerve, and the profunda brachii artery. The forearm is most often affected by compartment syndrome, and it is divided into four compartments: superficial volar, deep volar, dorsal compartment, and the mobile wad of Henry. The superficial volar compartment contains the FCU, FCR, pronator teres, palmaris longus, FDS muscle, ulnar nerve, and ulnar artery. The deep volar compartment consists of the flexor digitorum profundus, flexor pollicis longus, pronator quadratus muscle, median nerve, and the anterior interosseous artery and nerve. The dorsal compartment contains the extensor digitorum, EDM, ECU, supinator, extensor indicis, extensor pollicis longus and brevis, abductor pollicis longus muscle, and the posterior interosseous artery and nerve. The mobile wad of Henry contains the brachioradialis, extensor carpi radialis longus and brevis muscles, and the radial artery and nerve. The hand is divided into ten different anatomic compartments. These compartments include four dorsal interossei muscle compartments, three palmar interossei muscle compartments, a thenar and hypothenar compartment and the adductor pollicis muscle compartment.

The lower extremity is divided into three sections: the upper leg, the lower leg, and the foot. The upper leg has three compartments: the anterior, posterior and adductor compartments. The anterior compartment contains the quadriceps and sartorius muscle with the femoral nerve. The posterior compartment contains the semitendinosus, semimembranosus, and the biceps femoris muscles with the sciatic nerve. The adductor compartment contains the gracilis, obturator externus, adductor brevis, adductor longus and adductor magnus muscles with the obturator nerve. The lower leg is divided into four compartments: anterior, lateral, superficial posterior, and deep posterior. The anterior compartment contains the tibialis anterior, extensor hallucis longus, extensor digitorum longus, peroneus tertius muscles, the deep fibular nerve, and the anterior tibial artery. The lateral compartment contains the peroneus long and tertius muscles with the superficial fibular nerve and fibular artery. The superficial posterior compartment contains the gastrocnemius, soleus, and plantaris muscles with the sural nerve. The deep posterior compartment contains the tibialis posterior, flexor hallucis longus, flexor digitorum longus, and popliteus muscles. The tibial nerve and posterior tibial artery run along this compartment also. The foot is divided into nine main compartments. The medial compartment contains the abductor hallucis and flexor hallucis brevis muscles. The lateral compartment contains the abductor digiti minimi and flexor digiti minimi brevis muscles. There are four distinct interosseous compartments containing each interosseous muscle. The central compartment is further divided into three separate compartments. The superficial compartment contains the flexor digitorum brevis muscle. The central compartment contains the quadratus plantae muscle and the deep compartment contains the adductor hallucis muscle with the posterior tibial neurovascular bundle.

Etiology. When a patient presents with swelling in an extremity, the surgeon needs to determine if the swelling indeed caused compartment syndrome. The common signs of compartment syndrome are pain, pallor, paresthesia, pulselessness, and paralysis. If an extremity exhibits these symptoms, then a compartment pressure test is performed using a needle manometer system. For each compartment of the extremity, a needle is inserted in the muscle of each compartment to measure the intercompartmental pressure. Normal compartment pressure is 0 to 8 mm of mercury. A compartment pressure measuring 30 mm of mercury or higher is the standard threshold to diagnose compartment syndrome and a fasciotomy needs to be performed emergently to prevent irreversible limb ischemia.

Surgical Considerations of the Upper Arm. When the upper arm presents with compartment syndrome, a medial incision is created to access both the anterior and posterior compartments. After the skin incision, the medial intermuscular septum is identified and incised. The fascia of the biceps brachii muscle is incised to release the anterior compartment and the triceps brachii muscle fascia is incised to release the posterior compartment.

Depending on the compartment effected, a volar and/or dorsal incision is created to relived compartment syndrome of the forearm. For the volar incision, the skin is incised on the radial side of the FCU muscle and extended to the medial epicondyle of the humerus. The incision is completed distally across the wrist toward the hypothenar eminence, which completes a carpal tunnel release. Completing a carpal tunnel release is important to prevent injury to the median nerve from the increased pressure. The superficial fascial compartment is identified and incised. The ulnar neurovascular bundle and FDS muscle is retracted medially to expose the deep fascial compartment. To release the deep fascial compartment, an incision is made into the flexor digitorum profundus fascia. These fascial releases extend the length of the skin incision to ensure adequate release of the compartment. For the dorsal incision, a skin incision is made between the EDC and extensor carpi radialis brevis muscles from the wrist to the lateral epicondyle. The mobile wad of Henry fascia can now be released, and further dissection exposes the extensor retinaculum. Incising the extensor retinaculum allows for the release of the posterior compartment.

Surgical Considerations of the Hand. Because of the multiple compartments the make up the hand, many different approaches are available to correct the compartment syndrome. The interosseous compartments and adductor compartments are released using dorsal skin incisions. Two dorsal incisions are created, one over the second metacarpal and one over the fourth metacarpal. Both sides of each metacarpal bones are dissected to release all the interosseous compartments. To decompress the thenar compartment, an incision is created along the first metacarpal bone on the radial side. An incision created along the fifth metacarpal bone releases the hypothenar compartment.

Surgical Considerations of the Lower Extremity. When the upper leg presents with compartment syndrome, an anterolateral incision extending the length of the thigh is necessary. After the skin incision is completed, the tensor fascia lata is incised, which exposes the anterior compartment for decompression. The vastus lateralis muscle is retracted medially to uncover the lateral intermuscular septum. The septum is incised, which decompresses the posterior compartment. If the adductor compartment also needs release, then a medial incision may be added.

When the lower leg presents with compartment syndrome, a double incision fasciotomy is performed. A 20-cm anterolateral skin incision is created along anterior intermuscular septum located between the tibial crest and fibular. After the skin incision, the anterior intramuscular septum is incised which exposes the anterior and lateral compartments. To release the posterior compartment, a 20-cm posteromedial incision is made along the tibia beginning 2 cm superiorly to the medial malleolus. Dissection continues down to the posterior fascial compartment, careful to avoid the long saphenous vein and the saphenous nerve. The posterior fascial compartment is incised as well as the fascia overlying the flexor digitorum longus muscle.

When the foot presents with compartment syndrome, the standard release technique is to use a dual dorsal incision. A dorsal medial incision is created medial to the second metatarsal. This incision releases the first and second interosseous, medial, and deep central compartments. Next, a dorsal lateral incision is created lateral to the fourth metatarsal. This incision

releases the third and fourth interosseous, lateral, superficial, and middle central compartments. After each skin incision is created, the dorsal fascia of each interosseous compartment is incised, which alleviates the pressure in the compartments.

Postop Considerations. Following the fasciotomy, the incisions are dressed loosely with a wet to dry dressing. A loose dressing is necessary to avoid any external pressure on the compartments. After 48 hours, the fasciotomy incisions are evaluated for closure if the compartments are soft. Typically, surgeons will wait 1 to 2 weeks post-fasciotomy to ensure compartment pressures will stay normal after the closure. Primary closure of the incisions is the goal; however, skin grafting may occur if the extremity is too swollen for approximation of the incision edges. Primary closure involves a two-layer closure. The dermis being closed utilizing an interrupted deep buried suture technique with a 3-0 absorbable braided suture. The skin is then approximated with a 3-0 or 2-0 nonabsorbable monofilament. Alternating interrupted suture techniques of vertical mattress and simple interrupted are utilized. Delayed primary closure techniques may be utilized to avoid skin grafting. Silastic vessel loops anchored across the incision in a shoelace pattern creates tension on the skin edges which slowly allow the edges to come closer together. These loops are anchored using skin staples. Negative wound pressure therapy can also aide in approximating the skin edges. The delayed primary closure techniques require multiple trips to the OR and more time spent in the hospital. Ultimately, these techniques prevent the need to skin grafting in about 50% of fasciotomy patients, which helps the patient's cosmesis and overall healing from the compartment syndrome.

Postop Complications. Following the fasciotomy, patients are at risk of various complications depending on the severity of the compartment syndrome. Acute renal failure is common because of the muscle necrosis which can lead to rhabdomyolysis. Nerve damage and limb weakness may occur due to the swelling of the compartments and muscle death. Delayed or incomplete fasciotomies may lead to the amputation of the extremity. The patient also may have wound healing complications following fasciotomies. Muscle herniation, dehiscence, and infection are all potential complications. Cosmetically, fasciotomy incisions result in extensive scarring due to the size of the incisions are well as the need for skin grafting. The extremity will not look the same postoperatively and for some patients that is difficult to manage.

Bibliography

Andrews K, Rowland A, Pranjal A, Ebraheim N. Cubital tunnel syndrome: anatomy, clinical presentation, and management. *J Orthop.* 2018 Aug 16;15(3):832-836. doi: 10.1016/j.jor.2018.08.010. Erratum in: *J Orthop.* 2020 Dec 14;23:275. PMID: 30140129; PMCID: PMC6104141.

Anesthesia Considerations for Arthroscopic Shoulder Surgery. OBS Anesthesia Management Groups (radiusanesthesia.com). Ambulatory Anesthesia Services | OBS Anesthesia Management Groups (radiusanesthesia.com)

Arthur JR, Spangehl MJ. Tourniquet use in total knee arthroplasty. *J Knee Surg.* 2019 Aug;32(8):719-729. doi: 10.1055/s-0039-1681035. Epub 2019 Mar 1. PMID: 30822788.

Baker DK, Perez JL, Watson SL, et al. Arthroscopic versus open rotator cuff repair: which has a better complication and 30-day readmission profile? *Arthroscopy.* 2017 Oct;33(10):1764-1769. doi: 10.1016/j.arthro.2017.04.019. Epub 2017 Jul 5. PMID: 28688827.

Bankart Lesion. Health Jade Team. Bankart lesion causes, symptoms, diagnosis & treatment (healthjade.net)

Bankart Lesion. Physiopedia (physio-pedia.com). Bankart lesion - Physiopedia (physio-pedia.com)

Brislin KJ, Field LD, Savoie FH 3rd. Complications after arthroscopic rotator cuff repair. *Arthroscopy.* 2007 Feb;23(2):124-128. doi: 10.1016/j.arthro.2006.09.001. PMID: 17276218.

Chambers AR, Dreyer MA. Triple arthrodesis. [Updated 2022 Jan 9]. In: StatPearls [Internet]. Treasure Island (FL): StatPearls Publishing; 2022 Jan. Available from: https://www.ncbi.nlm.nih.gov/books/NBK551713/

Chandraprakasam T, Kumar RA. Acute compartment syndrome of forearm and hand. *Indian J Plast Surg.* 2011;44(2):212-218. https://doi.org/10.4103/0970-0358.85342

Chua MJ, Hart AJ, Mittal R, Harris IA, Xuan W, Naylor JM. Early mobilisation after total hip or knee arthroplasty: a multicentre prospective observational study. *PloS One.* 2017;12(6):e0179820. https://doi.org/10.1371/journal.pone.0179820

Cluett J. What you should know about Smith Fractures. Updated on March 25, 2021. Smith's Fracture, or Volar Displacement of Broken Wrist (verywellhealth.com)

Cluett J. Anatomy of the Knee. Updated on August 22, 2020. Knee Anatomy: Bones, Muscles, Tendons, and Ligaments (verywellhealth.com)

Cluett J. SLAP Repair Surgery for a Labral Tear. SLAP Repair Surgery for a Labral Tear (verywellhealth.com)

Cutts S. Cubital tunnel syndrome. *Postgrad Med J.* 2007;83(975):28-31. https://doi.org/10.1136/pgmj.2006.047456

Dawson-Amoah K, Raszewski J, Duplantier N, Waddell BS. Dislocation of the hip: a review of types, causes, and treatment. *The Ochsner J.* 2018;18(3):242-252. https://doi.org/10.31486/toj.17.0079

Del Buono A, Chan O, Maffulli N. Achilles tendon: functional anatomy and novel emerging models of imaging classification. *Int Orthop.* 2013;37(4):715-721. https://doi.org/10.1007/s00264-012-1743-y

Dermofasciectomy. Dupuytren Foundation. Dermofasciectomy | Dupuytren Research Group (dupuytrens.org)

Ejnisman B, Belangero PS. Patient Positioning and Anesthesia for Rotator Cuff Surgery. Musculoskeletal Key Patient Positioning and Anesthesia for Rotator Cuff Surgery | Musculoskeletal Key

Familiari F, Rojas J, Nedim Doral M, Huri G, McFarland EG. Reverse total shoulder arthroplasty. *EFORT Open Rev.* 2018;3(2):58-69. https://doi.org/10.1302/2058-5241.3.170044.

Fisher ES, Goodman DC, Chandra A. Disparities in health and health care among medicare beneficiaries: a brief report of the Dartmouth Atlas Project. Lebanon (NH): The Dartmouth Institute for Health Policy and Clinical Practice; 2008 Jun 20. PMID: 36454933.

Hoffman M. Picture of the Shoulder. Shoulder Human Anatomy: Image, Function, Parts, and More (webmd.com)

http://synthes.vo.llnwd.net/o16/Mobile/Synthes%20International/KYO/Trauma/PDFs/036.000.519.pdf. Accessed July 14, 2023.

http://www.osteosyntese.dk/LCP%20CONDYLAR%20PLATE%2045-50.pdf. Accessed July 14, 2023.

https://emedicine.medscape.com/article/824224-overview

https://surgicalreference.aofoundation.org/orthopedic-trauma/adult-trauma/tibial-shaft/simple-fracture-spiral/intramedullary-nail. Accessed July 14, 2023.

https://teachmeanatomy.info/lower-limb/bones/femur/. Accessed February 4, 2022.

https://teachmeanatomy.info/upper-limb/bones/radius/. Accessed July 14, 2023.

https://teachmeanatomy.info/upper-limb/muscles/upper-arm/ accessed January 23, 2022.

https://www.amputee-coalition.org/resources/limb-loss-statistics. Accessed July 14, 2023.

https://www.orthobullets.com/basic-science/9063/orthopaedic-implants. Accessed July 14, 2023.

https://www.orthobullets.com/hand/6034/scaphoid-fracture. Accessed July 14, 2023.

https://www.orthobullets.com/hand/6037/metacarpal-fractures. Accessed July 14, 2023.

https://www.orthobullets.com/knee-and-sports/3010/mcl-knee-injuries. Accessed July 14, 2023.

https://www.orthobullets.com/recon/12769/hip-anatomy. Accessed July 14, 2023.

https://www.orthobullets.com/recon/3001/ligaments-of-the-knee. Accessed July 14, 2023.

https://www.orthobullets.com/recon/5003/tha-implant-fixation. Accessed July 14, 2023.

https://www.orthobullets.com/recon/5009/tha-revision. Accessed July 14, 2023.

https://www.orthobullets.com/recon/5013/tha-periprosthetic-fracture. Accessed July 14, 2023.

https://www.orthobullets.com/recon/5021/tka-revision. Accessed July 14, 2023.

https://www.orthobullets.com/recon/5031/tka-approaches. Accessed July 14, 2023.

https://www.orthobullets.com/recon/9065/knee-biomechanics. Accessed July 14, 2023.

https://www.orthobullets.com/shoulder-and-elbow/12268/bankart-repair-with-capsular-plication-arthroscopic. Accessed July 14, 2023.

https://www.orthobullets.com/shoulder-and-elbow/3043/rotator-cuff-tears. Accessed July 14, 2023.

https://www.orthobullets.com/shoulder-and-elbow/3053/slap-lesion. Accessed July 14, 2023.

https://www.orthobullets.com/shoulder-and-elbow/3075/total-shoulder-arthroplasty. Accessed July 14, 2023.

https://www.orthobullets.com/trauma/1001/leg-compartment-syndrome. Accessed July 14, 2023.

https://www.orthobullets.com/trauma/1030/pelvic-ring-fractures. Accessed July 14, 2023.

https://www.orthobullets.com/trauma/1037/femoral-neck-fractures. Accessed July 14, 2023.

https://www.orthobullets.com/trauma/1038/intertrochanteric-fractures. Accessed July 14, 2023.

https://www.orthobullets.com/trauma/1039/subtrochanteric-fractures. Accessed July 14, 2023.

https://www.orthobullets.com/trauma/1040/femoral-shaft-fractures.

https://www.orthobullets.com/trauma/1041/distal-femur-fractures. Accessed July 14, 2023.

https://www.orthobullets.com/trauma/1044/tibial-plateau-fractures. Accessed July 14, 2023.

https://www.orthobullets.com/trauma/1045/tibial-shaft-fractures. Accessed July 14, 2023.

https://www.orthobullets.com/trauma/1046/tibial-plafond-fractures. Accessed July 14, 2023.

https://www.orthobullets.com/trauma/1062/proximal-third-tibia-fractures. Accessed July 14, 2023.

https://www.orthobullets.com/trauma/1063/thigh-compartment-syndrome. Accessed January 28, 2022.

https://www.orthobullets.com/trauma/1065/foot-compartment-syndrome. Accessed January 28, 2022.

https://www.orthobullets.com/trauma/12076/tibial-intramedullary-nail. Accessed July 14, 2023.

https://www.orthobullets.com/trauma/12184/proximal-humerus-fracture-orif. Accessed July 14, 2023.

https://www.orthobullets.com/trauma/12190/humerus-shaft-fracture-orif-with-anterolateral-approach. Accessed July 14, 2023.

https://www.orthobullets.com/trauma/12191/humerus-shaft-orif-with-posterior-approach. Accessed July 14, 2023.

https://www.orthobullets.com/trauma/12219/distal-humerus-fracture-orif. Accessed July 14, 2023.

https://www.orthobullets.com/trauma/12222/olecranon-fracture-orif-with-plate-fixation. Accessed July 14, 2023.

https://www.orthobullets.com/trauma/12223/distal-radius-intraarticular-fracture-orif-with-dorsal-approach. Accessed July 14, 2023.

https://www.orthobullets.com/trauma/12290/both-bone-forearm-fracture-orif. Accessed July 14, 2023.

https://www.uptodate.com/contents/acute-compartment-syndrome-of-the-extremities#H15. Accessed January 28, 2022.

https://www.uptodate.com/contents/complications-of-total-knee-arthroplasty. Accessed July 14, 2023.

https://www.uptodate.com/contents/total-knee-arthroplasty. Accessed July 14, 2023.

https://www.vastortho.com/herbert-screws/. Accessed July 14, 2023.

John Hopkins Medicine. Cubital Tunnel Syndrome. Cubital Tunnel Syndrome | Johns Hopkins Medicine

JOMI. Ulnar Nerve Transposition. Ulnar Nerve Transposition | Journal of Medical Insight (jomi.com)

Knight SR, Aujla R, Biswas SP. Total hip arthroplasty: over 100 years of operative history. *Orthopedic Rev.* 2011;3(2):e16. https://doi.org/10.4081/or.2011.e16

Kuroda S, Ishige N, Mikasa M. Advantages of arthroscopic transosseous suture repair of the rotator cuff without the use of anchors. *Clin. Orthop. Relat. Res.* 2018;471(11):3514-3522. https://doi.org/10.1007/s11999-013-3148-7

Li X, Orvets ND. Arthroscopic ACL reconstruction with bone patellar bone graft using anteromedial technique. *J Med Insight.* 2016,2016(45). https://jomi.com/article/45/arthroscopic-acl-reconstruction-btb-autograft-using-anteromedial-technique. Accessed July 14, 2023.

Li YS, Chen CY, Lin KC, Tarng YW, Hsu CJ, Chang WN. Open reduction and internal fixation of ankle fracture using wide-awake local anaesthesia no tourniquet technique. *Injury.* 2019 Apr;50(4):990-994. doi: 10.1016/j.injury.2019.03.011. Epub 2019 Mar 11. PMID: 30904247.

Longo U, Petrillo S, Loppini M. et al. Metallic versus biodegradable suture anchors for rotator cuff repair: a case control study. *BMC Musculoskelet Disord.* 2019;20:477. https://doi.org/10.1186/s12891-019-2834-3

Mak MF, Stern R, Assal M. Repair of syndesmosis injury in ankle fractures: current state of the art. *EFORT Open Rev.* 2018;3(1):24-29. https://doi.org/10.1302/2058-5241.3.170017

Marissa Selner. Congenital Hip Disorder. Updated on July 8, 2017. Congenital Hip Dislocation: Causes, Symptoms, and Diagnosis (healthline.com)

Mathews AL, Chung KC. Management of complications of distal radius fractures. *Hand Clinics.* 2015;31(2):205-215. https://doi.org/10.1016/j.hcl.2014.12.002

McClawhorn AS. What Is Congenital Hip Disorder?. Hip Dysplasia & SCFE Treatment & Surgery in Stamford, CT & NYC (drmclawhorn.com)

Moretti VM, Post ZD. Surgical approaches for total hip arthroplasty. *Indian J Orthop.* 2017;51(4):368-376. https://doi.org/10.4103/ortho.IJOrtho_317_16

Myers M, Chauvin BJ. Above-the-Knee Amputations. [Updated 2022 Jun 21]. In: StatPearls [Internet]. Treasure Island (FL): StatPearls Publishing; 2023 Jan. https://www.ncbi.nlm.nih.gov/books/NBK544350/. Accessed July 14, 2023.

Pandian G, Hamid F, Hammond M. Rehabilitation of the patient with peripheral vascular disease and diabetic foot problems. In: DeLisa JA, Gans BM, editors. Philadelphia: Lippincott-Raven; 1998.

Ranawat CS. History of total knee replacement. *J South Orthop Assoc.* 2002 Winter;11(4):218-226. PMID: 12597066.

Robbins JM, Strauss G, Aron D, Long J, Kuba J, Kaplan Y. Mortality rates and diabetic foot ulcers. *J Am Podiatr Med Assoc.* 2008 Nov;98(6):489-493.

Rossi LA, Rodeo SA, Chahla J, Ranalletta M. Current concepts in rotator cuff repair techniques: biomechanical, functional, and structural outcomes. *Orthopaedic J Sports Med.* 2019;7(9):2325967119868674. https://doi.org/10.1177/2325967119868674

Rotator Cuff Injury. Rotator cuff injury - Diagnosis and treatment - Mayo Clinic

Roussel R, Kelley D, Marek A, et al. Total Shoulder Arthroplasty. Physiopedia (physio-pedia.com). Total Shoulder Arthroplasty - Physiopedia (physio-pedia.com)

Sanchez-Sotelo J. Total shoulder arthroplasty. *The Open Orthopaedics J.* 2011;5:106-114. https://doi.org/10.2174/1874325001105010106

Scheer RC, Newman JM, Zhou JJ, et al. Ankle fracture epidemiology in the United States: patient-related trends and mechanisms of injury. *J Foot Ankle Surg.* 2020 May-Jun;59(3):479-483. doi: 10.1053/j.jfas.2019.09.016. PMID: 32354504.

Schroeder SM, Thomson JD. Triple Arthrodesis. Medscape. Triple Arthrodesis: Background, Indications, Contraindications (medscape.com)

Screws. Wheeless' Textbook of Orthopaedics. wheelessonline.com). https://www.wheelessonline.com/bones/hand/screws/. Accessed July 14, 2023.

Tantigate D, Ho G, Kirschenbaum J, et al. Timing of open reduction and internal fixation of ankle fractures. *Foot Ankle Spec.* 2019 Oct;12(5):401-408. doi: 10.1177/1938640018810419. Epub 2018 Nov 14. PMID: 30426777.

Tejwani N, Polonet D, Wolinsky PR. External fixation of tibial fractures. *J Am Acad Orthop Surg.* 2015 Feb;23(2):126-130. doi: 10.5435/JAAOS-D-14-00158. Epub 2015 Jan 21. PMID: 25613987.

Tibone JE. Anterior Shoulder Instability: Arthroscopic Suture Anchor Repair of the Bankart Lesion. https://musculoskeletalkey.com/anterior-shoulder-instability-arthroscopic-suture-anchor-repair-of-the-bankart-lesion/

Tjoumakaris FP, Herz-Brown AL, Bowers AL, Sennett BJ, Bernstein J. Complications in brief: Anterior cruciate ligament reconstruction. *Clin. Orthop. Relat. Res.* 2012;470(2):630-636. https://doi.org/10.1007/s11999-011-2153-y

Total Shoulder Arthroplasty. https://www.mayoclinic.org/tests-procedures/shoulder-replacement/about/pac-20519121

Tyagi A, Salhotra R. Total hip arthroplasty and peripheral nerve blocks: limited but salient role? *J Anaesthesiol Clinic Pharmacol.* 2018;34(3):379-380. https://doi.org/10.4103/joacp.JOACP_114_18

Ulnar Nerve Transposition at the Elbow. Neurosurgical Associates, PC. Ulnar Nerve Transposition at the Elbow - Birmingham, AL - Spine and Neurosurgery (neurosurgicalassociatespc.com)

UW Ortho and Sports Medicine. Bankart Repair. UW Orthopaedics and Sports Medicine, Seattle. Bankart Repair for Unstable Dislocating Shoulders | UW Orthopaedics and Sports Medicine, Seattle (https://www.uwmedicine.org/specialties/orthopedics-sports-medicine)

Vahldick Z. Shoulder Labral Injuries: SLAP and Bankart Lesions. Labral Tears: SLAP and Bankart Lesions : Branson Chiropractic and Rehab (https://www.uwmedicine.org/specialties/orthopedics-sports-medicine)

Varacallo M, Luo TD, Johanson NA. Total Knee Arthroplasty Techniques. [Updated 2021 Jul 31]. In: StatPearls [Internet]. Treasure Island (FL): StatPearls Publishing; 2021 Jan. Available from: https://www.ncbi.nlm.nih.gov/books/NBK499896/

Ward BD, Lubowitz JH. Basic knee arthroscopy part 1: patient positioning. *Arthroscopy Techniques.* 2013;2(4):e497-e499. https://doi.org/10.1016/j.eats.2013.07.010

Watson JT. External Fixation of the Tibia. Musculoskeletal Key. External Fixation of the Tibia | Musculoskeletal Key. Accessed July 14, 2023.

What Is Cubital Tunnel Syndrome? Medically reviewed by Klinefelter RD. OrthoNeuro. Ulnar Neuritis (Cubital Tunnel Syndrome) | Columbus, OH (orthoneuro.com)

Wilson C. Shoulder Pain Explained. Bankart Lesion. Bankart Lesion: Causes, Symptoms & Treatment (shoulder-pain-explained.com)

www.morthoj.org/2014/v8n2/cannulated-screw-fixation.pdf. Accessed July 14, 2023.

Ziegler-Graham K, MacKenzie EJ, Ephraim PL, Travison TG, Brookmeyer R. Estimating the prevalence of limb loss in the United States: 2005 to 2050. *Arch Phys Med Rehabil.* 2008;89(3):422-429.

20

Plastic and Reconstructive Surgery

Jessica Wilhelm

DISCUSSED IN THIS CHAPTER

1. The complexity of plastic surgery
2. Common cosmetic procedures
3. Cosmetic correction of birth defects
4. Breast surgery following cancer

INTRODUCTION

This chapter introduces the student to the complexity of plastic surgery and the important role surgical assistants (SAs) play during these procedures. The student will learn that plastic surgery involves all components of the body from the face to the feet. Plastic surgery solves cosmetic issues for the patient, as well as reconstructing defects for the patient caused by cancer or trauma. A highly trained SA allows for successful dissections and incision closures during plastic surgery procedures.

RHYTIDECTOMY

A rhytidectomy, or facelift as it is commonly referred to, is the surgical solution for the aging face. As a person ages, the skin and subcutaneous structures begin to drop giving the patient an older appearance. The facelift removes and suspends these structures to regain the patient's youthful appearance. In 2019 almost 70,000 facelifts were performed in the United States. Most facelift patients are female; however, males make up about 5% of the surgical patients.

The facelift procedure was first described in the early 1900s by Eugene von Hollander. Many other surgeons, including American Charles Miller, began publishing facelift techniques over the next 10 years. After World War I, the interest in rhytidectomy procedures increased due to war injuries requiring reconstructive surgery. Until the 1960s, the techniques focused primarily on the skin excision; however, Aufricht in 1960 described the need to suspend the deep tissues during the facelift. Further modifications of the techniques came over the next few decades and focus more today on minimally invasive techniques.

Anatomy of the Face

The face consists of multiple layers of tissue with the most superficial layer being the skin. Immediately following the skin is the superficial musculoaponeurotic system (SMAS). The SMAS consists of the platysma muscle, parotid fascia, and cheek fibromuscular layer and it connects the facial muscles to the dermis. This connection enhances facial muscle activity and expression. The SMAS is found superior to the platysma muscle and inferior to the zygomatic arch. The next layers are the superficial and deep temporal fascia, then the galea aponeurotic along the upper face. Retaining ligaments are found connecting the deep layers of the face to the superficial layers. These ligaments play a vital role in fixating facial movements and respond to the pull of gravity during the aging process.

Numerous facial muscles work together to perform various facial movements. Beginning superiorly, the frontalis muscle is found on the front bone, and the orbicularis oculi muscle is found around the eye. These muscles are key for the movement of the eyebrows. Laterally are the temporalis and masseter muscles, which are responsible for mandibular movement and chewing. Inferiorly is the platysma muscle. The platysma inserts at the base of the mandible and side of cheek, then extends down the neck. The platysma is responsible for lowering the mandible and stretching the lower face skin.

The neurovascular supply to the face consists mainly of the facial artery, vein, and nerve. The facial artery branches into the masseteric, superior labial, inferior labial, and lateral nasal artery. The superior face however is innervated by the superficial temporal artery and the maxillary artery, which are the terminal branches of the external carotid artery. The facial vein drains the face with branches that correspond with the arterial branches of the face. The facial nerve, also known as cranial nerve seven, arrives at the face below the tragus of the ear and then branches deep into the SMAS. The facial nerve branches consist of the temporal, zygomatic, buccal, marginal mandibular, and cervical, all of which cross through the parotid gland to innervate their respective areas of the face and neck. The greater auricular nerve is important to identify as it runs along the sternocleidomastoid muscle and branches superficially at the parotid gland to innervate the auricle.

Anesthesia

Depending on the complexity of the rhytidectomy, the patient may be placed under either general anesthesia or conscious sedation. If the patient needs general anesthesia, the endotracheal tube needs to be secured in the center of the chin and the circuit placed down the patient's chest. This allows the surgeon easier access to the bilateral sides of the patient's face. If the patient qualifies for conscious sedation anesthesia, the patient will be given a mild sedative and use a local anesthetic to anesthetize the surgical area. The patient under conscious sedation will not be intubated for the procedure, which can give the surgeon better access to the entirety of the face.

Patient Positioning and Skin Prep

After the patient is anesthetized, the patient's arms are tucked at their sides using padding at the elbow to protect the ulnar nerve. The head is placed on a gel ring pillow, which gives the surgeon better access to the lateral portions of the face. The operating room bed is then turned between 90 and 180 degrees away from anesthesia. Moving the bed gives the surgeon more access to the patient's head and prevents the anesthesia machine from being in the way during the procedure. Once positioned, the patient's entire face is prepped with a betadine solution. The prep is extended into the hairline and down to clavicles. Both ears down to the bed are also included in the prepped area.

Draping

Once an adequate prep is achieved, the surgical field is draped. The head is lifted by the circulating nurse which allows the SA to place a folded in half large drape with a blue towel underneath head. The towel and the top half of the large drape are then wrapped around the head, excluding the hair and scalp from the sterile field. This allows the surgeon to manipulate the head from right to left without potentially contaminating the field with unsterile hair. Next, two balled blue towels are placed at the top of each shoulder and three blue towels are placed around the face. The endotracheal tube is wrapped with a blue towel and one split sheet drape is used to complete the sterile field.

Surgical Procedure

Before incisions are made, the surgeon injects the surgical sites with a local anesthetic. The local anesthetic can be either lidocaine or marcaine; however, it needs to contain epinephrine. The epinephrine will constrict blood vessels to aid in hemostasis during the procedure, and the local anesthetic confers pain relief to the surgical sites. Injection occurs not only at the incision sites but also along the area of dissection of the bilateral cheeks.

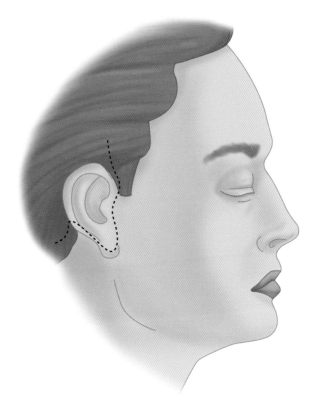

Figure 20-1 · Rhytidectomy incision. (Reproduced, with permission, from Brunicardi FC et al, eds. *Schwartz's Principles of Surgery.* 11th ed. New York, NY: McGraw Hill; 2019.)

- The surgical incisions are created on bilateral sides of the patient along the border of the ear. The incision starts below temporal hairline along the helix of the ear (see Figure 20-1). If the patient is female, the surgeon will make the incision behind the tragus; however, if the patient is male the incision is made in front of the tragus. Making the incision behind the tragus prevents the hairline to be pulled closer to the ear. The incision is extended downward along the tragus and around the ear lobe. If an extensive skin excision is necessary, the incision is continued along the postauricular sulcus to the mastoid and extended along the occipital hairline. The goal of the incision is to allow for adequate dissection, while hiding the incision in the natural lines of the face.

- After incisions are created, skin flaps are dissected from the zygomatic arch medially to the nasolabial folds then inferiorly to the mandible. The surgeon uses any combination of scalpel, electrocautery, and tenotomy scissors. The SA retracts the skin flaps upward using Freeman facelift retractors. As the dissection progresses, the SA switches to a lighted bladed retractor, like an Aufricht retractor. The light allows the surgeon better visualization while dissecting the medial face.

- Care is taken during the skin undermining to protect the facial nerve and greater auricular nerve. If the patient's anatomy qualifies for it, the SMAS is lifted and plicated using a 3-0 suture. Surgeon's preference dictates whether a permanent or absorbable suture is used during the plication.

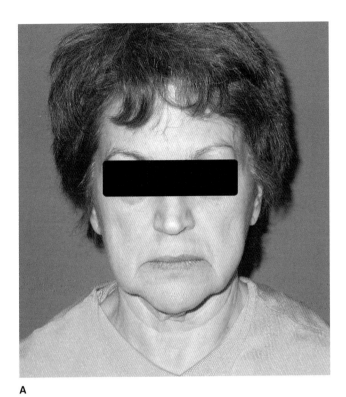

A

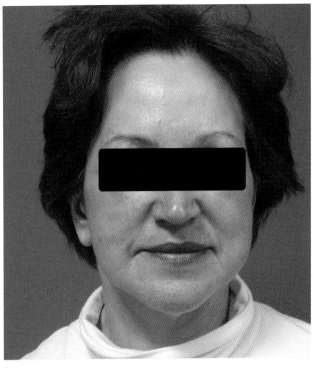

B

Figure 20-2 · Rhytidectomy before and after. (Reproduced, with permission, from Brunicardi FC et al, eds. *Schwartz's Principles of Surgery*. 11th ed. New York, NY: McGraw Hill; 2019.)

Plicating the SMAS addresses any deep tissue laxity and helps define the jawline.

- The platysma muscle also is manipulated during the dissection. The surgeon may choose to plicate any laxity of the platysma or transect the muscle.

- Once the undermining and plication are complete, the excess skin is excised. The surgeon will pull the skin over the ear to measure the amount of excess skin to remove, and marker is used to draw the excision line on the skin flap. Care is taken to ensure the direction the skin is pulled does not leave the patient with dog ears or bunching of the skin on the neck.

- The key is to avoid tension on the preauricular incision which will distort the ear anatomy.

- Drains are placed in the dissected region of the face and exit the postauricular region. The drains help prevent hematoma formation and are secured using a drain stitch. After the drain is placed, closure of the incisions begins.

- The incisions are closed using a 4-0 or 5-0 absorbable suture.

- Again, the surgeon's preferences will determine which closure technique is utilized. Some surgeons prefer simple interrupted sutures, whereas others prefer running techniques. Whichever closure technique is utilized, be sure to make small and deliberate bites to prevent extensive trauma to the skin near the incisions.

- Dressings vary based on surgeon's preferences. Surgeons may want minimal dressings with just bacitracin ointment covering the incisions. Some surgeons want compression over the surgical incisions. Four-by-four gauze and a four-inch

ace bandage wrapped around the face are used to achieve the compression. The drains are included in the wrap.

- Postoperatively, the patients experience minimal discomfort following the rhytidectomy. The patients have little pain; however, some bruising and swelling are expected. Complications of a rhytidectomy include hematoma, seroma, and facial nerve palsy. Patients may also experience hairline alterations, wound healing complications, and ear anatomy deformities. It is important to note that each patient's outcome is unique and appropriate patient counseling is necessary to tailor expectations (see Figure 20-2).

RHINOPLASTY

Rhinoplasty was first described by Sushruta in 600 B.C. to correct the defect left from criminal punishment in India. These patients had a rotational flap from the cheek placed over the raw nasal wound and allowed to heal over time. The modern description of a rhinoplasty is credited to John Orlando Roe in 1887. He published a paper "Correction of the Pug Deformity," which describes decreasing the volume of the nasal tip. Doctor Jacques Joseph is credited with being the "father of modern rhinoplasty" for continuing to develop techniques for improving the appearance of the nose as well as ensuring proper function of the nose. The American Rhinologic Society was founded in 1954 by Doctor Maurice Cottle who continued to pioneer nasal surgery with special interest in restoration of nasal physiology. Many other surgeons were involved in developing the modern techniques for rhinoplasty, notably Doctor Irving Goldman for the endonasal rhinoplasty and Doctor Jack Anderson for the external rhinoplasty.

Anatomy

The external nasal anatomy consists of the nasal root, dorsum, and tip. The nasal root runs continuously with the forehead and the tip is the rounded end of the nose. The dorsum connects the nasal root and nasal apex. Inferiorly to the nasal tip are the right and left nares. These form the openings into the nasal cavity, which is divided medially by the nasal septum and laterally by the nasal ala. The nasal ala is the external cartilaginous wing of the nose. The muscles that connect to the external nose are innervated by branches of the facial nerve. The nasalis muscle inserts into the major alar cartilage, which when contracted dilates the nares. At the most proximal portion of the nose, the procerus muscle originates at the nasal bone and lateral nasal cartilage then inserts into the inferior forehead. When the procerus muscle contracts, the medial eyebrows depress and the superior dorsum skin wrinkles. The skin and muscle of the external nose are supplied by branches of the maxillary and ophthalmic arteries. Branches of the facial artery, the angular and lateral nasal artery supply the septum and alar cartilages as well. The facial vein drains the external nose structures.

The skeletal anatomy of the nose consists of cartilage and bone. The most distal portion of the nose is comprised of cartilaginous structures. Nasal tip cartilage consists of upper lateral, lower lateral, middle crura, and medial crura cartilages. Behind the major alar cartilage sits the minor alar cartilages and the bridge of the nose consists of the septal cartilage. The septal cartilage connects the cartilaginous structures to the boney structures of the external nose. The boney structure of the external nose connects with paired nasal bones and paired maxillary bones. Internally, the septal cartilage connects with the ethmoid bone to complete the midline of the nose. Finally, the cribriform plate of the ethmoid bone creates the roof of the nasal cavity and the hard palate of the oral cavity creates the floor of the nasal cavity.

Rhinoplasty is traditionally considered a cosmetic procedure, where a patient seeks to change the shape and/or size of the nose. Some patients seek a rhinoplasty for medical reasons, such as a deviated septum, cleft lip, and cleft palate. Patients with a deviated septum will have difficulty breathing and will need a septoplasty to fix the breathing concerns. See the otolaryngology chapter for further description of the septoplasty. A cleft lip and cleft palate are birth defects that affect the child's ability to eat properly and must be repaired to have a better quality of life.

Anesthesia

Anesthesia options are reviewed with the patient prior to surgery. Most patients will be given general anesthesia with an endotracheal tube insertion. This allows the patient to be completely comfortable during the procedure with no risk of movement. Some patients however may qualify for sedation with local anesthesia. This form of anesthesia is given to patients with less complex rhinoplasties, and the local anesthesia will ensure the patient has a painless experience. Surgeons will typically use a 1% lidocaine with epinephrine for pain relief and hemostasis. Surgeons may utilize topical vasoconstriction of the septal mucosa by using 4% topical cocaine or 0.05% oxymetazoline (Afrin®) soaked onto a ½ x 3 neurosurgical pattie (Cottonoid®).

Skin Prep and draping

Once the patient has been given anesthesia, the entire face is prepped with a povidone-iodine solution. Povidone-iodine is the safest solution to use near the eyes. It is important to prep the entire face to be able to observe the symmetry of the nose in relation to the entire face during the procedure. The patient's face is then sterilely draped for surgery. The surgeon may use a large drape placed under the head and wrapped around the hairline of the patient. These two ends of the drape are secured with a towel clip. This is referred to as a head turban drape. Four sterile towels can be placed around the periphery of the face and a split sheet or U-drape is used to cover the body. The limbs of the split drape or U-drape are placed around the periphery of the face and connected at the top of the head.

Surgical Procedure. The open rhinoplasty begins with an incision made in the mid-columellar skin of the nose (see Figure 20-3). The surgeon will use a 15-blade to make an inverted-V or stair-step incision while the SA holds a wide double-pronged retractor called a Joseph double skin hook.

- After the skin incision is completed, an intranasal incision is created along the inferior or caudal edge of the lower cartilage from the nostril margins moving laterally.

- This intranasal incision is done bilaterally while the SA gives exposure with the Joseph double skin hook and connects to the columellar incision.

- Skeletonization is completed to expose the cartilaginous and boney structures of the nose. Skeletonization involves dissecting a skin flap in the cephalad (or superior) direction staying on the surface of the osteocartilaginous structures of the nose. This is completed by using small dissecting scissors like a Littler, tenotomy, or curved Metzenbaum scissor.

- After skeletonization is complete, the surgeon can proceed to alter the appearance of the nose for the desired outcome.

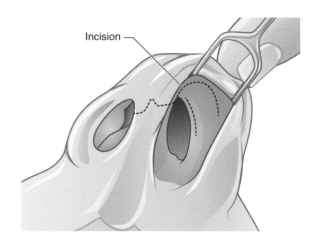

Figure 20-3 · Rhinoplasty incision options: Transdomal or interdomal. (Reproduced, with permission, from Lalwani AK, ed. *Current Diagnosis & Treatment in Otolaryngology—Head & Neck Surgery.* 4th ed. New York, NY: McGraw Hill; 2020.)

- The surgeon may begin with a tip-plasty. A tip-plasty consists of multiple suturing techniques and/or cartilage resection or grafting to alter the tip shape of the nose without compromising its structure. For a more bulbous nose, portion of the cephalic lateral crus is excised; however, this should not compromise the strength of the cartilage.

- To achieve the desired results, the surgeon can employ five different suturing techniques using a 5-0 absorbable monofilament suture. The first technique is a transdomal suture. The transdomal suture is placed in the center of the tip cartilage domes while beginning the horizontal mattress suture at the medial side of the dome. The next technique is an interdomal suture, which is placed between the cephalic middle crura to control the overall width of the nasal tip. The lateral crural mattress suture technique is used to flatten and strengthen the lateral crus. Next, a columella-septal suture can be used to connect the tip cartilages to the caudal nasal septum. A larger suture needle is needed for the columella-septal suture to ensure a full-thickness bite is achieved across the cartilage. Lastly, is the intercrural suture. This technique uses a horizontal mattress suture passing the suture medially from the middle crus on one side and then across to the other side. It is important to note that sufficient cartilage must be present for each suturing technique.

- If cartilage is not present or is too weak, grafting may be necessary using cartilage from behind the ear or rib.

- A strip of cartilage is removed from the donor site and is placed as either a columellar strut, septal extension graft or cap graft to increase the strength and to help with any tip deformities.

- The strut or graft is sutured during any of the above suture techniques by being included in the suture passes.

- If a patient has a large dorsal hump, the surgeon may need to decrease its size. The dorsum consists mainly of cartilage with a small boney component of the nasal bone.

- For the cartilaginous parts of the hump, the surgeon can use a 15-blade to cut away the unwanted cartilage.

- Then a surgeon may use a Fomon rasp to shave down small humps and contour the dorsum. For large dorsal humps, a Rubin osteotome can be used for excision. The osteotome is placed under the cut cartilage and a mallet is used to remove the excess bony hump.

- When using the mallet and osteotome, it is important to keep the hits evenly timed to avoid over excision of the cartilage and/or bone.

- Once the desired nasal shape is achieved, closure can begin. The intranasal incision is closed using interrupted 5-0 chromic gut sutures.

- The external skin incision on the columella is closed using a 6-0 permanent monofilament interrupted sutures. Care is taken to avoid a step deformity of the columella while closing the skin incision.

- With closure complete, the patient's face is cleaned of any blood and prep solution to prepare for dressing placement.

- Some surgeons may choose to place internal nasal splints in each nasal cavity. The internal splints are thought to prevent intranasal edema and adhesion formation. These splits may be removed anywhere from 24 hours to weeks after surgery, depending on the extent of the rhinoplasty.

- An external splint is also placed for 5 days to 1 week postoperatively. The nose is covered with tape or steri-strips to protect the skin and a thermoplastic stent is molded to fit over the taped nose. The external split applies pressure to the skin envelope to help the skin heal back to its original location. Also, the external split will help hold any bony structures in place that may have been modified.

- A nasal drip pad will also be placed around the patient's head to hold gauze at the nasal openings. The drip pad can be created by cutting a structured surgical mask into a strip, leaving the elastic in place to be passed around the patient's head.

Post-operatively, the patient is asked to avoid contact sports for up to 3 months as well as moderate sport activities for 1 month. The sutures will be removed around 1 week postoperation, and blood clots may be irrigated out at each postoperative visit (see Figure 20-4).

CHEILOPLASTY/PALATOPLASTY

An orofacial cleft is a congenital birth defect of the upper lip and/or palate. Orofacial clefts are the fourth most common birth defects and can be diagnosed through prenatal ultrasound around the 20th week of gestation. Although the causes of the orofacial clefts are unknown, research has shown that smoking while pregnant, having a diagnosis of diabetes prior to pregnancy and taking antiseizure medications can contribute to the genetic mutation.

Orofacial clefts have been long documented throughout history. Some cultures embraced the defect and sought ways to repair the clefts, whereas other cultures deemed the children possessed. The first documented cleft lip repair was in China in 390 B.C. on an 18-year-old boy. The first successful cleft palate repair was reportedly completed in 1766 by Le Monnier, who is a French dentist.

An orofacial cleft can develop between the fourth and ninth weeks of pregnancy due to the disruption of the frontal nasal prominence and the left and right maxillary prominences fusion. These prominences naturally grow toward the midline during development and should fuse together during the sixth to 13th weeks of pregnancy. When the fusion is disrupted, a cleft palate is the result. A cleft lip occurs when a skin bridge fails to form over the maxillary and nasal prominences (see Figure 20-5).

The classification of orofacial clefts varies depending on the extent of fusion disruption. The cleft can be unilateral or bilateral and complete or incomplete. A complete cleft involves the entire primary and secondary palate, whereas an incomplete cleft involved only the secondary palate. Multiple classification systems exist for orofacial clefts, but the Veau System is the most common. The Veau System divides orofacial clefts into four categories describing the extent of clefting. Veau Class I is

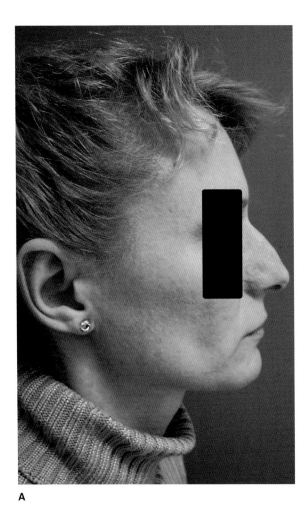
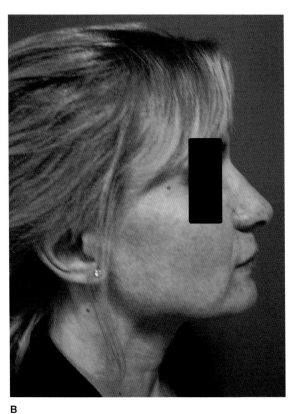

A   **B**

Figure 20-4 · Rhinoplasty before and after. (Reproduced, with permission, from Brunicardi FC et al, eds. *Schwartz's Principles of Surgery*. 11th ed. New York, NY: McGraw Hill; 2019.)

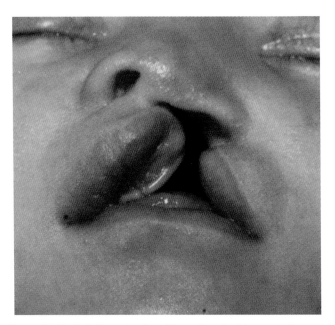

Figure 20-5 · Cleft lip and palate. (Reproduced, with permission, from Brunicardi FC et al, eds. *Schwartz's Principles of Surgery*. 11th ed. New York, NY: McGraw Hill; 2019.)

an incomplete cleft with only the soft palate involvement. Veau Class II involves the hard and soft palates with only secondary palate involvement. Veau Class III consists of a complete unilateral cleft including the lip and a Veau Class IV consists of a complete bilateral cleft.

Anatomy

The roof of the mouth contains the primary and secondary palate. The primary palate contains the alveolar arch with the four upper incisors. The secondary palate consists of the hard with the remaining dentition and soft palate. The hard palate continues from the alveolar arch and involves the palatine processes of the maxilla and horizontal lamina of the palatine bones. The hard palate is covered by oral and nasal mucosa, and the anterior palatine and nasopalatine nerves provide sensory innervation to the hard palate. Also covered by oral mucosa, the soft palate contains five muscles attached to the posterior portion of the hard palate. The muscles are the tensor veli palatini, levator veli palatini, palatoglossus, palatopharyngeus, and the musculus uvulae. These muscles work together to lift the nasopharynx during swallowing which prevents food from entering the nasopharynx. The soft palate is primarily innervated by the pharyngeal branch of the vagus nerve apart from the tensor veli palatini muscle which is innervated by the medial pterygoid nerve. The greater palatine arteries supply the hard and soft palate, and the pterygoid venous plexus provides the venous drainage.

The lip anatomy consists of oral mucosal membrane, vermillion, vermillion border, and skin (see Figure 20-6). The upper lip also includes the cupid's bow and philtrum. The vermillion is the external portion of the lip between the oral mucosal membrane and skin. Its color is dependent upon the patient's age and ethnicity. The vermillion is distinguished from the skin by the vermillion border also referred to as the white roll. The vermillion border has a paler appearance than the vermillion allowing for the demarcation. A unique anatomic feature of the upper lip is the cupid's bow. The cupid's bow is formed by two peaks of the vermillion that curve downward at the midline. This relates directly to the philtrum of the upper lip. The philtrum consists of a midline depression bordered by two philtral pillars. The pillars run between the nasal septum and peaks of the cupid's bow. The upper lip achieves movement by the orbicularis oris, the levator anguli oris, the levator labii superioris, and the zygomaticus major muscles. The orbicularis oris runs circumferentially around the lips and is directly affected by a cleft lip (see Figure 20-7). These muscles are innervated by the buccal branch of the facial nerve, and the sensory innervation of the upper lip is given by the infraorbital branch of the maxillary division of the trigeminal nerve. The lips are supplied by superior and inferior labial arteries, which are branches of the facial artery. Venous drainage is facilitated by the superior and inferior labial veins, which drain into the internal jugular vein.

Etiology

Orofacial defects cause a wide array of issues for the child's development. The main concern is difficulty eating. The cleft lip makes forming a seal around the breast or bottle difficult, and the cleft palate allows the food and/or liquid to enter the

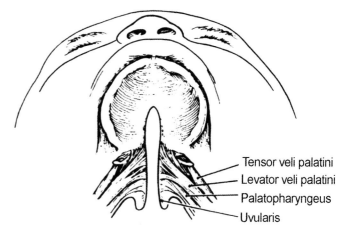

Figure 20-7 · Soft palate anatomy. (Reproduced, with permission, from Chan Y, Goddard JC. *K.J. Lee's Essential Otolaryngology: Head and Neck Surgery*. 12th ed. New York, NY: McGraw Hill; 2019.)

nasal cavity. Temporary palates may be used to help the child eat efficiently as well as specialized feeding apparatuses like a Habermann feeder or a Montgomery nipple may be used to aid in bottle feeding. It is also recommended the child is fed in a mostly upright position to help the fluid flow downwards into the stomach versus into the nasal cavity. Orofacial defects also affect the child's speech. The defects prevent the child from speaking certain sounds until the defects are repaired. Even after the repair, the child may benefit from speech therapy to help improve their articulation. Children with orofacial defects tend to have chronic otitis media due to eustachian tube dysfunction. This causes fluid to build up in the middle ear, which over time results in hearing loss. Tympanostomy tubes are often placed to relieve the fluid buildup. Dental problems are another concern for children with orofacial clefts. These children tend to have an alveolar ridge defect which prevents the upper incisor teeth to rupture. Other teeth may be malformed, and cavities tend to form more often in children with orofacial defects. Surgery performed around age 7 to 9 to replace or repair the alveolar ridge defect can help the permanent teeth to erupt.

Depending on the extent of the defect, orofacial clefts need surgical and nonsurgical intervention throughout the child's life. Though consistently debated amongst surgeons, most agree that the cleft lip is repaired around 3 to 6 months of age. This will aid in the child's feeding. Around 10 to 12 months, the cleft palate is repaired. Repairing the cleft palate during this time helps with speech development. Additional surgeries may be necessary as the child ages to assist in upper incisor teeth eruption and any revisions if needed.

Nonsurgical Treatments

Beginning with the first week of the child's life, nonsurgical treatments are employed to aid in the future closure of the cleft lip. The lip segments can be taped together to bring the two lip segments closer. A nasoalveolar molding (NAM) device can also be used to decrease the alveolar gap. The NAM and tape are adjusted weekly to guide the cleft closure. These nonsurgical treatments will ultimately lead to a surgical treatment with less tension.

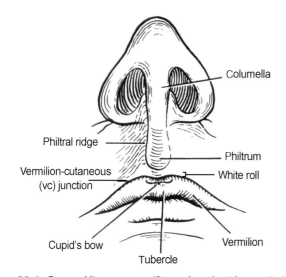

Figure 20-6 · External lip anatomy. (Reproduced, with permission, from Chan Y, Goddard JC. *K.J. Lee's Essential Otolaryngology: Head and Neck Surgery*. 12th ed. New York, NY: McGraw Hill; 2019.)

Anesthesia

For the surgical repair of the cleft lip and cleft palate, the patient is placed under general anesthesia with endotracheal intubation. The endotracheal tube is secured on the lower lip at the midline. This allows for ease of access to the upper lip and palate as well as prevents any distortion of the upper lip during the repair. The patient is positioned with a shoulder roll to extend the neck. The patient's arms are left at their sides or tucked using the draw sheet depending on age of the patient. This allows the easier access to the patient's mouth. After confirming the allergies, the patient's entire face is prepped using povidone-iodine. A large drape is placed under the head and wrapped like a turban around the patient's hairline. Four sterile blue towels are placed around the borders of the face and a split sheet or U-drape is used to complete the sterile field.

Surgical Procedure

- When repairing the cleft lip, multiple techniques may be utilized; however, the Millard rotation advancement flap is the most common (see Figure 20-8).

- Before an incision is made, the surgeon marks the key landmarks for the identification of the rotation flaps with methylene blue and a 30-gauge hypodermic needle. These landmarks are the peak of cupids bow on noncleft side, nadir of cupids bow, peak of cupids bow on cleft side, end of white roll on lateral lip, subnasale at columellar-lip crease, height of philtral column on noncleft side at lip-columellar crease, height of philtral column on cleft side at lip-columellar crease, noncleft side alar base, cleft side alar base, cleft side of oral commissure and noncleft side oral commissure.

- After these 11 key landmarks are marked, the surgeon can inject a local anesthetic into the lip area.

- An infraorbital nerve block can also be done at this time or later for postoperative pain relief. The local anesthetic typically has epinephrine mixed with it to aid in vasoconstriction during the surgery. While injecting the local, care is taken to not distort the anatomy by injecting too much fluid.

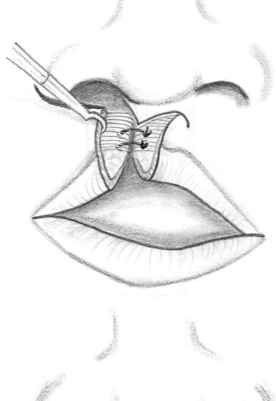

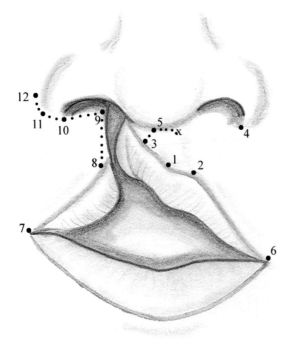

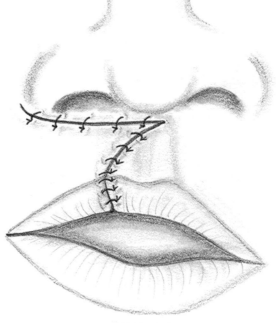

Figure 20-8 ∙ Millard rotation-advancement technique. (Reproduced, with permission, from Chan Y, Goddard JC. *K.J. Lee's Essential Otolaryngology: Head and Neck Surgery.* 12th ed. New York, NY: McGraw Hill; 2019.)

- A scalpel is used to create the medial lip incisions. The first incision begins at the cleft side's cupid's bow peak and extends toward the base of the columella in a curved direction. This incision creates the rotational flap, which will be referred to later as the "R" flap.

- The next incision is made from the cleft side's cupids bow peak along the vermillion border to the nasal base; then an additional incision is made perpendicular from the cleft side cupid's bow peak through the vermillion extending along the gingivobuccal sulcus. This incision creates the crossing flap, which will be referred to later as the "C" flap.

- The next incisions are made on the lateral side of the lip. From the end of the white roll, an incision is created along the vermillion toward the nasal sill.

- An additional incision can be made from the nasal sill to the alar base if more advancement is required.

- Lastly, an incision is made from the white roll traveling perpendicular through the vermillion to the gingivobuccal sulcus. These incisions create the advancement flap, which will be referred to later as the "A" flap.

- After all incisions are created, the orbicularis oris muscle is dissected off the skin and oral mucosa.

- The defect in the oral mucosa is now able to be closed using a 5-0 absorbable braided suture. Interrupted sutures are used to ensure strength across the cleft.

- After the mucosa is closed, the orbicularis oris muscle fibers are sutured in the correct orientation to complete the circle around the mouth. Using interrupted suture techniques, a 5-0 absorbable braided suture is used to secure the muscle fibers together.

- Now that all the internal layers have been reconstructed, the external lip cleft is repaired. The "C" flap crosses the nasal sill of the cleft and is secured to the cleft side alar base. This recreates the nasal opening on the cleft side.

- Next care is taken to realign the vermillion border. The "R" flap is rotated downward to align the cleft side of the peak of cupid's bow with the end of the white roll on the lateral lip. The "A" flap being advanced toward the nasal septum allows the lateral lip white roll to meet the cleft side peak of cupid's bow. The tip of the "A" flap is secured to the subnasale at columellar-lip crease.

- The dermis of the flaps is secured using a 5-0 absorbable braided suture, utilizing interrupted suture techniques.

- The skin can now be closed utilizing various techniques depending upon the patient and surgeon's preference. A running 5-0 permanent monofilament can reapproximate the skin edges, though some surgeons may prefer a fast-absorbable suture.

- If the dermis is approximated sufficiently, the skin can be approximated using cyanoacrylate skin adhesive instead of sutures.

- Dressings are minimal due to the location of the incision. If permanent sutures are used, then a topical antibiotic ointment is applied to the suture line. The other skin closure techniques do not require any ointment or additional dressing placed. The child can bottle or breastfeeding immediately post-surgery, and sutures are removed around day 5.

Cleft Palate Repair. Around 12 months of age, the child will have the cleft palate repaired. Many surgical techniques have been developed, but ultimately, the goal is a tension-free closure of the cleft.

- A common surgical technique being utilized is the Bardach two-flap palatoplasty (see Figure 20-9). For this technique, the surgeon creates incisions bilaterally at the edges of the cleft. Lateral incisions are also created where the hard palate and alveolus meet.

- The oral mucosa is then dissected away from the palate, careful to preserve the greater palatine artery and vein.

- This is safely done using blunt dissection with a periosteal elevator. With the oral mucosa flaps elevated, this exposes the tensor veli palatine and levator palatini muscles as well as the nasal mucosa.

- The muscles are elevated from the hard palate to allow for repositioning posteriorly as a muscle sling to reconstruct the soft palate. This muscle sling will close the velar opening preventing air from entering the nasal cavity through the pharynx.

- The tensor veli palatine and levator palatini muscles are secured to the pharynx using a 5-0 absorbable braided suture.

- Next the nasal mucosa is elevated from its attachments bilaterally to allow midline closure. The mucosa is closed using a 5-0 absorbable braided suture.

- The palatini muscles that were not used for the sling are then closed at the midline next with a 4-0 absorbable braided suture.

- The final layer closed is the oral mucosa. The midline oral mucosa incision is approximated using interrupted 4-0 absorbable braided suture then the lateral oral mucosa incisions are closed using the same technique.

- No dressings are utilized since all incisions are inside the mouth, and the patient is given water or diluted milk the night of surgery or next day.

Post-op Considerations. A team of specialists is involved throughout the child's life. These specialists consist of oral surgeons, otolaryngologists, plastic surgeons, speech pathologists, social workers, psychologists, orthodontics, and dentists. Once the initial surgeries are completed, the patient will work with speech pathologists to correct any speech impediments. Revision surgeries may be necessary as the patient ages and if any complications occur. The most common complication from a cleft lip and cleft palate repair is dehiscence of the incision line or fistula formation. This requires reoperation to close the incision or fistula. Dehiscence and fistula formation can be prevented by ensuring a tension-free closure as well as proper suturing techniques. Alevolar grafting may be needed as the child ages to help with teeth eruption. Collectively, these specialists work toward giving the child a successful outcome.

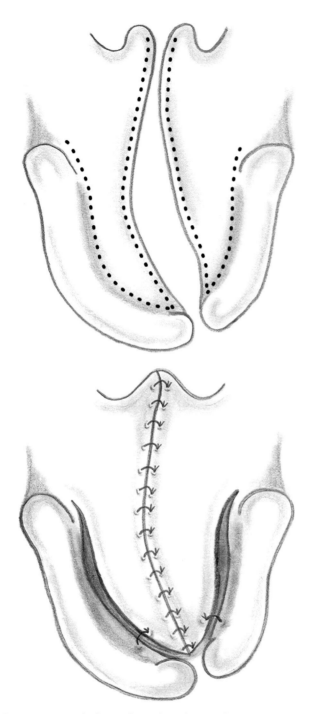

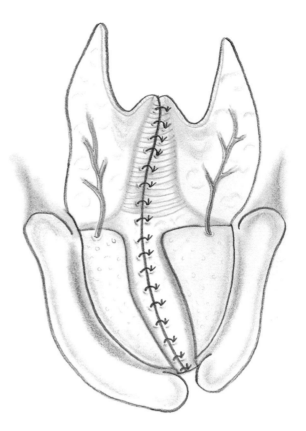

Figure 20-9 · Bardach two-flap palatoplasty technique. (Reproduced, with permission, from Chan Y, Goddard JC. *K.J. Lee's Essential Otolaryngology: Head and Neck Surgery*. 12th ed. New York, NY: McGraw Hill; 2019.)

REDUCTION MAMMOPLASTY

A reduction mammoplasty is a surgical procedure to decrease the size of the breast volume as well as improve the shape and position of the nipple-areolar complex. In some cultures, having small breasts are a sign of higher social status, so women were seeking the chance to change their appearance to assimilate easier into their society. The first documented surgery to reduce the size of a woman's breast was recorded in the late 19th century, and advancements continued to be made with the surgical technique well into the 20th century. Notably, in 1928, Biesenberger developed a technique using a wide skin undermining and a lateral superior rotation pedicle. This was the most popular technique until Wise in 1956 redesigned the skin excision pattern. He developed the Wise-keyhole pattern using the bra design from Fredricks of Hollywood. The Wise-keyhole pattern was more successful by emphasizing preoperative skin marking. The next 20 years was spent perfecting the pedicle technique to preserve the blood supply to the nipple-areolar complex. In 1977, Courtiss and Goldwyn developed the inferior pedicle technique which is the most popular to date.

Anatomy

The breast is a glandular structure located at the fourth intercostal space overlying the pectoralis major muscle. The breast contains 15 to 20 lactiferous glands surrounded by adipose tissue (see Figure 20-10). The lactiferous glands drain into the nipple via lactiferous ducts, and the nipple is surrounded by a darker area of tissue called the areola. The areola's purpose is to cover sebaceous glands used for lubrication. The breast maintains its structure through suspensory ligaments also known as Cooper's ligaments. These ligaments firmly attach the glands to the skin and loosely attach the glands to the deep fascia of breast. Sixty percent of the breast tissue is supplied by the internal mammary artery through medial perforators. The lateral thoracic artery supplies 30% of the blood supply through superior and lateral perforators. The inferior portion of the breast tissue is supplied by the intercostal arteries, namely the fourth

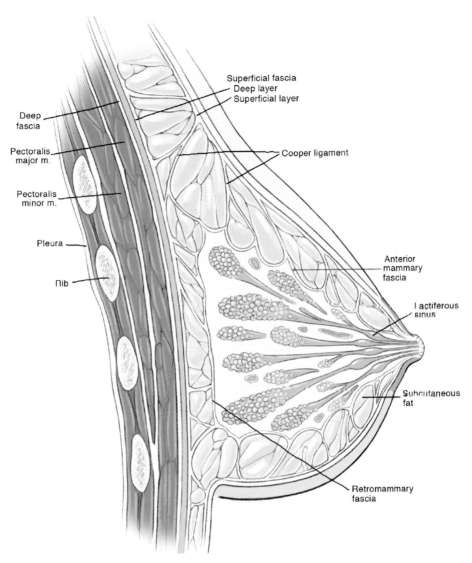

Figure 20-10 Breast anatomy. (Reproduced, with permission, from Harness JK, Wisher DB, eds. *Ultrasound in Surgical Practice—Basic Principles and Clinical Applications*. New York, NY: Wiley Liss; 2001:159-236.)

and fifth branches. These blood vessels combine centrally to supply the nipple-areolar complex. The breast's cutaneous innervation arises from the first through sixth intercostal nerves. These intercostal nerves branch into the anterior and lateral cutaneous nerves to innervate the skin and converge in the middle to innervate the nipple-areolar complex.

Etiology

Women choose to undergo a reduction mammoplasty to reduce the size of their larger breasts. The breasts typically cause chronic neck and back pain for the women, as well as skin issues like rashes in their inframammary crease. Having larger breasts may also cause headaches and deep skin grooves from the bra straps. Because of the large breasts, the women may have difficulty exercising, which perpetuates incidences of weight gain. This further exacerbates any psychosocial issues the women have due to embarrassment and feeling self-conscious about the way their body looks (see Figure 20-11).

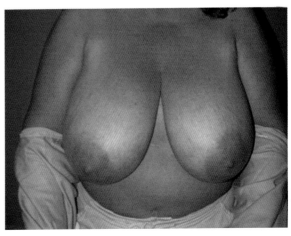

Figure 20-11 Macromastia. (Reproduced, with permission, from Morita SY, Balch CM, Klimberg VS, Pawlik TM, Posner MC, Tanabe KK, eds. *Textbook of Complex General Surgical Oncology*. New York, NY: McGraw Hill; 2018.)

A reduction mammoplasty may also be performed to correct gross asymmetry a woman may have due to breastfeeding or hormones. Lastly, a reduction mammoplasty can be used as a breast reconstruction technique following a partial mastectomy. The defect left from the partial mastectomy can be hidden by rearranging the tissue in a similar fashion to a reduction mammoplasty.

Surgical Approaches

The basis of the reduction mammoplasty technique relies on its pedicle. The pedicle is a mass of breast tissue with the nipple and areola attached. Within the pedicle is the blood supply that feeds the nipple and areola. Without an adequate pedicle, the patient risks nipple and/or areola necrosis. Four main pedicle techniques that are used today, the most common technique being the inferior pedicle. The inferior pedicle keeps a wedge of tissue at the base of the breast and is supplied by the deep internal mammary artery located at the fourth intercostal space. The next most commonly used pedicle technique is the medial pedicle. This pedicle utilizes the medial branches of the internal mammary artery. The superior pedicle technique offers the most fullness at the top of the breast and relies on the descending artery of the internal mammary artery arising from the second intercostal space. Last and least used is the lateral pedicle. This pedicle maintains the breast fullness on the lateral aspect of the breast which makes creating a natural breast mound more difficult. The lateral pedicle relies on superficial branches of the lateral thoracic artery to supply the nipple-areola complex.

To create the pedicle, breast tissue must be removed from the skin envelope. To determine how much breast tissue must be removed, the tissue is weighed intraoperatively. A scale is needed with two identical buckets tared onto that scale. Any amount of weight can be removed from each breast to achieve the correct breast size and symmetry of the breast. The insurance companies deem that at least 500 grams need to be removed from each breast to get reimbursement for the procedure. However, the amount of tissue removed is dictated by the vascular supply to the pedicle. If too much breast tissue is removed, then the vascular supply could be compromised causing nipple or areolar necrosis.

When a woman has extremely large breasts, the viability of the blood supply to the nipple-areolar complex may be compromised during a reduction mammoplasty. Either pre-planned or as a backup plan during the procedure, a surgeon may choose to do a free nipple technique. The free nipple technique removes the nipple and areola as a skin graft from the breast. After the breast is reshaped, the nipple-areolar complex is sutured back onto the breast mound. This technique must be discussed with the patient prior to surgery because the patient will no longer have sensation to the nipple and areola as well as be unable to breastfeed.

Another key component of a reduction mammoplasty is the skin resection pattern. The pattern chosen is decided preoperatively based on the size of the breast. The two most common skin patterns used are the wise or inverted T pattern and the vertical or lollipop pattern. The wise pattern is used for large ptotic breast that need a more extensive breast tissue excision. The wise pattern consists of an incision around the areola and an inframammary incision (see Figure 20-12). These two incisions are connected via a vertical incision. The final skin incision pattern will look like an inverted T or an anchor. The vertical skin resection pattern is used for breasts that need a smaller tissue excision, so less skin needs to be removed. The vertical pattern eliminates the inframammary incision leaving only the circumareolar and vertical incisions. Whichever pattern is needed to complete the reduction mammoplasty, it is key that the surgeon marks the patient preoperatively while that patient is in the upright position. Marking the patient in the upright position allows for a more natural breast mound after surgery.

Preparing the Patient for Surgery

Once the breast markings are complete, the patient will be taken to the operating room suite. The patient will be placed in the supine position with the arms extended on arm boards. The patient will be placed under general anesthesia and a Foley catheter may be placed if the surgery time extends longer than 2 hours. To ensure breast symmetry, the patient's arms will be placed at ninety degrees on the arm boards and the shoulders relaxed. If one shoulder or arm is raised higher than the other, then the breast shape for that side will be affected. The arms will be secured onto the arm boards with two pieces of foam and ace wraps. This ensures the patient's arms will remain safe while sitting the patient upright during the surgery. The patient will be prepped from chin to umbilicus and down to the operating room table bilaterally. Once prepped, two large drapes will be tucked slightly underneath each side of the patient. Sterile towels will be placed around the breasts: one at the clavicles, one above the umbilicus, and one lateral on each side of the operating room table. Be aware that some patients may need more than four sterile towels to complete the sterile field. Next, a chest or transverse laparotomy drape will be placed at the level of the breasts. Two split sheets may also be used to drape out around the breasts.

Surgical Procedure

- To start the procedure, the SA will use both hands to stretch the skin around the areolar to provide traction for the circumareolar incision (see Figure 20-13). If the patient's breast is too large to get adequate traction, a tourniquet can be made using a lap wrapped tightly around the base of the breast and a kocher clamp used to hold the lap in place.

- The surgeon will use a Freeman areola marker to mark a perfect circle around the areola, and then use a 15-blade to make the incision.

- After the circumareolar incision is made, the rest of the skin incisions are made down to dermis, and a skin incision is made for the preplanned area of the pedicle.

- Because the pedicle will be buried beneath the skin once the appropriate amount of breast tissue is excised, the epidermis overlying the pedicle needs to be removed. This process is called deepithelization.

- To properly deepithelize, the SA uses an Adson with teeth and a 10-blade or ridgeback scissors. The SA lifts the cut edge of the incision, angles the knife blade or scissors upward and begins to excise the epidermis from the dermis. The dermis is the white layer of tissue and should be left behind during deepithelization. If the subcutaneous fat is seen through the dermis then the SA has gone too deep during the excision. To correct this, the angle of the knife or scissors needs to face up more.

- After the pedicle is deepithelized, the skin flaps are created. The SA will use facelift retractors to lift the skin flaps upward while the surgeon excises the breast tissue away. Care is taken to not disturb the dermal connection of the pedicle.

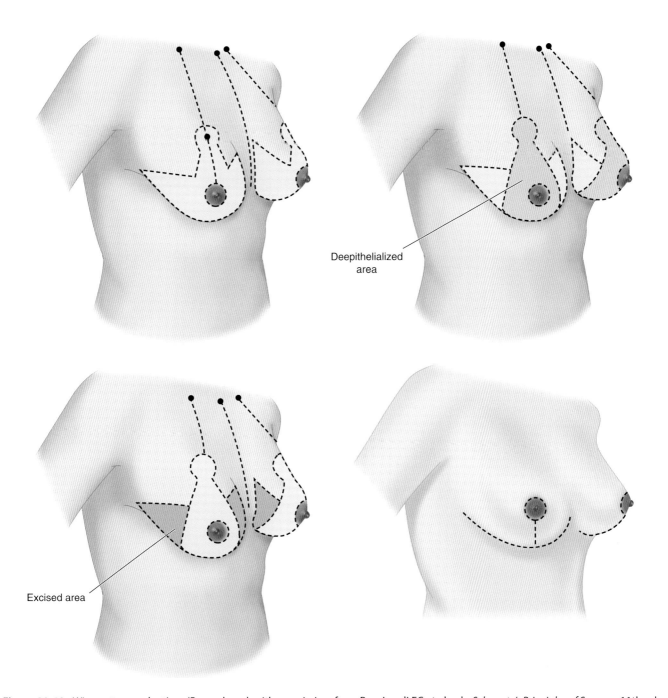

Deepithelialized area

Excised area

Figure 20-12 · Wise pattern reduction. (Reproduced, with permission, from Brunicardi FC et al, eds. *Schwartz's Principles of Surgery*. 11th ed. New York, NY: McGraw Hill; 2019.)

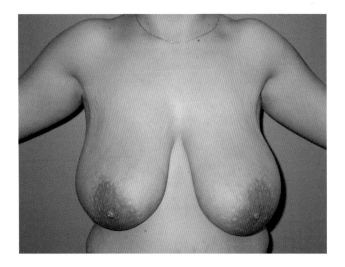
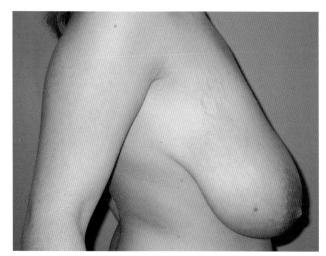
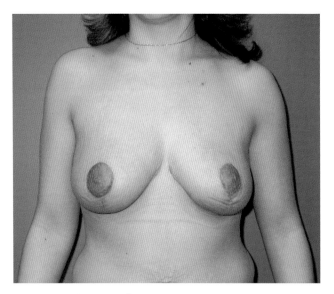
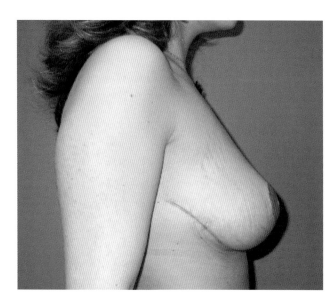

Figure 20-12 · (*Continued*)

- Now, the breast tissue can be removed surrounding the pedicle to achieve the desired breast mound. As the breast tissue is being removed, the tissue is placed into the nonsterile bucket on the scale to obtain a weight. Keeping the blood supply to the pedicle safe is the SA's number one job during this step.

- The SA will place one hand firmly on top of the pedicle while the surgeon excises the breast tissue. The SA must make sure pedicle stays in its designed spot to prevent undermining of the pedicle. If the pedicle becomes undermined, the vascular supply to the nipple and areola could be compromised.

- The SA should communicate with the surgeon if they feel the pedicle begin to shift while the surgeon is removing the excess breast tissue. This will allow the surgeon to pause the excision and place the pedicle back into its designed spot.

- After the predetermined weight of breast tissue has been removed from the breast, the surgeon will begin the skin closure. Suture preference changes depending on the surgeon, but all surgeons are concerned with achieving a strong closure without the knots spitting.

- To begin the closure, each apex of the skin flaps is sutured to the midline of the inframammary incision. This requires a three-point deep buried suture technique by passing the suture through the three points of dermis before tying the knot. The surgeon will use a 2-0 suture for this stitch.

- The skin will now be temporarily closed with staples, and the surgeon will begin the other breast reduction.

- When both breast mounds are completed, the nipple and areola need to be placed in its new position. To ensure the nipple and areola are placed in the most natural position, the back of the bed will be raised to a 90-degree position. This simulates the patient being in a standing position which allows the breasts to lie in the correct anatomical position.

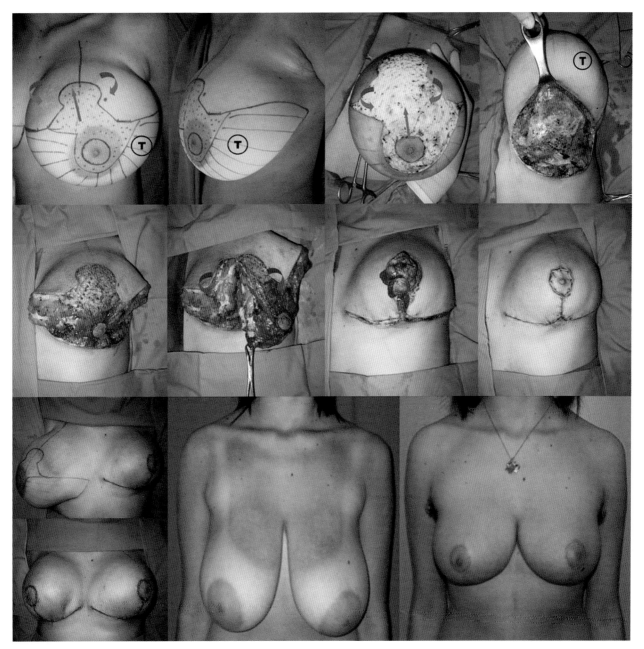

Figure 20-13 · Wise pattern breast reduction technique. (Reproduced, with permission, from Morita SY, Balch CM, Klimberg VS, Pawlik TM, Posner MC, Tanabe KK, eds. *Textbook of Complex General Surgical Oncology*. New York, NY: McGraw Hill; 2018.)

- The surgeon will use the Freeman areolar marker again to mark a perfect circle on the new breast mound. The SA may be asked to help decide where the nipple and areola should be placed. The nipple and areola look best toward the lower half of the breast, pointed a little outward and downward.

- After the position is decided, the circular incision will be made and deepithelized. This allows the nipple and areola that is attached to the pedicle to be sutured to the skin flaps.

- The dermis of the inframammary and vertical incision will be closed with interrupted 3-0 deep buried suture and the circumareolar incision will be closed with a 4-0 deep buried suture. Care needs to be taken when closing the dermis to ensure the apices of the incisions lay flat, so dog ears do not form.

- After the dermal closure, the skin of all the incisions is closed using a 4-0 intracuticular suture.

- After all incisions are sutured closed, the dressings are placed. Though dressings may change depending on surgeon's preference, the key is to have a simple noncompressive dressing that provides support to the breasts. This ensures the vascular supply to the nipple and areola will not become occluded. Many surgeons are using Prineo Dermabond© to seal incisions. Abdominal pads or 4 × 4s are placed over the incisions and the breasts will be wrapped with a kerlix. Over the kerlix, a 6-inch ace will be loosely wrapped around the breasts. If available, some surgeons prefer using a bra to hold the dressings in place instead of the wraps. When choosing the size of bra, always choose at least one size larger than the patient's normal size. This ensures the breasts will not be compressed.

Post-op Considerations. Complications can arise following a reduction mammoplasty. Some minor complications are hematoma, small wound dehiscence, or infection. Though rare, some major complications can arise after a reduction mammoplasty. Serious wound dehiscence may occur and will need surgical intervention to correct. Also, if the patient is a smoker or has a BMI over 30, vascular compromise may occur causing nipple/areolar or skin flap necrosis. Some surgeons will require the patient to quit smoking before the surgery will be performed because of the increased risk of vascular issues.

BREAST AUGMENTATION

Breast augmentation is the surgical enlargement of the breast using an implant. This surgery was first performed in 1962 by Cronin and Gerow and quickly gained popularity amongst women wanting larger breasts. Breast augmentation was the most common cosmetic surgical procedure performed in the United States in 2018 with a little over 313,000 performed. This procedure is traditionally done in the plastic surgeon's office operating room or an outpatient surgery center.

Since the creation of the first implant in 1961, breast implants have undergone many changes to better the surgical outcomes. Even though many changes have been made, the general characteristics of the breast implants have remained the same. Breast implants are made of a two-part system with a silicone shell and either silicone gel or saline filler inside. The silicone shell is made smooth or with texture. The texture helps stabilize the implant in the breast pocket. Recent studies have shown a correlation between textured implants and lymphoma, so these types of implants have fallen out of favor with the plastic surgery community. The saline-filled breast implants are filled at the time of surgery, which allows for an easier implant insertion and allows for a tailored volume fill within the manufacturer's volume recommendation. Saline breast implants are less costly but are becoming less used for cosmetic breast augmentations due to their unnatural feeling. Silicone breast implants have a more natural feel to them, so more surgeons are implanting these devices. Silicone breast implants come prefilled with an exact amount of silicone filler. This makes these implants slightly harder to place inside the breast through a small incision. Many adaptations of the silicone filler have been created throughout the decades with the latest version being more cohesive. The cohesive silicone gel filler has a "gummy bear" texture, which feels more natural and in case of rupture

will stay solidified in the breast pocket. Lastly, breast implants come in different shapes. Because no two breasts are the same, many breast implant companies have developed round- and anatomic-shaped breast implants to fit the needs of the patient. For a more natural look, anatomic breast implants have a teardropped shape to mimic the slope of the natural breast. The type of breast implant as well as size of breast implants are all discussed preoperatively with the patient. At the time of surgery, a few different size implants may be available to temporarily size in situ to determine and to ensure the best patient outcome.

Preparing the Patient for Surgery

Breast augmentation is usually performed under general anesthesia with the patient in the supine position. The patient's arms will be placed on arm boards at a 90-degree angle, careful not to overextend the shoulders. The arms need to be secured to the arm boards using ace wraps between two pieces of foam. This allows the patient to be safely lifted during the procedure to view the breasts in a more anatomical position. To sit the patient up, the bed is positioned to flex the patient at the waist. The patient will be prepped from chin to umbilicus and laterally to the edge of the operating room table on each side. Two large drapes will be placed slightly underneath the patient on each side to cover the operating room table then four sterile towels will be placed around the breasts. One towel is placed at the clavicles, one placed just above the umbilicus and one towel is placed laterally at the axilla. A chest or transverse laparotomy drape can be used to complete the draping of the patient or two split sheets can be used to complete the sterile field. Lastly, the surgeon may choose to place a sterile tegaderm over each nipple to create a barrier between the lacrimal ducts and incisions. Bacteria naturally inhabit the lacrimal ducts and while manipulating the breast, the incisions can potentially become contaminated.

Surgical Approaches

The surgeon has multiple incision options to choose from for a breast augmentation. Becoming more popular with plastic surgeons, the inframammary incision allows for a larger incision while being hidden in the patient's natural fold (see Figure 20-14). It also is associated with a reduced risk of capsular contracture, a complication of breast implants. This incision requires minimal dissection of the breast tissue and gives the surgeon access to either the subglandular or subpectoral plane.

- If the patient is requiring a mastopexy at the time of the breast augmentation, the implant is placed through the mastopexy incision. The size of the incision will be based on the size of the patient's areola, though even a small areolar incision can be stretched to 4 cm. Utilizing this incision comes with some risk of bacterial contamination from the lactiferous ducts as well as increased pain from dissecting through the breast tissue to create the implant pocket.

- As a less direct approach, the transaxillary and transumbilical incisions avoid creating an incision on the breast, which makes using an anatomical or silicone gel implant more

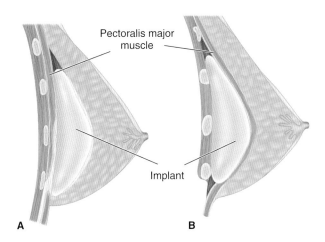

Figure 20-14 · Breast implant placement subglandular and subpectoral. (Reproduced, with permission, from Brunicardi FC et al, eds. *Schwartz's Principles of Surgery*. 11th ed. New York, NY: McGraw Hill; 2019.)

difficult. These approaches create the implant pocket without having to dissect the breast tissue but controlling symmetry and implant position is more difficult.

- Once the incision choice is made, the surgeon must choose which plane to place the implant. The implant pocket will be created in either the subglandular or subpectoral plane. When creating the subglandular plane, the implant pocket will sit above the pectoralis major muscle and just beneath the breast tissue. This plane is adequate for patients with ample native breast tissue but poses more risks for implant visibility and a less natural breast slope.

- The subpectoral plane is the more popular approach as the implant will sit below the pectoralis major muscle. The pocket between the pectoralis muscle and ribs is a relatively bloodless and easy field to dissect. The subpectoral plane provides enough implant coverage to prevent the rippling effect and allow for a more natural slope to the upper pole of the breast. This plane does have a risk of dynamic deformity when the pectoralis major is activated, which may require additional surgeries to achieve optimal patient satisfaction.

Surgical Procedure

- While the surgeon is creating the implant pocket, the SA is responsible for retracting the breast tissue and providing visualization for the surgeon.

- The SA begins with army navy retractors to retract the skin after the initial incision is made. As the surgeon dissects through the breast tissue using electrocautery, small Deaver retractors and/or lighted retractors are used to retract further into the breast implant pocket.

- At this point, the surgeon can continue to create the implant pocket with electrocautery or blunt dissection. The plane under the pectoralis major muscle is generally a bloodless plane, so blunt dissection is easier because visualization is minimal due to the small incision.

- If the surgeon continues to use the electrocautery, the SA needs to evacuate the smoke from the implant pocket. This can be achieved by placing the suction at the edge of the incision and then periodically dipping the suction into the implant pocket to evacuate the smoke.

- Care needs to be taken at this point to not disrupt the surgeon's visual field with the suction tip, but still evacuate the smoke.

- After the implant pocket is created, final preparations are made before placing the implant.

- The pocket will be irrigated with an antiseptic solution. Depending on the patient's allergies and surgeon's preference, the antiseptic solution could contain 1 g of cefazolin sodium, 80 mg of gentamicin and 50 cc of betadine mixed with 1 liter of normal saline. Irrigating the pocket helps remove any bacteria or debris from the tissue dissection as well as check for hemostasis.

- Antiseptic solution laparotomy sponges can be placed in the implant pocket while the surgeon moves to the second breast to begin the dissection.

- Once both breast implant pockets are dissected and irrigated, the surgeon may want to use an implant sizer to determine which size is best suited for the patient. Sizers are available for both saline and silicone gel-filled implants.

- The surgeon will sit the bed up to as close to 90 degrees as possible to assess the pocket shape and size with the breast implant sizer in place. When the patient is lying flat, the breasts fall laterally, so it is vital the surgeon evaluates the breast implant size and shape while the patient is in the most anatomically normal position.

- After the correct size is chosen, the SA pours betadine into the implant pockets as well as preps the incision sites. The betadine kills any native flora that survived the original prep to prevent implant contamination upon insertion. The surgeon will often change his or her sterile gloves prior to handling the implants to further prevent contamination.

- When inserting the implants, preventing contamination is of the utmost importance, so most surgeons have implemented the "no touch" technique for handling the implants. While on the back table, the implants will stay in their respective containers, soaking in the antiseptic solution. Because skin can never truly be rendered sterile, the surgeon wants to limit the contact the implant makes with the incision edges.

- To continue with the "no touch" technique, the silicone implant is placed in a Keller© Funnel. The end of the Keller© Funnel is cut to the correct size to allow the silicone implant to be passed into the breast pocket without the implant touching the incision edges.

- If inserting a saline-filled implant, the implant comes filled with air for shipping purposes. The implant must be deflated before insertion into the breast pocket. Once deflated, the implant is rolled on itself to prevent the implant from touching the incision edges.

- During the insertion process, the SA is responsible for retracting the skin incision open. Proper retraction will allow for an easier implant insertion as well as prevent skin flora contamination on the implant.

- Using two small Deaver retractors allows for adequate retraction deep into the breast pocket, especially when placing the implant subpectoral. Two army navy retractors may be adequate for retraction as well as a combination of Deaver and army navy.

- Avoid using any sharp retractors during insertion process to prevent tearing holes in the implant shell. The Deaver retractors are inserted into the implant pocket and lifted upwards to open the space.

- The surgeon will insert the end of the Keller© Funnel with the silicone gel implant into the incision, and then squeezes from the top of the funnel to insert the implant into the breast pocket. If inserting a saline implant, the implant pocket will be lifted open with the Deaver retractors, and the deflated implant is inserted into the implant pocket.

- After insertion, injectable saline is used to inflate the implant to the desired volume. After the implants are inserted, the final assessment of the breast implant size and shape is achieved while the bed is sitting at ninety degrees.

- The surgeon will rely on the SA's experience with breast augmentations to help make decisions about the final breast shape and size.

- The breast pocket is irrigated with the antiseptic solution one last time before closure begins.

- The deep fascia of each breast is closed using a 2-0 absorbable suture but be sure to avoid taking large suture throws that could puncture the underlying breast implant.

- The deep dermis is closed with a 3-0 interrupted absorbable suture, then the superficial dermis is closed with a 4-0 absorbable monofilament intracuticular suture.

- The incisions are dressed in half-inch steri-strips and the chest is wrapped circumferentially with a 6-inch kerlix and 6-inch ace wrap.

- The surgeon may choose to use a bra instead of the circumferential wrap. Four-by-four gauze and/or abdominal pads may be placed over the incisions as well to help with compression.

Post-op Considerations. Postoperatively, the patient is at risk for a variety of rare but potential complications. The most common complication of breast augmentation is capsular contracture. The body naturally forms a barrier or capsule around the breast implant and occasionally the body will create an increased inflammatory reaction to the implant. This causes pain as well as changes to the shape of the breast pocket. Reoperation of the affected breast is the solution to this complication. Infection is also a potential complication with breast augmentation surgery; however, avoidance of the circumareolar incision and the use of antibiotic irrigation helps limit the risk. Whenever placing any implant in a patient comes with an inherent risk

of infection, so it is critical that the team uses impeccable sterile technique during the procedure. Lastly, implant rupture is a known risk of breast implants. Over a 10-year life span of a breast implant, the rupture rate is approximately 5% for a saline implant and 8% for silicone gel implant. The patients are counseled to watch for signs of implant rupture and consider replacements around 10 years postoperatively.

ABDOMINOPLASTY

An abdominoplasty is the cosmetic removal of excessive skin and tissue from a patient's abdomen along with the tightening of the abdominal muscles. The excess skin and tissue can be from extensive weight loss or pregnancy. According to the 2019 Plastic Surgery Statistics Report, abdominoplasties were performed on 123,427 patients with 96% being female patients (see Figure 20-15).

The first reported abdominoplasty was credited to Doctor Demars and Doctor Marx of France in 1890. Then, in 1899, a gynecologist named Doctor Kelly performed the first abdominoplasty in America. These early abdominoplasties were completed only by also removing the umbilicus and little concern was given on scar placement. In 1905, surgeons in France performed the first abdominoplasty without removing the umbilicus, and in 1909 Doctor Weinhold established using a vertical and horizontal flap incision which allowed the umbilicus to survive the procedure. As abdominoplasty techniques continued to evolve, surgeons utilized abdominoplasties mostly to treat wounded World War I soldiers. Throughout the 1960s and 1970s, techniques became more refined focusing on scar placement, layers of suturing and contouring of the waist. In 1967, Doctor Ivo Pitanguy of Brazil developed the Pitanguy abdominoplasty where the transverse incision is made along the pubic line and Doctor Sinder further developed this technique in 1975 by describing the superior epigastric incision in relation to the circumferential incision around the umbilicus. Lastly, Doctor Baroudi-Keppke described the technique for choosing the new umbilical opening in the superior flap with suture stabilization of the umbilicus.

Anatomy

The abdominal wall is comprised of multiple layers of soft tissue that extend from the costal margins to the symphysis pubis and bilaterally to the iliac crest and midaxillary line. The outermost layers are the epidermis and dermis. Under the dermis is the subcutaneous fat layer also known as Camper's fascia and an additional pseudo fascial layer called Scarpa's fascia. Camper's and Scarpa's fascia are most prominent below the arcuate line which is located beneath the umbilicus. The umbilicus is in the midline of the abdomen about at the level of the superior iliac spines. Beneath these layers is the anterior rectus sheath covering the two bellies of the rectus abdominus muscles and a posterior rectus sheath under that. The rectus abdominus fascia combines to form the linea alba at the midline of the abdomen. Along with the paired rectus abdominus muscles at the midline, the abdomen laterally has three additional muscle

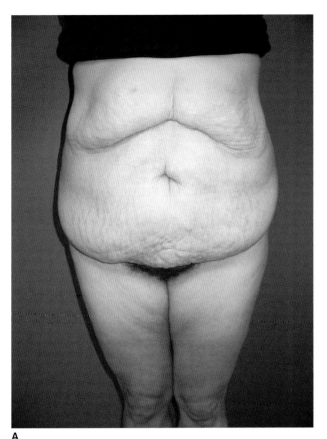

A

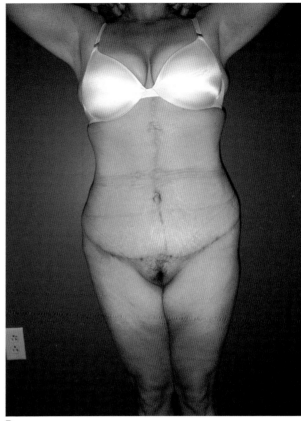

B

Figure 20-15 · Abdominoplasty before and after. (Reproduced, with permission, from Brunicardi FC et al, eds. *Schwartz's Principles of Sur*gery. 11th ed. New York, NY: McGraw Hill; 2019.)

layers: internal oblique, external oblique, and the transverse abdominus muscles. These four muscles provide support for the abdomen and allow for flexion and rotation of the trunk. The vascular supply to the abdominal wall consists of the superior and inferior epigastric arteries as well as the deep circumflex iliac arteries. The superior and inferior epigastric arteries run with the rectus abdominus muscle. The abdominal wall is innervated by the thoracoabdominal, iliohypogastric, and ilioinguinal nerves. The motor function of the rectus abdominus muscles is innervated by the intercostal nerves at T7-T11 and the subcostal nerves at T12.

Surgical Approach

Depending on the patient's anatomy, the surgeon has different abdominoplasty techniques to choose from. The first technique is called a miniabdominoplasty, and this technique requires the patient to only have infraumbilical laxity of abdominal skin. The most common technique is the Pitanguy abdominoplasty which is required for patients that have laxity above and below the umbilicus. The umbilicus will also be transposed during this technique. A modification of the Pitanguy abdominoplasty is to create an inverted-T incision by creating a vertical incision toward the umbilicus connecting to the transverse incision. The technique is utilized most often for patients that need extensive skin removal.

Preparing the Patient for Surgery

On the day of surgery, the surgeon will mark the patient's incision lines prior to entering the operating room. The surgeon will identify the inferior suprapubic incision while the patient is in the supine position. The incision will be marked midline at the suprapubic line extending bilaterally toward the inguinal crease ending at the anterior superior iliac spine. Then, the patient will stand, and the superior epigastric incision is drawn to connect to the lateral extent of the inferior incision. If liposuction will be used to aid in the abdominal contouring, the areas will be marked at this time as well.

Prior to the patient entering the operating room, the operating room bed needs to be positioned to allow the patient to flex at the waist during the surgery. This is to aid in the skin closure later. Because the patient will be sitting up during a portion of the procedure, it is important to secure the arms to the arm boards. This can be accomplished by wrapping the arms in foam padding and using six-inch elastic wrap or kerlix to secure the arms and padding to the arm board. The abdominal binder can also be placed preoperatively on the operating room bed beneath the patient to aid in dressing placement postoperatively. To protect the abdominal binder from fluids during the surgery, two chux pads can be used to cover the binder, which can then be removed once it is time to apply the binder.

Anesthesia

Patients undergoing an abdominoplasty will receive general anesthesia with endotracheal intubation to ensure intraoperative relaxation of the rectus abdominus muscles. If the patient is a proper candidate, sedation and local anesthetic at the incision site can be used for the miniabdominoplasty technique.

Prepping and Draping

Once the patient is anesthetized, the patient's skin will be prepped for surgery and the sterile drapes are placed. The antiseptic solution used will be based on surgeon's preference, as the only limitations for this surgery are based on the patient's allergies. The skin is prepped from the patient's nipples down to the mid-thighs, including the mons pubis. The lateral abdomen is prepped to the edge of the operating room bed on both sides. Occasionally, the lateral abdominal skin hangs too close to the edge of the operating room bed to be sterile prepped, so a member of the team will roll the patient laterally for the skin prep to extend far enough on the patient's side. Before the patient is rolled back, a sterile member of the team will place a large drape along the side, which will allow the patient's prepped skin to rest on sterile drapes. This same process will occur on the opposite side of the patient. With the large drapes placed along the sides of the patient, sterile blue towels are placed along the borders of the sterile field. One blue towel is placed at the xiphoid process, another blue towel is placed at the most inferior border of the mons pubis. Sometimes more than one towel is needed to span the distance across the patient. Blue towels are also placed on each side of the patient connecting the sterile field with the other blue towels placed. Lastly, two U-drapes or two additional large drapes can be used to cover the remaining unsterile portions of the patient.

Surgical Procedure

- After the sterile field has been established, the suprapubic incision is excised first using a 10-blade scalpel.

- While the surgeon is using the scalpel, the SA is keeping tension on the skin opposite the surgeon and using a laparotomy sponge to control any bleeding on the incision line.

- The surgeon will use the electrocautery to continue the dissection through the dermis, subcutaneous fat and Scarpa's fascia. Large superficial vessels may be present while the surgeon is dissecting, so the SA should have a curved hemostat ready to clamp any large bleeding vessels.

- Additional electrocautery could also be helpful during this procedure to facilitate hemostasis and allow for continued progress during the case. Dissection of the suprapubic incision ends at the rectus abdominus fascia then the abdominal skin flap is dissected cephalad toward the xiphoid process.

- When the cephalad dissection reaches the umbilical stalk, a circumferential incision is created around the umbilicus and dissection is carried through the skin flap around the umbilical stalk. The umbilicus is tagged with a nonabsorbable suture and hemostat to allow for easier manipulation.

- Once the umbilicus is completely free from the skin flap, the cephalad dissection using electrocautery can continue medially toward the xiphoid process.

- The SA can use a Yancoskie Abdominoplasty Retractor to aid in retracting the large abdominal skin flap cephalad. Care is taken to preserve the lateral attachments of the abdominal wall which contain the neurovascular bundles of the abdominal skin.

- The goal is to free the pannus and medial abdominal wall attachments from the anterior rectus abdominus fascia. The surgeon may also dissect the inferior skin flap toward the mons pubis to aid in incision closure later.

- The SA can use facelift retractors to reflect the inferior skin flap upward while the surgeon dissects the skin flap.

- The surgeon will focus on bringing the superior skin down more than bringing the inferior skin upward to avoid stretching the pubic hair out of the bikini line region.

- With the skin attachments free from the rectus abdominus, the patient is placed in Fowler's position by flexing the bed and lowering the leg portion of the bed. The Fowler's position will aid in pulling down the abdominal skin toward the suprapubic incision.

- The surgeon must ensure that the superior incision will easily meet the suprapubic incision without excessive tension. If the tension is too great between the incisions, then wound healing will be compromised.

- After assessing the superior skin incision, the surgeon will amputate the skin flap at the marked incision line.

- The SA will assist with the amputation by holding traction on the skin flap. Any bleeding from the superior abdominal skin flap is controlled using electrocautery.

- The surgeon will now focus on the rectus abdominus muscle plication. With excessive weight gain or pregnancy, the strain on the midline rectus abdominus attachments can cause a diastasis of the two bellies of the rectus abdominus muscles.

- Over time, the diastasis causes decreased core strength as well as the lack of the standard "six-pack" rectus abdominus appearance. To solve this problem, the surgeon will plicate the anterior rectus abdominus muscle fascia together. The plication technique uses either an absorbable or nonabsorbable suture, size zero on a large suture needle like a CT-1.

- Buried, interrupted vertical mattress sutures are used along the length of the diastasis to bring the splayed edges together. The SA can tie the sutures for the surgeon or start suturing at one end of the diastasis meeting the surgeon in the middle.

- Once the rectus abdominus muscle fascia is plicated, the incision closure begins. The surgeon may have the preference to place bilateral Jackson-Pratt drains at the hips during an abdominoplasty, and these need to be placed prior to the beginning of skin closure. The drains are secured to the skin using a nonabsorbable monofilament suture.

- Alternatively, the superior abdominal flap is sutured down to the rectus abdominus with a quilting suture using a 2-0 absorbable braided suture starting proximally working down toward the inferior incision line. These sutures close the dead space created during the skin flap dissection, which helps prevent hematoma and seroma formation making drain placement unnecessary.

- After the dead space is adequately closed, the superior and inferior incision lines are sutured together. Starting with an interrupted deep buried suture using a 2-0 absorbable braided suture, the Scarpa's fascia layer is sutured together. While suturing this layer, the Scarpa's fascia is attached to the rectus abdominus fascia directly under the incision line. This suturing technique helps add strength to the incision line as well as close dead space. The suture in this layer will be evenly spaced about three centimeters apart. It is best to start at the apex of the incision when suturing the deep layers.

- A complication of abdominoplasty is uneven apices or "dog-ears." This is prevented by lining up the superior and inferior incision lines to lay flat at the apex.

- Before closure of this layer is completed, the reattachment of the umbilicus will occur. The surgeon will mark on the abdominal wall where the umbilicus will sit and create a cross-incision through the skin and subcutaneous tissue. The choice of reattachment site needs to allow for minimal tension on the umbilical stalk to ensure successful wound healing.

- The SA can use a hemostat to reach into the new incision and grab the suture tag on the umbilicus to deliver it to the new attachment site.

- The umbilicus is sutured to the abdominal skin using a 4-0 absorbable suture, either monofilament or fast-absorbing gut suture.

- Next, the deep dermis of the lower abdominal transverse incision is closed using a 3-0 absorbable braided suture. The deep dermal layer is sutured in a continuous running pattern, and because of this some surgeons have adopted using a barbed suture in this layer.

- The final layer closed is the superficial dermal layer using a 4-0 absorbable monofilament suture. Because an abdominoplasty has an extensive amount of suturing involved, the surgeon and SA work simultaneously to complete all the closure.

- The closed incisions will be dressed using 1-inch steri-strips and approximately eight abdominal pads. If drains were used, then gauze and tape may be placed over the entrance sites. The abdominal binder is placed around the patient for compression and core support.

Post-op Considerations. Complications vary from patient to patient; however, seroma formation, umbilicus necrosis, wound dehiscence, and deep vein thrombosis are the most common complications following an abdominoplasty. Ensuring the incision is closed under just the right amount of tension to achieve the flattened abdomen look will help in preventing dehiscence as well as quality suturing. The umbilicus needs to be reattached also under minimal tension to ensure no necrosis, though the surgeons will counsel the patients of the risk for umbilical loss. The quilting sutures and abdominal binder will allow for the abdominal skin to adhere to the rectus abdominus fascia to avoid seroma formation. Deep vein thrombus is preempted with an injection of 5000 of heparin either preoperatively or postoperatively as well as the use of antithrombotic stockings and/or sequential compression devices intraoperatively and early ambulation during postoperative recovery.

SKIN GRAFT

The first documented use of a skin graft dates back almost 3000 years ago in India. Criminals were punished by having their noses amputated, so doctors repaired the defect using skin taken from the gluteal region. In modern times, the first full-thickness skin graft dates to 1817 by Sir Astley Cooper to cover an amputated thumb, and as more surgeons began to use full thickness skin grafts, Wolfe and Krause mainstreamed the use of the full-thickness skin graft. Modern split-thickness skin graft began in 1886 with Thiersch using a thin skin graft to cover a large wound. Recognizing the need to control the thickness of the harvested skin, Graham Humby developed the Humby knife, which allows the surgeon to control the depth of tissue harvested. In 1948, the first electric dermatome was developed by Harry Brown with many modifications throughout the years. The electric dermatome allowed the surgeon to rapidly remove long areas of skin which proved especially useful for burn patients. Meshing technology was developed in 1964 to expand the split-thickness skin graft up to 12 times the original size.

Anatomy

The skin is comprised of two layers of tissue: the epidermis and dermis. The thickness of the layers depends upon the location of the body. The face measures the thinnest of skin layers on the body, whereas the back measures the thickest skin layers of the body. Determining where to harvest a skin graft depends upon where the wound is that needs covering. Skin grafts are composed of the epidermis and either all or part of the dermis. The epidermis is a thin avascular layer of various cells that provides a physical barrier for the body. The thick dermal layer contains many structures within its collagen matrix. Sebaceous and sweat glands are in the dermis layer as well as a complex vascular network. Hair follicles originate in the dermis and grow through the epidermis layer. This plays an important role in determining where a donor graft will be harvested on the body. The harvested skin graft needs to match thickness, color, and hair density to the wound site as closely as possible to give the patient a cosmetic result.

Surgical Approach

Skin grafts are necessary to cover wounds that are not able to epithelialize. These wounds can be from excision sites, infections, or burns. Choosing to use a split- or full-thickness skin graft is based on the location of the wound and the surgeon's judgment. A split-thickness skin graft only contains the epidermis with the superficial portion of the dermis. A full-thickness skin graft contains both the epidermis and full dermis. Traditionally, full-thickness skin grafts are used on wounds that are small and/or located on the face. Full-thickness skin grafts blend in with the surrounding tissue easier, so the outcome is more cosmetic. Split-thickness skin grafts are used to cover large wounds on most areas of the body. The process of meshing the split-thickness skin graft allows the surgeon to take a small section of donor skin to cover a much larger wound area. A disadvantage to a split-thickness skin graft is that it can leave a large scar at the donor site; however, in some burn patient cases this is unavoidable.

When harvesting skin for a skin graft, donor site selection must be determined based on the size of defect that needs covering. Split-thickness skin grafts are harvested mostly from the lateral thigh, but the donor site can be taken from any large flat surface of the body. Some examples are buttocks or back. Since a portion of the dermis is left behind, the donor site is left

to heal. Epithelial cells advance from pilosebaceous units and migrate laterally to reconstitute a new epithelial layer, a process called epithelialization. A full-thickness skin graft needs to be taken from an area of the body that has enough laxity to allow for closure since the complete dermis is removed from the site. The groin, post-auricular area, supraclavicular area, and abdomen are common donor sites for full-thickness skin grafts.

Surgical Procedure

- To achieve a split-thickness skin graft, the skin is generally removed from the patient with an electric dermatome (see Figure 20-16). The dermatome has an adjustable depth gauge and a sterile disposable blade to achieve the desired thickness of graft.

- To use the dermatome, the electrical cord is passed off the field and connected to the motor box. The skin harvesting location is lubricated with mineral oil to decrease the friction against the dermatome.

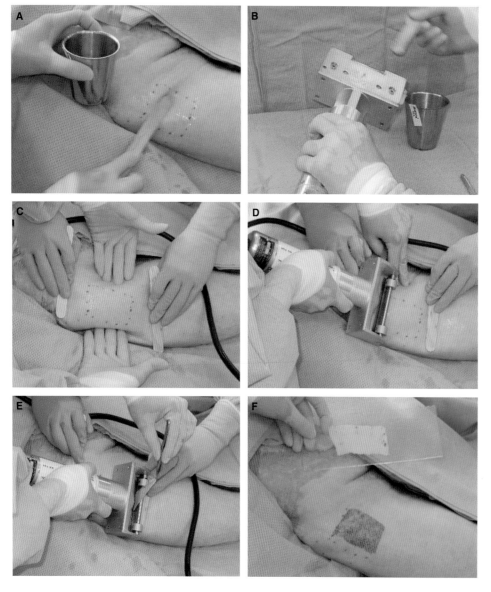

Figure 20-16 · Skin harvest site preparation using dermatome. (Reproduced, with permission, from Morita SY, Balch CM, Klimberg VS, Pawlik TM, Posner MC, Tanabe KK, eds. *Textbook of Complex General Surgical Oncology.* New York, NY: McGraw Hill; 2018.)

- The SA will pull traction against the skin using a laparotomy sponge and hold an Adson forceps with teeth in the other hand.

- The surgeon engages the dermatome against the skin and gradually pushes the dermatome forward. As the skin begins to lift off the donor site and into the dermatome, the SA will use the Adson forceps with teeth to hold the beginnings of the skin graft upward. This allows the surgeon to assess his or her progress.

- After the skin is fully removed from the donor site, the donor skin is placed on a skin graft carrier plate, and an epinephrine solution soaked on a laparotomy sponge is placed over the donor site. This aides in hemostasis of the raw donor site.

- The skin graft carrier plate allows the skin graft to be passed through a meshing device. The meshing device allows the harvested skin to expand its surface area by creating specific size holes in the harvested skin as well as allowing for fluid to exude through the meshed graft interfaces (see Figure 20-17).

- Subsequent graft fluid accumulations result in graft failure. The skin graft carrier plate comes in a variety of expansion ratios, ranging from 1:1.5 to 1:9. The choice of skin graft carrier plate is determined based on the size and number of wounds that need to be covered with the skin graft. The smaller the expansion ration means the smaller the holes are, so the harvest skin will not be able to stretch as wide.

- Extensive burn patients will typically need the large expansion ratio skin graft carrier plate to maximize the square footage of harvestable skin. The meshing device has a manual rachet handle and is sterile on the back table.

- The harvested skin is placed either epidermis down or epidermis up on the skin graft carrier plate. The SA uses the back end of a forceps and saline to unroll the edges of the harvested skin. The goal is to have the harvested skin as flat as possible to mesh the skin uniformly.

- Once the harvested skin lays flat on the carrier plate, the carrier plate is introduced into the meshing device and slowly advanced through the device.

- While the skin graft carrier plate is advancing through the meshing device, the SA uses an Adson forceps with teeth to ensure the skin does not wrap around the barrel of the meshing device. Once the carrier has fully passed through the meshing device, the harvested skin will be ready to be placed on the wound.

- To achieve a full-thickness skin graft, the skin is removed with a scalpel. The donor site is measured and drawn onto the patient to ensure enough skin is harvested.

- The SA holds tension on the skin while the surgeon excises through the epidermis and dermis in an ellipse pattern.

- The donor site is fully excised away from the underlying subcutaneous tissue, then hemostasis is achieved of the donor site. Any subcutaneous fat still attached to the dermis is removed using curved Metzenbaum scissors before it is transferred to the wound.

- Before the harvested skin is placed on the wound, the wound bed must be debrided of all necrotic and granulated tissue.

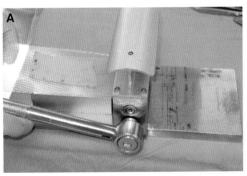
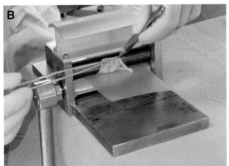
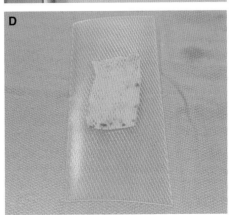

Figure 20-17 · Donor skin meshing technique. (Reproduced, with permission, from Morita SY, Balch CM, Klimberg VS, Pawlik TM, Posner MC, Tanabe KK, eds. *Textbook of Complex General Surgical Oncology.* New York, NY: McGraw Hill; 2018.)

- The surgeon may use a scalpel to achieve this or a hydrosurgical device, like a Versajet©. Careful hemostasis is achieved at the wound bed to ensure no hematoma formation once the skin graft is placed.

- If any bone or implant is exposed in the wound bed, the skin graft will not adhere so an alternative plan, like a pedicle flap, is needed.

- Once the wound bed is ready for grafting, the split- or full-thickness skin graft is secured to the wound bed. Handling the split-thickness skin graft can be difficult because of its thinness, so transferring the skin by flipping the skin onto the wound bed using the skin graft carrier is an effective transfer method. Full-thickness skin grafts have more tissue, so they are easier to manipulate by hand to the shape of the wound bed.

- The surgeon will choose the method to secure the skin graft based on location of wound and personal preference. The skin graft can be secured to the wound using sutures or staples. Staples are a quick option; however, using absorbable suture prevents the patient from needing to have the suture removed later.

- The skin graft donor and recipient site need to have dressing placed during this procedure. The split-thickness skin graft donor site has multiple options for dressing and the surgeon will determine his or her preference. Some surgeons will leave the donor site open to air or cover with a Vaseline-impregnated gauze stapled to the size of donor site.

- The full-thickness donor site is closed using a 3-0 braided absorbable suture in the dermis and a 4-0 monofilament absorbable suture using an intracuticular in the superficial dermis. This allows the full-thickness donor site to be dressed using steri-strips and gauze.

- Multiple dressing options are available for the recipient site, but the dressing should be nonadherent against the skin graft and allow for immobilization of the skin graft. Immobilization can occur using negative pressure wound therapy dressing or a cotton bolster dressing (see Figure 20-18). The negative pressure wound dressing or cotton bolster dressing helps the skin graft adhere to the underlying wound bed by preventing hematoma formation and maintaining compression between the two tissues.

- If the skin graft is near a joint, the surgeon may choose to place the extremity in a splint. The splint will help prevent shear forces against the graft by preventing excessive movement of the extremity.

Post-op Considerations. Complications involving split- or full-thickness skin grafts revolved around graft failure. The harvested skin does not have its own blood supply, so successful wound healing is reliant upon the graft adherence to the underlying wound bed. The skin graft can fail because of hematoma or seroma formation, which lifts the skin graft away from the wound bed. Shear forces against the skin graft can also prevent adherence to the wound bed and lead to a lack of revascularization.

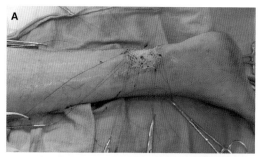
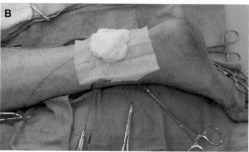
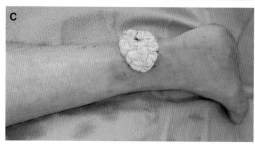

Figure 20-18 · Bolster dressing application over skin graft. (Reproduced, with permission, from Morita SY, Balch CM, Klimberg VS, Pawlik TM, Posner MC, Tanabe KK, eds. *Textbook of Complex General Surgical Oncology*. New York, NY: McGraw Hill; 2018.)

TRAM FLAP BREAST RECONSTRUCTION

For patients needing an autologous tissue breast reconstruction, a transverse rectus abdominus muscle (TRAM) flap is a viable option. A TRAM flap uses a portion of the abdominal wall with or without the rectus abdominus muscle attached to create a breast mound after mastectomy. Approximately, 14,000 patients chose TRAM flap reconstruction in 2019 making it the most popular autologous breast reconstruction technique. Patients may have a TRAM flap reconstruction immediately following a mastectomy or the reconstruction is performed at another time. This is due to surgeon availability or the patient's cancer treatment plan requiring priority.

Surgical Approach

Transverse rectus abdominus muscle flap reconstruction has a few variations depending on patient's anatomy and wishes. The first option is a pedicle transverse rectus abdominus muscle flap, which was first described by Hartrampf in 1982. The pedicle flap does not detach the superior portion of the rectus abdominus muscle, so the flap is vascularized through the superior epigastric vascular bundle. A tunnel is created from the abdomen into the breast pocket to pass the pedicle TRAM flap for the breast reconstruction. The other TRAM flap options utilize a free muscle flap that requires a microvascular anastomosis to provide the vascular supply for the breast reconstruction. A free TRAM flap removes a portion of the rectus abdominus muscle with the inferior epigastric vascular bundle. The free TRAM flap was first described in 1979 by Holmstrom, but slowly gained popularity as microvascular surgical techniques became more common. In 1992, Robert Allen further modified the free TRAM flap by creating a flap without removing any portion of the rectus abdominus muscle. A DIEP TRAM flap utilizes the deep inferior epigastric perforators to provide the vascular supply by dissecting the perforators away from the rectus abdominus muscle.

Anatomy

The abdominal wall is comprised of multiple layers of soft tissue that extend from the costal margins to the symphysis pubis and bilaterally to the iliac crest and midaxillary line. The outermost layers are the epidermis and dermis. Under the dermis is the subcutaneous fat layer also known as Camper's fascia and an additional pseudo-fascial layer called Scarpa's fascia. Camper's and Scarpa's fascia are most prominent below the arcuate line which is located beneath the umbilicus. The umbilicus is in the midline of the abdomen about at the level of the superior iliac spines. Beneath these layers is the anterior rectus sheath covering the two bellies of the rectus abdominus muscles and a posterior rectus sheath under that. The rectus abdominus fascia combines to form the linea alba at the midline of the abdomen. Along with the paired rectus abdominus muscles at the midline, the abdomen laterally has three additional muscle layers: internal oblique, external oblique and transverse abdominus muscles. These four muscles provide support for the abdomen and allow for flexion and rotation of the trunk. The vascular supply to the abdominal wall consists of the superior and inferior epigastric arteries as well as the deep circumflex iliac arteries. The superior and inferior epigastric arteries run with the rectus abdominus muscle. The abdominal wall is innervated by the thoracoabdominal, iliohypogastric and ilioinguinal nerves. The motor function of the rectus abdominus muscles is innervated by the intercostal nerves at T7-T11 and the subcostal nerves at T12.

Preparing the Patient for Surgery

Prior to the patient entering the operating room, special equipment and instruments must be available. The operating room bed must be positioned to allow it to flex at the waist. This is important for closure to offload the tension on the abdominal flaps. If the patient is undergoing a free TRAM flap, an operating microscope must be in the room and must be tested to ensure it is fully operational. Along with the microscope, a Doppler machine is utilized to find and monitor the vascular flap. Having a complete microvascular instrument set is also vital for a successful surgery. The operating room will also be warmed to at least 75° Fahrenheit. A patient that is normothermic will have dilated vessels, making the vasculature of the TRAM flap more viable. An underbody Bair Hugger

blanket may be utilized to warm the patient, since most of the patient will be exposed during the surgery.

Anesthesia

Once the patient has entered the operating room, the patient will undergo general anesthesia during her transverse rectus abdominus muscle flap breast reconstruction. An epidural may also be offered for postoperative pain relief. After the patient is intubated, a Foley urinary catheter is inserted since this procedure will be longer than 3 hours. The patient's arms are padded on the arm boards and secured using an ace wrap or Kerlix wrap. Since the patient will be flexed at the waist, it is vital that the arms are secured appropriately to avoid injury. A safety strap is placed just above the knees and a pillow is placed under the knees for support.

Prepping and Draping

The patient will be prepped from the chin down to the midthigh and down to the elbows. The prep will also include laterally down to the operating room bed as well as the mons pubis. The prep utilized is based on surgeon's preference as well as the patient's allergies.

After the patient is sterilely prepped, a large drape is placed on the lateral sides of the patient, tucking it slightly underneath the abdomen and thorax. Multiple blue towels are then used to mark the border of the sterile area. One blue towel is placed across the clavicles. Another blue towel is placed across the thighs at the base of the mons pubis. Towels are then placed laterally along the abdomen and thorax, and care is taken to include the axilla of the operative side. A split sheet drape is placed at the base of the mons pubis and extended laterally down to the operating room table. An additional split sheet drape is placed at the clavicle and extended laterally around the axilla down to the operating room table.

Surgical Procedure

- The transverse rectus abdominus muscle flap is created by ellipting the lower abdominal skin. A low transverse incision is made bilaterally from the anterior superior iliac spine to the pubis.

- The ellipse is completed by making a transverse incision at the supraumbilical level. The umbilicus is also isolated from the flap by creating a circular incision around the umbilicus and the umbilical stalk is dissected down to the rectus fascia.

- The dermis and subcutaneous tissue are dissected down to the underlying fascia. Then the flap is lifted laterally from the external oblique fascia until the inferior epigastric vascular perforators are found.

- Both sides of the abdominal flap are dissected to ensure the side with the strongest perforators is used for breast reconstruction. Typically, a pedicle TRAM flap utilizes the ipsilateral abdominal flap, whereas the free TRAM flap utilizes the contralateral abdominal flap.

- Once the perforators are identified, the lateral rectus fascia is incised exposing the rectus muscle. The deep inferior epigastric artery and vein are identified down to their insertion on the iliac vessels. The perforators are identified medially, and the medial rectus fascia is incised.

- While this dissection is occurring, care is taken by the SA to not pull too forcefully on the abdominal flap. This prevents shear forces from damaging or avulsing the perforators from the flap.

- The type of flap the surgeon chooses to use dictates how much of the rectus muscle and/or perforators are dissected. If the surgeon is using a pedicled flap, the rectus muscle is excised from its insertion at the pubis, and the inferior epigastric vascular pedicle is ligated.

- The rectus muscle is separated from its peritoneal attachments up to the costal margin. The rectus muscle is left attached at the costal margin and the superior epigastric vascular bundle stays intact.

- If the surgeon is using a free TRAM flap, the rectus muscle is excised superiorly and inferiorly ensuring that all the necessary perforators stay intact.

- For the free DIEP flap, the inferior epigastric artery vascular bundle is dissected away from the rectus muscle leaving the rectus muscle completely intact (see Figure 20-19).

- For both free flap techniques, the inferior epigastric vascular bundle is ligated at the iliac artery and vein using multiple clips. At this point, the flap is no longer receiving blood flow, so the start of ischemia time is noted. The longer the flap is without blood flow, the higher the risk is for flap death, so surgeons like to keep ischemia time to under 1 hour.

- After all the peritoneal attachments are released and the perforators are preserved, the flap is presented to the mastectomy defect for insetting.

- A pedicle TRAM flap is passed from the abdominal region into the mastectomy defect through a subcutaneous tunnel created. Utilizing the ipsilateral abdominal flap allows the TRAM flap is be tunneled into the mastectomy defect without leaving a large bulge in the patient's epigastric region.

- For a free TRAM and DIEP flap, the abdominal flap is completely lifted away from the abdominal and placed onto the mastectomy defect with the vascular bundle facing the vessels used for the anastomosis.

- The surgeon has two options for vascular anastomosis recipient: the internal mammary vessels or the thoracodorsal

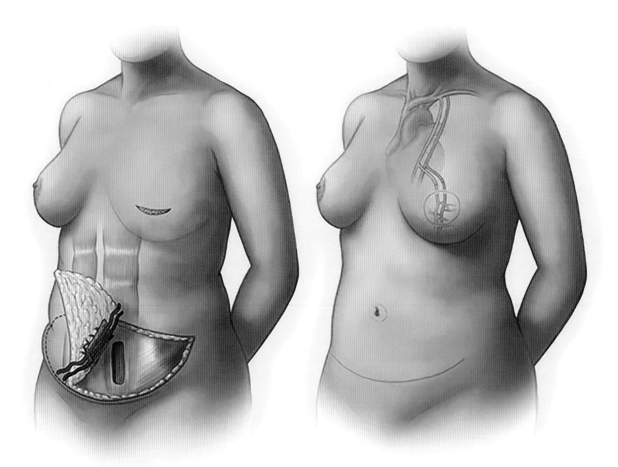

Figure 20-19 • Tram flap reconstruction. (Reproduced with permission from the Mayo Foundation for Medical Education and Research. All rights reserved.)

vessels. Choosing between these two vascular bundles is based on surgeon's preference as well as patient anatomy.

- It is important that the SA discusses the surgeon's preferences prior to beginning the surgery to ensure all specialty instruments are available. If the surgeon uses the internal mammary vessels, rib cutters will be necessary to access the vessels.

- Whichever vessel recipient is chosen, the artery and vein need to be dissected and exposed prior to the ligation of the inferior epigastric vascular bundle. This ensures flap ischemia time will not be wasted and the anastomosis can begin immediately following the ligation.

- Before the anastomosis begins, anchoring sutures using 2-0 suture are placed connecting the rectus muscle to the pectoralis muscle, as well as staples placed connected the TRAM flap skin to the mastectomy skin edges. These prevent the TRAM flap from drastically moving during vessel anastomosis.

- For revascularizing the flap, the inferior epigastric artery and vein are anastomosed to the recipient vessels utilizing an operating microscope. The inferior epigastric artery and vein are trimmed to the appropriate length to meet the recipient vessel. Too long of a vessel can cause kinking of the vessel after the anastomosis is completed and too short of a vessel puts too much tension on the anastomosis leading to leaking.

- The vessels are irrigated using a heparinized saline to flush any debris or clots from the lumen and any extra adventitia is removed from around the opening in the vessels.

- The arteries are sutured together using a 9-0 monofilament permanent suture. The surgeon places interrupted sutures connected the vessels being careful not to grab the opposite vessel wall when placing the suture needle.

- The suture tails can be left long for the SA to use as handles. This allows the SA to manipulate the artery without risking damaging the arterial walls.

- After the arterial anastomosis is completed, the micro bulldog placed on the recipient vessel is released, checking for leaks in the suture line.

- The veins are anastomosed utilizing a microvascular coupler device. The coupler device everts the vein's intima and joins the two veins with an interlocking ring. Suturing the veins with a 9-0 monofilament permanent suture is still a viable option; however, veins are inherently very friable and need to be handled delicately.

- Once the artery and veins are connected, blood flow is reestablished to the TRAM flap and a Doppler is used to find an arterial signal in the superficial skin portion of the flap. A dyed monofilament permanent suture is used to mark the site of the strongest Doppler signal for postoperative monitoring of the TRAM flap.

- With circulation reestablished through the TRAM flap, the flap insetting is completed. Additional interrupted sutures are placed anchoring the rectus muscle to the underlying pectoralis muscle being cautious to not ligate any perforators.

- The skin and subcutaneous tissue is shaped to fit the mastectomy defect.

- If needed, portions of the skin is deepithelialized to allow the dermis to be buried beneath the skin edges. This allows for maximum use of the flap for projection and defect coverage.

- The dermis is closed using an interrupted 3-0 braided absorbable suture, and then the skin is closed with an intracuticular 4-0 monofilament absorbable suture.

- After the TRAM flap is secured to the mastectomy defect, the abdominal closure begins. Regardless of the type of TRAM flap utilized for the reconstruction, the rectus fascial defect must be repaired.

- The fascial defect is primarily closed using a size 0 suture utilizing a buried interrupted suturing technique. The type of suture utilized varies depending on the surgeon's preference; however, surgeons typically chose a suture that is long lasting to give the fascia time to heal.

- While primarily closing the fascial defect, the contralateral side's rectus fascia may also need plicating to keep the umbilicus centrally located.

- After the defect is primarily closed, the surgeon may choose to secure mesh over the closed fascial defect. This gives the fascia support to prevent future herniation. The same suture utilized for the rectus fascia closure is used to secure the mesh. Once the fascial defect is repaired, the closure continues in the same manner as an abdominoplasty closure.

- The breast and abdominal incisions are dressed in a similar manner. Most surgeons are utilizing Prineo® dermabond skin closure mesh over the incision sites. An alternative is to use steri-strips. The umbilicus is covered in a petroleum jelly–impregnated gauze, and abdominal pads are used to cover the breast and the entire abdomen. The dressings are held onto the patient with a loose-fitting bra and an abdominal binder. Tape is avoided for risk of tape blisters due to swelling, and the abdominal binder applies pressure to prevent seroma or hematoma formation under the abdominal flap.

Post-op Considerations. A TRAM flap is contraindicated for patients that have undergone previous abdominoplasty or do not have adequate abdominal tissue to utilize for the flap. Also, patients who are morbidly obese have a higher risk of complications and active smokers have a higher risk of flap loss when utilizing the free TRAM technique. Careful consideration must also be given to patients needing bilateral breast reconstructions. Though not impossible to perform, a bilateral TRAM flap leaves the patient with a weaker abdominal wall, as well as being under anesthesia for a longer period. The most common complication following TRAM flap breast reconstruction is flap necrosis and abdominal bulging. Other potential complications include complete flap failure, seroma formation, hematoma, and abdominal hernia. Patients stay in the hospital for a minimum of 3 days postoperatively to monitor the flap and for pain control.

LATISSIMUS DORSI FLAP BREAST RECONSTRUCTION

The latissimus dorsi flap is a breast reconstruction technique that utilizes a portion of the latissimus dorsi muscle and skin paddle to add volume and coverage after a mastectomy. The pedicled flap reconstruction can also be combined with a tissue expander or breast implant. The latissimus dorsi flap is a dependable option for patients in need of breast reconstruction, especially those with radiated tissue (see Figure 20-20).

In 1906, Iginio Tansini first described utilizing the latissimus dorsi muscle with a skin paddle to cover the large skin defect after the standard radical mastectomy of that era. Due to the lack of anesthesia and resuscitation abilities during surgery in the early 1900s, this technique was rarely done. By the late 1970s, the muscle flap began to gain popularity for breast reconstructions for its ability to cover the breast implant with muscle and replace surface area lost during the mastectomy. In 1983, Papp and McCraw described a latissimus dorsi flap technique that allowed for the reconstruction to be completed without the use of a breast implant. Variations of these techniques have been developed throughout the past few decades; however, the basic concepts of the latissimus dorsi flap have remained the same.

Anatomy

The latissimus dorsi muscle is a large flat triangular muscle that is located on the posterior trunk. Its broad muscle belly structure has multiple origin points across the posterior trunk. The inferior border originates on the posterior superior iliac spine, and the superior border begins on the inferior angle of the scapula. The medial border originates on the

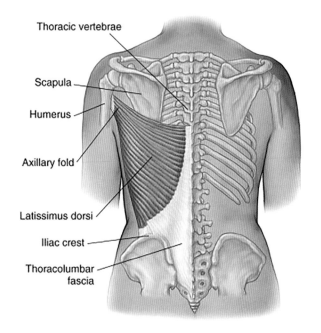

Figure 20-20 · Latissimus dorsi flap. (Reproduced, with permission, from Latissimus dorsi flap. *Pocket Dentistry.* https://pocketdentistry.com/latissimus-dorsi-flap/)

spinous processes of the sixth thoracic, lumbar, and superior sacral vertebrae, and the lateral border derives from the fourth rib's external surface. The latissimus dorsi muscle fibers travel toward the axilla where it fuses with the external surface of the serratus anterior muscle. The muscle fibers combine with the teres major muscle to form a large tendon, which inserts at the intertubercular groove of the humerus. The function of the latissimus dorsi muscle is to adduct, extend and medially rotate the humerus. When the latissimus dorsi muscle is transposed for a muscle flap, the shoulder girdle muscles take over those functions for the humerus. The latissimus dorsi muscle is supplied by the thoracodorsal trunk, which is found in the axilla. The thoracodorsal trunk contains the thoracodorsal artery, vein, and nerve. The thoracodorsal artery is a branch of the subscapular artery, and it inserts posteriorly into the latissimus dorsi muscle near the insertion point. The thoracodorsal vein drains into the circumflex scapular vein, which further empties into the axillary vein. The thoracodorsal nerve provides the motor innervation for the latissimus dorsi muscle, and it arises from the C6 to C8 roots of the brachial plexus. The nerve travels posterior to the axillary vein to join the thoracodorsal trunk in the axilla.

Preparing the Patient for Surgery

Preoperatively, the latissimus dorsi donor site as well as the breast recipient site is marked. If the mastectomy is completed immediately prior to reconstruction, the area of skin incision, usually around the nipple-areolar complex is identified. If the reconstruction is occurring secondarily, the surgeon follows the previous incisions for preparing the breast recipient site. For both instances, the inframammary crease is marked to allow the surgeon a guide for creating the new breast mound. The latissimus dorsi donor site is marked by identifying the borders of the latissimus dorsi muscle. Then, the size of skin paddle is chosen based on the amount of skin necessary to cover any defect on the mastectomy site. The skin paddle needs to be marked centrally over the latissimus dorsi muscle, and care is taken to hide the final scar where a swimsuit strap would lie.

Anesthesia

For a latissimus dorsi flap reconstruction, the patient is placed under general anesthesia due to the multiple position changes that occur to complete the reconstruction. The patient begins in the supine position to complete the mastectomy or to prepare the breast pocket due to a prior mastectomy. However, to access the latissimus dorsi muscle, the patient is placed in the lateral decubitus position using a vacuum pack surgical positioning system. The bottom leg is bent and padded with foam. Pillows are placed between the knees and ankles. The top leg is extended straight on top of the pillows. An axillary roll is placed along the nonoperative side's axilla to prevent a brachial plexus injury. The bottom arm is padded with foam and secured to an arm board. The operative side's arm will be draped into the field to allow for manipulation of the latissimus dorsi muscle tendon insertion site. To assist with holding the sterile draped arm for the procedure, a padded and sterile draped mayo stand can be placed across the lower arm after

(Figure labels: Thoracic vertebrae, Scapula, Humerus, Axillary fold, Latissimus dorsi, Iliac crest, Thoracolumbar fascia)

draping is completed. After the harvesting of the latissimus dorsi muscle and skin paddle, the surgeon may want to turn the patient back supine to inset the flap at the mastectomy site. Surgeon's preference as well as patient selection will determine if the surgical procedure is performed only in the lateral position or if multiple position changes are necessary. Communicating with the surgeon before the patient is brought to the operating room allows the SA to be prepared with multiple changes of sterile drapes.

Prepping and Draping the Patient

After the patient is anesthetized, the patient's first site is prepped using the surgeon's preferred antiseptic agent. The patient is prepped from chin to umbilicus, and laterally to the top of the operating room bed. A large sterile drape is placed laterally on each side of the patient. This drape covers the arm and is tucked slightly under the patient's side. Next, four sterile blue towels are placed around the breasts and a transverse laparotomy drape is used to complete the sterile field. At this time, the breast recipient site is prepared. If the patient requires it, the mastectomy will be completed at this time. If the mastectomy was completed at a previous date, then the skin flaps for the breast mound need to be dissected upward. The surgeon makes an incision over the previous scars and any damaged radiated skin is removed. The SA lifts the skin edge with facelift retractors while the surgeon uses electrocautery to dissect the skin flap off the underlying pectoralis major muscle. Once the breast recipient site is prepared, the area is temporarily sealed with an incise drape like Loban™. This allows the patient to be repositioned laterally without closing the breast incision.

Once the patient is repositioned lateral, the patient's posterior trunk and anterior chest well to the chin are prepped down to the operating room bed. The operative side's arm is also prepped to the wrist. After the prep is complete, a large drape is placed at the bottom of the posterior trunk to cover the operating room bed. Another large drape is placed on the opposite side of the patient to cover the lower arm and operating room table on the anterior chest side of the patient. Four sterile blue towels are placed at the chin, the anterior superior iliac spine, and on top of the large drapes. The arm is draped using an impervious stockinette and wrapped in Coban™. Two split drapes are used to complete the sterile field.

Surgical Procedure

- With the lateral sterile field complete, the surgeon begins the latissimus dorsi muscle harvest. The surgeon uses a scalpel to incise the preplanned incisions for the skin paddle over the latissimus dorsi muscle.
- The paddle's skin and dermis are dissected downward until the latissimus dorsi muscle comes into view, then the SA uses facelift retractors to create skin flaps on the posterior trunk. These skin flaps separate the latissimus dorsi muscle anteriorly from the posterior trunk's dermis.
- The superior skin flap is dissected cephalad toward the humerus and then the inferior skin flap is dissected to the posterior superior iliac spine.

- Once the skin flaps begin to form, the facelift retractors are switched to large, bladed retractors, like Eastman or Deaver. Lighted retractors are also useful during this dissection because the distance between the skin paddle and humerus is long.
- After the anterior latissimus dorsi muscle is released from the dermis, the posterior muscle is dissected off the trunk. To prevent shear forces affecting the perforators to the skin paddle, temporary sutures are placed between the muscle belly and the dermis of the skin paddle.
- Beginning at the posterior superior iliac spine, the latissimus dorsi muscle is dissected from the posterior attachments. Care is taken to control bleeding as the muscle belly is lifted cephalad toward the axilla.
- The SA retracts the skin flaps with the large-bladed retractors to allow the surgeon greater visualization. As the surgeon dissects the muscle belly closer to the axilla, the SA keeps a hand on the flap to ensure it does not separate from the thoracodorsal trunk. When the surgeon reaches the axilla, the draped operative arm is abducted to allow the surgeon more access to the latissimus dorsi muscle insertion site on the humerus.
- The surgeon will transect the tendon to allow the muscle flap to rotate through a tunnel in the axilla and onto the breast donor site.
- At this stage, the latissimus dorsi muscle flap is only connected to the patient via the blood supply of the thoracodorsal trunk. As the flap rotates through the axilla, the surgeon checks to ensure the blood vessels are intact without twisting. The surgeon may also decide to transect the thoracodorsal nerve in some instances to prevent any motor function of the latissimus dorsi muscle flap.
- Drains are placed in the harvest site to monitor hematoma and seroma formation. The drains exit the patient at the inframammary crease which will allow easier access for removal and more comfort for the patient.
- The surgeon has two choices at this point, which are to turn the patient supine to complete the insetting of the flap to the breast site or to inset the flap while the patient is still lateral. This decision is determined by surgeon's preference as well as patient size. If the surgeon chooses to turn the patient supine, the posterior trunk incision is closed and sterile dressed and the breast site is again covered with an incise drape for the change of position.
- The change of position will require an additional sterile prep and sterile drapes.
- Before the patient is repositioned, the posterior incision requires closure and dressings. The dead space created from the superior and inferior skin flaps is closed with a 2-0 absorbable suture using a simple interrupted closure technique.
- The number of interrupted sutures necessary to close the dead space is dependent upon the size of the flaps created; however, it is vital this space is closed to prevent seroma formation. After the dead space is closed, the deep dermis of the incision is sutured utilizing a 2-0 absorbable suture about every three centimeters.

- The simple buried interrupted suture grabs the deep dermis on either side of the incision as well as a deep bite down to the thoracolumbar fascia. This technique also helps close dead space to prevent hematoma and seroma formation.

- The rest of the deep dermis is closed using a running 3-0 absorbable suture.

- The final layer of the incision is closed using a 4-0 absorbable monofilament suture utilizing an intracuticular wound closure technique. The patient's back is thoroughly cleaned before dressings are placed. Dressings vary depending on surgeon's preference; however, Prineo™ is becoming a popular choice among surgeons.

- With the posterior incision completed, the insetting of the latissimus dorsi flap onto the mastectomy site begins. The skin paddle of the latissimus dorsi flap is aligned with the mastectomy defect to ensure proper coverage.

- Care is taken to check the thoracodorsal artery and vein to ensure they are patent without twists or kinks. If the artery or vein is obstructed, the flap must be repositioned.

- Once it is confirmed the flap has patent vascular flow, the borders of the latissimus dorsi muscle are secured to the pectoralis major muscle using a 2-0 absorbable suture. This step is to ensure that muscle movement will not cause shear forces on the vascular structures on the flap.

- A drain may be placed at this time between the flap and pectoralis major muscle to monitor for hematoma formation.

- The skin paddle dermis is then sutured using a 3-0 absorbable suture to the mastectomy site's dermis, and the skin is closed using an intracuticular suture technique with a 4-0 absorbable monofilament suture.

- Dressings for the incisions on the flap recipient site are usually the same as the donor site dressings with surgeon preference being the ultimate factor. A loose-fitting bra or six-inch ace wrap may be used to hold the dressing onto the reconstructed breast. The key is to ensure minimal compression on the flap to prevent ischemia.

- Before completing the skin closure, the surgeon may choose to place a tissue expander between the latissimus dorsi flap and the pectoralis major muscle. This is dependent upon the patient's postoperative desires for size of breast mound. The latissimus dorsi muscle flap may not create enough projection for the patient, so a breast implant is used to create this projection.

- The surgeon discusses with the patient preoperatively, which allows the operating room to be prepared with the correct breast implants for the patient.

- If the tissue expander is used, the expander tabs are secured to the pectoralis major muscle with a 2-0 suture. This prevents the tissue expander from flipping while in the new breast pocket.

- The tissue expander is then filled with sterile saline to the appropriate size determined by the surgeon. After the addition of the tissue expander, the incision closure is completed.

Post-op Considerations. Postoperatively, the patient is monitored for a few days in the hospital. The flap is assessed frequently during the first 24 hours to ensure vascular patency, which is critical to the survival of the flap. The patient's pain level is also monitored and controlled before the patient is discharged home. The patient will have shoulder discomfort for a few weeks and is asked to avoid strenuous arm activities like heavy lifting and driving for 6 weeks postoperatively. Removal of drains comes around 1 to 2 weeks after surgery, depending upon the amount of drainage during this time period. Seroma is one the most common complications following latissimus dorsi reconstruction, so the timing of drain removal is critical to prevent this. Due to transposition of the latissimus dorsi muscle, the patient will experience some range of motion and muscle strength deficits after a latissimus dorsi breast reconstruction. However, after 1 year postoperatively, most patients recover their preoperative strength and range of motion. An occasional complication of latissimus dorsi breast reconstruction is flap necrosis; however, this flap is highly reliable due to the thoracodorsal vascular trunk, so it has a high survivability rate. With the addition of tissue expander placement, the patient has additional risks of infection and implant failure.

Latissimus dorsi reconstruction is not always the final surgery for these patients. If the patient had a tissue expander placed, the patient will undergo expansion over a 3- to 6-month time frame; then the tissue expander is replaced with a permanent breast implant. The patient may also choose to have a nipple and areola reconstruction that also requires additional surgery. Patients however are generally satisfied with their postoperative outcomes from a latissimus dorsi reconstruction and have a significant quality of life improvement in comparison with mastectomy-only patients.

LEFORT FRACTURES

LeFort fractures are fractures of the maxillary bone. These fractures were first described by Rene LeFort in 1901 after experimenting on cadaver skulls. His experiments determined the patterns of weakness along the maxilla which become prone to injury after blunt force trauma. This blunt force trauma may be the result of a sports injury, assault, motor vehicle accident or fall from a significant height. About 10% to 20% of facial fractures are categorized as LeFort fracture.

LeFort fractures are characterized based on their fracture pattern. A LeFort type I fracture occurs along the horizontal plane at the base of the nose. The fracture extends from the nasal septum to the pterygomaxillary junction, then travels horizontally above the teeth apices. A LeFort type II fracture is a pyramidal fracture that extends from the nasal bridge through the lacrimal bones to the pterygoid plates. This fracture also includes hard palate, effectively disarticulating a pyramidal portion of facial skeleton. Lastly, the LeFort type III fracture goes from the nasofrontal and frontomaxillary suture to the base of the sphenoid. This fracture extends through the orbital bone and the zygomatic arch (see Figure 20-21).

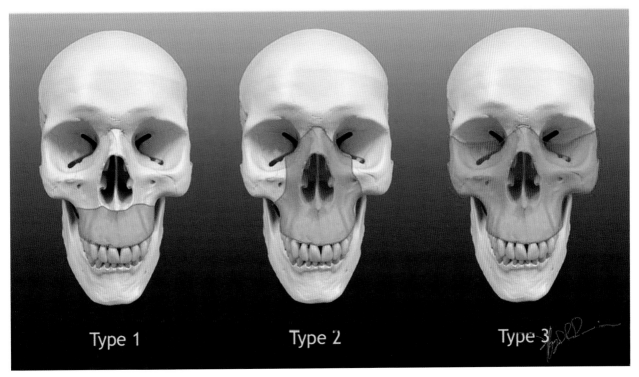

Figure 20-21 · LeFort fractures. (Reproduced, with permission, from LeFort classification of facial fractures. Trauma Radiology Reference Resource. University of Washington. Seattle, WA. 2017. https://sites.uw.edu/eradsite/trauma-radiology-reference-resource/2-hn/lefort-classification-of-facial-fractures/)

Preparing the Patient for Surgery

When a patient presents with a LeFort fracture, the first action must be to secure the airway. Loss of an airway is a potential threat due to excessive bleeding and anatomic distortions due to the fractures. Endotracheal intubation is necessary, but if the patient has extensive facial trauma, an emergency tracheotomy may be performed.

Prepping and Draping

After the airway is secured, the patient is prepared for surgery. The patient's arms are tucked bilaterally at the sides with foam padding the ulnar nerve. This allows the surgeon and SA to have better access to the face. Because these fractures are associated with high-impact trauma, care must be taken to not exacerbate any other injuries the patient may have while positioning. The whole face is prepped with betadine then the patient can be sterilely draped. A balled-up blue towel is placed on either side of the neck, and four towels are placed surrounding the patient's face. A split sheet is placed at the base of the chin then extended around the face meeting at the top of the head.

Surgical Procedure

- Regardless of the type of LeFort fracture, the goals of the repair stay the same. The surgeon seeks to disimpact the fracture, which reestablishes the correct facial projection and position of the nose and orbit.

- The surgeon uses a periosteal elevator or disimpaction forceps to realign the maxilla. Next the surgeon ensures the teeth line up properly in the patient's mouth.

- To maintain the appropriate occlusion of the teeth, the surgeon places arch bars to form mandibulomaxillary fixation.

- Lastly, the fractures are buttressed together using miniplates and screws. The size and number of plates used are dependent upon the patient's size and fracture patterns.

- To access the fracture sites, incisions are carefully chosen based on fracture location as well as cosmesis. For a LeFort type I fracture, gingivolabial incisions are utilized. For a LeFort type II fracture, a combination of gingivolabial and transconjunctival incisions is used. For a LeFort type III fracture, a bicoronal incision may be used to access the entire frontozygomatic buttress; however, multiple smaller incisions may be used.

- To access the complete fracture, a gingivolabial, transconjunctival, lateral brow, and/or glabellar fold incision may be utilized.

- The gingivolabial incisions are closed with a biologic suture, and the other incisions are closed using a 6-0 monofilament permanent suture.

Post-op Considerations. Patients with a LeFort fracture tend to have a higher mortality rate than other mid-face fractures. This is due to the LeFort fracture's typical pairing with other life-threatening injuries. Complications following a LeFort fracture repair consist of cerebrospinal fluid leak and epistaxis. For patients with mandibulomaxillary fixation, a liquid diet is necessary until the arch bars are removed around 6 weeks postoperatively. Also, a wire cutter is sent with the patient and always kept with patient, to access the oral cavity quickly in an emergency.

LeFort fractures are traumatic facial fractures that require a multidisciplinary team for the patient's recovery. Depending on the extent of the fractures, ophthalmology, otolaryngology, and dental surgeons may be involved with the patient's care.

Bibliography

American Society of Plastic Surgeons. 2018 Plastic Surgery Statistics Report. https://www.plasticsurgery.org/documents/News/Statistics/2018/cosmetic-procedure-trends-2018.pdf. Accessed September 7, 2023.

Baek WY, Lew DH, Lee DW. A retrospective analysis of ruptured breast implants. *Archives Plast Surg.* 2014;41(6):734-739. https://doi.org/10.5999/aps.2014.41.6.734.

Barrett DM, Casanueva FJ, Wang TD. Evolution of the rhytidectomy. *World J Otorhinolaryngol Head Neck Surg.* 2016;2(1):38-44. doi:10.1016/j.wjorl.2015.12.001.

Bhattacharya S, Khanna V, Kohli R. Cleft lip: the historical perspective. *Indian J Plast Surg.* 2009;42(Suppl):S4-S8. https://doi.org/10.4103/0970-0358.57180.

Braza ME, Fahrenkopf MP. Split-thickness skin grafts. [Updated 2019 Nov 24]. In: StatPearls [Internet]. Treasure Island (FL): StatPearls Publishing; 2020 Jan.

Campbell A, Costello BJ, Ruiz RL. Cleft lip and palate surgery: an update of clinical outcomes for primary repair. *Oral Maxillofac Surg Clin North Am.* 2010;22(1):43-58. doi:10.1016/j.coms.2009.11.003.

Chandawarkar RY, Miller MJ, Kellogg BC, Schulz SA, Valerio IL, Kirschner RE. Plastic and reconstructive surgery. In: Brunicardi F, Andersen DK, Billiar TR, et al. eds. *Schwartz's Principles of Surgery.* 11th ed. New York, NY: McGraw-Hill.

Crosara PF, Nunes FB, Rodrigues DS, et al. Rhinoplasty complications and reoperations: systematic review. *Int Arch Otorhinolaryngol.* 2017 Jan;21(1):97-101.

Daane SP, Rockwell WB. Breast reduction techniques and outcomes: a meta-analysis. *Aesthet Surg J.* 1999;19(4):293-303. https://doi.org/10.1053/aq.1999.v19.100635001.

Fernandes JW, Damin R, Holzmann MVN, Ribas GGO. Use of an algorithm in choosing abdominoplasty techniques. *Rev Col Bras Cir.* 2018;45(2):e1394. doi:10.1590/0100-6991e-20181394.

Fuller JC, Shaye DA. Unilateral cleft lip repair. *Oper Tech Otolaryngol.* 2020;31(1):55-61. https://doi.org/10.1016/j.otot.2019.12.011.

Gampper TJ, Khoury H, Gottlieb W, Morgan RF. Silicone gel implants in breast augmentation and reconstruction. *Annals Plast Surg.* 2007;59(5):581-590. doi:10.1097/01.sap.0000258970.31562.5d.

Gruber RP, Weintraub J, Pomerantz J. Suture techniques for the nasal tip. *Aesthet Surg J.* 2008;28(1):92-100. https://doi.org/10.1016/j.asj.2007.10.004.

Hall-Findlay EJ, Shestak KC. Breast reduction. *Plast Reconstr Surg.* 2015;136(4):531e-544e. doi:10.1097/PRS.0000000000001622.

Hashem AM, Couto RA, Duraes EFR, et al. Facelift part I: history, anatomy, and clinical assessment. *Aesthet Surg J.* 2020 Jan;40(1):1-18. https://doi.org/10.1093/asj/sjy326.

Kosowski TR, Weathers WM, Wolfswinkel EM, Ridgway EB. Cleft palate. *Semin Plast Surg.* 2012;26(4):164-169. https://doi.org/10.1055/s-0033-1333883.

Koudoumnakis E, Vlastos I, Parpounas K, Houlakis M. Two-flap palatoplasty: description of the surgical technique and reporting of results at a single center. *Ears Nose Throat J.* 2012;91(3):33-37.

Lee JC, Ishtihar S, Means JJ, Wu J, Rohde CH. In search of an ideal closure method. *Plast Reconstr Surg.* 2018;142(4):850-856. doi:10.1097/PRS.0000000000004726.

Lenventhal DD, Constantinides M. Rhinoplasty. In: Lalwani AK, ed. *Current Diagnosis & Treatment Otolaryngology-Head and Neck Surgery.* 4th ed. New York, NY: McGraw Hill.

Maxwell G, Gabriel A. The evolution of breast implants. *Plast Reconstr Surg.* 2014;134:12S-17S.

Nava MB, Rancati A, Angrigiani C, Catanuto G, Rocco N. How to prevent complications in breast augmentation. *Gland Surg.* 2017;6(2):210-217. https://doi.org/10.21037/gs.2017.04.02.

Park DM. Total facelift: forehead lift, midface lift, and neck lift. *Arch Plast Surg.* 2015;42(2):111-125. doi:10.5999/aps.2015.42.2.111.

Phillips BJ, Turco LM. Le Fort fractures: a collective review. *Bull Emerg Trauma.* 2017 Oct;5(4):221-230. doi:10.18869/acadpub.beat.5.4.499.

Piccinin MA, Zito PM. Anatomy, head and neck, lips. [Updated 2020 Aug 10]. In: StatPearls [Internet]. Treasure Island (FL): StatPearls Publishing; 2020 Jan. https://www.ncbi.nlm.nih.gov/books/NBK507900/.

Purohit S. Reduction mammoplasty. *Indian J Plast Surg.* 2008;41(Suppl):S64-S79.

Rose J, Puckett Y. Breast reconstruction free flaps. *StatPearls*; 2021 Jan.

Roumeliotis G, Ahluwalia R, Jenkyn T, Yazdani A. The Le Fort system revisited: trauma velocity predicts the path of Le Fort I fractures through the lateral buttress. *Plast Surg (Oakv).* 2015 Spring;23(1):40-42. doi:10.4172/plastic-surgery.1000899.

Schwartz MR. Evidence-based medicine. *Plast Reconstr Surg.* 2017;140(1):109e-119e. doi:10.1097/PRS.0000000000003478.

Sood R, Easow JM, Konopka G, Panthaki ZJ. Latissimus dorsi flap in breast reconstruction: recent innovations in the workhorse flap. *Cancer Control.* 2018 Jan-Mar;25(1):1073274817744638. doi:10.1177/1073274817744638.

Spear SL, Bulan EJ, Venturi ML. Breast augmentation. *Plast Reconstr Surg.* 2006 Dec;118(7 Suppl):188S-196S. doi:10.1097/01.PRS.0000135945.02642.8B.

Taylor EM, Chun YS. Plastic and reconstructive surgery. In: Doherty GM, ed. *Current Diagnosis & Treatment: Surgery.* 15th ed. New York, NY: McGraw Hill.

U.S. National Library of Medicine. *The Aesthetic Society's Cosmetic Surgery National Data Bank: Statistics 2019. Aesthet Surg J.* 2020 Jun 15;40(Suppl 1):1-26. https://pubmed.ncbi.nlm.nih.gov/32542351/.

Uebel CO. Lipoabdominoplasty: revisiting the superior pull-down abdominal flap and new approaches. *Aesthet Plast Surg.* 2009;33(3):366-376. https://doi.org/10.1007/s00266-009-9318-z.

Vincent A, Hohman MH. Latissimus dorsi myocutaneous flap. *StatPearls*; 2021 Jan.

Whitney ZB, Jain M, Zito PM. Anatomy, skin, superficial musculoaponeurotic system (SMAS) fascia. [Updated 2020 Oct 28]. In: StatPearls [Internet]. Treasure Island (FL): StatPearls Publishing; 2020 Jan. https://www.ncbi.nlm.nih.gov/books/NBK519014/.

Neurosurgery*
Jeanie Moran and Dana Klope

Neurosurgery focuses on diagnosing and treating the brain, spine, spinal cord, and peripheral nerves. Although it is a surgical discipline, neurosurgery requires knowledge and training in neurology, critical care, trauma care, and radiology.

Neurosurgery encompasses a broad scope of illnesses, from tumors of the nervous system and its supporting structures to neurovascular disorders, seizures, and infections.

Those privileged to assist a neurosurgeon will find it challenging, at times stressful, and also a most rewarding and fascinating area of medicine.

ANATOMY OF THE SKULL

Multiple bones form the human skull, which serves as a hard protective covering for the brain. These bones are: frontal bone, parietal bone, temporal bone, occipital bone, maxilla, nasal bone, sphenoid bone, zygomatic bone, lacrimal bone, ethmoid bone, mandible, coronal suture, sagittal suture, squamosal suture, lambdoid suture, occipitomastoid suture, zygomatico-temporal suture, zygomaticofrontal suture, sphenozygomatic suture, sphenofrontal suture, sphenoparietal suture, sphenosquamosal suture, inion, opisthion, asterion, and lambda.

*Special thanks to Drs. Roman Guerrero, Edward Santos, David Strothman, Trevor Wahlquist, and Nick Wills and all their PA's for their knowledge and experience.

ESSENTIAL LANDMARKS OF THE SKULL

Frontal Bone

The frontal bone is an unpaired, large bone that starts developmentally as two halves. At about 2 months of age, these bones begin to fuse along the **metopic suture**. This significant bone articulates with the right and left parietal, ethmoid, zygomatic, sphenoid, lacrimal, maxillary, and nasal bones.

The frontal bone has three sections, namely the squamous, orbital, and nasal parts.

- The **squamous** portion is the largest and is also smooth. On each side of the midline are two rounded elevations, called the **frontal eminences**. Under these are two **superciliary arches** linked in the middle by the **glabella**.

  On its cranial surface, the squamous portion of the frontal bone holds the **sagittal sulcus**, in which the **sagittal venous sinus** lives. The edges of the sulcus extend inferiorly, forming the **frontal crest**, where the **falx cerebri** joins.

- Laterally, the supraorbital margins make up the **orbital** rim and the **supraorbital notch**. Here the supraorbital vessels and nerves are conducted. The **orbital** area of the frontal bone forms from two orbital plates merged by the **ethmoidal notch**, and occupied by the **cribriform plate** of the ethmoid. The inferior surface of each orbital plate has a slight depression under the zygomatic process called the **lacrimal fossa**. The orbital portion of the frontal bone holds the **frontal** and the **frontonasal ducts**.

- Lower to the glabella lie the nasal notch and spine, which join with the nasal bones and the perpendicular plate of the ethmoid.

Ethmoid Bone

The ethmoid bone is a single thick bone with a cube-like shape. It has contact with 13 cranial and facial bones. The cranial bones it connects with are the frontal and sphenoid bones. The ethmoid has three sections: the cribriform plate, the ethmoidal labyrinth, and the perpendicular plate. The cribriform plate joins with the ethmoidal notch of the frontal bone. This articulation becomes the **foramen cecum** anteriorly.

The **crista Galli (Latin for roosters crest)** rises from the superior surface of the **ethmoid bone** at its midline and projects upward into the **anterior cranial fossa**. It also serves as an attachment to the **falx cerebral** anteriorly.

This thick triangular process is where the **perpendicular plate** and **crista galli** begin ossification approximately 2 months after birth. This area is commonly recalled as the soft spot on an infant's head.

This smooth, thick process separates the olfactory bulbs found in the **olfactory fossae** on both sides of the crista galli on the **cribriform plate**. Immediately lateral to the crista galli are the nasal slits, the area where the **anterior ethmoidal nerves** descend into the top part of the nasal cavity.

Spreading inferiorly from the cribriform plate at the midline is the **perpendicular plate**. This flat bone forms the largest bony section of the nasal septum. The plate is mostly smooth aside from several grooves on each side which house the **olfactory nerves**. Beneath the cribriform plate laterally sits the **ethmoidal labyrinth,** which holds a system of thin-walled cavities, the **ethmoidal cells**.

Fragile, smooth plates that protect the adjacent surfaces of the labyrinth are called the **lamina papyracea**. Posterior areas of the medial surfaces of the labyrinth contain thin, curved bones that form the **superior nasal conchae** and have a superior meatus. Another curved projection includes the **middle nasal conchae**, also having an associated meatus.

Just inferior to the middle concha is the **uncinate process**, a small, bony projection forming a section of the medial area of the maxillary sinus.

Sphenoid Bone

The **sphenoid bone** is also unpaired and sits in the middle of the **cranial base**. It is contiguous with the temporal, parietal, frontal, occipital, ethmoid, zygomatic, palatine, and vomer bones. It contains many tiny foramina.

Surgical Landmark: In endonasal skull base surgery, this bone is at the center of the procedure.
The sphenoid is comprised of several parts, including a central body where the **sella turcica** is contained.

Additionally, two greater wings and two lesser wings sit laterally. The greater wings make up the front portions of the **middle cranial fossae,** and the lesser wings comprise the posterior part of the **anterior cranial fossa.**

The **anterior clinoid processes** are very noticeable ends of the lesser wing of the sphenoid bone and spread toward the **Sylvian fissure.**

Surgical Landmark: These are essential features of the sphenoid bone in skull base surgery.

The middle clinoid processes form the anterior border of the sella turcica. The **dorsum sellae** are formed from the posterior clinoid processes, and their size and shape vary in individuals.

Attached to the **posterior clinoids** is the **tentorium cerebelli**. Situated at the intersection of the body are the **optic canals**, which pass on the optic nerves and the ophthalmic arteries.

The **optic groove** is found in the midline of the **sphenoid body**, behind which **tuberculum sellae** will be found.

The cleft fashioned between a greater and lesser wing creates the **superior orbital fissure**. This area is a communication center for the following:

- Oculomotor nerve
- Trochlear nerve (IV)
- Lacrimal
- Nasociliary
- Frontal divisions of the ophthalmic nerve (V1)
- Abducens (VI)
- Ophthalmic vein, superior and inferior divisions
- Sympathetic fibers from the cavernous sinus

Each greater wing presents the **foramen rotundum**, necessary for transmitting the maxillary nerve (V2), and the **foramen ovale**, which conducts the mandibular nerve (V3), accessory meningeal artery, and the lesser petrosal nerve.

The **foramen spinosum**, responsible for transmitting the middle meningeal vessels and the recurrent branch of the mandibular nerve, is also found here.

Inferiorly, the sphenoid bone holds two **pterygoid processes** formed from a medial and lateral plate. The medial and lateral pterygoid muscles attach here and give movement to the jaw.

The pterygoid or **Vidian's canal** is seen when viewing the sphenoid bone from the front. Located below and medial to the foramen rotundum, Vidian's nerve, artery, and vein are transmitted through this canal which is formed by the connection of the greater petrosal nerve and the deep petrosal nerve inside the canal.

Temporal Bone

The temporal bones are distributed into the squamosal, mastoid, tympanic, styloid, and petrous segments. Each part connects with the sphenoid bone (sphenosquamosal suture), the zygomatic bone (zygomaticotemporal suture), the parietal bone (parietosquamous suture), and the occipital bone (occipitomastoid suture).

Surgical Landmark: Several critical open skull base approaches use this bone as a landmark as it houses important neurovascular structures, including the seven lower cranial nerves and the major vessels to and from the brain, temporal and transverse bone.

Superficially, the squamous portion of the temporal bone has a smooth surface. This area serves as an attachment point for the temporalis fascia and muscle at the superior and inferior temporal lines, individually.

With both anterior and posterior roots, the zygomatic process runs anteriorly to connect with the zygomatic bone. At the bottom of the anterior root of the zygomatic process is the **articular tubercle.**

The articular tubercle is near the anterior root of the zygomatic process, and just behind it is the **glenoid fossa**. Here is the location of the **temporomandibular joint** resides.

Posteromedial to the glenoid fossa is the **petro tympanic fissure** through which the **chorda tympani** and the tympanic branch of the **maxillary artery** run.

Inside the tympanic portion of the temporal bone sits the **external auditory meatus** covered by the **tympanic membrane.** Also, the medial wall of the tympanic cavity, which houses the **oval window** (fenestra vestibule), is shielded by the **stapes bone, footplate,** and the **round window** (fenestra cochleae), covered by its **secondary tympanic membrane.**

Inferiorly, the **vaginal process** is found laterally and the **styloid process** is found medially. Behind the styloid process sits the **stylomastoid foramen,** needed for transmission of the facial nerve and stylomastoid branch of the **posterior auricular artery**.

Behind, and near the mastoid bone, is the **tympanomastoid fissure** conducting the auricular nerve of CN X.

A considerable prominence in the latter part of the temporal bone is the **mastoid process.** Located inferior and posterior to the ear canal, lateral to the styloid process, it has a conical shape and sits behind and below the ear. It is filled with mastoid cells or sinuses. This bony prominence serves as attachment to the posterior auricular occipitalis and sternocleidomastoid, posterior belly of the digastric, longissimus capitis, and splenius capitis muscles.

On the bottom surface is the **carotid canal** that runs the internal carotid artery and the sympathetic nerve plexus. Neighboring the carotid canal are the **cochlear** and **tympanic canaliculi.** The tympanic canaliculus sends both the tympanic branch of CN IX and the inferior tympanic artery. The cochlear canaliculus transmits the perilymphatic vein and duct.

The mastoid bone is located at the back part of the temporal bone. It has a rough surface allowing attachment to muscles via tendons. It also has openings for blood vessels, a hollow for the sigmoid sinus, and small foramen that typically transmit an emissary vein to the sinus on the cranial surface. The petrous portion contains an impression for the superior petrosal sinus, and from this sinus blood drains from the cavernous sinus to the transverse sinus.

Surgical Landmark: The arcuate eminence, marking the location of the superior semicircular canal, is another important landmark in neurosurgery.

Anterior and lateral to the arcuate eminence is a fragile bone segment named the **tegmen tympani,** which divides the cranial cavity from the tympanic cavity.

All inner ear structures, including the ossicles, cochlea, and semicircular canals, are found inside the petrous section of the temporal bone. A noticeable foreman called **the internal acoustic meatus** transmits the facial nerve (CN VII), vestibulocochlear nerve (CN VI), and the internal auditory branch of the basilar artery. Just above and to the side of this is the **aqueduct of the vestibule**. Through this aqueduct, the endolymphatic duct and a small artery and vein project. Beneath and slightly lateral to the internal acoustic meatus is the **cochlear aqueduct** through which the perilymphatic duct runs.

Just lateral to the front portion of the carotid canal anteromedial to the temporal bone is the bony part of the eustachian tube. Above the eustachian tube extends a shallow groove laterally and posteriorly called the **hiatus of the facial canal.** This opening transmits the greater petrosal nerve.

Surgical Landmark: The temporal bone has importance to many approaches utilized in neurosurgery.

- Presigmoid (supra- and infra-tentorial) approach to the posterior and middle fossa
- Subtemporal anterior transpetrosal (Kawase approach)
- Subtemporal preauricular infratemporal
- Translabyrinthine
- Transcochlear
- Postauricular transtemporal

Parietal Bone

At the sagittal suture, a pair of parietal bones form the sides and roof of the skull. Not only do they articulate with each other, but the parietal bones also connect with the frontal (coronal suture), temporal (squamosal suture), occipital (lambdoid suture), and sphenoid bones.

Externally, the parietal bone's surface is marked near the center by a point called the **parietal eminence.** Beneath this are two curving lines, called the **superior** and **inferior temporal lines.** The **superior temporal line** is where the temporalis muscle fascia attaches. The upper attachment site of the temporalis muscle is at the **inferior temporal line.**

Located on the inner surface of the parietal bone is the sulcus for the superior sagittal sinus and its associated foveolae granulares, indentations for the arachnoid granulations. Inferiorly, there is a groove for the middle meningeal artery.

Occipital Bone

At the rear portion of the cranium and the skull base, the occipital bone sits. Containing three parts, namely the squamous, basilar, and lateral parts, the occipital bone articulates with the temporal (occipitomastoid suture), parietal (lambdoid suture), and sphenoid bones. Superficially, the most noticeable portion of the squamous part of the occipital bone is an external occipital protuberance, called the **inion**. Here, the trapezius muscles and the nuchal ligament attach. The smooth superior portion of the bone is called the **planum occipital.**

A series of nuchal lines, named **superior** and **inferior,** are found lesser and transversely angled to the planum occipital. They join medially with the external occipital protuberance.

This median nuchal line extends from the external occipital protuberance to the foramen magnum.

In the interior surface of the squamous part is the internal occipital protuberance, where the Torcular Herophili serves as the junction of the sagittal sulcus and occipital sulcus, and grooves the transverse sinuses.

In the posterior part of the foramen magenum sits the **vermian fossa**. Extending upward from the foramen magnum is the basilar part of the occipital bone forming the **clivus,** which articulates with the sphenoid bone at the dorsum sellae. The outer exterior of the basilar part holds the **pharyngeal tubercle**.

The sides of the foramen magnum form from the lateral parts of the occipital bone. Beneath the surface is the **occipital condyles**. Behind the occipital condyle are the **condyloid canal fossa** and **condyloid fossa**, which transmit an emissary vein. The hypoglossal nerve (XII) and meningeal branch of the ascending pharyngeal artery send through a tunnel called the hypoglossal canal

The hypoglossal canal is a significant landmark for far lateral approaches to the ventral brainstem in neurosurgery.
Extending laterally from the condyle on the external surface of the hypoglossal canal is the **jugular process** with the **jugular notch** frontal to it. The posterior part of the **jugular foramen** is crested from the jugular notch. The lateral aspects of the upper surface form the **jugular tubercle,** which covers the hypoglossal canal.

The largest foramen of the occipital bone is the **foramen magnum** which communicates with the medulla, the spinal accessory nerve (XI), vertebral arteries, anterior spinal arteries, posterior spinal arteries, and alar ligaments.

Soft Tissues of the Skull

Just inside the skull, three layers of tissue called meninges surround the brain. **Dura mater** is the thick outermost layer. The middle tissue layer is the **arachnoid mater,** and the **pia mater** is the innermost layer.

Between the arachnoid and pia mater is **subarachnoid space.** This space contains a clear fluid called **cerebrospinal fluid** and many blood vessels.

Blood vessels called **bridging veins** connect the dura mater with the surface of the brain. Additional vessels called **cerebral arteries** bring blood to the brain inside the skull.

Intracranial Pressure

The brain requires a balance of pressure between the blood vessels and cerebrospinal fluid (CSF) surrounding the brain and its tissue to function normally. This is referred to as **normal intracranial pressure**. Certain conditions can increase intracranial pressure, putting pressure on the brain and causing it to swell or change shape inside the skull. Some of these conditions are brain tumors, head injuries, problems with blood vessels, or infections in the brain or spinal cord.

Circulatory System of the Brain

Blood is returned to the brain by two paired arteries, namely the vertebral and the internal carotid arteries (see Figure 21-1).

Internal carotid arteries return blood from the body to the brain. **The internal carotid** supplies the anterior (front) areas, and the **vertebral arteries** supply the brain's posterior (back) regions. After entering the skull, the left and right vertebral arteries join together to form the single **basilar artery**. The

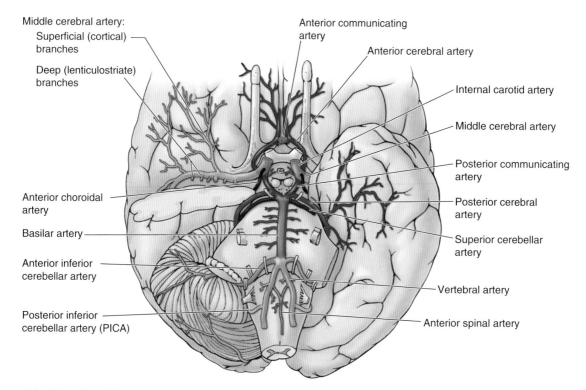

Figure 21-1 · Blood supply to the skull. (Reproduced, with permission, from Martin JH. *Neuroanatomy: Text and Atlas*. 5th ed. New York, NY: McGraw Hill; 2021.)

internal carotid and basilar arteries "communicate" with each other in a ring called the **Circle of Willis** at the brain's base.

Anterior Cerebral Circulation. The following arteries supply blood to the anterior portion of the brain.

- **Internal carotid arteries** are large arteries of the common carotid arteries that run on the left and right side of the neck and enter the skull, where they continue to branch into the anterior cerebral artery and forms the middle cerebral artery.

- The **External carotid** branches supply blood to the facial tissues.

- **Anterior cerebral artery** (ACA) supplies blood to much of the midline portions of the frontal lobes and superior medial parietal lobes of the brain.

  - Anterior communicating artery connects both anterior cerebral arteries, within and along the floor of the cerebral vault.

- **Middle cerebral artery** (MCA) develops from the internal carotid artery and continues into the lateral sulcus to branch off into the lateral cerebral cortex. It supplies blood to the anterior temporal lobes and the insular.

Posterior Cerebral Circulation. These posterior arteries supply blood to the rear portion of the brain, including the occipital lobes, cerebellum, and brainstem.

Vertebral Arteries. These smaller arteries that branch from the subclavian arteries supply the shoulders, lateral chest, and arm. The two vertebral arteries fuse into the basilar artery within the skull.

Posterior Inferior Cerebellar Artery (PICA). The posterior inferior cerebellar artery (PICA), is often the largest branch of the vertebral artery and anastomoses with several arteries.

- Basilar artery: Supplies the midbrain, cerebellum, and usual branches into the posterior cerebral artery

- Anterior inferior cerebellar artery (AICA)

- Pontine branches

- Superior cerebellar artery (SCA)

- Posterior cerebral artery (PCA)

- Posterior communicating artery

Veins of the Brain

Veins are thin-walled vessels that lack a muscular wall. They drain blood after it has passed through tissues or organs and lost oxygen. Veins are under very little pressure, returning blood to the heart to get pumped to the lungs. Veins outside the brain are usually more visible as blue vessels near the skin's surface (see Figure 21-2).

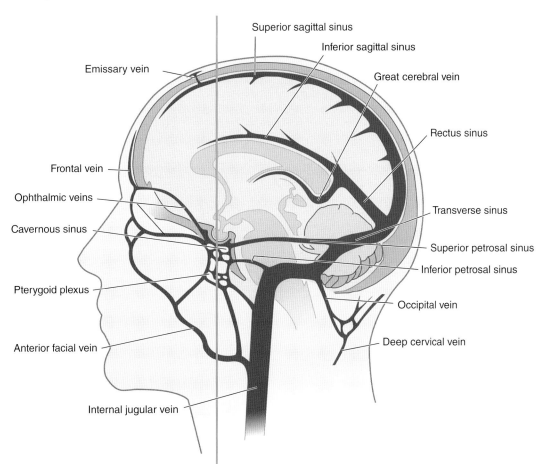

Figure 21-2 · Veins of the brain. (Reproduced, with permission, from Waxman SG. *Clinical Neuroanatomy.* 29th ed. New York, NY: McGraw Hill; 2020.)

DIAGNOSTIC MODALITIES IN NEUROSURGERY

Neurological Exam

The first step in diagnosis and symptom assessment is the neurological exam. A neurological exam is very comprehensive and includes checking vision, hearing, balance, coordination, strength, and reflexes, among other things. Various symptoms will provide clues about the part of the brain and nervous system that could be affected by different neurological conditions. Upon completion of a neurological examination, the doctor will order additional testing based on his findings. There is blood work, but diagnostic imaging will often be the first step in determining where the symptoms originate.

Diagnostic Imaging

Neuroimaging has evolved in tandem with neurosurgery. The specialty is highly dependent on diagnostic imaging. The neurosurgeon must become proficient in interpreting various imaging studies, including x-ray, computed tomography (CT), magnetic resonance imaging(MRI), and angiography.

The surgical assistant (SA) is expected to have a general ability to recognize essential brain and nervous system structures on various intraoperative imaging modalities.

Computed Axial Tomography (CT Scan). Usually the first ordered is a CT scan to diagnose common pathologies in neurosurgery. This specialized x-ray machine uses electromagnetic radiation to create two-dimensional pictures of a body part. These "slices" of the brain can be sorted into approximately 4000 various tissue densities into 16 different groups of the brain to help locate bleeding and other common pathologies in the brain.

Plain CT. A CT scan without intravenous contrast ("plain CT") is usually quickly ordered when an intracranial pathology is suspected. CT is more accurate than MRI to diagnose acute brain bleeding due to its speed and the fact that it provides easy visualization of acute blood and boney detail.

Common Uses for Plain CT: Often used in emergencies to quickly rule out acute abnormalities such as:

- Detection of masses
- Hydrocephalus and pneumocephalus (fluid in skull cavity)
- Epidural or subdural hematoma
- Subarachnoid and intraparenchymal hemorrhage
- Aneurysm
- Fluid in skull cavity in cases of pneumocephalus
- Fractures of skull

CT with Contrast/Infusion (CT Angiography Cerebral Angiogram, or Cerebral Arteriogram)

- When used intravenously during a CT scan, the contrast absorbs into damaged tissues of the brain, causing the damaged areas to appear bright on the CT scan.

- Dye is also used to observe blood flow in the brain and diagnose and locate a ruptured aneurysm.

Common Uses for CT with an Infusion:

- The first choice to diagnose Intracranial hemorrhage
- Vasospasm and hypoperfusion
- Neoplasms and vascular malformations

All CT contrast agents contain iodine.
A patient allergic to shellfish or iodine may have an adverse reaction to iodine-based media.

They are typically ordered for suspected skull fractures when a patient cannot undergo an MRI due to a previously implanted metal device. *Although the resolution will be lower, CT with contrast can replace contrast-enhanced MRI.*

Cerebral Angiogram or Cerebral Arteriogram. Dye injected using a thin, flexible tube (catheter) is fed into a large artery usually located in the groin region and threaded past the heart to the arteries in the brain. X-ray images reveal details about the artery's location and site of a ruptured aneurysm. This invasive exam is used after other diagnostic tests don't provide enough information.

Magnetic Resonance Imaging (MRI). When intraparenchymal lesions are suspected, MRI is the gold standard. An MRI uses a magnetic field with radio waves to create detailed images of the brain. The pictures can either be present in two-dimensional or three-dimensional slices Also used to detect brain or spine tumors or infections. Many specialized MRI scan components can help evaluate the tumor and plan treatment.

MRI can distinguish between distinct components of lesions, such as calcifications, cysts, fat, and the absence or presence of contrast media, helping surgeons distinguish between various lesions. *The SA will need to understand MR because the neurosurgeon will often refer to them in the OR.*

Functional MRI: MRI without infusion

Perfusion MR: Contrast media is injected through the patient's IV to show tumors and infection. The contrast solution used in MRI is not iodine-based, so it is safe for patients with iodine allergies.

Magnetic Resonance Angiography (MRA). MRA helps to locate areas of reduced vascular blood flow because of its ability to visualize the condition of the blood vessel walls. This test examines vessels leading to the kidneys, brain, and legs. MRA can distinguish blood flow and is highly effective when screening for aneurysms. With an injected contrast material, MRA can enhance images of blood vessels around the site of an aneurysm rupture. It is also effective for the diagnosis of carotid stenosis and follow up assessment of coiled aneurysms.

Magnetic Resonance Spectroscopy (MRS). MRS is an additional tool to differentiate a brain tumor from an abscess, postoperative enhancement, or recurrent MS plaques.

This diagnostic exam can show peaks in proton MRS, commonly seen in lipids, lactate, *N*-acetyl aspartate (NAA), creatinine (Cr), and choline (Cho). A normal brain will not have the presence of lactate. This marker of anaerobic metabolism is present in ischemia, infection, tumor necrosis, radiation necrosis, and demyelinating disease (see Figure 21-3).

fMRI. The fMRI is performed before surgery for preop planning of the resection of gliomas near the language and sensorimotor cortices and provides a functional assessment of cortical activity by causing stimuli alterations in blood flow. Multiple tasks that call on speech, visual, memory, and motor paradigms are reached using stimuli to elicit cortical activity.

The fMRI is not reliable if an arteriovenous malformation (AVM) is near the functional cortices because of the effect the AVM has on regional blood flow.

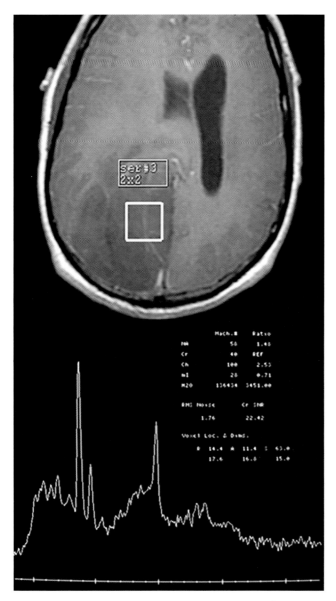

Figure 21-3 · MRS test. (Reproduced, with permission, from *Magnetic resonance spectroscopy*. Cincinnati, OH: Mayfield Brain & Spine; 2010.)

DTI Tractography. Diffusion tensor imaging (DTI) is an MRI-based method used to map tracts of white matter according to the physical makeup of the axons and surrounding matter of the tracts in the brain.

DTI is most useful when removing a mass or glioma that potentially impinges on or lies near an important white matter tract.

Digital Catheter Angiography (Arteriography). Catheter angiography is the gold standard study used to evaluate blood flow, arrangement, and distribution when diagnosing and treating AVMs and aneurysms.

This procedure is more invasive than CT angiography or MRA; but it is essential and allows for treatment during imaging.

Most AVMs and some patients with complex aneurysms undergo arteriography. Though CT angiograms detect aneurysms, the 3D reconstruction images of the arteriogram are beneficial for operative planning.

Positron Emission Tomography (PET Scan). It is suspected that a brain tumor may result from cancer that has spread from another area of the body. In that case, PET uses a radioactive isotope injected into the patient, which attaches to cancer cells and shows up on imaging.

Electroencephalography (EEG). An EEG is a test used to record the measurements of the electrical activity of the brain and measure changes in electric potentials to detect abnormalities in brain waves or the electrical activity of the brain. The EEG is used to evaluate many different brain disorders. In the case of epilepsy, seizure activity will occur as rapid spiking waves on an EEG.

Brain lesions resulting from tumors or stroke often have abnormally slow EEG waves. Of course, this depends on the lesion's size and location.

The EEG can also help diagnose other disorders that influence brain activity, for example, Alzheimer's disease, narcolepsy, and certain psychoses.

CSF Test (Lumbar Puncture). The procedure using a needle to draw CSF from the spine is called a lumbar puncture or spinal tap. This test can be helpful when there are symptoms of a ruptured aneurysm without CT confirmation of bleeding. Red blood cells will typically appear in the CSF around the spine and brain in a subarachnoid hemorrhage (SAH).

Chemotherapy (Targeted Drug Therapy). Targeted drug treatments (chemotherapy) work by focusing on specific abnormalities within the cancer cells. When these abnormalities can be blocked, as in the case of chemotherapy, targeted drug treatments can cause cancer cells to die.

Many targeted therapy drugs are available for specific brain tumors, and many more are constantly being studied in clinical trials. The most commonly used chemotherapy drug is **temozolomide (Temodar),** which is taken as a pill. Many other chemotherapy drugs are available and are used depending on the type of cancer.

Side Effects of Chemotherapy: Chemotherapy can cause nausea, vomiting, and hair loss depending on the type and dose of drugs received.

PERIOPERATIVE DUTIES OF THE SURGICAL ASSISTANT

Considerations

Ensuring the room is set up and everything is ready when the surgeon arrives will set the tone for the case. Though a surgical technologist and circulator will complete most of the preoperative setup, the SA is expected to go through the room before surgery and be sure nothing has been missed.

- Position lights to the surgeon's preference.
- Ensure images are uploaded before the surgeon enters the room.
- The microscope (if being used) is set up for the surgeon's specific settings and is turned on and ready to be moved in at a moment's notice.
- Check-in with scrub tech and offer to grab gloves, especially if they are new.
- If there is an implant rep, they must be there in the operating room. Has an x-ray been called? Will neuromonitoring be used for this case? Is the technologist there and ready to go?
- If cell saver is going to be needed, have they been set up?
- Will the craniotome be used for this case; is it set up?
- Is the foot pedal on the surgeon's side of the bed? If not, then it likely has not been tested yet.
- Be sure everything is clipped firmly in place.
- Test the foot pedal before starting the case to make sure it is turning smoothly. If the scrub tech has already done so, then obviously, there is no need to do it twice.

The SA is always conscious of the many moving pieces that occur before starting any case. With many different people involved and a systematic list of presurgical steps in place, it is not unusual for an action to be misplaced from time to time, making it essential for everyone involved to work as a team and not be afraid to speak up.

- The patient's name is printed on all neuroimaging films and then cross-checked with the identification band. Miscommunications due to a language barrier can lead to wrong-sided surgery.
- The attending neurosurgeon needs to be present during the induction and positioning of the patient to confirm the surgical site and side.
- This may not always be possible; therefore, preoperatively, the patient's scalp is marked with an indelible imprint by the surgeon. An arrow is used to indicate the right side of craniotomy.
- These procedures are confirmed by verbal agreement and signature documentation among the circulating nurse, neurosurgeon, and anesthesiologist.

- Some hospitals require cross-checking of consent forms, radiology films, and the patient's chart for the correct hemisphere of surgery.
- During the time out, the surgical team, including the anesthesiologist, will verbally agree on the approach, medications given, patient allergies, fire risk, and any other concerns to be addressed.

Surgical Skin Prep

Often the circulator and/or SA will begin the process of prepping the patient. In neurosurgery, it is widespread for the surgeon to take on this role.

Have alcohol-soaked 4x4s bedside to pass to the surgeon before the final preparation. Some surgeons will even prefer their marker wiped with an alcohol pad before giving it to them to mark the incision site. In this case, be prepared to wipe the pen with a fresh alcohol-soaked pad each time before passing the marker. The same goes for when surgeon asks for something to mark the spot with for the initial x-ray.

SURGICAL APPROACHES AND PATIENT POSITIONING FOR CRANIOTOMY AND NEUROSURGICAL PROCEDURES

Supine Position(Dorsal Decubitus)

This is the most frequently utilized position in neurosurgery and is often used for cranial procedures, carotid endarterectomies, and anterior approaches to the cervical and lumbar spine.

It is also used for endoscopic transnasal, pterional, frontal, temporal, interhemispheric, and anterior parietal craniotomies, anterior and middle skull base osteotomies, and anterior and middle fossa craniotomies.

Risks. Head rotation or flexion often is required to create optimal surgical conditions.

- Endoscopic transnasal, pterional, frontal, temporal, interhemispheric and anterior parietal craniotomies, anterior and middle skull base osteotomies, and anterior and middle fossa craniotomies

Three types of supine positioning are utilized in neurosurgery.

Horizontal Position or Supine

- Patients lie on their back on a straight table.
- Avoid skin-to-metal contact; arms must be padded, restrained along the body, or positioned on arm boards.
- Bony contact points at elbows and heels require padding.

Lawn Chair (Contoured) Position or Semi-Fowlers: Modification of horizontal position with 15-degree angulation and flexion at the trunk-thigh-knee.

Advantages of This Position

- This provides physiological positioning of the lumbar spine, hips, and knees.

- A blanket, pillow, or soft (gel) cushion under the knees will keep them flexed.
- Slight head elevation can improve venous drainage from the brain.
- Slight elevation of legs can improve venous return to the heart.

Head-Up Tilt or Reverse Trendelenburg Position: About 10 to 15 degree repositioning from the horizontal axis for optimal venous drainage from the brain.

Modified Park-Bench or Lateral Oblique

- This position is followed for posterior parietal, occipital, posterior fossa and skull base corridors, craniocervical junction operations and may cause significant postoperative neck pain.
- Standard position for morbidly obese or patients with significant cervical degenerative stenotic changes if any neck turn is necessary.
- Patients with lesions near the parietal eminence are also frequently placed in the modified park-bench position.

The Park-bench position **is a modifi**ed lateral position.

Benefits of Park-Bench Position

- Better access to the posterior fossa, than the lateral position
- The best approach of temporal lobe craniotomy and skull base
- Interhemispheric approach (the anterior interhemispheric route) for a third ventricular tumor
- Posterior interhemispheric route for a splenial AVM
- Posterior fossa procedures and the retroperitoneal approach to the thoracolumbar spine

Sitting Position

- Resection of acoustic neuromas
- Morbidly obese patients undergoing posterior fossa operations

Prone Position

This is commonly utilized for approaches to the posterior fossa, suboccipital region, and posterior approaches to spine.

Benefits. Good position for posterior approaches and lower incidence of venous air embolism compared to the sitting position.

Risks of Prone Position

- Logistically difficult positioning for anesthesia due to the challenges of maintaining hemodynamics, ensuring adequate oxygenation, and providing adequate ventilation
- Poor access to patient's airway
- Difficult to secure IV lines and tracheal tube
- Vascular compression, air embolism, brachial plexus injuries, blindness, quadriplegia

OPERATIVE PROCEDURES

Craniotomy

There is evidence that various forms of a craniotomy procedure can be traced back to the late Paleolithic and early Neolithic periods (8000-5000 BCE). Trephination was thought to be used for treatment related to trauma. Or perhaps openings in the skull were part of ritual practice relating to ancient supernatural beliefs. The craniotomy procedure was standardized only in the 20th century, resulting in improved surgical outcomes. Simultaneously medical imaging and stereotactic navigation systems were evolving, giving doctors the ability to correlate the findings of images with surgical approaches.

After a cut is made in the skull, a flap of bone is taken to access the brain underneath. This procedure is used for several different brain diseases, injuries, or conditions and can be performed on any part of the skull.

At first, most neurosurgical approaches utilized extended craniotomies. There were several reasons why large cranial openings were used in the past. It was impossible to determine the size of pathological lesions without modern imaging, which meant that intracranial lesions were not typically diagnosed until they had grown large. Also, lighting in operating theaters was not good, creating the need for a sizeable cranial opening that could allow the proper amount of light into the field.

Through evolving approaches to craniotomy surgery, as well as stereotactic navigation, neurosurgery has developed. Craniotomies can be localized over the specific lesion site, leading to fewer complications and improved outcomes.

Advanced diagnostic imaging greatly aided the development of neurosurgical techniques and approaches. The use of high-definition computed tomography images with MRI has given surgeons more ability to pre-plan procedures.

Image-guided navigation started as frame-based stereotactic systems in the early 19th century. Today, frameless systems are used in most craniotomy operations. Surgeons can now select the safest, most approachable surgical corridor for vascular, tumor, or functional surgery, providing adequate exposure to a cranial lesion while protecting the normal brain and vascular tissues.

Positioning for Craniotomy

Head Positioning: Two options for head positioning are unfixed and fixed. Unfixed is used when stabilization of the head is not needed or not advised, as in children younger than 3 years. Pins are not recommended because of the risk of a depressed skull fracture. There are different frames for head fixation. The Mayfield head holder is the most common, with skull fixation pins not placed close to the operative site.

Body Positioning: There are many positioning options including supine, prone, lateral, sitting, and semi-sitting position. The most commonly used in neurosurgery is **supine,** which allows frontal, temporal, and parietal craniotomies. Posterior fossa approaches for cerebellopontine angle masses and pterional approaches also make use of the supine position. There are also variations of approaches.

Prone is the preferred position for occipital and suboccipital craniotomy. It is also helpful for craniectomy access to posterior occipital and fossa regions.

Lateral positioning is good for the retrosigmoid approach, the far lateral approaches, and the supratentorial craniotomies involving the occipital and parietal lobes.

Fowler's-sitting position is occasionally used for posterior fossa access or access to the pineal region. The sitting position has become associated with venous air embolism and spinal cord infarction risks.

Semi-Fowler's or semi-sitting position is helpful for occipital lesions, the supracerebellar infratentorial approach, and pineal and parietal region tumors.

A Brief Overview of the Most Common Types of Craniotomies

Frontal Craniotomy: This is either unilateral or bilateral (bifrontal).

- Used for access to the large midline, anterior, and middle skull base lesions.
- Approach lesions of the planum sphenoidal, olfactory groove, and tuberculum sella, as well as pituitary and falcine lesions.
- Access to anterior interhemispheric lesions.
- Exposure to repair the lesion and its vascular supply with minimal frontal lobe retraction, reducing the risk of injury to nearby neurovascular structures.

Burr Holes

- Two burr holes posteriorly on each side of the sagittal sinus.
- Two anterior burr holes are adjacent to the superior sagittal sinus.
- Additional spots over the lateral temporal region or the pterion are based on the patient's age, exposure needed, and the doctor's preference.
- Positioning of additional burr holes may be where the superior temporal line and orbital rim meet posteriorly to the sphenoid wing.

Anatomical Landmarks

- The bone is cut just above the frontal sinus, creating a front lateral or unilateral subfrontal approach to access the anterior cranial fossa, the sellar region, and the olfactory fossa.
- Other areas accessed are lamina terminalis, lesions associated with the optic chiasm, and the anterior third ventricle.

Risks to Avoid

- Cosmetic deformity
- CSF leak
- Because of this, the surgeon will be meticulous about the reconstruction of the calvarium
- Superior sagittal sinus injury
- Damage of the bilateral frontal lobes secondary to retraction

Patient Position: Supine

Temporal Craniotomy

Common Exposure of Temporal Craniotomy

- Middle cranial fossa, including extra-axial and trigeminal nerve lesions and intra-axial lesions that include the mesial temporal lobe.

Incision

- Linear or question mark.

Burr Hole Placement

- Posterior to insertion of the zygomatic arch and upper anterior portion of the zygomatic bone.

Variations of Temporal Craniotomy

Subtemporal Craniotomy

Common Exposure of Subtemporal Technique

- Petroclival areas
- Basal cisterns
- Superior clivus
- Anterior superior brainstem
- Trigeminal and petroclival lesions (ie, chondrosarcomas or meningiomas)
- Smaller vestibular schwannomas
- Anterior superior brainstem
- Basilar aneurysms
- Semicircular canal to repair dehiscence of the superior semicircular canal

Subtemporal Approach Combined with Anterior Petrosectomy

- Common exposure of subtemporal approach combined with anterior petrosectomy
- Lesions involving the middle clivus above the auditory canal and lesions at the petrous bone tip.

Landmarks

- Essential to preserve the vein of Labbe
- Avoid the superficial temporal artery and vein upon incision

Patient Position: Supine with the head rotated to expose the lateral and temporal scalp.

Additional Considerations: Adipose tissue often is used during the closure as a CSF leakage barrier.

Parietal Craniotomy

Common Exposure of Parietal Craniotomy

- Middle and posterior hemispheres
- Anterior exposure provides access to the motor and sensory cortex
- Posterior direction offers access to the visual cortex
- Ability to expose the mid to posterior cerebral hemisphere while avoiding the motor and sensory cortices.

- Intra-axial and extra-axial lesions (ie, gliomas, metastasis, vascular malformations, and meningiomas).

Variations of Parietal Craniotomy

Interhemispheric

- Medial parietal lesions
- Parafalcine lesions
- Splenial lesions

Transcortical Route

- Intra-axial lesions by way of the superior parietal lobule

Important Anatomical Structures

- Two groups of veins along the medial and lateral surfaces of the parietal lobe.
- Medial and lateral surface drains into the superior sagittal sinus **superiorly** and *from* the superior sagittal sinus **inferiorly.**
- Vein of Trolard (the superior anastomotic vein).
- The lateral vein crosses at the Sylvian fissure to the superior sagittal sinus.
- Intra-axial lesions can be localized using cortical mapping.

Patient Position

- Three-quarter prone position
- Head positioned with parietal scalp toward the ceiling

Complications to Avoid

- Many venous lakes in this area have numerous tributaries into the superior sagittal sinus.
- Can result in bleeding during drilling.
- Avoid injury to the superior sagittal sinus and overlying cortical veins.
- Can result in bleeding and cortical/sinus vein thrombosis.

Pterional or Frontotemporal Craniotomy

Common Exposure Approach

- Standard craniotomy for anterior Circle of Willis aneurysms and cavernous sinus
- Most widely used approach for supratentorial lesions
- Visualization of microvasculature lesions in the suprasellar cistern
- Access to the temporal and frontal lobes and Sylvian fissure

Variants of Pterional Craniotomy

- Pterional used in conjunction with subfrontal approach
- For access to the anterior cranial fossa

Important Anatomical Structures

- Optic nerves and chiasm
- Sellar and parasellar lesions
- Basal cisterns

- Frontal, temporal, and parietal operculum
- Temporal lobe
- Sylvian fissure

Patient Position: Supine with head turned away from the side of the approach. The degree of the head angle depends on the pathology location and is determined by the surgeon.

Complications to Avoid

- Avoid temporal artery and temporalis fascia injury during scalp dissection.
- Avoid frontal sinus, if large enough, which can be injured and require vascularized pericranial graft repair.
- Identify and preserve the frontalis branches of the facial nerve to prevent frontalis palsy.
- Unintentional fracture of the sphenoid wing during osteotomy extending into the optic canal and leading to blindness.

Additional Considerations

- The frontal lobe can be accessed using gentle retraction following dural opening.
- For lateral exposure, the Sylvian fissure opened around the opercular frontal gyrus.
- Further dissection is needed for medial lesions such as basilar tip aneurysms or anterior communicating artery access.

Orbitozygomatic (OZ) Craniotomy

- A modern approach to craniotomy frequently referred to as the OZ craniotomy.
- First, the zygomatic, temporal, and fronto-orbital craniotomies were combined with the removal of the rear wall of the major sphenoid wing and orbital bone.

Variants of OZ

Supraorbital

- The OZ was modified into a supraorbital variation in 1982 to extend to the lateral and supraorbital rim and zygoma.
- Extends to the lateral and supraorbital rim and zygoma.
- Allows better access to the subfrontal corridor, reducing the need for frontal lobe retraction while accessing the inferior anterior and middle cranial fossa.
- "Deeper" access is designed to reach high-riding basilar tip aneurysms and aneurysms of the large posterior communicating artery.
- An additional variant of OZ approach is performed in one or two-piece osteotomies.

One-Piece Osteotomy

- To remove the complete supraorbital and frontotemporal osteotomy as one bone flap.

Two-Piece Osteotomy

- To remove traditional pterional bone flap and supraorbital craniotomy.

Both craniotomies are used for:

- Lesions within the orbital apex
- Parasellar and paraclinoid areas
- Basal cisterns
- Cavernous sinuses
- Upper clivus
- Superiorly extending cranial base masses.

Patient Positioning: Similar to pterional approach.

Complications to Avoid

- Fracture of the orbital roof and rim, which can injure the optic nerve within the optic canal.
- Fractures of the sphenoid and ethmoid sinuses may lead to CSF leaks.

Retrosigmoid Approach (Lateral Suboccipital): Became popular in the early 1900s. Various modifications have evolved into the modern retrosigmoid approach. This approach uses a lateral suboccipital craniotomy in combination with a partial mastoidectomy.

Common Exposures

- Optimal access to cerebellopontine and cerebellomedullary cisterns.
- Access to the dorsolateral aspect of the posterior fossa.
- Vestibular schwannoma and other lesions requiring exposure of cranial nerves and brainstem.
- Neurovascular decompression of the trigeminal nerve.
- Aneurysms of the PICA, anterior inferior cerebellar artery, and basilar trunk.
- Excision of small-to-medium size tumors of the internal auditory canal.
- Resection of large tumors to relieve compression of the brainstem and adjacent neurovascular structures.
- One main advantage of the retrosigmoid approach is for resection of vestibular schwannoma treatment.
  - The trans-labyrinthine approach sacrifices structures of the inner ear.

Patient Positioning

- Sitting, supine, or lateral decubitus, with lateral decubitus being the most common.

Complications to Avoid

- Preserve lesser occipital and greater auricular nerves to prevent headache and postoperative dysesthesia.
- The mastoid emissary vein should be located during craniotomy exposure to avoid because substantial bleeding and air embolism.
- Avoid vertebral artery injury during exposure at the occipital bone during osteotomy of the lower part of the exposure.

- Other complications may include retraction injury to the cerebellum, cranial nerves and brainstem damage, and postoperative CSF leaks.

Common Diagnoses for Craniotomy

Neurological

- Removal of brain tumor.

Cerebrovascular

- Clipping of a ruptured aneurysm (ie, SAH)
- Clipping an unruptured aneurysm
- Resecting a vascular malformation (CVM, AVM)
- Hematoma evacuation (subdural, epidural, intracerebral hemorrhage)
- Intracranial or extracranial bypass
- Hemicraniectomy for decompression to cerebral edema after malignant MCA ischemic stroke

Neoplasms of the Brain

- Resection of malignant or benign CNS neoplasms (eg, glioblastoma, meningioma, multiforme)
- Metastatic lesion resection
- Stereotactic or open-needle biopsy
- Tumor-associated cyst aspiration

Infection

- Stereotactic needle drainage or resection for brain abscess

Functional

- Placement of epilepsy electrode grids
- DBS placement
- Hydrocephalus secondary to tumor
- Trigeminal neuralgia (microvascular decompression)
- Ventriculoperitoneal or ventriculoatrial
- Ommaya reservoir insertion
- Trauma

A craniotomy helps to relieve brain swelling, stops bleeding, clips or repairs an aneurysm, removes blood clots from a leaking blood vessel (hematoma), and improves an abnormal mass of blood vessel formation (AVM), repairs skull fractures or damaged meninges. Finally, a craniotomy can also help treat brain conditions such as epilepsy, deliver medication to the brain, or aids in the implantation of a medical device such as a deep brain stimulator.

Risks of Craniotomy

- Brain swelling
- Seizures
- CSF leak
- Bleeding
- Infection

- Blood clot
- Lung infection (pneumonia)
- Unstable blood pressure
- Muscle weakness
- Risks of general anesthesia

Complications are rare and generally specific to specific areas in the brain. These incude:

- Memory or speech problems.
- Paralysis or coma.
- Abnormal balance or coordination.
- Less than 1% of patients will experience some cerebellar mutism.

Intraoperative Steps

The following procedure is a general guide.

- Local anesthetic with epinephrine is infiltrated into the scalp before incision to minimize bleeding.
  - The SA will be applying digital pressure along the edges of the skin as the surgeon incises the skin and galea.
- Apply Raney scalp clips to skin edges.
- SA will help the surgeon in placing the self-retaining retractors if needed. The surgeon uses electrical surgical unit (ESU) on significant scalp vessels for bleeding.
- The surgeon will reflect the scalp flap subperiosteal plane using periosteal elevators and monopolar devices to divide muscle attachments.
- Towel clips, sutures, or rubber bands typically will be used to support a scalp roll. The SA will aid the surgeon as he requests.
- Curettes and Kerrison rongeurs are used to expand the width of Burr holes.
  - *SA performs continuous water/saline irrigation at the drilling site to prevent the accumulation of bone dust in the intracranial cavity to prevent sterile or infected meningitis/ granulomas and abscesses.*
- When operating near the midline, be aware of the **superior sagittal sinus,** and this sinus is a big Venus Lake of blood. *The surgeon will stay a couple of centimeters away because damage to that sinus can be very difficult to repair, in some instances proving fatal.*
- When coming around over contours in the skull, the blade can get a little stuck.
  When this occurs, the surgeon may change the blade angle slightly and wiggle a little bit to regain gentle control of the saw for smooth nonforceful cutting.
- Especially important when coming down through these angles, **especially around the sphenoid,** where there is a ridge which is big on thick bone mass.
- The surgeon's left hand (*or the assistants*) will be resting on the bone flap to prevent bone from falling on the floor if the saw jumps.

- Woodson, Penfield, or Adson dissector is used to dissect the dura from the skull.
- The surgeon continues craniotomy with footplate attachment on the craniotome as the assistant irrigates to cool the bone.
- Placement of bone flap and irrigation solution on the back table.
- The SA will irrigate bone dust away from the wound and assist the surgeon in establishing hemostasis.
- Bone wax is applied to the bleeding edges of the bone.
- Bleeding vessels in the dura are electro-coagulated with the bipolar ESU or occluded with thrombin-soaked Gel foam and patties. *An assistant typically helps with the application.*
- After the surgeon places hemostatic agents and patties around the craniotomy edges, permanent dural tacking sutures will be set by the surgeon to prevent postoperative epidural hematoma formation.
- After hemostasis is achieved, the surgeon opens the dura with a #11 or #15 blade.
- A dural suture may be placed in the dura before incising it. This tents the dura, ensuring that the surface of the brain is not inadvertently nicked.
- A Woodson dissector and blade or metzenbaum scissors are used for extending the dural incision.
- Bleeding from transected dural vessels can be prevented by coagulating them with the bipolar ESU before cutting them. To avoid shrinking the dura, hemoclips can be placed, or vessels can be compressed with a hemostat.
- A self-retaining retractor system is placed if necessary.
- Cortical dissection is achieved using the bipolar ESU, micro scissors, and suction, and the specific surgical procedure is completed.
- **Specific surgical procedure is completed.**
- Samples of tumors are sent for pathological study if applicable.
- Hemostasis is established. Irrigation can be used to find bleeding sites in the brain.
- A resection cavity is lined with *Surgicel* and filled with irrigation.
- Valsalva's maneuver can be produced with the ventilator to verify hemostasis.
- The surgeon closes the dura with a 4-0 suture (braided nylon or silk).
- Gaps in the dura can be repaired using muscle, pericranium, dural substitute, or pericardium.
- A central dural tacking suture may be placed, and *Gel foam* may be placed over the dura.
- The bone plate is fitted with titanium plates and screws and reconnected to the cranium, or it may be wired into place depending on the surgeon's preference.

- Muscle/fascia is reapproximated, and the galea is closed with interrupted absorbable sutures. Skin is closed with sutures or staples.

Suboccipital Craniectomy

Posterior Fossae Approach

Standard treatment for Chiari 1 malformation.

In the early 20th century, cerebellar lesions and Posterior fossa lesions were both considered risky and inoperable.

This is commonly used for exposure of the following:

- Removal of the caudal part of the occipital bone.
- Provides broad exposure of the posterior fossa.
- It can be approached early in treatment to minimize or avoid brainstem compression during surgery and allow decompression of the posterior fossa.
- Access to the posterior fossa through the suboccipital approach allows treatment of the cerebellar hemispheres, medulla, vermis, cerebellar tonsils, and fourth ventricle.
- Craniocervical junction and foramen magnum lesions.
- During treatment for Chiari 1 malformation, resection of the C1 posterior arch takes place.

Patient Positioning

Prone, lateral decubitus, or sitting position.

Important Surgical Landmarks

- Be aware of transverse sinuses during burr hole placement and occipital sinus during dura dissection.

Craniectomy

A decompressive craniectomy is a surgical procedure used to remove part of the skull. This is most often necessary to relieve brain swelling and decrease pressure within the brain. Pieces of bone may be taken from either one or both sides of the skull based on diagnoses and reasons for a craniectomy.

Positioning and Skin Prep. Follow guidelines as explained in the above "Craniotomy" section, approach section, positioning section, or per surgeon's direction.

Intraoperative Steps

The following is a basic outline, as many steps overlap with craniotomy; reference proper section for specific details.

- General anesthesia.
- Positioning, prepping, and draping are carried out in a similar manner to various craniotomy instructions.
- The surgeon will place an incision along one or both sides of the patient's head.
- The skin and muscle layers pulled back.
- Burr holes are drilled in the skull along the incision line.
- Midas Rex saw is used to connect the holes and cut the piece of the skull.
- Piece of the skull, called "bone flap," will be kept on the back table during surgery.
- The dura is cut.

- For drainage of excess CSF, a drain may be placed.
- A dural substitute will be gently placed over exposed brain tissue that will allow the brain to expand.
  - Possible dural substitutes
    - Lyoplant™, bovine pericardium and
    - Neuro-Patch™, made from polyesterurethane.
- The duraplasty will create a "pouch" for the intracranial volume to fill while intracranial pressure (ICP) is elevated.
- The bone flap will be preserved in one of the two ways.
  - An abdominal wall pouch is surgically created or bone flap may be frozen in an antibiotic solution.
  - *If the bone is too damaged from trauma, cancer, etc., an artificial skull cap will be made later and used in place of the skull cap.*
    - Depending on recovery, the bone flap will typically be left out of the patient's head for 6 weeks to 5 months.
- The outer layer of muscle is pulled back over the brain
- Sutures are used to close the skin.
- Bandages are wrapped around the patient's head

Postop. The patient will leave the operating room (OR) connected to several machines. They may have swelling in their eyes, requiring cool compresses to decrease swelling. Pain medicine is given to stave off mild to severe headaches after surgery. The bed will be elevated to prevent an increase in brain pressure.

After brain swelling has decreased, surgery may replace the skull. Either the piece of skull previously removed or a manufactured material is used.

Risks of Craniectomy

- Hydrocephalus
- Bleeding and infection
- Meningitis or a bone infection
- Delayed wound healing
- Seizures

Cranioplasty

After a craniotomy or craniectomy, the bone flap may be left off, allowing the brain room to swell.

Usually, several months later, the bone flap will be replaced during an operation called cranioplasty.

If the patient's bone flap has been saved either in a belly pouch or in the freezer, it can be reattached, though, often due to trauma or infection, this isn't possible.

There are options for skull replacement materials, including mesh.

The following is a sample of a typical cranioplasty using a 3D printed patient-specific bone, using a CT scan of the patient; the implant is designed to recreate the skull's original shape, allowing for a precise fit and cosmetic appearance.

The skull cap is made from regenerative calcium phosphate with 3D printed titanium reinforcement. The regenerative material is designed to encourage new bone growth and integrate with the patient's bone.

Anesthesia, Positioning, and Skin Prep

It will be the same as for craniotomy or craniectomy or as per the doctor's preference.

- The doctor will open the old incision along the same scar using a Colorado cutting tool to burn through the layers and seal them. (Scalp is vascular and will bleed profusely.)
- The SA will be suctioning plume and blood to aid with exposer.
  - Remember that during exposure to cranioplasty, there will be just skin overlying the brain.
- It is essential to remove all of the scar tissue away from the bone edges so that the cranioplasty plate will fit in place.
- As scar tissue is dissected, the delicate layers covering the brain and the skull will come into view.
- Be very careful here so as not to damage the brain as it that might be just beneath this scar tissue which has most likely had several months to form.
- Scar tissue can be stuck down toward the brain and its coverings now.
- The dura is exposed along with other materials that would have been placed during the original operation.
- The surgeon will start methodically teasing the scar tissue away from the bone edges, so the screws and the cranioplasty plate sit flush against the skull.
- At this point, the doctor will likely place a finger beneath the temporalis muscle, which has fused to this covering of the brain.
- Temporalis muscle will be carefully cut away and stitched over the top of the cranioplasty plate to give an excellent cosmetic result.
  - *if the temporalis muscle is not stitched over the top of the cranioplasty plate, it can fall back down towards the cheek and create a lump in the side of the face.*
- The bone edges reveal, and the scar tissue is removed to the doctor's satisfaction that bone edges are transparent for the plaits to sit on.
- Swabs are soaked in betadine to help prevent infection.
- The cranial fitting template will be tested for a flush fit.
- The cranioplasty plate can now be removed from the packaging.
- Titanium screws are used to fix cranial implants into the defect.
- The doctor will check to make sure that the temporalis muscle can fit over the implant.
- If needed, the doctor will shave away bone to make sure this fits well.
- Sutured material or stitches are passed through the plate to attach the temporalis muscle to it once the plate is attached.

- After the desired fit is achieved, titanium screws are drilled through prefabricated templates screw holes pre-designed carefully, bearing in mind how much access there is to those points.
- With hand ties, the temporalis muscle is stitched over the top of the plate, helping to reconstruct the shape of the head.
  An excellent SA will learn and be skilled at standard neurosurgical hand tie methods.
- A drain will be placed to prevent the risk of blood pooling after the operation.
  The drain sits over the top and is tunneled out towards the top of that skull.
- The skin is sutured back together.
- Regenerative calcium phosphate matrix over the top of the titanium reinforcement should encourage new bone growth and integration with the patient's bone.

CRANIOTOMY FOR TUMOR REMOVAL

What Causes Brain Tumors?

A brain tumor is caused by uncontrolled cell multiplication, which has led to abnormal growth. Brain tumors can cause pressure on the brain because of the brain's expansion limits within the skull.

Classification of Tumors

Classification by Origin. Primary tumors are located at the site where cancer began to grow or originated.

Metastatic, or secondary tumors, have spread to other parts of the body from the original tumor site.

Classification Based on the Growth Trend

Malignant, or cancerous, tumors:

- Keep growing despite treatment.

Benign, or noncancerous, tumors:

- Slow growing, potential to be cured by treatment.
- Cause problems due to pressure on surrounding brain tissue.
- Benign tumors can be life-threatening.

Symptoms of Brain Tumors

- Headaches with or without vomiting
- Numbness, weakness, or neck pain
- Seizure
- Personality or behavior changes
- Mental decline, ie, memory loss, confusion, speech difficulty, impaired concentration or reasoning
- Sleepiness
- Loss of movement or sensation in arms or legs, and gait problems
- Speech and comprehension problems
- Changes in vision

Diagnostics

- Neurological exam to assess the function of eyes, ears, nose, muscles, sensations, balance, coordination, mental state, and memory.
- Imaging studies such as MRI or CT scans will be quickly ordered based on observations, and symptom list.
- Biopsy to examine tissue samples from the tumor. (Biopsy of brain lesion requires craniotomy.)

Treatment Options for Brain Tumors

Nonsurgical Treatment Options for Brain Tumors

Slow-growing or static tumor that does not cause pressure on the brain may first be treated with conservative therapy and observed over time.

Aggressive growing or life-threatening tumors are often initially treated with such techniques as radiation therapy, chemotherapy, and biopsy (surgical treatment of brain tumors generally requires a craniotomy).

Radiation Therapy

Ionizing radiation is in the form of high-energy beams coming from a machine outside of the body. Other names for radiation therapy are radiation oncology, radiotherapy, or therapeutic radiation. By interfering with their metabolic activity, radiation kills cells—radiation administered with a beam that passes through tissue or with an implantable radiation source.

Ionizing Radiation: Works to target and kill cancer cells by displacing electrons from atoms and molecules. The sources of this energy usually come from x-rays or protons. This radiation method is applied to cause breaks in the double-stranded DNA molecule, which resides in each cell nucleus. In turn, this causes the cancer cells to die and, as a result, prevent or slow the progression of malignant disease.

Particle Beam Therapy: Allows charged particles (**proton beams**) and more relatively heavy ion beams (**carbon ions**) to deposit more energy by traveling deeper into the body resulting in a higher dose of absorbed radiation. These beams can increase to a sharp maximum at the end of their range. Then the residual energy is lost over a short distance, causing a rise in the absorbed dose with a rapid fall off of the amount to zero, resulting in the Bragg peak event.

Particle beam therapy is sometimes the preferred method of radiation therapy because of the minimal damage to surrounding healthy structures adjacent to the tumor (eg, the spinal cord).

Brachytherapy: Brachytherapy is another technique used to deliver radiation directly to the tumor or tissue which contains it. The radioactive sources are encapsulated and inserted directly into the affected tissue or body cavity surrounding it through catheters or needles. Catheter placement is often used after tumor resection to implant the radiation into the tumor bed. Brachytherapy has the ability of its use to deliver high doses of radiation to tumor tissue or tumor bed and still spare the healthy surrounding tissue.

Stereotactic Radiosurgery (SRS)

- Stereotactic radiosurgery was first created and named by a neurosurgeon named Dr. Lars Leksell in 1951. Seventeen years later, a team of neurosurgeons and physicists in Sweden developed a way to put SRS into use by inventing the Gamma Knife. This new technology could be used to deliver radiation to target exact locations in the brain while causing minimal damage to nearby tissue. This stereotactic radiosurgery requires using a frame on the patient's head to focus radiation on targeted tissue sights of the brain. In 1991, John Adler, a Stanford neurosurgeon, completed a year-long fellowship with Dr. Leksell and became determined to find a way to make SRS functional on any part of the human body. Because the rigid frame could not be used other than on the head, he invented the Cyberknife, the first mask-based tool for SRS or any stereotactic procedure. By 2000, the Cyberknife had become practical and easy to acquire.
- SRS works by altering and destroying the DNA of tumor cells, causing cells to lose the ability to replicate and die.
- Often divided into several smaller doses of stereotactic radiation on separate days of treatment, there will usually be two to five treatments. The thought process is that the healthy cells have time to repair in between treatments and lessen the patient's side effects by giving a smaller dose.
- This is also called staged radiosurgery, also known as fractionated stereotactic radiosurgery (FSR).
- Generally, SRS is used for treating tumors that are smaller than three centimeters in maximal diameter. Most commonly, SRS is used for the treatment of metastatic brain tumors. SRS is also very effective in treating small tumors ascending from the vestibular nerve, known as vestibular schwannoma (or acoustic neuroma).
- This is considered a noninvasive treatment option for various conditions, including AVMs, arteriovenous fistulas, trigeminal neuralgia, and many intracranial tumors.

Stereotactic Radiosurgery (SRS) Procedure: With a framework approach to SRS, the frame is placed on the patient's head after a local anesthetic has been injected into the scalp. Four sterile pins secure the frame to the patient's skull. When using one of the more recent alternative frameless systems, fiducial markers are attached to the skin or implanted onto the outside of the head. These markers are used in imaging modality to register the physical; location of the fiducials, which align with the surgical target and help precisely deliver radiation.

- Medications administered: Additional pain-relieving medicines, such as morphine may be given intravenously to aid in the patient's comfort during the procedure. Children typically receive general anesthesia for this procedure. Decadron may be given intravenously.
- Once the frame is secured, or fiducial markers are attached, the patient is taken for a CT with contrast which will then be merged with the MRI. Together, the two studies improve the precision of the procedure.

- Once returned to the OR, the patient is positioned onto an MRI or CT table, and the frame or fiducials are secured.
- The neurosurgeon and radiation oncologists study the images and together plan the radiation treatment. They will both be in attendance during the procedure. In addition, several other specialized medical professionals will be helping: a medical radiation physicist, dosimetrist, therapist, and radiation therapy nurse.
- The stereotactic coordinates are entered into the computer, and the procedure is performed through a burr hole. The computer directs the stereotactic probe.
- Instruments may be guided through the burr hole to the precise location of treatment.
- The radiation is then administered.
- The average time to treat one tumor or lesion is 30 to 45 minutes. It will take longer if more than one tumor is being targeted.
- Afterward, the frame and any external markers are removed, and a clean dressing is applied.

Alternative Uses for SRS Approaches:

- Stereotactic biopsy of brain tissue: a needle is guided into an abnormal area and a piece of tissue removed for exam under a microscope.
- Stereotactic aspiration: to remove fluid from abscesses, hematomas, or cysts.
- Catheter placement to plant electrodes in regions of the brain to find the origin of seizure.
- Chemical and mechanical treatment or electrical

Stereotactic Radiotherapy (SRT)

- Stereotactic radiotherapy is reserved for patients with more than four metastatic tumors in the brain. This procedure is also known as **whole-brain radiation therapy**. Generally, SRT is only used when SRS is not an option because, though it is effective at killing tumor cells, it can also damage normal brain cells causing cognitive and decline.
- Sometimes, SRS is used along with whole-brain radiation in order to boost its effects. Suppose SRS is desirable, but the location of the tumor is near a critical structure, such as the optic nerves. In that case, the radiation will often be divided into portions and delivered in segments. This is known as stereotactic radiotherapy (SRT).

   Another difference between SRT and SRS is that with SRT, a custom mask made of thermoplastic material is often used instead of the frame since the patient has to undergo several sessions of treatment.
- After a tumor has been targeted using stereotactic CT, MRI, positron emission tomography (PET), magnetoencephalography, or cerebral angiography, depending on the indication, the unit directs gamma radiation very precisely to a target point, allowing an effective radiation dosage to be delivered in one treatment session, often used successfully for patients with benign or malignant brain tumors or vascular malformations.

- The Gamma Knife is mainly to deactivate benign brain tumors (meningiomas acoustic neuromas, craniopharyngiomas, pituitary adenomas, and other tumors of the brain and skull base).
- In addition, to malignant tumors, Gamma Knife is used to treat chronic pain conditions such as trigeminal neuralgia, treatment-resistant epilepsy, and movement disorders such as tremors.
- For certain engrained tumors or AVMs, the Gamma Knife may be more desirable to conventional surgery because it can modify radio surgical doses to lesions of appropriate size.
- Gamma is sometimes used as an alternative microsurgical or endovascular embolization.

Side Effects of Radiation Therapy

- Fatigue, headaches, memory loss, and scalp irritation.

Intraoperative Steps

- After positioning, prepping, and draping.
- Craniotomy, craniectomy, and keyhole placement based on surgical approach is carried out. (See appropriate section for specifics.)

About Burr Holes

The surgeon will then make burr holes in different places.

- Using one hand is relatively unstable, so he will usually try and fix one hand down in place or support it with the other hand as a precaution to prevent the saw from sliding while drilling.
- The clutch system detects pressure changes in the drill bits as an additional safety measure to prevent plunging into the brain.
- Should it fail, which is very unlikely, the other hand will stop it.
- The surgeon will always start perpendicular to the bone to perfect the burr hole and ensure access to the cranium underneath.
- Expect this step to take a bit of time
- Next, a cranial feed is fit into the footplate. If turned upside down, it looks like a foot hence the name.
- The footplate will strip the dura off the underside of the bone. The dura is leathery, covering the brain.
- The surgeon will likely angle it back and then make sure they are not tearing the dura.
- The footplate may be angled down into a burr hole to see that the dura is untethered from the skull.

   Surgical assistant: Check that everything is locked together before drilling.
- The handle rotates, allowing the doctor to follow different curves around the skull.
- The surgeon may seem to be leaning back slightly so that while connecting the burr holes, he can be assured that he is cutting up and away from the dura.

- It is essential to control the footplate as it comes out of the burr hole to prevent it from suddenly coming out and catching things in the blade-like surgeon or assistant's finger.
- Peeling the bone off the dura is usually done with instruments like an Adsen smooth elevator or sometimes a finger.
- The surgeon usually will expect the assistant to keep a hand near the bone flap if it drops.
- The dura is peeled from the bone using care not to rip it, which is sometimes unavoidable.
- Specialized tools are used to remove the section of bone called the bone flap.
- The bone flap is temporarily removed for replacement after the brain surgery is complete.
- The bone flap will be stored on the back table in a basin by the surgical technologist or, in prolonged cases, may be refrigerated.

Stereotactic Needle Biopsy. Performed for brain tumors in hard-to-reach areas or susceptible areas within the brain that a more extensive operation might otherwise damage. The neurosurgeon will drill a small hole into the skull. Frequently guided by CT or MRI, a thin needle is inserted through the hole, and a tissue sample is removed.

Typically sent as a cold sample during surgery, a microscope viewing determines if the biopsy sample is cancerous or benign. The lab will call up to the operating suite with the results.

VENTRICULOPERITONEAL SHUNT PLACEMENT

Surgical implantation of drainage tube to relieve the pressure of hydrocephalus, which is excess the CSF within the ventricles of the brain.

The term "hydrocephalus" literally means "water brain." This condition of ventricular enlargement is a result of obstruction to the normal flow of CSF. The sites of obstruction can occur at the third ventricle, at the medullary foramina (Luschka and Magendie), aqueduct of Sylvius, or in the basal or convexity subarachnoid spaces. Due to obstruction or overproduction, the CSF accumulates within the ventricles, causing increasing pressure, which enlarges the ventricles and expands the brain's hemispheres.

Non-communicating: Hydrocephalus results from an **obstruction** within the ventricular system. Ventricular fluid may not communicate with other ventricles or the with the subarachnoid fluid.

Communicating: An increase in the amount of CSF normally produced, or the improper absorption of CSF by the arachnoid villi causing increase cranial pressure.

The causes of hydrocephalus are still not completely understood, and it is thought to result from inherited developmental disorders. Other complications include from premature birth, intraventricular hemorrhage, meningitis, traumatic brain injury, tumors, or SAH.

Symptoms

The symptoms of hydrocephalus vary from patient to patient based on factors such as age, progression of the disease, and individual differences in tolerance to the condition.

Pediatric Symptoms

- The most typical indication of hydrocephalus in infancy is a considerable head size or increase in head circumference as pediatric skull sutures extend to take on CSF buildup.
- Sleepiness, vomiting, irritability.
- Seizures and downward deviation of the eyes (also called "sunsetting").
- Older children and adults may experience different symptoms than an infant.

Adult Symptoms

- Headache followed by nausea and vomiting
- Blurred or double vision
- Coordination, gait disturbance problems with balance, sunsetting of the eyes
- Urinary incontinence
- Loss of or slowing of developmental progress
- Drowsiness, lethargy, irritability
- Memory loss or other changes in personality or cognition

Some of these symptoms overlap with other disorders such as Parkinson's disease, Alzheimer's disease, and Creutzfeldt-Jakob disease resulting in incorrect diagnoses of normal pressure hydrocephalus and improper treatment.

Diagnostic Imaging and Tests

Doctors use various tests to diagnose normal pressure hydrocephalus and rule out other conditions accurately.

- Brain scans such as CT
- MRI of the brain
- Spinal tap or lumbar catheter
- Intracranial pressure monitoring
- Neuropsychological tests

Surgical Procedure for Ventriculoperitoneal Shunt Placement

For demonstrative purposes, this case will outline a standard procedure using a 1-week old infant.

The patient is undergoing a right occipitoparietal ventriculoperitoneal shunt placement.

The shunt is most commonly placed in the right frontal horn of the lateral ventricle through a parieto-occipital entry point (see Figure 21-4).

After the location for the proximal ventricular catheter is selected, the surgeon will select a **distal terminus**. While there are several acceptable locations, the peritoneum is the most commonly selected. Accessing the peritoneum is safe.

- The peritoneal cavity absorbs CSF well.

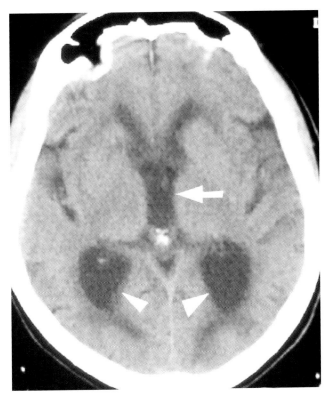

A

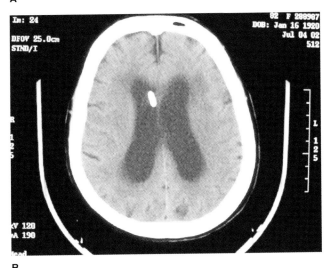

B

Figure 21-4 · Ventriculoperitoneal shunt. (Reproduced, with permission, from Brunicardi FC, Andersen DK, Billiar TR, et al., eds. *Schwartz's Principles of Surgery*. 11th ed. New York, NY: McGraw Hill; 2019.)

- Excess catheter can be placed in anticipation of future growth in the patient.
- The right heart atrium is also acceptable as a distal site.
- CSF typically absorbs into the venous system, making the atrium ideal due to risk of endocarditis, thrombosis, nephritis, myocardial injury, and arrhythmias. The distal catheter of the Ventriculoatrial (VA) shunt is a fixed length. A growing child might need lengthening of this distal catheter with age.
- Pleural space is also an accepted distal site.

Disadvantages of Pleural Space

- Pleura is sensitive, and pain may be felt from the distal catheter.
- Low lung capacity in children may prevent handling the amount of CSF.
- Many surgeons will not place a Ventriculoperitoneal (VPl) shunt in children under 7 years of age for this reason.
- The pleural space creates negative pressure on the shunt system. Every inspiration subjects the shunt to a "suck" that can lead to a situation of low or negative resistance.
- The gallbladder is used infrequently as distal terminus.
- Used in patients with intolerance of other locations. Additional sites that have been described include the transverse sinus and bone marrow.
- Other possible distal sites options include the transverse sinus and bone marrow.

Preoperative antibiotics are given.

Patient Positioning

- **An infant will be positioned at the very end of the table; the head turned and a shoulder bump in place to keep the mastoid process and the clavicle on the same plane.**
- Modified supine with shoulder roll.
- Head is turned opposite the side of the proximal catheter.
- Head rotated 45° to 60° away from the surgeon with a slight posterior tilt.
- Extra rotation for occipitoparietal shunt.
- Place bump under shoulders to form a straight line between the neck, thorax, and retroauricular region.
- The clavicle and mastoid processes should be close to the same horizontal plane, in order to facilitate safe tunneling.
- The surgical team should all double glove, as this practice has been shown to reduce the risk of shunt infection.

Skin Prep and Draping

- The entire length of the shunt path must be exposed and surgically prepared.
- Only enough hair is clipped to make room for a clean incision. and skip incisions if necessary.
- Hair removed from burr hole site to behind ear and down to the neck length of shunt path is to be surgically prepared and exposed.
- Clean burr hole site, neck, chest, and abdomen; the site of shunt insertion are prepped.
- The most common placement for the proximal catheter is the frontal horn of a lateral ventricle from either a frontal or occipitoparietal approach. Ideally, the catheter rests in front of the foramen of Monro, away from the choroid plexus.
- The skin incision is curvilinear and should be fashioned such that it is away from the shunt hardware.

Key anatomic landmarks for placing a frontal catheter include:

- Medial canthus of ipsilateral eye.
- Tragus of ipsilateral ear.
- Kocher's point, located 1 to 2 cm anterior to the coronal suture and 3 cm lateral from the midline, is used for placement of the burr hole.
- Corner of the anterior fontanelle in infants good site for entry.
- A retroauricular skip incision is generally required for frontal shunts.
- *The entire length of the shunt path should be exposed and surgically prepared.*
- The patient is draped to provide access to all parts of the shunt system in case of shunt failure.
- The shunt will be soaked in normal saline with an antibiotic solution on the back table and primed just before insertion
  - *Avoid trapped air in valve assembly and check that valve is aligned correctly to allow CSF to flow from the ventricle to the peritoneum*

Anatomic Landmarks for Frontal Catheter

Image guidance is frequently used for mapping the incision:

- The shunt may be inserted via the frontal, parietal, or occipital lobe.
- Medial canthus of the ipsilateral eye.
- Tragus of the ipsilateral ear.
- Kocher's point about 1 to 2 cm ventral to the coronal suture and 3 cm lateral to the midline for burr hole placement.
- For infants, the corner of the anterior fontanelle is a common entry point.
- Preoperative antibiotics are given.
- Frazier's point is a familiar anatomic landmark when placing the burr hole for an occipitoparietal shunt which is 3 cm lateral from the midline and 6 cm superior to the inion.
- An additional method used to estimate the burr-hole placement for an occipitoparietal shunt is as follows:
  - The surgeon measures a mark halfway between the external acoustic meatus and the inion.
  - A second measurement is made halfway between this mark and the vertex of the skull to locate the flatter area of the head that exists just superior and posterior to this mark. *This makes an ideal entry point for an occipitoparietal shunt catheter.*

Surgical Steps

- Horseshoe-shaped, curvilinear cranial incision made right or left of midline, along papillary line. A retroauricular skip incision is typically required for frontal shunts.
- The skin incision is curvilinear and fashioned away from the shunt hardware.

- Scalp bleeding is controlled.
- Skin and periosteum are elevated.
- The galea needs to be identified in an infant to keep it attached to the skin because the galea is the only layer to hold a deep stitch consistently. The incision opens through the galea and into the periosteum of the skull.
- The galea is separated easily from the peritoneum with blunt dissection within the loose areolar plane.
- The galea is the only layer that will reliably hold a deep stitch. The incision should be opened through the galea and into the periosteum of the skull. The galea should separate easily from the peritoneum with blunt dissection within the loose areolar plane.
- A 6- to 10-mm burr hole is created using Midas Rex, Anspach burr, or Hudson brace, and D'Errico bit.
- Dura is incised after being coagulated using bipolar ESU to control bleeding of the pia at the catheter insertion site.
  - A valve pocket between the periosteum and the galea is created with a hemostat in the plane of the loose areolar tissue without detaching the galea from the skin layer.
- The proximal catheter is most often placed in the frontal horn of a lateral ventricle either from a frontal or occipitoparietal approach. The best placement for the catheter will be in front of the foramen of Monro, away from the choroid plexus.
  Most neurosurgeons will insist that the shunt be soaked in an antibiotic saline mixture before use.
- Some valves or antisiphon devices differ in their specific placement or orientation space requirements.
- The surgeon and the assistant must understand the differences between each valve.
- Once penetrated, the introducer is removed.
- CSF flow is verified, and a small amount is taken as a specimen
- The reservoir and valve are attached and secured with 2-0 silk ties.
  For temporary catheter placement, external end of the catheter is connected to a drainage system which allows the CSF drainage to be controlled and for the measurement of ICP.
- When CSF treatment is long term, an internal ventricular shunt may be placed. The neurosurgeon will determine the size and type.

Peritoneal Abdominal incision

Three common ways to access the abdomen:

- **Minilaparotomy:** The most common method for accessing the peritoneal space. Multiple sites for the incision.
- **Laparoscopically:** The laparoscope-assisted method is often used in obese patients and is often performed by a general surgeon.

- **Lateral subcostal incision:** Advantageous for entering the peritoneal space over the liver to minimizing the risk of bowel perforation. The surgeon will have three layers of muscle to navigate with this incision.
- **Midline vertical incision:** Advantageous for cutting through the avascular linea alba. Superior and lateral to the umbilicus is common for insertion; either side is acceptable. When a patient needs a gastrostomy tube, the right side is preferred. A benefit of this simple exposure is that the muscle and fascia act together as support of the distal tubing and prevent CSF leakage.

Procedure

- A transverse minilaparotomy incision is made superior to the umbilicus, and just to the right of the midline, approximately 1.5 cm in a small child.
- The incision is carried through the fat and Scarpa's fascia to the anterior rectus sheath. The anterior rectus sheath is opened transversely. The rectus abdominus muscle is visualized, and a hemostat is used to split these fibers vertically, in line with their orientation.
- The surgeon will carefully pull the sheath toward oneself.
- One hemostat will be used to grab the sheath, and a second hemostat is used to sweep away the rectus muscle.
- The back and forth motions of the two hemostats expose a section of the posterior sheath.
- Gentle superior traction on the sheath allows the intra-abdominal contents to fall away.
- The posterior rectus sheath is cut with scissors and the peritoneal space is directly entered.

  The surgeon should handle the scissor tips under direct vision through the tissue before cutting, helping them avoid inadvertently cutting the bowel.
- The undersurface of the abdominal wall will be very smooth, and the surgeon will be able to use his finger to verify that the abdominal cavity has been entered.
- If left in the peritoneal space, the catheter will generally fail quickly, therefore, fluoroscopy is usually used to ensure the catheter enters freely into the appropriate area.
- If the catheter remains tightly coiled (generally determined via C-arm imaging) this is unacceptable.
- Subcutaneous tunneling is performed next.
- A subcutaneous tunnel is created from the burr hole to abdominal incision.
- Tunneling is accomplished by using a tunneling device such as a long-curved sarot or plastic tunneler *avoiding the nipples and umbilicus.*
- Catheter is passed through a tunneling device to the abdominal incision.
- The spontaneous flow of CSF is checked.
- Using a purse string suture, the catheter is secured to the peritoneum.

- The surgeon connects both catheters to the valve beneath the scalp.
- Incisions are sutured closed, and bandages are applied.

Postop

- A hospital stay of a few days.

Risks of Ventriculoperitoneal Shunt Placement

- Shunt failure caused by obstruction, disconnection, infection, or malfunction.
- Approximately 1% chance of clinically relevant intracranial hemorrhage.
- Approximately 1% chance of damaged abdominal viscera.
- About 5% to 8% risk of shunt infection.
- Approximately half children who undergo shunt placement will require a shunt revision within 2 years.

TRANSSPHENOIDAL HYPOPHYSECTOMY

The central skull base, where the pituitary gland is located is challenging for surgeons to access. Over the last century, pituitary surgery, also called hypophysectomy, has evolved from an open surgery, requiring a craniotomy, to a fully endoscopic endonasal procedure performed through the sphenoid sinuses. In 1910, the transsphenoidal approach was described and popularized by Harvey Cushing and Oskar Hirsch, as a method to access this location of the brain, utilizing sublabial and transnasal routes. Although the popularity of the transsphenoidal approach went down when Cushing began using transcranial approaches, Dott and Guiot continued to use it, and Hardy refined it by introducing microsurgical approaches.

Two Main Surgical Approaches

There are two main surgical approaches: transcranial and extracranial.

Transcranial Approach

- Microscopic approach.
- Used when transsphenoidal approaches are contraindicated.
- Involves pterional and anterior subfrontal approaches.

Pterional

- Involves removing the sphenoid wing with minimal brain retraction.
- Shortest trajectory to the parasellar region.
- Excellent visualization of the pituitary gland.
- Less risk of damage to olfactory nerves and frontal sinuses.

Anterior subfrontal approach

- The advantage is straight visualization of the pituitary tumor between the optic nerves.
- Risk of damage to frontal sinuses and olfactory nerves.

Extracranial Approaches

- Transsphenoidal microscopic approaches (transnasal or sublabial)

- Endoscopic transnasal transsphenoidal approach (along with modifications)

- EEEA (expanded endoscopic endonasal approach)

- CTTA (combined transsphenoidal trans axillary approach).

- Transsphenoidal microscopic approaches (sublabial or septal incisions)

- Wide dissection of the mucoperichondrium/mucoperiosteum of the septum and the nasal floor with partial resection of the vomer, the sphenoid rostrum, and the perpendicular plate of the ethmoid.

With a self-retaining speculum, the nasal contents were pushed laterally, allowing bimanual instrumentation and an operative microscope. Because of the many poor side effects of this technique, endoscopic pituitary surgery was created as recently as the early 1990s.

With the natural medial nasal corridor used for access to the sphenoid sinus, this method has become more popular over transsphenoidal microscopic approaches due to its shorter hospital stay, wider view, and ease of mobility with angled views.

Relevant Anatomy and Physiology

Located in a saddle-shaped depression of the sphenoid bone, sella turcica, and pituitary fossa sits the pituitary gland. The floor of the pituitary fossa creates the posterior roof of the sphenoid sinuses. The anterior wall of the pituitary fossa ends at the tuberculum sellae and is bounded laterally by the middle of the clinoid process, as well as the posterior boundary being the dorsum sella (a vertical projection of bone). The posterolateral angles of the dorsum sellae create the posterior clinoid processes. Anterior to the tuberculum sellae sits the grooved sulcus chiasmatic, leading laterally to the optic canals. The optic chiasma sits posterior to the sulcus chiasmatic and anterior to the pituitary stalk. Anterior to the sulcus chiasmatic lies the planum sphenoidal, a smooth roof of the sphenoid body.

Related Endoscopic Anatomy. The sphenoid sinuses can be accessed with an endoscope through the medial corridor, between the middle turbinate and the nasal septum.

Medial to the superior turbinate, at the same level as the superior border of the natural ostium of the maxillary sinus, are the sphenoid ostia. It sits 1 to 1.5 cm from the choanal roof, about 7 cm from the nasal sill at a 30° angle, and about 11 mm from the base of the skull. The amount of sphenoid pneumatization varies, with the most common type being sellar, and pneumatization extends posteriorly to the sella turcica and then the sellar and post-sellar type patterns.

The sphenoid sinus can also be pneumatized laterally into the pterygoid root causing a lateral recess that leads to exposure of the V2 and the vidian nerve.

The main structures easily seen in the sinus are the optic nerve, the sella turcica, and the carotid artery.

After removing the inter-sinus septum, the remaining structures are easily located. The pituitary fossa is in the middle. Surrounding are the cavernous sinus and the anterior genu of the cavernous segment of the carotid artery.

At the roof and sidewall, the optic nerve is located. The carotid arteries follow superiorly. Above the pituitary is the tuberculum sella, at the roof of the sphenoid sinus (planum sphenoidal) and junction of the anterior face of the pituitary fossa.

A triangular bony depression called the lateral opticocarotid recess (OCR) represents the ventral surface of the optic strut. The medial OCR is a teardrop-shaped depression at the medial junction of the paraclinoid carotid and optic canal. Its lateral end (tail) connects with the medial aspect of lateral OCR. This is where the paraclinoid carotid artery and the optic canal come together.

So many anatomical variations make endonasal transsphenoidal access difficult. The deviation of the nasal septum or a pneumatization of the middle turbinate can make the nasal passage narrow.

Previous nasal surgery or gross deviation of the septum or prior septal surgery can negatively impact the ability to harvest a nasoseptal flap. This a common reconstructive technique in sellar surgery. The presence of nasal polyps or sinonasal disease can cause harm to the nasal passage and warrants sinus surgery.

For a critical evaluation of the sphenoid sinus and adjacent structures, CT scan is helpful. The surgeon will use this to determine the extent of sphenoid sinus and its anatomy including location of the optic nerve and carotid artery.

Common Indications for Transsphenoidal Hypophysectomy

- Pituitary adenomas (both micro and macroadenomas) are the most frequent indications for transsphenoidal hypophysectomy.

- Nonsecreting adenomas causing vision disorders, hypopituitarism, and pituitary apoplexy, which show progression on serial imaging.

- Secreting adenomas unresponsive to treatment.

- Rathke's cyst, meningiomas, craniopharyngiomas, chordomas, metastatic lesions, and other sellar lesions can be approached similarly.

- Contraindications for transsphenoidal approach.

- Sphenoid sinusitis.

- Intrasellar vascular anomalies.

- Ectatic midline carotid arteries.

- Significant lateral suprasellar tumor extension of tumor, especially when the epicenter is lateral to the carotid artery.

- Poor pneumatization of the sphenoid sinus.

- Suprasellar adenoma extension and constrictive diaphragma sellae.

- Hardy self-retaining bivalve speculum

Revision Procedures and Parasellar Extension Distorted Anatomy

- Image guidance navigation (IGN) system for revision procedures, parasellar extension, or cases with distorted anatomy.

- Intraoperative MRI for pituitary surgery for updated images to measure tumor volume, the dura, and normal pituitary.

- Endoscopic surgery of pituitary tumors can require two surgeons or a CSFA to assist with a four-handed technique.

- The CSFA holds the endoscope to provide an optimal view for the surgeon while performing bimanual dissection.

- Some surgeons will operate as a team with an endoscopic sinus surgeon when safe fast access to the sella.

- It is more common today for neurosurgeons to operate independently, utilizing an SA who has been trained. An otolaryngologist can greatly enhance the speed of surgery and provide access in cases with difficult anatomies, such as the deviated nasal septum, nasal polyps, or non-pneumatized sella.

- Usually, the otolaryngologist exposes the dura over the sella, and then the neurosurgeon opens the dura, followed by removing the tumor. Often, the assistance of a skilled endoscopic sinus surgeon can help tackle cases with extrasellar extensions, such as cavernous sinus and retrocarotid extension, as well as in postoperative management of complications such as nasal synechiae and atrophic rhinitis. Hence, close coordination between the neurosurgeon and otolaryngologist is vital.

Clinical Work-Up

- Comprehensive history, including a full head and neck examination.

- Vision examination, for visual acuity, gaze restriction, and perimetry. Preoperative nasal endoscopy to rule out anatomical obstruction or sinonasal disease.

- Evaluation of pituitary function and hormone status by an endocrinologist.

- Lack of pituitary reserve prior to surgery increase the risk of hypopituitarism after surgery. The interprofessional team should have been made be aware of secretory or nonsecretory nature of the tumor.

- Baseline pituitary function to evaluate if the patient is a candidate for medical therapy prior to surgery. Measurement of growth hormone (GH), serum prolactin, cortisol, triiodothyronine, follicle-stimulating hormone (FSH), thyroxine, and luteinizing hormone (LH).

Most important are thyroid and cortisol hormone levels. Exogenous glucocorticoids or thyroid replacement supplements will be administered prior to surgery.

Imaging Studies

- CT scan
- MRI

- MRI of T1W, with and without contrast, in coronal and sagittal planes is critical for any skull base surgery.

- Important for defining sellar pathology.

- Soft-tissue contrast allows the distinction of vital structures such as optic chiasm, optic nerves, intracavernous carotid arteries, and cavernous sinuses.

- Helps to understand the exact extension of tumor as well as tumor composition, and to differentiate the lesion from another obstruction by fluid or mass. It will also provide information concerning involvement or invasion of dura.

- **Past nasal surgery:** Scarring of mucosa from previous surgery or the presence of perforated septum can make the harvest of a nasoseptal flap more difficult and require the use of alternate reconstruction methods after sellar surgery. Nasal endoscopy is useful to identify residual septal deviations or synechiae (post-surgery), which may be corrected earlier or concomitantly with pituitary surgery.

Preparation and Positioning

Position: Supine with head secured in Mayfield head holder.

The patient will be catheterized to maintain proper fluid balance. Topical vasoconstrictive agents are used for decongestion of both nasal cavities. The abdomen or thigh is prepared as a graft site. For endoscopic cases, a navigation transmitter is attached to the forehead, and the patient is registered.

Nasal Stage Endoscopic Endonasal Transsphenoidal Approach

Decongestion of nasal cavities from anatomical obstructions, a deviated nasal septum or concha bullosa, and correction of those issues.

A medial corridor between the nasal septum and middle turbinate is widened by lateralizing the latter.

A pedicled septal flap, popularly known as Hadad Bassegastegay flap and based on the posterior nasal artery, can be raised if extended pituitary approaches are anticipated.

The sphenoid ostium is identified and widened to lamina papyracea.

The mucosa of the sphenoid sinus should be elevated in a medial to lateral fashion to leave two laterally based mucosal flaps for reconstituting the anterior wall of the pituitary fossa.

About 1 to 1.5 cm of the posterior edge of the septum is usually removed for ease of instrumentation.

Microscopic Sublabial Transsphenoidal Approach

The gingival and nasal mucosa are infiltrated with local anesthetic containing a vasoconstrictor.

Sublabial incision is made from one canine fossa to the other.

Subperiosteal dissections expose the piriform aperture and the rostrum of the maxilla.

Elevation of mucoperichondrium and mucoperiosteum from one side of the nasal septum and nasal floor.

Disarticulation of the quadrangular cartilage from the vomer and perpendicular ethmoid plate of the ethmoid.

A hand-held retractor is introduced to elevate mucosa with lateral retraction exposing the rostrum of the sphenoid.

After the sphenoid ostia are identified, a self-retaining Hardy bivalve speculum is introduced, making space for bimanual instrumentation.

The microscope is introduced to improve magnification.

Rongeurs are used to resect the rostrum for access to the sphenoid sinus.

Microscopic Transnasal Transsphenoidal Approach

This approach is through a single nostril to reach the sphenoid sinuses.

The surgeon will incise the posterior and inferior margins of the quadrangular cartilage.

After submucosal dissection, the quadrangular cartilage is disarticulated at its posterior margin.

A bivalve speculum is now inserted.

Subsequent steps are similar to the sublabial approach.

Benefits of Approach

- Less dissection of soft tissue
- Cosmetic lower postoperative morbidity, no upper jaw numbness

Risks of Approach

May be difficult in patients with a small nostril.

Sphenoid Stage

Mucosa of sphenoid sinus is stripped off to prevent further mucosal bleeding and postoperative mucocele formation.

Diamond drill or rongeur is used for careful Inter-sinus septation removal.

The surgeon will be observing the location of the medial and lateral OCRs, the optic nerves, and the anterior genu of carotid arteries, as their location limits sellar exposure.

Diamond burr will be used for "egg-shell" fracture of the bone over the sella.

The bone is removed with a Kerrison punch.

The underlying dura will be removed from one carotid artery canal to the opposite canal to expose the underlying dura and also from the planum sphenoidale to the clivus.

Sellar Stage

The surgeon will perform a U-shaped or cruciate incision to open the dura and expose the fossa.

Important Landmarks

The healthy pituitary gland will appear yellow and solid; the tumor will appear amorphous and white.

The tumor will be resected using an extracapsular resection.

CSF pulsations through an intact arachnoid will typically be used to help deliver the tumor. An angle between the arachnoid and the carotid artery needs to be determined.

A 30-degree endoscope is used to ensure total clearance in the case of the parasellar extension to avoid the limits of the arachnoid (diaphragma sellae) in superior and posterior dissection.

Gelfoam is used to fill the pituitary fossa.

The dura is repositioned back.

The mucosal flaps are replaced over the dura with surgical cellulose product and a layer of fibrin glue for fixation.

Reconstruction Options

Regardless of the reconstructive material, a multilayer closure and complete defect coverage are critical. The edges of the defect must be denuded of mucosa to prevent mucocele formation and promote graft revascularization. Free tissue grafts are commonly used to reconstruct small to moderate skull base defects (ie, <1 cm) and for low-flow CSF leaks. Fascia lata or collagen matrix is used as a subdural or epidural inlay graft as the first layer of closure. A subsequent layer of onlay graft is then bolstered with a free fat graft, harvested from the abdomen, or a free fascial graft. These layers are finally supported with a nonabsorbable gelatin sponge or the balloon of a Foley catheter.

Postoperative Complications

The most common complications are CSF leak, sinusitis, and meningitis. CSF leaks, occurring in six in every 100 cases, are usually prevented by a multilayer closure at the end of surgery. In the occurrence of a leak in the postoperative period, the patient is advised bed rest, and a lumbar drain is placed. If the leak does not improve in 24 hours, exploration and closure of the defect are to be done. Worsening of vision as a result of bleeding or manipulation and arterial hemorrhage are other immediate complications. A detailed study of preoperative imaging is essential to avoid catastrophes like optic nerve and carotid artery injury. Suspected injury to the optic nerve would entail a full gamut of measures, from observation, intravenous high-dose steroids to optic nerve decompression, depending on the degree of suspicion, time since the injury, and loss/progressive deterioration of vision. Control of such arterial bleeding can be achieved using muscle patches or direct vascular repair using endovascular clamps and clip appliers. In situations where intraoperative hemostasis could not be achieved, immediate transfer for endovascular interventions, such as stenting, balloon occlusion, or coiling, is critical.

Long-Term Complications

Nasal congestion and mild nasal bleeding are predicted in the immediate first 1 to 2 weeks after surgery. Other expected complications include pain over the nasomaxillary region, nasal crusting, mucosal scarring, periorbital edema, and numbness of the upper incisors. Mucosal damage can impair ciliary function and lead to sinusitis.

Postoperative Management

Patients are monitored in an intensive care unit in the immediate postoperative period with monitoring for neurological deterioration, epistaxis, visual dysfunction, diabetes insipidus (DI), and hypotension secondary to acute hypocortisolism. Desmopressin and/or steroid replacement need to be continued postoperatively if the patient was already on it, along with strict electrolyte surveillance. If the preoperative pituitary function was normal, serum cortisol and prolactin levels are measured on the morning after the procedure. In the case of a secretory tumor, non-stimulatory hormone levels (cortisol, prolactin, or GH) are obtained on postoperative days 1 and 2. Serum sodium and urine output are serially monitored for the next 48 hours. If the cortisol levels are low, then steroid replacement is initiated. If new onset DI is suspected, oral fluid management with water may suffice if the patient is awake and stable. If desmopressin is started, then it requires close monitoring by an endocrinologist. Usually, patients are discharged by postoperative day 2 or 3.

The need for nasal packs is dependent on the type of reconstructive technique and the surgeon's choice (used only in a minority of cases). The nasal pack will be removed on postoperative day 1. Septal splints are warranted in traditional sublabial-transeptal-transsphenoidal approaches and removed on postoperative days 5 to 7. The first follow-up visit is 1 week after the procedure, where postoperative day 7 serum sodium levels are reviewed to rule out occult hyponatremia.

ARTERIOVENOUS MALFORMATION (AVM)

An AVM is a complicated knot-like tangle of abnormal veins and arteries which are connected directly by one or more shunts or fistulas. This tangle of arteries and veins is often referred to as a nidus.

Normally, as high-pressure arterial blood pumps through a capillary bed, there will be a decrease in blood pressure before reaching the venous system. In the case of an AVM, the capillary bed is missing causing the high-pressure arterial blood to bypass normal brain tissue instead of pumping it directly into the venous system, which is normally at low pressure.

Blood flow through the nidus of the AVM is usually high. This could be due to the high-pressure blood from the arterial system gravitating toward a low-resistance path. It is also thought that an AVM recruits blood vessels. It is not known whether the high flow is a cause or effect of the abnormal blood vessels or both.

Ultimately, instead of working through capillary beds which feed surrounding brain tissue, the arterial blood rushes through the AVM, increasing blood flow through the nidus.

This re-direction of arterial blood away from the brain tissue and through the AVM is referred to as shunting. Over time, this high blood flow and the shunting of high-pressure arterial blood through the AVM will cause the feeder arteries and veins that make up the AVM to dilate or expand. This weakens the veins, and they become susceptible to hemorrhage, and the arteries become susceptible to aneurysms. This leakage causes the

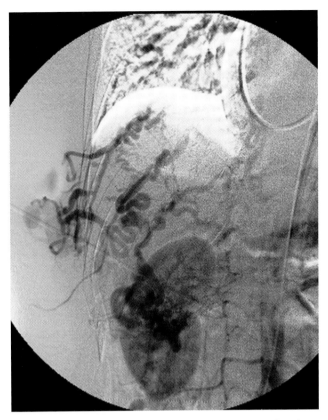

Figure 21-5 · Arteriovenous malformations. (Reproduced, with permission, from Dean SM, Satiani B, Abraham WT, eds. *Color Atlas and Synopsis of Vascular Diseases*. New York: McGraw Hill; 2014.)

flow of blood to the brain to become reduced, often resulting in a blood clot which can damage the brain (see Figure 21-5).

What Causes AVM?

AVMs are thought to be congenital and also to arise from developmental derangements at the embryonic stage of vessel formation, at the fetal stage. This is a theory that has not been clearly established. They may also arise after birth. Typically AVMs remain single unless the patient has hereditary hemorrhagic telangiectasia (HHT).

- AVMs occur in <1% of the population.
- The average age of AVM rupture is 17 years old.
- About 12% of people with an AVM experience symptoms.
- Each year, 2% to 4% of people with an AVM have a hemorrhage.
- About 2% of hemorrhagic strokes are related to an AVM.
- More than 50% of people with an AVM will have an intracranial hemorrhage.

Symptoms of AVMs

An AVM may or may not exhibit any symptoms. Depending on the size and location of the AVM, the patient may experience seizures, bleeding, headaches, and stroke-like symptoms.

Diagnostic Tests for AVM

Most AVMs are detected with either CT brain scan, an MRI brain scan, or a cerebral angiogram.

Cerebral Arteriography (Cerebral Angiography). is the most detailed test to diagnose an AVM. This reveals location, size, and characteristics of the feeding arteries and draining veins.

- A long, thin tube (catheter) is inserted into an artery in the groin and threads it to the brain using fluoroscopy to inject dye into the brain's blood vessels, making them visible under x-ray imaging.

Treatment Options

Using a grading system called "The Spetzler-Martin Grading System," scores are assigned based on the size of AVMs, the eloquence of adjacent brain, and venous drainage, either superficially or deep cerebral venous drainage. The scores from each feature are totaled, and a grade is determined.

Class A combines Grades I and II AVMs.

Class B are all Grade III AVMs.

Class C combines Grades IV and V AVMs.

The Spetzler Martin Grading Scale helps the doctor and patient estimate the risk of open neurosurgery AVM. A Grade 1 AVM is considered small, superficial, and located in the non-eloquent brain, and therefore a low risk for surgery. Grade 4 or 5 AVMs are large, deep, and adjacent to eloquent brain, a medium risk. Grade 6 AVM is considered non-operable.

- Size of nidus
  - Small (<3 cm) = 1
  - Medium (3-6 cm) = 2
  - Large (> 6 cm) = 3
- Eloquence of adjacent brain
  - Non-eloquent = 0
  - Eloquent = 1
- Venous drainage
  - Superficial only = 0
  - Deep = 1
- Using every sequence of the preoperative angiogram and MR images, the surgeon will develop a pre-surgical planned strategy.
- The doctor will be memorizing sequences of feeding vessels, their location, and serpentine routes of aneurysms.
- Surface landmarks, embolic material, and large draining veins will be used as guides to localize feeding arteries.
- The border of the AVM containing the predominant feeding arteries will be mapped so that they know where to begin dissection and disconnection.
- CT angiogram scans and MR images will be observed to plot the dissection approach relating to the hematoma cavity. Functional cortices are anatomically planned relative to the nidus and the hematoma.

- Deep white matter feeder locations are noted.
- CT angiogram sequences offer high resolution of vascular anatomy in relation to brain surface landmarks and are often the preferred pre-surgical planning method of some neurosurgeons.

AVM Treatment Options

AVMs are challenging to treat. The most positive result is from total removal depending on the size and location of the AVM; embolization or radiation therapy may be attempted. Most often, near the brain, surgical removal or clipping is the best option.

Other options used separately or in conjunction with surgery include preoperative embolization; stereotactic radiosurgery with Gamma knife is more commonly used now. Surgical glue is sometimes delivered through a catheter into the blood vessels before surgery, and the glue is removed during surgery along with the AVM. Serial embolization is also used to reduce the size of AVM.

Most often, AVMs in the brain will require a craniotomy to treat them.

Surgical Approach

Based on the location of the lesion, either a supratentorial or infratentorial craniotomy is done.

Surgical Procedure

- Standard skin prep and positioning for craniotomy procedure.
- The head is positioned just above the heart level with the neck slightly extended while avoiding extreme rotation of the head to either side.
  - These considerations prevent intracranial venous hypertension, which can be problematic for cranial surgery in general and AVM surgery in particular.
- The surgeon will use free surfaces to access the lesion and maximize natural retraction obtained from gravity.
  - This may prevent the need for fixed retractors which increase the risk of cortical injury and death.
- Due to the risk of intraoperative bleeding and technical challenges associated with AVM surgery, the operative field must be generous and provide numerous flexible working angles for the timely handling of subcortical bleeding.
- The dura is incised, and the blood vessel with the AVM is found.
- The brain tissues around the AVM are separated from the AVM, then removed as a single piece.
- The surgeon closes the dura and places the bone flap back in its original position. Tiny plates and screws are used to secure the bone flap and keep it in place.
- The skin is approximated and sutured.
- Dressings are applied.

Risks of AVM Surgery

- Bleeding
- Damage to nearby brain tissue
- Stroke to other areas of the brain

BRAIN ANEURYSM

Brain aneurysms are a cerebrovascular disease in which a weakening of a cerebral artery causes an abnormal focal dilatation. Microsurgical and endovascular treatment aims to eliminate brain aneurysms from cerebral circulation and prevent rupture. Despite rapid advances in the development of endovascular treatment, complete and long-lasting aneurysm occlusion remains a challenge, and the biological mechanisms that predispose brain aneurysms to grow and recanalize are not yet fully understood.

Aneurysms can appear anywhere in the body with an artery; however, they often occur in the brain, called cerebral or intracranial aneurysms. A ruptured brain aneurysm is deadly. About 10% of patients will die before receiving any medical care. If left untreated, 50% more will die within a month. There is also a 20% risk of rebleed within 2 weeks. Those who survive an initial aneurysm rupture are at risk for continued brain damage due to artery spasms leading to stroke.

Early treatment at a hospital increases survival rates. Rapid diagnosis, aneurysm repair, and control of blood vessel spasms with medications all increase survival rates (see Figure 21-6).

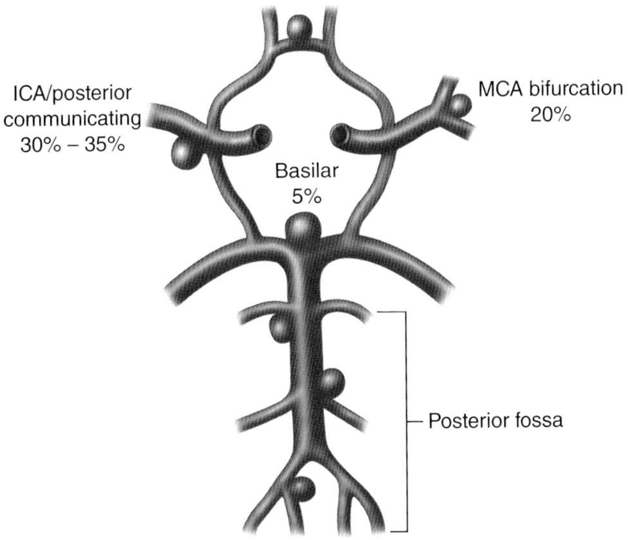

Intracranial aneurysums

Anterior communicating artery
30% – 35%

ICA/posterior communicating
30% – 35%

MCA bifurcation
20%

Basilar
5%

Posterior fossa

Miscellaneous sites distal to circle of Willis
1% – 3%

Figure 21-6 · Cerebral aneurysm. (Reproduced with permission from Osborn AG. *Handbook of Neuroradiology: Brain and Skull*, St. Louis-Mosby: Elsevier; 1991.)

Relevant Anatomy

The artery wall is made of several layers. Arteries of the brain only have one elastic layer, whereas elsewhere in the body, there are two elastic layers in arteries, which tend to have many regular openings (perforations), and anything that damages this layer will increase the likelihood of a brain aneurysm forming in this area of the artery.

The smooth muscle layer of brain arteries has naturally occurring defects that may present as isolated regions where layers may be thinned out or missing; this commonly occurs at arterial bifurcations, making aneurysms more likely to happen in these regions. Also, at arterial bifurcations, the flow of blood exerts (hemodynamic forces) is increased compared to other segments along the artery. Any condition that increases blood flow pressure and turbulence (such as high blood pressure and high cholesterol) will aggravate the tendency for this part of the artery to expand as a brain aneurysm.

An aneurysm is considered to be any bulging, weakened middle layer of a blood vessel wall.

Frequent Aneurysm Locations

- Internal carotid artery
- Middle cerebral artery
- Anterior cerebral artery
- Basilar artery
- Vertebral basilar
- Posterior communicating artery
- Cavernous carotid artery

Cause of Aneurysms

Aneurysms have different causes, including high blood pressure, atherosclerosis, heredity, abnormal blood flow at the junction where arteries come together, and trauma. Some aneurysms are present at birth and stay very small, never causing problems throughout the patient's lifetime. Most brain aneurysms remain small, only diagnosed incidentally during an autopsy. Incidental aneurysms are found in over 1% of patients who died from another cause.

In most cases, aneurysms are sporadic; however, certain medical conditions such as polycystic kidney disease, fibromuscular dysplasia (FMD), and Ehlers–Danlos syndrome are associated. In rare cases, cerebral aneurysms run in families.

Lifestyle choices contribute to aneurysm formation and growth. High blood pressure, atherosclerosis, and cigarette smoking are common in the patient history of aneurysms. In rare cases, infections of the artery wall cause mycotic aneurysms. Drug abuse, especially the overuse of cocaine, can cause artery walls to become inflamed and weaken. Tumors and trauma also contribute to aneurysm formation.

Types of Aneurysms

True Aneurysm

When the blood vessel expands and involves all layers of the vessel's wall.

The most commonly recognized true aneurysms are:

- Fusiform and saccular

  Less common presentation of true aneurysms are:

- Pseudo
- Blister
- Mycotic

Berry Aneurysm (Saccular)

- Most common aneurysm type.
- Resembles a sack protruding from the side of a blood vessel wall.
- Usually has a neck area that is sometimes difficult to locate.
- Berry aneurysms are commonly found to grow and rupture.
- Saccular aneurysms, the most common cause of nontraumatic SAH, are attached to a dome (a more significant portion).
- Develops along with a weak spot in the artery wall.

Fusiform "Dissecting" Aneurysm

- Less common form of aneurysm is called the "fusiform" (dissecting) aneurysm. Looks as if the blood vessel has expanded in all directions.
- Commonly the result of injuries to the blood vessel's innermost layers, and traumatic injury or atherosclerotic (fatty plaque) are contributors.
- Has no "neck" region; these aneurysms rarely rupture or present with SAH.
- Can cause strokes when they reach a specific size.

Mycotic Aneurysm

- Very rare.
- Like saccular aneurysm, arises from an artery that has been affected by a source of infection in a specific part of the wall.
- The condition usually originates somewhere else in the body (eg, the heart) and spreads to the brain's blood vessels through the bloodstream.
- Often associated with subacute bacterial endocarditis, caused by infectious agents.
- It is common to find multiple mycotic aneurysms along the distal (superficial) portions of the brain arteries.

False "Pseudoaneurysm"

- Occurs when a blood vessel wall expansion that does not involve all wall layers occurs.
- Most often—involving the outermost layers of the brain artery only—these aneurysms usually follow injury or tearing of a blood vessel wall. Referred to as a "dissection" or "laceration."
- Often present in regions where the falx or tentorium is near the cerebral arteries. Ballooning can happen on one side of the artery wall or block off and obstruct arterial blood flow.
- Traumatic injury is the most common cause of pseudoaneurysm.
- Can also form spontaneously.
- Treatment will be determined based on the shape and location of the aneurysm.

Symptoms Associated with Brain Aneurysm (Also called Cerebral Aneurysm or Intracranial Aneurysm)

When a brain aneurysm grows, it will often exert pressure on brain tissue and nerves, causing symptoms. When a brain aneurysm leaks or ruptures, blood may leak into one of the membranes (meninges) that covers the brain and spinal canal. This is known as an SAH. Blood is irritating to the brain and its surrounding tissues and causes inflammation of the meninges.

Symptoms (Sudden Onset)

- "The worst headache of their life"
- Nausea and/or vomiting
- Vision changes
- Pain and stiffness of the neck
- Diplopia (double vision)
- Back pain
- Photophobia
- Phonophobia
- Loss of consciousness or seizure

Some symptoms suggestive of a brain aneurysm are also indicative of other diagnoses. These other conditions are migraine headaches, tumors, meningitis, and stroke caused by blood leaking into the brain's ventricles. A leaking aneurysm is the first thing doctor will rule out.

Related Diagnostic Modalities

CT Scan

CT scan performed within 72 hours of the onset of the headache will find 93% to 100% of all aneurysms.

Lumbar Puncture

When CT is inconclusive and the aneurysm is still suspected, a lumbar puncture may be performed to identify blood in the CSF running to the subarachnoid space.

CT Angiography

Angiography with a catheter threaded into the brain's arteries with dye injection will illustrate arterial anatomy and confirm the presence and location of an aneurysm.

Formal Angiogram

CT angiography or MRA can also be performed without threading catheters into the brain with a formal angiogram. The doctor decides which type of angiogram to use based on each patient's condition and symptom set.

Special care is taken to protect the brain and blood vessels from further damage when an aneurysm is present.

- Vital signs will need frequent monitoring, including heart monitors for abnormal heart rhythms.
- Medications prevent high blood pressure and blood vessel spasm, agitation, seizure, and pain.

Surgical Treatment of Aneurysm

Clipping and **coiling** are two treatment options most commonly used to repair the blood vessels of asymptomatic aneurysms.

Coiling

This procedure is often but not always done with the aid of an interventional neurologist. Like an angiogram, a tube will be threaded through the arteries, to identify the aneurysm; coils of platinum wire or latex are used to fill it. This prevents additional blood from entering the aneurysm and resolves the problem.

Clipping

During aneurysm clipping, the neurosurgeon will operate on the brain through a craniotomy of the skull. After identifying the damaged blood vessel, a clip is applied across the aneurysm to prevent blood from entering the aneurysm and causing additional blood leakage or aneurysm growth.

Clipping has been used for several decades, though recently, coiling has been accepted as an alternate approach to clipping in the treatment for ruptured SAH.

Still, as an invasive procedure, this clipping procedure requires a longer recovery period than the coiling procedure. The treatment will be selected by the surgeon based on whether the aneurysm has ruptured, its size, location, and shape.

Coiling

Performed using angiogram.

- After the patient has been anesthetized, the doctor will insert a femoral catheter) into the femoral artery and threads it, with the guidance of angiography, through the body to the aneurysm site.
- Additional catheters are navigated through blood vessels toward the blood vessels of the brain and eventually into the aneurysm.

  When coiling involves the assistance of a stent, the stent is permanently placed into the vessel just beside the aneurysm to provided support and scaffolding to keep the coils within the aneurysm sac.

  Balloon remodeling requires temporary placement of a removable balloon adjacent to the aneurysm while the coils are being positioned in the aneurysm.

- Next, a guide wire is used to assist in placing detachable coils (platinum wire spirals) or small latex balloons are passed through the catheter and then released directly into the aneurysm. The balloons or coils fill the aneurysm and block it from circulation, causing the blood to clot, which destroys the aneurysm.
- This procedure may need to be performed additional times during the lifetime of the patient.

Flow-Diverting Embolization Devices

The major advance in endovascular techniques over the last few years is the flow diverting embolization devices. Similar to a stent, these devices are placed into the main vessel adjacent to an aneurysm. They divert flow away from the aneurysm and provide a scaffolding for healing of the vessel wall to occur. Over time, the aneurysm will disappear. This technology allows the doctor to treat aneurysms that were previously considered untreatable or that were high risk by other methods. New devices are under development, including a stent that can bridge two vessels.

Postop

- Patients must remain in bed until the bleeding stops.
- Other conditions, such as high blood pressure, must be controlled.
- Anticonvulsants are often used to prevent seizures when cerebral aneurysm is symptomatic.
- Analgesics are given to treat headache.
- Calcium channel–blocking drugs and sedatives may be given to prevent vasospasm when the patient cannot rest.
- A shunt may need to be surgically inserted into a ventricle several months following rupture CSF pressure has built up causing pressure on the tissues.
- Rehabilitative, occupational, and speech therapy may be needed for patients who have suffered an SAH help regain function that was lost and learn to cope with any permanent disability.

Sometimes a bypass involves combining an **occlusion** to reroute the blood flow around the occluded artery. The procedure involves the doctor taking a small blood vessel from another area of the body, usually the leg, and grafting it to a section of the brain artery where it is needed to bring blood to the area of the brain that had been fed by the damaged artery.

Considerable advances in open surgery techniques have been made.

Mini craniotomies, or eyebrow incisions, are now used to clip an aneurysm.

In some patients, a small incision over the eyebrow followed by a small 2-inch window in the bone over the eye is used to place a small clip across the opening of the aneurysm.

Risks of Aneurysm Repair

Each of these treatments come with the risk of further damage to the blood vessel, more bleeding, damage to nearby brain tissue, and causing spasm to blood vessels near the aneurysm. If blood is prevented from reaching the brain, a stroke may be caused.

Surgical Procedure

Cranio-orbitozygomatic Approach of MCA Aneurysm

- In a hybrid angio/OR suite which allows for ease of intraoperative angiography

Surgical Procedure

- Standard skin prep and positioning for craniotomy procedure.

- Angiography table is used.

- The head will be placed in a radiolucent Mayfield headrest.

- The head is positioned just above the level of the heart with.

- At final positioning, the patient's head is turned 30° and slightly.

  Extended while avoiding extreme rotation of the head to either side.

- The femoral sheath is accessed before the start of surgery for speed of intraoperative angiography.

  The surgeon will use free surfaces to access the lesion and maximize natural retraction obtained from gravity.

  - This may prevent the need for fixed retractors which increase the risk of cortical injury and death.

- Electrodes applied for neurophysiological monitoring.

- Due to the risk of intraoperative bleeding and technical challenges associated with MCA surgery, the operative field must be generous and provide numerous flexible working angles for timely handling of subcortical bleeding.

- The incision is made in a curved linear fashion behind the hairline.

- Steps of craniotomy are performed in the usual fashion.

- If the aneurysm is extensive, both branches of the superficial temporal artery are harvested during exposure to allow for potential bypass if required during the procedure.

- First, the anterior branch is dissected away and rotated posteriorly and a small wet clip is placed on the end.

- The skin flap is rotated anteriorly superficial to the temporalis muscle fascia.

- Temporalis fascia is cut through both shallow and deep layers along with the skin flap to protect the facial nerve's frontalis branch.

- The incision is made directly behind the fat pad, within the temporalis fascia. Then, the orbital nerves are identified in a foramen within the orbital rim. Subperiosteal dissection continues along the anterior of the zygomatic process along the zygomatic arch in order to expose the front of the zygomatic process.

- The wedge of bone is cut in the orbital rim to allow the supraorbital nerve to be reflected anteriorly along with the periorbital and the skin flap to protect it from damage during.

- The zygomatic arch is cut in two places:

  - First, along the route of the zygoma;

  - second, adjacent to the malar eminence.

- With the ultrasonic bone scalpel, the zygomatic angle is reflected inferiorly to allow space for the temporalis muscle to be exposed.

- The temporalis muscles are dissected, preserving the deep temporalis fascia muscle down to the area provided by the zygomatic arch.

- An osteotomy McCarty keyhole borough is performed using a high-speed drill and half within the frontal lobe region and the periorbital is protected using a brain blade.

- Additional burr holes are performed as needed.

- Surgeon may elect to perform a cranial orbit or zygomatic approach for this if aneurysm is large in size and based on location along the floor and tip of the temporal fossa.

- This allows exposure of the entire aneurysm as well as easy access toproximal control of the M1 segment is sphenoidal or horizontal segment without any retraction.

- The frontal portion of the craniotomy is carried through the orbital rim.

- An additional osteotomy is performed along the front of the zygomatic process.

- This osteotomy is connected to the orbital portion of the McCarty keyhole per hole.

- Final cuts are made within the orbital rim along the lateral orbit as well as in the orbital roof.

- Patties are placed on both the orbital and the dural side of the orbital roof to protect it during the final cut.

- The previous osteotomies are now used for elevation of a one-piece cranial orbit and zygomatic bone flap.

- Additional osteotomy performed along the lateral and superior orbit.

- This different piece can later be replaced along with the remainder of the bone flap.

- The microscope is brought in.

- Under the microscope, the periorbital dura are visualized.

- The dura is opened in a C-shape fashion reflecting along the sphenoid wing.

- Dural tack-up sutures allow reflection of the periorbital anteriorly.

- Sylvian fissure is opened in a standard fashion, first opening the superficial arachnoid.

  - Sharp dissection is used throughout the dissection.

- The M1 branch is identified and followed approximately to the carotid bifurcation into the carotid optic cistern. The arachnoid over the optic nerve is also opened using a sharp arachnoid knife.

- Sylvian fissure is split widely to allow access to the middle cerebral branches the carotid bifurcation and the A1 branch.

- The larger M2 branch coming out of the aneurysm dome is identified and dissected free from the aneurysm dome and is now separated from the temporal lobe to provide wide exposure the giant dome of the aneurysm.

- Here the second M2 branch coming from the management dome is identified distally and followed approximately down to the aneurysm neck.

- A perforator-free segment of the middle cerebral M1 branch is then identified to allow for temporary clipping; temporary clip is required to soften the dome and to allow for safe clipping of the aneurysm.
- Here once again the M2 branches are visualized.
- The neck of the aneurysm is firm with atheroma although no significant calcified second M2 branch take-off is identified on the opposite side of the aneurysm dome.
- Temporary clip is applied to the M1 segment allowing softening of the dome of the aneurysm.
- A large fenestrated straight pin is then used to finish right around the proximal atheroma; the distal blades are carefully placed to avoid the takeoff of the temporal M2 branch once the first clip is on the temporary clip is removed.
- The micro Doppler is used to confirm flow within the two branches.
- The second clip is placed within the fenestration to illuminate the portion of the aneurysm that was fenestrated.
- Ultrasonic Doppler fee is used to confirm flow patency within the branches.
  - Additional fenestrated bolster and the clip is placed at the junction of the previously placed penetrated clip and the second clip to prevent flow within that segment.
  - The Doppler once again is used and demonstrates good flow within the M1 and bilateral M2 segments.
- The segment can also be inspected with ICG video images.
- Once the head is covered; the table is rapidly rotated into position to allow the angiography equipment to be brought in.
- An intraoperative angiogram is performed, with the preferred result demonstrating complete obliteration with an excellent blood flow within both M1 and M2, two branches, and distal filling.
  The quality of the interrupted angiography is significantly improved in the hybrid angio suite.
- Standard dural closure is performed.
- A small pair of cranial flap is harvested to cover a small opening on the frontal sinus that was created during the craniotomy.
- The frontal sinus on the bone flap side is cranialized.
- Plating screws are attached to the previous osteotomies.
- Lateral orbit is reattached to the bone flap to minimize the cranial gap.
- Holes are made to allow tacking of the temporalis muscle and central tack up for the dura.
- The bone flap is then replaced and plated.
  Care is taken for precise alignment of both lots to allow the orbital rim to align appropriately to optimize cosmetic appearance and healing.
- Fish hooks are removed from the temporalis muscle.
  - The zygomatic arch is returned to normal anatomic position and replaced using plates and screws for these plates and screws.

- Often neurosurgeons will pre-drill the holes to allow for ease of drilling screws are placed both in the malar eminence as well as the ruda zygoma.
- An additional tack-up screw is replaced within the zygomatic arch to allow for armor plating.
- The temporalis must be tacked up to the previously placed holes using vicryl sutures to offer an anatomic re-approximation.
- After irrigation, the gallea is closed in a standard fashion.
- Three-dimensional reconstruction of postop CT demonstrates the rebuilding of the cranial orbital zygomatic bone flap.
- The dura is incised, and the blood vessel with the AVM is located.
- The brain tissues around the AVM are separated from the AVM and removed as a single piece.
- Dura is closed, and bone flap is replaced to its original position with tiny plates and screws to secure and keep it in place.
- The skin is approximated and sutured.
- Dressings are applied.

Risks of Cerebral Aneurysm Surgery

- Bleeding
- Damage to nearby brain tissue
- Stroke to other areas of the brain

Relevant Imaging Studies

Images must be displayed before the surgeon enters the room. They will be running through many things during this pre-surgical time and looking for the patient's most recent imaging studies. Often the neurosurgeon will ask the assistant to point out or confirm a finding, so it is essential to at least grasp a basic understanding of what is shown on various images.

ULNAR TRANSPOSITION

The cubital tunnel is created by the cubital tunnel retinaculum which spans between the medial epicondyle and the olecranon. The floor of the tunnel is formed by the capsule and the posterior band of the medial collateral ligament of the elbow joint and contains the ulnar nerve. The ulnar nerve is a single nerve that emerges from a set of nerves known as the brachial plexus. It runs down the inner side of the arm, behind a bony prominence on the inner surface of the elbow called the medial epicondyle, and down to the hand, providing feeling to the muscles of the forearm and hand along the path. The ulnar nerve conducts electrical signals to muscles in the forearm and hand. The ulnar nerve is also responsible for feeling in the fourth and fifth digits of the hand, section of the palm, and the underneath of the forearm. Cubital tunnel syndrome is the second most common peripheral nerve entrapment neuropathy affecting the upper limb. Decompression of the ulnar nerve is a common approach in treating cubital tunnel syndrome, and it can be performed both openly or endoscopically.

There are three approaches to ulnar nerve transposition: subcutaneous, intramuscular, and submuscular. Subcutaneous transposition was first described by Benjamin Curtis in 1898. It is preferred to do a subcutaneous transposition over the other two approaches whenever possible. However, if the patient presents with excessive nerve instability, then an intramuscular or submuscular transposition may be a better option. An advantage of the submuscular transposition is that there is an additional layer of protection over the ulnar nerve with the muscle.

Etiology

Ulnar transposition is indicated when there is excessive pressure on the elbow where the ulnar nerve exists. Leaning on the elbow for many hours, fracturing of the medial epicondyle or rheumatoid arthritis and cubital tunnel syndrome can cause entrapment of the ulnar nerve.

With compression of the ulnar nerve, the function is compromised. Patients may experience pain at the medial epicondyle or weakness of the muscles supplied by the ulnar nerve. Other symptoms produce tingling and numbness in the fingers. More serious cases display irreversible muscle atrophy, hand contractures, and loss of function.

Common anatomical sites for ulnar nerve compression are:

- C8 radiculopathy
- Thoracic outlet syndrome
- The cubital tunnel itself
- Compression within Guyon's canal

Diagnostics

- A detailed history and physical exam.
- An electromyography (EMG) or nerve conduction study (NCS) may be ordered. This will aid in identifying how the muscles and nerves are functioning.
- The EMG will measure muscle activity and muscle response to nerve stimulation. An NCS measures the amount and speed of conduction of electrical impulses through the nerve.
- An MRI neurography may be ordered to deliver enhanced images of nerves. An ultrasound may also be ordered.
- Froment's sign is a special test that measures the palsy of the ulnar nerve and action of the adductor pollis.
- Wartenberg's sign will highlight the persistent adduction of the fifth digit during attempted adduction of all digits.
- Tinel's sign can also help identify the diagnosis when slight percussion over the nerve elicits a tingling sensation.

Nonsurgical Treatment

- Occupational therapy will strengthen the ligaments and tendons in the hands and elbows.
- Medications that include aspirin, ibuprofen, and other pain relievers to reduce pain and inflammation.
- Splints may be indicated to immobilize the elbow.

- If the diagnosis is early, your physician may suggest an anti-inflammatory medicine, such as ibuprofen, to help reduce swelling around the nerve.
- You may be prescribed a padded brace or splint to wear at night to maintain your elbow in a straight position.
- Physical therapy employs exercises that help the ulnar nerve slide through the cubital tunnel at the elbow and the Guyon's canal at the wrist to manage symptoms. These exercises may also help prevent stiffness in the arm and wrist.

Surgical Approach

Positioning

The patient is positioned supine with the affected extremity slightly flexed on a hand table. A tourniquet is placed on the upper arm and the entire arm is prepped and draped. A soft tissue set will be utilized. Bone instruments should be on hand for the procedure.

The procedure is commonly performed with the patient under a general anesthetic or regional anesthesia augmented with Marcaine with epinephrine to aid in minimizing bleeding and postop pain control. A simple cubital tunnel release is performed by cutting and dividing the roof of the cubital tunnel to decrease the pressure on the nerve.

Intramuscular Procedure

- An incision is made on the lateral aspect of the elbow close to the epicondyle.
- The medial antebrachial cutaneous nerve is identified and preserved.
- The fascia and the flexor carpi ulnaris muscle are separated.
- Blunt dissection is made posterior to the medial epicondyle until the ulnar nerve is freed and the medial intermuscular septum is mobilized.
- The cubital tunnel is closed before transposing the ulnar nerve to prevent subluxation or dislocation of the nerve.
- The nerve is re-positioned and is placed deep into where the brachialis flexor muscle originates.
- A mattress suture is used to attach the fascial sling to the anterior skin flap.
- The wound is irrigated, checked, and closed in layers.
- A short arm posterior splint is applied postoperatively.

Postoperative

The operative arm may be raised using pillows. Ice may be applied to combat swelling. The wound is dressed with a splint, bandages, and dressings. The bandages will be removed in 24 hours. Stitches will be removed in 10 days. Full activity can be resumed in 4 to 6 weeks. A submuscular transposition requires a longer time in a splint.

Possible Complications

- Sore throat
- Nausea and vomiting
- Reaction to anesthesia

- Bleeding or blood clots
- Infection
- Nerve injury

SPINE SURGERY

Operative spine surgery began in the seventh century by Paulus Aegina. He performed the first lumbar laminectomy to decompress a spinal cord injury after a fall. From its infancy until now spine surgery has evolved from a relatively unknown to a highly specialized field of practice. Treatment of operative spinal issues can be performed by surgeons from the field of either neurosurgery or orthopedic spine surgery. Regardless of the field, the training required to become a spine surgeon is as detailed and delicate as the subject matter itself. This section is designed to introduce the basic anatomy, imaging, and surgical procedures of the spine to serve as a building block for future use.

Anatomy of the Spine

The spine consists of the vertebral column, connective tissues, and muscles. The primary purpose of the spine is to protect and support the spinal cord from its exit at the base of the skull to its exit into the peripheral nervous system. The vertebral column consists of 33 vertebrae and the intervertebral discs. The vertebrae are separated into five separate regions and each region has its anatomical variations that make identification of the vertebral levels unique.

Bony Structures

The levels of the vertebral column are illustrated in Figure 21-7 and are the cervical, thoracic, lumbar, sacral, and coccygeal. There are 7 cervical, 12 thoracic, 5 lumbar, 5 sacral, and 4 coccygeal vertebrae. The sacral and coccygeal vertebrae are mainly fused together, but the cervical, thoracic, and lumbar vertebrae have individual numbered bones numbered from the skull down within their region. Cervical levels are C1 through C7, thoracic are T1 through T12 and lumbar are L1 through L5. The labeling of the vertebrae is important and locating the levels is a crucial part of the SA's role. At the beginning of each surgery, the proper spinal level is confirmed using C-arm to ensure the correct level is being operated on. These levels are counted from either the sacrum or the base of the skull. A surgery performed on the L2-L3 disc would be on the intervertebral disc between the second and third lumbar vertebrae.

As illustrated in Figure 21-7, the cervical, thoracic, and lumbar vertebrae have differences in their vertebral body, spinous process, vertebral foramen, and transverse processes. These differences all contribute to the varying pathophysiologic changes of the spine.

The vertebral body is the most anterior portion of the vertebrae and it is the largest weight-bearing surface of the bone. From the body two bony processes called the pedicles extend posterolaterally and connect and flatten to become the posterior lamina. At the most posterior aspect of the vertebrae is the spinous process, which joins the lamina to complete a ring. This ring-like structure is called the vertebral foramen, which is where the spinal cord lays. On this ring at the lateral portion, there are two bony wings called the transverse processes. The vertebral bodies form a joint composed of the intervertebral disc anteriorly and posteriorly the vertebral arches join at the superior and inferior articular processes. The formation of joints between the vertebral arches creates the intervertebral foramen, which is where the spinal nerve exits the vertebral column (see Figure 21-8).

Ligamentous Structures

The intervertebral disc is a joint between the vertebrae composed of two different layers. The first layer is the outermost called the annulus fibrosis, which is firmer and more protective and composed of mostly collagen tissue. The inner layer is called the annulus pulposus; it is the inner gel-like layer, which is composed of loose connective tissue in a mucous-like gel. Disc herniations develop when the fibrosis layer weakens and the pulposus extrudes into the vertebral column.

The anterior longitudinal ligament (ALL) covers the anterior portion of the vertebral body and functions to prevent hyperextension of the spine. It is the only spinous ligament that does this and can become problematic if specific pathologies or disruptions develop. The posterior longitudinal ligament (PLL) is inside the vertebral canal on the posterior side of the vertebrae and is important for preventing hyperflexion, and may need to be removed as part of certain procedures. The ligamentum flavum, yellow ligament, helps to hold the lamina of the vertebrae together and is frequently encountered and removed during discectomies, laminectomies, and decompression surgeries of the spine.

Blood Supply

Blood supply to the vertebral canal is via the spinal artery, vertebral artery, and numerous perforating divisions. Blood is drained via the corresponding veins. The vertebrae are well supplied and surgeries requiring extensive bone work such as fusions and multiple-level laminectomies may require consideration of intraoperative blood-saving measures. Meticulous hemostasis is required for visualization of the anatomy during surgery as well and there are many options for hemostatic agents available to spine surgeons for this reason.

Nerve Supply

The nerve supply of the spine is via the spinal cord and direct branches. The spinal cord runs from the medulla oblongata to the L1-L2 level where it terminates into the cauda equina (see figure 21-9). It rests within the vertebral foramen of the column and is protected by three levels of covering the outermost of which is the dura mater. The dura protects the spinal cord, brain, cauda equina, and also encloses the spinal fluid, which also covers and protects the cord. Spinal nerve roots are formed at each vertebral level and exit the column at the intervertebral foramen formed by the vertebrae above and below its level. For example the L1 nerve root exits at the L1-L2 intervertebral foramen. This helps the surgeon clinically correlate what level the patient is having symptoms with due to the specific distribution of the nerve roots. Patients will have specific patterns of numbness and tingling on the skin, called a dermatome, and specific patterns of muscle weakness, called myotomes,

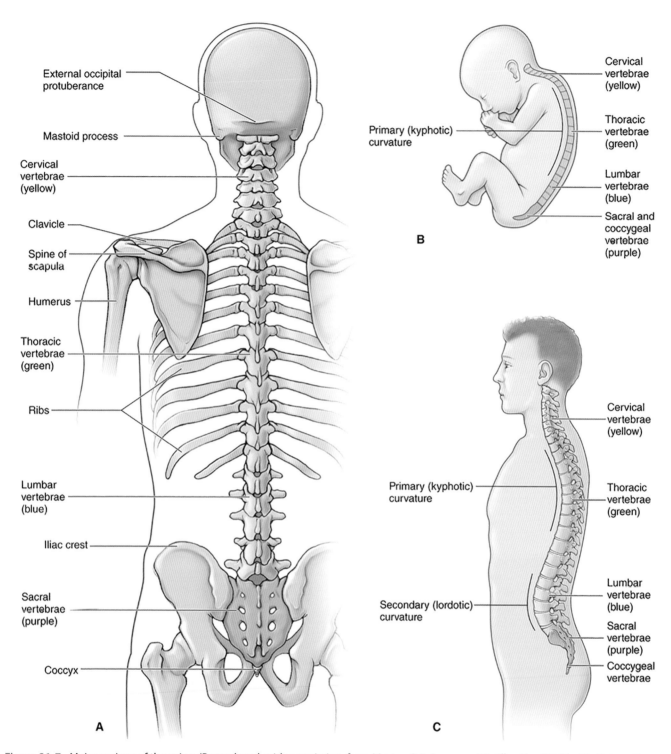

Figure 21-7 · Major regions of the spine. (Reproduced, with permission, from Morton DA, Foreman KB, Albertine KH. *The Big Picture: Gross Anatomy*. 2nd ed. New York, NY: McGraw Hill; 2019.)

depending on the nerve root involved. Clinical exams testing muscle strength, sensation, and reflexes are an important piece of the diagnosis of pathology (see Figure 21-10).

Diagnostic Imaging

X-ray provides the ability to locate bony abnormalities, and is used widely in spine surgery. It is used in both the clinical and the operative setting. In the OR it is useful to locate the proper spinal levels and confirm proper location of instrumentation. MRI is useful to diagnose soft tissue injury and can be used to show disc herniation and spinal cord impingement. CT scans are helpful to assess bony injury in better detail. Both MRI and CT scans can be used for preoperative planning by the surgeon. CT is used intraoperatively as a part of stereotactic guiding during the placement of instrumentation in fusions.

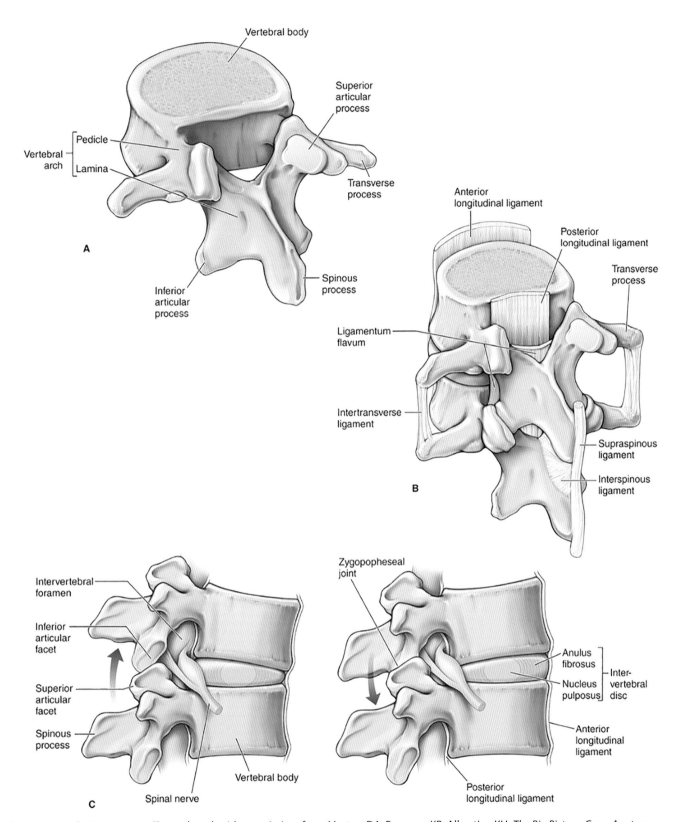

Figure 21-8 · Spine anatomy. (Reproduced, with permission, from Morton DA, Foreman KB, Albertine KH. *The Big Picture: Gross Anatomy*. 2nd ed. New York, NY: McGraw Hill; 2019.)

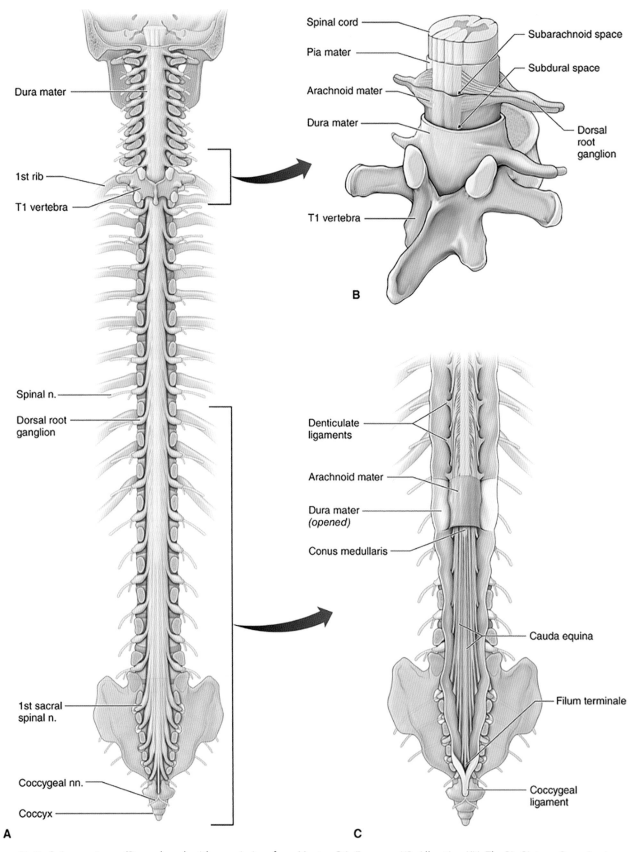

Figure 21-9 · Spine anatomy. (Reproduced, with permission, from Morton DA, Foreman KB, Albertine KH. *The Big Picture: Gross Anatomy*. 2nd ed. New York, NY: McGraw Hill; 2019.)

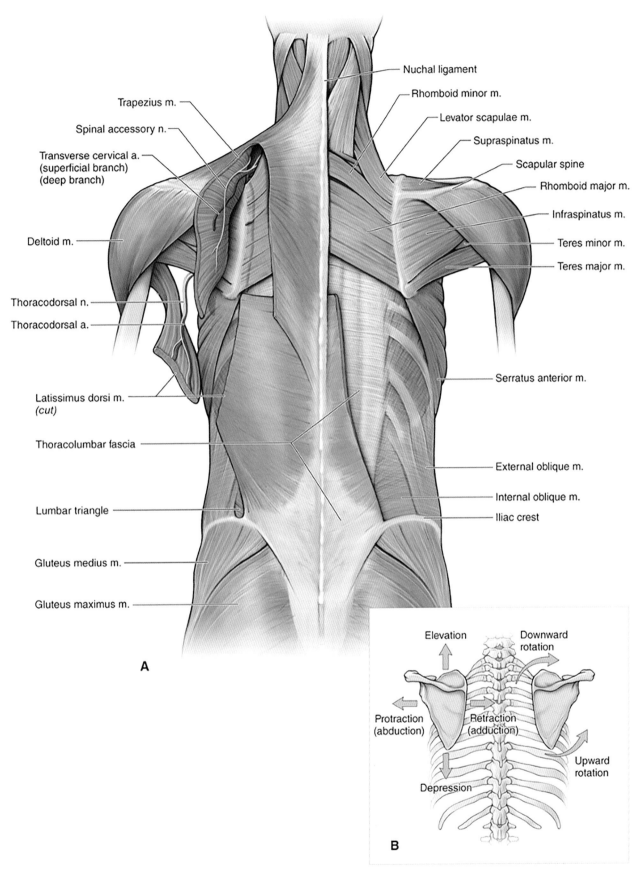

Nuchal ligament
Rhomboid minor m.
Levator scapulae m.
Supraspinatus m.
Scapular spine
Rhomboid major m.
Infraspinatus m.
Teres minor m.
Teres major m.
Serratus anterior m.
External oblique m.
Internal oblique m.
Iliac crest

Trapezius m.
Spinal accessory n.
Transverse cervical a.
(superficial branch)
(deep branch)
Deltoid m.
Thoracodorsal n.
Thoracodorsal a.
Latissimus dorsi m.
(cut)
Thoracolumbar fascia
Lumbar triangle
Gluteus medius m.
Gluteus maximus m.

A

Elevation
Downward rotation
Protraction (abduction)
Retraction (adduction)
Upward rotation
Depression

B

Figure 21-10 · A. Superficial muscles of the back. B. Movements of the scapula. (Reproduced, with permission, from Morton DA, Foreman KB, Albertine KH. *The Big Picture: Gross Anatomy*. 2nd ed. New York, NY: McGraw Hill; 2019.)

Surgical Considerations

Positioning

Surgery of the spine is either in the supine or prone position depending on the approach. Anterior approach to the spine is done with the patient in the supine position, while the posterior approach requires the patient to be prone. Most hospitals and surgery centers will have specialized beds for prone spine cases. These beds can be placed in numerous configurations depending on surgeon preference. Care must be taken in either position to avoid injuries such as pressure, falls, ischemia, and wrong-site surgery. During certain procedures or if the surgeon prefers neural monitoring may be needed to watch the patient's responses to correction during surgery. Neural monitoring requires electrodes to be placed on the patient and special coordination with anesthesia to make sure that sensory and motor responses can be watched throughout the case.

Anesthesia

Anesthesia for spinal surgery is general anesthesia with endotracheal tube placement. Paralytics are required during spine cases for the surgeon to be able to reach the spine, due to the musculature surrounding it. The type and duration of the paralytic will depend on the surgeon as well as if neural monitoring is required for the case. Patients will frequently receive steroids to decrease swelling during the case as well. Anesthesia will carefully monitor blood pressure throughout the case. They are careful to maintain lower pressures to decrease blood loss during the case.

Hemostasis

Hemostasis during a spine case is critical not only for visualization but also after the surgery as well. The formation of hematomas in the operative area can have devastating consequences due to the very tight space the spine is in. Hematomas of the thoracic and lumbar spine can cause compression of the spinal cord and nearby structures. Cervical hematomas are emergent in that they can compress the spinal cord and nearby airway. Typical hemostatic agents in a spine case are topical thrombin, cottonoids, bipolar cautery, and bone wax. The agents are applied as needed throughout the case and if the patient has a higher blood loss, oozing tissues, or had multiple levels worked on the surgeon can always elect to leave a drain in place.

Other Equipment

Spine surgery ORs can become quickly congested with the instrumentation required for them and will usually take place in larger rooms for this reason. Typical needs for a spinal procedure include a larger spine bed and C-arm at a minimum. Depending on the surgeon or procedure other equipment such as stereotactic equipment, neural monitoring equipment, robots, and microscopes may be added. As an SA, it is important to have a working knowledge of the specific equipment the surgeon uses and how to work with the facility and nursing staff to accommodate these needs within the confines of the OR.

Spine Procedures

Lumbar Laminectomy

The lumbar laminectomy is one of the fundamental procedures in spinal surgery. It can be performed by itself to relieve compression of the spinal cord and spinal nerves, or it can be performed in conjunction with a procedure such as a fusion. A laminectomy may be performed as the removal of one-sided, hemi-laminectomy, or both. The procedure also has the potential to be performed either open or minimally invasive depending on the patient, the procedure being performed, and the surgeon's preference.

Lumbar Laminectomy with Discectomy Procedure

Positioning

- The patient is brought to the OR and anesthetized on the stretcher. The SA will help turn the patient prone onto the chosen spine table. Care must be taken to ensure that the hips and neck are in alignment, arms are properly padded, and either male genitals or female breasts are not being crushed between the patient and the table. The patient's feet will be elevated on one to two pillows and the knees should also be properly padded. Depending on the surgeon the patient will be adjusted with the table crank into optimal kyphosis or lordosis for the level to be worked on.

- The patient is then prepped and draped in a sterile fashion and the surgeon is called to the room.

Surgical Procedure

- The surgeon will use an 18-gauge spinal needle and the C-arm to confirm the proper levels and will mark the area of incision.

- A skin incision is made in the midline and is carried down to the supraspinous ligament. The SA may provide traction with a lap sponge and aid in hemostasis with either cautery or clearing with a sponge.

- The surgeon will then use the cautery, Cobb elevators, and rongeurs to dissect the muscles away from the vertebral spines and laminae. The SA will help by suctioning smoke, retracting tissue with small cerebellars and progressing as needed. Depending on the level of trust the assistant may also assist in exposure of the opposite side of the spine the surgeon is working on.

- When dissection is complete the surgeon usually will place a self-retaining retractor such as a McCulloch. The assistant can help preselect the blade length based on the depth of the incision. Also, the retractor should be preassembled and the end of the retractor that fits in the blades can be pre-coated with patient fat to help the retractor slide through the blades more easily.

- The surgeon will then use a curette to identify the ligamentum flavum and carefully peel it from the lamina. Then the surgeon will use kerrisons and a bone burr to remove inferior portion of the lamina.

- The surgeon will then use the bone burr and kerrisons to complete the bone removal and smooth rough bone edges.

The SA will clean the kerrison after each time the surgeon uses it and will also facilitate the surgeon changing his grip on the kerrison as needed. The surgeon also may need the assistant to hold suction for them as they work. The assistant also should be prepared for the need to switch to the bipolar or the bone burr at any point as needed.

- The surgeon will use the pituitary forcep to remove disc material from the disc space without going farther than the anterior annulous space. The surgeon will use a nerve hook or probe to carefully explore the nucleus pulposus for any further remaining disc fragments and ensure that the space is clean. The assistant will hold the nerve root retractors until they are no longer needed and then will help clean the pituitary while being careful to save disc pieces if that is the surgeon's preference (see Figure 21-11).

- The surgeon will then inspect the area and use a combination of bipolar cautery, topical thrombin, and electrocautery to achieve hemostasis.

- After hemostasis has been achieved either the surgeon or the assistant will close the supraspinous ligament with absorbable interrupted sutures. The assistant will then close the subcutaneous layer with absorbable sutures and the skin according to the surgeons preference.

- Dressings are usually gauze and Tegaderm. Adhesive strips may be used if a subcuticular skin closure was made.

Minimally Invasive Lumbar Laminectomy

The basic procedural steps of a minimally invasive lumbar laminectomy are very similar to an open procedure. The key difference is that the surgeon will now be performing the tasks down a tube that is either 18 mm or 22 mm wide. The tubes allow for the patient's tissues to be spread to the sides rather than sharply dissected. In addition the initial incision is smaller for a minimally invasive approach than an open approach. The instruments used for a minimally invasive approach are the same as with a regular approach until the tube length exceeds 80 mm. At this length special long kerrisons, suction tips, Penfield, and retractors are added to the field. This section will highlight the key differences in the set-up of the procedure; however, once the surgeon has located the correct position for the tubes, the assistant's role is fairly limited to cleaning the kerrison and pituitary rongeurs until it is time to retract the dura and nerve root.

- Positioning: Prior to the patient being rolled onto the spine table the SA should ensure that the special bed adaptor for the minimally invasive retractor is on the bed rail, on the side preferred by the surgeon, usually the assistant's side, and is tightened. The patient can then be rolled, positioned, and draped the same as an open procedure.

- After the patient is draped, the assistant will attach the sterile portion of the retractor to the adaptor through the drapes and tighten this into position. The assistant will then change outer gloves since the bedrail is below waist level.

- Surgical Procedure: The surgeon will then begin by identifying the level of surgery and proceed with the incision as described in the open procedure. A small weitlaner is generally used to retract skin edges since the incision is too small for larger retractors and the depth of dissection is much less.

- While the surgeon is performing the dissection the assistant will be suctioning smoke from the cautery and working with the technologist to ensure the retractor is properly set up for use.

- The surgeon will then place the smallest tube in the dilation set toward the operative level and x-rays will be taken to confirm proper level. The surgeon will then dilate the sequentially larger tubes until they reach the desired width tube, one below the size they would like to use. The surgeon will then use markings on the side of the dilators to determine the appropriate length of the tube and the technologist will present the surgeon with the correct tube. The tube for use will then slide into position over the final dilator and fit into position.

- The assistant and the surgeon will then work together to fit the tubes on the retractor and place the retractor arm in the appropriate place for use. Once the retractor is set it is important not to bump the retractor. Doing so will disrupt the placement and the view of the operative field of the surgeon.

- The surgeon will remove the dilators and continue the case in a manner as described in the open case. The assistant in this case should be aware that the surgeon will be looking down the tubes the entire case and the more the assistant can facilitate instruments being given to the surgeon in a position where they do not have to change their field of vision will be extremely helpful.

- After the surgeon completes the case they will obtain hemostasis and the tubes will be removed. The assistant will close the incision as described above, but may need the assistance of a Cobb elevator to retract the tissue to see enough to properly place the deep sutures.

- Dressings are also 4 × 4s and Tegaderm or tape.

Spinal Fusion

There are many reasons why a patient may need a posterior spinal fusion. Fusion may be indicated for patients with instability as a result of degenerative disc disease, osteoarthritis, rheumatoid arthritis, isthmic spondylolisthesis, fracture of a vertebral body, or spinal deformities. The patient may or may not require the presence of an interbody cage. The patient also may be able to utilize a bone graft from their iliac crest or donated graft. There are many surgical considerations as to the best surgical approach for the patient such as anterior lumbar interbody fusion (ALIF), posterior with bilateral laminectomy (PLIF), transforaminal (TLIF), posterior with unilateral laminectomy, and lateral (XLIF). Many of these depend on surgeon's preference, surgeon's comfort, and the level affected. Any spinal fusion procedure has many pieces to it and the SA plays a vital role in helping the case to run smoothly.

Spinal disc herniation

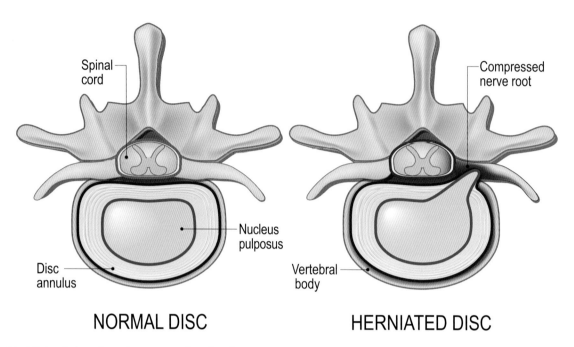

Figure 21-11 · Minimally invasive spine surgery. (Used with permission from Designua/Shutterstock)

Posterior Spinal Fusion Surgery

The most commonly used type of posterior fusion is the posterolateral gutter approach. With the use of an interbody for degenerative disc disease and other causes, the most popular fusion is the TLIF. This is the posterior fusion with a unilateral lumbar laminectomy. This is the lumbar fusion that will be discussed here.

Transforaminal Lumbar Interbody Fusion (TLIF)

Postioning

- The patient is brought to the OR and anesthetized on the stretcher. The SA will help turn the patient prone onto the chosen spine table. Care must be taken to ensure that the hips and neck are in alignment, arms are properly padded, and either male genitals or female breasts are not being crushed between the patient and the table. The patients' feet will be elevated on one to two pillows and the knees should also be properly padded. Depending on the surgeon, the patient will be adjusted with the table crank into optimal kyphosis or lordosis for the level to be worked on.

- The patient is then prepped and draped in a sterile fashion and the surgeon is called to the room.

Surgical Procedure

- The surgeon will use an 18-gauge spinal needle and the C-arm to confirm the proper levels and will mark the area of incision.

- A skin incision is made in the midline and is carried down to the supraspinous ligament. The SA may provide traction with a lap sponge and aid in hemostasis with either cautery or clearing with a sponge.

- The surgeon will then use the cautery, Cobb elevators, and rongeurs to dissect the muscles away from the vertebral spines and laminae. The SA will help by suctioning smoke, retracting tissue with small cerebellars and progressing as needed. Depending on the level of trust the assistant may also assist in exposure of the opposite side of the spine the surgeon is working on.

- When dissection is complete the surgeon will place a self-retaining retractor usually large cerebellar retractors initially, which are eventually replaced by deep gelpies.

- The surgeon will then use a curette to identify the ligamentum flavum and carefully peel it from the lamina, and then the surgeon will use rongeur to remove the spinous process and lamina of the side they are planning on inserting the interbody. The assistant must save all of the bone and give it to the technologist as this will be turned into bone graft.

- The surgeon will then use the bone burr and kerrisons to complete the bone removal and smooth rough bone edges. The SA will clean the kerrison after each time the surgeon uses it and will also facilitate the surgeon changing his grip on the kerrison as needed. The surgeon also may need the assistant to hold suction for them as they work. The assistant also should be prepared for the need to switch to the bipolar or the bone burr at any point as needed.

- At this point in the procedure the surgeon has two choices, they can proceed with placing the interbody or can place the pedicle fixation screws. This procedure will continue with interbody placement first.

- The ligamentum flavum is then removed from where it fuses with the interspinous ligament. This exposes the dura.

- After exposing the dura the surgeon will retract it medially by using a Penfield four. The nerve root is identified and retracted with a nerve root retractor as needed by the assistant to allow the surgeon easy access to the PLL. As the assistant, at this point in the surgery it is very important not to move once the surgeon places you and your retractors. The assistant may or may not be able to see at this point in the procedure and they are holding both the nerve root and the dura away from the surgeon as they work.

- The surgeon will then use a knife to incise the PLL over the intervertebral space in a cruciate fashion. The surgeon will then use a pituitary forcep to enter the space.

- Using a series of large curettes and pituitaries the surgeon will remove all remaining intervertebral disc and ensure that the space is cleaned to the bony vertebral body in preparation for the graft. The surgeon may use a lamina spreader to facilitate this process as well. The assistant may still need to protect the dura with dural retractors at this point.

- The surgeon will use a series of graft sizers to spread the vertebral bodies apart and C-arm shots will be taken until the surgeon is satisfied that the appropriate height of the intervertebral space has been achieved. The size graft is identified and passed onto the field. At this point in the procedure the assistant may need to assist the technologist with packing the graft according to the surgeon's preference. Usually the interbody is filled with autograft from the patient and as much auto graft as possible is placed into the intervertebral space. Depending on the amount of autograft available allograft may also need to be added. The assistant will help the surgeon with visualization within the intervertebral space and retract the dura and nerve root as needed.

- When the surgeon is satisfied with the bonegraft, the interbody is placed in the intervertebral space and proper placement is confirmed with C-arm. The assistant may need to hold the interbody inserter until placement is confirmed.

- After the interbody is successfully placed the surgeon will then begin the preparation for pedicle screw placement and fixation. The assistant will want to make sure the bone burr, gear shift, and probe are readily available while the technologist is preparing the rest of the equipment.

- The surgeon will then identify the pedicles and remove the posterior cortical wall at the entrance of the pedicle using the burr.

- The surgeon will then use the Penfield or nerve hook to identify the entrance to the pedicle and place the gearshift in the path to the vertebral body. The C-arm is used to verify the correct placement and the gearshift is malleted into place. During this part of the procedure, the assistant is providing lateral traction to provide the surgeon with good exposure to the site.

- The surgeon will then remove the gearshift and use a Holt probe to feel the placement and verify that he has not breached the intervertebral foramen. The surgeon may use a snap and ruler to measure the length of the screw at this point. The surgeon will then use the appropriate-sized tap for the level they are working on. After the hole has been tapped the appropriate size screw is placed and placement is again verified using the C-arm.

- This process is repeated for the pedicle below the fusion and then the surgeon and the assistant will switch sides and repeat the procedure for the opposite side.

- After successful placement of the pedicle screws, the surgeon will utilize the remaining allograft and autograft to form the posterolateral gutter graft. The assistant will help the surgeon with exposure as well as ensure the graft is the correct size.

- The surgeon will then select the appropriate length and contoured rods to achieve the proper physiologic curve. The rods are then placed and locked in the correct position with set screws. Once proper placement and compression are achieved the set screws are broken off flush with the rods. The C-arm is then used to confirm placement of the screws and rods and final films are taken (see Figure 21-12).

- The surgeon will then obtain hemostasis utilizing bipolar cautery, topical thrombin, gelfoam, and electrocautery. The surgeon may elect to place a suction drain.

- Either the surgeon or the assistant will then close the incision beginning with the supraspinous ligament with interrupted absorbable sutures. The subcutaneous space is then closed in multiple layers usually one interrupted layer and a continuous layer both with absorbable suture. Skin may be closed with staples and absorbable or nonabsorbable sutures depending on the surgeon's preference. The drain is fixed in place with either nylon or adhesive strips.

- Dressings are 4 × 4s and tape to form a pressure dressing.

The TLIF may also be performed as a minimally invasive procedure following the same technique except that the 22-mm tubes are used. Other exciting technologies in the field of fusions are the use of stereotactically guided equipment and robotics. Stereotactic-guided equipment has been around for a little bit now and uses an O-arm to create a 3D CT scan in the OR of the patient. Using a specialized retractor and surgical equipment with a tracker designed to navigate movements, the surgeon can see on the computer screen precisely where they are on the spine. They are also able to use the computer to project pathways for the gearshift, taps, burr, and screwdrivers prior to use so that optimal placement can be made.

Robotic technology is just now starting to be used. The specialized robotic arm is guided by the surgeon's input for the exact spot for drill, tap, and screw placement to even further enhance the accuracy of equipment placement in the spine.

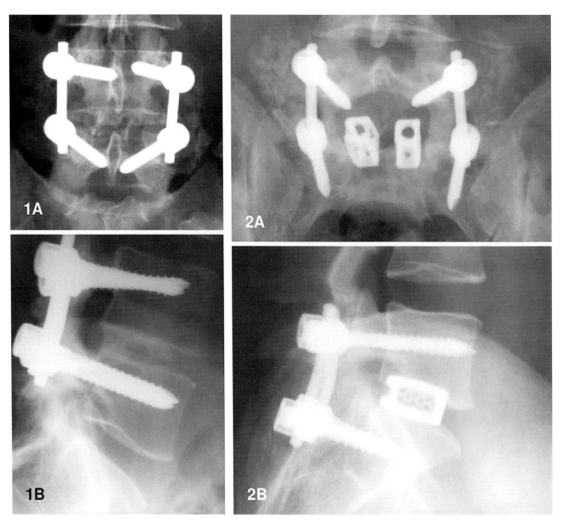

Figure 21-12 · Posterior lumber interbody fusion combined with instrumented posterolateral fusion: 5-year results in 60 patients. (Reproduced with the permission from Freeman B, Licina P, and Mehdian S. Posterior lumbar interbody fusion combined with instrumented postero-lateral fusion: 5-year results in 60 patients. *Eur Spine J.* 2000;9:42-46; Figure 1a-b, Figure 2a-b.)

Cervical Spine

The cervical spine is another area of the body that is particularly sensitive to wear and tear. Degenerative disc disease, cervical disc herniation with subsequent nerve pain (radiculopathy) and muscle weakness (myelopathy), and cervical spondylolisthesis are all potential indications of a cervical fusion. The cervical discectomy and fusion can be done from either the anterior or posterior approach, but the anterior approach is the more commonly used approach.

Anterior Cervical Discectomy and Fusion

Anesthesia

- The patient is brought to the OR and is transferred to a regular OR table in the supine position. The patient is placed under general anesthesia, but anesthesia may need an endoscopic-assisted intubation due to the patient's neck stiffness. The SA should be aware of the anesthesia's potential needs and be prepared to assist them.

Positioning

- After induction the patient will be positioned with the arms tucked and a shoulder roll placed beneath the patient's neck to reach proper neck extension. Depending on the patient's size and the cervical level being operated on, the patient's shoulders may need to be taped to the foot end of the bed for adequate exposure for both the surgeon and the C-arm.
- The patient is then prepped and draped in the usual sterile fashion and the surgeon will begin.

Surgical Procedure

- A transverse horizontal skin incision will be made on one side of the neck over the cervical level being operated on.
- A small weitlaner or springs are used to retract the skin edges and the surgeon will divide the platysma with sharp dissection.
- The surgeon will then identify the medial edge of the sternocleidomastoid muscle and use a combination of sharp and

blunt dissection to clearly define the tissue plane.

- The surgeon will then use gentle finger dissection to dissect the plane between the carotid artery on the lateral side and the esophagus and trachea on the medial side. They will then place retractors such as clowards or langenbecks to hold the carotid and the trachea and esophagus out of the operative field. The assistant should be very careful to replicate the exact amount of tension and placement of the retractors due to the very sensitive tissue they are retracting.

- The surgeon will then identify the anterior spine and will use either peanut dissectors or elevators to carefully peel away the long muscle of the neck from the anterior surface of the spine giving adequate exposure to complete the procedure. The surgeon will use bipolar cautery and cottonoids for hemostasis.

- The surgeon will then place a spinal needle or Penfield on the intervertebral space and C-arm is used to confirm the level.

- The surgeon will usually place a self-retaining retractor such as the trimline or invuity-bladed retractor to retract the muscle, carotid, esophagus, and trachea out of the operative field. The surgeon will also place Caspar pins into the vertebral bodies above and below the intervertebral space being worked on. This retractor allows the surgeon to gently open the disc space for ease in clearing the disc material and preparing the disc space for the new interbody graft. The assistant will help the surgeon with tapping in the Caspar pins, and proper placement of retractors to give the surgeon the best view of the operative field.

- The surgeon will then use a fresh blade to incise the disc space and a pituitary ronguer is used to remove the disc. A series of kerrisons, pituitaries, curretes, and bone spurs are used to clear the intervertebral space of any remaining disc, and bony spurs that may impede the placement of the interbody. The surgeon will also use a nerve hook, Penfield, and Murphy probes to ensure proper decompression of the nerve roots is completed.

- The size of the interbody graft is determined by using graft sizers and c-arm. Once the surgeon has selected the size that he likes the graft is passed to the field and the assistant will help pack the graft to the surgeon's preference.

- The graft is placed with the assistance of the C-arm to verify proper vertical and horizontal placement.

- After the graft has been properly placed the anterior plate is selected and placed over the vertebrae above and below the disc space with screws (see Figure 21-13). The C-arm is used to verify proper placement, distraction, and alignment of the graft and plate.

- Hemostasis is obtained with a combination of bipolar, topical thrombin, and electrocautery. The platysma is then closed with absorbable suture and the skin is closed in a subcuticular fashion. The surgeon may or may not elect to place a drain.

- Dressings are typically adhesive strips, 4×4s, and Tegaderm.

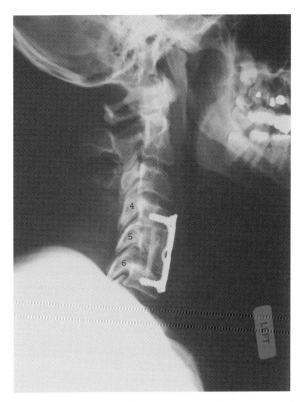

Figure 21-13 Lateral cervical spine x-ray post C5 corpectomy for cervical spondylotic myelopathy. (Reproduced, with permission, from Brunicardi FC, et al., eds. *Schwartz's Principles of Surgery.* 11th ed. New York, NY: McGraw Hill; 2019.)

Post-op Complications

Of all the spinal surgeries patients with anterior cervical fusions must be watched for postoperative complications most closely. Like other surgeries, there is a chance for hematoma formation. Unlike other surgeries, the hematoma for an ACDF patient forms over the esophagus, trachea, and carotid. A hematoma of even a small size can become a surgical airway emergency quickly. For this reason, patients with an ACDF stay at least overnight in either a hospital or surgery center setting.

Bibliography

AANS Neurosurgeon. *Stereotactic Radiosurgery: A Neurosurgical Technology.* 2019. http://aansneurosurgeon.org/feature/stereotactic-radiosurgery-a-neurosurgical-technology.

Bowen B. Orthopedic Surgery. In Rothrock JC, McEwen DR, eds. *Alexander's Care of the Patient in Surgery.* 14th ed. St. Louis, MO: Mosby Elsevier; 2011: 809-814.

Cohen-Gadol A. *Introduction and Review of Imaging Modalities.* The Neurosurgical Atlas; July 13, 2021. Retrieved September 18, 2021, from https://www.neurosurgicalatlas.com/volumes/neuroradiology/introduction-and-review-of-imaging-modalities.

Cohen-Gadol A. *Surgeon's Philosophy and Operating Position.* The Neurosurgical Atlas; March 24, 2021. Retrieved September 18, 2021, from https://www.neurosurgicalatlas.com/volumes/principles-of-cranial-surgery/surgeons-philosophy-and-operating-position.

Cutts S. Cubital tunnel syndrome. *Postgrad Med J.* 2007;83(975): 28-31. https://doi.org/10.1136/pgmj.2006.047456.

Davies BM. Does chlorhexidine and povidone-iodine preoperative antisepsis reduce surgical site infection in cranial neurosurgery? *Ann R Coll Surg Engl.* 2016;98(6):405-408. https://doi.org/10.1308/rcsann.2016.0143

Disturbances of cerebrospinal fluid, including hydrocephalus, pseudotumor cerebri, and low-pressure syndromes. In Ropper AH, Samuels MA, Klein JP, Prasad S, eds. *Adams and Victor's Principles of Neurology. 11th ed.* New York, NY: McGraw Hill; 2019. https://neurology.mhmedical.com/content.aspx?bookid=1477&sectionid=145989641.

Ferrara-Hoffman D, Krizman S. Neurosurgery. In Rothrock JC, McEwen DR, eds. *Alexander's Care of the Patient in Surgery.* 14th ed. St. Louis, MO: Mosby Elsevier; 2011: 876-877.

Gadol E. *Surgeon's Philosophy and Operating Position.* Neurosurgical Atlas; 2021. https://www.neurosurgicalatlas.com/volumes/principles-of-cranial-surgery/surgeons-philosophy-and-operating-position.

Greenberg M. *Handbook of Neurosurgery.* 9th ed. New York, NY: Thieme; 2019.

Hendricks BK, Patel AJ, Hartman J, Seifert MF, Cohen-Gadol A. Operative anatomy of the human skull: A virtual reality expedition. *Oper Neurosurg (Hagerstown).* 2018 Oct 1;15(4):368-377. Retrieved September 18, 2021, from https://pubmed.ncbi.nlm.nih.gov/30239872/.

Johns Hopkins Medicine. *Electroencephalogram (EEG).* https://www.hopkinsmedicine.org/health/treatment-tests-and-therapies/electroencephalogram-eeg.

Moore KL, Dalley AF, Agur AMR. *Clinically Oriented Anatomy.* 6th ed. Baltimore, MD: Lippincot Williams & Wilkins; 2010: 440-481.

Phillips N. *Berry and Kohn's Operating Room Technique.* 12th ed. St. Louis, MO: Mosby; 2013: 804-821.

Phun J, Ilyas AM. Subcutaneous Ulnar Nerve Transposition. Sidney Kimmel Medical College, Rothman Institute at Thomas Jefferson University. https://jomi.com/article/296/Subcutaneous-Ulnar-Nerve-Transposition.

Rao D, Le RT, Fiester P, Patel J, Rahmathulla G. An illustrative review of common modern craniotomies. *J Clin Imaging Sci.* 2020;10:81. https://www.ncbi.nlm.nih.gov/pmc/articles/PMC7771396/.

Rhoton AL Jr. The anterior and middle cranial base. *Neurosurg.* 2002;51(4 Suppl): S273-S302.

Rhoton AL Jr. The orbit. *Neurosurg.* 2002;51(4 Suppl):S303-S334.

Rozet I, Vavilala MS. Risks and benefits of patient positioning during neurosurgical care. *Anesthesiol Clin.* 2017;25(3):631-653. https://doi.org/10.1016/j.anclin.2007.05.009.

Sampson HM, Montgometry JL, Henryson GL. *Atlas of the Human Skull.* 2nd ed. Lewis St, TX: Texas A&M University Press; 1991.

Singh G. Positioning in Neurosurgery. In Prabhakar H, ed. *Essentials of Neuroanesthesia.* Academic Press; 2017:Chapter 10, 183-205. https://doi.org/10.1016/B978-0-12-805299-0.00010-5

Singh, G. *Positioning in Neurosurgery.* Essentials of Neuroanesthesia. Published on March 31, 2017. Retrieved September 18, 2021, from https://www.sciencedirect.com/science/article/pii/B9780128052990000105.

Steris. *Patient Positioning Instructions Quick Reference Guide.* https://www.steris-healthcare.com/medias/docs/9c8c5ea19ec8b-51de54550fc8a35aea2bc2a87f7.pdf.

Tay B, Freedman B, Rhee J, Boden S, Skinner H. Disorders, Diseases, and Injuries of the Spine. In Skinner H, McMahon P, eds. *Current Diagnosis and Treatment Orthopedics.* 5th ed. New York, NY: McGraw Hill; 156-229.

Taylor BS, Kellner CP, Connolly Jr. E. Postcraniotomy complication management. In Lee K, ed. *The NeuroICU Book. 2nd ed.* New York, NY: McGraw Hill; 2017. https://neurology.mhmedical.com/content.aspx?bookid=2155&sectionid=163965349.

Truven Health Analytics. *Decompressive Craniectomy.* CareNotes, Gale Health and Wellness; 2019. link.gale.com/apps/doc/A587018190/HWRC?u=uphoenix&sid=bookmark-HWRC&xid=f05bb162. Accessed June 17, 2021.

Ulnar Nerve Entrapment. John Hopkins Medicine. https://www.hopkinsmedicine.org/health/conditions-and-diseases/ulnar-nerve-entrapment.

Ulnar Transpostion at the Elbow. Neuroassociates PC. https://neurosurgicalassociatespc.com/ulnar-nerve-transposition-at-the-elbow/.

Ventriculo-Peritoneal Shunt. The Neurosurgical Atlas. https://www.neurosurgicalatlas.com/volumes/csf-diversion-procedures/ventriculo-peritoneal-shunt.

Wedro B. *Brain Aneurysm (Cerebral Aneurysm).* Medicinenet.com; 2019. https://www.medicinenet.com/brain_an.

What Is an aneurysm? Joe Niekro Foundation; March 8, 2017. Retrieved September 18, 2021, from https://www.joeniekrofoundation.com/understanding/what-is-an-aneurysm/.

Zubair A, M Das J. Transsphenoidal Hypophysectomy. [Updated 2021 Jul 26]. In: StatPearls [Internet]. Treasure Island (FL): StatPearls Publishing; 2021 Jan. Available from: https://www.ncbi.nlm.nih.gov/books/NBK556142/.

Cardiac Surgery

Michael W. Morrison

THE FIELD OF CARDIAC SURGERY

The world of cardiac surgery is ever evolving, especially the role as a cardiac surgical assistant (SA). Cardiovascular surgery, or better termed cardiac surgery, is the field of surgical procedures, including open and minimally invasive procedures performed on the heart, lungs, and the great vessels. The most common procedures are coronary artery bypass surgery, or CABG for short, which treats ischemic heart disease.

Cardiac surgeries are performed on all types of patients ranging from infants (congenital heart problems) to geriatric populations. Surgery is also performed on the structural heart to treat various valve-related diseases including endocarditis, rheumatic heart disease, and atherosclerosis. Cardiac surgery also includes thoracic (heart and lung) transplantation.

This chapter will touch on a few cardiac procedures, as well as give some insight into the role of the SA.

FUNCTIONS OF THE HEART

The main functions include:

- Managing/transmitting blood supply
- Producing blood pressure
- Securing one-way blood flow

The cardiovascular system is a muscular pump that is comprised of four one-way valves and major arteries and veins which allow the heart to pump oxygenated and deoxygenated blood to the pulmonary and systemic systems. The heart itself is weighs less than a pound and is about the size of a person's fist (see Figure 22-1).

ANATOMY AND PHYSIOLOGY

The sternum and ribs make up the thoracic cavity and act as a protective agent to the mediastinal cavity. The sternum has three distinct parts: the manubrium, the body, and the xyphoid process. The manubrium is the upmost part of the sternum, the body is the middle section, and the xyphoid process is the lower portion of the sternum. The ribs are attached laterally to the sternum. The place where the ribs connect to the sternum is called costal joints and can easily be identified after sternotomy by visual and feel. In between the ribs themselves are called intercostal spaces.

The mediastinum, which is the medial cavity of the thorax, is where the heart is situated, between the right and left lungs. The apex of the heart points toward the left hip and sit approximately around the fifth intercostal space. The pericardium, a protective sac surrounding the heart, is composed of multiple layers. The exterior layer is dense fibrous tissue which is used to protect the heart and anchors the diaphragm and the sternum. The interior of the pericardium is comprised of a serous tissue.

Layers of the Heart

The heart muscle is composed of three defining layers which are the epicardium, myocardium, and endocardium. The epicardium is considered the outermost layer of the heart.

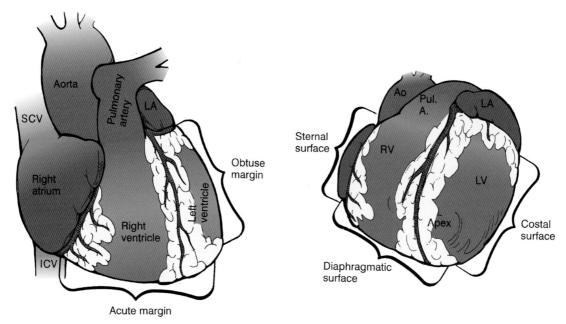

Figure 22-1 · Anatomy of the heart. (Reproduced, with permission, from Cohn LH, Adams DH, eds. *Cardiac Surgery in the Adult*. 5th ed. New York: McGraw Hill; 2018.)

The myocardium consists of cardiac muscle and is the layer that contracts. The endocardium is the innermost layer of the heart and is the thin endothelium that lines the heart.

Chambers of the Heart

The heart has four chambers which is comprised of two atria and two ventricles. The two atria are considered the receiving chambers, whereas the two ventricles (pumps of the heart) are considered the discarding chambers. When the ventricles contract, blood is ejected out of the heart to either the pulmonary system or systemically. The septum is the structure that extends the length of the heart and separates the left and the right side of the heart (see Figure 22-2).

Heart Valves

The heart is equipped with four valves, which allow blood to flow in only one direction through the heart chambers. The mitral valve and tricuspid valve are located between the between the atria (upper heart chambers) and the ventricles (lower heart chambers). The aortic valve and pulmonic valve are located between the ventricles and the major blood vessels leaving the heart.

- Tricuspid valve: Located between the right atrium (RA) and the right ventricle (see Figure 22-3)
- Pulmonary valve: Located between the right ventricle and the pulmonary artery (PA) (lungs)
- Mitral valve: Located between the left atrium and right ventricle
- Aortic valve: Located between the left ventricle and the major artery of the body (aorta)

The Pathway of the Conduction System

The conduction system occurs systematically through:

- SA node: sino-atrial node (SA)
- AV node: atrio-ventricular node (AV)
- AV bundle: atrio-ventricular bundle (AVB)
- Bundle branches and Purkinje fibers

The cardiac conduction system is a group of specialized cardiac muscle cells in the walls of the heart that send signals to the heart muscle causing it to contract. The main components of the cardiac conduction system are the SA node, AV node, bundle of His, bundle branches, and Purkinje fibers.

The SA node (anatomical pacemaker) starts the sequence by causing the atrial muscles to contract. From there, the signal travels to the AV node, next through the bundle of His, down the bundle branches, and through the Purkinje fibers, causing the ventricles to contract. This signal creates an electrical current that can be seen on a graph called an electrocardiogram (EKG or ECG). Doctors use an EKG to monitor the cardiac conduction system's electrical activity in the heart (see Figure 22-4).

Cardiac Cycle

In a healthy heart, the atria contract simultaneously, then, as they start to relax, contraction of the ventricles begin.

At the beginning of the cardiac cycle, both the atria and ventricles are relaxed (diastole). Blood is flowing into the RA from the superior and inferior venae cava and the coronary sinus. Blood flows into the left atrium from the four pulmonary veins. The two atrioventricular valves, the tricuspid and mitral valves, are both open, so blood flows unimpeded from the atria and

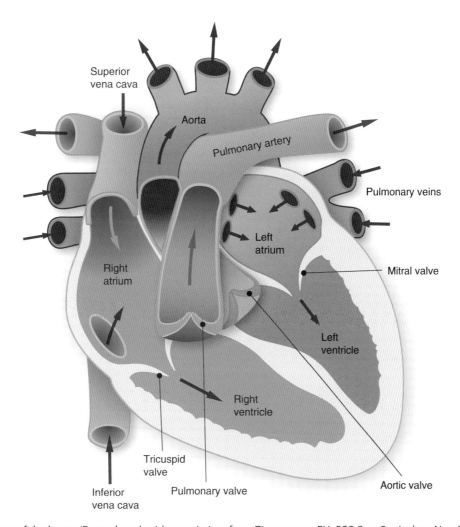

Figure 22-2 · Chambers of the heart. (Reproduced, with permission, from Zimmerman FH. *ECG Core Curriculum*. New York, NY: McGraw Hill; 2023.)

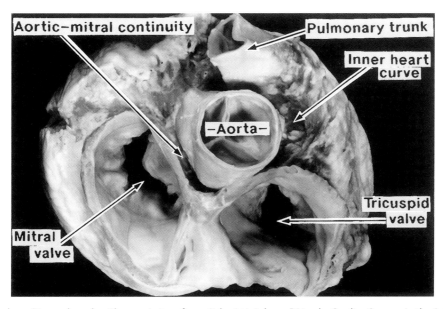

Figure 22-3 · Heart valves. (Reproduced, with permission, from Cohn LH, Adams DH, eds. *Cardiac Surgery in the Adult*. 5th ed. New York, NY: McGraw Hill; 2018.)

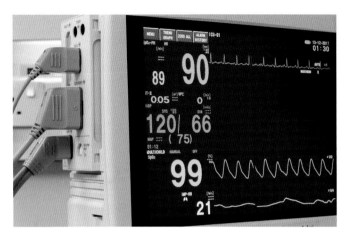

Figure 22-4 · ECG monitor. (Used with permission from Laksamon-But/Shutterstock)

into the ventricles. Approximately 70% to 80% of ventricular filling occurs by this method. The two semilunar valves, the pulmonary and aortic valves, are closed, preventing backflow of blood into the right and left ventricles from the pulmonary trunk on the right and the aorta on the left.[1]

Atrial Systole and Diastole. Contraction of the atria follows depolarization, represented by the P wave of the ECG. As the atrial muscles contract from the superior portion of the atria toward the atrioventricular septum, pressure rises within the atria and blood is pumped into the ventricles through the open atrioventricular (tricuspid, and mitral or bicuspid) valves. At the start of atrial systole, the ventricles are normally filled with approximately 70% to 80% of their capacity due to inflow during diastole. Atrial contraction, also referred to as the "atrial kick," contributes the remaining 20% to 30% of filling. Atrial systole lasts approximately 100 ms and ends prior to ventricular systole, as the atrial muscle returns to diastole.[1]

Ventricular Systole. Ventricular systole follows the depolarization of the ventricles and is represented by the QRS complex in the ECG (see Figure 22-4). It may be conveniently divided into two phases, lasting a total of 270 ms. At the end of atrial systole and just prior to atrial contraction, the ventricles contain approximately 130 mL blood in a resting adult in a standing position. This volume is known as the end diastolic volume (EDV) or preload.

Initially, as the muscles in the ventricle contract, the pressure of the blood within the chamber rises, but it is not yet high enough to open the semilunar (pulmonary and aortic) valves and be ejected from the heart. However, blood pressure quickly rises above that of the atria that are now relaxed and in diastole. This increase in pressure causes blood to flow back toward the atria, closing the tricuspid and mitral valves. Since blood is not being ejected from the ventricles at this early stage, the volume of blood within the chamber remains constant. Consequently, this initial phase of ventricular systole is known as isovolumic contraction, also called isovolumetric contraction.

In the second phase of ventricular systole, the ventricular ejection phase, the contraction of the ventricular muscle has raised the pressure within the ventricle to the point that

it is greater than the pressures in the pulmonary trunk and the aorta. Blood is pumped from the heart, pushing open the pulmonary and aortic semilunar valves. Pressure generated by the left ventricle will be appreciably greater than the pressure generated by the right ventricle, since the existing pressure in the aorta will be so much higher. Nevertheless, both ventricles pump the same amount of blood. This quantity is referred to as stroke volume. Stroke volume will normally be in the range of 70 to 80 mL. Since ventricular systole began with an EDV of approximately 130 mL of blood, this means that there is still 50 to 60 mL of blood remaining in the ventricle following contraction. This volume of blood is known as the end systolic volume (ESV).[1]

Ventricular Diastole. Ventricular relaxation, or diastole, follows repolarization of the ventricles and is represented by the T wave of the ECG. It is divided into two distinct phases and lasts approximately 430 ms.

During the early phase of ventricular diastole, as the ventricular muscle relaxes, pressure on the remaining blood within the ventricle begins to fall. When pressure within the ventricles drops below pressure in both the pulmonary trunk and aorta, blood flows back toward the heart, producing the dicrotic notch (small dip) seen in blood pressure tracings. The semilunar valves close to prevent backflow into the heart. Since the atrioventricular valves remain closed at this point, there is no change in the volume of blood in the ventricle, so the early phase of ventricular diastole is called the isovolumic ventricular relaxation phase, also called isovolumetric ventricular relaxation phase.

In the second phase of ventricular diastole, called late ventricular diastole, as the ventricular muscle relaxes, pressure on the blood within the ventricles drops even further. Eventually, it drops below the pressure in the atria. When this occurs, blood flows from the atria into the ventricles, pushing open the tricuspid and mitral valves. As pressure drops within the ventricles, blood flows from the major veins into the relaxed atria and from there into the ventricles. Both chambers are in diastole, the atrioventricular valves are open, and the semilunar valves remain closed. The cardiac cycle is complete.[1]

Blood Circulation Through the Heart. The right and left sides of the heart work together in achieving a smooth flowing blood circulation.

- Entrance to the heart:
  - Blood enters the heart through two large veins, the inferior and superior vena cava (SVC), emptying oxygen and poor blood from the body into the RA of the heart.
- Atrial contraction:
  - As the atrium contracts, blood flows from the RA to the right ventricle through the open tricuspid valve.
- Closure of the tricuspid valve:
  - When the ventricle is full, the tricuspid valve shuts to prevent blood from flowing backward into the atria while the ventricle contracts.

- Ventricle contraction:
  - As the ventricle contracts, blood leaves the heart through the pulmonic valve, into the PA and to the lungs where it is oxygenated.
- Oxygen-rich blood circulates:
  - The pulmonary vein empties oxygen-rich blood from the lungs into the left atrium of the heart.
- Opening of the mitral valve:
  - As the atrium contracts, blood flows from your left atrium into your left ventricle through the open mitral valve.
- Prevention of backflow:
  - When the ventricle is full, the mitral valve shuts. This prevents blood from flowing backward into the atrium while the ventricle contracts.
- Blood flow to systemic circulation:
  - As the ventricle contracts, blood leaves the heart through the aortic valve, into the aorta and to the body.

Coronary Arteries

Arising off the aorta, there are two main coronary arteries: right coronary artery (RCA) and left coronary artery (LCA) (see Figure 22-5).

The LCA, which supplies oxygenated blood to the left side of the heart, include the left atria and ventricle as well as the interventricular septum. The LCA then branches off into two main branches: The left anterior descending (LAD) and the circumflex (LCX). Occasionally, in some patients, an extra artery arises from the LCA, called a Ramus or Intermediate Artery.

The RCA supplies oxygenated blood to the right side of the heart, which include the RA and ventricle, as well as portions of the left ventricle. The RCA branches off into the posterior descending artery (PDA) and the right marginal artery. The artery that supplies the posterior third of the interventricular septum—the PDA—determines the coronary dominance.[2]

- If the PDA is supplied by the RCA, then the coronary circulation can be classified as "right-dominant."
- If the PDA is supplied by the CX, a branch of the left artery, then the coronary circulation can be classified as "left-dominant."
- If the PDA is supplied by both the RCA and the CX, then the coronary circulation can be classified as "co-dominant."

Approximately 70% of the general population are right-dominant, 20% are co-dominant, and 10% are left-dominant. A precise anatomic definition of dominance would be the artery which gives off supply to the AV node, ie, the AV nodal artery. Most of the time this is the RCA.

Nonsurgical Treatments

Most cardiac related issues, if severe, need surgical intervention. This is in no way a substitute for severe cardiac procedures. There are, however, a few modalities that are available.

Some cardiac conditions that can be managed with medications such as beta blockers. Beta blockers are a type of medication that is used to block stress hormones. They are typically used for irregular/abnormal heartbeats. Beta blockers can also affect high blood pressure and are typically given after a patient experiences a heart attack. Thrombolytic agents are also given to break down and dissolve blood clots which cause heart attacks. Other medications, such as statins, can be given to slow down the progression of atherosclerosis.

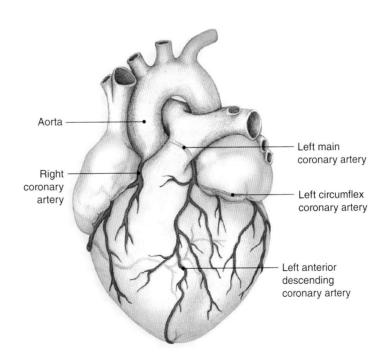

Figure 22-5 · Coronary arteries. (Reproduced, with permission, from Zimmerman FH. *ECG Core Curriculum*. New York, NY: McGraw Hill; 2023.)

Also, there are percutaneous options for heart disease. A patient can have a balloon angioplasty where a balloon is utilized in opening a blocked or clogged coronary artery. Also, at that time, a metal stent can be placed into the open coronary to help the blockage stay open. This is an alternative for a coronary artery bypass.

Alternative therapies such as cardiac rehabilitation is a considerable option. This helps a patient with a specialized, tailored exercise and an education to have a better prognosis. Rehabilitation has shown signs of slowing the progression of heart disease and reducing the risk of future heart problems.

Most facilities have an electrophysiology lab available. These labs preform minor procedures which will help correct atrial fibrillation and arrhythmias without having major open-heart surgery. Cardiologists can often identify these fast, irregular heartbeats and treat them with an ablation. Other small procedures, like a pacemaker insertion, are performed on patients that have an abnormally slow heartbeat.

Most patients consider diet and exercise as a preventative as well as alternative method of reversing heart disease. If nonsurgical treatments do not return patients to an acceptable quality of life, then surgery may be their only option. Numerous preoperative tests are performed to gain an accurate picture of the patient as they prepare for surgery.

Surgical Preoperative Preparation
Non-Invasive Tests
- Blood work
- CBC (complete blood count)
- BMP (basic metabolic panel)
- CMP (complete metabolic panel)
- Lipid panel
- Thyroid panel
- Coagulation panel
- Enzyme markers
- DHEA sulfate panel
- C-Reactive protein test
- Pregnancy test
- STD tests
- MRSA
- Antibody resistance
- COVID-19 nasal swab
- Chest x-ray
- EKG or ECG: Additional conditions of heart (conduction disorders, arrhythmias, valve disease, etc.)
- Pulmonary function test (PFT): Lung function
- Carotid Doppler/ultrasound study: Blockage or narrowing of carotid arteries for signs and symptoms of possible stroke
- Transthoracic echocardiogram: Assesses heart valves and function of the heart and could be done on skin

- Vein mapping: Assesses greater saphenous vein in both legs for CABG
- Arterial duplex: Assesses radial artery and flow to patient's hand if radial; conduit is usable in CABG procedures

Invasive Tests
- Transesophageal echocardiogram (TEE): Echocardiogram performed by passing probe into Esophagus (see Figure 22-6)
- Heart catheterization (CATH): Assesses coronary blood flow and to determine blockages. Occasionally, blockages may be treated with angioplasty and stenting
- Computed tomography (CT) scan: Assesses aorta (largest blood vessel in the body), lungs, and thoracic structures
- Cardiac magnetic resonance imaging (MRI): Detailed function of heart muscle and may also be used to determine myocardial viability

Additional consults for heart/lung transplants include: financial planning, psychology consult, nutrition, weight loss (if obese past recommended guidelines), smoking secession classes (if currently smoking), pharmacy consult, transplant coordinator's consult, transplant physician clinic, cardiologist clinic, and others if indicated.

Anesthesia
General anesthesia with an endotracheal tube (ET Tube) is utilized for all cardiac surgery procedures.

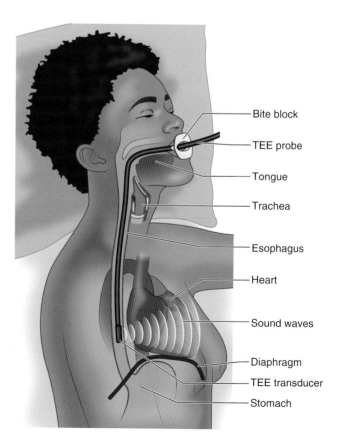

Figure 22-6 · TEE procedure.

Positioning

All patients for the procedures listed below are positioned supine. The arms, once all invasive lines and IVs are inserted, should be tucked in the correct manner, to prevent any nerve damage. This is accomplished with the patient's arms extended, and their thumb pointing directly to the ceiling. A draw sheet is then used to go over the patient's arm and then tucked underneath the patient's side. Sleds and blankets are also recommended for more obese patients whose arms extend past the bed padding.

It is important to note that all bodily hair is then removed once the patient is asleep. Hair is removed from the patient's neck extending down to the ankles, and from the most visible lateral right side extending to the patients lateral left side, using a clipper and not a razor. The patient's ankles/heels and bottom are padded with an adhesive, padded dressing to prevent any skin breakdown.

The temperature Foley, once inserted, is placed underneath either leg and the drainage bag is then given to anesthesia to record urine output.

The electrocautery pad is placed over non-bony prominences, usually posterior thigh, or buttocks.

A shoulder roll is to be placed horizontal underneath the shoulders extending from left to right. Care is taken that the neck is not hyper extended.

An attachment to the head of the bed, also called a monster or mayo table, is connected securely to the bed. This is a small, working table the assistant's instruments and other necessities are placed on during surgery.

For procurement of conduits, it is the preference of the assistant in their positions of legs/arm. Normally, blankets or a "frogger" pillow is used to position the legs suitable for endoscopic saphenous vein harvest. The legs are then placed in a frog position.

A folded towel may be used underneath the wrist for extension of the Radial Artery along with a tourniquet when using the endoscope to procure the radial artery. The arm is left on an arm board, prepped, and draped.

Prepping

Prepping of the patient is done after all positioning requirements are completed. The chest is prepped in normal standard fashion starting from the sternum and working out to the periphery. The prep should extend from the chin to waist, and equally bilateral on both sides extending to the tucked arms. The groins are then prepped.

The legs are lastly prepped circumferentially, starting at the incision site, and working away from incision.

Hospital and departmental protocols are followed in which specific solution is used. Drying time is allotted before applying surgical drapes.

Draping

Normal cardiac draping incudes access above the Manubrium, draping wide enough to access the Axillary Artery and both groins and legs. This will allow access to both groins if the patient needs to be converted to bypass and allows access to saphenous vein procurement.

Procedure

Creating a Sternotomy

- To access the thoracic cavity, the surgeon and their assistant are tasked to make a median sternotomy incision onto this chest. The landmarks which are first established is the manubrium and the xiphoid process. Once these two structures are located, an incision is made from the top of the manubrium to the bottom of the xiphoid process (see Figure 22-7). Some surgeons' preferences are tailored to a smaller median sternotomy incision.

- Electrocautery is then used to incise the subcutaneous tissue down to the anterior table of the sternum. Marking the sternum with the Electrosurgical unit (ESU) pencil to establish true midline is crucial to making the appropriate sternotomy. The surgeon or the assistant will then find the manubrium and mark the true center of the sternum. The marking

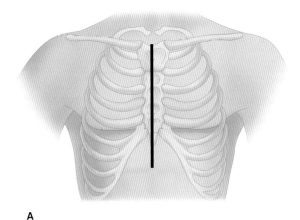

A

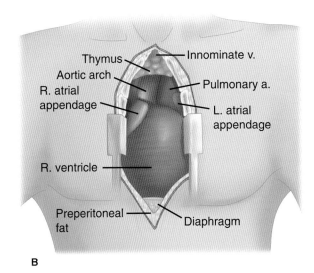

B

Figure 22-7 · Sternotomy. (Reproduced, with permission, from Brunicardi FC et al., eds. *Schwartz's Principles of Surgery.* 11th ed. New York, NY: McGraw Hill; 2019.)

will continue distally feeling the rib spaces to make sure they are centered accordingly. Once marked, the surgeon will ask for the lungs to be depleted of air (lungs down), and a sternal saw with a guard is used to separate the sternum. Once a sternotomy is completed, the patient will be placed back on the ventilator to resume normal respiratory function.

- Attention is now placed on the sternal edge, to minimize any type of additional bleeding from the sternal edges. Marrow bleeding is minimalized using a hemostatic agent of the surgeon's preference. Once hemostasis is controlled, a sternal retractor is used to retract the divided sternum. Anterior mediastinal fat is exposed and is divided, taking consideration to vessels which are inside of the fat, and are ligated with clips.

- Once cleared, the dense fibrous sac visible is the pericardium. An anterior longitudinal small incision is made into the pericardium. It is noted that the assistant, at that time, will retract the pericardium with forceps and suction any pericardial fluid that enters the field. The pericardium is divided distally and then attention is focused on dividing it proximally. At the superior pericardial reflection is the innominate vein. The left and right brachiocephalic veins (or innominate veins) are formed by the union of each corresponding internal jugular vein and subclavian vein.

- Care is taken to prevent damage to the structure. Once completely dissected, the pericardium is then "tacked up" with sutures and a cradle is created so direct visualization of the heart is exposed. The responsibility of the SA is to aid the surgeon during these steps and assist with direct visualization.

- Once this step is complete, the appropriate procedure can then begin. The above mentioned is the standard opening procedures for all non-minimally invasive heart procedures requiring a sternotomy.

Cannulation

- Once the surgeon isolates one or both mammary arteries and the assistant has procured their respective conduits (if CABG), focus now goes to preparing the patient to go on cardiopulmonary bypass. Preparation is needed before the surgeon can initiate bypass. Systemic heparin is given before the cannulation process is started.

- Two purse-string sutures, 3-0/4-0 nonabsorbable monofilament or braided sutures, are placed in ascending aorta (AO) with tourniquets for securing. Attention is now focused on the RA. A single purse-string suture (same as listed above) is placed around the appendage of the RA and secured with a tourniquet. The SA is responsible for cutting the needles and applying tourniquets. Distally on the atrial free wall, another purse-string is placed for retrograde perfusion cannula. Attention is then returned to the anterior AO and a single purse-string stitch is placed and tourniquet applied on the Antegrade perfusion cardioplegia cannulation site. Once all sutures are placed, appropri-

ate cannulas (aortic cannula, venous cannula, antegrade and retrograde cardioplegia cannula, are opened on the sterile field.

- Starting with the aorta, a small hole is made with an #11 blade and the surgeon inserts the cannula. The assistant then retrieves the tourniquets and snares down the cannula, sealing the aorta around it. The cannula is secured using the surgeon's preference and then the cannula is de-aired by allowing blood to fill the cannula. A wet connect is established between the cannula and the pump tubing assuring that there are no air bubbles circulating in the tubing. The SA is responsible for also monitoring the tubing to make sure no air bubbles are present (see Figure 22-8).

- Once the tubing is secured to the drape, normally with a towel clip, attention is back to the atrium. The SA grabs the tissue with two forceps and exposes the purse-string for the surgeon. Again, a small stab is made in-between the purse-string and a tonsil is used to dilate the opening. The venous cannula of choice is inserted and the assistant, again, grabs the respected tourniquet and snares down and secures with a hemostat. A silk tie is placed around the cannula and the snare to prevent slipping of the cannula. Once secure, the surgeon connects the venous cannula to the venous tubing which is connected to the bypass machine.

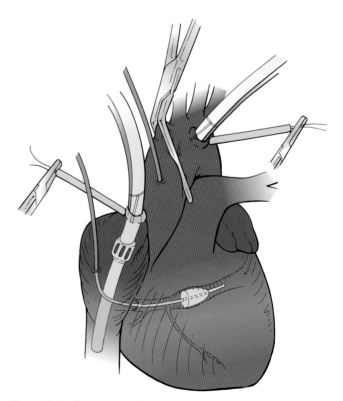

Figure 22-8 • Aortic cannulation. (Reproduced, with permission, from Cohn LH, Adams DH, eds. *Cardiac Surgery in the Adult.* 5th ed. New York, NY: McGraw Hill; 2018.)

There does not need to be a wet connect done on the venous line, as the air in the tubing will be drained at the pump reservoir.

- The next cannula that will be placed is the retrograde cardioplegia cannula. As the same steps as before, a small incision is made inside the purse string or the free wall of the atrium and then dilated with a tonsil. The retrograde cannula is then inserted through the wall of the RA into the mouth of the coronary sinus. This will allow for cardioplegia to be perfused retrograde through the venous system of the heart. Once placed, the SA grabs the tourniquet and snares down the previously placed purse-string and secures the tourniquet with a hemostat. A silk tie is also used to secure the cannula.

- The last cannula to be placed is the antegrade cardioplegia cannula into the anterior wall of the aorta. The cannula comes with a sharp needle tip so an incision does not need to be made. The surgeon places the needle tip in the aorta, inside the purse-string, and then removes the needle. Blood is allowed to bleed back into the cannula and a cardioplegia line is established for another wet-connect." A silk tie is used to secure the cannula and snare.

- Space is left between the aortic cannulation site and the antegrade cannula. This space where the cross-clamp is applied to ejection of the heart. The aortic cannula is cranial to the clamp, as the blood entering the body from the cannula, perfuses the whole body. The antegrade cardioplegia cannula is caudal to the cross-clamp, providing cardioplegia solution to arrest the heart down the RCA and LCA.

Decannulation

- Once the arrested heart part of the procedure is complete, the aortic cross-clamp is removed, and the heart re-perfuses and starts beating. Normal sinus electro-mechanical activity is often achieved automatically, however, direct current cardioversion may be necessary to obtain normal sinus rhythm. Epicardial pacing wires, which can supplement the heart's rhythm, are placed on the ventricular and atrial epicardium.

- The heart is examined in the field and via a TEE. TEE can evaluate myocardial wall motion, valvular structures, and the integrity of surgical intervention (eg, myocardial function of bypassed territories if CABG procedure is done, or to visualize the structural integrity of a valve if repaired or replaced). TEE is also used to evaluate air in the heart. Air in the heart can be detrimental, as it can escape to the coronary circulation, brain, and lungs in the form of an air embolism. Care is taken by opening the antegrade cannula to suction, on the bypass machine, to facilitate air removal from the aorta and the heart.

- Once the TEE has been reviewed, and it is safe to proceed, the heart lung machine is weaned, and the heart and lungs resume normal functions without mechanical assistance. The removal of cannulas is a structured and order event as indicated by the numbers below:

1. Venous return cannula
2. Retrograde coronary sinus cannula

3. LV vent (if present)
4. Air evaluation
5. Antegrade/Root vent
6. Protamine administration
   - The assistant carefully ties one of the sutures while the surgeon removes each of the cannula. This process is established because of high pressure of blood in the Aorta and necessary hemostasis that is maintained by the assistant during the removal of the cannula. Protamine is given to counteract the loading dose of Heparin.

Closing a Sternotomy Incision

- Once all cannulas are out, the surgeon and the assistant evaluate all surgical sites, including distal, and proximal anastomosis (if CABG), aortotomy, atriotomy, or ventriculotomy (if present), and cannulation sites for bleeding. Any surgical bleeding is repaired, placing appropriate simple or figure-of-eight sutures. Once hemostasis is ensured, the pericardium and any residual thymus fat is closed with interrupted suture.

- The next plane of closure is the sternum. Both hemi-sternums are typically closed in the adult patient with #6, or #7 stainless steel wire. Often sternal closure is performed by the assistant. Three or four sternal wires are placed in the manubrium, and the remaining wires are either placed in the rib spaces or the rib heads themselves of the sternum. Once all wires are placed, the chest wall, wire sites, and sternum is checked for bleeding. Electrocautery or suture are used to control bleeding. Once hemostasis is controlled, the sternum is approximated by crossing the wires, which are then twisted, trimmed, and tuned down into the sternum.

- A 0-braided absorbable suture is then used to close the inferior fascia below the xiphoid. This can be performed in an interrupted or continuous running fashion. The chest tubes are connected to pleura-vac containers, and outside suction, to measure drainage from the pericardium and pleural spaces. A 0-braided suture is then used to close the fascia above the sternum from the manubrium to the xiphoid.

- A 2-0 braided absorbable suture is used to close the subcutaneous layer. The final closure is the skin, which is used in a subcuticular fashion, with a 4-0 braided or absorbable monofilament.

Surgical Modifications Intra-Op

There are times when an incidental finding may call for additional procedures.

- Ex1: Patient consented for a CABG, and it is found on TEE that there is a significant patent foramen ovale (PFO); the surgeon may need to open the heart and close the PFO.

- Ex2: Patient consented for aortic valve replacement, and it is noticed upon opening, the aorta is aneurysmal. The aorta may need to be replaced.

- Ex3: Patient consented for aortic valve replacement, and an incidental finding of tricuspid valve regurgitation present. The tricuspid valve may need to be addressed.

CORONARY ARTERY BYPASS GRAFTING (CABG)

Coronary artery bypass grafting is among the most commonly performed major surgical procedures, with approximately 400,000 operations occurring annually in the United States. During the past decade, however, there has been nearly a 30% decline in CABG procedures in the United States, despite an aging population and growing evidence to support the effectiveness and safety of the operation. This can be related to an increase in percutaneous coronary intervention that can correct coronary artery stenosis.

Coronary artery disease involves the reduction of blood flow to the myocardium due to buildup of plaque in the arteries of the heart.[3,4] It is the most common of the cardiovascular diseases.[1] Acute coronary syndrome is defined by increasing severity including stable angina, unstable angina, myocardial infarction, and sudden cardiac death.[3] In 2015, CAD affected 110 million people and resulted in 8.9 million deaths, making it the most common cause of death globally.[5,6]

A common symptom is chest pain or discomfort which may travel to the shoulder, arm, back, neck, or jaw. Occasionally, it may feel like heartburn. Often symptoms occur with exercise or emotional stress, last less than a few minutes, and improve with rest. Shortness of breath may also occur. Sometimes no symptoms are present. In many cases, the first sign is a heart attack. Complications of CAD include heart failure (HF) or arrhythmias.

Revascularization is crucial to restore blood flow to restricted myocardium. The SA and the cardiac surgeon evaluate the left CATH films together, to determine which vessels meet criteria for intervention. Once established which vessels will need bypasses, a surgical plan is determined on what conduit will be used to bypass the blockages in the respective arteries. With the exception of LIMA and RIMA, normally the SA is tasked with harvesting the appropriate conduit.

Common Conduit Choices

The common conduit choices include:

- Left internal mammary artery (LIMA; also left internal thoracic artery) is the gold standard in coronary revascularization. The LIMA is most often used "in-situ," to bypass blockages of the LAD coronary artery. The LAD is the longest coronary artery that arises as a branch of the LCA and travels down the anterior surface of the heart to the apex. This is the gold standard due to superior long-term patency rate over all other conduits to when grafted to the LAD, generally the most important vessel, clinically, to revascularize.[7]

- Right internal mammary artery (RIMA; also right internal thoracic artery). This is used either "in-situ," meaning still attached proximally, or used as a free graft, where it is transected proximally and distally and sutured proximally on the aorta or as a "Y" off another conduit.

- Radial artery. The radial artery in the arm is another option for arterial conduit selection. An open incision is made (preferably on the patient's nondominant hand) and carefully harvested by either open or endoscopic techniques. Non-invasive evaluation, with arterial duplex and the Allen's test, is performed to ensure the radial artery is of good quality; and that the patient will still have adequate blood flow to the hand.

- Saphenous vein. Ancillary vein in the leg extending from the saphenofemoral Junction to the lower ankle. Vein is harvested, normally by the assistant, endoscopically with a camera and a harvesting system, or using an open technique, which include small bridge incisions, or a full incision extending the full length of the leg. For each conduit, the assistant must know where each bypass is planned, and the size of the heart, to remove the appropriate length accordingly.

Bypass Grafts

Surgical Procedure: CABG

- During a CABG, before the aortic cross-clamp is applied, the surgeon and the assistant take a close examination of the heart. They evaluate all major arteries in the heart, feeling them for calcification, and determine targets for bypassing. A #15 blade is used for dissecting epicardial tissue around the coronary, to better visualize the anastomotic target. Close examination of the harvested conduits will be inspected for length and quality.

- Once the cross-clamp is applied, the patient's temperature is regulated to the surgeon's specifications, for systemic hypothermia. Some surgeons do not like to lower the patient's body temperature, but to drift to a lower temperature and then slowly warm the patient's core temperature. Ice or cold saline is poured on the heart to help induce local hypothermia and therefore lower myocardial metabolism.

- Once full arrest is achieved, the surgeon positions the heart in the ideal position to expose the coronary artery, where the bypass will be sewn. As the assistant exposes the area with fine forceps, the surgeon opens the coronary with a scalpel, and extends the incision with forward and reverse Potts scissors. The assistant then positions and manages the conduit, as the surgeon performs bypass grafting. Most often, a small diameter polypropylene suture is used in a running fashion. While there are many approaches to coronary micro-anastomosis, all are used to create a watertight connection between the conduit and the coronary artery. Blood or saline is often injected through the conduit to make sure there are no significant leaks. The performance of all distal anastomoses followed by all proximal anastomoses, versus completing bypasses individually, is surgeon and patient anatomy specific. The aorta is examined and, depending on how many conduits need to be attached proximally, the surgeon makes an aortotomy for each proximal anastomosis. A round aortic punch is used to make each aortotomy. The conduit is inspected in its entirety for leaks, bends, or twists to eliminate the possibility of compromised flow. Once again, the assistant then positions and manages the conduit, as the surgeon performs bypass grafting (see Figure 22-9).

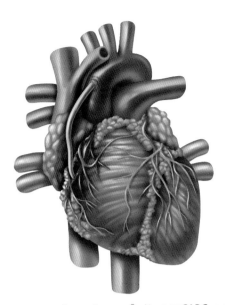

Figure 22-9 · Coronary Artery Bypass Grafting or CABG as an obstruction of plaque in the coronary artery or arteries as a vein from a leg that is grafted to a heart bypassing a blockage in a 3D illustration style. (Used with permission from Lightspring/Shutterstock.)

OP-CABG (Off-Pump Coronary Artery Bypass Graft)

Surgical Procedure

- After a median sternotomy incision, the left internal thoracic artery, or better termed LIMA, was dissected in its entirety from the chest wall. Careful dissection with tenotomy scissors and the use of small clips are used to isolate branches off the LIMA, to harvest the conduit safely.

- The patient is given systemic heparin. The distal left portion of the LIMA is divided and prepared for use as an in-situ conduit. The pericardium was opened, and the location of the LAD is then identified.

- Retracto-tapes (or sylastic tapes) are utilized as an aid in exposure, as well as temporary occlusion the LAD.

- A stabilizing device is used to minimalize the movement of the LAD. Should a bypass be needed behind the heart, an apex suction device can be used to manipulate the heart to expose the coronary with limited hemodynamic compromise. Care needs to be given to the patient's pressure. Lifting the heart can cause limited cardiac return and output, as well as arrhythmia. The SA needs to constantly be aware of this and monitor it continuously.

- Often, during OP-CABG, a coronary intravascular shunt is used to prevent ischemia during performance of the anastomosis.

Pericardial Window

As noted, the pericardium is a sac that encapsulates and protects the heart. This sac has two thin layers and contains a small amount of physiologic fluid. The fluid aids in reduction of friction when the heart beats. Excess fluid in the pericardial sac compresses the heart, reduces pre-load, and prevents proper cardiac function.

There are different pathologies that cause fluid buildup around the heart. Patients that have had injury to the pericardium, previous or active cancer and radiation, and infection (pre- or post-cardiac surgery) are more susceptible to have this type of surgery.

The pericardium does vary in the response with regard to inflammation of all layers. Chronic inflammation can cause the pericardium to be fibrotic and calcified, which can become thickened and calcified. Untreated, this can lead to pericardial constriction.

There are other ways to drain pericardial fluid from around the heart. This procedure is called a pericardiocentesis. This is where a needle is inserted through the pericardium and a wire is advanced in through it. A catheter, or drain, is placed over the wire and into the pericardium to help unload some of the fluid. Should a patient have multiple attempts with unsuccessful results, a pericardial window is indicated. There are some instances in which the fluid returns. In more extreme cases, a patient may need to have a pericardiectomy.

A pericardial window is a surgical procedure to incise the pericardium and to drain fluid from the pericardial sac. A pericardial window is one method of draining excess fluid and preventing future fluid buildup.

There are numerous incisions and approaches to a pericardial window. The classic traditional approach is through a midline subxiphoid incision. A pericardial window can also be performed through an anterior mini-thoracotomy, or video-assisted thoracoscopy (VATS).

Surgical Procedure

- A small lower midline incision, or subxiphoid incision, is made over (or just below) the xiphoid process. In a patient who has had a sternotomy, the lower portion over the xyphoid is incised and accessed. With the subxiphoid approach, the surgeon will be accessing the pericardium anteriorly, over the right ventricle. Electrocautery is used until the base of the sternum is found and xyphoid is noted. The xyphoid is routinely excised if found to be a hinderance to exposure. A handheld or self-retaining retractor is used to expose the cardio phrenic fat which should be visible.

- The pericardium may or not be visible, depending on the patient's size. Careful dissection through the cardio phrenic fat pad is performed until the pericardium is fully visible. In some instances, this fat pad is excised to better visualize the pericardium. The SA is a key link to ensure communication between the surgical and the anesthesia members, to make everyone aware when the pericardium is about to be entered. Anesthesia providers may need to intervene and manage hemodynamics after pericardial entry, especially is tamponade is present.

- Once the pericardium is visible, a #15 blade is used to gently make an incision through the pericardium. Care is taken while incising the pericardium to not damage the heart on the posterior side. Once a small incision is made, the surgeon and the assistant will use suction to remove the excess fluid and forceps to retract upwards the pericardium. A tonsil or hemostat can be used, as well as tacking sutures.

- The surgeon will then excise enough pericardium to make a "window" for fluid to drain effectively. Pericardium is excised and sent to pathology for examination. Lastly, a small chest tube or drain is inserted into the pericardial space, through a separate counter incision. Routine fascial, soft tissue, and skin closure is performed (see Figure 22-10).

Pericardectomy

The pericardium is a double-walled membrane sac that covers the heart. Inside of the pericardium is pericardial fluid, which is a lubricant for the heart and is approximately 50 mL in volume.

A pericardectomy is a surgical treatment for a patient with a diseased pericardium. This is also diagnosed as restrictive pericarditis. The pericardium is the sac like structure that surrounds the heart. A successful pericardiectomy is deemed as an adequate resection and removal of the diaphragmatic pericardium and the anterior pericardium. Removal of this thickened, fibrous sac will allow for the heart to beat without compression.

Surgical Procedure

- A traditional median sternotomy incision is performed for a pericardectomy. A left anterolateral thoracotomy incision can also be utilized. After the median sternotomy incision is performed, the pericardium is then visualized, opened carefully, and excised meticulously. Dissection is then directed over the anterior and lateral portions of the heart. Care is taken to not dissect into the heart itself. It is the responsibility of the SA to carefully retract the dissected edges and lift the pericardium with forceps while the surgeon dissects the plane between the heart and the pericardium. The phrenic nerve is a structure that is identified by both the surgeon and the SA and to carefully be preserved during the removal of the surrounding pericardium.

- This procedure is routinely done without the use of cardiopulmonary bypass. The beating of the heart is occasionally

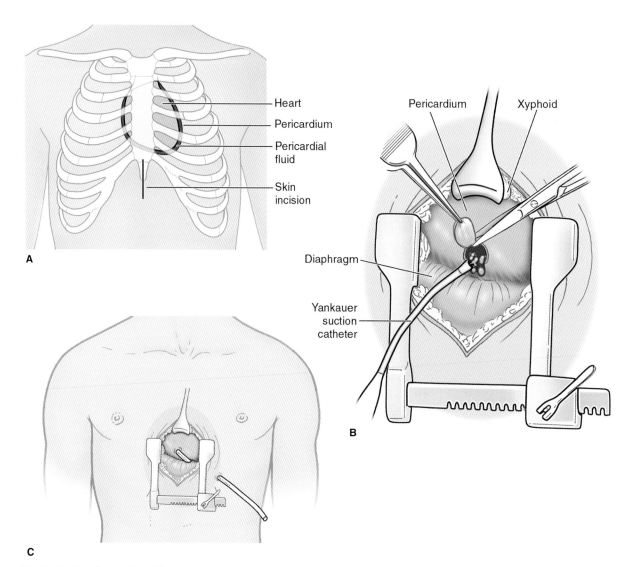

Figure 22-10 · Pericardial window. (Reproduced, with permission, from Reichman EF. *Reichman's Emergency Medicine Procedures*. 3rd ed. New York, NY: McGraw Hill; 2019.)

needed for thorough removal of the affected tissue. This also allows for clearer boarders to be dissected and removed, as well as, to determine if there are any additional areas of compression of the heart that are not visibly noted.

- Cardiopulmonary bypass, however, can be useful in this operation. With the use of bypass, the heart is able to be lifted or compressed for adequate dissection of the pericardium. Again, not all cases require the use of the heart-lung machine.

- Once all pericardium is safely and adequately removed, the patient is closed in routine fashion.

Pacemaker Insertion

A pacemaker insertion inserted just below the clavicle to help regulate the heartbeat of the patient. Pacemakers are normally placed for patients who have complex arrhythmias. This procedure is done to correct a slow or irregular heartbeat. Pacemakers also aid patients with HF.

Arrhythmias can affect blood distribution to the entire body. Symptoms of this include, but not limited to, active or nonactive chest pain, rapid heartbeat, weakness, fatigue, and shortness of breath. More severe cases could cause the organ damage and could possibly result in cardiac death.

There are different types of pacemakers that serve different functions. The different types are single chamber pacemakers, dual chamber pacemaker, and biventricular pacemaker.

- A single chamber pacemaker affects the right ventricle and the electrical pulses delivered to it.

- A dual chamber pacemaker sends electrical pulses to the RA and the right ventricle. This aids in for contractions between the chambers themselves.

- A biventricular pacemaker affects both the right and the left ventricles of the heart to maximize blood flow. Patients with electrical rhythms in HF need this device. Another term for a biventricular pacemaker is called cardiac resynchronization therapy.

General or local anesthesia is administered for the procedure, however, local anesthesia is more commonly utilized.

Surgical Procedure

- A small incision is made roughly one fingerbreadth beneath the clavicle. The SA will help maintain exposure with forceps, handheld retractors, or a self-retaining retractor. A small plane underneath the subcutaneous fat, above the muscle, is created as a pocket for the future site of the generator.

- Access to the subclavian vein is then obtained. Once isolated, a needle is inserted into the subclavian vein. A small guidewire is then placed into the needle. Multiple wires will be used to gain access to areas in the heart to establish proper placement. The leads, one at a time, will then be threaded through the entrance, traveling down to the desired spot via fluoroscopy, until they reach the RA where they are attached.

- The surgeon will use fluoroscopy again to view proper placement of the leads. Once placed, they will be intraoperatively tested and analyzed to make sure they function properly. Once checked and confirmed all leads are active, a generator, or pacemaker is opened, and the leads will be properly connected. The generator (pacemaker) is placed into the small pouch pocket created earlier by dissection, underneath the collarbone. Routine closure is then performed only on subcutaneous tissue, and skin. Monitoring will be utilized before leaving the OR and while the patient is in the hospital to make sure pacemaker is working properly. Before leaving the hospital, final adjustments will be made to the pacemaker.

- Another type of procedure for pacemaker insertion is the application of epicardial leads. An incision is made via a small, lateral mini thoracotomy, just below the patients left nipple to gain access to the apex of the heart. In some instances, the epicardial leads need to be placed while other procedures are performed on the heart, so a median sternotomy can be an alternative incision.

- Once the heart is exposed the epicardial leads are held down and tested in various areas on the surface of the heart.

- Once a viable, active spot is found, the surgeon will sew on an epicardial pacing lead. The SA is responsible for holding the leads in place while the surgeon secures them onto the heart. This is accomplished with a polypropylene suture, which holds the lead firmly against the heart. Once the epicardial leads are placed and then tested again, the leads are then tunneled throughout the subcutaneous fat up to the incision just below the collarbone where the generator is located. Again, as aforementioned, the leads will be tested, to make sure it did not come dislodged or cracked during tunneling, before hooking up to the generator. Routine closure is done for the small incision below the collarbone and ancillary incisions.

Aortic Valve Replacement

The aortic valve separates the left ventricle from the aorta. After every contraction, the aortic valve closes to allow blood to fill the left ventricle and open to eject blood systemically. The valve closes to prevent any blood leaking back into the ventricle. When this process is disrupted, the aortic valve becomes insufficient, which leads to the valve to be replaced.

The aortic valve is made up of three coronary cusps and three leaflets of the aorta. The left coronary cusp gives rise to the LCA. The right coronary cusp gives rise to the RCA. The non-coronary cusp, does not have any coronary arteries arise, thus called non-coronary cusp.

Aortic stenosis is when there is a narrowing of the aortic valve. This restricts the blood flow through the valve. With restricted flow, the heart must contract more forcefully to pass blood through the valve. This is normally due to calcified leaflets. Aortic valve replacement (AVR) remains the standard therapy for severe aortic stenosis.

Bicuspid aortic valve is a congenital defect that affects the aortic valve. This is where instead of three leaflets, there are two leaflets. Occasionally, there are three leaflets that are fused together to make two leaflets total. This, like aortic stenosis, causes narrowing over time and blood to leak backwards. When blood returns to the ventricle, this is termed aortic regurgitation. Aortic regurgitation, if left untreated, can lead to HF. Aortic valve, or valvular heart disease, is inherited and/or acquired.

The replacement valves fall into two categories:

- Tissue: Animal tissue (bovine, porcine, etc.). Most likely lasts for around 10 to 15 years before possibly needing replacement.

- Mechanical: Plastic. Should not need replacement but requires patient to be on anti-coagulation therapy to prevent clot formation on leaflets for the rest of their life.

Surgical Procedure

- Once the heart is cannulated and arrested, the aortic cross-clamp is applied. Antegrade and retrograde cardioplegia is given to totally arrest and decompress the heart. Retrograde cardioplegia can be given semi-continuously during the operation when it does not interfere with the operation. Tacking sutures are then placed on the right ventricular outflow tract to retract and expose the aortic root. Dissection is carried out between the aorta and the PA. The SA is then tasked with exposure as this is a deep structure to expose. A peanut on a Kelly clamp is ideal, but the same exposure can be obtained with digital manipulation, with the use of a sponge to protect the heart. After adequate dissection, attention is brought back to the aorta.

- The aorta is then transected above the pericardial reflection. Carbon dioxide is then placed near the incision level to displace any air that may be entrapped in the open heart. The aortic valve is then exposed. Attention is then brought to the anatomy of the valve. First, the coronaries are assessed and made sure that there is no surrounding damage, either anatomically or surgically. The valve is then assessed. The leaflets of the native aortic valve are then removed, as well as any calcium that has formed on the annulus of the Aortic Valve. The SA will be tasked with paying careful attention to any calcium that may break off. Any pieces that break off are then removed with suction.

- Once the valve is completely resected and the calcium is removed safely, the valve area is then flushed with normal saline multiple times to remove any debris. The annulus is then sized with the appropriate sizers (mechanical or tissue, vendor-specific). The valve is announced, opened to the sterile field, and if applicable, rinsed to the manufacture's standards.

- Nonabsorbable sutures (pledget vs. non-pledget sutures depending on the surgeon's specifications) are evenly placed in the annulus and brought out to the level of the skin and either tagged with a hemostat or placed in a suture divider. The valve is then brought up to the surgical area from the back table and then each suture is placed, again, evenly spaced, in the new aortic valve.

- Once all sutures are placed and the needles cut off, the valve is then parachuted down to the native annulus and checked for appropriate fit. Sutures are then hand tied with approximately 6 to 8 knots per suture strand and excess cut a millimeter from the knot. A dental mirror is passed below the aortic valve to demonstrate good seating of the new aortic valve.

- The valve is then again checked that it was in the normal position and fully competent. The LCA and RCA are visualized and examined for a wide-open, nonobstructive passage of blood.

- The aortotomy is then closed with 4-0 running polypropylene suture. Care is given to not incorporate the running stitch into the valve, which will cause complications. Once the aortotomy is closed, the left heart is then de-aired, and the cross-clamp is removed. An ECG is then done to access the functionality of the new valve, which should show a normal functioning valve with no regurgitation. A normal ejection fraction should be visualized.

Aortic Aneurysm Replacement

The aorta is the main artery in the body. Its function is to carry blood from the heart to the rest of the body. When the Aorta becomes enlarged, and bulging out in an area, this is known as an aortic aneurysm. There are two types of aortic aneurysms:

- Thoracicaortic aneurysms: Type A: ¼ aneurysms are Type A.

- Abdominal aortic aneurysms: Type B: ¾ aneurysms are Type B.

Type A is when the ballooning of the aorta in the thoracic cavity, normally just distal to the great vessels that arise off the aorta. Type B is when the aneurysm is in the descending aorta or past the great vessels and in the abdomen, respectively.

Should either of those rupture, this can cause catastrophic bleeding and be fatal. Most cases of Type A aneurysms can be caught early and treated with various medications. Medications are used to decrease blood pressure to prevent a rupture. Surgical intervention is also needed in the most severe cases and can be treated via percutaneous and open surgical intervention. When surgical intervention is needed, the diseased aorta is removed, and a new aorta is constructed and replaced.

In most cases, aortic aneurysms produce little to no symptoms and are normally caught accidentally by another incidental finding, normally by CT scans. Surgery is most likely course of treatment if aneurysm is large or near rupture. For Type A aneurysm, the walls of the aorta are weak and normally arise from a small tear in the aortic lining. Blood then enters this small tear creating a false lumen or opening in the aorta. The blood filling this false lumen begins to enlarge. Adversely as this false lumen grows, the pressure then slowly collapses the true lumen, or native flow. As the compression happens, the wall of the false lumen begins to swell or balloon outwards, which will cause the aortic wall to rupture, causing immense bleeding and more often, become fatal.

Other Indications for Type A Aneurysms. The other indications for Type A aneurysms include:

- Atherosclerosis, a build-up of fatty deposits in the arteries
- Obesity
- High blood pressure
- Smoking (you are eight times more likely to develop an aneurysm if you smoke)
- Family history of aortic aneurysm and heart-related issues
- Marfan syndrome (connective tissue disorder)
- Trauma, such as a blow to the chest in a car accident
- Stimulant drugs

Symptoms. As mentioned before, symptoms are occasionally not present. Some symptoms to be cautious of are: pain in your chest, neck, upper back, jaw, trouble breathing, hoarseness and coughing.

Additional Diagnostic Tests and Procedures Relating to Type A Aneurysms

- Chest x-ray
- Ultrasound
- CT scan
- MRI
- Angiography/Aortogram

Treatment

- Diameter < 3 cm, no symptoms present, the patient will be watched, medically treated, and followed.
- Diameter 3 to 4 cm, no symptoms present, yearly routine follow-up, medically treated and followed.
- Diameter 4 to 4.5 cm, testing every 6 months, medically treated, and followed.
- Diameter >5 cm and/or actively growing more 1 cm/year, surgery is considered.
- Surgery may also be recommended if an aneurysm is large and likely to rupture.

Surgical Procedure

- Once cannulated and bypass initiated, the cross-clamp is applied and one dose of antegrade or retrograde cardioplegia is given. This allows for the heart to be totally arrested. The heart will remain arrested and can maintain arrest with intermittent doses of retrograde cardioplegia and antegrade by the coronary ostium's every 15 minutes.
- Once the heart is arrested, the next step is to transect the dissected portion of the AO and completely remove all the dissected tissue. This resection is from the level of the coronary ostium all the way to the emergence of the innominate trunk. During this time, the SA is holding the dissected tissue and protecting the surrounding structures. The use of scissors is utilized to transect and dissect tissue adhered to the posterior side of the aorta. A bovie is used in conjunction

to safely remove tissue adhered to prevent future bleeding that is not easily accessible behind the aorta.

- After complete removal of the dissected tissue, the aortic valve is approached and meticulously inspected. Should the dissection reach to the aortic root, then additional procedures would need to be done, such as a Bentall procedure, which replaces the whole aortic root and reattachment of coronaries. If the root was clean and free of dissection, but the valve needed replaced, then an Aortic Valve Replacement would need to be done. (See section "Aortic Valve Replacement").
- Proceeding forward, a Gelweave tube graft is utilized as the new conduit in reconstruction of the AO. The graft is sized to the appropriate diameter of the distal and proximal aorta. Once sized, the graft is carefully sewn on with a 4-0 running polypropylene suture to the proximal aorta. Once that anastomosis is completed, the graft is then measured and cut to the size required. The distal anastomosis is performed with 4-0 running polypropylene suture.
- A 4-0 polypropylene purse string stitch with a pledget is placed in the tube graft. This is for direct access cannulation into the graft with an antegrade root vent cannula. This is then connected to the cardiopulmonary bypass machine and used as a suction to remove excess air from the heart. Once all air is removed, the cross-clamp is taken off and the function of the valves are assessed by TEE.

CONGESTIVE HEART FAILURE: LVAD AND HEART TRANSPLANT

Heart Failure and Respective Diagnosis

This section discusses the complications that include:

- Congestive HF, chronic HF
- Left- or right-sided HF
- Systolic HF
- Diastolic HF or HF with preserved systolic function

According to the American Heart Association, about 6.5 million U.S. adults have HF, and nearly half of patients die within 5 years of diagnosis. HF and congestive heart failure (CHF) are serious conditions and remain without a cure. As mentioned above, the heart is responsible for delivering oxygen- and nutrient-rich blood to the body's cells. When a normal heart is functioning properly, the body receives enough oxygen and nutrients. In HF patients, the supply and demand f blood and nutrients are not sufficiently met. The heart is not able to pump enough blood, thus making it hard to keep up with the workload demanded on it. The blood begins to back up and, as a result, the veins, tissues, and lungs become congested with fluid. The most common symptom of HF is shortness of breath, fatigue, and coughing.

In short, since the heart cannot undertake the workload, it ties to compensate in various ways. The heart begins to stretch and enlarge for contractions to become stronger. This compensation maneuver tries to contract stronger and supply the body with enough blood. Another maneuver is the heart tries to pump faster and try to increase the hearts output. Lastly, the heart being enlarged and pumping faster, produces more muscle mass. When the heart muscles increase in size, it compensates by pumping stronger, and the heart enlarges even more.

The body also tries to compensate for the lack of oxygen- and nutrient-rich blood. Some of the body's blood vessels become narrowed for an elevated blood pressure to be obtained. The body also shunts blood away from other organs. The compensation in numerous ways is taxing on the heart, which then CHF becomes worse. It then becomes a point where nothing seems to work anymore.

Heart failure develops because of reduced function of the left ventricle (left-sided HF). Reduced function of the right ventricle (right-sided HF or pulmonary heart disease) can also occur in HF. As blood begins to back up behind the failing left ventricle and into the lungs, it becomes harder for the right ventricle to pump returning blood through the lungs. The right ventricle will then weaken and begin to fail.

As mentioned, HF can involve the heart's left side, right side or both sides. For left-sided HF, there are two types:

- Systolic HF: The left ventricle is unable to contract normally, thus making systemic circulation difficult.
- Diastolic HF: The left ventricle is unable to relax after contraction because of muscle stiffness, which making filling of the LV difficult.

Right-sided HF, also called right ventricular HF, is a direct result of left-sided HF. When the left ventricle fails and cannot eject blood, there is an increase of pressure back to the lungs, which directly affect the right side of the heart. Because of this back up of blood, there is also backup of blood in the body's venous system. When all of this occurs, this is deemed CHF.

CHF has numerous signs and symptoms which include, but not limited to, edema/pulmonary edema, shortness of breath, fatigue, coughing/wheezing, loss of appetite, nausea, confusion, and increased heart rate.

Additional Medical Conditions

The additional medical conditions that contribute to HF include:

- Coronary artery disease
- Past heart attack (myocardial infarction)
- Uncontrolled high blood pressure (hypertension or HBP)
- Abnormal heart valves
- Diseased heart muscle (dilated cardiomyopathy, hypertrophic cardiomyopathy) or inflammation (myocarditis)
- Heart defects present at birth (congenital heart disease)
- Severe lung disease
- Diabetes
- Obesity
- Sleep apnea

The other less common conditions, but still related to CHF, include:

- Low red blood cell count (severe anemia)
- An overactive thyroid gland (hyperthyroidism)
- Abnormal heart rhythm (arrhythmia or dysrhythmia)

Treatment of heart failure from a surgical aspect is by three ways:

- Manage with medication, diet, and exercise.
- Additional circulatory support (LVAD, left ventricular assist device): Assist with pumping blood throughout the body.
- Heart transplantation.

Left Ventricular Assist Device (LVAD)

An LVAD or VAD is a pump that is surgically placed inside the body to treat HF and improve blood flow to viable organs. The pump has a Dacron graft which is anastomosed to the Aorta, which aids in pumping blood from the Left Ventricle to the Aorta systemically. Also attached to the pump is a driveline, or power source, that is tunneled under the skin, brought out from a small incision in the abdomen, and connected to batteries outside of the patient. Patients will always remain connected to this. Once the patient leaves the hospital, batteries are utilized which make this portable and they can continue throughout their daily lives.

There are two types of therapies for heart failure patients with LVADs:

- Destination therapy (DT): When a patient is not eligible for a heart transplant, but has severe HF. They are presented with this option as a therapy for their HF. They will have this pump for the rest of their life.
- Bridge to transplant (BTT): An LVAD is placed into a patient that will be listed for transplant. This mechanical support device is placed because the patient HF is worse and cannot survive without it, but still meet the criteria for transplantation. With the use of mechanical support, occasionally, this places them higher on the transplant list (see Figure 22-11).

Surgical Procedure

- A median sternotomy incision performed. Bypass is initiated. Bypass can either be initiated by femoral arterial and venous cannulation or direct cannulation by means of aorta and left atrium.
- The LVAD and all components are open and prepped on a separate table. The left ventricular apex is the assessed. A felt sewing ring is placed on the apex and fixed with a running 3-0 polypropylene suture. This can be accomplished by multiple sutures, both running and interrupted sutures. The apex is then cored out with a coring device from the LVAD accessory kit. Once the tissue is removed, inspection of the apex is done to make sure no internal structures would be impeding the flow of blood. The use of pump suckers, or suctions that directly connected to the cardiopulmonary machine, are utilized for better visualization inside the heart and reduce the total blood loss.

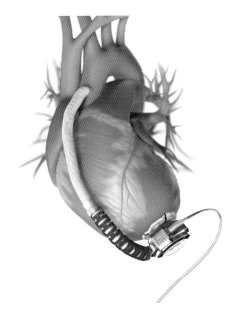

Figure 22-11 BTT, HVAD system. (Reproduced with permission from Medtronic.)

- The LVAD is prepped on a separate table and then brought up to the OR table. It is then attached to the sewing ring and fixed in place with an LVAD clip, which is also in the accessory kit. The outflow graft, which is pre-connected, is then cut to length to reach the aorta. With the use of a partial occluding clamp, the outflow graft is anastomosed to the AO using 4-0 polypropylene suture in a routine fashion. The partial occluding clamp is then removed, and hemostasis is obtained by checking for small leaks in the suture lines. The outflow graft is then thoroughly de-aired by placing small needle holes in the graft for air to escape.

- The next step is to tunnel the power supply, or better known as a driveline. A driveline connects the LVAD to an external power source. The power source is batteries. The batteries fit into a vest that the patient will wear postoperatively. For operative procedures and in-house management, the patient's driveline is connected to an LVAD machine power supply, allowing for adjustments to the LVAD internally, which later will be disconnected from the LVAD Machine power supply and connected to batteries once the procedure is over and/or patient is discharged from the intensive care unit.

- The drive line is tunneled in such a manner that a small umbilical incision is made and brought out through this incision. It is reintroduced into that incision and brought out through a small, cored incision. Preoperatively, this is discussed with the patient as to which side of the body is preferred. Routinely, it is well received on the patient's right side, lateral to the umbilical incision.

- Once the LVAD driveline was brought out through the two separate incisions, the driveline is then connected to the controller and pumping of the LVAD is initiated.

- After appropriate reperfusion of the LVAD, patient was weaned off cardiopulmonary bypass. Careful attention is brought to the LVAD, making sure adequate flow is established Adjustments are made accordingly. A TEE is performed to assess the structural integrity of the heart and to confirm the proper position of the inflow cannula. All cardiopulmonary bypass cannulas are then removed, and hemostasis is maintained. Chest tubes are placed, and the patient is closed in standard fashion.

Heart Transplant

A heart transplant is a treatment for end stage CHF. This is considered after all other modalities have been discussed and all other forms of treatment have been utilized. All other organs must be in good health to be considered for a transplant. Heart transplants, simply put, is removing a diseased heart from the recipient, procuring of a viable heart from a donor, and then implanting the new donor heart into the recipient.

Reasons such as coronary artery disease, cardiomyopathy, hypertensive heart disease, and congenital heart defect are also diagnoses that could warrant a heart transplant.

When examining the procedures for heart transplant, it primarily revolves around timing. The timing of donor's and recipient's cardiectomy is crucial in minimizing the ischemic time on the donor heart, as well as the length of bypass time for the recipient. Ischemic time should be less than 4 hours.

Precise communication between both the procurement and the transplant teams is crucial in planning a timeline. The recipient exposure should be started before the donor heart arrives.

Surgical Procedure

- A median sternotomy is made in standard fashion. The following structures are then dissected: aorta, PA, SVC, and inferior vena cava (IVC). If the patient is a redo sternotomy, which means they have had previous heart surgery before the transplant, dissection is minimal around the structures just enough to access for cannulation. Further dissection can be done once the patient is on bypass.

- Cannulation is differentiated using bicaval cannulation. Bicaval cannulation is when two venous cannulas are utilized for drainage when the left side of the heart is opened for a procedure (eg, mitral valve surgery). In this case, the diseased heart will be removed so cannulas will need to be placed above and below the atrium. Normally, the SVC and the IVC are cannulated. Once cannulated, umbilical tapes, or also called caval snares, and a Rummel tourniquet are then used to snare the SVC and IVC for total occlusion. Alternatively, the femoral vein and the SVC can be cannulated. Once cannulated in either fashion, both cannulas are connected with a "Y" connector and tubing and then connected to the venous line.

- For a patient that has had previous redo sternotomy, the groins are then accessed. Per surgeon's directive, an SA may perform open cutdown to the femoral artery and vein. Alternatively, a percutaneous approach may be utilized. This is done to decompress the heart, since scar tissue will be present. This also allows for any attachment of the scar tissue to the sternum to be decompressed as well. Care is taken by the SA and surgeon when preforming a redo sternotomy to not cut into the heart accidentally and cause significant blood loss.

- Once the procurement team has landed (or is leaving procurement facility if it is local), the aorta is cross-clamped. The aorta and PA are transected at the level of the semilunar valves. The SVC and then the IVC are transected. The atrium is opened and transected toward the mitral valve and then continued circumferentially until the native heart is then removed. This is referred to as a cardiectomy.

- The aorta, PA, IVC, and SVC are then trimmed for an adequate fit for the new donor heart. When the heart arrives and is removed from its respective packaging, it is thoroughly examined.

- The donor heart is then inspected and found to be anatomically normal. This means that there were no signs of a PFO and there was no visible valvular abnormality/disease. Once inspected, the new heart is then flushed with cardioplegia to preserve it until the cross-clamp is removed and blood flow is re-established. This is done after each anastomosis. It should be noted that when the heart comes out of the container, 1 L of cardioplegia is given antegrade. Another 300 cc is given after the second anastomosis and their after until cross-clamp is removed.

- The donor heart is then implanted with the following sequences of anastomosis: left atrium, PA, aorta, IVC, and SVC.

- The first anastomosis, which is the left atrium, is performed using a 3-0 polypropylene suture. The SA in this procedure is to carefully hold the donor heart while the stitches are placed and make sure that the suture is lining up with the donor heart and the recipient tissue.

- After the anastomosis is completed, a vent cannula is placed in the right PV (pulmonary vein) to remove air and any venous blood that could enter the lungs.

- The PAs are then addressed. If the recipient tissue needs trimmed, it is done at this time for correct sizing. The anastomosis is completed with a 4-0 polypropylene suture.

- Once secured and tied, the aorta is then addressed. The anastomosis of the aorta is also completed with a 4-0 polypropylene suture. Once finished, a pledged vent stitch and respective cannula are then placed into the new aorta to allow venting of the heart.

- Once placed, the cross-clamp is removed, and focus is now on the SVC and IVC. The SVC and IVC anastomosis can be done on a beating heart, as the patient is still on bypass. This also aids the warming of the patient and allows the heart to naturally start beating and perfusing, respectively. The IVC anastomosis is performed with a 4-0 polypropylene suture. The SVC anastomosis is performed with a 4-0 polypropylene suture.

- Once all structures have been anastomosed, time is given for the donor heart to perfuse adequately. Typically, the data shows that you allow roughly 15 minutes for every hour the heart was ischemic. Once the time allotted for reperfusion, the patient is slowly taken of the bypass machine. Once off bypass, the patient is then carefully monitored.

- The patient is then rewarmed, and a TEE assessment is done. This is to access the function of the heart, valves, and measure ejection fraction. After confirmation, a routine closure is performed.

Postop. After the sternotomy is closed, dressings are applied in a sterile fashion to all incisions and around chest tube sites. Dressings are determined by surgeon's preference. Patients are then connected to monitors to measure vitals and then moved over to the patient's ICU bed and subsequently transferred to the ICU for postoperative management. Once in the unit, the patient is cared for by the ICU staff and an x-ray is ordered.

In rare cases that the sternum cannot be closed primarily, the pericardium is packed with gauze, and or lap sponges and covered with a wound vac. The patient will then go to the intensive care unit with their chest open and will be brought back to the OR for closure at a later date. These situations are determined on a case-by-case basis and may be caused by numerous factors. Cardiomegaly post procedure, fluid overload, and excessive bleeding are some of the more prominent reasons why a patient's chest will need to be left open. Also, if the patient had an extended time on bypass and hypercoagulated or if a major redo surgery occurred and raw surfaces of the heart are continuing to bleed, medical correction of the labs may be needed. This process will take more time to correct, so transferring them to the unit is appropriate. This also allows time for the heart to rest after such an extensive operation.

Postop ICU. The first 48 hours are the most crucial after cardiac surgery. Directly after the procedure, there is always risk for bleeding. This is one of the main potential complications. Care is taken in the unit to monitor the drainage from the chest tubes. Any substantial bleeding should be addressed. First, the patient will be given blood, platelets, and any other prescribed medication to alter the bleeding rate. Should the patient output still increase, the patient may need to be brought back to the OR for exploration for bleeding. Bleeding can also cause the patient to tamponade or collect blood and fluid on and/or around the heart. Tamponade compresses the heart so it will not function and will eventually cause the patient to arrest.

Another complication to any cardiac surgery is an air leak in the thoracic space, or better termed pneumothorax. Normally, this is found after on the postop x-ray. A small pigtail catheter is placed bedside by the ICU attending or the attending surgeon to relieve the air.

Discharge Planning. Before leaving the hospital, patients will have a discharge summary and a pamphlet/handout on their instructions when leaving the hospital. Discharge for most patients will be within 5 to 7 days but will ultimately vary between patients. For someone who underwent cardiac surgery, it will take around 4 to 6 months to fully recuperate and go back to their normal life. The patient will be on various prescribed medicines with restrictions to such activities like driving, lifting, etc. Patients are encouraged to walk frequently and strategize on how to live a healthier lifestyle. They will be tasked with controlling their blood pressure and monitoring their blood sugar, exercise regularly, decrease stress, and control their weight. Lastly, a follow-up appointment will be scheduled in the office/clinic about 1-week postop and then another appointment 2 to 3 months out. It is strongly encouraged during this visit, and subsequent visits, to see how they are healing. Also, during these visits, it is strongly advised that the patient notify their immediate family and future generations to get screened for heart disease as it is hereditary.

References

1. Biga LM, Dawson S, Harwell A, et al. 19.3 Cardiac Cycle. http://library.open.oregonstate.edu/aandp/chapter/19-3-cardiac-cycle/. Accessed on September 5, 2023.

2. Fuster V, Alexander RW, O'Rourke RA. *Hurst's The Heart.* 10th ed. New York, NY: McGraw-Hill; 2001:53.

3. Coronary Artery Disease (CAD). Published 12 March 2013; archived from the original on 2 March 2015; retrieved 23 February 2015. Accessed on September 5, 2023.

4. Wong ND. Epidemiological studies of CHD and the evolution of preventive cardiology. *Nature Reviews. Cardiology.* May 2014;11(5):276-289. doi:10.1038/nrcardio.2014.26.

5. GBD 2015 Disease and Injury Incidence and Prevalence, Collaborators. Global, regional, and national incidence, prevalence, and years lived with disability for 310 diseases and injuries, 1990–2015: a systematic analysis for the Global Burden of Disease Study 2015. *Lancet.* Oct 2016;388(10053):1545-1602. doi:10.1016/S0140-6736(16)31678-6.

6. GBD 2015 Mortality and Causes of Death, Collaborators. Global, regional, and national life expectancy, all-cause mortality, and cause-specific mortality for 249 causes of death, 1980–2015: a systematic analysis for the Global Burden of Disease Study 2015. *Lancet.* Oct 2016;388(10053):1459-1544. doi:10.1016/S0140-6736(16)31012-1.

7. Cohen G, Tamariz MG, Sever JY, et al. The radial artery versus the saphenous vein graft in contemporary CABG: a case-matched study. *The Annals of Thoracic Surgery.* 2001;71(1):180-185, discussion 185-186. doi:10.1016/S0003-4975(00)02285-2.

Bibliography

Alexander JH, Smith PK. Coronary-Artery Bypass Grafting. *N Engl J Med.* 2016;374(20):1954-1964. doi: 10.1056/NEJMra1406944.

The A.D.A.M. Medical Encyclopedia. MedlinePlus. Updated by Michael A. Chen and reviewed by David Zieve, and the A.D.A.M. Editorial team. https://medlineplus.gov/encyclopedia.html. Accessed October 17, 2023.

23

Thoracic Surgery

Jason Ryu

DISCUSSED IN THIS CHAPTER

1. Anatomy Patient Considerations
2. Diagnostics and Indications for Surgery
3. Surgical Procedures Affecting The Thorax Cavity

MEDIASTINOSCOPY

Introduction

As the name suggests, mediastinoscopy is a procedure where a scope (-scopy) is utilized to enter into the mediastinal space. The procedure was first described in 1954 by Harken and his group[1] who inserted the laryngoscope through supraclavicular incision. Since then, this procedure went through modifications to become the "gold standard" in oncologic staging we know today. It has low mortality (0.5%) and morbidity (2.5%).[2]

The space explored, the mediastinum, comes from the Latin word "mediastinus" meaning "midway." As the name suggests this space lies in the center of the thoracic cavity. Specifically, this location is the space between the lungs and the sternum. The main purpose of this procedure is to retrieve lymph nodes to properly stage the cancer. Lung cancer tends to spread through our body's lymph system and these nodes are sites to check how far it has spread. It also has other uses such as looking for other cancers that may grow around mediastinum such as tracheal cancer, lymphoma, or thymoma. Lastly, this method can be utilized to look for any inflammation in the area for diseases, such as Sarcoidosis or infections. There are two main classifications of mediastinoscopy: cervical mediastinoscopy and transthoracic mediastinoscopy (AKA Chamberlain's procedure).

Anatomy and Physiology

Due to the nature of this procedure and location of the scope, understanding of the anatomical structures may be initially difficult. It is imperative to first understand the anatomy of the mediastinal spaces (see Figure 23-1). Mediastinum is an area bordered by five sides. Laterally lies the two pleural cavities, and in the posterior border lies the vertebral column, and is between thoracic inlet and the diaphragm. This area contains many structures, mainly the heart and its great vessels, trachea, esophagus, thymus gland, and lymph nodes. The main nerves that exist in this area are the phrenic nerve, vagus nerve, and the left and right recurrent laryngeal nerve. Furthermore, mediastinal space is divided into superior and inferior mediastinum at the level of thoracic vertebral space T4 and T5. The inferior mediastinum is further divided into anterior, middle, and posterior mediastinum.

Because the main purpose of this procedure is to obtain the lymph nodes, the numbering system should be understood. The lymph nodes in the mediastinal spaces are numbered superior to inferior, and then follow the tracheal divisions. Also, at the top is the supraclavicular node station 1. Then within the superior mediastinal zone, there are nodes numbered 2, 3, and 4. Node stations 5 and 6 are surrounding the aorta. Station 7 is located on the carina of the trachea. The node stations then follow down the bronchi which is not explored through mediastinoscopy.

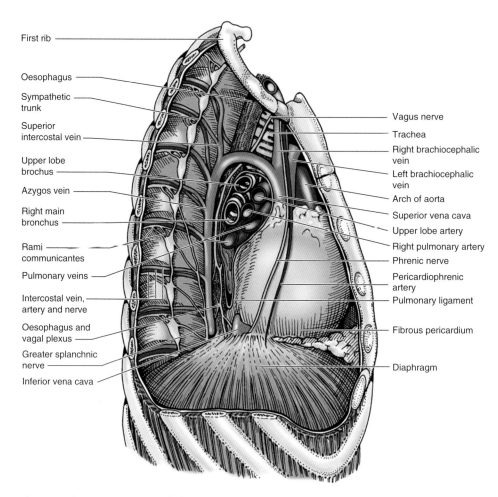

First rib

Oesophagus

Sympathetic trunk

Superior intercostal vein

Upper lobe brochus

Azygos vein

Right main bronchus

Rami communicantes

Pulmonary veins

Intercostal vein, artery and nerve

Oesophagus and vagal plexus

Greater splanchnic nerve

Inferior vena cava

Vagus nerve

Trachea

Right brachiocephalic vein

Left brachiocephalic vein

Arch of aorta

Superior vena cava

Upper lobe artery

Right pulmonary artery

Phrenic nerve

Pericardiophrenic artery

Pulmonary ligament

Fibrous pericardium

Diaphragm

Figure 23-1 · The mediastinum human anatomy with detailed information on a white background. (Reproduced with permission from Chummy S. Sinnatamby. Last's Anatomy E-Book. Elsevier Health Sciences; 2011.)

As the function of the lymph system is to bring the interstitial fluid back into the bloodstream, the lymph nodes act as a checkpoint allowing us to locate how far the metastatic tumor has spread. Then the patient's care plan can be decided among the oncologist, the radiologist, and the thoracic surgeon.

Diagnosis (Modalities)

The indication for mediastinoscopy is to stage metastatic lung cancer, tissue biopsy of tumors, or removal of any mediastinal masses. Lymphoma (Hodgkins and non-Hodgkins) can be diagnosed via mediastinoscopy along with sarcoidosis. Masses such as thymoma and benign mediastinal cysts can also be excised. It can be used to diagnose and treat mesothelioma.

There are several major contraindications for this procedure, such as any anterior mediastinal mass, previous recurrent laryngeal nerve injury, ascending aortic aneurysm, previous mediastinoscopy, and an inoperable tumor. It is up to the surgeon's discretion whether to proceed with mediastinoscopy if the patient has superior vena cava syndrome, severe tracheal deviation, thoracic inlet obstruction, or history of radiation therapy.

Common physical examination includes palpation of cervical and supraclavicular lymph nodes. Neck extension should be evaluated for proper positioning for the procedure. Close attention should be given for any respiratory symptoms that may be exacerbated with exercise or positioning.

There are no specific lab tests required for this procedure. Pulmonary function test, EKG, chest x-ray with posteroanterior and lateral views, and CT scan of chest and the neck are needed.

Surgical Approaches

There are two main approaches depending on which lymph node sites are needed. Cervical mediastinoscopy gives access to pre-tracheal, paratracheal, and anterior subcarinal lymph nodes. The transthoracic mediastinoscopy or Chamberlain's procedure gives access to aortopulmonary lymph nodes.

Anesthesia Considerations. General anesthesia is used for this procedure (see Figure 23-2).

Position. Patient will be positioned supine with a scapular roll under the shoulders to extend the neck. Head should be

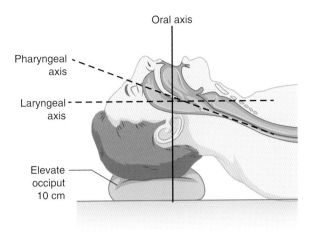

Oral axis
Pharyngeal axis
Laryngeal axis
Elevate occiput 10 cm

Figure 23-2 · Example of neck extension needed not only for intubation but also for mediastinoscopy. (Reproduced, with permission, from Tintinalli J, Stapczynski J, Ma O, Cline D, Cydulka R, Meckler G. *Tintinalli's Emergency Medicine: A Comprehensive Study Guide.* 8th ed. New York, NY: McGraw Hill; 2016.)

positioned as high as possible for maximum extension. Arms may be tucked.

Specifics for Surgical Skin Prep. Surgical prep that will not cause any allergic reaction may be used. Prep from chin down to the entire anterior chest/upper abdomen. This is in case an emergency sternotomy is required.

Procedure Including the Role of the Assistant (SA, PA, and Resident)

Cervical Mediastinoscopy:

- The surgical assistant's (SA) role is to assist in the exposure of the mediastinal space so that the scope can be entered.
- Incision is made transversely 1 to 2 cm above the sternal notch.
- The platysma is divided transversely.
- The strap muscles are then separated in the midline.
- Dissection is carried down to pretracheal fascia.
- Incise the fascia and enter the pretracheal space.
- Important note is that this space is avascular.
- Use blunt finger dissection along anterior trachea into the mediastinum.
- In most cases, one should be able to reach the carina as well as R and L mainstem bronchi.
- Locate the vascular landmarks at this point by digital palpation.
- Insert the mediastinoscope and stay within the dissected pretracheal plane.
- Do not lose sight of trachea and bronchi as it is important in maintaining orientation.
- Use the suction device to perform blunt dissections as needed.

- Dissecting along the right and left main stem bronchi will also help maintain orientation.
- Lymph nodes can be dissected and freed as much as possible using suction devices.
- The sample can be obtained with laryngeal biopsy forceps.
- Usually the upper paratracheal stations are sampled first, followed by lower paratracheal stations.
- Subcarinal space is sampled last as it is most prone to bleeding.
- Check for any bleeding and utilize cautery for hemostasis as needed.
- The layers are then closed starting with the platysma (usually 2-0 vicryl, deep dermal interrupted) and then the skin (can utilize quill or 4-0 monocryl for closure).

Chamberlain's Procedure: The alternative procedure is known as Chamberlain's procedure or simply anterior mediastinoscopy.

- Incision is over the second rib at the junction with the sternum.
- Some surgeons use a vertical incision to allow extension of the dissection to another interspace as needed.
- Pleura is pushed laterally using blunt dissection until aortopulmonary (AP) window lymph nodes are reached.
- A scope can be inserted through interspace for dissection rather than removing costal cartilage.

Steps Highlighted, Key Landmarks, Core Nerves/Arteries to Be Identified. If the team is on the right plane, it should be pretty bloodless surgery. Major vascular landmarks to watch for are the innominate artery, azygos vein, arch of the aorta, and the right (R) main pulmonary artery. Be careful not to injure the recurrent laryngeal nerve. Left side injury is most common and usually results from traction during dissection. About 5% to 10% of patients may develop hoarseness following the procedure. Use of cautery is discouraged when taking biopsy from 4L station as the left recurrent laryngeal nerve is close by.

Modifications/Additional Associated Procedures Commonly Seen

- If there is excessive bleeding, packing with raytac may be used for 2-10 min.
- If a patient becomes hypotensive, this constitutes an emergency situation and quick recognition of the situation is crucial. A major vessel injury has occurred.
- Most likely sites of injury are the azygos vein and the right main pulmonary artery.
- Median sternotomy offers most flexibility in dealing with the injuries.
- This is preferred for any injuries to azygos vein, aortic arch, innominate artery, main pulmonary artery, and the superior vena cava. Selection of sternotomy or thoracotomy is a decision made by the surgeon's assessment of the most likely area of injury.
- Primary goal is to achieve vascular control. This could require cardiopulmonary bypass.

• Any hilar injuries often require intrapericardial access. Vascular clamps are placed proximally and distally from the injury and then the repair can be performed (check vascular section for vascular repairs). If unable to gain control of the injury, giving a full dose of heparin and bypass is necessary.

Postop
Drains Used/Dressings:

• Drains are unnecessary unless the pleural space is entered.

• Many different types of dressing may be utilized on the incision per surgeon's preference (steri-strips, primapore, dermabond, etc.).

Potential Complications Common to This Procedure

• Compression of the innominate artery can occur when the mediastinoscope is inserted. This could affect the readings of the art line and pulse ox if placed on the right arm.

• As the patient is positioned in reverse Trendelenburg, there is a possibility that vascular injuries could lead to air being introduced to the vascular system.

• Left recurrent laryngeal nerve injury is at most risk due to its position. Bilateral recurrent laryngeal nerve injury can lead to complete respiratory failure and the need for a surgical airway.

THORACOTOMY

Wedge Resection

Introduction. Initially, pulmonary resections were performed to treat tuberculosis back in late 1890s.[3] Many following studies were done taking smaller sections such as lobectomy and even segmentectomy and wedge resections. Wedge resections are favorable with patients with lesser pulmonary function and thus would suffer greatly from removing a larger portion of the lung. With the advancement of radiographs, we are able to notice even smaller lung nodules that can be removed through wedge resection. The procedure is considered nonanatomical as the location of removal is solely dependent on the location of the nodules or tumors. The function of this operation is to remove a small wedge of lung that contains the tumor identified through radiographs so that it can be analyzed pathologically (see Figure 23-3).

Anatomy and Physiology. The thoracic cavity contains the mediastinal space and the two pleural cavities. The left lung is divided into two lobes whereas the right lung is divided into three lobes. Airway from trachea is divided into primary, secondary, and tertiary bronchi and then into bronchioles where the CO_2 and O_2 exchange occur within the capillary walls. Important landmarks in the lungs include the cardiac notch in the left lung, oblique and horizontal fissures that divide the lobes, the hilum, pulmonary ligament, and the costomediastinal recess (see Figure 23-4).

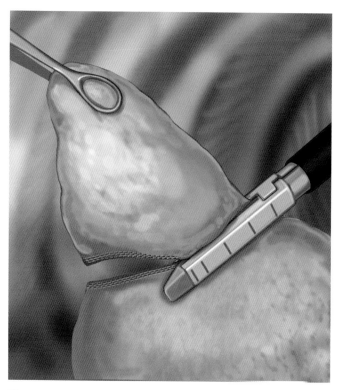

Figure 23-3 · Wedge resection. (Reproduced with permission from Sugarbaker DJ, Bueno R, Burt BM, Groth SS, Loor G, Wolf AS, eds. *Sugarbaker's Adult Chest Surgery*. 3rd ed. New York, NY: McGraw Hill; 2020.)

Muscles that are affected during this procedure are latissimus dorsi, anterior serratus, and rhomboid muscles. These muscles cover the outer layer of the rib cage.

Core Anatomical Organ(s) Affected. The lung mass to be removed can be located within any of the lung segments.

Etiology. Lung tumors and inflammation can be caused from smoking, secondhand smoke, exposure to radiation, chemicals, and can be idiopathic.

Diagnosis (Modalities). Indications for wedge resection include patients with multiple synchronous tumors, inability to tolerate lobectomy due to insufficient pulmonary reserve, metastasectomies, and resection of undiagnosed lesions for pathological review.

Diagnostic Tests

• Chest x-ray posteroanterior and lateral views

• CT scan of the chest to identify the nodules

• Pulmonary function test

Procedural Considerations (Nonsurgical Treatment, Surgical Treatment, List of Surgical Approaches such as Open, Laparoscopic, and Robotic)

Open thoracotomy is not a preferred method for wedge resections. Minimally invasive video-assisted thoracoscopic surgery (VATS) is preferred. If desired, the procedure may also be done through the use of robotic instruments.

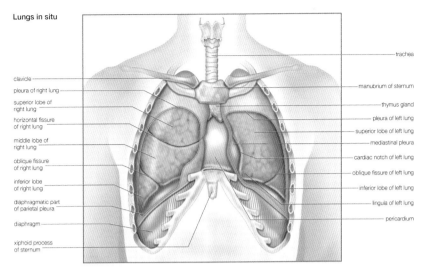

Lungs in situ

clavicle
pleura of right lung
superior lobe of right lung
horizontal fissure of right lung
middle lobe of right lung
oblique fissure of right lung
inferior lobe of right lung
diaphragmatic part of parietal pleura
diaphragm
xiphoid process of sternum

trachea
manubrium of sternum
thymus gland
pleura of left lung
superior lobe of left lung
mediastinal pleura
cardiac notch of left lung
oblique fissure of left lung
inferior lobe of left lung
lingula of left lung
pericardium

Figure 23-4 · Overview of the lungs in-situ. (Used with permission from Encyclopaedia Britannica/UIG/Getty Images)

Treatment Options. Depending on pathological findings, combination therapies such as chemotherapy, radiation therapy, and surgical resection can be utilized.

Anesthesia Considerations. General anesthesia is used. Insertion of double-lumen endotracheal tube, arterial line, and central venous line is placed. An epidural catheter is considered for postop pain management.

Position

Lateral Decubitus Position:

- Patient's xiphoid should be at the level of the bed break/flex point.
- Patient will be positioned lateral decubitus with the side of wedge resection up.
  - NOTE: The naming convention can be confusing. Right lateral decubitus position is with the right side of the body *lower* than the left and thus left side up, and vice versa.
- There are many methods to achieve this. Some may use bean bags that suctions and can be shaped into a hard positioning aid and some use gel rolls. Whatever the method the patient should be properly secured.
- Axillary roll should be placed to get the pressure off the shoulders.
- Flex the bed so that the hips are lowered and proper access can be made to the chest cavity. Use the reverse Trendelenburg position to adjust so that the patient's chest is parallel with the floor if necessary.
- Arm board is necessary to hold both arms out.
- Pillows should be placed between the legs in a T fashion and the bottom leg bent to avoid any pressure injuries.
- Secure the patient's hips to the bed utilizing straps or a strong tape (see Figure 23-5).

Specifics for Surgical Skin Prep. Check to see if the patient has any shellfish or betadine allergies before deciding on the prep material. Patient should be prepped at least from neck to hips and from middle of sternum in the front to middle of the back (vertebral column).

Procedure Including the Role of the Assistant (SA, PA, Resident)

- Wedge resection can be conducted either through the utilization of VATS or thoracotomy (open procedure). VATS procedure is described later in the chapter and specific thoracotomy procedure will be discussed in the next segment as it is more relevant with lobectomy procedure.
- Once the pleural space has been entered through either VATS or thoracotomy, the ventilation on the side of the lung for the procedure is turned off and suctioned down if needed.
- Once the nodule has been identified, with the use of laparoscopic stapler the section of the lung is cut out.
- The section is then sent for frozen pathological analysis and checked for clear margins before proceeding to close the

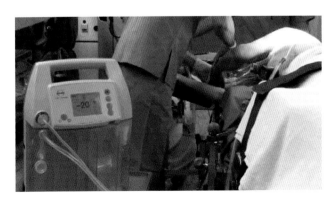

Figure 23-5 · Example of lateral decubitus position.

incision. If the margins are not clear, a bigger section needs to be taken.

Postop

Drains Used/Dressings:

• See the section on thoracotomy or VATS.

• Prognosis with treatment, eg, PT, radiation.

Potential Complications Common to This Procedure:
Air leaks after a resection is a well-known problem. There will be some degree of postoperative air leak. Majority of air leaks originating from the periphery of the lung will stop within 24 to 48 hours after surgery (see Figure 23-6).

Lobectomy

Introduction. Lobectomy has been the standard for lung cancer surgery for a long time. This is where a whole lobe of the lung is removed along with the tumor. Lesser resections such as segmentectomies or wedge resections are not recommended due to a randomized trial that was conducted in 1980s showing higher death rate and a higher locoregional recurrence rate associated with limited resections without any benefits.[4] If the patient is able to tolerate a lobectomy for removal of the diseased lung, it is preferred. This operation can be completed through

thoracotomy incision or with the use of VATS (see section VATS; Figure 23-7).

Anatomy and Physiology. Depending on the side of the operation, there are slight anatomical differences. Right side of the lung contains three lobes: upper, middle, and lower. The right main pulmonary artery is longer, the azygos vein runs posterior to anterior and lies on top of the right mainstem bronchus. The venous branches vary greatly from patient to patient and special care should be taken during dissection not to damage them unknowingly.

Diagnosis (Modalities). Indications for this surgery include persistent lung abscess, chronic tuberculosis (see Figure 23-8), emphysema, benign tumor, untreatable fungal infections, and lung cancer.[5]

Similar imaging and clinical tests should be performed for lobectomy that was performed for the wedge resection (see Figure 23-9).

Procedural Considerations (Nonsurgical Treatment, Surgical Treatment, List of Surgical Approaches such as Open, Laparascopic, and Robotic). Many times, VATS is preferred choice of operation due to faster recovery time and studies that show adjuvant therapy can be safely delivered quicker with a

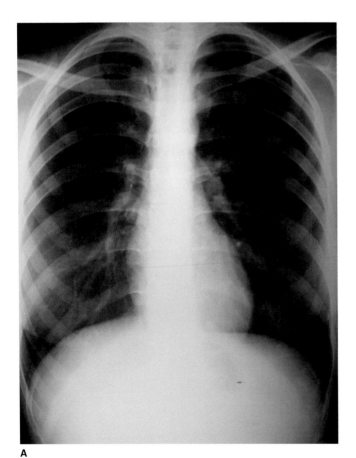
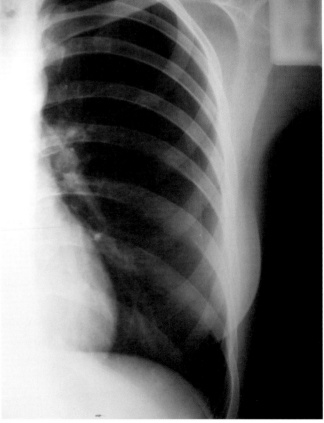

A   **B**

Figure 23-6 · Example of a complication, pneumothorax. (Reproduced, with permission, from Tintinalli J, Stapczynski J, Ma O, Cline D, Cydulka R, Meckler G. *Tintinalli's Emergency Medicine: A Comprehensive Study Guide.* 8th ed. New York, NY: McGraw Hill; 2020.)

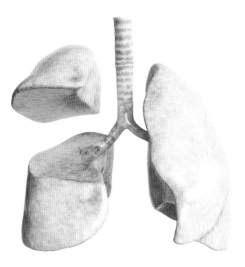

Figure 23-7 · Three-dimensional rendered image of lobectomy. (Used with permission from CreVis2/Getty Images.)

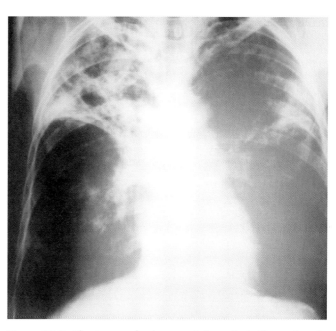

Figure 23-8 · Chest x-ray of pulmonary tuberculosis. (Reproduced, with permission, from Tintinalli J, Stapczynski J, Ma O, Cline D, Cydulka R, Meckler G. *Tintinalli's Emergency Medicine: A Comprehensive Study Guide*. 8th ed. New York, NY: McGraw Hill; 2020.)

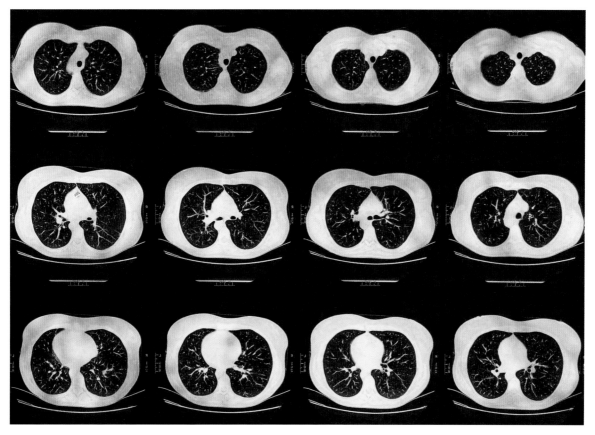

Figure 23-9 · MRI slices of the chest. (Used with permission from Bunyos/Getty Images.)

minimally invasive approach.[5] However, this is not always possible and open thoracotomies are still being performed.

Requirements for Procedure (No Smoking, Lose Weight, Psychological Counseling, Nutritional Aspects, Etc.). Smoking cessation can greatly increase procedural outcome and should be encouraged with the patient.

Anesthesia Considerations. General anesthesia is used. Insertion of double-lumen endotracheal tube, arterial line, and central venous line is placed. An epidural catheter is considered for postop pain management.

Position. Lateral decubitus position previously described in wedge resection is used.

Specifics for Surgical Skin Prep. Check to see if the patient has any shellfish or betadine allergies before deciding on the prep material. Patient should be prepped at least from neck to hips and from middle of sternum in the front to middle of the back (vertebral column).

Procedure Including the Role of the Assistant (SA, PA, Resident). Posterolateral thoracotomy is most commonly used in incision as it provides excellent access to the anatomical structures and safe control of pulmonary blood vessels (see Figure 23-10).

Thoracotomy:

- The skin incision is from the anterior axillary line over fifth or sixth intercostal space and curved around posteriorly to medial aspect of the scapula.
- The latissimus dorsi muscle is transected with the use of cautery. Care should be taken to transect the muscle perpendicular to the fibers so that it can be approximated easily at the end of the procedure.
- Serratus anterior muscle is usually spared. The muscle is elevated and retracted anteriorly. This muscle can be used to remedy the postop complication of bronchopleural fistula.

- If needed, the anterior portion of trapezius and rhomboid muscle can be divided.
- Most operations are conducted through the fifth intercostal space. The ribs can be counted starting with the first rib by reaching underneath the scapula.
- It is important to note that the intercostal vein, nerve, and artery are hidden under the intercostal groove and access should be acquired above the ribs.
- Depending on the need of the exposure, a large segment of the rib can be removed, or a small 1-cm segment removed, or a periosteal elevator can be used to just spread the ribs.
- No matter what the need, care should be taken not to break the ribs as they are extremely painful and could cause postoperative respiratory complications.
- Endothoracic fascia and parietal pleura is opened and the pleural space is now entered.
- Rib spreader retractor is utilized and if desired suture can be placed on serratus anterior muscle to retract it away from the field. The ribs need to be spread slowly to avoid fractures (see Figure 23-11).

Lobectomy Specific Procedure:

- The lung is freed from peripheral adhesions with scissors, cautery, blunt dissection, or sponge on a stick.
- The hilum is then entered.
- The branches of pulmonary arteries and veins are identified for the lobe to be removed.
- They are ligated and divided with scissors. Based on the surgeon's preference, staples or nonabsorbable ties can be used.
- After identifying the bronchus branch, it is clamped and the lung is inflated to clearly visualize the margins of the lobe.
- The bronchus can be divided with scissors and closed with staples or mattress sutures.

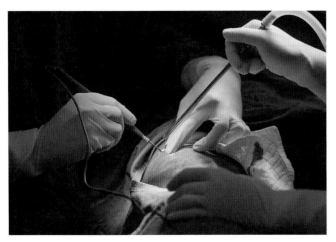

Figure 23-10 · First incision of thoracotomy. (Used with permission from ChaNaWiT/Getty Images.)

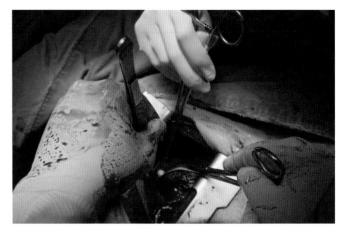

Figure 23-11 · Thoracotomy incision and entering of the pleural space. (Used with permission from ChaNaWiT/Getty Images.)

- Pleural flap or other methods of securing bronchus may be used.
- The pleural space is explored for hemostasis and the remaining lobes are inflated to check for air leaks.

Thoracotomy Closure:

- Chest tubes can be inserted. They are usually placed in line with anteriosuperior iliac spine on skin and pointing towards the apex of the pleural space.
- Use of drills to make holes into the upper and lower ribs for the suture is recommended for closure as it prevents damage to the neurovascular bundle. Absorbable interrupted sutures are utilized to close the intercostal space.
- Then the muscle layer, subcutaneous tissue and skin are closed.

Modifications/Additional Associated Procedures Commonly Seen:

- Depending on the patient's clinical presentation and the preference of the surgeon, an anterolateral thoracotomy approach may be used.
- This positioning is where the patient is supine but elevated approximately 30° to 45° on the ipsilateral side. The thoracotomy incision is made between the third and fourth intercostal spaces.
- During this incision, it is important to recognize the location of the mammary artery and care should be taken not to damage the vessel.

Postop
Drains Used/Dressings:

- Straight chest tube drain is usually used with the tip pointing at the apex (see Figure 23-12).
- Several different dressings can be utilized per surgeon's preference such as 4 × 4 with tegaderm, primapore, medipore tape, and dermabond.

Potential Complications Common to This Procedure:

- Some of the complications are bleeding, infection, pneumothorax, pleural effusion, shoulder dysfunction, and pain.
- More specific complications may include persistent air leaks, bronchopleural fistula, ischemic necrotizing pneumonia, nonobstructive atelectasis, pulmonary edema, dehiscence, hemothorax, esophagopleural fistula.[6]

Pneumonectomy

Introduction. The first pneumonectomy was performed in 1933 for lung carcinoma by Evarts Graham.[7] Initially this procedure was popular for TB emphysema but is more commonly used for mesothelioma nowadays. Pneumonectomy is a radical procedure where one side of the lung is completely removed. Lungs play a very important physiological role not only with gas exchange but also functions as a defense against outside infections. They are always exposed to a wide variety of carcinogens and microorganisms. These exposures could lead to lung deterioration which could ultimately need a pneumonectomy (see Figure 23-13).

Diagnosis (Modalities). The procedure is usually utilized to remove malignant lung cancer. Additional reasons may include extensive unilateral bronchiectasis, chronic pulmonary abscess affecting more than one lobe, and mesothelioma.

Similar imaging and clinical tests should be performed for pneumonectomy that was performed for the wedge resection.

Procedural Considerations (Nonsurgical Treatment, Surgical Treatment, List of Surgical Approaches such as Open, Laparascopic, and Robotic). Someone requiring a pneumonectomy may not have any other options. Many patients will have other comorbidities that may affect the surgical outcome.

This procedure has a mortality rate of 3% to 12%;[7] hence, preoperative staging should assess the true need for the

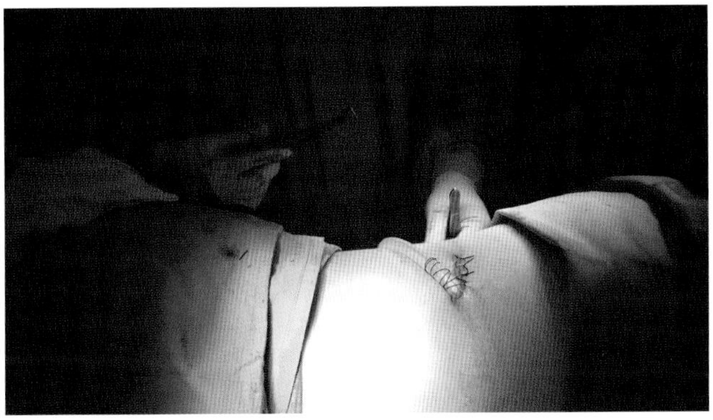

Figure 23-12 • Chest tube postoperation. (Used with permission from Casa nayafana/Shutterstock.)

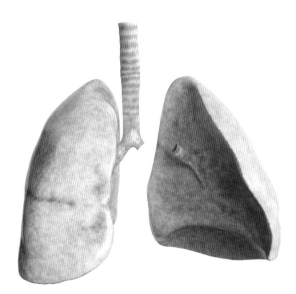

Figure 23-13 • Three-dimensional rendered image of pneumonectomy. (Used with permission from Crevis/Shutterstock.)

operation when possible. VATS can be used but thoracotomy is the most often used method for pneumonectomies.

Anesthesia Considerations. General anesthesia is used. Insertion of double-lumen endotracheal tube, arterial line, and central venous line is placed. An epidural catheter is considered for postop pain management.

Position. Lateral decubitus position previously described in wedge resection is used.

Specifics for Surgical Skin Prep. Check to see if the patient has any shellfish or betadine allergies before deciding on the prep material. Patient should be prepped at least from neck to hips and from middle of sternum in the front to middle of the back (vertebral column).

Procedure Including the Role of the Assistant (SA, PA, Resident)

- Thoracotomy and the access to pleural space is obtained through the process described previously with lobectomy.
- The peripheral adhesions are removed and the lung is mobilized with the use of cautery, blunt dissection, and scissors.
- The pulmonary ligament is also divided and the hilum is dissected.
- The superior pulmonary vein is retracted and pulmonary artery is dissected.
- The branches of the pulmonary artery and vein is ligated with right angle vascular clamps and sutures. Alternatively, staples can be used.
- The inferior pulmonary vein is exposed and also ligated.
- Bronchus is clamped and cut near tracheal bifurcation. Mattress sutures or staples can be used.
- Transecting mainstem bronchus near the carina is necessary to decrease residual bronchial stump length. The stump should be covered with autologous tissue such as pleura, pericardial fat, or intercostal muscle to prevent bronchopleural fistula.
- The pleural space is explored for hemostasis and air leaks.
- Chest tubes are inserted. They are usually placed in line with anteriosuperior iliac spine on skin and pointing toward the apex of the pleural space.
- The lung is inflated to ensure proper inflation and placement of the chest tube.
- Use of drills to make holes into the upper and lower ribs for the suture is recommended for closure as it prevents damage to the neurovascular bundle. Absorbable interrupted sutures are utilized to close the intercostal space.
- Then the muscle layer, subcutaneous tissue and skin are closed.

Modifications/Additional Associated Procedures Commonly Seen. For patients with extensive advanced malignant lung disease, extrapleural pneumonectomy may be performed. This is an expanded procedure that resects the parietal and visceral pleura, hemidiaphragm, pericardium, and mediastinal lymph nodes.[6]

Postop
Drains Used/Dressings:

- Straight chest tube drain is usually used with the tip pointing at the apex.
- Several different dressings can be utilized per surgeon's preference such as 4 × 4 with tegaderm, primapore, medipore tape, and dermabond.

Potential Complications Common to This Procedure:

- Some of the complications are bleeding, infection, pneumothorax, pleural effusion, shoulder dysfunction, and pain.
- More specific complications may include persistent air leaks, bronchopleural fistula, ischemic necrotizing pneumonia, nonobstructive atelectasis, pulmonary edema, dehiscence, hemothorax, and esophagopleural fistula.[6]

Lung Decortication

Introduction. Lung decortication is a process of removing fibrous capsule that had formed around the lung due to chronic inflammation or bleeding that had occurred. First lung decortication was probably conducted in 1895 by Dr. Delorme, who is known to be the pioneer of chest surgery. Post World War I, the need for lung decortication for inflammatory diseases were widely accepted.[8] It was not until much later that lung decortication was established as a procedure to treat tuberculosis emphysema and clotted hemothorax.

This case can cause a significant amount of blood loss and trauma to the patient. The goal is to allow the lungs to fully expand once again.[9]

Etiology. Persistent inflammation, tumor, and hemothorax can lead to thick capsule formation around the lungs requiring decortication.

Similar imaging and clinical tests should be performed for pneumonectomy that was performed for the wedge resection.

Procedural Considerations (Nonsurgical Treatment, Surgical Treatment, List of Surgical Approaches such as Open, Laparascopic, and Robotic). Open thoracotomies are the preferred method for lung decortication. However, there have been some reports of successful decortication with VATS.

Anesthesia Considerations. General anesthesia is used. Insertion of double-lumen endotracheal tube, arterial line, and central venous line is placed. An epidural catheter is considered for postop pain management.

Position. Lateral decubitus position previously described in wedge resection is used.

Specifics for Surgical Skin Prep. Check to see if the patient has any shellfish or betadine allergies before deciding on the prep material. Patient should be prepped at least from neck to hips and from middle of sternum in the front to middle of the back (vertebral column).

Procedure Including the Role of the Assistant (SA, PA, Resident)

- Thoracotomy is performed.
- One deviation might be that the pleural fascia might be tightly attached to lungs.
- Care must be taken not to damage the lungs. Blunt dissection is preferred.
- When dissecting near mediastinum, it is important to identify the pericardium so that it can be avoided.
- The lung and its capsule is separated from the chest wall, mediastinal surface, and pericardium.
- The fibrous membrane is then carefully incised and separated from the lung enclosed within.
- Once the capsule is removed, lungs are reinflated and checked for hemostasis, leaks, and other trauma to the area.
- Chest tubes are inserted and closed similarly to other procedures utilizing thoracotomy.

Postop

Drains Used/Dressings:

- Chest tube for the pleural space entered, straight; make sure that the tip is pointing to the top toward the head.

Potential Complications Common to This Procedure:

Similar complications with all the thoracotomy and VATS procedures.

Pectus Excavatum/Carinatum

Introduction. Pectus deformities are the most common congenital chest anomalies; pectus excavatum (PE) occurs in 23 per 10,000 births.[10] Pectus carinatum (PC) is a chest deformity where the chest is pushed forward, opposite of PE. PE is more common in men and constitutes about 90% of congenital chest deformities. PE is when the anterior chest wall is depressed into the thoracic cavity. It could present minor symptoms and cosmetic issues or it could present with disabling cardiopulmonary symptoms such as right-sided heart compression and restrictive pulmonary deficits. Up to 43% of patients have family history.[10] It is caused by unbalanced growth of costochondral regions during development. Studies show shorter ribs on the more depressed side of the defect. At current state, the exact genes responsible are unknown. It has shown to be associated with scoliosis and connective tissue disorders such as Marfan syndrome, Ehlers-Danlos syndrome, and Noonan syndrome.[11] Although this is an inherited disease, many patients will not present until early adolescence (see Figures 23-14 and 23-15).

Anatomy and Physiology. Understanding of the anatomy of the anterior chest wall is crucial for this procedure.

Etiology. The cause of PE and PC are both unknown.

Diagnosis (Modalities)

PE:

- Cardiac auscultation may reveal a murmur as sunken chest might affect cardiac function.

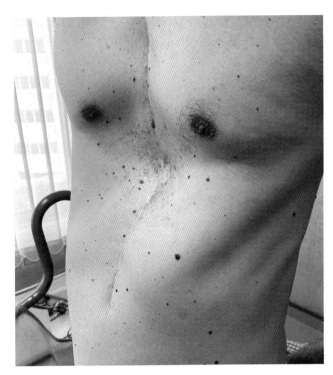

Figure 23-14 · Patient with severe pectus excavatum. (Used with permission from Douglas Olivares/Shutterstock)

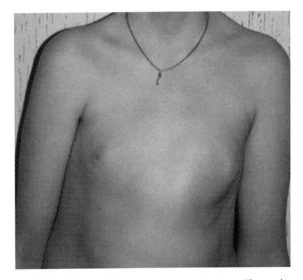

Figure 23-15 · Patient with severe pectus carinatum. (Reproduced with permission from Heide ST, Curtis RR, Deborah W, et al. Marfan Syndrome (MFS): Visual Diagnosis and Early Identification. *J Pediatr Health Care.* 2017;31(5):609-617; Figure 2.)

- Imagining can detect a leftward shift of the heart.
- Patients show greater symptoms as they age.
- Adolescent patients can be susceptible to psychological stress and trauma from peers.
- Imaging studies include noncontrast CT or MRI. CT is needed on both inspiration and expiration.

- To assess the extent of the deformity, Haller index or correctional index may be used. Exact mathematical analysis is beyond the scope of the practice of SAs.

- ECHO should be performed to rule out substantial anatomic abnormalities.

- In many cases, PE does not seem to substantially affect pulmonary function but pulmonary function tests should be performed.

PC:

- Generally does not have symptoms other than cosmetic defects.

Procedural Considerations (Nonsurgical Treatment, Surgical Treatment, List of Surgical Approaches such as Open, Laparascopic, and Robotic)

PE: There are two procedures used to correct the deformity: Ravitch procedure or Nuss procedure. Nuss procedure is the current preferred method of treatment.

PC: Three methods of treatment are available for PC: nonsurgical bracing, surgical correction, and cosmetic concealment.

Surgically, the patient can be treated with Ravitch procedure or reversed Nuss procedure.

Anesthesia Considerations. General anesthesia is used. Insertion of double-lumen endotracheal tube, arterial line, and central venous line is placed. An epidural catheter is considered for postop pain management.

Position. Patient will be supine.

Specifics for Surgical Skin Prep. Check to see if the patient has any shellfish or betadine allergies before deciding on the prep material. Patient should be prepped at least from neck to hips and from middle of sternum in the front to middle of the back (vertebral column).

Procedure Including the Role of the Assistant (SA, PA, Resident)

PE—Nuss Procedure:

- Incision is made for the scope.

- Another incision made to introduce the tunneling device.

- With the use of the device, anterior mediastinum is dissected.

- The device exits the chest on the other side at the same level of the introduced site.

- Then a long passer material is passed to the hook and through the chest.

- The passer is then tied to the pre-bent pectus bar, and is guided through the chest.

- The bar is rotated 180 degrees slowly making sure that it is flat against the sternum and is able to lift the sternum without issue.

- The area is checked for any severe bleeding or lacerations that might have occurred (see Figure 23-16).

- Chest drain is placed and the lungs are inflated.

- Incisions are then closed.

- Patient returns after 6 to 10 months to have the bar removed.

PE and PC—Ravitch Procedure: NOTE: This procedure is much more invasive and has higher chance of complications. It is usually reserved for older groups of patients (see Figure 23-17).

- Incision is made right under the rib cage, subcostal incision.

- Pectoralis major is split and dissected away toward top and bottom.

- A U-shaped cut is made around the sternum.

- Piece by piece, each costal cartilages are cut out.

- A wedge of sternal angle is cut and nonabsorbable suture such as 2-0 proline is used to connect and elevate the body and the manubrium of the sternum together.

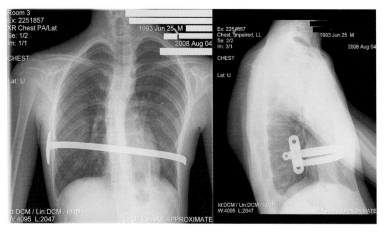

Figure 23-16 · X-ray of chest post-Nuss procedure.

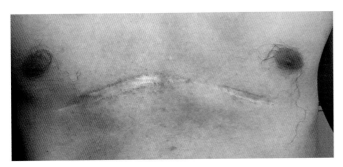

Figure 23-17 · Typical scar left post-Ravitch procedure.

- Stainless steel struts elevate the sternum.
- Two hemovac drains above and below pectoralis muscle.
- Pectoralis muscle is repaired/re-approximated.

PC—Abramson Procedure aka Reversed Nuss Procedure (Relatively New)

- Steel bar is placed subcutaneously *in front* of the sternum and anchored bilaterally to the ribs.

Modifications/Additional Associated Procedures Commonly Seen. The examples include CBDE for a lap chole and conversion to open procedure.

Any damage to the heart or its great vessels during anterior mediastinum dissection requires a quick conversion to thoracotomy or sternotomy to gain hemodynamic control.

Postop

Drains Used/Dressings:

- Hemovac drain or chest tubes may be needed depending on the procedure.

Potential Complications Common to This Procedure:

- Some of the complications include persistent pain, migration of the metal bar, hemothorax, pneumothorax, damage to critical organs such as the heart or the lungs, and return of the PE or PC.

Video-Assisted Thoracoscopic Surgery (VATS)

Introduction. The very first thoracoscopic examination described was in 1910 by Jacobaeus.[12] Ever since, the minimally invasive endoscopic procedures have evolved to handle many different procedures. Today, the vast majority of thoracic surgery can be completed with the use of an endoscope. It can be utilized to perform anywhere from a wedge resection to pneumonectomy. As the technology advances, more and more procedures are becoming minimally invasive and VATS is definitely here to stay.

Diagnostic Modalities Relevant to Condition/Procedure. Similar imaging and clinical tests should be performed for VATS that was performed for the wedge resection.

Preoperative Preparation

Anesthesia Considerations: General anesthesia is used. Insertion of double-lumen endotracheal tube, arterial line, and central venous line is placed. An epidural catheter is considered for pos op pain management.

Position: Patient may be in supine or lateral decubitus position depending on the operation (see Figure 23-18).

Specifics for Surgical Skin Prep: Check to see if the patient has any shellfish or betadine allergies before deciding on the prep material. Patient should be prepped at least from neck to hips and from middle of sternum in the front to middle of the back (vertebral column).

Procedure Including the Role of the Assistant (SA, PA, Resident)

- Initial 2- to 3-cm camera port incision is made between fifth and seventh intercostal spaces, usually the trocar size is 10 or 12 mm.
- The field is then assessed to make sure that the thoracoscopic procedure can proceed.
- Additional port sites are created so that graspers and other instruments can be inserted (see Figure 23-19).
- The insufflation, if desired, can be used to shrink the lungs further.
- The number and the size of port sites vary greatly depending on the procedure.
- Once the operation is complete, the port sites can be used as a chest tube site.
- When closing the layers, close attention should be taken to approximate each muscle layer before tending to subcutaneous tissue and skin.

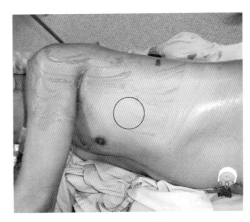

Figure 23-18 · Lateral positioning for VATS and the circle marks the usual location for the first camera port site. (Reproduced, with permission, from Chen CH, Lee SY, Chang H, Liu HC, Chen CH, Huang WC. Technical aspects of single-port thoracoscopic surgery for lobectomy. *J Cardiothorac Surg.* 2012;7:50.)

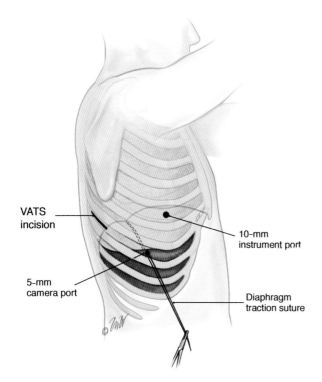

Figure 23-19 · Ideal port placement for direct repair with VATS. (Reproduced, with permission, from Sugarbaker DJ, Bueno R, Burt BM, Groth SS, Loor G, Wolf AS, eds. *Sugarbaker's Adult Chest Surgery*. 3rd ed. New York: McGraw Hill; 2020.)

Modifications/Additional Associated Procedures Commonly Seen: The examples include CBDE for a lap chole and conversion to open procedure.

If any major vessels are damaged or if the hemodynamic control is lost, the operation needs to be converted into open thoracotomy or sternotomy.

Postop

Drains Used/Dressings:

- Straight chest tube drain is usually used with the tip pointing at the apex.

- Several different dressings can be utilized per surgeon's preference such as 4 × 4 with tegaderm, primapore, medipore tape, and dermabond.

Potential Complications Common to This Procedure:

- VATS carry similar complications to the procedure such as air leaks, atelectasis, abnormal heart rhythms, excessive bleeding, pneumonia, emphysema, wound infection, and blood clots.

LUNG TRANSPLANTATION

Introduction

The lung transplant attempts have been recorded as early as 1946 on dogs.[13] It was not until 1980s we started to see hope of success. Today, with a careful donor matching system, organ preservation, and advancement in immunosuppressants, lung transplant is a possible therapy for patients with end-stage lung diseases. There are now more options to prolong the life of the donor organ through *ex vivo* lung perfusion.

Today there are 1019 people waiting on a lung donor and the average wait time is anywhere between 80 and 1000 days depending on the condition.[14] Many times, the procedure will be completed as heart and lung transplant *en bloc*. Depending on the patient's needs, it may also be single or double lung transplant. The process to gain access for the procedure should be similar in all three cases.

Studies show that lung transplantation can improve quality of life and prolong survival. However, there still are lot of challenges facing postoperative complications. This section will briefly discuss the process of lung transplant pertaining to the SA (see Figure 23-20).

Anatomy and Physiology

It is important to have an understanding of the lung and its hilar structures covered in previous sections.

Diagnosis (Modalities)

Indications for lung transplantation are broad and include many end-stage lung diseases: Chronic obstructive pulmonary disease (COPD), Cystic Fibrosis (CF), pulmonary fibrosis, and pulmonary malignancy.

There are many other factors to consider, such as age, life expectancy, rehabilitation potential, and both emotional and psychological support postoperation.

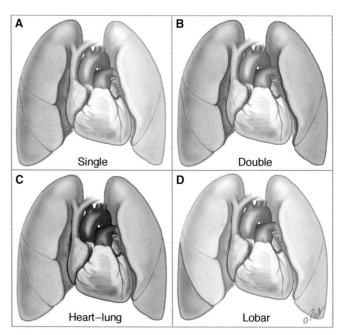

Figure 23-20 · Anatomy of lung transplant. (Reproduced, with permission, from Sugarbaker DJ, Bueno R, Burt BM, Groth SS, Loor G, Wolf AS, eds. *Sugarbaker's Adult Chest Surgery*. 3rd ed. New York: McGraw Hill; 2020.)

Anesthesia Considerations

- General anesthesia is used for this procedure.

Position

- Patient will be positioned supine. Arms may be tucked or abducted depending on the procedure.
- Surgical prep that will not cause any allergic reaction may be used. Prep from chin down to the entire anterior chest/upper abdomen.

Procedure Including the Role of the Assistant (SA, PA, Resident)

Sternotomy Approach

- Median sternotomy incision, covered in cardiac surgery section, is made (see Figure 23-21).
- Mediastinal pleura is opened exposing the pulmonary vein and arteries.
- At this location, phrenic nerve is close by and must be protected.
- For double lung transplant, the procedure can be completed sequentially.
- This is to allow one lung to support the body while the other is being replaced.
- Many times the surgeon will opt to utilize Cardiopulmonary bypass (CPB) for the procedure instead.
- Pneumonectomies are then performed.
- The vascular structures can be stapled.
- Sutures through the cartilage of broncus can be used to aid in retraction during anastomosis.

- Pericardium around pulmonary artery (PA) and left atrium can be opened to lengthen the structures if needed.
- Now the donor lung can be prepared and brought in.
- The pulmonary vein and artery are divided from the en bloc donor organs and the bronchus is divided two rings above the secondary carina.
- End to end anastomosis is completed starting with the bronchus then the pulmonary vein and artery.
- Hemostasis is then achieved before closing of the sternotomy.

Clamshell/Hemiclamshell Approach

- Clamshell approach is associated with much greater postoperative pain and complications.
- However, due to its great exposure of the chest cavity, it is warranted in certain patient populations.
- Hemiclamshell incision is made for single lung transplant.
- Some surgeons might prefer abducting the arms instead of tucking them for this procedure.
- The incision is made from a midaxillary line following the submammary fold, usually around the level of fifth or sixth rib.
- Pectoralis major is separated and lifted up exposing the chest wall.
- Serratus muscle is divided, and incision is completed toward the sternum.
- Pleura is then entered.
- Intercostal muscles are divided to maximize rib spreading.
- Internal mammary vessels are ligated.

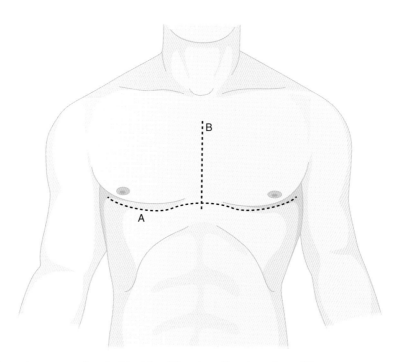

Figure 23-21 · Incisions in thoracic surgery: clamshell incision (A) and median sternotomy (B).

- Bilateral rib spreaders are used.
- Internal thoracic pedicle should be ligated to avoid bleeding.
- Now the lung transplant can proceed with the exposure of hilar structures.
- For closure, pericostal stitches are placed.
- The muscle and subcutaneous tissue are closed sequentially.

Postop

Postoperative period is very crucial to the lung transplant procedure. Immediately after, there is a large focus on ventilatory and hemodynamic support. The biggest fear is the body's rejection of the organ or failure of the new lung's function. A major cause of morbidity and mortality within the first 72 hours is primary graft dysfunction. The patient will be on immunosuppression. Even though lung transplant techniques have improved drastically, the 5-year survival rate still remains at only about 50%.[13]

References

1. Harken DE, Black H, Clauss R, Farrand RE. A simple cervicomediastinal exploration for tissue diagnosis of intrathoracic disease; with comments on the recognition of inoperable carcinoma of the lung. *N Engl J Med*. 1954;251(26):1041-1044.

2. Migliore M, Nardini M, Rogers L, Vidanapathirana P, Dunning J. *A Pragmatic View of the Usefulness of Video-Mediastinoscopy in the Modern Era*. 2000 [online]; Jovs.amegroups.com. http://jovs.amegroups.com/article/view/20378/20111. Accessed on September 12, 2023.

3. Asamura H, Aokage K, Yotsukura M. Wedge resection versus anatomic resection: extent of surgical resection for stage I and II lung cancer. *Am Soc Clin Oncol Educ Book*. 2017;37:426-433.

4. Ginsberg RJ, Rubinstein LV. Randomized trial of lobectomy versus limited resection for T1 N0 non-small cell lung cancer. Lung Cancer Study Group. *Ann Thorac Surg*. 1995;60(3):615-622.

5. Samson PC. Indications for lobectomy and pneumonectomy in pulmonary tuberculosis. *Ann Surg*. 1940;112(2):201-211.

6. Chang B, Tucker WD, Burns B. Thoracotomy. [Updated 2020 Jul 31]. In: StatPearls [Internet]. Treasure Island (FL): StatPearls Publishing; 2020 Jan. https://www.ncbi.nlm.nih.gov/books/NBK557600/. Accessed on September 12, 2023.

7. Baue AE. Evarts A. Graham and the first pneumonectomy. *JAMA*. 1984;251(2):261-264. doi:10.1001/jama.1984.03340260065032.

8. Lynn RB, Wellington JL. Decortication of the lung. *Can Med Assoc J*. 1963;89:1260-1265.

9. Andrade-Alegre R, Garisto JD, Zebede S. Open thoracotomy and decortication for chronic empyema. *Clinics (Sao Paulo)*. 2008;63(6):789-793.

10. Rajabi-Mashhadi MT, Ebrahimi M, Mobarhan MG, Moohebati M, Boskabady MH, Kazemi-Bajestani SM. Prevalence of chest wall deformities in a large sample of Iranian children aged 7-14 years. *Iran J Pediatr*. 2010;20(2):221-224.

11. Meester JAN, Verstraeten A, Schepers D, Alaerts M, Van Laer L, Loeys BL. Differences in manifestations of Marfan syndrome, Ehlers-Danlos syndrome, and Loeys-Dietz syndrome. *Ann Cardiothorac Surg*. 2017;6(6):582-594. doi:10.21037/acs.2017.11.03.

12. He J. History and current status of mini-invasive thoracic surgery. *J Thorac Dis*. 2011;3(2):115-121. doi:10.3978/j.issn.2072-1439.2010.03.01.

13. Yeung JC, Keshavjee S. Overview of clinical lung transplantation. *Cold Spring Harb Perspect Med*. 2014 Jan 1;4(1):a015628. doi:10.1101/cshperspect.a015628.

14. *2020 Current U.S. Waiting List*. Department of Health and Human Services, Health Resources and Services Administration, Healthcare Systems Bureau, Division of Transplantation, Rockville, MD; United Network for Organ Sharing, Richmond, VA; University Renal Research and Education Association, Ann Arbor, MI.

24

Peripheral Vascular Disease

Steve Noyce

DISCUSSED IN THIS CHAPTER

1. Peripheral vascular anatomy and physiology
2. Peripheral vascular disease
3. Diagnostics and indications for intervention
4. Arterial and venous insufficiency
5. Nonsurgical and surgical treatments for peripheral vascular disease.

SURGICAL ANATOMY

Vascular system is made up of two individual systems: the venous system and the arterial system. Figure 24-1 shows the two systems.

Arteries

Each artery, no matter what its size, has walls with three distinct layers, also known as coats. The delicate innermost layer, the tunica intima, consists of a lining, a fine network of connective tissues, and a layer of elastic fibers bound together in a membrane pierced with many openings. The middle layer, the tunica media, is made up principally of smooth (involuntary) muscle cells and elastic fibers arranged in roughly spiral layers. The outermost layer, the tunica adventitia, is a tough layer consisting mainly of collagen fibers that act as a supportive element. The large arteries differ structurally from the medium-sized arteries in that they have a much thicker tunica media and a somewhat thicker tunica adventitia.

Arteries are muscular elastic tubes that must transport blood under a high pressure exerted by the pumping action of the heart. The pulse, which can be felt over an artery lying superficial to the surface of the skin (epidermis), results from the alternate expansion and contraction of the arterial wall as the beating heart forces blood into the arterial system via the aorta. Large arteries branch off from the aorta and in turn give rise to smaller arteries until the level of the smallest arteries, or arterioles, is reached. The threadlike arterioles carry blood to networks of microscopic vessels called capillaries, which supply nourishment and oxygen to the tissues and carry away carbon dioxide and other waste products of metabolism by way of the veins. The carotid artery commences at the aorta in the chest as the common carotid and progresses up through the neck to the head. Adjacent to the larynx, the common carotid divides into the external and internal carotid arteries. The external carotid arteries provide blood to the face and scalp. The internal carotid arteries provide blood to the brain. The largest artery in the human body is the aorta, which arises from the left ventricle of the heart. The aorta arches briefly upward before continuing downward close to the spine; the arteries that supply blood to the head, neck, and arms arise from this arch and travel upward. As it descends along the spine, the aorta gives rise to other major arteries that supply the internal organs of the thoracic cavity. After descending to the abdomen, the aorta divides into two terminal branches, each of which supplies blood to one leg.

Veins

As in the arteries, the walls of veins have three distinct layers, or coats: an inner layer, tunica intima; a middle layer, tunica media; and an outer layer, tunica adventitia. Each layer has several sub layers. The tunica intima differs from the inner layer of an artery: many veins, particularly in the arms and legs, have valves to prevent backflow of blood, making blood flow unidirectional and the elastic membrane lining the artery is absent in the vein, which consists primarily of endothelium and scant connective tissue. The tunica media, which in an artery is composed of muscle and elastic fibers, is thinner in a vein and contains less muscle and elastic tissue, and proportionately more collagen fibers (collagen, a fibrous protein, is the main supporting element in connective tissue). The tunica adventitia consists

Human circulatory system

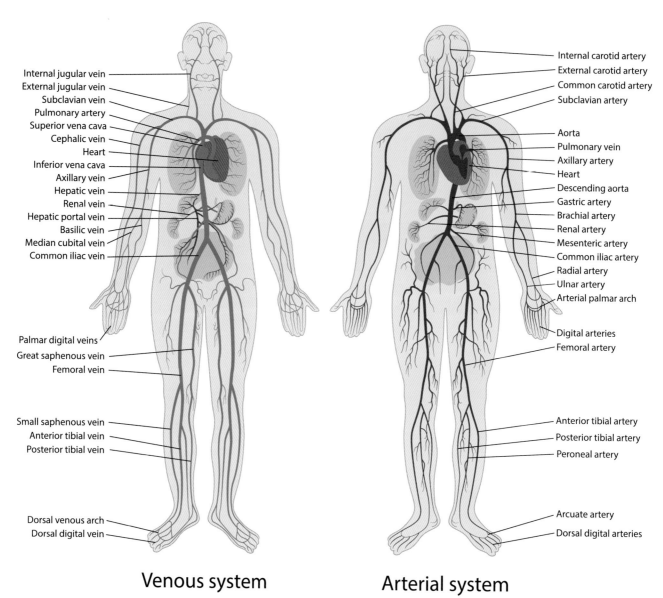

Venous system

- Internal jugular vein
- External jugular vein
- Subclavian vein
- Pulmonary artery
- Superior vena cava
- Cephalic vein
- Heart
- Inferior vena cava
- Axillary vein
- Hepatic vein
- Renal vein
- Hepatic portal vein
- Basilic vein
- Median cubital vein
- Common iliac vein
- Palmar digital veins
- Great saphenous vein
- Femoral vein
- Small saphenous vein
- Anterior tibial vein
- Posterior tibial vein
- Dorsal venous arch
- Dorsal digital vein

Arterial system

- Internal carotid artery
- External carotid artery
- Common carotid artery
- Subclavian artery
- Aorta
- Pulmonary vein
- Axillary artery
- Heart
- Descending aorta
- Gastric artery
- Brachial artery
- Renal artery
- Mesenteric artery
- Common iliac artery
- Radial artery
- Ulnar artery
- Arterial palmar arch
- Digital arteries
- Femoral artery
- Anterior tibial artery
- Posterior tibial artery
- Peroneal artery
- Arcuate artery
- Dorsal digital arteries

Figure 24-1 · Human circulatory system. (Used with permission from Olga Bolbot/Shutterstock.)

chiefly of connective tissue and is the thickest layer of the vein. As in arteries, there are tiny vessels called vasa vasorum that supply blood to the walls of the veins and other minute vessels that carry blood away. Veins are more numerous than arteries and have thinner walls as a result to lower blood pressure. They tend to parallel the course of arteries.

PERIPHERAL VASCULAR DISEASE

Peripheral vascular disease (PVD) is a slow and progressive circulatory disorder. Narrowing, blockage, or spasms in a blood vessel can cause PVD. PVD may affect any vessel outside of the heart and brain including the arteries, veins, or lymphatic vessels. PVD in arteries is referred to as arterial insufficiency or peripheral artery disease (PAD).

PAD affects over 200 million adults worldwide and the incidence of PAD increases to as high as 20% in people over the age of 70. Although PAD has traditionally been perceived as a disease affecting men, the prevalence of PAD appears to be equal among senior men and women (see Figure 24-2). PAD usually involves atherosclerotic disease in the abdominal aorta, iliac, and femoral arteries. Atherosclerotic plaque builds up slowly on the inside of arteries. In the early stages of PAD, the arteries compensate for the plaque buildup by dilating to preserve flow through the vessel. Eventually, the artery cannot dilate any further, and the atherosclerotic plaque starts to narrow the arterial flow lumen. In some cases, the cause of sudden ischemia may be emboli either of cardiac origin or from atherosclerotic disease of the aorta. Emboli tend to be most common at sites of arterial bifurcation or where vessel branches have an

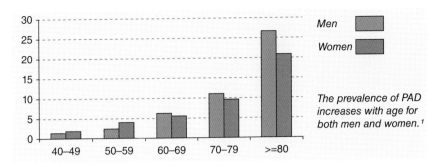

Figure 24-2 · The prevalence of PAD increases with age for both men and women.

abrupt takeoff. The most common site of atherosclerotic plaque buildup is the carotid bifurcation where the common carotid divides into the internal and external carotid arteries. The femoral artery is the most common site for emboli, followed by the iliac arteries, aorta, and the popliteal arteries.

Both men and women are affected by PAD; however, African Americans have an increased risk of PAD. Hispanics may have similar to slightly higher rates of PAD compared with non-Hispanic white people. Approximately 6.5 million people aged 40 and older in the United States have PAD.

Arterial Insufficiency

Arterial insufficiency is decreased blood flow or lack of blood flow through the arteries. Arterial insufficiency occurs when the arteries become narrowed or blocked by an underlying disease or condition. Narrowing of an artery is also called *stenosis*. This decreases blood flow and oxygen delivery to the cells, tissues and organs being supplied by your arteries. Without adequate blood flow and oxygen, cells and tissues may not function properly and may even begin to necrose. The most common cause of arterial insufficiency is atherosclerosis or hardening of the arteries. Atherosclerosis is a condition in which fatty material, such as fats and cholesterol in the bloodstream, collects along the walls of arteries. The fatty material thickens and hardens into deposits called plaques. Plaques narrow your arteries and may eventually block blood flow through them.

Arterial insufficiency or PAD can affect many regions of the body. The symptoms of arterial insufficiency will depend on the arteries and the areas of the body that are affected. When arteries to the brain are affected, you may experience symptoms of a transient ischemic attack (TIA) or stroke. This includes dizziness, numbness, drooping facial muscles, vision problems, slurred or inability to speak, numbness in arms or legs particularly on one side of the body (see figure 24-3). Arterial insufficiency or PAD that affects arteries supplying the kidneys (renal arteries) causes kidney problems and eventual kidney failure. Symptoms related to the renal arteries include malaise, nausea, headaches, fatigue, loss of appetite, high blood pressure with decreased kidney function, unexpected weight loss (see Figure 24-3 and Table 24-1).

Arterial insufficiency or PAD that affects arteries supplying intestines (mesenteric arteries) causes abdominal pain,

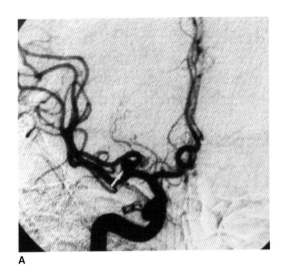

A

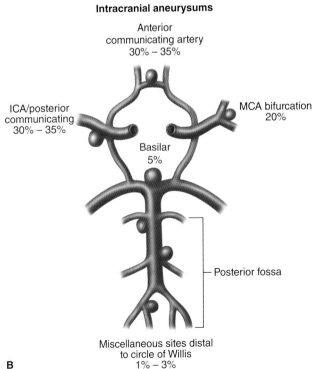

B

Figure 24-3 · Blood supply to the brain. (Reproduced with permission from Osborn AG. *Handbook of Neuroradiology: Brain and Skull.* St. Louis, MO: Elsevier, 1991.)

TABLE 24-1 • DIAGNOSTICS FOR PAD

Test	Method	Looks at
Doppler ultrasound	Sound waves for imaging	Blood flow in your vessels
Ankle-brachial index (ABI)	Ultrasound and blood pressure cuff around your ankle and arm, measured before and during exercise	Comparison of blood pressure readings in your leg and arm, as lower pressure in your leg could indicate a blockage
Angiography	Injected dye in a catheter that is guided through the artery	The flow of dye through blood vessels to diagnose the clogged artery
Magnetic resonance angiography (MRA)	Magnetic field imaging	Image of blood vessels to diagnose blockage
Computerized tomography angiography (CTA)	X-ray imaging	Image of blood vessels to diagnose blockage

diarrhea, acute mesenteric ischemia. Symptoms associated with mesenteric arteries include abdominal pain after eating, constipation, diarrhea, flatulence, nausea, vomiting, and unexpected weight loss.

PAD in lower extremities is the most prevalent. About half the people diagnosed with PAD are symptom free. For those with symptoms, the most common first symptom is painful leg cramping that occurs with exercise and is relieved by rest (intermittent claudication). During rest, the muscles need less blood flow, so the pain disappears. It may occur in one or both legs depending on the location of the clogged or narrowed artery. Other symptoms of PAD are:

- Changes in the skin, including decreased skin temperature, or thin, brittle, shiny skin on the legs and feet.
- Hair loss on the legs or toes, non-healing wounds, and gangrene.
- Weak pulses in the legs and feet.
- Pain, burning, or aching at rest commonly in the toes at night while lying flat.
- Numbness, weakness, and heaviness in muscles.
- Toenails can thicken or become opaque.
- Males can become impotent.

Arterial insufficiency and PAD treatments include lifestyle changes.

Nonsurgical Treatment

Non-surgical lifestyle changes that are treatment plans for some patients include getting regular physical activity, controlling cholesterol levels in a healthy range, maintaining a healthy body weight, maintaining a normal blood pressure, smoking cessation, and incorporating a healthy diet. A healthy diet reduces the amount of cholesterol and fat in the diet. Drug therapy is another non-surgical approach to treating PAD and includes vasodilators, rheological agents, hemodilution agents and antithrombotic therapy.

Surgical Treatments

Surgical treatments can consist of but are not limited to angioplasty, intra-arterial thrombolysis, atherectomy, endarterectomy, and even bypass.

Aneurysm

An aneurysm is an abnormal widening or ballooning of an artery due to weakness in the wall of the blood vessel (see Figure 24-4). Aneurysms are dangerous because they may rupture causing uncontrolled blood loss. An aneurysm can occur in any artery or vein in the body but commonly occurs in the aorta, intracranial arteries, and peripheral arteries (see Figure 24-5). Aneurysms in veins (venous aneurysm) are rare.

Aortic aneurysms are mostly found in the abdominal cavity abdominal aortic aneurysm (AAA) below the diaphragm and before the bifurcation. May also occur in the chest or thoracic cavity thoracic aortic aneurysm (TAA). Brain aneurysms (cerebral aneurysms or intracranial aneurysms) occur in any vessel in the brain. Peripheral artery aneurysms are found in the groin, legs, intestines, and spleen.

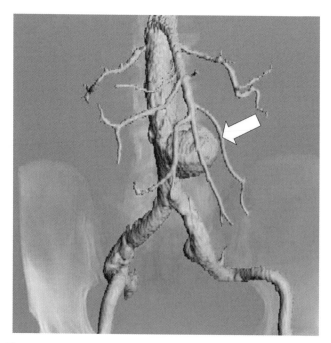

Figure 24-4 • Vessel aneurysm. (Reproduced with permission from Brunicardi FC, Andersen DK, Billiar TR, et al. *Schwartz's Principles of Surgery,* 10th ed. New York, NY: McGraw Hill; 2015.)

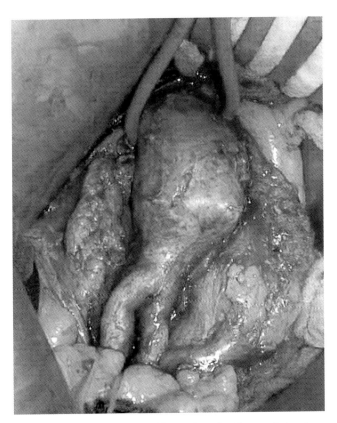

Figure 24-5 · In situ aneurysm. (Reproduced with permission from Brunicardi FC, Andersen DK, Billiar TR, et al. *Schwartz's Principles of Surgery,* 10th ed. New York, NY: McGraw Hill; 2015.)

Aneurysms are caused by a weakness in the wall of a cerebral artery or vein, aortic artery, or peripheral artery. The disorder may result from defects present at birth, from underlying conditions, such as hypertensive vascular disease and atherosclerosis, or from previous trauma to the area of the aneurysm. Pregnancy is often associated with the development and rupture of splenic artery aneurysms. Men 65 years and older are at a higher risk for aneurysm (Table 24-2).

The symptoms of an aneurysm vary with each type and location. Aneurysms that occur in the body or brain generally do not present signs or symptoms until they rupture or

TABLE 24-2 • FACTS ABOUT AORTIC ANEURYSMS IN THE UNITED STATES
Aortic aneurysms or aortic dissections were the cause of 9,904 deaths in 2019.
In 2019, about 59% of deaths due to aortic aneurysm or aortic dissection happened among men.
A history of smoking accounts for about 75% of all abdominal aortic aneurysms.
The U.S. Preventive Services Task Force recommends that men 65 to 75 years old who have ever smoked should get an ultrasound screening for abdominal aortic aneurysms, even if they have no symptoms.

Source: https://www.cdc.gov/heartdisease/aortic_aneurysm.htm

dissect. AAA symptoms include sudden and severe pain in the abdomen or lower back, rapid heart rate, dizziness, shortness of breath, or cold sweats. TAA symptoms include sudden and severe chest pain or back pain, drop in blood pressure, or numbness in the limbs. The symptoms of an intracranial aneurysm begin with a sudden and excruciating headache, vision problems, nausea, and loss of consciousness.

A dissecting aneurysm occurs when part of the aortic wall splits into two separate layers creating a false lumen. Blood pooling into this cavity can occlude branches of the aorta at that site. The most affected artery is the thoracic aorta.

Venous Insufficiency

Chronic venous insufficiency occurs when the leg veins do not allow blood to flow back up to the heart. The valves in the veins make sure that blood flows toward the heart. But when these valves do not work well, blood can also flow backwards. This can cause blood to collect in the legs. Several factors can cause venous insufficiency, though it is mostly caused by blood clots, deep vein thrombosis (DVT) and varicose veins. DVT (see Figure 24-6) is a serious condition in which a blood clot called a thrombus develops in a vein located deep within the body. A DVT usually forms within a large vein in the thigh or calf area, or sometimes the pelvic region. DVT can also develop in the arm, but this is rare. DVT can lead to a dangerous, potentially life-threatening

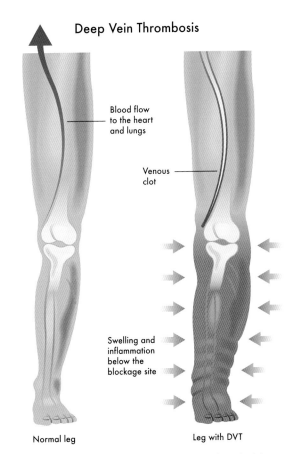

Figure 24-6 · Normal anatomy and DVT signs. (Used with permission from rob9000/Shutterstock.)

complication known as a pulmonary embolism (PE). This occurs when a blood clot breaks off and travels through the bloodstream and lodges in the lungs, obstructing the flow of blood.

DVT can develop without any obvious symptoms. When symptoms do occur, they can include extremity pain, warmth, redness, or swelling. You can have a PE without any symptoms of DVT. PE symptoms include difficulty breathing, faster/irregular heartbeat, chest pain worsens with deep breaths, coughing up blood, low blood pressure, or fainting.

Diagnostics. The most common diagnosis of venous insufficiency and DVT is a duplex ultrasound. The duplex ultrasound checks the speed and direction of blood flow. MRI and CT are also used to get detailed images of the blood vessels. Venogram, intravenous contrast injected into the vein with a series of x-rays, may be performed to pinpoint the location of the thrombosis, A D-dimer blood test is a test that can determine a blood clotting disorder and can be used to measure fibrin proteins; high levels of fibrin proteins suggest DVT.

The treatment of venous insufficiency depends on severity of symptoms. Treatments can range from prescribing compression stockings, and/or anticoagulants, to more invasive treatments. Vein stripping, phlebotomy, sclerotherapy, and venous ablation are all treatments for superficial veins. DVTs depending on severity may require additional treatments such as thrombectomy and thrombolytics. A vena cava filter system may be implanted to prevent blood clots from traveling to the lungs and causing a PE.

Surgical Interventions

Abdominal Aortic Aneurysm Repair: Aneurysmal disease can affect any segment of the aorta, from the aortic root to the aortic bifurcation. The treatment of aortic aneurysms has evolved dramatically in the past three decades, with the introduction of endovascular aneurysm repair using stent grafts. While the technical details of the management of aortic aneurysms vary greatly depending on the location of an aneurysm, the principles remain the same. Successful aortic aneurysm treatment depends on either open replacement or endovascular repair of the aneurysmal segment (see Figure 24-7). Long-term results of endovascular repair suggest that younger patients with long life expectancy and low perioperative risk may benefit more from open repair. Aortic disease is the direct cause of close to 10,000 deaths annually in the United States. The goal of aortic aneurysm repair is to prevent the high morbidity and mortality associated with aneurysm rupture.

The goal of elective AAA repair is to prevent rupture, given the severe morbidity and mortality associated with ruptured aneurysms. Therefore, the decision to treat AAA is based on the associated risk of treatment, the risk of aneurysm rupture, the patient's life expectancy, and patient preference. The primary determinant of rupture risk is maximum aneurysm diameter. Other factors independently associated with rupture include female sex, active smoking, and chronic obstructive pulmonary disease. The Society for Vascular Surgery recommends repairs for all patients of acceptable perioperative risk with AAA greater than or equal to 5.5 cm in diameter as well as

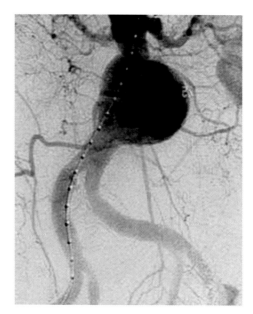

Figure 24-7 · Aortic aneurysm. (Reproduced with permission from Brunicardi FC, Andersen DK, Billiar TR, et al. *Schwartz's Principles of Surgery*, 10th ed. New York, NY: McGraw Hill; 2015.)

TABLE 24-3 • AORTIC RUPTURE RISK	
AAA Diameter (cm)	**Rupture Risk (%/y)**
<4	0
4-5	0.5-5
5-6	3-15
6-7	10-20
7-8	20-40
>8	30-50

Source: Reproduced with permission from Brewster DC, Cronenwett JL, Hallett JW, Johnston KW, Krupski WC, Matsumura JS; Joint Council of the American Association for Vascular Surgery and Society for Vascular Surgery. Guidelines for the treatment of abdominal aortic aneurysms. Report of a subcommittee of the Joint Council of the American Association for Vascular Surgery and Society for Vascular Surgery. *J Vasc Surg.* 2003;37:1106-17.

all patients with saccular and symptomatic aneurysms. These guidelines also suggest repair for women at a diameter of 5.0 to 5.4 cm (Table 24-3).

Open AAA repair consists of replacement of the aneurysmal segment with a synthetic graft. In most cases, a tube graft from the infrarenal neck to the bifurcation is sufficient. However, if the bifurcation or proximal common iliac artery (CIA) are diseased, a bifurcated graft can be used. Successful repair relies on exposure of the abdominal aorta and proximal and distal vascular control.

Transperitoneal Approach

Patient Position and Prep: The patient is positioned in the supine position. With arms out on arm boards. The patient will need to have a Foley catheterization pre-surgery. The surgical assistant (SA) should keep in mind that all pressure points and contact points must be padded as blood flow will be clamp to the lower body during the procedure. No Heating device can be used while cross clamped. Hair removal from nipples to knees should be performed per hospital policy. Skin prep from nipple to knees performed per surgeon preference. Draping will be performed to expose the patient from xiphoid process to above knees. Genital region needs to be covered and protected, to protect from cross contamination.

Anesthesia: Standard monitoring of the patient will include a five-lead ECG and invasive arterial pressure monitoring, which are placed before anesthesia. The patient is placed under general anesthesia often using a balanced combination of fentanyl, remifentanil, and morphine. A central venous line will be placed after the induction of anesthesia. A thoracic epidural catheter may be placed near T8 or T10 for postoperative analgesia.

Surgical Procedure

- Time out is performed per hospital policy.
- Incision: midline laparotomy incision from xiphoid process to the pubis symphysis.
- The SA will help with incisional hemostasis and provide exposure.
- The surgeon preference of self-retaining retractor will be inserted.

- The surgeon and SA will free up and move all the small bowel into the right quadrant.
- Once aneurysm exposure is complete the surgeon using Metzenbaum scissors and DeBakey pickups will incise the retroperitoneum superiorly above the aneurysm and distally past the bifurcation exposing the CIA (Figure 24-8).
- Blunt dissection of the aorta above the aneurysm infrarenal cross-clamp location should be used, when possible, not to interrupt blood flow to the renal arteries.
- The surgeon will determine clamp placement.
- The surgeon and SA should identify and protect the ureters during dissection.
- The surgeon then will work distally to expose and choose a location in the CIA.
- Heparin should be administered by anesthesia provider prior to cross-clamping.
- The SA should be aware at this point to make sure no patient warming devices below cross-clamp are present to prevent ischemic injury.
- The surgeon applies a cross-clamp to the aorta. Anesthesia should be notified, and the SA should take note of the clamp time; eg, DeBakey Fogarty or Satinsky clamp.

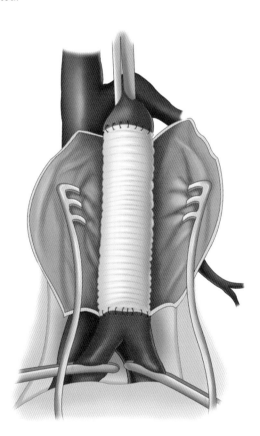
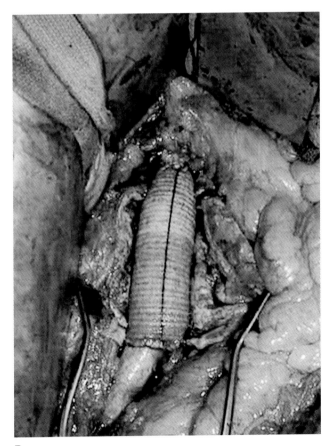

A   **B**

Figure 24-8 · Intraoperative aneurysm repair. (Reproduced with permission from Brunicardi FC, Andersen DK, Billiar TR, et al. *Schwartz's Principles of Surgery,* 10th ed. New York, NY: McGraw Hill; 2015.)

- Distal control will be obtained by clamping bilateral CIAs or with balloon occlusion.
- Aneurysm sac will be opened with scalpel or heavy scissors.
- The SA will assist with removal of thrombus and blood. Cell Saver should not be used at this time to avoid debris.
- Aneurysm walls may be excised but are often left to cover the prosthesis.
- Lumber vessels will have to be controlled, the surgeon will over sew these vessels.
- The surgeon will prepare the aortic cuff by removing calcified plaque.
- Using a double armed vascular suture, the surgeon will sew the anastomosis with through-to-through continuous technique.
- The SA should properly follow the suture keeping the suture tight to ensure a watertight closure.
- Clamps will need to be placed distally on the graft.
- Flashing the aortic clamp, the surgeon will inspect anastomosis for leaks and place interrupted stitches (rescue stitches) where needed.
- Working distally the surgeon will check for back bleeding of distal vessels.
- Each limb of the graft will be anastomosed to CIAs with a double-armed vascular suture with a through-and-through technique.
- The surgeon will open flow to the first limb when anastomosis is completed. Anesthesia must be notified.
- After the distal anastomosis is completed, the surgeon may close the aneurysm sac around the graft preventing a bowel fistula formation.
- The SA should assist the surgeon with an abdominal sweep to ensure no foreign bodies are left in the abdominal cavity.
- The surgeon will close the retro peritoneum and peritoneal cavity.
- Under the direction of surgeon's preference, the SA will close the abdominal wound.
- Dressing will be placed using the surgeon's preference.

Postop Recovery: The patient will go to ICU for recovery. Early postop mobilization and physiotherapy as soon as the patient can tolerate it is important to a successful outcome. Prophylaxis to prevent DVT, hydration, compression stockings, and heparin therapy is standard care and continued until the patient is fully mobile and no longer at risk of developing DVTs.

Complications
- Cardiovascular complications
- Myocardial ischemia
- Pneumonia
- Atelectasis
- Respiratory complications
- Cerebrovascular complications
- Carotid insufficiency
- Renal complications
- Gastrointestinal complications
- Abdominal compartment syndrome
- Neurological complications

Endovascular Abdominal Aortic Aneurysm Repair (EVAR)

EVAR excludes an aneurysm from blood flow through placement of a bifurcated stent graft, most commonly introduced through the femoral arteries. Sac exclusion is dependent on adequate proximal and distal seal between the graft fabric and the vessel wall. For infrarenal AAAs, the proximal seal zone is the aneurysm neck—healthy aorta distal to the lowest renal artery and proximal to the start of an aneurysm. The distal seal zone is most commonly in the CIA. Femoral access may be achieved percutaneously or via femoral artery cutdown (Figure 24-9A and B and Table 24-4).

Patient Position and Prep: The patient is positioned supine with arms out on arm boards less than 90°. A Foley catheter is inserted once the patient is anesthetized. Hair removal is accomplished from nipples to knees and should be performed per hospital policy. Skin prep from nipple to knees is performed as per the physician's preference. Draping will be performed to expose the patient from xiphoid process to above knees. Genital region is covered and protected, to prevent cross-contamination.

Anesthesia: The type of anesthesia utilized is based on a conversation between the patient, anesthesiologist, and takes into consideration of the vascular team, the approach, the complexity of the aneurysm, and the ASA class of the surgeon. Endovascular procedures can be performed under a local with sedation, regional or general anesthesia. Regional anesthesia can be spinal, epidural or a combined spinal/epidural (CSE) anesthesia. Advantages of a regional anesthetic include reduced inflammatory response, less stress response and possibly avoiding mechanical ventilation with cardiovascular insufficiency, and postop analgesia.

Surgical Procedure
- Time out is to be performed per hospital policy.
- Access to the femoral artery is gained using ultrasound guidance with a micro puncture needle.
- Percutaneous closure device will be deployed at this time to be used at the end of the procedure.
- Surgeon preference of access sheath will be placed.
- Glide wires will be passed superior to the aneurysm.
- A flush catheter will be passed over wire and wire removed.
- Angiogram runoff is performed.
- The SA will need to keep in mind once this runoff is performed the table and x-ray equipment cannot be moved.

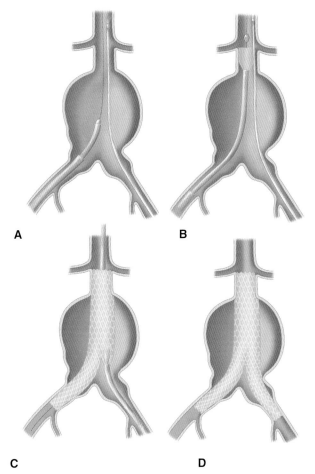

A. During an EVAR, the endograft is inserted through the femoral artery. **B.** The device is deployed in the aorta just below renal arteries. **C.** A contralateral device is inserted through a gate opening. **D.** Completion of the deployment of the graft device should fully exclude the aortic aneurysm while preserving the flow of the renal and hypogastric arteries. (Reproduced with permission from Brunicardi FC, Andersen DK, Billiar TR, et al. *Schwartz's Principles of Surgery,* 10th ed. New York, NY: McGraw Hill; 2015.)

Figure 24-9 ·

TABLE 24-4 • ADVANTAGES OF EVAR
Possible Advantages of EVAR over Open Surgical Repair
Minimally invasive
Less blood loss and fewer transfusions
Less fluid shifts
Minimal cardiovascular and metabolic stress response intraoperative
No cross-clamp
Less distal tissue ischemia
Less end-organ damage
Fewer complications
Earlier ambulation
Shorter hospital stays

- After determining the length of the endograft the surgeon will pass the main body of graft to the determined placement.
- The surgeon will deploy the main body of graft precisely not to cover the renal arteries.
- Another angiogram will be performed to ensure placement of graft is correct.
- The surgeon will perform another angiogram runoff to identify the distal seal zone.
- Identifying the hypogastric artery is important not to occlude.
- The surgeon will deploy bilateral limbs.
- Deploying a conformable balloon inflating with 60-cc syringe through the graft expanding graft into the wall of the vessels.
- Using a flush catheter again for a final angiogram to look for endo leaks.
- The surgeon removes sheath and uses the percutaneous closure device previously deployed to close the vessel.
- The SA will close the skin and dress the wounds per the surgeon preference.
- It is recommended that the SA monitor the incisions sites for bleeding or formation of hematoma.

Postop Care: Patients require ICU care for invasive blood pressure monitoring, measurements of blood gases, hemoglobin, serum electrolytes, and coagulation parameters. Lower Limb arterial assessment with a Doppler is an important aspect of post op care. Patients can eat or drink the same day. IV fluid therapy will reduce the possibility of contrast induced neuropathy (CIN). Pain is managed with oral analgesics.

Complications: Complications such as multiorgan failure and coagulopathy may occur but are rare. Post-implantation syndrome is a common complication and presents with pyrexia, leukocytosis, and elevated inflammatory markers. However, it usually resolves within 2 weeks of surgery.

Percutaneous Transluminal Angioplasty and Stenting

Angioplasty (ballooning) and stenting is a procedure to treat narrowed or blockages of the peripheral arteries (see Figure 24-10).

These are image guided procedures under x-ray control carried out under local anesthetic and minimal sedation. The surgeon accesses the femoral artery in the groin using a micro puncture needle under ultrasound guidance. Once access is achieved the surgeon will exchange over a wire to a larger access sheath. An angiogram will be performed locating the narrowed or blocked artery. Through the access sheath the surgeon will pass a very fine wire through the diseased segment. At this point the wire will be used like a *railroad* for the balloon and/or stent. The balloon will be inflated, to manufacture specifications) once or multiple times in all areas needed. In some areas the addition of a stent will hold the artery open and improve the results. Another angiogram will be performed to verify effectiveness. Once satisfied the surgeon will remove the

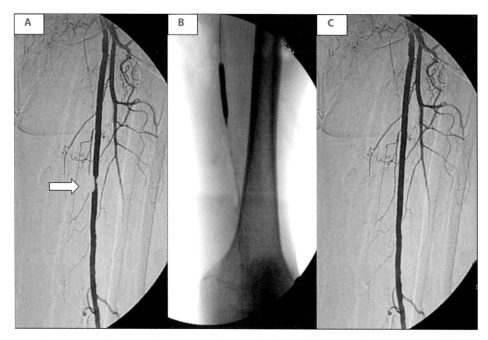

Figure 24-10 · Intraoperative angiography demonstrating stenosis of the left superficial femoral artery (SFA) and the result after angioplasty and stenting. (Reproduced with permission from Brunicardi FC, Andersen DK, Billiar TR, et al. *Schwartz's Principles of Surgery,* 10th ed. New York, NY: McGraw Hill; 2015.)

wire and deploy a closure device of their choice to manufacture specifications. These techniques can be used in many different arteries. The arteries to the arms, bowel, and kidneys can be treated this way.

Femoropopliteal Bypass

Femoral popliteal (also called femoropopliteal or Fem-Pop) bypass surgery is a procedure used to treat femoral artery disease. It is performed to bypass the blocked portion of the Femoral artery in the leg using a graft (vein or artificial material). Vein grafts can be taken from anywhere but most common is the legs (see Figure 24-11).

Indications

- Lifestyle changes and medicine have not improved symptoms, or symptoms are worse
- Leg pain that interferes with daily life or ability to work
- Wounds that do not heal
- Infection or gangrene
- Leg pain at rest
- Danger of losing the limb due to decreased blood flow

Procedure Overview
Position and Prep

- The patient is positioned supine with arms out on arm boards less than 90°.
- Operative leg is externally rotated, knee bent at approximately 30° and elevated.
- The patient will need to have a Foley catheterization.
- Hair removal from umbilicus to toes should be performed per hospital policy.

- Skin prep from umbilicus to toes circumferentially and bilaterally performed per physician preference.
- Draping will be performed to expose the patient from umbilicus to toes bilaterally (nonoperative leg should be prepped and draped into the field to allow possible saphenous vein harvest).
- Genital region needs to be covered and protected, to prevent cross contamination.

Anesthesia: The procedure is typically done under general anesthesia but in some cases the procedure can be done under local anesthesia.

Surgical Procedure

- Time out is to be performed per hospital policy.
- Incision: longitudinal incision made slightly above inguinal crease extended distally to below the femoral artery bifurcation.
- The SA will help with incisional hemostasis and provide exposure.
- The surgeon preference of self-retaining retractor will be inserted.
- The SA will provide countertraction on the tissues to help provide optimal exposure.
- Once the femoral artery exposure is complete the surgeon using Metzenbaum scissors and DeBakey pickups the surgeon will mobilize the common femoral artery (CFA) and superficial artery (SFA).
- The surgeon will elevate the CFA and SFA slighting exposing the origin of the profunda femoris artery (PFA).
- The surgeon will carefully expose the PFA.

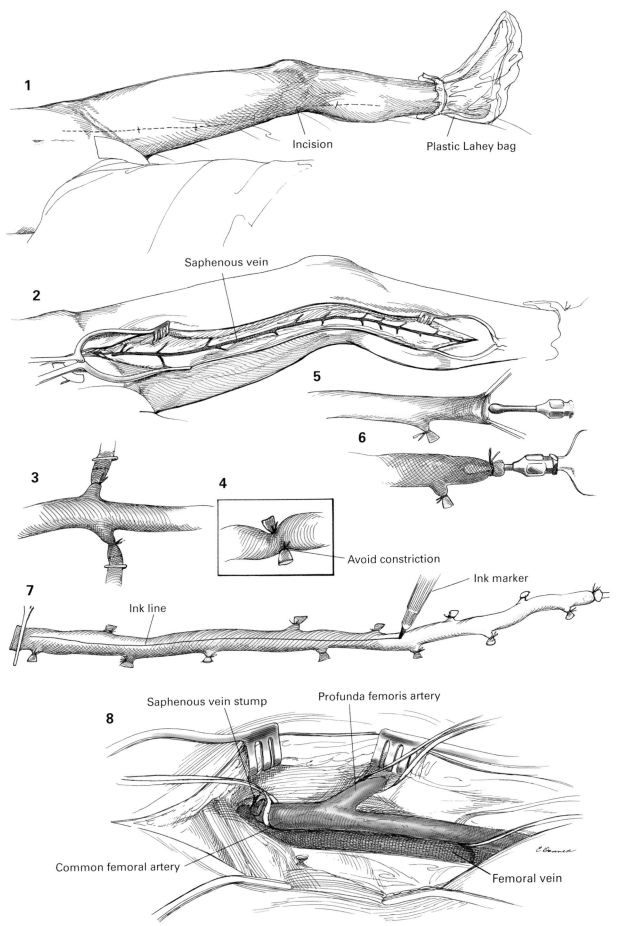

Figure 24-11 · Femoral popliteal bypass. (Reproduced with permission from Ellison EC, Zollinger Jr. RM, Pawlik TM, Vaccaro PS, Bitans M, Baker AS. *Zollinger's Atlas of Surgical operations,* 11th ed. New York, NY: McGraw Hill LLC; 2022.)

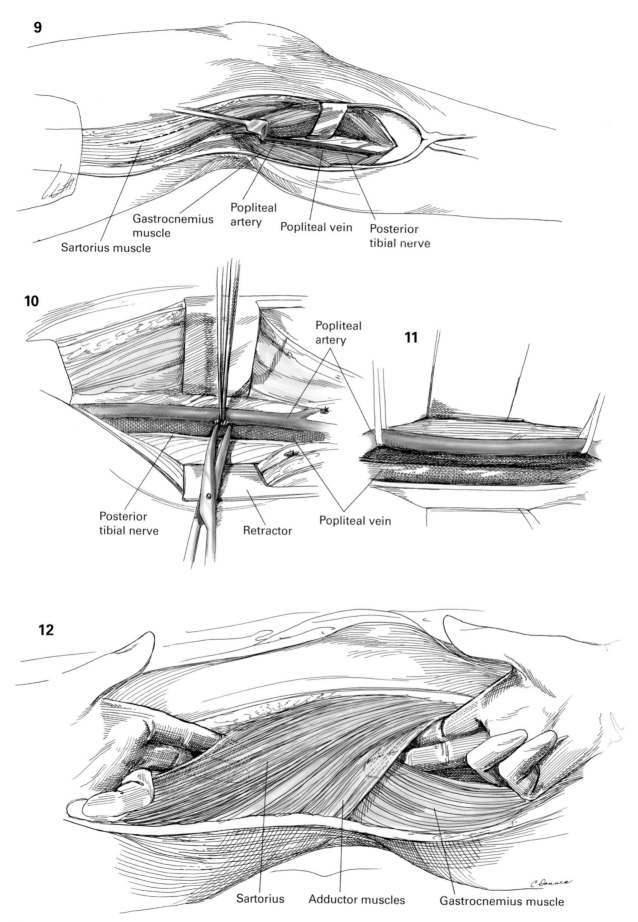

9

Sartorius muscle

Gastrocnemius
muscle

Popliteal
artery

Popliteal vein

Posterior
tibial nerve

10

Popliteal
artery

11

Posterior
tibial nerve

Retractor

Popliteal vein

12

Sartorius

Adductor muscles

Gastrocnemius muscle

Figure 24-11 · (*Continued*)

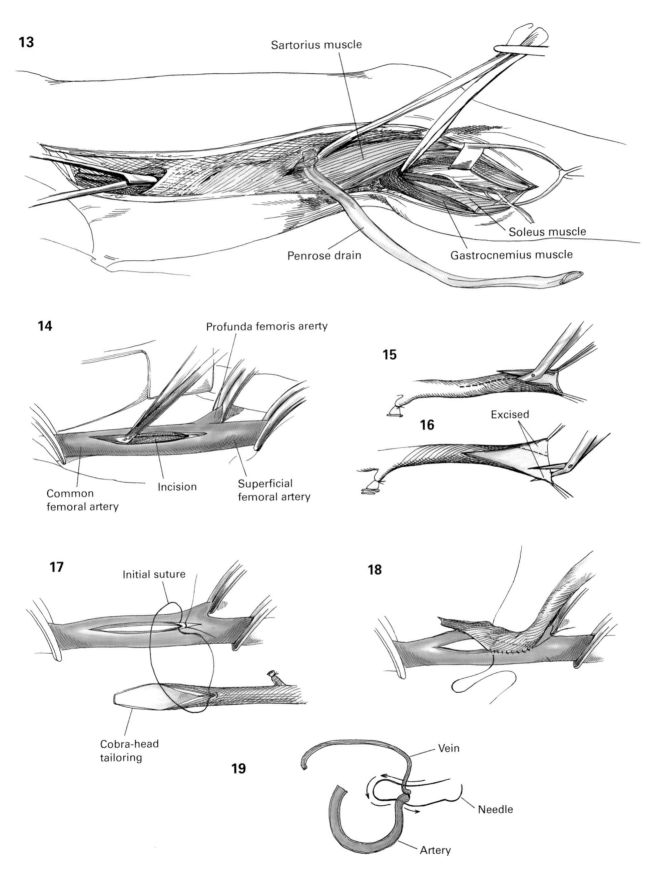

13

Sartorius muscle

Penrose drain

Soleus muscle

Gastrocnemius muscle

14

Profunda femoris arerty

Common femoral artery

Incision

Superficial femoral artery

15

16

Excised

17

Initial suture

Cobra-head tailoring

18

19

Vein

Needle

Artery

Figure 24-11 · (*Continued*)

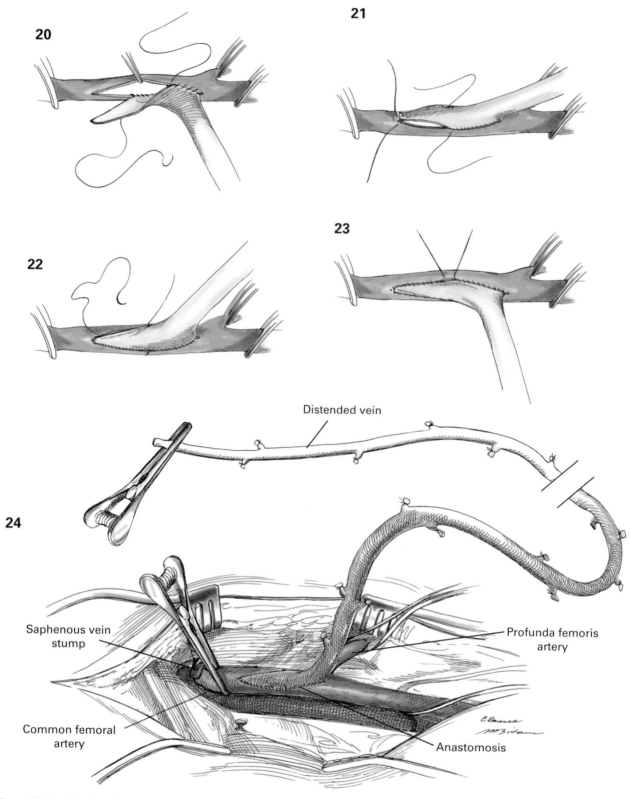

Figure 24-11 · (*Continued*)

- The surgeon and SA will pass vessel loops around CFA, SFA, and PFA.
- The SA will pack a moistened lap sponge into the wound.
- The surgeon will now make an incision in the lower thigh over the adductor canal.
- The saphenous vein will be identified and protected.
- The surgeon will dissect between the sartorius and the vastus medialis muscles.
- Use of a self-retaining retractor to expose the vascular bundle containing the popliteal artery (PA) and vein.
- The surgeon will separate the PA from the vein.
- The surgeon and SA will pass vessel loops around the PA.
- The SA will pack a moistened lap sponge into the wound.
- The surgeon will now perform autograph harvest commonly of the saphenous vein, which would have been predetermined via diagnostic testing to ensure proper length and size.
- The surgeon's preference of continuous/discontinuous incisions directly over the vein are performed.
- The vein is immobilized, and collateral branches ligated.
- Preparation of the autograph can be performed by the surgeon or SA by heparinized saline flush through the autograph to insure patency.
- The surgeon will now use a tunneling instrument to create the tunnel between femoral arteries and popliteal artery.
- The surgeon will occlude the PA with clamps both proximal and distal of the arteriotomy location.
- Arteriotomy is made with scalpel and/or Potts scissors.
- Using a double armed vascular suture, the surgeon will sew the end to side anastomosis with through-to-through continuous technique.
- The SA should properly follow the suture keeping the suture tight to ensure a watertight closure.
- Clamps will need to be placed proximal on the graft.
- Flashing the PA clamp, the surgeon will inspect anastomosis for leaks and place interrupted stitches (rescue stitches) where needed.
- The surgeon ensuring the graft is not twisted will tunnel the graft using the previously placed tunneling instrument to the femoral incision.
- The surgeon will occlude the CFA, SFA, and PFA arteries and make an arteriotomy in the CFA.
- Using a double armed vascular suture, the surgeon will sew the end to side anastomosis with through-to-through continuous technique.
- The SA should properly follow the suture keeping the suture tight to ensure a watertight closure.
- Flashing the CFA clamp, the surgeon will inspect anastomosis for leaks and place interrupted stitches (rescue stitches) where needed.

- The surgeon will close the fascia in both femoral and popliteal wounds.
- The SA will close the wounds according to the surgeon's preference.
- Dressing will be placed using the surgeon's preference.

Postop Care: The patient will recover in ICU and will be continually monitored. Pulses will be checked often with a Doppler probe to ensure blood flow to the limb. The limb is observed for color, sensations of pain and movement. Oral analgesics may be prescribed for incision site pain.

Complications

- Myocardial infarction
- Cardiac arrhythmias
- Hemorrhage
- Wound infection
- Leg edema
- Thrombosis
- Pulmonary edema
- Nerve injury
- Graft occlusion

Carotid Endarterectomy

Stroke is a leading cause of death in the United States and is a major cause of serious disability for adults. About 795,000 people in the United States have a stroke each year. Carotid endarterectomy is a procedure to treat carotid artery disease. This disease occurs when fatty, waxy deposits build up in one of the carotid arteries. The procedure is typically done under general anesthesia but in some cases the procedure can be done under local anesthesia. The surgeon makes an incision exposing the artery and performs an endarterectomy (surgical procedure to remove the atheromatous plaque material). Then repairs the artery with a patch graft (patch of vein or artificial material) (see Figure 24-12). Another technique a surgeon can use is an eversion carotid endarterectomy. This involves cutting the carotid artery and turning it inside out, then removing the plaque. The surgeon then reattaches the artery.

Anatomy. The arch of the aorta lies within the superior mediastinum at the level of the sternal angle. Three large vessels come off the aorta: the brachiocephalic trunk or innominate artery, the left common carotid artery, and the left subclavian artery. The common carotid artery arises as the first branch of the brachiocephalic trunk on the right side of the aorta. The left and the right common carotids bifurcate into the internal and external carotid arteries, in the neck at the level of the fourth cervical vertebra, near the superior border of the thyroid. The carotid sheath is formed from cervical fascia and surrounds the carotid arteries, internal jugular veins, and vagus nerve, and recurrent laryngeal nerve. The carotid sheath lies medially to the sternocleidomastoid muscle. The internal carotid artery continues into the skull to form part of the Circle of Willis and supplies blood to the brain and eyes. The external

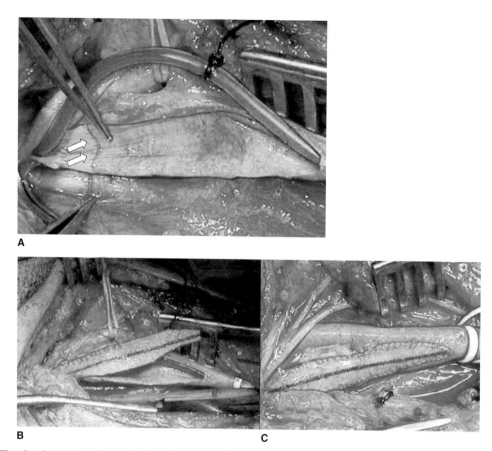

Figure 24-12 · A. The distal transition line (left side of the picture) in the internal carotid artery where the plaque had been removed must be examined carefully and should be smooth. Tacking sutures (arrows) are placed when an intimal flap remains in this transition to ensure no obstruction to flow. **B.** An autologous or synthetic patch can be used to close the carotid arteriotomy incision, which maintains the luminal patency. **C.** A completion closure of carotid endarterectomy incision using a synthetic patch. (Reproduced with permission from Brunicardi FC, Andersen DK, Billiar TR, et al., eds. *Schwartz's Principles of Surgery,* 10e. New York, NY: McGraw Hill; 2015.)

carotid artery supplies blood to the neck and face. The carotid sinus, or carotid bulb, is where the carotid artery widens at its main branch point. The carotid sinus contains sensors that help regulate blood pressure.

Patient Position and Prep. The patient is positioned in the supine position. Head turned opposite of the surgical site. Shoulder roll to extend the neck, careful consideration not to hyperextend the neck. Arms to be tucked to the patients' sides. Reverse Trendelenburg the bed and airplane the bed 20° to 40° to the opposite of the surgical site. Keep in mind to use extra restraints so the patient does not slide. Hair removal from earlobe to midline of chin to sternal notch and the skin is prepped from earlobe to midline of chin to sternal notch. Draping should expose landmarks of earlobe, midline of chin, and sternal notch.

Anesthesia. The procedure can be performed under general anesthesia or local with sedation.

Surgical Procedure

- Timeout is performed per hospital policy.
- Incision: longitudinal anterior border of sternocleidomastoid (SCM).
- The SA will help with incisional hemostasis and provide exposure.

- The surgeon preference of self-retaining retractor will be inserted. The medial blade of retractor should be placed in the superficial layers to refrain from damage to the superior laryngeal nerve.
- The surgeon will continue dissection with Metzenbaum scissors.
- The SA will provide countertraction on the tissues to help provide optimal exposure. (The SA should be mindful of tissues as there are several facial nerves reside in this region and reporting any movements to the surgeon.)
- The internal Jugular vein will need to be retracted out of the surgical site.
- The carotid sheath is exposed and incised.
- The surgeon will dissect out the external carotid artery passed the first branch identified as thyroid artery.
- The common carotid artery is dissected carefully from the vagus nerve.
- The surgeon will dissect out the internal carotid artery paying attention to the hypoglossal nerve.
- The surgeon and SA will pass vessel loops around the External and Internal carotid arteries and a Rummel tourniquet around the common carotid artery.

- The surgeon clamps the internal artery first so any debris cannot travel to the brain.
- Next the common carotid, external carotid, and the thyroid artery are clamped.
- An arteriotomy into the common carotid with scalpel and extend into the internal carotid artery with Potts scissors.
- The surgeon's preference if shunt to be placed.
- The surgeon will remove the plaque, ensuring they leave a smooth vessel wall. The surgeon may use a vascular suture to secure any damage to the vessel.
- The surgeon will use a patch of their preference to close the artery with a vascular suture. This is done to prevent narrowing of the carotid artery.
- Before the final suturing the internal carotid artery clamp is flushed allowing backflow to flush debris from lumen.
- Clamps are removed. Thyroid artery then the external carotid followed by common carotid and last internal carotid. This sequence ensures any embolic material is flushed into the external carotid.
- The surgeon will close the fascia.
- The SA will close the wound according to surgeon preference.
- Dressing will be placed using the surgeon's preference.

Major Complications

- Myocardial infarction
- Hyper perfusion syndrome
- Nerve injury
- Perioperative stroke
- Restenosis
- Death

Minor Complications

- TIA
- Bleeding
- Infection
- Greater auricular nerve injury
- Dysphagia

Carotid Stenting and Transcarotid Artery Revascularization (TCAR)

Carotid stenting and TCAR are alternatives to the carotid endarterectomy surgery. Carotid stenting can be done from three common access sites. Femoral artery, brachial artery, or the common carotid artery are the access sites used. Depending on access location determines the length of products needed. If access is in the femoral or brachial the surgeon will use longer wires and catheters.

Surgical Procedure:

- The surgeon will use a crossing wire and catheter to navigate through the aortic arch into the common carotid artery.

- Once the surgeon has wire access to the common carotid, they will pass a sheath of appropriate length and diameter. Care should be taken during these steps to avoid disruption to the stenosis to not dislodge any plaque sending it to the brain.
- The surgeon will place an embolic protection device (EPD), three types of EPD are distal occlusion balloon, distal filter device or proximal flow diversion.
- The surgeon may choose to pre-dilate the common carotid artery (CCA) and internal carotid artery (ICA) at this time.
- The surgeon will determine according to angiography the appropriate length and diameter of the stent that is needed. Stent will be a self-expanding stent, and post-dilation will be performed to ensure the stent expands adequately.
- A post stent placement angiography will be performed to ensure adequate stent placement and to also evaluate the EPD. If significant embolic load in EPD an aspiration catheter should be used to clear debris.
- The surgeon will remove all access sheaths closing the artery with the surgeon's preference closure device (see Figure 24-13).

TCAR

Surgical Procedure:

- TCAR procedure is performed with two surgical sites.
- A small open incision between the heads of the sternocleidomastoid muscle.
- Dissection to the CCA is made circumferential and umbilical tape with a Rummel tourniquet is placed.
- The surgeon will sew a purse string suture in the CCA for closure at the end of the procedure.
- The surgeon will make access using a micro puncture system into the femoral vein under ultrasound guidance.
- Using a 0.035 wire the surgeon will advance a venous return sheath (VRS), the VRS will be secured with a silk suture.
- Access to the CCA is performed using a micro puncture system through the previous purse string suture.
- Angiography is performed through the micro puncture to identify the location of the lesion, also noting where the bifurcation of external and internal carotid arteries.
- The surgeon will pass a 0.035 wire into the CCA not disrupting the lesion. Removal of micro puncture and insertion of arterial access sheath (AAS) is advanced to a predetermined sheath stopper.
- Sheath position placement will be confirmed using fluoroscopy. The sheath is suture into place with gentle forward tension. The flow controller is connected to the AAS.
- The surgeon will occlude inflow to the CCA with Rummel tourniquet previously placed. The flow controller is tested to verify that flow is reversed.
- The surgeon will pass a 0.014 wire across the lesion.

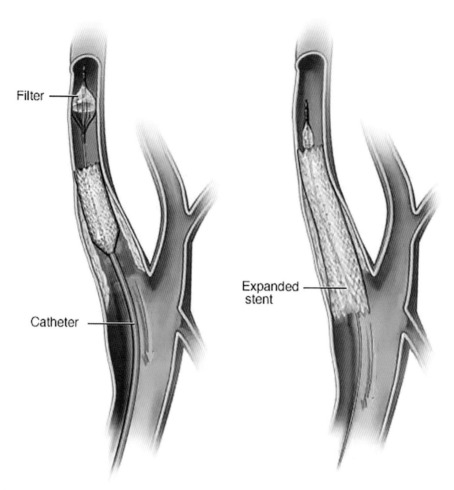

Figure 24-13 · Carotid stenting. (Used with permission of Mayo Foundation for Medical Education and Research, all rights reserved.)

- The stent will be placed into position determined by the previous angiography. The surgeon will deploy the stent, post-dilation may be performed.
- Antegrade flow is restored by closing off the stopcock to the flow controller and losing the Rummel tourniquet.
- The AAS is removed, and the artery closed with the preclosure suture tied.
- The surgeon will remove the VRS from the femoral vein and pressure applied per surgeon preference.

Arteriovenous Fistula and Shunt. An arteriovenous shunt, also referred to as an arteriovenous fistula (AVF), is a connection between an artery and a vein that allows blood to flow between the two. AVF surgery creates a place to access the body's circulatory system to perform dialysis. An AVF allows blood to flow from your body to the dialysis machine and back into your body after filtering (see Figure 24-14).

Patient Position and Prep. The patient is positioned in the supine position. The operative arm is placed on an arm table. The contra side arm is placed on an arm board. Hair removal should be performed to surgeon preference. Skin prep of operative arm circumferentially performed per surgeon preference.

Draping per the surgeon's preference, the SA should keep in mind to cover the fingers to protect from gross contamination. Time out is performed per hospital policy.

Surgical Procedure

- Location of the AVF will be predetermined by the surgeon using vein mapping done pre-surgery or can be chosen under ultrasound at this point.
- Incision will be made above the vein choosing.
- The SA will help with incisional hemostasis and provide exposure.
- The surgeon and SA will pass a vessel loop around the vein.
- The surgeon will dissect enough of the vein to ensure enough length to attach to the artery.
- The SA will provide countertraction on the tissues to help provide optimal exposure.
- The surgeon will now perform arterial exposure.
- The surgeon and SA will pass vessel loops around the artery.
- The surgeon will ligate the vein as per the preferred method, using clip and/or free ties, ensuring proper length was achieved.

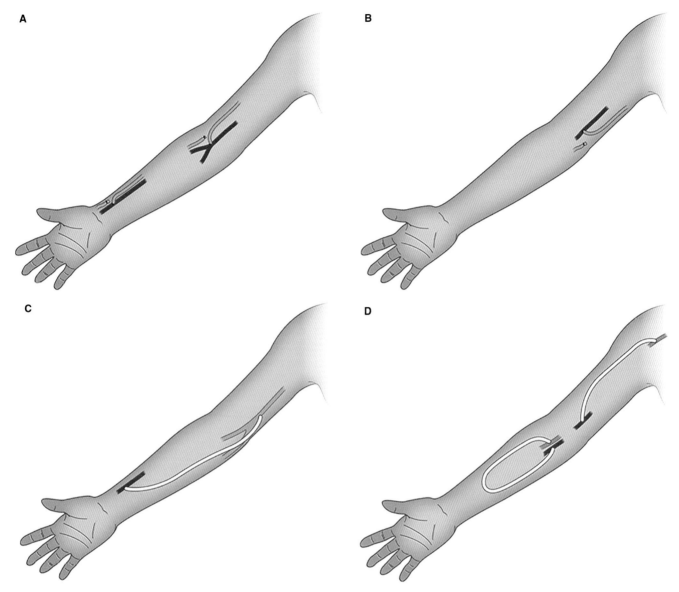

Figure 24-14 · Different fistula formations. (Reproduced with permission from Ahmed A, Ahmed A. Hemodialysis access. In: Nazzal M, Blebea J, Osman M.F. (eds.), *Vascular and Endovascular Surgery: Clinical Diagnosis and Management.* New York, NY: McGraw Hill; 2023.)

- The surgeon might pre-dilate the vein with vessel dilators.
- The artery is occluded with either vascular clamps or by tightening the vessel loops previously placed.
- An arteriotomy is performed with scalpel and extended with Potts scissors.
- Using a double armed vascular suture, the surgeon will sew the end to side anastomosis with through-to-through continuous technique.
- The SA should properly follow the suture keeping the suture tight to ensure a watertight closure.
- Blood flow is restored by releasing the vascular clamps or vessel loops.
- The SA will close the wounds according to the surgeon's preference.
- Dressing will be placed using the surgeon's preference.

Inferior Vena Cava Filter Placement

Inferior vena cava (IVC) filter placement, a filtering device, is placed within the IVC. Blood clots in the veins of the legs and pelvis can occasionally travel to the lungs where they may cause a pulmonary embolism or blockage. IVC filters help reduce the risk of pulmonary embolism by trapping large clots and preventing them from reaching the heart and lungs.

Patient Position and prep. The patient will be supine on the bed. Two common access areas are a femoral vein or the jugular vein. Prep and drape the access site as per the surgeon's preference.

Surgical Procedure

- Under ultrasound guidance, percutaneous venous access is performed with a micro puncture catheter.
- The surgeon will swap to a larger working access sheath.

- A wire is passed into the inferior vena cava under fluoroscopy guidance.
- A venogram will be performed for visualization of appropriate placement. IVC filter kit is opened, and an operating sheath is passed over the wire.
- Wire will be removed, and the filter system passed through sheath and deployed.
- Finalization venogram is performed for placement and deployment confirmation.
- Sheath is removed and manual pressure is performed per Surgeon preference.

Vein Ligation and Stripping

Varicose veins are twisted, distended blood vessels that are visible just under the skin's surface common in lower extremities. When the vein walls are weak and the valves are not working correctly, blood backs up in your vein. Spider veins, which may surround varicose veins, are minor red or purple lines that appear close to your skin's surface.

Phlebectomy is one of the oldest recorded methods to treat varicose veins. It was described by Aulus Cornelius Celsus, a Roman historian of medicine, in AD 45. The first description of a phlebectomy hook is detailed in a surgery textbook published in 1545. A Swiss dermatologist named Robert Muller developed ambulatory phlebectomy and since 2003 the surgical approach to vein ligation is performed less often.

Etiology

- **Age:** Veins often lose elasticity and stiffen as one ages.
- **Gender:** Pregnant females, those on birth control pills or someone going through menopause due to changes in hormone levels.
- **Family History:** This condition may be inherited.
- **Lifestyle:** Sedentary lifestyle or restrictive clothing can exacerbate the issue.
- **Overall Health:** Health anomalies such as severe constipation or certain tumors, increase pressure in the veins leading to varicose veins.
- **Tobacco use:** People who utilize tobacco products are more prone to develop varicose veins.
- **Weight:** Excess weight puts pressure on blood vessels.

Symptoms

- Bulging veins
- Heavy legs
- Itching
- Swelling
- Skin discolorations and ulcers

Nonsurgical Treatments

- Elevation of lower legs above the waist
- Compression stockings to stop the veins from stretching
- Sclerotherapy to scar the vein tissue
- Laser therapy to close off damaged veins

Diagnostics. Direct observation during a health evaluation due to the bulging skin as well as ultrasound that will show blood clots and the effectiveness of the valves.

Complications of Varicose Veins

- Superficial thrombophlebitis
- DVT
- PEs

Ambulatory Phlebectomy. This is also known as stab avulsion or a micro-extraction phlebectomy. This procedure is performed under straight local anesthesia. After the administration of anesthesia, the surgeon will make small micro incisions 1 to 3 mm in length. The surgeon will use a phlebectomy hook through each incision and using a mosquito clamp will pull the vein out through the incision. Once all the vein segments are removed, the leg is washed with hydrogen peroxide. The leg is dressed in foam wrap, several layers of cotton and an adhesive bandage. A compression stocking is drawn up over the wrapping. Dressings are removed between 3 and 7 days, but the compression stocking is worn for another 2 to 4 weeks to minimize bruising and swelling. Mild activities like walking will minimize the risk of blood clots.

Transilluminated Powered Phlebectomy. Transilluminated powered phlebectomy (TIPP) is performed with an illuminator and a motorized resector. Once the patient is placed under a light general anesthesia, the surgeon makes two small incisions: one for the illuminating device and the other for the resector. After making the first incision and introducing the illuminator, the surgeon uses tumescent fluid to fill the tissues around the veins and this makes the veins easier to remove. The second incision is used for the resector, which draws the vein by suction toward an inner blade. The suction removes the small pieces of venous tissue left by the blade. Once the procedure is complete, a single suture or steri-strip is used to close the incisions. Gauze dressing is placed over the incisions and the leg is wrapped in a sterile compression dressing.

Surgical Approach

Position and Prep: The surgeon will mark the varicose veins in the pre-op area while the patient is in a standing position.

The patient is placed in a supine position with legs slightly abducted. The patient's extremity is prepped in a circumferential manner. Drapes are placed that enable lifting and flexing of the knee.

Anesthesia: The patient will be placed under general anesthesia.

Surgical Procedure

- The surgeon makes an incision in the upper thigh, parallel to the abdominocural crease, clamps and ligates any bleeders.

- The saphenous vein is identified.
- The SA places a Weitlaner retractor separating the incision.
- The surgeon double ligates the saphenous vein branches with silk ties, or they are transfixed, clamped, and divided.
- The proximal stump is dissected upward toward the femoral vein, where it is ligated and disconnected from the femoral vein.
- The surgeon will make an incision at the distal end of the saphenous vein if it is being excised.
- The vein is identified, ligated, and divided at the distal point.
- A vein stripper is inserted and advanced to the proximal end of the vein near the groin.
- The stripper is secured with heavy suture and the tip is attached.
- The surgeon will pull the stripper up the leg.
- The SA will apply external compression.
- Tributaries are excised through numerous micro incisions along the vein.
- The surgeon will close the groin wound in layers.
- The SA will close all other micro incisions with suture or staples.
- Dressing and a compression stocking are applied.

Postop Complications

- Allergic reactions
- DVTs
- Infection

Bibliography

Al-Hashimi M, Thompson J. Anaesthesia for elective open abdominal aortic aneurysm repair. *Continuing Education Anaesth Crit Care Pain.* 2013;13(6):208-212. https://doi.org/10.1093/bjaceaccp/mkt015.

Britannica, T. Editors of Encyclopedia. *Artery.* Encyclopedia Britannica; January 14, 2016. https://www.britannica.com/science/artery.

Britannica, T. Editors of Encyclopedia. *Vein.* Encyclopedia Britannica; August 7, 2013. https://www.britannica.com/science/vein-blood-vessel.

Bruce DF. *Pictures of the Carotid Artery.* Medically Reviewed by Carol DerSarkissian. June 23, 2021. https://www.webmd.com/heart-disease/carotid-artery-disease-causes-symptoms-tests-and-treatment. Accessed on September 23, 2023.

Centers for Disease Control and Prevention. *Stroke.* CDC, 2021. https://www.cdc.gov/stroke/. Accessed on September 23, 2023.

DaCosta M, Tadi P, Surowiec SM. Carotid Endarterectomy. [Updated 2021 Sep 29]. In: StatPearls [Internet]. Treasure Island (FL): StatPearls Publishing; 2022 Jan-. Available from: https://www.ncbi.nlm.nih.gov/books/NBK470582/.

de Fraga Guimarães J, Angonese CF, Gomes RK, Miranda V, Farias C. Anesthesia for lower extremity vascular bypass with peripheral nerve block. *Brazilian J Anesthesiol* (English Edition). 2017;67(6):626-631. https://doi.org/10.1016/j.bjane.2014.07.020.

John Hopkins Medicine. Femoral Popliteal Bypass Surgery. https://www.hopkinsmedicine.org/health/treatment-tests-and-therapies/femoral-popliteal-bypass-surgery. Accessed on September 23, 2023.

Kothandan H, Haw Chieh GL, Khan SA, Karthekeyan RB, Sharad SS. Anesthetic considerations for endovascular abdominal aortic aneurysm repair. *Annals Cardiac Anaesth.* 2016;19(1):132-141. https://doi.org/10.4103/0971-9784.173029.

Sharma A, Sethi P, Gupta K. Endovascular abdominal aortic aneurysm repair. *Interv Cardiol Clin.* 2020 Apr;9(2):153-168. doi:10.1016/j.iccl.2019.12.005.

Swerdlow NJ, Wu WW, Schermerhorn ML. Open and endovascular management of aortic aneurysms. *Circulation Res.* 2019;124(4):647-653. https://doi.org/10.1161/CIRCRESAHA.118.313186.

The Johns Hopkins University, The Johns Hopkins Hospital, and Johns Hopkins Health System. *Peripheral Vascular Disease.* Hopkinsmedicine.org; 2022. https://www.hopkinsmedicine.org/health/conditions-and-diseases/peripheral-vascular-disease. Accessed September 23, 2023.

Varicose Veins. Cleveland Clinic. https://my.clevelandclinic.org/health/diseases/4722-varicose-veins. Accessed on September 23, 2023.

Vein Ligation. Encyclopedia of Surgery. https://www.surgeryencyclopedia.com/St-Wr/Vein-Ligation-and-Stripping.html. Accessed on September 23, 2023.

Virani SS, Alonso A, Aparicio HJ, et al. Heart disease and stroke statistics—2021 update: a report from the American Heart Association. *Circulation.* 2021;143:e254–e743.

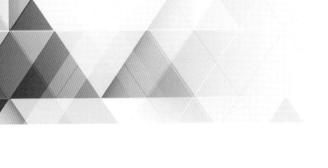

25

Pediatric Surgery

Brandy Farrington and Deborah Klaudt

DISCUSSED IN THIS CHAPTER

1. The pediatric surgical patient
2. Common pediatric anomalies
3. Pediatric obstructions
4. Pediatric tumors
5. Pediatric cardiac and neurological procedures

Pediatric patients are 18 years of age and under, encompassing care for neonates, infants, children, and adolescents. This chapter will outline common pediatric surgeries. It is important as a surgical assistant (SA) to understand the unique needs and special considerations of the Pediatric patient in the OR. It is not an adult surgery performed on "little adults" or scaled down to pediatric patients. The need for surgery often results from congenital anomalies that threaten life or ability to function and trauma. Special care is required to safely perform surgical procedures on the pediatric patient. Multiple psychologic and physiologic changes occur with age. The major physiologic areas include pulmonary status, cardiovascular status, temperature regulation, metabolism, and fluid management.

Classification of pediatric patients is as follows:

Newborn or Neonate: infant up to 1 month

Infants: 1 to 18 months of age

Toddler: 18 to 30 months of age

Preschool: 2.5 to 5 years of age

School-age: 6 to 12 years of age

Adolescent: 12 to 18 years of age

Considerations when dealing with Pediatric patients begin with **cognitive development** and **psychosocial development**. Communication barriers and ability to comprehend preoperative, operative, and postoperative care can be challenging. Separation from parents can increase anxiety. Often a favorite toy or parent can accompany a child back to the operating suite. Occasionally children may be carried back by the Operating room staff or parent. Careful consideration of using medical terminology and surgical instrumentation within the view of a child may be upsetting. Excessive noise should be avoided. Pediatric patients are easily excitable during anesthesia induction.

Pulmonary status changes dramatically from infancy to adulthood due to increasing airway size, changes in the rigidity of the airway, and neuromuscular changes. A child becomes hypoxic much faster than an adult if the airway is lost. Small airways have higher resistance and can become compromised with small amounts of swelling. Loose teeth are also a potential airway risk in children 5 to 14 years of age.

Important changes occur in the **cardiovascular status** at birth with the transition from fetal circulation. Young children are predisposed to increased vagal tone which is induced by painful stimuli and can affect heart rate and cardiac output. Control of blood loss is important in pediatric patients because the total blood volume is quite small. Any murmurs found on exam should be investigated because anesthetic agents cause vasodilation and potentially cardiac dysrhythmias.

Children will require different **temperature regulation** than an adult. Pediatric patients have a higher body surface-to-weight ratio and can be sensitive to thermal change. Often the operating room thermostat is raised to warm the room temperature. Warming blankets, bed warmers, and warm fluids may also be used to aid in maintaining a child's body temperature. Neonates have an increased risk for hypothermia. Special consideration must be given to surgical neonates. The risk for hypothermia is increased because of transporting and time in the surgical suite.

Nutritional needs and preoperative fasting will be different than for adults. Metabolic rate is much faster for Pediatric

TABLE 25-1 • NORMAL VITAL SIGNS BY AGE			
Age	Heart Rate/Min	Respirations/Min	Systolic Blood Pressure
Newborn	100-150	30-55	60-90
Infant to 2 years	110-160	25-40	85-105
Toddler 2-6 years	70-110	22-34	90-110
School-age 6-10 years	60-105	18-30	97-120
Adolescent 10-16 years	60-100	12-18	110-130

Source: Adapted from MAVCC, Surgical Procedures, Part B; pp. 13-19.

patients, which will affect medication and anesthetic doses. Immature blood-brain barrier and decreased protein binding increases sensitivity to sedatives, opioids, and hypnotics. Nutritional needs vary between pediatric classifications. Challenges occur in maintaining proper nutrition with neonates and infants. Often gastric feeding tubes may be needed.

Fluid management is a critical component for successful pediatric care. Blood volume to body size ratio is lower in children than in adult patients. Special attention is given to accurately measuring irrigation solutions, weight of sponges for blood loss, and urine output. Replenishing lost fluids will help prevent hypovolemia and dehydration.

Children require surgery for congenital anomalies, acquired diseases, and trauma. Pediatric surgery is subdivided into all specialties. See Table 25-1 for normal vital signs by age.

COMMON PEDIATRIC GENERAL ANOMALIES

What Is Intestinal Atresia and Stenosis?

Intestinal atresia and stenosis involve narrowing or closure of the intestine. Food is blocked from passing through the intestine, which prevents normal feeding and intestinal function. Intestinal atresia and stenosis usually involve the small intestine but can affect any part of the gastrointestinal tract.

Intestinal stenosis is a partial obstruction that causes the center opening of the intestine to become narrower, while intestinal atresia is a complete closure of the intestine.

Intestinal Atresia Types

There are different types of intestinal atresia, depending on where the closure occurs.

Pyloric Atresia. The obstruction is at the pylorus, which is the passage linking the stomach and the first portion of the small intestine (duodenum). Pyloric atresia is rare and tends to run in families. Children with pyloric atresia vomit the contents of their stomachs; they also develop a swollen upper abdomen because of an accumulation of intestinal contents and gas.

Duodenal Atresia. The duodenum is obstructed. This is the first portion of the small intestine; it receives contents emptied from the stomach. Half of the infants with this condition are born prematurely; about two-thirds also suffer from cardiac, genitourinary, or other intestinal tract problems. Nearly 40% have Down syndrome. Infants with duodenal atresia usually vomit within hours after birth and may develop a distended abdomen.

Jejunoileal Atresia. This involves an obstruction of the middle region (jejunum) or lower region (ileum) of the small intestine. The part of the intestine that is blocked off expands, which lessens its ability to absorb nutrients and push its contents through the digestive tract. There are four subtypes of jejunoileal atresia:

Intestinal Atresia Type I: A web-like membrane forms inside the intestine while the baby is forming in the uterus. The membrane blocks the intestine, but the intestine itself usually develops to a normal length.

Intestinal Atresia Type II: The dilated section of intestine forms a blind end. It is connected to a smaller segment of the intestine by scar tissue. The intestine develops to a normal length.

Intestinal Atresia Type III: Two blind ends of intestine are separated by a flaw in the intestinal blood supply. This significantly reduces the length of the intestine, which may result in long-term nutritional deficiencies or short gut syndrome.

Intestinal Atresia Type IV: Multiple sections of the intestine are blocked. This may result in a very short length of useful intestine.

Infants with any of the four types of jejunoileal atresia usually vomit green bile within a day of their birth. However, those with obstructions farther down in the intestine may not vomit until 2 to 3 days later. A baby with jejunoileal atresia may develop a swollen belly, and not have a bowel movement during the first day of life the way most babies do.

Colonic Atresia. Less than 15% of babies with intestinal atresias experience this form. The bowel becomes massively dilated, and patients develop signs and symptoms similar to those associated with jejunoileal atresia. Colonic atresia may occur in conjunction with small bowel atresia, Hirschsprung's disease, or gastroschisis.

Intestinal Atresia and Stenosis Diagnosis

The methods used to diagnose intestinal atresia and stenosis vary depending on the type (or location) of the obstruction in the intestine. In newborns with the symptoms listed above, an abdominal x-ray is usually all that is needed to establish a diagnosis, sometimes accompanied by an x-ray contrast enema. More and more, intestinal obstructions are detected with prenatal ultrasonography. Using this imaging technique, doctors may find excess amniotic fluid, a sign that the intestine cannot properly absorb the fluid. If excess amniotic fluid is found on an ultrasound, infant will be examined for intestinal atresia and stenosis after his or her birth using these methods: lower GI series, upper GI series, and abdominal ultrasound.

Because many newborns with intestinal atresia also have other life-threatening problems, echocardiography and other imaging studies of the heart and kidneys may also be performed after the infant is stabilized.

Intestinal Atresia and Stenosis Treatment

Children with intestinal atresia and stenosis need surgery to correct the problem. The type of operation they require depends on where the obstruction is located. Before the operation, a tube is placed into the stomach (through the mouth) to remove the excess fluid and gas. This prevents vomiting and aspiration, as well as provides babies with some relief from the discomfort caused by a swollen abdomen. Nutrients are provided intravenously, to replace what was lost through vomiting.

Babies with intestinal atresia feed through a tube that goes through their nasal passages directly into the stomach. This is left in place until their bowel function returns, a period of time which may vary from a few days to several weeks. Once the intestines can function normally, nutrition is given orally or through a feeding tube passed into the small intestine. During the period of bowel inactivity, nutrition is provided intravenously.

After the surgery, parents can expect their child's hospital stay to last from one to several weeks until the child's diet is enough to provide a good level of nutrition. However, the hospital stay is often longer for premature infants.

Children will require continued regular follow-up to make sure they are growing and developing normally, and to ensure that their intestine is absorbing enough of the nutrients they need.

If a baby has a sufficient length of intestine, and there are no other associated problems, he or she generally does well after recovery. Complications after surgical therapy are rare but may occur. During the immediate postoperative and early recovery period, intestinal contents may leak at the suture line. This can cause an infection in the abdominal cavity and require additional surgery. Possible long-term complications include short gut syndrome, malabsorption syndromes, and segments of intestine that cannot function properly because they are dilated or paralyzed.[1]

Esophageal Atresia

It is a congenital condition diagnosed at infancy, usually between 3 and 6 weeks of life. Symptoms are excessive salivation, coughing, or choking during the initial oral feeding. These secretions spill over from the closed esophageal pouch possibly causing aspiration and respiratory distress. Immediate management is required. An anteroposterior chest x-ray will display an air column in the upper thorax, failure to see air below the diaphragm confirms esophageal atresia.

Tracheoesophageal Fistula

It is common with esophageal atresia. Video esophagography with contrast may be needed for diagnosis, or bronchoscopy with esophagoscopy. These anomalies affect 1 in 4000 live births, males slightly predominate with approximately one-third having low-birth weight. About 60% to 70% will also have associated congenital anomalies referred to as the VACTERL—**V**ertebral, **A**norectal, **C**ardiac, **T**racheo**E**sophageal, **R**enal and **L**imb. This condition is formed in the 4th week of gestation with failure of the esophagotracheal diverticulum of the foregut to divide completely to form the esophagus and trachea.

Surgical Treatment. It is performed via a right thoracotomy in the 4th intercostal space using a retropleural approach. This procedure can also be done thoracoscopically. The fistula is located at the level of the tracheal bifurcation. After isolating and dividing the fistula, a portion of the esophagus is left on the trachea to aid in closure and reduce narrowing of the trachea. Dissecting the upper esophageal pouch free up into the mediastinum for additional length, a tension-free, single-layer repair is performed. A gastrostomy is performed to bolus gastric feeding over several months to enlarge the stomach.

Biliary Dyskinesia

Obesity has also become a significant health problem for adolescents. In conjunction with this, we are witnessing an ever-increasing number of pediatric patients with cholelithiasis and biliary colic as a result of dyskinesia. Biliary dyskinesia has become more common. Pediatric surgeons are frequently consulted to evaluate the need for surgical intervention by performing a cholecystectomy, which is determined by low ejection fraction. An ejection fraction below 35% to 40% is linked to typical biliary colic.

OBSTRUCTIVE DISORDERS

Hirschsprung's Disease

Hirschsprung's disease is a developmental disease that affects an estimated 1 in 5000 infants. There is a higher prevalence among males than females, approximately 4:1. It is common for infants with Hirschsprung's disease to have associated anomalies such as numerous cardiac anomalies and 3% to 5% have Down syndrome.

This disease affects the motility of the proximal bowel and rectum. The absence of ganglion cells occurs during embryonic development from the decrease or lack of rostrocaudal migration of enteric neurons. If the complete gastrointestinal tract is aganglionic the disease is generally fatal; however, enterocolitis is the leading cause of death in pediatric patients. A contrast enema study and rectal biopsy will confirm the diagnosis.

Surgical Approaches. Currently, there are three surgical procedures for Hirschsprung's disease. Duhamel, Swenson, and Soave procedures are all endorectal pull-throughs. The Duhamel procedure, a retrorectal approach, avoids extensive dissection anterior of the rectum and retains the affected rectal stump. The healthy normal colon is brought rectrorectal and anastomosed. The advancement of stapling devices has simplified this procedure. The Swenson procedure, a full-thickness rectosigmoid dissection, is the original procedure for treatment. This technique is a near-total bowel excision with a low oblique colorectal anastomosis. Special care is taken to preserve the parasympathetic pelvic splanchnic nerves.

Finally, the Soave procedure, an endorectal dissection, is done laparoscopically and is the most prevalent. This procedure benefits from being done completely transanal and eliminates the need for a colostomy. It also reduced the risk of pelvic structural damage associated with the Swenson procedure. The Soave technique dissects the endorectal mucosa and submucosa within the aganglionic distal rectum, pulling the normal colon through the remaining muscular cuff and anastomosing.

Imperforate Anus

Imperforate Anus is a birth defect occurring in the 5th to 7th week of fetal development. Imperforate is the abnormal development of the anus and rectum inhibiting stool from being passed. It occurs more often in males than females with 1 in 5000 babies affected and has three classifications. Classification of anatomic variants is based on the rectum and puborectalis muscle. Translevator lesion or malformation is low and supralevator malformation is a high lesion. Additionally, Cloaca is a complex malformation with the rectum, urethra, and vagina draining into a common pouch that connects with the perineum (see Figure 25-1). Boys tend to have high lesions where the colon is higher in pelvis connecting the rectum to the bladder and urethra by fistula. Girls significantly have low lesions with the colon near the skin and stenosed or absence of the anus. A colostomy is often needed for more severe imperforate anus defects. This allows the baby to grow for 3 to 6 months before complete repair. The colostomy will likely be left in place for 2 to 3 more months.

Surgical Intervention for Low Imperforate Anus in a Female

- The infant is placed in lithotomy position with Foley catheter inserted and perineum prepped and draped. An electrical stimulator is used to find the midline of the anus so neuromuscular blocking agents must not be used.

- Equal amounts of innervated tissue should be left on each side to ensure function of the anus. The fistula, if present, is excised with an oval incision followed by dissection of the bowel from surrounding structures.

- With the dissection complete, a vertical midline incision is made at the opening of the true anus and fibers of the external sphincter are identified.

- The mobilized rectum is then pulled down to the new location.

- The end of the fistula is amputated and the external sphincter is sutured to the rectal serosa. The new anus is constructed using interrupted sutures and Hegar dilators to size the new anus.

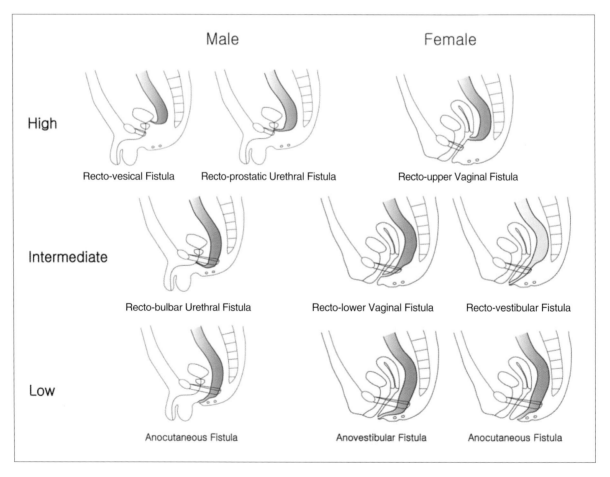

Figure 25-1 · Imperforate anus. (Reproduced with permission from Choi YH, Kim IO, Cheon JE, Kim WS, Yeon KM. Imperforate Anus: Determination of Type Using Transperineal Ultrasonography. Korean J Radiol. 2009;10(4):355-360.)

Surgical Intervention for High Imperforate Anus—Posterior Sagittal Anorectoplasty

Posterior Approach

Presentation of Posterior Sagittal Anorectoplasty (PSARP) requires surgical intervention within 24 to 48 hours of birth. A sigmoid colostomy is necessary to allow for irrigation of the hiatal lumen and removal of meconium plugs as well as maintaining proximal colon function. Further studies such as cystograms and vaginograms should be performed after colostomy. PSARP is performed around 1 year of age or when the condition and size of the child allow.

- With the patient in a jackknife position, electrostimulation is used to locate the true anus, and a midsagittal incision is made from the midsacrum to the anterior border of the anal site.
- Dissection continues until the external sphincter muscles are identified. Electrostimulation is used to dissect the fibers exactly midline.
- The coccyx is split midsagittally and the muscle complex is split sagittally along the visceral endopelvic fascia.
- The rectal pouch and urethra are identified and the bowel is incised vertically, exposing the fistula.
- The fistula is closed and the rectum is mobilized and tapered to allow for placement within the muscle complex.

- Sutures are used to reconstruct the muscles and keep the bowel securely positioned within the muscle complex.
- Electrostimulation is used to identify innervated tissue. External sphincter muscles and the coccyx are reapproximated and excess bowel is trimmed.
- Bowel is then secured to the skin edges of the anus and the skin is closed (see Figure 25-2).

Abdominal Approach

An abdominal approach may be necessary for very high rectal pouches and fistulas.

- After the midsagittal incisions and dissections are done, a drain is placed through the pelvis.
- One end is placed in the peritoneal cavity and the other end through the center of the anus and sutured to the skin.
- The patient is turned supine, an abdominal incision is made, the rectal pouch is mobilized, and the fistula is closed.
- The bowel is tapered and the terminal portion is sewn to the drain and pulled down through the rectum and the anal orifice.
- The bowel is sutured to the muscle and reapproximation of the coccyx and sphincter muscle is performed as previously described.

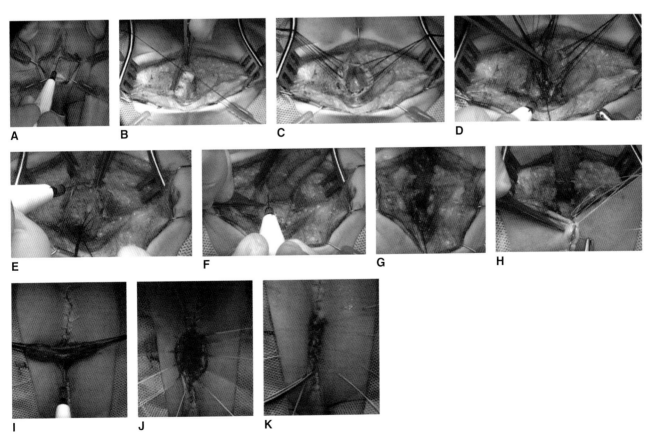

Figure 25-2 · Posterior sagittal anorectoplasty. (Reproduced with permission from Speck KE, et al. "Posterior Sagittal Anorectoplasty." Pediatric Surgery NaT. American Pediatric Surgical Association; 2018.)

TUMORS

Wilms' Tumor

Wilms' tumor is a rare cancer and is the most common cancer of the kidneys in children. Also known as nephroblastoma, Wilms' tumor most often affects children ages 3 to 4 and becomes much less common after age 5. Wilms' tumor most often occurs in just one kidney, though it can sometimes be found in both kidneys. Infrequently, Wilms' tumor may extend into the inferior vena cava and the atrium of the heart. Signs and symptoms of Wilms' tumor vary widely, and some children are asymptomatic. Signs and symptoms include an abdominal mass you can feel, abdominal swelling, abdominal pain, fever, blood in the urine, nausea, vomiting, constipation, loss of appetite, shortness of breath, and high blood pressure.

Surgical Intervention

- Children are positioned supine with a roll under the affected side.
- The chest and abdomen should both be included in the surgical prep. A separate sterile setup should be used to inspect the contralateral kidney.
- A transabdominal approach is used to inspect the abdomen and clamp the renal pedicle. If needed, the transabdominal incision may be extended to the thoracic cavity.
- Before tumor resection, suspicious lymph nodes are removed. If no suspicious nodes are present, biopsies are taken in the adjacent areas.
- The contralateral kidney is explored before resection of the tumor. The tumor is removed to the extent that it does not place the child in jeopardy and hemostatic clips are placed around the area to facilitate radiation therapy.
- The adrenal gland is usually removed and the abdomen and viscera are inspected for metastasis.
- Tumor extension may also require partial colectomy or partial resection of the diaphragm.

Neuroblastoma

Neuroblastoma is the third most common childhood cancer after leukemia and brain cancer. It occurs in approximately 7.4% of children. Neuroblastoma develops from immature nerve cells (neuroblasts) and can develop anywhere sympathetic nerve tissue is found. It most commonly arises in and around the adrenal glands, however, it can also develop in other areas of the abdomen and in the chest, neck, and near the spine, where groups of nerve cells exist. Neuroblastoma in the abdomen is the most common form and may include signs and symptoms such as abdominal pain, a nontender mass under the skin, and changes in bowel habits, such as diarrhea or constipation. Neuroblastoma most commonly affects children age 5 or younger, though it may rarely occur in older children. It is a silent tumor in its early stages but can metastasize rapidly. Treatment includes surgery, chemotherapy, and radiation.

Sacrococcygeal Teratoma

A sacrococcygeal teratoma is a tumor that grows at the base of the spine in a developing fetus. It occurs in 1:40,000 newborns and girls are four times more likely to be affected than boys. Teratomas are usually benign but may undergo malignant changes if not treated early in life. Teratomas often present as a large protuberance in the sacrococcygeal area but may extend into the pelvis and abdomen. Early surgical resection is important since these tumors are not sensitive to radiation therapy and are only temporarily responsive to chemotherapy. If not all the tumor is removed during the initial surgery, the teratoma may recur and additional surgeries may be needed. Studies have found that sacrococcygeal teratomas recur in up to 22% of cases.

GENITOURINARY TRACT CONDITIONS

Testicular Torsion

The most common genitourinary tract emergency is testicular torsion. Testicular torsion is a twisting of the spermatic cord and its contents. Immediate surgical intervention is required to relieve testicular ischemia. This is most common in early adolescents. The Initial symptom of scrotal discomfort can occur gradually or abruptly. Additional symptoms may be edematous, extremely tender, and abnormal placement of the teste. Accompanied by urination urgency, fever, and dysuria. Intervention whether it be manual or surgical is most effective within 6 hours of the torsion. Delayed treatment over 12 hours drastically reduces the viability of the testis, with a 75% chance it will need to be removed. In all cases, surgery will be necessary to stabilize the testis in the scrotum to prevent reoccurrence.

The surgical procedure is minimally invasive. A trans-scrotal surgical approach is predominately used to access the affected testicle. Once the torsion is relieved and blood flow is returned to the testis, it is secured within the scrotal sack. Postoperatively strenuous activity should be limited with pain management.

Cryptorchidism

Cryptorchidism is the absence of one or both testicle from the scrotum. It is the most common birth defect involving the male genitalia.

Treatment. Surgical correction is generally required. Gentle manipulation of the testicle into the scrotum and performing an orchiopexy may be done open or laparoscopically. This is generally done between 5 to 15 months of age.

Surgical Intervention

- If the testicle is in the groin, an inguinal incision is used to release the testicle. The testicle is then tunneled through the inguinal canal into the scrotum. An additional incision is made in the scrotum to perform an orchiopexy.
- A camera may be used if the testicle cannot be palpated in the inguinal canal.

- A small incision is made in the abdomen and a laparoscopy is performed to locate the testicle. It may be necessary to stage this procedure depending on the difficulty of locating and releasing the testicle.
- Once free the testicle can be left in the abdomen for up to 6 months, returning for the second stage of surgery to complete transcending the testicle into the scrotum and being secured.

Hypospadias

Hypospadias is the failure of tubularization and fusion of the urethral groove. It is most prevalent in boys. The urethral opening is located on the underside of the penile shaft by the penoscrotal junction, in the scrotal folds, or in the perineum. The foreskin is not circumferential and gives the impression of a dorsal hood. Methods of hypospadias repair include meatoplasty and glanuloplasty, orthoplasty, urethroplasty, skin cover, and scrotoplasty. Common complications of hypospadias repair are urethral fistulas and strictures.

Meatoplasty and Glanuloplasty Incorporated (MAGPI)

The MAGPI procedure is routinely performed on an outpatient basis without any urinary diversion. A circumferential incision is made approximately 8 mm proximal to the meatus and corona. The skin is subcutaneously dissected away from the phallus. A bridge of tissue is made between the meatus and glanular groove with a transverse closure of the upper meatal edge to the distal glanular groove. Three traction sutures are placed at the apex of the ventral meatus and the lateral areas of the glans. The glans are sutured together ventrally and redundant tissue is excised. Vertical mattress sutures are used to approximate the glans beneath the meatus. Excessive foreskin should be removed and the penile skin reapproximated.

Orthoplasty

Orthoplasty, also known as chordae repair, is performed to straighten the penis. Artificial erection is achieved by injecting preservative-free injectable saline into the corpus cavernosum making it possible to determine the degree of curvature of the penis. An incision is made around the corona and distally to the urethral meatus and below the glans. Dissection is carried to the level of the tunica albuginea. Proximally, the fibrous plaque is freed and the urethra is elevated. The chordae are freed completely along the entire penile shaft to the penoscrotal junction. The glans penis is closed and excess skin is removed. If urethroplasty is not required, the incision is closed along the dorsal midline.

Urethroplasty

Surgical Approaches

Urethroplasty is a surgery where the urethra is reconstructed to correct problems like urethral strictures. There are two general types of urethroplasty procedures: primary anastomotic repairs and substitution repairs. Primary anastomotic repairs involve excision of the stricture with reconnection of the healthy ends of urethra. Substitution urethroplasty involves tissue transfer techniques typically using buccal mucosa grafts or genital skin flaps to build on to the stricture and increase its caliber. When possible, anastomotic repairs are preferred as they are less complex and carry excellent durable success rates. There are certain situations, usually when the stricture is too long, where substitution techniques are required. Certain cases require a combination of techniques, typically when there are multiple severe strictures present. All of these procedures require temporary urinary diversion.

- Adjacent skin flaps can be created by tubularizing the skin adjacent to the meatus to create a neourethra. Graft material can also be supplied by transfer of the dorsal skin to the ventrum. This thin rotational flap is less than ideal due to decreased vascularity and the results are prone to complications.
- Free skin grafts should be full thickness and need to be revascularized. It is important to have full skin cover of the dorsal preputial penile skin that is well vascularized.
- The ventral preputial skin is used as a free graft and anastomosed proximally to the urethra.
- The middle glans are fixed to the corpora and meatoplasty with the dorsal glans is completed. The meatus, glans, and dorsal penis shaft are then sutured in place.
- Vascular flaps of preputial penile skin may also be used. It is mobilized to the ventrum and left attached to the outer surface of the prepuce or used as an island flap. Preputial skin is preferred due to its rich blood supply.
- The ventral preputial skin is dissected and used to create a neourethra.
- A glans channel is created just above the corpora, and the neourethra is spiraled to the ventrum.
- It is anastomosed proximally to the urethra and carried to the tip of the glans.
- The dorsal penile flaps and transposed laterally to the midline and excess skin is excised.
- Closure around the glans and the penile shaft is completed (see Figure 25-3).

Hydrocelectomy

A hydrocelectomy is a surgical procedure to repair a hydrocele, which is a buildup of fluid within the scrotum. The fluid is contained within the tunica vaginalis. Often a hydrocele will resolve itself without treatment. However, as a hydrocele grows larger, it can cause swelling, pain, and discomfort in the scrotum and may need surgical repair. This is often due to infection or trauma. During hydrocelectomy, an anterolateral incision is made in the scrotum over the mass. The fascial layers are incised and the tunica vaginalis exposed. The fluid sac is freed and opened. Contents are aspirated and the sac is inverted to cover the testis, epididymis, and distal cord. The tunica vaginalis is sutured behind the testicle and returned to the scrotum. A drain is placed if necessary and the scrotal layers are closed in the appropriate fashion.

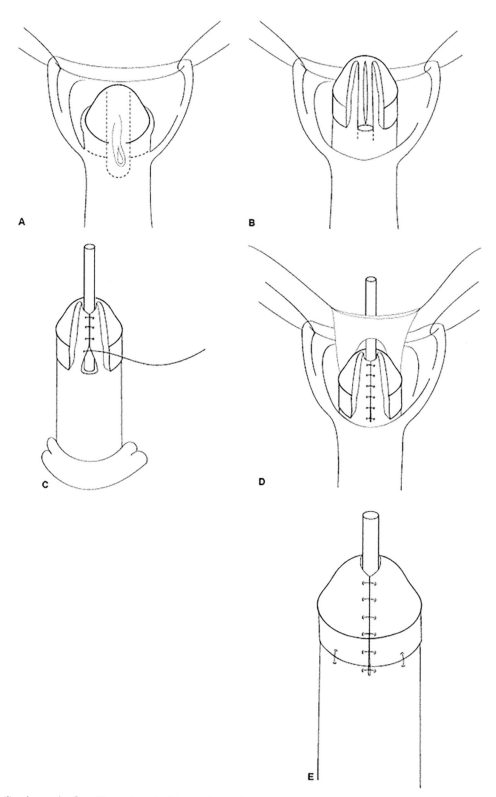

Figure 25-3 · Mobilized vascular flap. (Reproduced with permission from Ziegler MM, Azizkhan RG, von Allmen D, Weber TR. *Operative Pediatric Surgery,* 2nd ed. New York, NY: McGraw Hill; 2014.)

GASTROINTESTINAL DISORDERS

Congenital Diaphragmatic Hernia

The diaphragm forms over the course of the 6th through 12th weeks' gestation in the fetus. When it does not form completely, a defect, called congenital diaphragmatic hernia (CDH), is created (see Figure 25-4). The hernia is repaired by replacing the displaced viscera into the abdominal cavity and closing the diaphragmatic defect. Intra-abdominal abnormalities are high in infants with CDH; therefore, an abdominal approach is preferred. Intrusion of the abdominal viscera into the thoracic cavity can cause significant cardiovascular and pulmonary compromise. The repair is not emergent but is considered urgent and usually takes place within the first week of life. A chest tube may be needed to prevent tension pneumothorax, as well as a gastrostomy tube for feeding and hernia mesh or silastic sheeting for complex repairs.

Surgical Intervention

- A subcostal incision is made on the side of the defect. The abdominal contents are withdrawn from the thorax and held downward.

- Due to concurrent abdominal abnormalities, such as malrotation, the contents of the abdomen are closely inspected and repairs are completed as needed.

- The diaphragmatic defect is inspected and resection of the hernia sac, if present, is performed.

- Primary closure of the anterior and posterior rim of the diaphragm is performed. If the diaphragmatic tissue is insufficient, hernia mesh or silastic sheeting may be used to reinforce the closure.

- Gastrostomy tube placement is then performed.

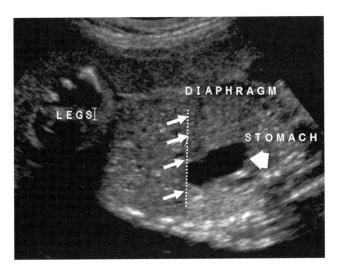

Figure 25-4 · Prenatal ultrasound of a fetus with a congenital diaphragmatic hernia. (Reproduced with permission from Brunicardi FC, Andersen DK, Billiar TR, Dunn DL, Hunter JG, Matthews JB, Pollock RE. *Schwartz's Principles of Surgery,* 10th ed. New York, NY: McGraw Hill; 2015.)

- If the musculature allows, the abdominal wall is closed. If the abdomen cannot accommodate the viscera, a ventral hernia is left with the skin closed over the top, with the child returning later for ventral hernia repair.

Nissen Fundoplication

Nissen fundoplication is a procedure which is done to restore the function of the lower esophageal sphincter by wrapping the stomach around the esophagus. This procedure creates a new functional valve between the esophagus and the stomach and prevents reflux of acid and bile from the stomach into the esophagus. This procedure can be done through a left subcostal incision or laparoscopically (minimally invasive). Nissen fundoplication is indicated for infants and children who experience severe reflux. The major cause of this reflux is an inadequate anti-reflux barrier caused by inadequate strength and amount of muscle fibers, length of the abdominal esophagus, and high-pressure zone in the lower esophagus. Inadequate anti-reflux barrier can lead to obstructive apnea, aspiration pneumonia, esophagitis, and failure to thrive.

Open Nissen Fundoplication Repair

Surgical Procedure

- With the patient in supine position, an esophageal dilator is placed into the esophagus to prevent the wrap from being too tight.

- A left subcostal incision is made, the esophagus is mobilized and the crural opening is identified.

- The stomach is mobilized to allow for a loose wrap of the fundus around the gastroesophageal junction (GE junction).

- Sutures are placed through the muscular layers of both the stomach and esophagus to fix the wrap in place.

- The fundus wrap is secured to the crural edges as well. Sometimes a gastrostomy tube will also be placed to allow for feeding after the surgery (see Figure 25-5).

ABDOMINAL WALL DEFECTS

Anterior abdominal wall defects are a common condition. During normal embryonic development, the midgut herniates through the umbilical ring and continues to develop. At the 11th week of embryonic development, the midgut returns to the coelomic cavity, allowing the closure of the umbilical ring. Failure of the midgut to return and allow proper rotation and fixation of the midgut causes an omphalocele (see Figure 25-6A).

Gastroschisis is represented by an abdominal wall defect, without a sac covering the abdominal viscera to the right of the umbilical cord (see Figure 25-6B).

Omphalocele

Omphalocele is a midline hole in the abdominal wall. The defect is usually greater than 4 cm in diameter with a membranous pouch. The outside layer of tissue is amnion, with the

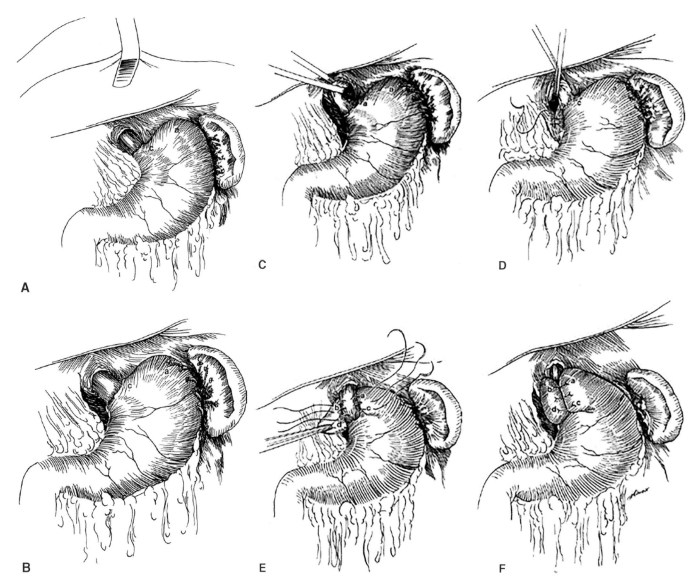

Figure 25-5 · Nissen fundoplication. (Reproduced with permission from Ziegler MM, Azizkhan RG, von Allmen D, Weber TR. *Operative Pediatric Surgery,* 2nd ed. New York; NY: McGraw Hill; 2014.)

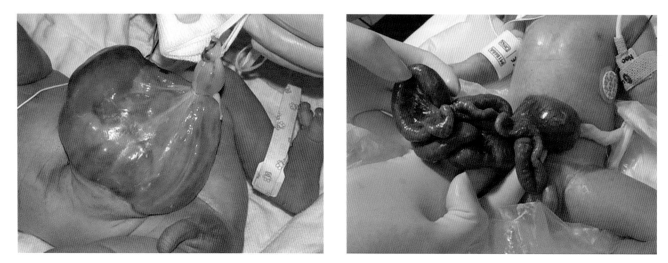

Figure 25-6 · **A.** Omphalocele with intact sac. **B.** Gastroschisis with bowel to the right of the umbilical cord. (**A**: Reproduced with permission from Zinner MJ, Ashley SW, Hines OJ. *Maingot's Abdominal Operations,* 13th ed. New York, NY: McGraw Hill; 2019. B: Reproduced with permission from Doherty GM. *Current Diagnosis & Treatment: Surgery,* 15th ed. New York, NY: McGraw Hill; 2020; Figure 45-34. ISBN 9781260122213. Used with permission from Craig W. Lillehei, MD.)

interior layer being peritoneum. Newborns with an omphalocele have a 50% prevalence of correlated irregularities. A complete diagnostic examination must be conducted to determine any related anomalies.

Surgical correction of omphaloceles is primary closure of the defect. Hypothermia is a risk, and the infant should be monitored. Additionally, a graft may aid in primary closure. Graft material may be synthetic or autologous. Giant omphaloceles are treated by applying caustic agents to the sac, encouraging thickening and epithelialization. Such topical agents are silver nitrate, betadine, or mercurochrome. Infant mortality will be determined by the severity of the defect and associated anomalies.

Gastroschisis

Gastroschisis is a defect that also presents during embryonic development. This anomaly is found to the right of the umbilical cord, generally creating a 4-cm-diameter defect. Unlike the Omphalocele there is not a protective sac around the intestines. Causing the intestine to thicken, be edematous, and altered by exposure to the amniotic fluid. Gastroschisis does not have the associated anomalies like the Omphalocele. However, there is a 15% stricture rate. Newborns must be handled with care so as to not cause damage to the bowel.

Primary closure can be achieved when the intestines can be safely reduced. Skin and fascia can successfully be closed. Larger defects may require a prosthetic patch or biomaterial alternatives. Dysfunctional intestine or short gut syndrome remains one of the most difficult challenges with gastroschisis.

OTORHINOLARYNGOLOGIC PROCEDURES

Foreign Body Removal

Pediatric foreign body ingestion is accidental, although deliberate ingestion can also occur. In addition to the mouth, children may also place objects in their noses and ears. Most swallowed foreign bodies will harmlessly pass through the GI tract, but some will lead to health problems if they become lodged, are sharp, or caustic. Removal may be necessary by esophagoscopy or open procedures. Objects placed in the ears and nose can cause bleeding, difficulty with hearing, rhinorrhea, nasal crusting, and air outflow obstruction.

Aspiration is the most significant risk of foreign body ingestion. Children have immature laryngeal sphincters and lack molars to chew food. The most common aspirated foods in children are candy, gum, nuts, popcorn, vegetables, hotdogs, and fish bones. The most common non-food items are coins, toys, crayons, pen tops, tacks, and beads. Aspiration can cause partial or complete airway obstruction and may require rigid or flexible bronchoscopy.

Myringotomy with Tube Placement

Surgical Procedure

Myringotomy is a surgical procedure of the tympanic membrane. The procedure is performed by making a small incision with a myringotomy knife through the layers of tympanic membrane. This surgical procedure permits direct access

to the middle ear space and allows the release of middle-ear fluid, which is the end-product of otitis media (OM), whether acute or chronic. The fluid is suctioned from the middle ear through the incision and, if indicated, sent for bacterial or viral cultures. Bilateral myringotomy is often used in conjunction with placement of middle-ear ventilation tubes, which permits the incised drum to remain open and allows better drainage of middle-ear fluid. This approach facilitates instillation of antibiotic otitic drops and ultimately results in faster resolution of the OM.

Risk factors for the development of OM include exposure to bacteria and viruses in daycares, exposure to second-hand smoke, bottle feeding, cleft palate, and Down syndrome. Hearing loss caused by fluid in the middle ear can have a negative impact on speech development and performance in the classroom.

Surgical Intervention

- General anesthesia is required for children to prevent movement during the procedure. An aural speculum is inserted into the ear canal.

- The microscope is positioned, and excess cerumen is removed with a wax curette.

- A radial incision is made in the anterior quadrant of the pars tensa using a myringotomy knife.

- Fluid is suctioned from the middle ear and a tube is inserted into the incision (see Figure 25-7).

- The lumen of the tube is gently suctioned and antibiotic drops are instilled.

Tonsillectomy and Adenoidectomy

Tonsillectomy and adenoidectomy are performed for either recurrent infections or upper airway obstruction. Recurrent infections may contribute to asthma, OM, and sinus problems. Upper airway obstruction can cause obstructive sleep apnea.

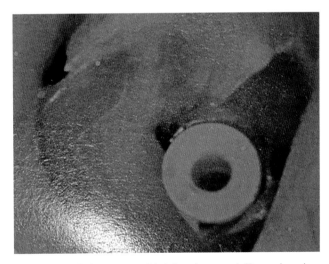

Figure 25-7 · Myringotomy with tube placement. (Reproduced with permission from Brunicardi FC, Andersen DK, Billiar TR, et al. *Schwartz's Principles of Surgery*, 11th ed. New York, NY: McGraw Hill; 2019.)

Surgical removal of the tonsils and adenoids is particularly painful for the first 5 to 7 days postop. Parents should keep a daily log of the child's eating, drinking, voiding, and medication intake until the child's activity level returns to normal. There is a small risk of bleeding postoperatively that may require emergent electrocoagulation. Postoperative complications also include velopharyngeal insufficiency, nasopharyngeal stenosis, and pharyngeal stenosis.

Surgical Intervention

- A mouth gag with tongue blade is inserted and held by a mayo stand placed over the patient's chest. The posterior and lateral walls, as well as the hard palate, are palpated for abnormalities and defects.
- Adenoids should not be removed if a submucous cleft is found in order to avoid velopharyngeal insufficiency.
- Red rubber catheters are threaded through the nose and out the mouth and clamped to retract the soft palate.
- The nasopharynx is inspected with a mirror and the adenoids are removed with adenotomes, curettes, or microdebrider.
- The eustachian tube orifices and the torus tubarius should be avoided. The adenoid bed is then packed with wet tonsil sponges.
- A tonsil suction is used to suction the plume from the electrocoagulation pencil and the escaped oxygen from the endotracheal tube.
- The superior pole of the right tonsil is grasped and the anterior and posterior tonsillar pillars are outlined with the electrocoagulation pencil.
- Dissection continues to the tonsillar capsule and the tonsil is removed.

Residual bleeding vessels are coagulated and the procedure is repeated on the left side.

NEUROSURGICAL PROCEDURES

The most common neurologic problems in infants and children include myelomeningocele, encephalocele, cranio-synostosis, hydrocephalus, brain tumors, and traumas.

Myelomeningocele/Meningocele

Myelomeningocele is a severe form of spina bifida in which the meninges, spinal cord, and nerve roots develop outside of the body and are contained in a fluid-filled sac that is visible outside of the back (see Figure 25-8). The exposed spinal cord is known as the neural placode. These babies typically have weakness and loss of sensation below the sac. This can result in muscle weakness and/or paralysis, bowel and bladder problems, hydrocephalus, Chiari Malformation, seizures, and orthopedic conditions such as scoliosis, hip problems, and foot deformities. The extent of disability depends on the vertebral level of the spina bifida. Myelomeningocele affects about 1 in every 1000 babies. Most cases of myelomeningocele

are treated surgically with a repair soon after birth. In some cases, the repair is done while still in the womb prior to delivery. Children with hydrocephalus will likely require a Ventricular Peritoneal shunt. Meningoceles are similar to myelomeningoceles, but less devastating in that meninges and cerebrospinal fluid (CSF) protrude into the defect, but not the spinal cord.

Surgical Intervention

- Children with this defect are at high risk of developing latex allergy. All procedures should be performed in a latex-free environment.
- An elliptical incision is made around the defect. The epithelial tissue is removed from the neural placode.
- Dissection is performed on the ventral side of the placode following the nerve tissue down to the spinal cord.
- The dura is then separated from the fascia and closed over the neural placode.
- The fascia is freed from the muscle layer and closed over the dura.
- The muscle layer is closed and the skin is approximated.

Craniectomy for Craniosynostosis

Craniosynostosis is the premature fusion of the cranial sutures and can be characterized by the number of sutures involved (see Figure 25-9). One fused suture line is simple while more than one is compound. Cranial sutures allow for brain growth and for the calvaria to bend during the birthing process. The sutures usually begin to fuse around age 2 and are completely fused by 8 years of age. Sagittal synostosis occurs in approximately 50% of all synostosis and affects males more than females. Premature closure results in elongation of the skull in the anterior-posterior plane. Surgery usually occurs between 6 weeks and 6 months of age with the best cosmesis occurring at the earlier age.

Surgical Intervention

- A sinusoidal incision is made halfway between the anterior and posterior fontanelles from ear to ear, posterior to the pinna.
- The scalp is elevated anteriorly and posteriorly to expose the fontanelles and asterion. A burr hole is made on each side of the sagittal suture on the lambdoidal suture.
- A craniotome is used to cut anteriorly to the anterior fontanelle on each side of the sagittal suture.
- Rongeurs are used to connect the burr holes across the sagittal suture. The sagittal suture is gently elevated off the dura.
- A burr hole is placed in the asterion on each side and a craniotome makes a curvilinear cut posterior to the coronal suture.
- The parietal bone is then fractured laterally leaving the periosteum intact.
- The skin is then closed.

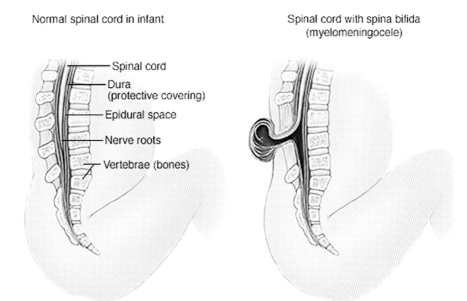

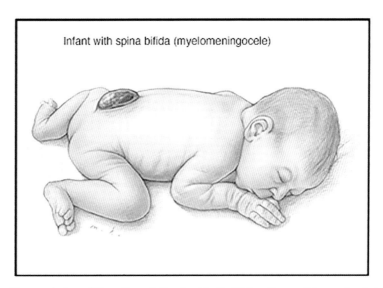

Figure 25-8 · Spina bifida. (Used with permission of Mayo Foundation for Medical Education and Research, all rights reserved.)

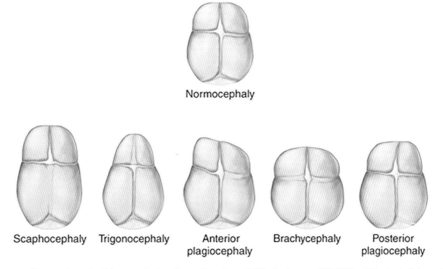

Figure 25-9 · Cranial sutures. (Reproduced with permission from Brunicardi FC, Andersen DK, Billiar TR, et al. *Schwartz's Principles of Surgery,* 11th ed. New York, NY: McGraw Hill; 2019.)

ORTHOPEDIC PROCEDURES

Developmental Dysplasia of the Hip (DDH)

DDH is an abnormality of the hip joint where the acetabulum does not fully cover the femoral head, resulting in an increased risk for joint dislocation, simple dysplasia, and dysplasia with subluxation. Eighty percent of DDH cases occur in females and in all cases, 60% involve the left hip. The goal of DDH management is to achieve and maintain a concentric reduction of the femoral head in the acetabulum to provide for optimal development of the structures. A Pavlik harness is the most commonly used nonsurgical treatment. If this fails, the infant is brought to surgery for a closed hip reduction and application of a spica cast. Failure of closed reduction will result in open reduction with an adductor tenotomy to allow abduction to reduce the femoral head. Children under 2 will then be placed in a spica cast. Children over 3 years of age may need a shortening varus femoral (derotational) osteotomy to facilitate reduction. A pelvic osteotomy may also be needed in some cases.

Surgical Intervention

DDH Open Reduction: The hip joint is opened and the soft tissue in the acetabulum is excised. The femoral head is then reduced and the capsule closed.

Derotational Osteotomy: The femur is internally rotated and divided. The distal fragment is rotated externally to place the knee and foot straight ahead. The osteotomy is frequently done in the subtrochanteric region and the osteotomized fragments are held in place with plates and/or screws.

Pelvic Osteotomy: A complete osteotomy is made in the wing of the ilium from the sciatic notch to the anterior margin of the ilium. The ilium is then wedged to increase the depth of the acetabulum when the osteotomy site is opened and bone grafted. The capsule is closed and a spica cast is applied.

PLASTICS AND RECONSTRUCTIVE SURGERY

Cleft Lip Repair

Sugical Techniques

There are many techniques to repair unilateral cleft lip deformity. Three basic techniques for unilateral cleft lip repair are the straight-line technique, the triangular flap technique, and the rotation-advancement technique. Each has its advantages and limitations; therefore, no individual technique has gained universal acceptance. This method is conceptually the simplest method to understand and perform. The basic concept of the straight-line technique involves the use of angled incisions made at the opposing cleft margins. The lateral cleft segment is mobilized to join the medial segment creating a philtral column where the scar lies. Limitations of this technique are the creation of a short upper lip. The triangular flap technique recruits tissue from the lateral cleft by creating a triangular flap and inserting this flap into the medial segment. This is a Z-plasty technique. This method corrects the common problem of a short lip typical of straight-line closure. The downfall of this technique is that it creates an unnatural scar that crosses the philtrum in a highly visible portion of the lip. Rotational flap advancement is the most common used technique for unilateral cleft lip repair. This technique involves the rotation of the medial cleft element into the back cut near the columellar-labial junction. It is important to establish symmetry to the lip and nose at the time of the initial lip repair. This is done by establishing normative measurements between anatomic landmarks and emphasizing adherence to these measurements. However, these landmarks are often arbitrary and require considerable time and experience to master.

Cleft Palate Repair

Cleft palate is a condition in which the two plates of the skull that form the hard palate are not completely joined. The soft palate is in these cases cleft as well. In most cases, cleft lip is also present. Palate cleft can occur as complete (soft and hard palates) or incomplete (soft palate). When cleft palate occurs, the uvula is usually split. It occurs due to the failure of fusion of the lateral palatine processes, the nasal septum, or the median palatine processes. The hole in the roof of the mouth caused by a cleft connects the mouth directly to the inside of the nose. The major function of the soft palate is to aid in speech. The hard palate is necessary to prevent air escape while speaking and prevent the egress of liquid and food to the nose. Cleft palate repair usually occurs around 6 months of age (see Figure 25-10).

Surgical Intervention

- A mouth gag and throat pack are inserted.
- The outlines of the palatal flaps are marked and the palate is injected with lidocaine with epinephrine.
- The flaps are incised and elevated.
- A three-layer closure involves the nasal mucosa, muscle, and the palatal mucosa. A mattress suture may be placed in the tongue to aid in airway management postoperatively and the throat pack removed.
- The V-Y palatoplasty technique is frequently used to correct cleft palate.
- A V-shaped incision is made on the oral side of the palate. Mucoperiosteal flaps are elevated on both the oral and nasal side.
- Care is taken to preserve blood supply. A three-layer Y-shaped closure closes the cleft and lengthens the palate.
- A secondary procedure, a pharyngeal flap, may be necessary to improve speech after cleft palate repair. In this procedure, tissue from pharynx is added to the soft palate.
- A pharyngeal flap repair is usually done before the patient is 14 years of age.

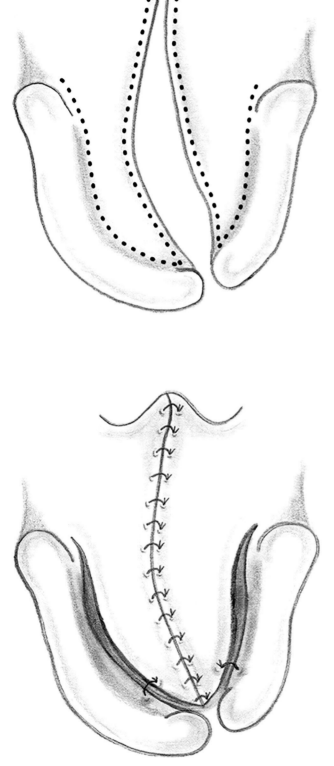

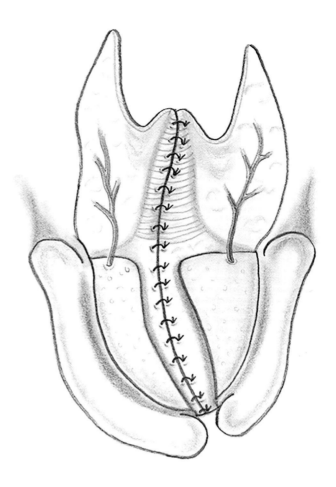

Figure 25-10 · Cleft palate. (Reproduced with permission from Tibesar RJ, Black A, Sidman JD. Surgical repair of cleft lip and palate. *Otolaryngol Head Neck Surg*. 2009; 20(4): 245-55.)

Syndactyly

Syndactyly is a term used to describe webbed or conjoined fingers or toes. It may occur as an isolated finding or may be a symptom of a genetic syndrome. It is occasionally seen in conjunction with polydactyly and other bony abnormalities. The most common form of syndactyly involves normal digits with a web of skin adjoining the digits (see Figure 25-11). Each digit has its own tendons, vessels, nerves, and phalanges. Plans for full-thickness skin grafting should be made since a deficiency in the skin is always present when separation is performed.

Surgical Intervention. Skin incisions are marked, and the tourniquet is inflated.

- The skin is incised and flaps at the sides of the fingers and in the web are elevated.
- Patterns of the areas of absent skin are transferred to the skin graft donor site.
- The graft is taken and sutured in place.
- Stent dressings are placed over the skin grafts and the hand is immobilized.

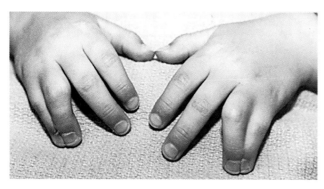

Figure 25-11 • Syndactyly. (Reproduced with permission from Patrick J. McMahon, Harry B. Skinner. *Current Diagnosis & Treatment in Orthopedics,* 6th ed. New York, NY: McGraw Hill; 2021.)

OPHTHALMIC PROCEDURES

Children will almost always need general anesthesia in order to have any surgery in or around their eyes.

Correction of Strabismus

Strabismus is a condition in which the visual axes of the eyes are not parallel and the eyes appear to be looking in different directions. In exotropia, the visual axes diverge. In esotropia, the visual axes converge. The danger with strabismus is that the brain may come to rely more on input from one eye than the other, and the part of the brain circuitry that is connected to the less-favored eye may fail to develop properly, leading to amblyopia in that eye. The initial treatment for mild-to-moderate strabismus is to cover the stronger eye with a patch, forcing the weaker eye to do enough work to catch up. However, severe strabismus may require surgery.

Surgical Intervention. The eye muscles attach to the sclera. The muscles are covered by a thin layer of transparent tissue called the conjunctiva.

- The eyelids are held open by a lid speculum.
- The surgeon incises the conjunctiva to access and isolate the eye muscles. A recession weakens function by altering the attachment site of the muscle on the eyeball.
- Once the muscle has been identified, a suture is placed through the muscle at the attachment site to the eye.
- The muscle is detached from the surface of the eye and reattached further back from the front of the eye, loosening the resting tension of the muscle.

A resection strengthens muscle function by reattaching a muscle to the eyeball at the original insertion site after a portion is removed. A suture is placed through the muscle at the intended new attachment site. The segment of muscle between the suture and the eyeball is removed and the shortened muscle is reattached to the eye.

Standard strabismus surgery uses a permanent knot tied during the surgical procedure. Adjustable suture technique uses a bow-knot or slip-knot in an accessible position. After surgery, the eye alignment can be altered by adjusting the temporary knot. The adjustment is typically done with the patient awake and the operated eye numbed. Adjustable suture surgery may only be offered to patients who are able to fully cooperate with the adjustment process. This adjustment may be done in the postoperative room, the next day, or later in the week, depending upon the surgeon's preference.

CONGENITAL HEART DEFECTS

Congenital heart anomalies are classified as cyanotic or acyanotic and their effect on pulmonary blood flow. Acyanotic defects increase pulmonary blood flow and include but are not limited to patent ductus arteriosus (PDA), septal defects, and atrioventricular (AV) canal defects. These defects cause left-to-right shunting of the blood and can lead to congestive heart failure (CHF), increased pulmonary vascular resistance, and thickened pulmonary vessels. Acyanotic obstructive defects include but are not limited to aortic stenosis, pulmonary stenosis, and coarctation of the aorta. Obstructive defects increase the afterload on the heart causing cardiomegaly, ventricular hypertrophy, and in severe cases, heart failure. Cyanosis implies right heart obstruction with right to left shunting, mixing of arterial and venous blood, or transposed great vessels. Defects include but are not limited to Tetralogy of Fallot (TOF), pulmonary atresia with an intact septum, tricuspid atresia, transposition of the great arteries (TGA), total/partial anomalous pulmonary venous return (TAPVR/PAPVR), and hypoplastic left heart syndrome (HLHS).

Atrial Septal Defects (ASD)

There are three common types of ASDs. Secundum defects, the most common, are located in the central portion of the atrial septum. Primum defects, the second most common, are located in the lower portion of the atrial septum and are associated with AV canal defects. Sinus venosus defects, the least common, are located in the right atrium at the superior vena cava junction and are associated with anomalous veins. If left untreated, patients may develop right heart hypertrophy, atrial dysrhythmias, CHF, embolic events, and pulmonary vascular disease.

Surgical Intervention. A median sternotomy and cardiopulmonary bypass (CPB) are required.

- The right atrium is incised and the defect is identified.
- The defect is closed primarily with suture or with a patch of pericardium.
- The right atrium is closed.

Ventricular Septal Defects (VSD)

There are four basic types of VSDs. A perimembranous VSD is an opening in a particular area of the upper section of the ventricular septum (membranous septum), near the valves. This type of VSD is the most commonly operated on. Perimembranous VSDs do not usually close spontaneously. A muscular VSD is an opening in the muscular portion of the lower section of the ventricular septum. This is the most common type of

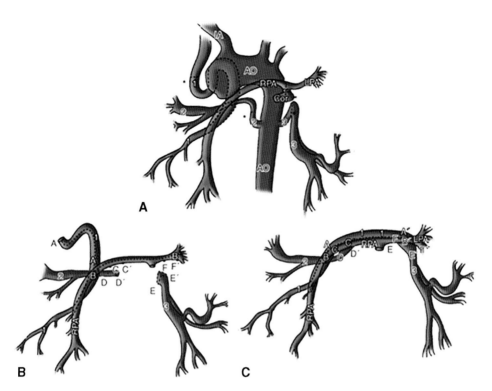

Figure 25-12 · Tetralogy of Fallot. (Reproduced with permission from Reddy VM, Liddicoat JR, Hanley FL. Midline one-stage complete unifocalization and repair of pulmonary atresia with ventricular septal defect and major aorto-pulmonary collaterals. *J Thorac Cardiovasc Surg.* 1995;109:832–45.)

VSD. A large number of these muscular VSDs close spontaneously and do not require surgery. Inlet VSDs are associated with atrioventricular canal defect. The VSD is located underneath the tricuspid and mitral valves.

Conal septal VSDs are the rarest of VSDs and occur in the ventricular septum just below the pulmonary valve. Large VSDs may contribute to CHF and pulmonary hypertension.

Surgical Intervention. A median sternotomy and CPB are required.

- For perimembranous and Inlet VSDs, an incision is usually made in the right atrium.
- Conal VSDs may need to be repaired through the pulmonary artery.
- Muscular VSDs can usually be repaired through the right atrial incision but may require a ventriculotomy.
- A patch repair of either synthetic material or pericardium is usually used to close the VSD. The defect is rarely closed primarily.
- The tricuspid valve is tested for regurgitation and the right atrium is closed.

Tetralogy of Fallot (TOF)

Four anatomic findings are consistent with TOF. These include an overriding aorta, a VSD, subpulmonary stenosis, and right ventricular hypertrophy. In patients with minimal pulmonary stenosis, physiology and hemodynamics are similar to that of a VSD. These patients are labeled as "pink tets" and have

right-to-left shunting and are not cyanotic. Patients with severe pulmonary stenosis exhibit significant right-to-left shunting, hypoxemia, and are labeled "blue tets." These patients experience increased incidence of hypercyanotic events or "tet spells" (see Figure 25-12).

Surgical Intervention. A median sternotomy and CPB are required.

- The VSD is closed in the fashion previously described.
- A ventriculotomy is made in the infundibulum.
- Hypertrophied infundibular muscle is excised from the right ventricular outflow tract.
- Pulmonary valvulotomy may be needed as well as patch closure of the infundibulum.
- CPB is discontinued and the sternum closed.

Patent Ductus Arteriosus (PDA)

In fetal life, blood bypasses the fetal lungs directly to the systemic circulation through the PDA. The vessel normally closes shortly after birth as a result of the onset of respiration. The ductus arteriosus connects the pulmonary artery to the aorta. If the ductus does not close, a shunt is created from the aorta to the pulmonary circulation (see Figure 25-13). This is common in premature babies. Isolated PDA should be closed to prevent hypertrophy and enlargement of the left heart. PDA in association with other heart defects is a life-sustaining structure and should not be closed until time of complete defect repair.

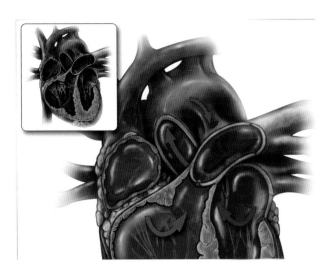

Figure 25-13 • Patent ductus arteriosus. (Used with permission from Evan Oto/Science Source.)

Surgical Intervention. Newborn PDAs are ordinarily closed bedside in the intensive care unit.

- The patient is placed in the right lateral position.
- A left posterior lateral approach is usually used.
- The chest wall is entered through the third or fourth intercostal space.
- The pleura is incised and the lung retracted out of the way.
- The mediastinal pleura is opened to expose the ductus.
- The recurrent laryngeal nerve is identified.
- The aortic arch, pulmonary artery, and ductus are dissected.
- The ductus may be divided using ties or suture or ligated using ties or hemostatic clips.
- The mediastinal pleura is closed, the lung re-expanded, and the ribs closed.

CHEST WALL DEFORMITIES

The most common congenital chest wall deformities are pectus excavatum and pectus carinatum. Pectus excavatum is five times more common than pectus carinatum. Approximately 1 in 100 children will have chest wall deformities. The male-to-female ratio of 3 or 4 males to 1 female. The deformation is usually present at birth and steadily becomes more pronounced between 8 and 10 years of age. Kyphosis and scoliosis are also commonly associated with chest wall deformities. Associated anomalies with pectus excavatum include congenital heart disease, mitral valve prolapse, Marfan syndrome, and Ehlers-Danlos syndrome. Therefore, an in-depth preoperative evaluation should be performed to diagnose the severity of the pectus excavatum. Indications for surgery require two or more pathologies: (1) abnormal pulmonary function test, (2) Haller index ratio 3:2, (3) mitral valve prolapse, murmurs with conduction, (4) progression of documented deformity.

Surgical Management

Surgical intervention for pectus excavatum is recommended while the chest is at the most malleable, primarily between 10 and 14 years of age. This age group tends to recover faster and have a better understanding of their health issue. There are two common procedures. The Nuss and the Ravitch procedures.

The Nuss procedure is a minimally invasive technique. Insertion of 1 to 3 curved metal bars posterior to the sternum guides the chest to the correct anatomical anatomy. Approximately 2- to 3-year postoperation the bars are removed.

The Ravitch procedure was developed in 1949. It is not minimally invasive. A transverse inframammary incision across the chest with bilateral subchondral resection of the costal cartilages, includes sternal osteotomies. Anterior fixation is done with metal bars. The fixation is removed after subsequent healing. The Nuss procedure is the surgery of choice, with minimal incisions, easy pain control, and successful results.

PEDIATRIC TRAUMA

Trauma affects children more so than adults, leading to surgical intervention. Pediatric trauma causes more deaths in children than all other causes combined. Blunt trauma is the leading injury type, with an increase in violent injuries among teenagers. The basic trauma ideologies are the same as with adults, but it's important to remember pediatric patients have different emotional and physical needs.

As with the ABCs of trauma, the pediatric patient's airway is paramount. Infants and toddlers may not be able to vocalize, so observations for choking, coughing, drooling, or crying can aid in diagnosis. Endotracheal intubation may be necessary. To determine the correct endotracheal size, compare to the child's 5th digit. The trachea is narrower and shorter than in adults. It's important to identify the variances between adults and pediatric patients. Small mouth with a larger tongue and short neck name are just a few of the challenges in maintaining an airway in children. The glottis is substantially anterior relative to an adult and the vocal cords are angled anterior. The epiglottis in children is more supple and rounded. Children are at high risk for hypoxia because of the smaller pulmonary functional residual capacity.

After securing the airway and breathing, evaluate circulation to confirm sufficient oxygenation. Once again age may challenge verbalization so observation of general color, presence of peripheral pulses, and presence of capillary refill. Parasympathetic hypertonia is prone in children and can be triggered by any painful stimuli. Awareness of blood loss is critical because pediatric patients have a low blood volume. After the preliminary ABCs, a secondary evaluation should be implemented. Hypothermia should be avoided to prevent difficulties of acidosis and coagulopathy.

Head and Spine Injuries

The leading cause of death among pediatric patients is traumatic brain injury (TBI). Shaken baby syndrome in toddlers 2 years and under is the most common cause of serious head injury. Hemorrhages of the subdural, subarachnoid, and retina are symptoms. Motor vehicle accidents, falls, bicycle and pedestrian accidents are the leading cause for majority of traumatic brain injuries in toddlers 3 years and older. Other symptoms of mild head injury include nausea, headache or possible amnesia, minor behavioral issues, or trouble concentrating.

THORACIC TRAUMA

The second leading cause of death with pediatric trauma is thoracic trauma. Primarily blunt trauma caused by motor vehicle accidents. It is possible for children to have major thoracic trauma without evidence of rib cage fractures. Children have more cartilaginous rib cage and therefore more pliable. Abuse is often suspected in children under 3 with rib fractures. Pulmonary contusions, tachypnea, hypercarbia, and hypoxemia may be substantial and require intubation and surgical intervention. Radiographic results may be variable, therefore undependable for diagnosis.

ABDOMINAL TRAUMA

Bruising of the mid anterior abdominal wall is called the seat belt sign, common in children involved in a motor vehicle accident. These injuries may present subtle signs of bowel injury or the presence of free peritoneal fluid. Perforation of the greater curvature is seen in blunt force injuries to the abdomen such as a handlebar impact, skateboarding, or being hit by a vehicle. A CT scan will display free fluid in the abdomen, as well as organ trauma.

Organ Injuries

The intra-abdominal solid organs are particularly vulnerable to blunt trauma in children. Nonoperative management is the standard therapy for hemodynamically stable children with blunt solid organ injury. Those who fail to respond to nonoperative management usually do so within the first 12 hours. The American Pediatric Surgical Association has detailed guidelines regarding the management of isolated liver and spleen injuries based on initial CT findings; these have been shown to reduce the length of hospital stay significantly, without adverse outcomes (Table 25-2). Splenic injuries are relatively common in pediatric trauma. Splenic injuries are managed conservatively unless there is evidence of hemodynamic instability. CT scan can delineate the extent of splenic injury. The role of splenic artery embolization in the treatment of pediatric blunt splenic injury remains uncertain, unlike in adult patients. An isolated hepatic injury without involvement of the hepatic vein, IVC, or portal vein can also be managed conservatively. Some have reported that 85% to 90% of patients can successfully be treated with nonoperative management. However, those who fail to

TABLE 25-2 • CLASSIFICATION OF INTRA-ABDOMINAL SOLID ORGAN INJURIES			
Grade	Liver	Spleen	Kidney
I	Hematoma: <10% subcapsular surface area	Hematoma: <10% subcapsular	Contusion: microscopic or gross hematuria
	Laceration: capsular tear <1 cm	Laceration: capsular tear <1 cm	Hematoma: subcapsular, nonexpanding, no parenchymal tear
II	Hematoma: 10%-50% subcapsular surface area, <10 cm intraparenchymal hemorrhage	Hematoma: 10%-50% subcapsular surface area, <5 cm intraparenchymal hemorrhage	Hematoma: nonexpanding perirenal hematoma confined to retroperitoneum
	Laceration: capsular tear 1-3 cm deep, <10 cm length	Laceration: capsular tear, 1-3 cm parenchymal depth not involving a trabecular vessel	Laceration: <1 cm parenchymal depth of renal cortex without collecting system rupture or urinary extravasation
III	Hematoma: >50% expanding subcapsular surface area, ruptured subcapsular hematoma with active bleeding, or intraparenchymal hematoma ≥2 cm or expanding	Hematoma: ruptured subcapsular or parenchymal hematoma; intraparenchymal hematoma >5 cm or expanding	Laceration: >1 cm parenchymal depth of renal cortex without collecting system rupture or urinary extravasation
	Laceration: >3 cm parenchymal depth	Laceration: >3 cm parenchymal depth involving trabecular vessels	
IV	Hematoma: ruptured parenchyma with active bleeding	Hematoma: ruptured parenchyma with active bleeding	Laceration: parenchymal laceration extending through the renal cortex, medulla, and collecting system
	Laceration: parenchymal disruption involving 25%-75% of hepatic lobe	Laceration: hilar vessels with major devascularization (>25% of spleen)	Vascular: main renal artery or vein injury with contained hemorrhage
V	Laceration: parenchymal disruption involving >50% of hepatic lobe	Laceration: completely shattered spleen	Laceration: completely shattered kidney
	Vascular: juxtahepatic venous injuries (retrohepatic vena cava, central major hepatic veins)	Vascular: hilar vascular injury with total devascularization	Vascular: avulsion of renal hilum with devascularization of kidney
VI	Vascular: hepatic avulsion		

respond do so because of hemodynamic instability, changes in clinical examination findings, or transfusion requirements of more than half of blood volume (roughly 40 mL/kg/day). Delayed bleeding after liver injury has been reported as late as 6 weeks after injury and may be seen in 1% to 3% of patients. As is the case with splenic lacerations, one should proceed with definitive surgical treatment whenever there is hemodynamic instability despite adequate resuscitation.

PANCREATIC INJURY

Pancreatic injuries occur from blunt trauma, such as falling into bicycle handlebars. An elevated amylase or lipase level is present. CT scan is a useful diagnostic modality for evaluation of most pancreatic trauma, although it is not as sensitive or specific for determination of pancreatic ductal injuries. There is little role for ERCP in acute settings of pediatric pancreatic injury. When presented acutely, transection of pancreas from blunt trauma is best managed with operative intervention of distal pancreatectomy. For those with delayed presentation, a conservative management is more appropriate. This may include TPN and bowel rest. ERCP is considered to evaluate for ductal injuries. External drainage procedure may be required.

References

1. Intestinal Atresia & Stenosis.| Types, Diagnosis & Treatment. cincinnatichildrens.org. Accessed September 12, 2023.

Bibliography

Duckett JW, Snyder HM 3rd. The MAGPI hypospadias repair in 1111 patients. *Ann Surg.* 1991;213(6):620-625. https://pubmed.ncbi.nlm.nih.gov/2039293/. Accessed September 5, 2023.

Genetic and Rare Diseases Information Center. Sacrococcygeal Teratoma. https://rarediseases.info.nih.gov/diseases/319/sacrococcygeal-teratoma. Accessed September 5, 2023.

Healthline. Hydrocelectomy: What You Need to Know. https://www.healthline.com/health/hydrocelectomy#candidates. Accessed September 5, 2023.

Hesgaard HB, Wright KW. Principles of strabismus surgery for common horizontal and vertical strabismus types. In: Pacheco PA, ed. *Advances in Eye Surgery.* London, UK: InTech; 2016. https://www.intechopen.com/books/advances-in-eye-surgery/principles-of-strabismus-surgery-for-common-horizontal-and-vertical-strabismus-types. Accessed September 5, 2023.

Meara JG, Andrews BT, Ridgway EB, Raisolsadat MA, Hiradfar M. Unilateral cleft lip and nasal repair: techniques and principles. *Iran J Pediatr.* 2011;21(2):129-138.

Medline Plus Medical Encyclopedia. Imperforate Anus Repair. https://medlineplus.gov/ency/article/002926.htm#:~:text=Imperforate%20anus%20repair%20is%20surgery%20to%20correct%20a,all%20stool%20from%20passing%20out%20of%20the%20rectum. Accessed September 5, 2023.

Memorial Hermann. (2021). Laparoscopic Nissen Fundoplication. https://memorialhermann.org/services/treatments/laparoscopic-nissen-fundoplication. Accessed September 5, 2023.

Reilly BK, Patel NJ. Myringotomy. Medscape. 2021. https://emedicine.medscape.com/article/1890977-overview. Accessed September 5, 2023.

Rothrock JC. *Alexander's Care of the Patient in Surgery.* 13th ed. Canada: Mosby Elsevier; 2007.

The Mayo Clinic. Wilms Tumor. https://www.mayoclinic.org/diseases-conditions/wilms-tumor/symptoms-causes/syc-20352655. Accessed September 5, 2023.

Wikipedia. https://en.wikipedia.org/wiki/Neuroblastoma. Accessed September 5, 2023.

UCSF Dept of Surgery. Congenital Diaphragmatic Hernia https://surgery.ucsf.edu/conditions—procedures/congenital-diaphragmatic-hernia.aspx. Accessed September 5, 2023.

Washington University Physicians. Myelomeningocele. https://www.ortho.wustl.edu/content/Patient-Care/6885/Services/Pediatric-and-Adolescent-Orthopedic-Surgery/Overview/Pediatric-Spine-Patient-Education-Overview/Myelomeningocele.aspx#:~:text=Myelomeningocele%20is%20a%20severe%20form,of%20sensation%20below%20the%20sac. Accessed September 5, 2023.

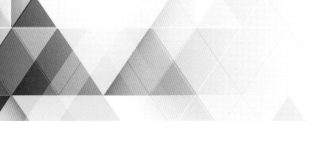

Organ Procurement

Maria Storer

ORGAN PROCUREMENT & TRANSPLANTATION FOR THE SURGICAL ASSISTANT

As technological and medical advancements continue to emerge, organ procurement and transplantation become more prevalent in our profession each day. Knowledge of the many steps required before procurement and transplantation happen will give you a better understanding of the entire process. The gift of life from one person to another is immensely generous and deserves to be honored. The best way to do so is to be knowledgeable during these procedures to ensure the best possible outcome. Both procurement and transplantation are extremely amazing breakthroughs in surgery.

Once the possibility of procuring organs became a reality, laws and organizations needed to be established to carry on this tremendous endeavor. The National Organ Transplant Act of 1984 (NOTA) was passed to ensure the organ allocation process would be carried out in a fair and efficient way, leading to an equitable distribution of donated organs. The legislature established a national computer registry, The Organ Procurement and Transplantation Network (OPTN), to match donor organs to waiting recipients. OPTN is managed by the United Network for Organ Sharing (UNOS), and all 58 organ procurement organizations use the UNOS computer system to match and place organs equitably and efficiently to save more lives.

The procurement process begins when a potential organ donor is identified. As a surgical assistant (SA), it is important to know the guidelines throughout the entire process. There are two main types of donors which differentiate which organs and/or tissues can be donated. An individual who is brain dead, is on a respirator, and has a beating heart is an acceptable donor

for the heart, liver, pancreas, eyes/corneas, kidneys, intestines, heart valves, skin, bone, and lungs. An individual who has no cardiac or respiratory activity is an acceptable donor for eyes/corneas, blood vessels, cartilage, skin, bone, pericardium, and soft tissues.

The nature of the injury leads a physician to determine what organs or tissues can be procured. The patient is declared brain dead or a potential donor after circulatory death candidate. Each designation has a different route throughout this process.

The hospital zone assigned Organ Procurement Organization (OPO) is notified of all imminent patient deaths. Information is provided on the patient's medical status and the organ recovery coordinator evaluates the situation. The evaluation includes a medical and social history, and physical examination of the patient.

Once the patient is determined to be a candidate for organ and/or tissue donation, the legal next-of-kin is approached about the prospect of donation. If a donor designation or individual authorization by the decedent cannot be identified, the family must give their consent. Should the family agree, the legal next-of-kin signs a donor consent form. The OPO clinical coordinator, in coordination with the hospital staff, proceeds to medically maintain the patient.

The OPO clinical coordinator must provide the information on the organs available for donation, in addition to the donor's blood type and body size. The UNOS computer then matches the donated organs to potential recipients. Recipient selection is based on blood type, body size, medical urgency, and length of time on the waiting list. The heart, liver, and lungs are matched by blood type and body size. In matching the pancreas and kidneys, genetic tissue type is also considered.

The coordinator's role is ultimately to match organs with recipients in the donation service area. A digital list of waiting patients in the matching blood group is used for the match. If a match cannot be made for a specific organ within this area, the organ is offered on a regional basis, then nationally thereafter.

The next step is for the coordinator to call the transplant center when an organ and recipient have been matched. The patient's transplant surgeon is responsible for making the decision whether to accept the organ. If the surgeon declines the organ for their patient, the coordinator contacts the transplant surgeon of the next patient on the list. The process continues for each organ until each one has been appropriately matched with recipients. The coordinator arranges for the operating room (for the recovery of the organs), and the arrival and departure times of the transplant surgery teams. When the surgical team arrives, the donor is taken to the operating room where the organs and tissues are recovered through a dignified surgical procedure.

Once the recipients have been identified, they are called by their transplant surgeons for the final pre-operative preparations while the organ recovery process is occurring at the donor hospital. Upon the organs' arrival at the transplant hospital, the recipients are taken to surgery and the transplants are performed. The coordinator takes a sample of the lymph node tissue to a laboratory for tissue typing and subsequent matching with recipients. Other organs are taken directly to the recipients by the surgical recovery teams.

The surgical procurement of organs is where the SA comes into play. The teams consist of surgeons, coordinators, circulating nurses, surgical technologists, and SAs. Anesthesiologists, transplant teams, and other ancillary staff are all part of the process. Knowledge of each step of this surgical procurement prepares the SA for readiness during the procedure, anticipating any needs or potential challenges.

MULTIORGAN SURGICAL PROCUREMENT PREPARATORY PROCEDURAL STEPS

- A complete midline incision is made from the suprasternal notch to the pubis.
- The gallbladder is incised and washed free of bile to prevent later autolysis.
- Left triangular ligament of the liver is incised, and the esophagus is held to the left with a retracting finger and a longitudinal incision in the diaphragmatic crura between the retrohepatic inferior vena cava and the esophagus.
- The aorta is encircled with a tape. Intercostal or lumbar branches are ordinarily not encountered in this location.
- Turning more distally, the inferior mesenteric artery is ligated and divided, and the aorta is encircled with tape.
- The final preparatory step is isolation, ligation, and cannulation of the inferior mesenteric vein.
- The cannula is advanced superiorly for approximately 5 cm in adults and for lesser distances in children so that the tip is in or just entering the portal vein.

MULTIORGAN PROCUREMENT SURGICAL STEPS

After all preparatory steps have been set in place, no further dissection is needed for removal of either the kidneys or liver. At this time, the cardiac team can proceed with their portion of the procedure. Most cardiac team members are in the operating room ready to begin. SAs are crucial at this time where quick, yet efficient delicate work must take place. A well-trained, cohesive cardiac team can remove the heart in approximately 5 or 10 minutes using a variety of core cooling techniques. These heart procurement times vary among the surgical expertise of each cardiac procurement team. The cardiac team then discontinues circulation by occluding the vena cava inflow or by cross-clamping the aorta, and the previously encircled aorta is cross clamped at the diaphragmatic site.

The cold-infusion starts through both the inferior mesenteric venous cannula and through the terminal aortic cannula. The preferred solution for this double infusion is chilled lactated Ringer's, even though some surgeons prefer to use one of the potassium-rich Collin's solutions. The utilization of each one is chosen by cost or surgeon preference.

Infusate outflow is then provided by transecting the vena cava at the level of the diaphragm. The cardiac team can also choose to cross-clamp or staple the inferior vena cava within the pericardium. The vena cava is cut off near its abdominal bifurcation allowing more distal fluid outpour. During the course of the procurement, as the cardiac team conducts a gentle cardiectomy, the liver must also be closely observed while it blanches.

Once the cardiectomy has been completed, the surgical team must wait until the liver is free of blood and hypothermia before they begin their dissection. A patch of diaphragm is then removed around the lumen of the suprahepatic inferior vena cava. Once a bloodless field is accomplished, dissection of the hepatic hilum begins. The gastroduodenal, right gastric, splenic, and left gastric arteries can be cut or ligated to the celiac axis and common hepatic artery. The portal vein is dissected and then followed inferiorly to the splenic and superior mesenteric veins.

This dissection occurs with the liver inset and divided at the back table in the operating room. During most multiorgan procurements, there are many team members in the field. At this time, an SA may choose to join the surgeon and help during this dissection. The recently cut portal tributaries are folded superiorly while a finger examination is conducted. This exam will show an anomalous right hepatic artery passing posterior to the portal vein originating from the superior mesenteric artery that will require a patch. Some length of the superior mesenteric artery is removed with a Carrel patch from the aorta, covering some of the celiac-axis origin artery. The celiac-axis origin can also be removed with a Carrel patch. Next, the specimen is moved to a basin on the back table. A cannula is then inserted into the portal vein through which ice-cold Collin's solution is flushed. Now the liver is ready to be cleaned, bagged in ice, packed, and labeled by procurement techs and prepared for transplantation.

During this time, the kidneys receive continuous cold perfusion in situ. The next step is to remove both kidneys which are then immersed in an ice bath and perfused with Collin's solution once more. This can be done individually through the aorta if they have not been separated at this point. Sometimes there are several teams in the room waiting for specific organs. Each team has everything ready because the procurement procedure and transportation to the potential recipient are both strictly time-constricted.

LIVER TRANSPLANT SURGERY

As with every transplantable organ, United Network of Organ Sharing (UNOS) has the task of allocating which patients will be receiving a needed organ. They have different procedure guidelines for adults and for pediatric patients. Once a liver becomes available for transplant, the OPO, region, medical urgency, points, and waiting time of the patient are factors for consideration. These points are measured by Status 1 which means, "has fulminant liver failure with a life expectancy without a liver transplant of less than 7 days." if a patient did not qualify under a Status 1, they are assigned a "probability of pre-transplant death derived from mortality risk score." The model for end-stage liver disease scoring system (MELD) measures the continuous function of total bilirubin, creatine, and prothrombin time. This determines the status of the liver disease and predicts the risk model in a prognosis of liver cirrhosis.

MELD scores = $10 \times [0.957 \times \ln(\text{creatinine mg/DL}) + 0.378 \times \ln(\text{bilirubin mg/DL}) + 1.120 \times \ln(\text{INR}) + 0.643 \times \text{Ic}]$

Stages of Liver Donation

Donated Liver, Status 1 patients in the OPO, Status 1 patients in the region, Non-status 1 patients in the OPO, Non-status 1 patients in the region, Status 1 Patient in the United States, Non-status patients in the United States.

Even though UNOS uses the MELD scores to allocate organ sharing, it "will remain the prerogative of the transplant surgeon and/or the physician responsible for the care of the patient." An organ may be declined due to low quality or health problems the donor may have had. Any patient who declines an organ will not be penalized and will have access to future livers.

Once the liver is accepted, the OPO and operating room team collaborate to get everything in motion. The call team is advised at what time to come in and set up the room. Once the team arrives, the case cart is checked, and all supplies are brought into the room. SAs joining the transplant team should review the preference sheet and become familiarized with any surgeon-specific details to ensure that integrating your role will be a seamless and smooth process.

The ergonomics of the operating room are important, as there will be lots of equipment and the flow should not be blocked in any way. There will be two back tables. One will be your back table and the other will be used for "benching" or getting the donor liver clean, flushed, and ready to transplant. Make sure the slush machine is on and ice is made before the patient gets in the room.

The circulating nurses and anesthesia team get the patient ready for the procedure. Once the patient is prepped, the team will drape the patient and hand off the Bovie, suction and connect to the cell saver.

At the benching table, one of the surgeons begins to prep the donor liver with an assistant while the rest of the team is at the patient's side beginning the case.

Liver Transplant Procedure Steps (See Figures 26-1 and 26-2)

- Inverted "T" incision is made, dissected, and maintained hemostasis, a Thompson self-retractor is then placed.
- Dissection on the right and then left side of the liver
- Dissection of vena cava
- Dissection of portal vein
- Dissection around cystic duct
- Clamp—either piggy-back of 2, incision on SVC and IVC

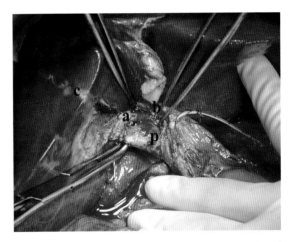

Figure 26-1 · Donor hepatectomy with landmarks. (Reproduced, with permission, from Brunicardi FC, Andersen DK, Billiar TR, et al., eds. *Schwartz's Principles of Surgery*. 11th ed. New York: McGraw Hill; 2019.)

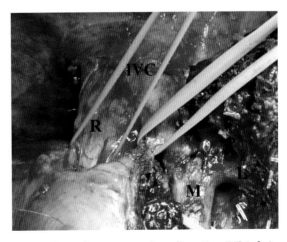

Figure 26-2 · Donor hepatectomy liver dissection. IVC, inferior vena cava; R, right hepatic vein; L, left hepatic vein; M, middle hepatic vein. (Reproduced, with permission, from Brunicardi FC, Andersen DK, Billiar TR, et al., eds. *Schwartz's Principles of Surgery*. 11th ed. New York: McGraw Hill; 2019.)

- Donor liver taken out of ice onto the field
- First anastomosis—vein
- Vein reperfusion
- Second anastomosis—artery
- Artery reperfusion
- Third anastomosis—cystic duct
- Apply drains/complete hemostasis
- Test with flow probes
- Close incision

KIDNEY TRANSPLANT SURGERY

It is important for SAs to have a general understanding of a procedure before taking part beside a transplant team. Kidneys can be shared by a living donor or a deceased organ donor. Both are transplanted similarly; however, the process before each one is different, and the timelines vary. The living donor and recipient are both admitted to the hospital. A series of tests must be performed on the donor to meet all criteria for donation. Physical exam, blood work, chest x-ray, and EKG are among the tests required before the procedure. Any health issues found will cause the transplant surgery to be postponed until the donor patient is completely healthy or another viable kidney is found.

Once the donor and recipient have passed all of the physical requirements, they are both brought to the operating rooms. For living donors, a separate operating room is set up and the kidney is excised and prepped to be taken to the next room for the recipient to receive the kidney transplant. The living donor nephrectomy will begin before the recipient in the next room. This procedure can be performed open or laparoscopically depending on surgeon preference. The nephrectomy is performed by dissecting, stapling, and removing the donor kidney. It is then taken to a benching table for the surgeon to have it analyzed, flushed, and prepared for transplant. It is then packaged in ice slush and custodial HTK solution. The recipient procedure will have been started in the next room. At this time, the team would be ready to transport the donor kidney to the next room for transplant.

When a kidney from a deceased donor is being transplanted, it comes in ice. It is turned in and checked by transplant team leaders and all documents are signed. Once the Kidney is brought into the room, the team must make sure all of the UNOS numbers are correct before opening the package.

Kidney Transplant Procedure Steps (See Figures 26-3 to 26-6)

- Patient is placed under anesthesia.
- Team places the patient on a bean bag in lateral Kidney position with the break of the bed at the hip. All team members should be on board at this time helping place lateral arm holders, pillows, foam, and straps to ensure patient safety.
- Incision is made and dissection begins. The SA helps the surgeon cauterize and retract.
- Self-retaining retractor is put in place to help maximize exposure.
- Dissection and hemostasis are done, Iliac vein and artery are identified.
- Vascular clamps are placed proximally and distally for anastomoses to begin.
- During this time, all irrigations must be cold.
- The vein is anastomosed first, then the artery.
- Re-perfusion begins and all irrigations must be warm.
- The ureter is then transplanted to the bladder.
- Doppler test is performed, and levels checked to ensure the transplanted kidney is working properly.
- Drains placed and closing of the patient begins.

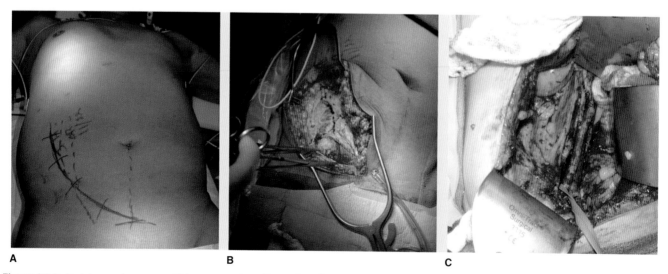

Figure 26-3 · Incision and exposure kidney transplant. (Reproduced, with permission, from Brunicardi FC, Andersen DK, Billiar TR, et al., eds. *Schwartz's Principles of Surgery.* 11th ed. New York: McGraw Hill; 2019.)

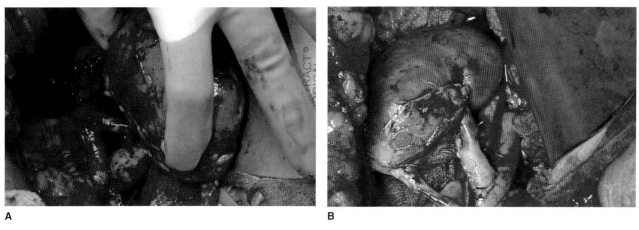

Figure 26-4 Vascular anastomoses of kidney transplant. (Reproduced, with permission, from Brunicardi FC, Andersen DK, Billiar TR, et al., eds. *Schwartz's Principles of Surgery*. 11th ed. New York: McGraw Hill; 2019.)

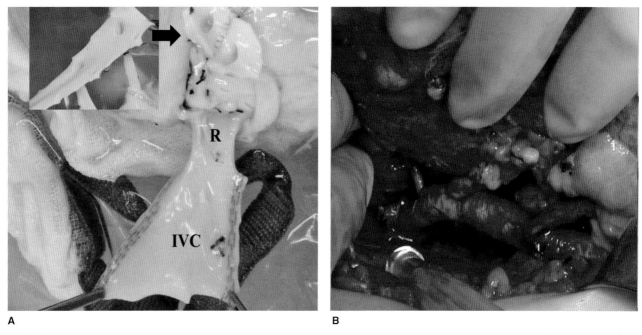

Figure 26-5 Arterial and venous reconstruction. **A.** Two renal arteries combined into a single Carrel patch (arrow). Right renal vein extension conduit constructed with stapled caval patch. IVC, inferior vena cava; R, right renal vein. **B.** Three renal arteries anastomosed to external iliac artery separately. (Reproduced, with permission, from Brunicardi FC, Andersen DK, Billiar TR, et al., eds. *Schwartz's Principles of Surgery*. 11th ed. New York: McGraw Hill; 2019.)

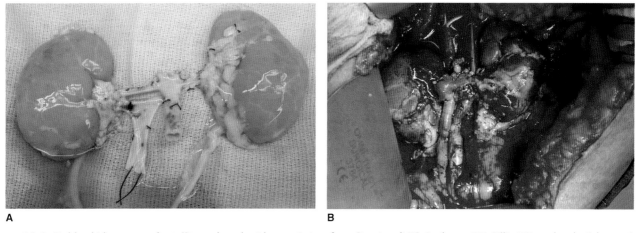

Figure 26-6 En bloc kidney transplant. (Reproduced, with permission, from Brunicardi FC, Andersen DK, Billiar TR, et al., eds. *Schwartz's Principles of Surgery*. 11th ed. New York: McGraw Hill; 2019.)

PANCREAS TRANSPLANT SURGERY (SEE FIGURES 26-7 TO 26-10)

- Incision made and retractors placed
- Pancreatectomy done
- Donor pancreas comes to the field
- First anastomosis: Renal vein—use Lambert K Clamp
- Second anastomoses: Renal artery—use Satinsky Bulldog Clamp
- Third anastomoses: Ureter
- Fourth anastomoses: Bladder
- Placement of drains is necessary, check hemostasis
- Close incision
- Place dressings

OPEN HEART TRANSPLANT SURGERY (SEE FIGURE 26-11)

Once a donor heart becomes available, the procurement and transplant teams are quickly activated. The donation and delivery of the heart must be done in a precise manner to ensure both teams have ample time for their procedures. As an SA, it is important to know the different stages during this transplant in order for things to run smoothly. Most teams fly to and from hospitals transferring the heart because they have a small window in which to get it to its destination.

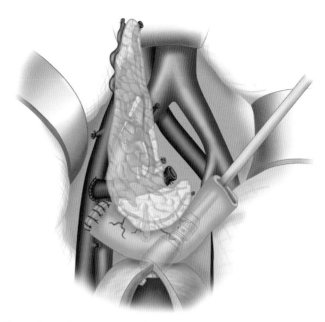

Figure 26-8 ⋅ Pancreas transplant. (Reproduced, with permission, from Gruessner RWG, Sutherland DER. *Transplantation of the Pancreas.* New York: Springer; 2004.)

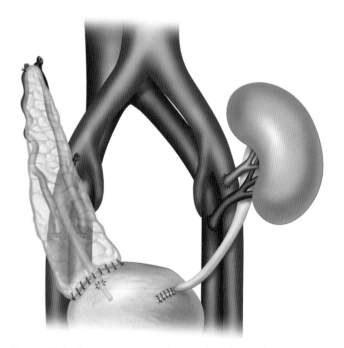

Figure 26-9 ⋅ Pancreas segmental transplant. (Reproduced, with permission, from Gruessner RWG, Sutherland DER. *Transplantation of the Pancreas.* New York: Springer; 2004.)

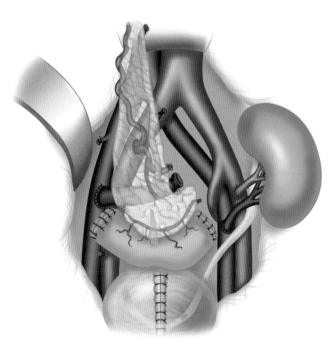

Figure 26-7 ⋅ Pancreas whole organ transplant. (Reproduced, with permission, from Gruessner RWG, Sutherland DER. *Transplantation of the Pancreas.* New York: Springer; 2004.)

Heart Transplant Procedure Steps

- Patient is put under anesthesia.
- Sternal saw is used to open sternal notch to xiphoid.
- Retractor is put into place.

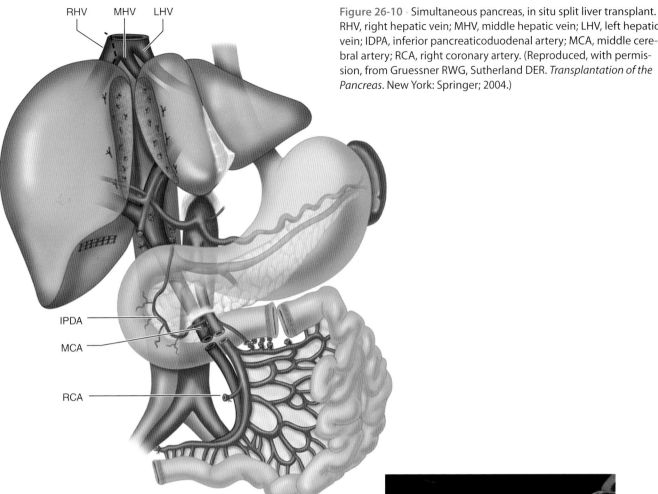

RHV   MHV   LHV

IPDA

MCA

RCA

Figure 26-10 · Simultaneous pancreas, in situ split liver transplant. RHV, right hepatic vein; MHV, middle hepatic vein; LHV, left hepatic vein; IDPA, inferior pancreaticoduodenal artery; MCA, middle cerebral artery; RCA, right coronary artery. (Reproduced, with permission, from Gruessner RWG, Sutherland DER. *Transplantation of the Pancreas.* New York: Springer; 2004.)

- Pericardial stitches are applied for retraction.
- Aortic, venous, LV vent, and antegrade cannulation to go on bypass.
- Cross clamps are applied and cardiectomy is performed.
- Removal of the deceased heart and irrigation are done.
- Donor's heart comes up to the field.
- Anastomosis begins with five vessels:
    a. Left atrium
    b. Inferior vena cava
    c. Superior vena cava
    d. Pulmonary artery
    e. Aorta
- Decannulation begins, clamps are taken off, the patient is warmed again.
- Hemostasis and function are checked.
- Drains and chest tubes are placed.
- Incision is closed with wires and sutures.

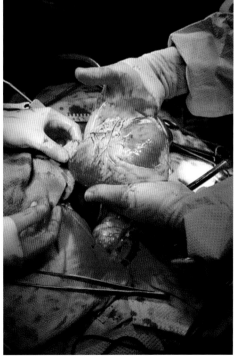

Figure 26-11 · Donor heart brought forth for anastomoses. (Reproduced, with permission, from Brunicardi FC, Andersen DK, Billiar TR, et al., eds. *Schwartz's Principles of Surgery.* 11th ed. New York: McGraw Hill; 2019.)

LUNG TRANSPLANT

Lung Transplant Procedure Steps (See Figures 26-12 to 26-15)

- Make sternotomy.
- Irrigate chest with warm saline.
- Place retractor of choice with towels on either side.
- Pericardial stitches are then used to retract pericardium.
- Cannulation begins and sutures are placed.
- Tourniquets are applied and joined together by Silk ties.
- Cannulas are inserted and bypass commences.
- Lungs are then excised.
- Donor lungs brought up to field.
- Bronchus, pulmonary artery, and vein are anastomosed.
- Chest tubes are placed and hemostasis checked.

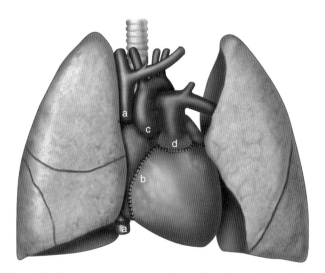

Figure 26-12 · Lung anastomoses. Suture lines for: a = bicaval anastomosis; b = biatrial anastomosis; c = aortic anastomosis; d = pulmonary artery anastomosis. (Reproduced, with permission, from Brunicardi FC, Andersen DK, Billiar TR, et al., eds. *Schwartz's Principles of Surgery*. 11th ed. New York: McGraw Hill; 2019.)

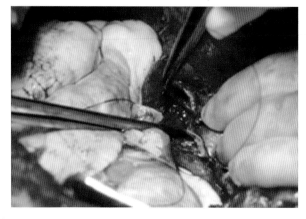

Figure 26-13 · Bronchial anastomoses. (Reproduced, with permission, from Brunicardi FC, Andersen DK, Billiar TR, et al., eds. *Schwartz's Principles of Surgery*. 11th ed. New York: McGraw Hill; 2019.)

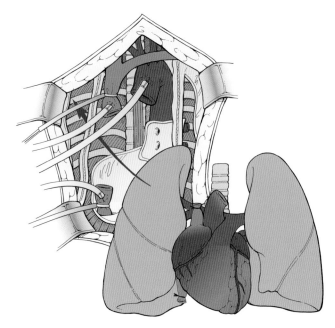

Figure 26-14 · Lung excised and explanted. (Reproduced, with permission, from Cohn LH, Adams DH, eds. *Cardiac Surgery in the Adult*. 5th ed. New York: McGraw Hill; 2018.)

- Chest is closed with wires.
- Incision is then closed.
- Dressings are done according to surgeon preference.

ARTERIAL AND SAPHENOUS VEIN GRAFTING

Coronary artery disease (CAD) is a prevalent condition affecting many patients. Treatment for CAD using a greater saphenous vein (GSV) is used as invasive coronary revascularization. The GSV is an accessible and reliable conduit with a significant length and is the conduit of choice today.

However, the left internal mammary artery (LIMA) has been shown to be a superior vessel to revascularize the left anterior descending artery (LAD) while near the myocardium. This graft demonstrates a visible increase in patency and patient survival. When working on revascularizing the LAD, the LIMA may be used. It may be anastomosed to various vessels and additional vessels may be needed.

In cases where multi-vessel CAD is present, the saphenous vein is usually the conduit of choice due to its length and flexibility. In cases where the GSV may not be an option, the short saphenous vein (SSV) might become a viable second option to be used.

There are two ways to harvest GSV, open or endoscopically. This will determine what equipment is needed for the case. Whether it is an open vein harvest (OVH) or endoscopic vein harvest (EVH), all equipment and supplies need to be in the room before the patient arrives.

Trays and Equipment

1. Tray of vascular standard surgical instruments
2. Ultrasound guidance: used to find the location of the vein

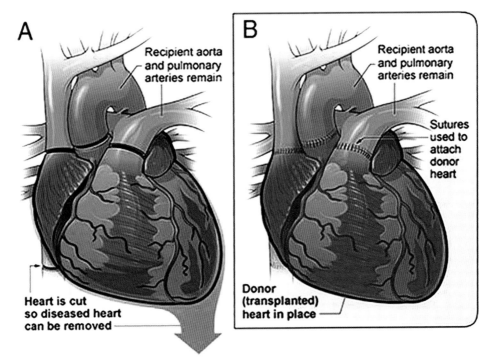

Figure 26-15 · Donor heart transplanted. (Reproduced with permission from Patel JK, Kobashigawa JA. Heart Transplantation. *Circulation.* 2011;124(4):e132-e134.)

3. Nonabsorbable and monofilament sutures and clips

4. Heparinized saline and a vessel cannula

5. Carbon dioxide insufflator

6. Balloon tip trocar with a camera for videoscopic dissection

7. Bipolar cautery to achieve endoscopic hemostasis

Several techniques have been described using a reverse valvulotome negating the function of the venous valves inherent to the saphenous vein.

Initial identification of the saphenous veins can be performed by identifying anatomic landmarks and palpating a thrill with one hand while milking the vein with the other hand.

Preoperative ultrasonography can directly visualize and mark the saphenous vein. Anatomical landmarks are marked for incision and dissection.

During open approach to SVG harvest, an incision is made following the course of the saphenous vein and continued down until the identification of the vein. Dissection continues along the length of the vein with care to manipulate the vein as minimally as possible.

Tributaries are identified and clipped or tied. When obtaining a suitable length of vein, the proximal and distal aspects of the vein are clamped. The vein is ligated and removed.

The vein is carefully cannulated to avoid endothelial damage, and heparinized saline is used to insufflate the vein to assess for any points where clips or ties may be needed. It can also be oversewn with monofilament suture. This specimen is then placed in a heparinized saline bath until used for implantation.

As a secondary choice, there is a less invasive approach to saphenous vein harvesting. Endoscopic vein harvesting (EVH) of the saphenous vein begins by making a small incision just above the medial aspect of the knee to obtain a graft roughly 35 cm and by making an additional incision 2 to 3 cm above the medial malleolus to capture the entire 70 cm length of the vein.

A balloon tip trocar is inserted through the incision in the direction of the groin. This creates a tunnel around the saphenous vein by insufflating the fascial canal along the length of the vessel.

The dissection cone is then advanced toward the groin along the anterior aspect of the vessel.

This creates a circumferential dissection of the vein carefully identifying any tributaries along the lateral and posterior aspects of the wall. These then undergo ligation with bipolar electrocautery.

Once the vessel is isolated entirely, a small incision is made at the groin to remove the vessel. The same steps as the open harvest are then taken (see Figures 26-16 and 26-17).

Tissue donation refers to a process by which a deceased person donates parts of his/her body (eg, skin, heart valves, ligaments, bones, veins, corneas) for use in transplant procedures to repair various defects or injuries.

TEN THINGS YOU NEED TO KNOW ABOUT TISSUE DONATION

1. Tissue donation is the process by which a deceased person donates parts of his/her body including skin, heart valves, ligaments, bones, veins, and corneas. These are used during transplant procedures to repair various defects.

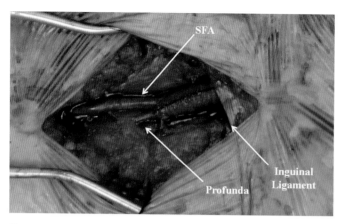

Figure 26-16 · Femoral artery graft. (Reproduced, with permission, from Dean SM, Satiani B, Abraham WT, eds. *Color Atlas and Synopsis of Vascular Diseases*. New York: McGraw Hill; 2014.)

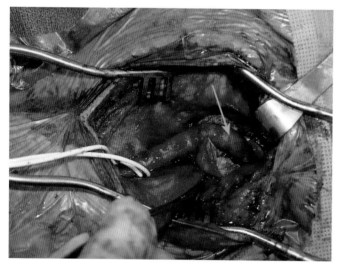

Figure 26-17 · Saphenous vein graft. (Reproduced, with permission, from Dean SM, Satiani B, Abraham WT, eds. *Color Atlas and Synopsis of Vascular Diseases*. New York: McGraw Hill; 2014.)

2. Donated tissue such as heart valves, connective tissue, or skin can improve a recipient's quality of life, and in many cases, it can mean the difference between life and death.

3. There are over 1 million tissue transplant surgeries performed each year in the United States. The number continues to rise yearly as it becomes more common practice.

4. People of all ages can; and have donated tissue if they are medically suitable at the time of death.

5. Through the gift of just one donor, the lives of up to 75 individuals can be positively impacted through tissue donation. Many lives can be saved, and individuals who had to live a life of laborious and expensive routine medical treatments can enjoy a dramatically improved quality of life.

6. Here are some amazing examples of how donated tissue can save or enhance an individual's life:
    - Donated bone can be used for various reconstructive procedures.
    - Donated skin can bring relief and healing to burn victims or individuals with serious infections.
    - Donated veins can help restore circulation.
    - Donated bones can help prevent the need for an amputation to be performed.
    - Donated heart valves can repair various cardiac defects.
    - Donated corneas can give the gift of sight to the visually impaired.
    - Donated ligaments and tendons can restore mobility and hope to Armed Forces personnel who have suffered life-altering injuries in combat.

7. Donated tissue can be stored for longer periods of time, providing more versatility to medical professionals who can use them for various cases such as severe burns, bone replacement, or ligament repair.

8. Each year, more than 25,000 tissue donors provide tissue for transplant operations.

9. The various tissues that are commonly used in transplant operations such as skin, heart valves, veins, and ligaments can normally be recovered up to 24 hours after the donor's death has occurred.

10. According to recent surveys, 95% of Americans believe that it is important to be a tissue and/or organ donor, but only 54% have actually registered to become donors. This needs to change! We must all share our knowledge to help others better understand the process.

References

Altshuler P, Nahirniak P, Welle NJ. Saphenous vein grafts. StatPearls [Internet]. https://www.ncbi.nlm.nih.gov/books/NBK537035/. Accessed December 14, 2023.

Starzl TE, Miller C, Broznick B, Makowka L. An improved technique for multiple organ harvesting. *Surg Gynecol Obstet.* 1987;165(4):343-348. https://www.ncbi.nlm.nih.gov/pmc/?term=PMC2674231.

Life Center. Ten things you need to know about tissue donation. https://lifepassiton.org/10-things-need-know-tissue-donation/. Accessed December 14, 2023.

National Kidney Foundation. www.kidney.org. Accessed December 14, 2023.

Optimizing organ allocation and acceptance. University of Pittsburgh. https://sites.pitt.edu/~schaefer/papers/OrganOptimizationChapter.pdf.

UNOS. Increasing organ donations. https://unos.org/transplant/opos-increasing-organ-donation/. Accessed December 14, 2023.

Understanding the organ/tissue procurement process. https://www.onelegacy.org/newsroom/presskit/organ_stepbystep.html. Accessed December 14, 2023.

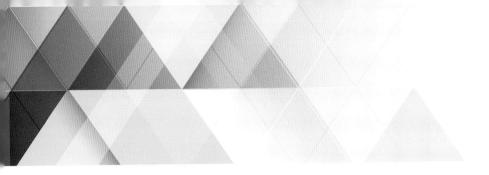

Index

Page numbers in **"bold"** refer to tables and page numbers in *"Italics"* refer to figures.